Operative Techniques in Upper Extremity Sports Injuries

Operative Techniques in Upper Extremity Sports Injuries

EDITOR

FRANK W. JOBE

ASSOCIATE EDITORS

MARILYN M. PINK, PhD, PT

RONALD E. GLOUSMAN, MD

RONALD S. KVITNE, MD

NORMAN P. ZEMEL, MD

THE KERLAN-JOBE ORTHOPAEDIC CLINIC

AND

CENTINELA HOSPITAL MEDICAL CENTER

INGLEWOOD, CA

Janice A. Schwegler, MS, CMI, Illustrator

with 1250 illustrations, 156 color

Mosby

St. Louis Baltimore Boston Carlsbad Chicago Naples New York Philadelphia Portland

London Madrid Mexico City Singapore Sydney Tokyo Toronto Wiesbaden

Mosby
Dedicated to Publishing Excellence

A Times Mirror
Company

Publisher: Anne Patterson
Editor: Robert Hurley
Developmental Editor: Lauranne Billus
Project Manager: Linda McKinley
Production Editor: Aimee E. Loewe
Production Assistant: Ginny Douglas
Designer: Elizabeth Fett
Manufacturing Manager: Theresa Fuchs

Printed in the United States of America
Composition by Graphic World, Inc.
Printing/binding by Von Hoffmann Press

Mosby-Year Book, Inc.
11830 Westline Industrial Drive
St. Louis, Missouri 63146

Library of Congress Cataloging in Publication Data

Operative techniques in upper extremity sports injuries / editor, Frank W. Jobe ; associate editors, Marilyn M. Pink ... [et al.] ; Janice A. Schwegler, illustrator.
p. cm.
Includes bibliographical references and index.
ISBN 0-8016-7207-4
1. Arm—Wounds and injuries. 2. Sports injuries. 3. Shoulder—Wounds and injuries. 4. Hand—Wounds and injuries. I. Jobe, Frank W. II. Pink, Marilyn M.
[DNLM: 1. Athletic Injuries. 2. Arm Injuries. WE 805 0613 1995]
RD557.064 1995
617.5′7—dc20
DNLM/DLC
for Library of Congress 95-7921
CIP

95 96 97 98 99 / 9 8 7 6 5 4 3 2 1

Contributors

Jerry L. Barron, MD
Associate, Miller Orthopaedic Clinic,
Charlotte, North Carolina

James R. Boatright, MD
Associate, Miller Orthopaedic Clinic,
Chief, Hand Service,
Carolinas Medical Center,
Charlotte, North Carolina

James P. Bradley, MD
Director, Sports Medicine Center,
St. Margaret Memorial Hospital,
Clinical Assistant Professor,
University of Pittsburgh Medical Center,
Team Physician, Pittsburgh Steelers,
Pittsburgh, Pennsylvania

Clive E. Brewster, MS, PT
Director, Department of Physical Therapy,
Kerlan-Jobe Orthopaedic Clinic,
Inglewood, California,
Physical Therapy Consultant,
Los Angeles Lakers, Los Angeles Kings,
Los Angeles, California,
California Angels,
Anaheim, California

Thomas D. Cahalan, PT
Staff Physical Therapist,
Physiotherapy Associates,
Cedar Rapids, Iowa

Robert W. Chandler, MD
Associate, Kerlan-Jobe Orthopaedic Clinic,
Inglewood, California,
Associate Clinical Professor,
University of Southern California,
School of Medicine,
Los Angeles, California
Assistant Clinical Professor,
University of California—Irvine,
School of Medicine,
Irvine, California

Michael G. Ciccotti, MD
Associate Clinical Professor,
Department of Orthopaedics,
Rothman Institute, Pennsylvania Hospital,
and Thomas Jefferson University,
Orthopaedic Consultant,
Philadelphia Flyers, Philadelphia Eagles,
Philadelphia, Pennsylvania

John E. Conway, MD
Associate, Orthopedic Specialty Associates,
Clinical Instructor, Fort Worth Affiliated Hospitals,
Orthopedic Residency Program,
Team Orthopedic Consultant, Texas Rangers,
Fort Worth, Texas

William P. Cooney, MD
Chair, Division of Hand Surgery,
Department of Orthopedic Surgery,
Mayo Medical School,
Professor of Orthopaedic Surgery,
Mayo Medical School,
Rochester, Minnesota

Donald F. D'Alessandro, MD
Associate, Miller Orthopaedic Clinic,
Chief, Sports Medicine and Shoulder Service,
Carolinas Medical Center,
Team Physician, Carolina Panthers,
Charlotte, North Carolina

Philip A. Davidson, MD
Tampa Bay Orthopaedic Specialists,
St. Petersburg, Florida

Nick M. DiGiovine, MD
Medical Director,
The Pittsburgh Center for Sports Medicine,
Shady Hospital,
Clinical Instructor,
University of Pittsburgh Medical Center,
Assistant Team Physician,
Pittsburgh Steelers,
Pittsburgh, Pennsylvania

Neal S. ElAttrache, MD
Associate, Kerlan-Jobe Orthopaedic Clinic,
Inglewood, California,
Assistant Clinical Professor of Orthopaedics,
University of Southern California, School of Medicine,
Orthopaedic Consultant, Los Angeles Rams,
Los Angeles, California

Ralph A. Gambardella, MD
Associate, Kerlan-Jobe Orthopaedic Clinic,
Inglewood, California,
Associate Clinical Professor,
Department of Orthopaedics,
University of Southern California, School of Medicine,
Orthopaedic Consultant,
Los Angeles Dodgers,
University of Southern California Athletics,
Loyola Marymount University Athletics
Los Angeles, California

Ronald E. Glousman, MD
Associate, Kerlan-Jobe Orthopaedic Clinic,
Inglewood, California,
Associate Clinical Professor,
University of Southern California, School of Medicine,
Los Angeles, California
Orthopaedic Consultant, Anaheim Mighty Ducks,
Anaheim, California

Stephen M. Gryzlo, MD
Assistant Professor of Clinical Orthopaedic Surgery,
Northwestern University Medical School,
Chicago, Illinois

Herndon P. Harding, Jr. MD
Team Physician—Psychiatry, Los Angeles Dodgers,
Los Angeles, California
Medical Director, ComCare,
Phoenix, Arizona

Christopher M. Jobe, MD
Associate Professor, Orthopaedic Surgery,
Loma Linda University, School of Medicine,
Loma Linda, California,
Orthopaedic Consultant,
San Bernardino Spirit,
San Bernardino, California

Frank W. Jobe, MD
Associate, Kerlan-Jobe Orthopaedic Clinic,
Inglewood, California,
Clinical Professor,
Department of Orthopaedics,
University of Southern California, School of Medicine,
Orthopaedic Consultant,
Los Angeles Dodgers,
Los Angeles, California
PGA Tour,
Senior PGA Tour

Steve E. Jordan, MD
Orthopedic Surgeon,
Tallahassee Orthopedic Clinic,
Orthopedic Consultant, Florida State University Athletics,
Orthopedic Consultant, Florida A & M University Athletics,
Tallahassee, Florida

Darryl M. Kan, MD
Assistant Professor of Surgery,
University of Hawaii, School of Medicine,
Orthopaedic Consultant,
University of Hawaii Athletics,
Honolulu, Hawaii

John T. Kao, MD
Department of Orthopaedics,
Kaiser Permanente Group,
San Francisco, California,
Clinical Instructor,
Division of Hand Surgery,
Stanford University Medical Center,
Stanford, California,
Orthopaedic Consultant,
Division of Orthopaedic Surgery,
Veterans Administration Hospital,
Palo Alto, California

John D. Kelley, MD
Associate, New Haven Orthopaedic Group,
Clinical Instructor, Department of Orthopaedic Surgery and Rehabilitation,
Yale University, School of Medicine,
New Haven, Connecticut

Robert K. Kerlan, MD
Associate, Kerlan-Jobe Orthopaedic Clinic,
Inglewood, California,
Clinical Professor,
Department of Orthopaedics,
University of Southern California, School of Medicine,
Orthopaedic Consultant,
Los Angeles Lakers, Los Angeles Rams,
Jockeys' Guild Medical Advisor,
Los Angeles, California

Scott Kingston, MD
Director of Magnetic Resonance Section,
Centinela Hospital Medical Center,
Inglewood, California,
Assistant Clinical Instructor,
University of Southern California, School of Medicine,
Los Angeles, California

Ronald S. Kvitne, MD
Associate, Kerlan-Jobe Orthopaedic Clinic,
Inglewood, California,
Assistant Clinical Professor,
Department of Orthopaedic Surgery,
University of Southern California,
Team Physician, Los Angeles Kings,
Los Angeles, California

Stephen J. Lombardo, MD
Associate, Kerlan-Jobe Orthopaedic Clinic,
Inglewood, California,
Associate Clinical Professor of Orthopaedics,
Department of Orthopaedic Surgery,
University of Southern California, School of Medicine,
Orthopaedic Consultant, Los Angeles Lakers,
Los Angeles, California

Walter J. McCarthy, MD
Associate Professor of Surgery,
Division of Vascular Surgery,
Northwestern University Medical School,
Chicago, Illinois

Edward G. McFarland, MD
Director of Section of Sports Medicine,
Assistant Professor, Department of Orthopaedic Surgery,
The Johns Hopkins University,
Orthopaedic Consultant, The Baltimore Orioles,
Baltimore, Maryland

Diane R. Moynes Schwab, MS, PT
Champion Rehabilitation,
San Diego, California

Gordon W. Nuber, MD
Associate Professor of Orthopaedic Surgery,
Vice Chairman, Department of Orthopaedic Surgery,
Northwestern University Medical School,
Team Physician, Chicago Bears,
Orthopaedic Consultant, Chicago Cubs,
Chicago, Illinois

Jacquelin Perry, MD
Chief of Pathokinesiology Laboratory,
Rancho Los Amigos Hospital,
Downey, California,
Professor of Orthopaedic Surgery,
University of Southern California, School of Medicine,
Los Angeles, California,
Consultant, Biomechanics Research Laboratory,
Centinela Hospital Medical Center,
Inglewood, California

Marilyn M. Pink, PhD, PT
Director, Biomechanics Research Laboratory,
Centinela Hospital Medical Center,
Inglewood, California,
Director, Research,
Department of Physical Therapy,
Mount St. Mary's College,
Los Angeles, California

Scott E. Powell, MD
Chief, Shoulder Service,
Department of Orthopaedics,
Kaiser Permanente,
Panorama City, California

Patrick M. Screnar, PT
Chief Physical Therapist,
Los Angeles Dodgers,
Los Angeles, California

Judy L. Seto, MA, PT
Assistant Director, Department of Physical Therapy,
Kerlan-Jobe Orthopaedic Clinic,
Inglewood, California

Benjamin Shaffer, MD
Director, Division of Sports Medicine,
Department of Orthopaedics,
Georgetown University Medical Center,
Team Physician,
Georgetown University,
Washington, DC

Clarence L. Shields, MD
Associate, Kerlan-Jobe Orthopaedic Clinic,
Inglewood, California,
Associate Clinical Professor of Orthopaedics,
University of Southern California,
Associate Clinical Professor,
Charles Drew School of Medicine,
Orthopaedic Consultant,
Los Angeles Rams,
Los Angeles, California,
Orthopaedic Consultant Medical Staff,
Rancho Los Amigos Hospital,
Downey, California

James E. Tibone, MD
Associate, Kerlan-Jobe Orthopaedic Clinic,
Inglewood, California,
Associate Clinical Professor,
Department of Orthopaedics,
University of Southern California, School of Medicine,
Medical Director,
University of Southern California Athletics,
Team Physician,
University of Southern California Football Team,
Los Angeles, California

Kevin D. Tollefson, PT
Champion Rehabilitation,
San Diego, California

Lewis A. Yocum, MD
Associate, Kerlan-Jobe Orthopaedic Clinic,
Inglewood, California,
Assistant Clinical Professor,
University of Southern California, School of Medicine,
Los Angeles, California
Orthopaedic Consultant, California Angels,
Anaheim, California

Norman P. Zemel, MD
Associate, Kerlan-Jobe Orthopaedic Clinic,
Inglewood, California,
Associate Clinical Professor,
Department of Orthopaedic Surgery,
University of Southern California, School of Medicine,
Hand Surgery Consultant,
California Angels, Los Angeles Dodgers,
Los Angeles Lakers, Los Angeles Rams,
Los Angeles Kings,
Los Angeles, California,
California Angels, Anaheim Mighty Ducks,
Anaheim, California

None of us produce our work in a vacuum. If it were not for our families and their solid support, we would not be able to contribute to our professions. Thus it is with much gratitude that this book is dedicated to the families of all who have contributed to this book.

Foreword

In this volume you will read work written by clinicians who are eminently rational scientists, technically expert surgeons, and patient, observant clinicians. All of them share an expertise in dealing with the intricate problems presented by upper extremity pathology. Because it treads the fine line between mobility and stability, the upper extremity is prey to injury from the repetitious strains induced by athletic participation.

The authors have included not only information about the most effective surgical procedures for athletes, but also, and perhaps more importantly, have adopted considerable effort to understanding the biomechanics of the upper extremity during athletic activity. With a rigorous grounding in the basic principles of upper extremity function, pathomechanics as the antecedent factor and its efficient treatment become a logical extension of the discussion.

The intensity of training, the extremes of motion and the fervor of participants render the anatomically vulnerable upper extremity to disruption, either acutely or chronically. Of course, the ultimate goal of any understanding of athletic upper extremity injuries and their treatment is to use that understanding and work backward along the deductive path to eliminate both the proximate and the more distant causes of these injuries.

A sports medicine physician must not only operate meticulously, but also listen carefully to the subtext of the patient's complaints, responding definitively to these problems and devising a plan to prevent recurrence.

Robert K. Kerlan

Preface

The world of sports medicine is rapidly moving forward. Part of the forward momentum has to do with technological progress. The technology, which supports us diagnostically and surgically, has been burgeoning and will continue to do so. The other component to the forward momentum has to do with concepts. The theories and concepts that enable accurate diagnosis and effective treatments have been surging forward. A factor contributing to this progress is the volume of excellent cutting edge research carried on throughout the world. This research is rapidly disseminated and built upon. To our patients, the advantage of this forward motion is that our ability to deliver optimal care is constantly being upgraded. Medical practitioners are challenged to sort out this new information and accurately apply it. As authors, our challenge is to get this book written before the concepts and methods become outdated!

Throughout time, the field of sports medicine has expanded on innovation, which has then been transferred to other medical disciplines. Hippocrates developed the first documented surgical technique for shoulder instability in his athletic patients. Paré's recommendation for wound care evolved from his experiences on the battlefield. After all, aren't our warriors indeed athletes? More recently, the field of arthroscopy imbued itself in sports medicine and has transferred into other surgical areas. As those of us in sports medicine work with athletes who want to push the envelope of what is possible, we are actually helping pave the way for that possibility in all patients.

The goal in sports medicine today is to return injured athletes to their preinjury levels of performance; in previous years the expectations were much lower. For example, in the recent past, professional baseball pitchers with shoulder instability would have had to terminate their athletic careers. A surgical procedure would have been able to take care of the instability, but the athletes could not have resumed their professional athletic careers. Another possibility exists today. It is possible for athletes to undergo surgical intervention and, with proper rehabilitation, to resume their prior level of competitive play.

Numerous treatment options are available to medical practitioners. As a member of the craft of sports medicine, I am aware that in different hands, different methods work better. This book offers one perspective of treatment options. That perspective represents the philosophy and methods used at Kerlan-Jobe Orthopaedic Clinic in Inglewood, California. The intent of this homogenous philosophy is to offer a comprehensive and common thread to an approach for treating the upper extremity in overhead athletes.

You will find an outline at the beginning of each chapter. You will notice the clinical assessment and treatment chapters follow a similar format. First the mechanism and incidence of injury are discussed. Then the clinical presentation is examined. These are followed by the definitive diagnosis and classification, special assessments, complications or advancing process of the condition, nonsurgical treatment, preferred surgical treatment, and postoperative rehabilitation. The outline provides some continuity, and it enables you to easily find the desired information.

I hope this book will stimulate you to continue building your thoughts regarding the treatment of the upper extremity in athletes. We welcome the decade before us; it will invariably bring new technology and research information enabling all of us to push the envelope of excellence further.

Acknowledgments

No work of this magnitude is possible without the dedication of an intelligent and cooperative team. I am very proud to work with such a team.

First and foremost, I would like to thank each contributing author. These men and women made time in their busy schedules to pull together their respective chapters. Not only did these people make time, but they did so with incredible, positive energy and devotion.

Along with "those who wrote," I'd like to thank "she who drew." I'm certain you've already noticed the fine illustrations in this book, and that credit goes to Janice A. Schwegler, MS, CMI. Throughout the two years we have worked on this book, Jan has been there every step of the way with wonderful suggestions. At the onset, it was obvious that her core values matched ours. She clearly had the talent, initiative, and dedication to produce exceptional, quality artwork for this book.

Drs. Jeffrey Bechler, John Kao, and Patrick Ruwe also contributed to this book by reviewing manuscripts. Since I do not want reviewing of the manuscripts to be a thankless job, I would like to publicly acknowledge their input.

Another behind-the-scenes, positive force was Cirila David, the administrative assistant who typed these manuscripts and helped organize this project. All of us involved with "the book" know Cirila and appreciate how much she did.

The work leading to the completion of this book would not have been possible without the foresight and insight of Russell S. Stromberg, President of Centinela Hospital Medical Center. Throughout the years, Russ has demonstrated an acute understanding of how technology and science affect patient care. He has consistently supported both technology and science, and therefore he has advanced the cutting edge of patient care.

I would also like to thank the editorial staff at Mosby-Year Book, Inc. When I began this project, I did not know the difference among editors, developmental editors, and production personnel. I now know the unique contribution each of them makes, and I thank them for it.

In one of the great books of all time it says "the first shall be last and the last shall be first." Thus in closing I'd like to thank all of the applied scientists who came before us to pave the way, and all who will come after us as they improve our works. In the hands of these men and women lie the progress and the outcome of our patients. Thank you.

Frank W. Jobe, MD

Contents

PART FOUR The Wrist and Hand

Operative Techniques in Upper Extremity Sports Injuries

PART ONE

Basic Principles

CHAPTER 1

Injury Prevention and Rehabilitation in the Upper Extremity

MARILYN M. PINK
PATRICK M. SCRENAR
KEVIN D. TOLLEFSON
FRANK W. JOBE

INTRODUCTION

The primary mission of sports medicine specialists is to prevent injury. A successful injury-prevention program must include the judicious balance of stretching and strengthening exercises, sport activities, and rest. The flexibility and strengthening program focuses on the soft-tissue structures, which are the primary tissues at risk. Bones usually are injured as a result of a specific traumatic event. The time spent in sports activity is divided between practice and competition. Rest prevents further trauma by allowing the tissues sufficient time to heal. As expected, talent also plays a role in this delicate balance. The athlete with relatively less talent may try to make up for this deficiency with high-volume workouts. In this case, increased volume multiplies the stress, diminishes the rest, and may increase the propensity for injury. Therefore consideration must be given to proper stretching and strengthening and to an appropriate balance between sport activity and rest to prevent injury.

If injuries do occur, the second mission is to rehabilitate athletes and return them to prior levels of competition. The components of a rehabilitation program are rest from the sport activity, modalities, and stretching and strengthening exercises. The priorities here are different from those in the preventive exercise program. The rehabilitation program has three phases. The goal of the first phase is to decrease or eliminate pain and swelling. This is done through modalities, stretching, and rest from the offending sport activity. The modalities most frequently used include ice, contrast baths, ultrasound, phonophoresis, and electrical stimulation. The contractile tissue stretching is very gentle in this phase and only within the available pain-free range. Joint-capsule mobilization also can be very effective. Rest from the offending activity is recommended if there is pain related to the sporting activity.

The goal of the second phase is to increase range-of-motion (ROM) and strength. Muscle stretching and soft-tissue mobilization during this phase are a bit more rigorous than in phase I. Muscle strengthening is injury specific and sport specific.

During phase III, the athlete initiates easy sport-mimicking activities. Throughout the rehabilitation process the active motion is constantly observed and the muscles are trained to fire in a coordinated, sequential pattern that is called *synchrony.*

In general, the last choice for treatment is surgery.

The purpose of this chapter is to discuss the prevention of injury and rehabilitation of the shoulder, elbow, wrist, and hand in the athlete. Concepts and philosophies of treatment are first introduced. Next, exercises for the shoulder, elbow, and wrist and hand are identified. In closing, the issue of sport-specific exercise and retraining is addressed. This unifying approach enables the sports rehabilitation specialist to dynamically solve problems and advance the care of the athlete.

CONCEPTS

To treat the athlete successfully the therapist must ask, "What is normal?" The "normal" requirements for a given athlete are based on the demands and requirements of the sport. For example, a baseball pitcher needs more humeral external rotation than a nonoverhead athlete. Most competitive pitchers exhibit external rotation beyond the normal value of 90°; the pure active glenohumeral external rotation may be as much as 135°. This degree of external rotation is innate to pitching mechanics and essential to athletic performance. It is erroneous to consider the "excessive" external rotation ROM as pathologic merely because it is different from that of the nonoverhead athlete. Likewise, the internal rotation may be decreased in that the athlete does not function in the extremes of internal rotation. Unless the athlete shows clinical symptoms related to these ROMs, the ranges need not be considered pathologic and the athlete is not treated for them. Thus to successfully treat the athlete, the sports medicine practitioner must rethink the concept of what is normal based on the demands and requirements of the athlete and the sport.

Just as physicians and therapists must understand what is normal, so must they grasp the concept of which tissues are at risk. The concept of tissues at risk also implies knowledge of anatomy and the mechanics of the sport. By thinking of the anatomy undergoing the kinetics and kinematics of the sport, the clinician begins to develop a dynamic thought process that allows for a better understanding of the ways to optimize, reestablish, or maintain proper function. This philosophy demonstrates the inextricable union of injury prevention and rehabilitation with biomechanics. Thus this chapter is followed by chapters on biomechanics of the shoulder, elbow, and wrist.

By using the previously mentioned thought process (anatomy undergoing kinetics and kinematics), the specialist can more easily identify the core of a problem. For example, the core of shoulder problems in the young competitive pitcher is typically glenohumeral joint instability. Treating just the symptoms of bursitis, tendinitis, impingement, or rotator cuff tear does not guarantee that further problems will not occur. Wise sports medicine practitioners constantly challenge themselves and ask whether the "diagnosis" is really the core of the problem or just a secondary effect.

The earlier the core problem is identified, the more efficient and successful the rehabilitation program is. However, early intervention demands attention to very subtle symptoms. In the earliest stages, athletes are actively competing and competing well enough to win. Athletes usually are unable to accurately identify the source of any inconsistencies. They may notice that something "just doesn't feel quite right" or that it takes longer to "get loose" or "get into the groove." The description of the problem is vague or attributed to "stiffness." The injury usually is due to muscular weakness, lost endurance, and/or asynchronous muscle action and is easily corrected with exercise. The best tool for detection at this stage is the sharp eye and ear of the practitioner, along with a thorough understanding of the mechanics of a specific sport.

The next level of progression of injury occurs when athletic performance begins to diminish, even though the athlete may be unable to pinpoint the reason. The astute clinician realizes that something is amiss and that the player must cease the athletic activity for a time. Typically and unfortunately, the problem is not recognized until pain and secondary symptoms occur. The pain may be either capsular or muscular, and often it is difficult to differentiate the two. Within a few weeks a muscular problem responds to treatment. A capsular problem may not respond so quickly because anatomic damage or stretching of noncontractile tissue already may have occurred. Obviously, the earlier the detection, the less time the athlete will need to abstain from the sport.

A sport-specific exercise program is a critical component of injury prevention as well as a measure to prevent the progression of injury. In addition, the program may enhance athletic performance. The next section includes general guidelines for developing such a program.

EXERCISE PROGRAM

The Shoulder

The shoulder is the most mobile joint in the body and the most frequently injured area of the upper extremity in sports. Because it is so mobile, stretch must be applied judiciously. As stated earlier, an overhead athlete's

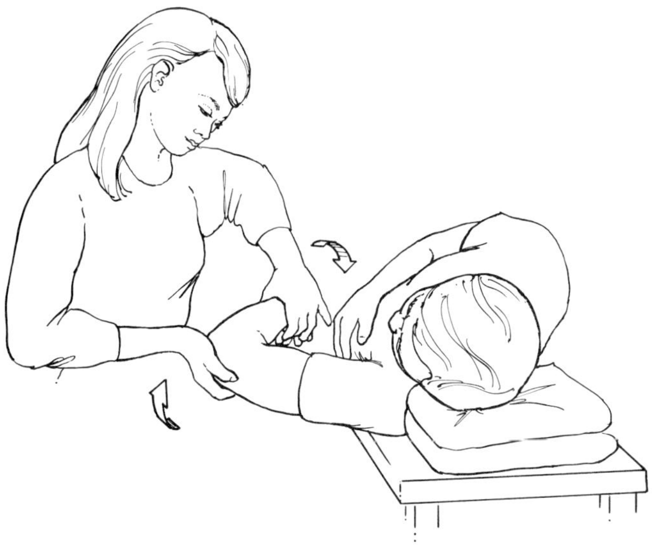

FIGURE 1-1 Stretching of the posterior contractile tissue.

humeral ROM is different from a nonoverhead athlete's. The functional increases in external rotation usually result in increased laxity of the anterior capsule. Thus further stretching of the anterior capsule may lead to instability. The posterior capsule, however, must be checked for restrictions. Sometimes the posterior capsule is tight. A restricted posterior capsule may not allow the humeral head to be positioned in an optimal or neutral position in the glenoid. Instead, it may position the head slightly forward in the glenoid, which encourages anterior subluxation and concomitant impingement. In addition, a tight posterior capsule can lead to a tight teres minor or adhesions beneath the posterior deltoid. Thus a tight posterior capsule must be mobilized and overlying contractile tissue must be stretched (Fig. 1-1). Contractile tissue stretching is best performed in a position of scapular stability.

An easy way to remember the concepts of strengthening is to think "E^3 and the 4 *P*'s." An effective and efficient exercise (E^3) program is focused on the four *P*'s: the glenohumeral "protectors" (rotator cuff muscles), the scapulohumeral "pivotors" (scapular rotator muscles), the humeral "positioners" (three heads of the deltoid), and the "power" drivers (pectoralis major and latissimus dorsi). The exercises recommended herein for the 4 *P*'s are considered effective and efficient because they have demonstrated an intensity and a duration of high-level EMG activity.[14,29] In addition, because the sport-specific critical muscles have been identified through EMG, that knowledge can be applied to the exercise program to better focus the treatment.

The glenohumeral protectors and scapular pivotors are strengthened first because they are most intimately involved in providing stability. Humeral positioners are strengthened next because they are associated with synchronous motion. The power drivers are strengthened after the other three groups have achieved at least a grade of "good" strength. If the power drivers are strengthened too early, they will overpower the balance of the protectors and pivotors and asynchronous motion results. The muscles first undergo isotonic strengthening, and then isokinetic strengthening. Strengthening these muscles in this logical sequence enables the therapist to focus on the weak links that most likely led to the problem. Because none of the muscle groups function in isolation, the exercises themselves will work more than one isolated muscle group. Thus the "art" of sequencing the exercises from each of these four groups is to balance the exercises of one group against the patient's progress with the entire sequence.

Glenohumeral Protectors

The rotator cuff muscles are responsible for humeral head depression and approximation into the joint. Each portion of the cuff provides protection as posterior (infraspinatus, teres minor), anterior (subscapularis), and superior (supraspinatus) stability is achieved. The true rotators of the rotator cuff (infraspinatus, teres minor, and subscapularis) also fine-tune the humeral rotation and provide maximum joint surface area contact and congruency of the humeral head within the glenoid.* The supraspinatus actually is not a true rotator of the humeral head; it is much more functionally akin to the deltoids. It does serve to protect the glenohumeral joint, however, by affording approximation of the humerus into the glenoid and a superior compressive and humeral depressive force.

The humeral rotation exercises are initiated with the patient lying on the side. For external rotation, the athlete lies on the opposite side, with a small pillow between the thorax and exercising arm. The abduction afforded by a pillow allows circulation to the rotator cuff[22] while not precariously positioning the glenohumeral joint in an unstable position. The patient first rotates the arm away from the body (Fig. 1-2) and then back to the starting position to repeat the exercise. For internal rotation, the individual lies on the side to be exercised. The arm is positioned slightly forward of the trunk and is rotated toward the body (Fig. 1-3). These exercises are progressed by adding weights and adding the exercises of prone horizontal humeral abduction with external rotation (Fig. 1-4) and supine horizontal humeral adduction with internal rotation (Fig. 1-5). The teres minor needs specific attention in the baseball pitcher because EMG studies have shown it to have very high levels of activity.[4] It can be strengthened separately from the infraspinatus by using arm positions with more humeral abduction (about 70°) while blocking the arm to prevent it from excessive rotation (Fig. 1-6) or humeral extension.

*References 4, 8, 19, 21, 26, 27.

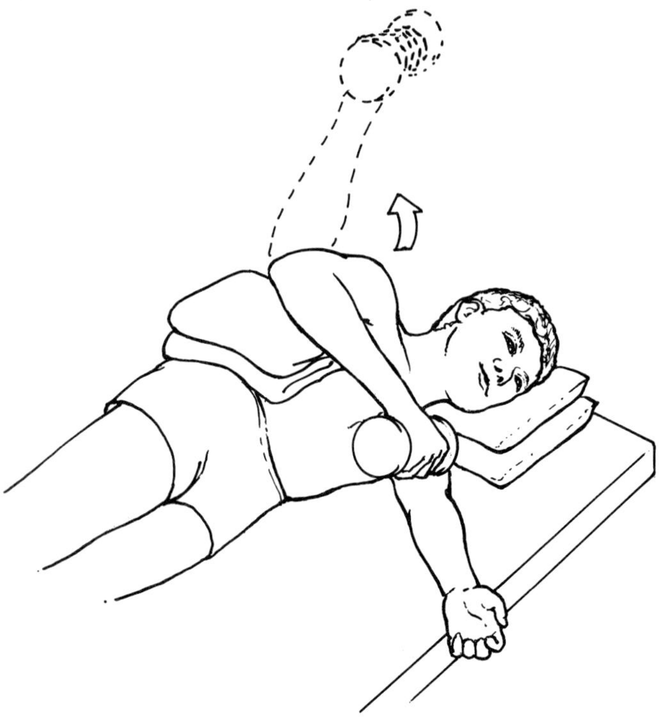

FIGURE 1-2 External rotation.

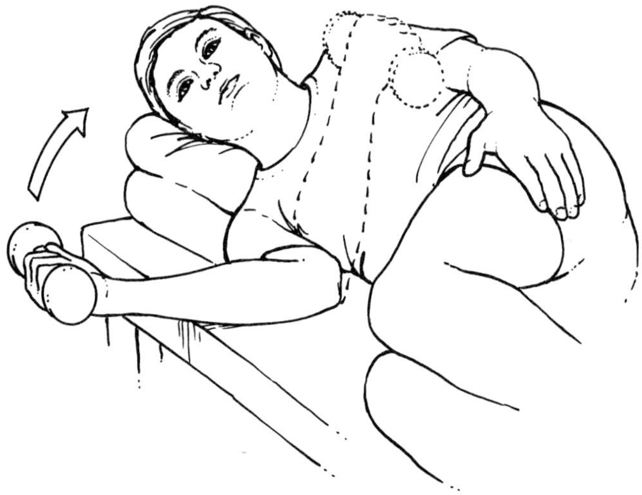

FIGURE 1-3 Internal rotation.

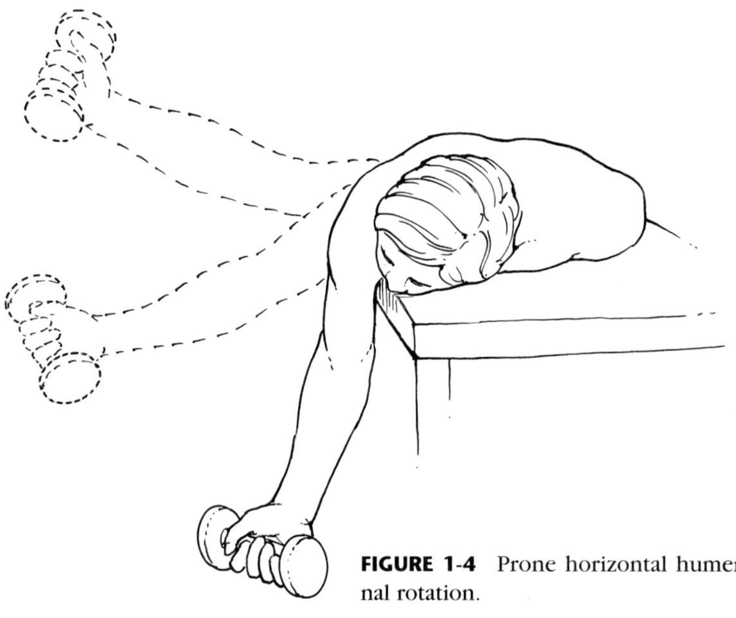

FIGURE 1-4 Prone horizontal humeral abduction with external rotation.

Synchrony of scapulohumeral motion is tested bilaterally. One way to do this is to abduct the humerus to 90° in the scapular plane with elbow flexion to 90° and have the patient internally and externally rotate the humerus (Fig. 1-7). The scapula must be stable when doing this exercise. Another way is to slowly and repeatedly elevate the arms (in sagittal, coronal, or scapular planes). When exercising in any plane, the motion should be smooth, without scapular eccentricities. Eccentric exercise with a resistance band is an advanced strengthening progression (Fig. 1-8). In this exercise the therapist places the humerus in a position of 90° abduction in the scapular plane and 90° external rotation. One end of a stretched exercise band is placed in the athlete's hand. The other end of the band is fixed at a set distance in front of the athlete. Tension of the stretched exercise band offers an

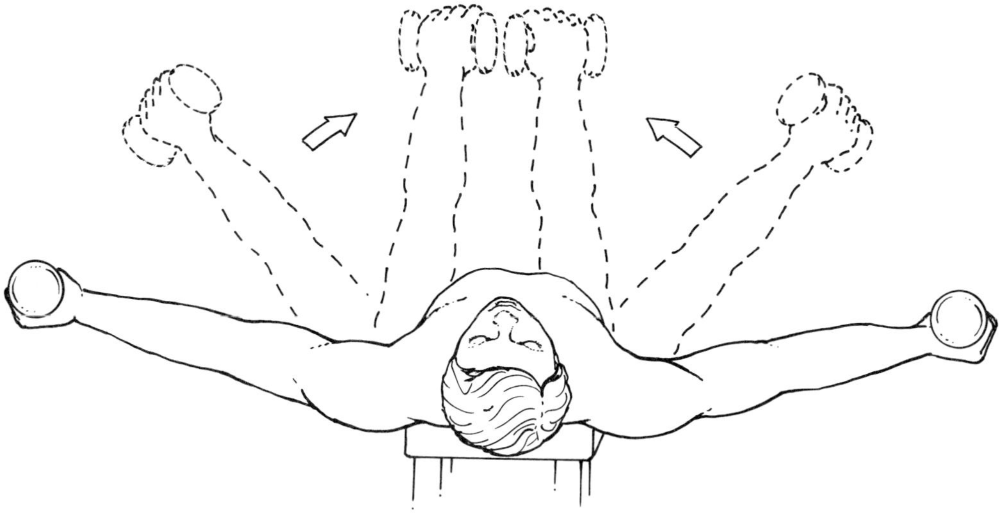

FIGURE 1-5 Supine horizontal humeral adduction with internal rotation.

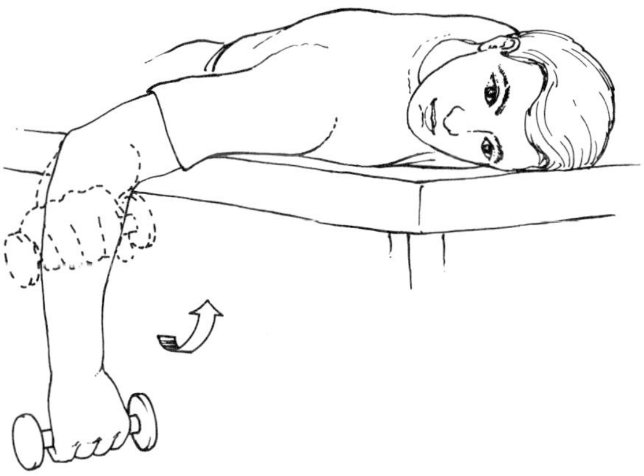

FIGURE 1-6 External rotation to isolate the teres minor.

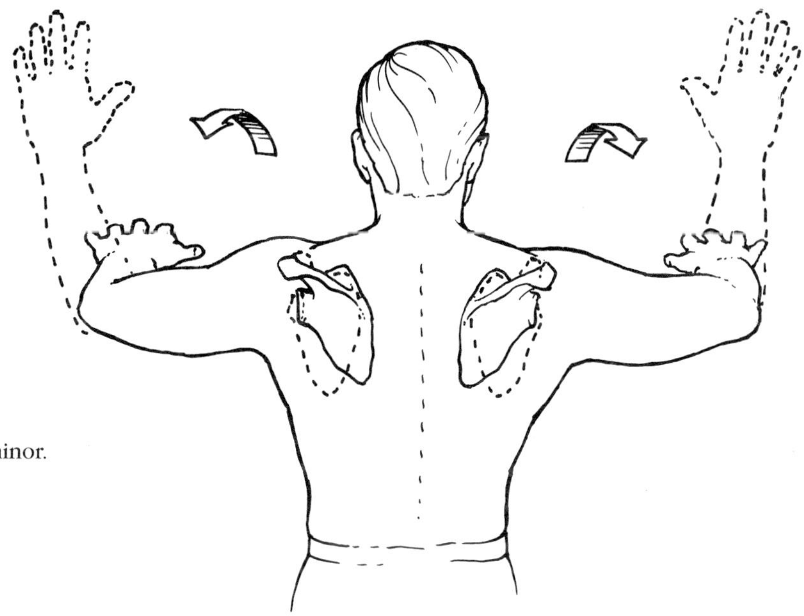

FIGURE 1-7 Synchrony of motion.

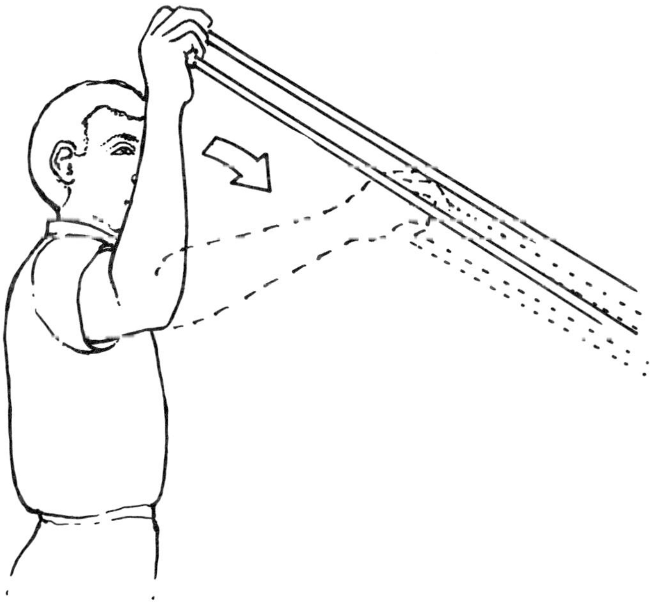

FIGURE 1-8 Eccentric exercise for the rotator cuff.

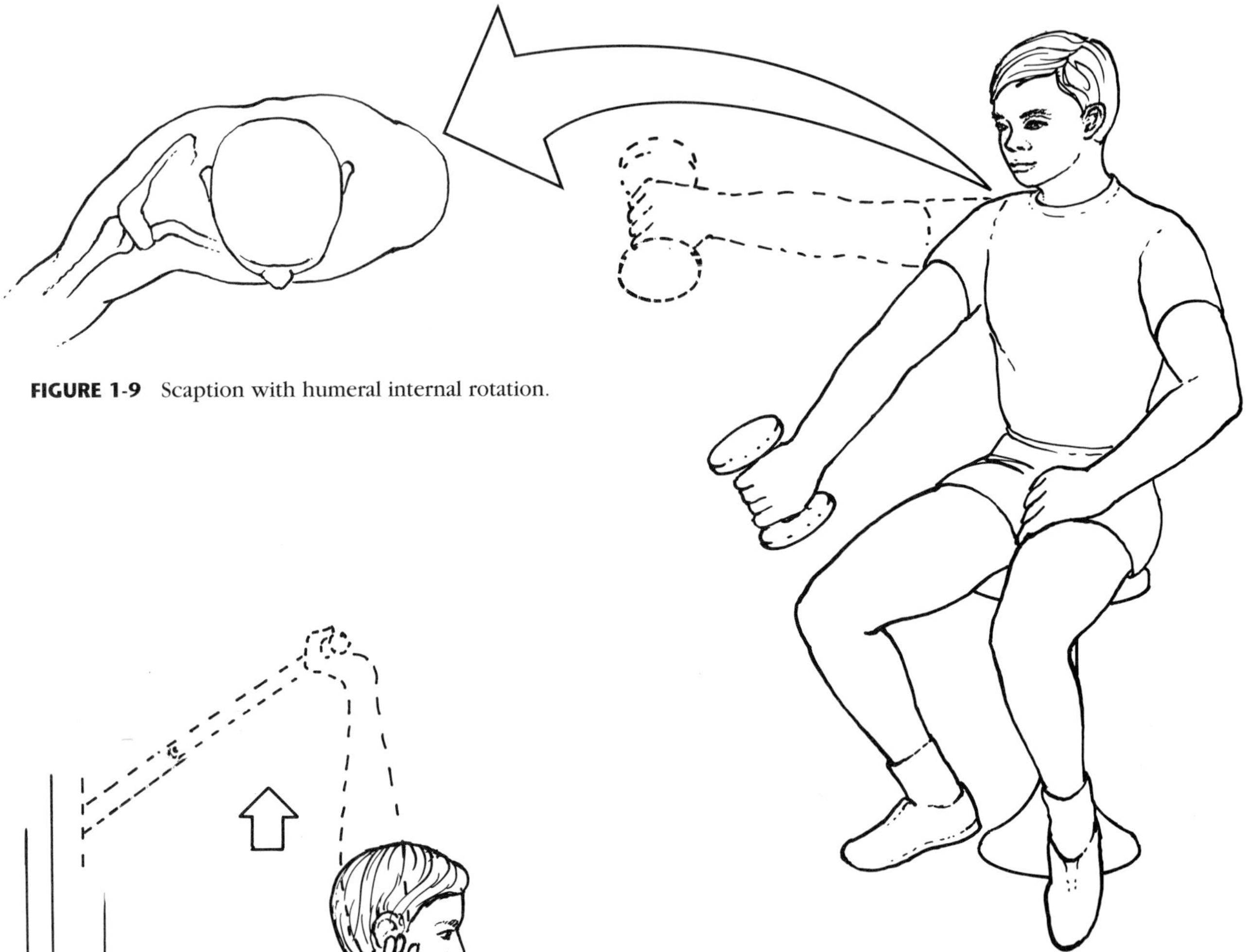

FIGURE 1-9 Scaption with humeral internal rotation.

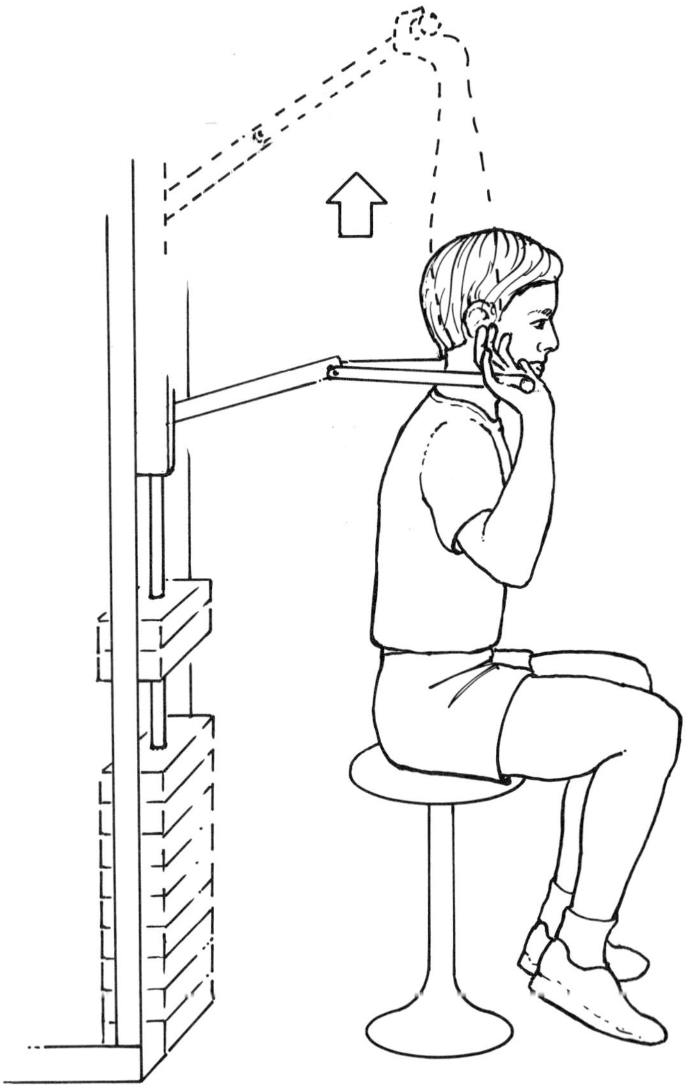

FIGURE 1-10 Military press.

eccentric force to the rotator cuff muscles. The athlete eccentrically controls the humeral internal rotation to about 25°. The athlete again places the arm in 90° abduction and 90° external rotation while the therapist positions the band, and the exercise is repeated.

The patient also can progress to isokinetic training of humeral internal and external rotation with the arm at the side (between 0° and 30° abduction). This exercise starts with low speeds at submaximal effort and progresses to high speeds. In the past, advanced rotator cuff isokinetic training was performed with the arm elevated to 90°. However, this may lead to glenohumeral joint instability. Therefore this position is no longer recommended.

The supraspinatus muscle is isolated when the humerus is elevated in the scapular plane. This motion, "scaption," is an abbreviation for scapular plane elevation. In the starting position, the arm is 30° forward of coronal plane abduction with the thumbs pointing downward; the arm is then raised to just below shoulder height (Fig. 1-9). Even the strongest of patients typically starts with very low weights (1 to 3 lb) for this exercise and builds up to 8 to 10 lb. The clinician must pay close attention to scapulohumeral rhythm and synchrony because this dictates the progression of the weight. If there

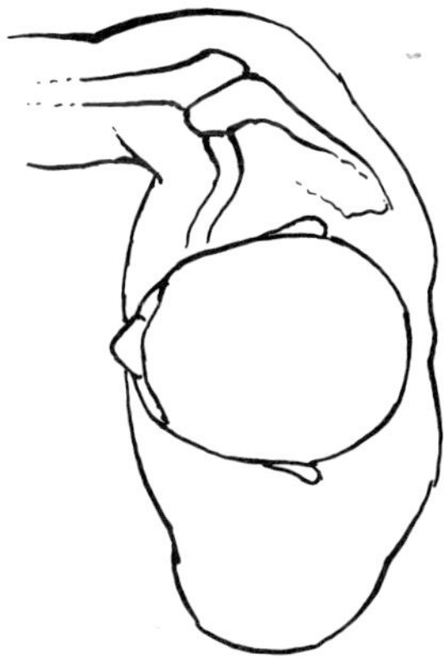

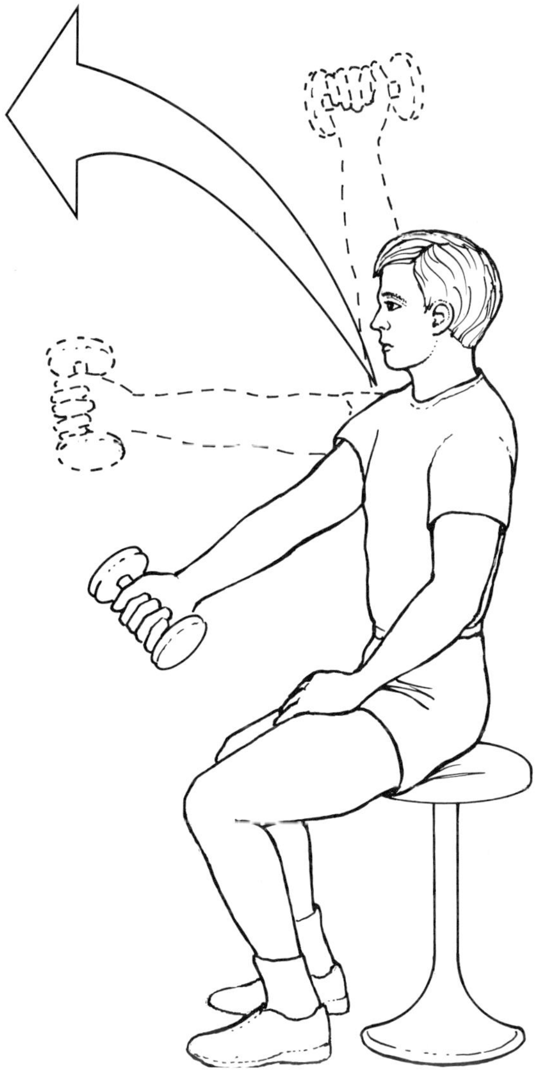

FIGURE 1-11 Arm flexion with neutral rotation

is no impingement pain, scaption can be performed while externally rotating the humerus. With external rotation, the patient can safely elevate beyond 90° without pinching the supraspinatus tendon under the coracoacromial arch. Other studies[2,31] have recommended different exercises for the supraspinatus; however, those studies evaluated the exercises during the isometric hold at the end of the range. Although these exercises are not harmful, scaption is the preferred exercise because consistent high-level EMG activity throughout the range can be sustained.

Additional exercises that require substantial input from the rotator cuff are the military press (Fig. 1-10) and arm forward flexion with neutral rotation (Fig. 1-11).

Scapular Pivotors

Full active scapular motion is very important to the overhead athlete and unfortunately easy to overlook. The muscles responsible for this include the trapezius (upper, middle, and lower portions), levator scapulae, rhomboids, serratus anterior, and pectoralis minor. These muscles function as force couples to optimally position the glenoid, thus providing maximal stability for the humeral head without causing impingement. For example, scapular upward rotation entails three complementary forces: upward rotation, retraction, and an anterolateral force from the inferior angle.[8] The upward rotation is supplied by the upper and lower trapezius and the serratus anterior, the retraction by the middle trapezius and rhomboids, and the anterolateral force by the serratus anterior. Muscles from all three borders of the scapula function in unison to rotate the scapula. A "weak link" at any one of these borders could result in asynchronous and/or limited motion.

The exercise that mimics the rowing motion (Fig. 1-12) and horizontal shoulder abduction both are excellent for all portions of the trapezius, levator scapulae, and rhomboid muscles. Flexion and scaption exercises also

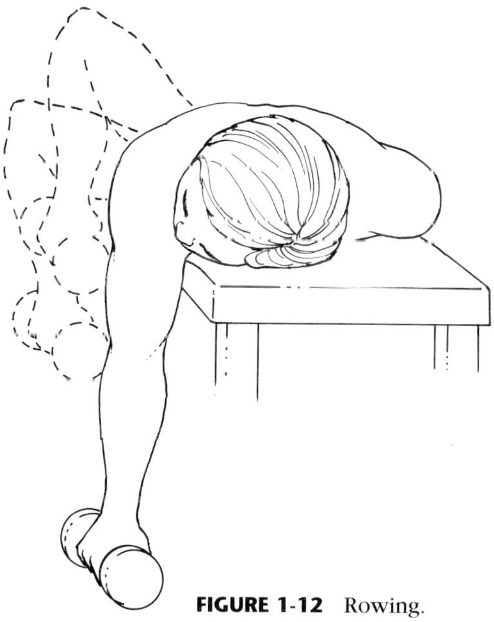

FIGURE 1-12 Rowing.

are valuable for most of the scapular muscles.[14] In addition, the shoulder shrug, the press-up (Fig. 1-13), and the push-up with a "plus" exercise are critical for the serratus anterior, pectoralis minor, levator scapulae, and upper trapezius muscles. The "plus" exercise during the push-up is performed by emphasizing scapular protraction and has been proven through electromyography to be the most beneficial arc of the exercise. The push-up with a plus is performed in the early stage of a rehabilitation program with the patient on the knees and forearms. The patient must be careful to lower the chest only as far as the shoulder during the push-up. To lower further would displace the humeral head anteriorly, thus aggravating the anterior structures and possibly increasing the likelihood of further instability. As the athlete progresses, the plus is added to the push-up by placing the palms of the hand on the floor and extending the elbows. Ultimately, this exercise is performed with weight on the toes and the knees extended (Fig. 1-14). This exercise frequently is performed poorly and must be carefully monitored. A bench press with a plus exercise accomplishes the same goal as the plus motion used with the push-up because of the closed kinetic chain. Again, however, the athlete must be instructed to bring the bar down only to the point where the elbows are in line with the shoulder to prevent the humeral head from displacing anteriorly.

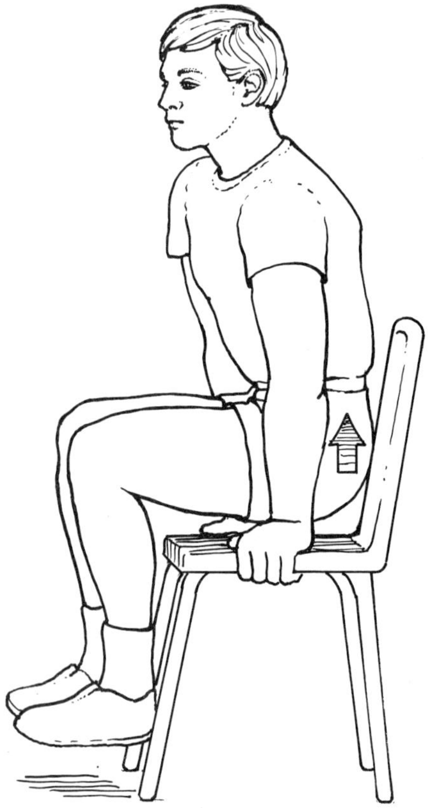

FIGURE 1-13 Press-up.

During athletic activities, most of these muscles fire briefly, then the muscle activity drops to resting levels.[4,6,17,21] The one exception is the serratus anterior. Frequently the serratus anterior fires over a prolonged time with a relatively high level of activity. When the athlete swims the freestyle stroke, for example, the serratus anterior fires at a significant level with no rest period[21] and therefore is highly susceptible to fatigue. In addition, a competitive swimmer often practices most of the year, 6 to 7 days a week, and covers 8000 to 20,000 meters a day.[23] Thus it is important not only to strengthen the serratus anterior, but also to introduce endurance exercise (such as an upper-extremity ergometer) into the exercise

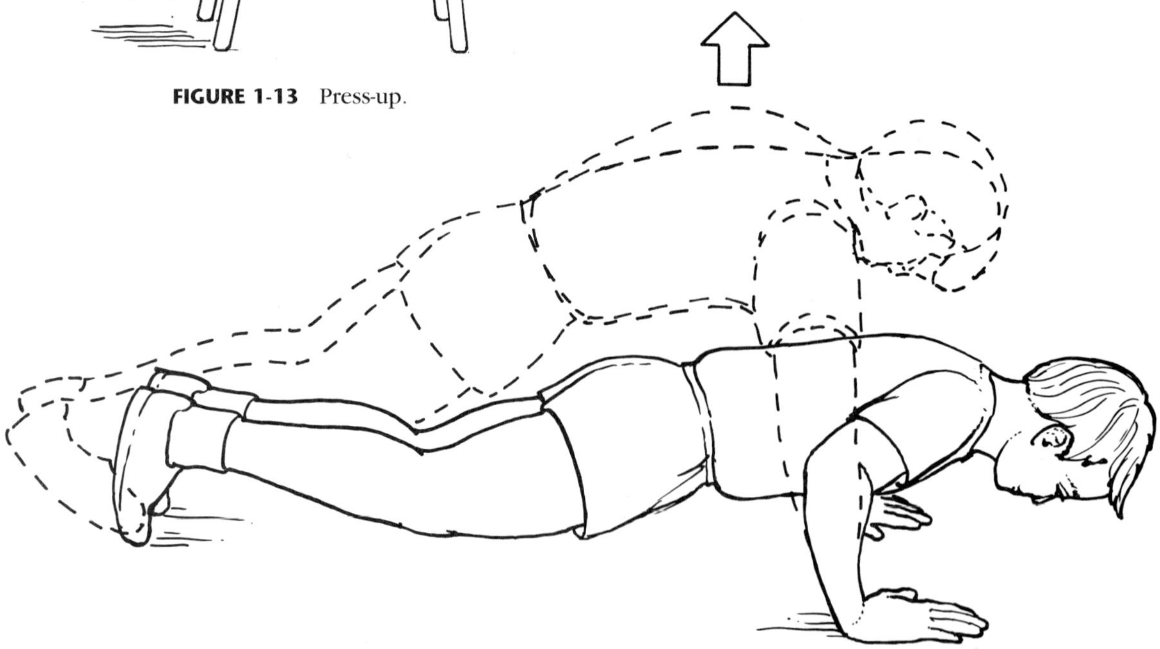

FIGURE 1-14 Push-up plus.

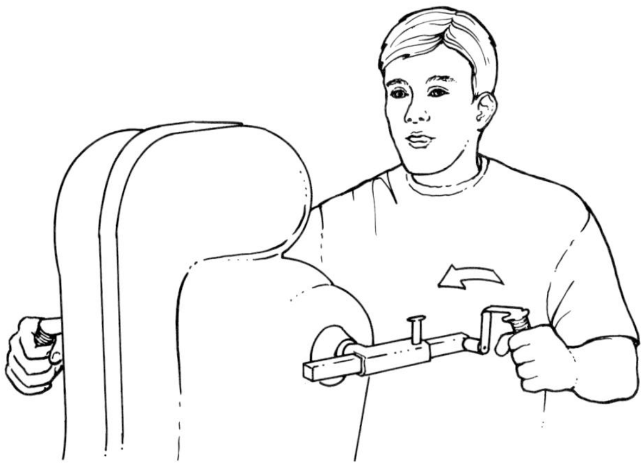

FIGURE 1-15 Upper-extremity ergometer.

program (Fig. 1-15). The height of the hand pedals on the ergometer must be varied to ensure optimal training to all of the broad-based fibers of the serratus anterior.

Humeral Positioners

The anterior, middle, and posterior deltoids are muscles that grossly position the humerus in space. These muscles are incorporated into the exercise after the protectors and pivotors are adequately strengthened. If the deltoids were strengthened and the protectors and pivotors were weak or ignored, the scapula would lag behind the humeral motion or there would be no fine-tuning of the humeral head within the glenoid. Either of these would result in pathologic motion.

Scaption, forward flexion, and prone horizontal abduction are good exercises for the positioners, as they are for the rotator cuff muscles. When the time comes to integrate the positioners a bit more, the rotator cuff muscles should be strong enough to add more weight to the exercise. Additional exercises to augment the program include the exercise that mimics the rowing motion (see Fig. 1-12) and the military press[13] (see Fig. 1-10). The typical deltoid muscle exercise of abduction in the coronal plane can be detrimental to the shoulder unless the rotator cuff muscles are strong enough to depress the humeral head. The theory is that abduction in the coronal plane can place tremendous forces on the glenohumeral joint and cause impingement of the rotator cuff muscles. Therefore significant cuff strength is essential before this maneuver is attempted. If applied correctly, abduction in the coronal plane to 90° is very effective in retraining scapulohumeral synchrony. Scaption activates the deltoid muscles with an intensity similar to abduction without jeopardizing the joint. When adding weights to the scaption exercise, the trainer must avoid encouraging scapular substitution. If the athlete substitutes by shrugging the shoulder, the rotator cuff muscles probably are not functioning normally.

Power Drivers

The pectoralis major and latissimus dorsi are the last muscles to be incorporated into an exercise program. Overall, the upper extremity contributes very little power to sports in which the feet are fixed to the ground. Typically, the power comes from the legs and is transferred through the trunk up to the arms and out to the projectile object (e.g., golf ball, baseball).[9,20,28,30] Research has demonstrated that the pectoralis major and latissimus dorsi are the only muscles in the upper extremity to have a positive correlation between peak torque developed in isokinetic testing and pitching velocity.[1] These muscles also have high activity during the propulsive phase of the freestyle and butterfly swim strokes.[19,21]

In addition to propulsion, the pectoralis major and latissimus dorsi muscles can help to grossly place and internally rotate the arm. When the rotator cuff muscles are not functioning in the painful shoulder, the pectoralis major and latissimus dorsi attempt to substitute with gross humeral head depression and internal rotation.[16] However, because they insert more distally on the humerus, and because they are much larger muscles, they are not as effective or efficient as are the finely tuned rotator cuff muscles. Thus the power drivers should be strengthened only after there is adequate strength and synchrony from the other glenohumeral and scapulothoracic muscles. The press-up (see Fig. 1-13), bench press,[29] and latissimus pull-down all are good exercises to strengthen the power drivers.

Thus an effective and efficient exercise program for either injury prevention or rehabilitation considers the role and the progression of the 4P's:

Protectors, Pivotors → Positioners → Power drivers

The Elbow

The elbow is a less common site of injury than the shoulder. This is largely because the elbow has less mobility and more inherent bony stability than the shoulder; thus it has fewer degrees of freedom for directions of motion. The four areas from which problems are likely to arise are the elbow flexors, the medial aspect of the joint, the lateral aspect of the joint, and the posterior compartment.

Elbow Flexors

During throwing, tremendous deceleration forces control the elbow extension encountered immediately after ball release.[15] Most of these forces are absorbed by the brachialis, brachioradialis, and biceps. Thus most competitive pitchers exhibit stiffness and soreness, especially within the flexor muscles. Over years of competition, many pitchers develop elbow flexion contractures of 20° or more. Because many pitchers and most throwers have these signs and symptoms, it is very difficult to determine which elbows actually may develop more serious problems. The logical solution is to prophylactically treat all throwers for flexor muscle soreness.

The treatment for throwers is to ice the elbow muscles after a throwing session and to gently stretch the muscles routinely. If the pitcher has a chronic elbow flexion contracture, gentle stretching is performed only to the point of the contraction. After years of competitive play, most pitchers exhibit a contracture that fortunately does not interfere with their performance. Forceful stretching of a chronic elbow flexion contracture may break off some of the bony overgrowth and result in loose bodies floating within the joint. Intraarticular loose bodies usually will interfere with performance and often must be surgically removed. Thus attempting to stretch the chronic elbow flexion contracture is ill-advised. Rather, an emphasis is placed on full elbow extension exercises. Strengthening exercises for both the acute and chronic elbow problem include elbow and wrist flexion and extension along with forearm pronation and supination.

Medial Aspect

The medial aspect of the elbow is particularly vulnerable to injury caused by large valgus forces generated during throwing.[5] There are two separate presentations of injury to this area. One is the gradual progression of soreness. In this situation, rehabilitation may be able to return the athlete to the prior level of competition. The second presentation is that of a spontaneous rupture of the medial collateral ligament (MCL) during a single pitch. In this instance, surgical intervention usually is recommended as soon as it is determined that the athlete cannot pitch with the injury and is mentally prepared to be out of competition for 1 year. Most likely, the athlete will not be mentally prepared for surgery immediately after the injury. If this is the case, an intense rehabilitation program begins. It may take only 2 to 4 weeks of rehabilitation for the patient with a spontaneous rupture to realize that surgery is the best option.

The rehabilitation program consists of icing and gentle stretching and strengthening of the elbow, wrist flexors, and extensors as well as the forearm pronators and supinators. If the severity of symptoms increases to the point of persistent MCL pain during throwing, and if performance is diminished by approximately 25% or more, the player is removed from competition while aggressively continuing with the aforementioned program. After approximately 3 months of intense rehabilitation, the player can begin a graduated return to throwing. If the pain at the distal attachment of the MCL or posterior compartment persists and the player cannot improve performance beyond 75%, the player again is removed from play and rehabilitation continues. After two unsuccessful attempts at conservative management, surgical intervention should be considered.

Lateral Aspect

The lateral aspect of the elbow joint also is vulnerable to injury caused by the lateral compressive forces about the elbow. These forces are compounded by improper mechanics of the tennis backhand[6,11,13] and, to a lesser degree, by the forces transmitted in golf from the club up through the arm during ball impact. Because the core of the problem for the tennis player with lateral elbow pain is improper mechanics,[11] the treatment of choice is to correct the poor mechanics. In the case of the golfer, the core of the problem may be mechanics (thus the obvious treatment recommendation) or may be partially related to the choice of metals of the club shaft (e.g., graphite, stainless steel, or titanium). At any rate, palliative treatment entails reduction of practice time, gentle stretching and strengthening of the elbow and forearm musculature, and the use of ice after exercise.

Posterior Compartment Syndrome

The posterior compartment of the elbow may incur injury in the throwing athlete resulting from the repetitive forces during forced, terminal elbow extension. Pitchers who throw the split-finger fastball or the slider are particularly vulnerable to this injury. The athlete will note tenderness in the area of the olecranon fossa. On examination, there will be effusion in the posterior compartment. The athlete may have palpable tenderness at the MCL and/or pain with valgus stress. Most likely the athlete will have a positive bounce test as the elbow moves into extension. Unfortunately, strengthening and stretching programs are of little benefit for this injury. Pain-reducing modalities can be used, as can antiinflammatory medication. If the symptoms persist, surgery may be necessary. Thus an effective exercise program for both injury prevention and rehabilitation of the elbow considers mechanics of the sport and the tissues at risk.

The Wrist and Hand

The strength of forearm and hand muscles may be important to performance in sports that require swinging an object to hit a projectile (e.g., batting, tennis swing, golf swing). In her book *The Complete Golfer,* Nancy Lopez mentioned that the PGA Tour professionals have better short games than do the women pros, conceivably because of the strength in the men's hands.[12] EMG studies on pitching reveal that forearm muscles are quite active.[4] However, EMG studies on batting have demonstrated relatively low levels of muscular activity in the wrist muscles.[28] The fact is that almost all injuries to the wrist and hand are traumatic. Thus in terms of injury prevention, there may be very little to be done.

Depending on the specific traumatic event, treatment may consist of immobilization (with cast, splint, or taping); modalities to decrease pain, inflammation, or adhesions; manual mobilization to decrease adhesions; stretching to increase ROM; and strengthening. The treatments for traumatic injuries are discussed in the chapters covering the specific injuries.

SPORT-SPECIFIC EXERCISE

Given the aforementioned basic information on exercise, the next step is to assimilate known information about key muscles for specific sports and integrate that information into the exercise program to focus on the tissues at risk.

During the freestyle and backstroke swimming strokes, as well as during the tennis serve and baseball pitch, the subscapularis and serratus anterior are key muscles for both strengthening and endurance training.[4,18,21,25] In addition, the teres minor requires specific attention for baseball pitchers.[4] Swimmers who consistently use the backstroke benefit from focusing on the teres minor and subscapularis.[18] Swimmers who engage in the breaststroke are at lower risk for shoulder injury[24] than swimmers who perform the other strokes, but the subscapularis and teres minor are important to evaluate to ensure optimal strength and endurance.

Pilot studies have demonstrated similarities between the volleyball and tennis serves[25]; thus volleyball players also need to consider strengthening the subscapularis and serratus anterior. The football pass and javelin throw are qualitatively similar to the baseball pitch; thus athletes who perform these maneuvers can focus on the serratus anterior, subscapularis, and teres minor.

The golfer does not elevate the arm above 90°[9]; thus golf is not officially considered an overhead sport. However, the scapular retractors and subscapularis do play important roles in protecting the shoulder joint during the golf swing.[10,17]

In the elbow, the EMG activity in both the biceps and brachialis is more than doubled immediately after ball release in the baseball pitch to control deceleration. In addition, the EMG activity in the brachioradialis is higher after ball release than during any other time of the pitch.[4] The medial muscles have demonstrated significantly reduced muscle activity in throwers with MCL-deficient elbows,[7] and thus this muscle group demands a focus in exercise. In particular, cadaver studies have demonstrated that the flexor carpi ulnaris (FCU) is the only muscle in line with the MCL when the elbow is flexed between 30° and 120°; thus the FCU specifically needs to be strengthened.[3] The lateral muscles have revealed significantly enhanced muscle activity during the tennis backhand in players with elbow problems,[6,11] which reinforces the improper mechanics to be corrected.

RETRAINING SYNCHRONY OF MOTION

Throughout a rehabilitation program, all active motion is constantly observed to ensure synchronous movement. At first this is performed by observing bilateral upper-extremity movements of elevation for any scapular or humeral asymmetries. Another excellent functional check for synchrony is to abduct the humerus to 90° and repetitively internally and externally rotate the arms (see Fig. 1-7). The scapula must remain stable bilaterally. The athlete then progresses to gentle, sport-specific movements under supervision. These movements may include an easy ball toss with a gradual progression to throwing, exercise on a swim bench, or a slow golf swing. It must be carefully explained that even though the athlete is continually getting stronger, this still is a time for evaluation, treatment, or reevaluation—not a "green light" to go "all out" to get into shape for competition. The words of Robert Frost are applicable: ". . . you must learn to work easy in the harness." When strong and synchronous sport-specific motion is achieved, the athlete is allowed to begin a graduated competition training program.

SUMMARY

In the ideal world, injury prevention and rehabilitation of the upper extremity in sports encompass an understanding of what is normal, the tissues at risk, functional anatomy, and the mechanics of motion. The prevention and rehabilitation program requires a judicious balance of sport activity, sport-specific stretching and strengthening exercise, and rest. The athlete benefits from early detection of an impending injury and intervention focused at the core of the problem. An injured athlete requires a retraining of the muscles to restore the synchrony of motion before returning to competition. This formula for injury prevention and rehabilitation produces a dynamic thought process that not only optimizes performance, prevents injury, and effectively rehabilitates the athlete, but also stimulates professionals to constantly improve care. This dynamic thought process enables the sports medicine practitioner to make the ideal world a reality for the athlete.

References

1. Bartlett LR, Storey MD, Simons BD: Measurement of upper extremity torque production and its relationship to throwing speed in the competitive athlete, *Am J Sports Med* 17:89-91, 1989.
2. Blackburn TA et al: EMG analysis of posterior rotator cuff exercises, *Athl Train* 25:40-45, 1990.
3. Davidson PA et al: Functional anatomy of the flexor pronator muscle group in relationship to the medial collateral ligament of the elbow, *Am J Sports Med* 23(2):245-250, 1995.
4. DiGiovine N et al: An electromyographic analysis of the upper extremity in pitching, *J Shoulder Elbow Surg* 1(1):15-25, 1992.

5. Feltner M, Dapena J: Dynamics of the shoulder and elbow joints of the throwing arm during a baseball pitch, *Int J Sports Biomech* 2:235-259, 1986.
6. Giangarra C et al: EMG and cinematographic analysis of elbow function in tennis players using single and double-handed backhands, *Am J Sports Med* 21(3):394-399, 1993.
7. Glousman RE et al: An electromyographic analysis of the elbow in normal and injured pitchers with medial collateral ligament insufficiency, *Am J Sports Med* 20(3):311-317, 1992.
8. Inman VT, Saunders M, Abbott LC: Observations on the function of the shoulder joints, *J Bone Joint Surg* 26:1-30, 1944.
9. Jobe FW et al: *Exercise guide to better golf,* Inglewood, Calif, 1993, Champion Press.
10. Kao J et al: EMG analysis of the scapular muscles during a golf swing, *Am J Sports Med* 23(1):19-23, 1995.
11. Kelley J et al: EMG and cinematographic analysis of elbow function in tennis players with lateral epicondylitis, *Am J Sports Med,* 22(3):359-363, 1994.
12. Lopez N: *Nancy Lopez's the complete golfer,* Chicago, 1987, Contemporary Books.
13. Morris M et al: Electromyographic analysis of elbow function in tennis players, *Am J Sports Med* 17(2):241-247, 1989.
14. Moseley B et al: EMG analysis of the scapular muscles during a shoulder rehabilitation program, *Am J Sports Med* 20(2):128-134, 1992.
15. Pappas AM, Zawacki RM, Sullivan TJ: Biomechanics of baseball pitching: a preliminary report, *Am J Sports Med* 13:216-222, 1985.
16. Perry J et al: The painful shoulder during the backstroke: an EMG and cinematographic analysis of 12 muscles, *Clin J Sport Med* 2:13-20, 1992.
17. Pink M, Jobe FW, Perry J: Electromyographic analysis of the shoulder during the golf swing, *Am J Sports Med* 18(2):137-140, 1990.
18. Pink M et al: The normal shoulder during the backstroke: an EMG and cinematographic analysis of 12 muscles, *Clin J Sport Med* 2:6-12, 1992.
19. Pink M et al: The normal shoulder during the butterfly swim stroke: an EMG and cinematographic analysis of 12 muscles, *Clin Orthop* 288:48-59, 1993.
20. Pink M, Perry J, Jobe FW: Electromyographic analysis of the trunk in golfers, *Am J Sports Med* 21(3):385-388, 1993.
21. Pink M et al: The normal shoulder during freestyle swimming: an EMG and cinematographic analysis of twelve muscles, *Am J Sports Med* 19:569-575, 1991.
22. Rathbun JB, MacNab I: The microvascular pattern of the rotator cuff, *J Bone Joint Surg* 52B(3):540-553, 1970.
23. Richardson AB, Jobe FW, Collins HR: The shoulder in competitive swimming, *Am J Sports Med* 8:159-163, 1980.
24. Ruwe P et al: The normal and painful shoulder the breaststroke: an EMG and cinematographic analysis of 12 muscles, *Am J Sports Med* 22(6):789-796, 1994.
25. Ryu RK et al: An electromyographic analysis of shoulder function in tennis players, *Am J Sports Med* 16(5):481-485, 1988.
26. Saha AK: *Theory of shoulder mechanism,* Springfield, Ill, 1961, Charles C Thomas.
27. Saha AK, Chakravarty BG: Studies on electromyographic changes of muscles acting on the shoulder joint complex, *Calcutta Med J* 53:409-413, 1956.
28. Shaffer B et al: Baseball batting: an electromyographic study, *Clin Orthop* 289:166-175, 1993.
29. Townsend H et al: Electromyographic analysis of the glenohumeral muscles during a baseball rehabilitation program, *Am J Sports Med* 19(3):264-272, 1991.
30. Watkins R et al: Dynamic EMG analysis of torque transfer in professional baseball pitchers, *Spine* 14(4):404-408, 1989.
31. Worrell TW et al: An analysis of supraspinatus EMG activity and shoulder isometric force development, *Med Sci Sports Exer* 24(7):744, 1992.

CHAPTER 2

Unusual Problems of the Upper Extremity in the Athlete

JAMES P. BRADLEY
FRANK W. JOBE

INTRODUCTION

The cornerstone of appropriate treatment of upper-extremity problems in the athlete is an accurate diagnosis. Attaining this goal requires a systematic approach to the athlete's complaint. A complete history and physical examination are the most useful tools to achieve this goal. In the vast majority of cases, applying these principles yields a solid working diagnosis. Fortunately, most athletes' injuries are predictable based on the history (macrotrauma versus microtrauma) and the biomechanics of the stresses applied by the specific sport. However, there are a few "zebras," and a high index of suspicion must be maintained regarding these unusual conditions.

This chapter presents uncommon causes of upper-extremity pain and dysfunction in the athlete that may masquerade as common athletic problems. This chapter also should engender a high index of suspicion concerning these rare disorders.

The chapter is separated into three sections, which divide the upper extremity into shoulder, elbow, and wrist. Each of these sections is subdivided into etiologic categories that include (1) traumatic, (2) neurovascular, (3) neoplastic tumor, (4) infectious, (5) metabolic, (6) rheumatoid and rheumatoid-like, and (7) miscellaneous. The conditions presented were chosen specifically because of their ability to mimic typical upper-extremity problems in athletes. The sports physician should recognize most of these rare problems, which will enable the physician to triage these problems for definitive treatment.

SHOULDER

Shoulder pain is an extremely common complaint in athletes. However, specialists must not be "lulled" into assuming that all shoulder pain is mechanical or glenohumeral in nature. Rather, there must be a vigilant search for subtle nuances in presentation or physical examination that suggest a possible rare malady. Other chapters in this book highlight the history and physical examination specifically applying to that individual condition. When the work-up does not correlate with the suspected pathology, the physician should be alerted to other infrequent pathologic conditions that can mimic these common conditions.

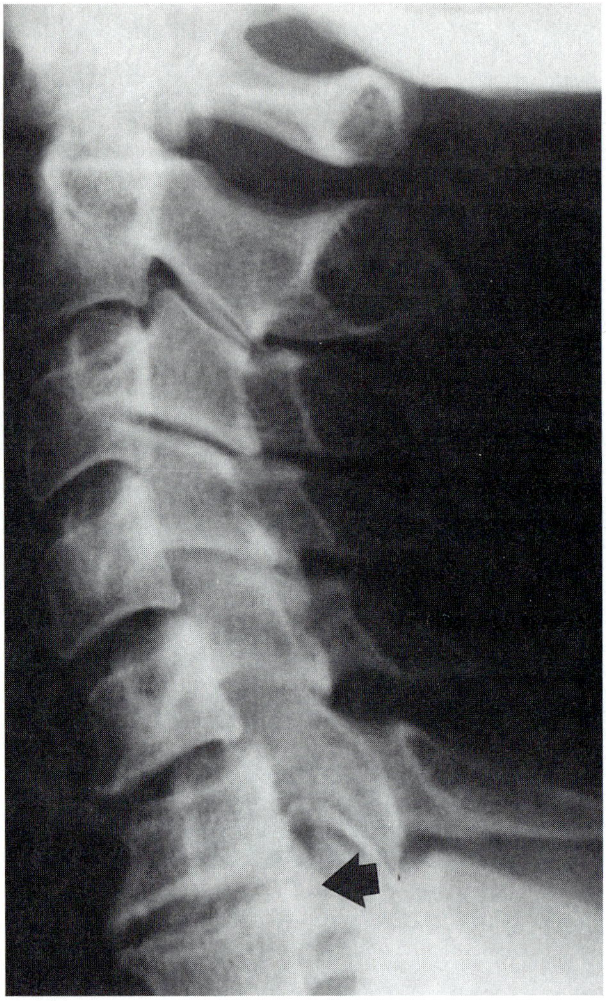

FIGURE 2-1 Cervical disc disease illustrating isolated narrowing of the C6-C7 interspace.

Neurovascular Problems

The shoulder often is the site of referred pain, most commonly from the cervical spine. Intradural, preforaminal, foraminal, and postforaminal lesions of the neck all can cause shoulder pain.[4] Ruptured intervertebral discs (preforaminal lesions) remain a common source of pain in the athletic population.

Cervical Spine Pathology

Shoulder pain secondary to cervical spine pathology has broad and complex sources. Generally, the neural element elicits typical pain characteristics, while the specific anatomic area produces typical patterns of distribution. Cervical spine pain by history is characterized by a deep burning pain localized to the insertion of the levator scapulae muscle at the superior medial border of the scapula.[65] Radicular pain is experienced down the arm to the fingers, associated with paresthesias in the fingers and less commonly in the forearm. Patients frequently hold the neck in one position to avoid the posterior pain, with the position depending on the site of the lesion.[4] Neck motion, especially extension, tends to exacerbate the posterior shoulder pain. Sometimes the patient will be more comfortable with the shoulder abducted, permitting the forearm to rest on the top of the patient's head. Presumably, this position decreases some of the tension on the cervical roots.[65] A good guideline is to identify the site of maximal pain. If the patient localizes the pain proximal to the lateral acromion, the cervical spine or other proximal sites are likely.

On physical examination, the Spurling test has been very helpful in uncovering cervical root irritation. The test is performed in a stepwise fashion of cervical spine extension, extension with rotation toward the painful shoulder, and finally axial cervical compression. Increasing posterior shoulder pain and radiculopathy are positive findings.[27] Obviously, a complete neurologic and vascular examination is mandatory to delineate any weakness or reflex changes. Most commonly, the radicular symptoms occur in the C5, C6, or C7 distribution. Symptoms other than at the C5, C6, or C7 level should alert the practitioner to the possibility that the cause of the root irritation is other than disc or spondylitic disease.

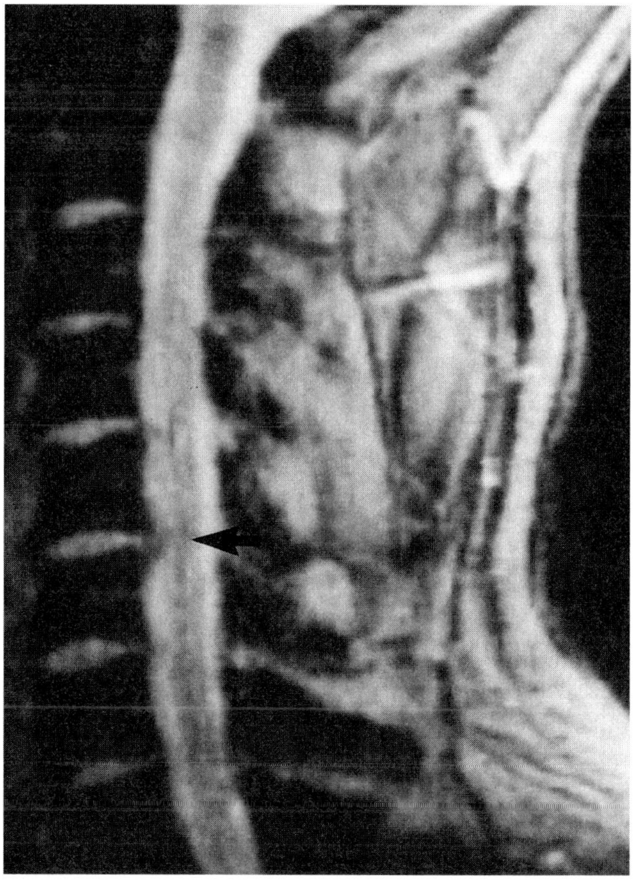

FIGURE 2-2 MRI of cervical spine demonstrating herniation of the C5-C6 disc.

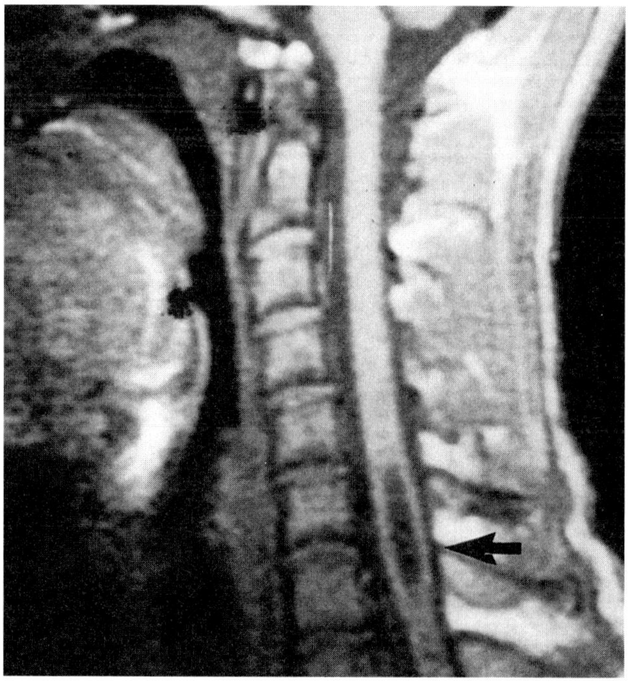

FIGURE 2-3 Syringomyelia of the cervical spine.

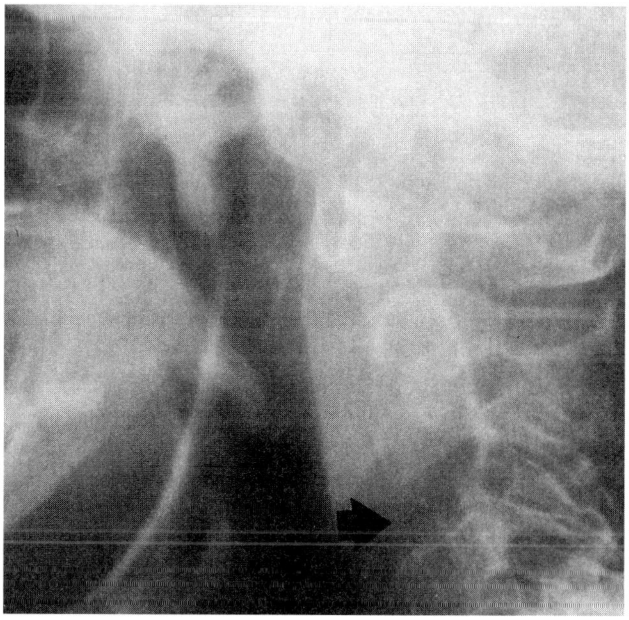

FIGURE 2-4 Complete destruction of C3 secondary to metastatic disease of the breast.

Symptomatic cervical disease is rarely seen without one or several abnormalities on the plain radiographs.[59] Typical findings include: (1) narrowing of the interspace (Fig. 2-1), (2) vacuum disc sign (air in disc space), (3) loss of normal lordotic curve, (4) foraminal encroachment, and rarely, (5) cervical instability. Magnetic resonance imaging (MRI) also is becoming more accepted in defining cervical spine pathology, especially with the introduction of high-resolution techniques (Fig. 2-2).

Just as not all shoulder pain is caused by underlying shoulder pathology, referred cervical spine pain does not always represent cervical disc or spondylitic disease. Essentially, four zones must be suspected when referred cervical spine pain is encountered. Intradural, preforaminal, foraminal, and postforaminal lesions of the cervical spine all are possible sources. Two intradural lesions must be ruled out: syringomyelia and cord tumor. Syringomyelia may present with a "boring" upper-extremity pain that can be mistaken for nerve root irritation[19] (Fig. 2-3). The pain commonly occurs at the shoulder level and the inside of the forearm and hand. Prominent physical signs usually are noted, such as muscle atrophy, weakness, and paresthesias in a dermatomal distribution[10] (see Fig. 2-3). Cord tumors also present with shoulder pain. In fact, the first successful identification of a spinal cord tumor recorded in North America was in a patient who complained of shoulder pain.[4] The triad of shoulder pain, distal radiation of pain, and profound sensory loss, usually anesthesia, can be caused by an intradural neoplastic lesion.[4]

Preforaminal lesions arising in a zone between the dura and the intervertebral foramen are common (Fig. 2-4) and generally produce cervical and brachial pain.

Acute herniation of an intervertebral disc is associated with neck stiffness, radiating pain (from discomfort to severe arm and finger pain) and, commonly, sensory loss and/or motor weakness. This is in contrast to degenerative disc lesions, in which the onset is much more insidious. Extradural neoplasms, usually of the meninges, are slow growing and hard to identify but produce significant motor and sensory changes while producing nerve-root irritation. Osseous tumors are grouped into primary and secondary lesions. They may produce nerve-root compression, usually caused by partial vertebral-body collapse. Osseous neoplastic pain usually is manifested in a distinctive manner that is nonmechanical, persistent, more intense at night (interfering with sleep), and sometimes exacerbated by periods of inactivity. Neurologic involvement depends on the anatomic location of the neoplasm.

Foraminal lesions represent the most common cause of persistent shoulder and radiating arm pain. Degenerative changes within the intervertebral discs may cause foraminal encroachment by osteophytic formation with resultant nerve-root irritation. The most commonly involved levels are C4-C5, C5-C6, and C6-C7. Classic symptoms include neck stiffness, shoulder/neck pain, and pain between the shoulder blades, often with extension to the upper arm and deltoid muscle insertion. Hypoesthesia is frequent, usually correlating with the zone of peripheral radiating pain. Late findings include diminished biceps and triceps reflexes and motor weakness.

Postforaminal Lesions (Acute Brachial Neuropathy)

Multiple problems can arise in the neurologic elements after they exit the foramina, and some tend to be more common in an athletic population. Acute brachial neuropathy (Parsonage-Turner syndrome) is of unknown etiology and appears occasionally. The main symptomatic finding is pain localized to the shoulder. Classically, the pain is intense and may continue for a few hours or 2 to 3 weeks, despite analgesics and rest.[9,21] The onset may be preceded by viral illness, immunization, or strenuous exercise. Usually no history of direct trauma to the limb is elicited.[22] Motor findings dominate and typically develop as the pain recedes. The motor involvement is often diffuse, encompassing the deltoid, supraspinatus, infraspinatus, serratus anterior, biceps, and triceps. In comparison, sensory loss is usually minimal and generally limited to the axillary distribution over the lateral deltoid. The problem is that significant pain predominates initially and neurologic findings lag; therefore the physician may be fooled into a diagnosis of acute calcific bursitis. The diagnosis frequently is confirmed by EMG evaluation.[64] Associated EMG findings may include (1) involvement of muscles that are not innervated by brachial plexus, (2) major denervation limited to muscles innervated by one or two peripheral nerves, (3) severe denervation of a single muscle, and (4) major motor involvement in a plexus or peripheral nerve distribution, with sparing of the sensory component.[22] EMG abnormalities have been reported up to 7 years after initial presentation. Therefore return to athletic activity is determined by the clinical return of strength.[22]

Postforaminal Lesions (Thoracic Outlet Syndrome)

The signs and symptoms of thoracic outlet syndrome (TOS) often are obtuse and vague, and the pathology often is difficult to define. In TOS the intimate proximity of nerves and vessels produces varying degrees of brachial plexus and subclavian vessel compression. This proximity accounts for the plethora of symptoms common to TOS: pain (in the face, neck, head, arm, chest, shoulder, or axilla) and upper-extremity symptoms of paresthesias, numbness, weakness, heaviness, fatigability, swelling, discoloration, ulceration, and sometimes Raynaud's phenomenon.[29] The most common symptom complex is caused by compression of the lower trunk of the brachial plexus.[33] This compression causes pain and paresthesias localized along the medial aspect of the brachium and ulnar aspect of the forearm, terminating at the ring and small fingers. Patients with motor findings may present with weakness of grasp caused by intrinsic muscle involvement. Discrete etiologic factors have been associated with TOS, including (1) cervical ribs (found in less than 1% of the population), (2) fibrous bands originating from the end of a prominent C7 transverse process or from the end of a short cervical rib, (3) anomalous scalene muscle development, and (4) body habitus consisting of a long neck and round back or endomorphic individuals with pendulous breasts.[29]

The diagnosis is difficult and sometimes one of exclusion; however, four classic tests have been described, including Adson's test, Wright's maneuver, and the costoclavicular maneuver.[32] The problem is that the reliability of these tests is variable, and there is a high incidence of false-negatives and false-positives.[33]

Anterior/posterior cervical spine radiographs may be helpful if a cervical rib or a long transverse process projects from C7. Other than these two conditions, x-ray tests are usually negative.

Although TOS overall is uncommon among athletes, its presentation of shoulder pain associated with a myriad of other symptoms may initially mimic several upper-extremity problems in athletes.

Neurofibromatosis

Neurofibromatosis is one of the neurocutaneous syndromes that are congenital disorders (autosomal dominant) characterized by abnormal growth of ectodermal tissues and demonstrating distinctive skin lesions and malformations or tumors of the nervous system. This is a very common genetic disorder, with an estimated frequency of 1 in 3000 births.[14,31] Upper-extremity pain and dysfunction may be an early finding, depending on the sites of the disease.

Although the disease is congenital, clinical manifestations usually appear gradually during childhood and adult life. Café-au-lait spots are common, and six or more macules of 1.5 cm or greater are considered reliable evidence of neurofibromatosis.[7] Other skin abnormalities include axillary freckles, soft cutaneous neurofibromas, and firm subcutaneous neurofibromas.[31] Plexiform neuromas may cause grotesque overgrowth of soft tissues and bones about the upper extremity. Scoliosis (with or without kyphosis) appears in 60% of cases, demonstrating either idiopathic or dysplastic curve patterns.[14] Radiographs of the upper extremity and chest show undulating ribbonlike or widened and angulated ribs. Pseudarthrosis of the clavicle as well as the tibia also is possible.[14] Because of the gradual onset in childhood and adult life, a vigilant search for the typical skin manifestation is helpful in early detection to allow for appropriate treatment.

Vascular Lesions

Venous Occlusion

Probably the most common vascular lesion presenting in athletes is axillary/subclavian venous thrombosis; however, it represents only 2% of all venous thrombosis in the general population.[2] In athletes, primary axillary/subclavian thrombosis occurs secondary to high-velocity repetitive activity or blunt trauma. The vessel typically is injured by repetitive microtrauma against anomalous structures, such as cervical ribs, hypertrophied scalenus anterior muscle, and normal structures (first rib or clavicle). Thrombus formation is secondary to reactive changes within the vessel wall. The history includes an insidious onset of swelling and pain in the upper extremity associated with numbness and heaviness. The pain usually is described as a dull ache with easy fatigability during activity. The most notable finding on physical examination is nonpitting edema of the entire upper extremity. Prominent superficial veins and cool, mottled skin are other significant findings. Distal arterial pulses are normal. Nondermatomal hyperesthesia is sometimes noted, but usually the neurologic exam is normal.[62] Venography localizes the lesion and confirms the diagnosis.

Axillary Artery Occlusion

Axillary artery occlusion is rare in athletes, although it has been reported in a baseball pitcher by Tullos et al.[66] and in a wind-surfer by Sadat-Ali.[57] In both cases the mechanism of injury was attributed to repetitive overhead activity. Symptoms are varied because of differing degrees of ischemia caused by the specific lesion. Coolness and ischemic pain about the upper extremity depend on the extent of the lesion and collateral flow. They may be present, diminished, or absent. Although palpation of the involved artery and Doppler flow studies help to localize the lesion, arteriography confirms the diagnosis.

Malignant Neoplasms

The overall incidence of primary sarcoma in the shoulder is approximately 15%, which is the third most common neoplasm after hip and pelvis (first) and knee (second).[11] The proximal humerus is the site of the majority of shoulder tumors (72%).[11] The age of the patient is very important in overall tumor occurrence because most malignant tumors of the skeleton have a peak incidence in adolescents and middle-aged adults.[11] Unfortunately, this age distribution coincides with the highest incidence of musculoskeletal injuries seen in athletes. Because of the relative rarity of neoplasms in the shoulder, there is usually a lag of several months before an accurate diagnosis can be established.

The diagnosis of neoplasm of the shoulder requires a high index of suspicion and attention to a few distinguishing characteristics in the presentation. Historically, these lesions have a subtle onset, with shoulder pain as the most common complaint. The problem is differentiating pain caused by a malignant neoplasm from musculoskeletal pain resulting from other much more common causes. The classic symptoms of an intraosseous malignancy are significant night pain (disrupts sleep) and rest pain. Some patients with degenerative or inflammatory shoulder disease also complain of night pain; however, night pain typically is not the dominant complaint of their pain pattern. Other salient findings include weight loss, poor appetite, and general malaise. The physical examination is variable, depending on the site of the tumor, the presence of soft-tissue extension, and the presence of neurologic compression. Meticulous inspection of the plain radiographs is an important step in the early diagnosis of tumors, specifically noting location, density, and margin of any lesions. It is beyond the scope of this chapter to discuss individual neoplasms; however, an awareness of certain lesions is necessary. Benign chondroblastomas and giant cell tumors tend to appear in the epiphysis, whereas osteosarcomas, chondrosarcomas, and benign simple bone cysts occur within the metaphysis (Figs. 2-5 and 2-6). Diaphyseal lesions include malignant round cell tumors. Most of these neoplasms have distinctive radiographic characteristics that are very helpful in the early diagnosis (Figs. 2-7 and 2-8). A neoplasm of special interest is the Pancoast tumor (adenocarcinoma) of the upper lobe of the lung, which typically presents with referred pain to the anterior or posterior aspect of the shoulder and scapular area. The pain sometimes radiates down the medial aspect of the brachium. Horner's syndrome (ptosis, miosis, anhidrosis,

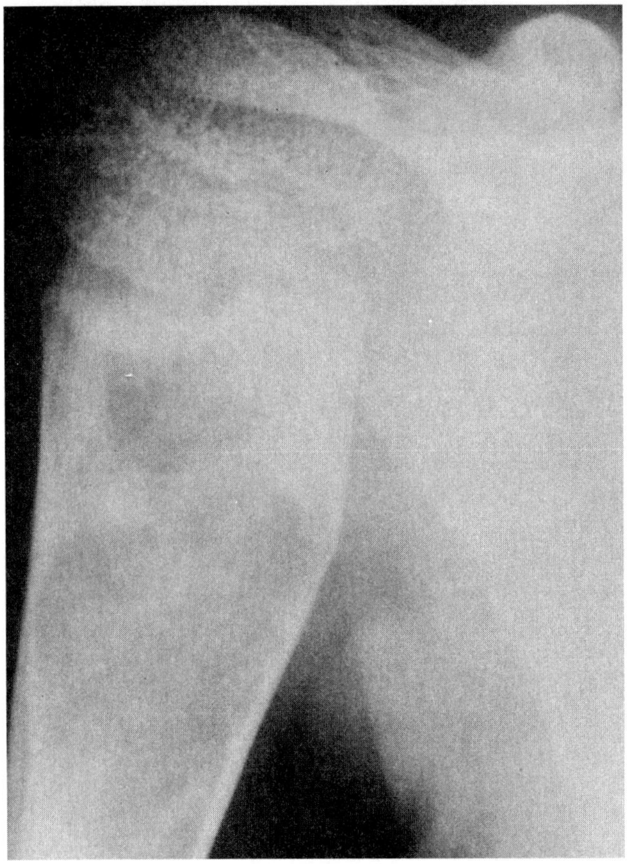

FIGURE 2-5 Simple bone cyst of the proximal metaphysis of the humerus.

and enophthalmos) caused by paralysis of the cervical sympathetic chain may be apparent. Special attention should be given to the superior pulmonary sulcus on the plain films.

Infectious Conditions

Herpes Zoster (Shingles)

Herpes zoster is a recrudescence of latent varicella virus that can cause severe burning pain in the shoulder, down the arm, and around the chest. Presentation keys are dermatomal radicular pain, patients over 50 years of age, and bitter complaints of clothing rubbing the area. The most useful signs are hypesthesia of a dermatomal zone, no deficits of range of motion, and no aggravation of pain by arm motion.[16,43] Rarely, herpes zoster can be associated with muscular weakness of the upper extremity.[16] Failure to recognize these signs and symptoms can delay the diagnosis until the typical erythematous base and clusters of hemorrhagic vesicles appear over the involved dermatome. Frequently, several adjacent dermatomes also are involved.

Lyme Disease

Lyme disease is a tick-borne inflammatory disorder, secondary to the spirochete *Borrelia burgdorferi.* Although named after Lyme, a city in Connecticut, it has been reported in 43 states, with the largest concentrations in the Northeast (Massachusetts to Maryland), the Midwest (Wisconsin and Minnesota), and the West (California, Oregon, and Nevada). Because the disease vector is a deer tick, *Ixodes dammini,* special attention should be given to outdoor athletes in the aforementioned areas of

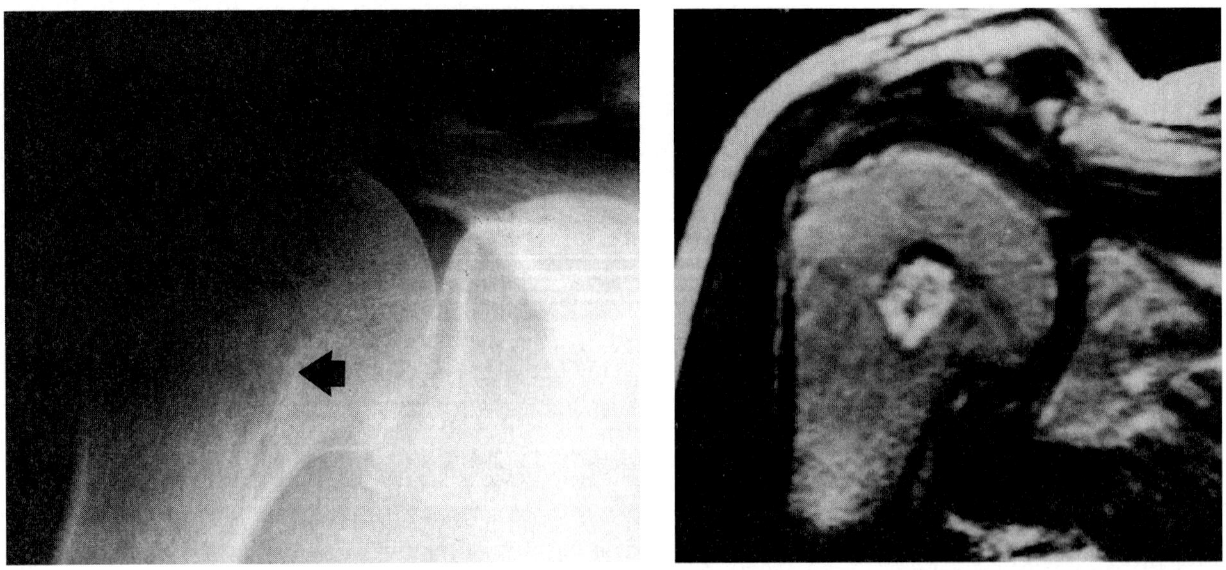

FIGURE 2-6 Shoulder radiograph and corresponding MRI exhibiting an enchondroma of the proximal humerus.

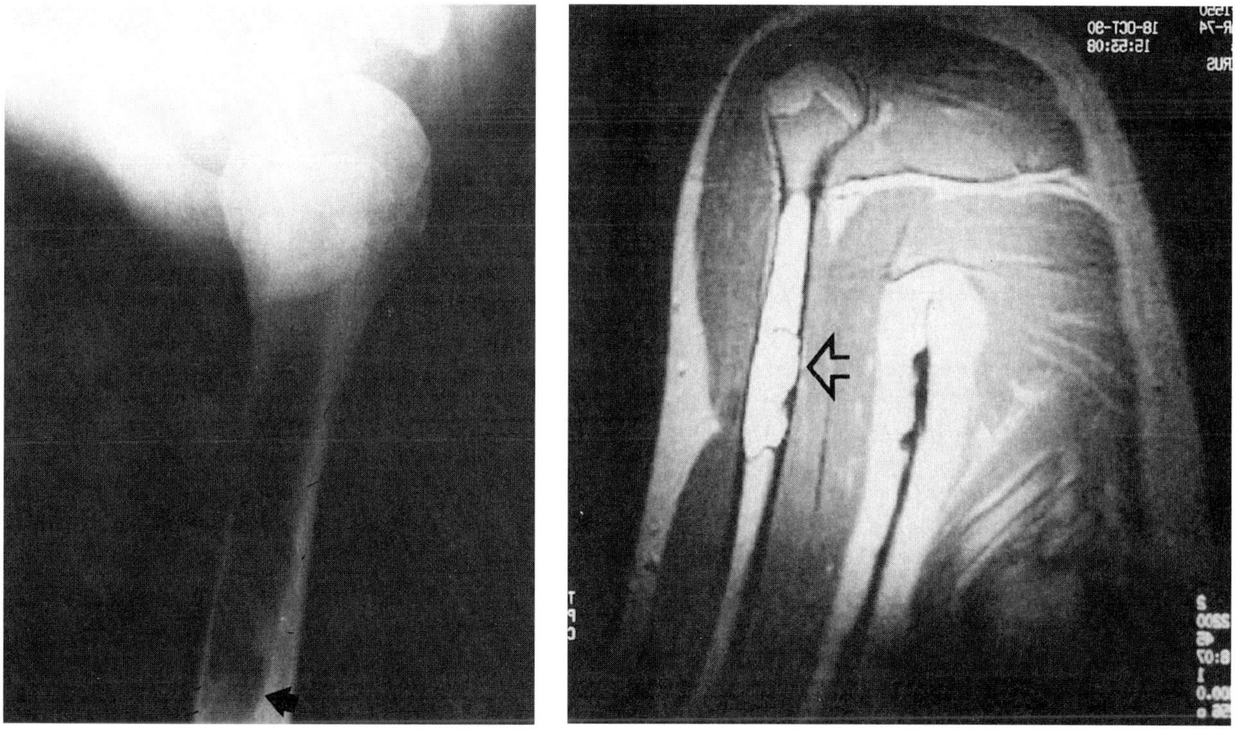

FIGURE 2-7 Shoulder radiograph and corresponding MRI of the diaphysis of the humerus showing fibrous dysplasia.

the country. The five most common symptoms are malaise (80%), headache (64%), fever and chills (59%), neck stiffness (18%), and arthralgias (48%).[35] The clinical hallmarks are an early skin lesion and erythema chronicum migrans, which begins as a red macule at the site of the bite and then expands to about 15 cm with usual central clearing. Orthopedic interest focuses on the 60% of patients who develop frank arthritis from weeks to as long as 2 years after the onset of the illness. Failure to uncover this syndrome early may lead to a troublesome diagnostic dilemma after the typical skin lesion has abated. The arthritis is characterized by intermittent episodes of asymmetric joint swelling and pain, primarily in large joints, including the shoulder. The joints are swollen, hot, and rarely red but can mimic a septic shoulder. The joint-fluid white cell counts can vary from 500 to 110,000 cells per millimeter, mostly made up of polymorphonuclear leukocytes. The bouts usually last from weeks to months and typically recur for several years, decreasing in frequency with time. Approximately 10% of patients become chronic, with pannus formation and associated erosion of cartilage and bone.[35] The polyarticular nature of the disease is helpful in determining that Lyme disease is not a typical athletic inflammatory or degenerative process; however, monoarticular involvement is possible, and without a thorough history, this diagnosis may be overlooked.

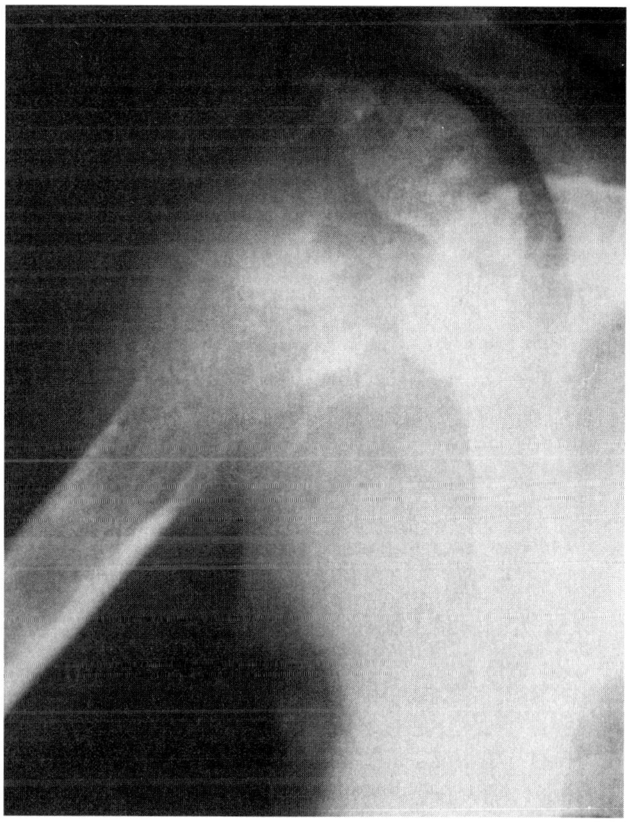

FIGURE 2-8 Ewing's sarcoma involving both the metaphysis and diaphysis of the humerus.

Rheumatoid Arthritis and Rheumatoid-Like Disease

Rheumatoid Arthritis

The orthopedist may be the first physician many patients with rheumatoid arthritis (RA) encounter. The clinical course of RA is highly variable, ranging from a mild pauciarticular illness of brief duration to a progressive destructive polyarthritis, but some prodromal symptoms are common. These symptoms include fatigue, anorexia, weakness, and generalized aching and morning stiffness. The joint symptoms generally emerge gradually and insidiously over weeks to months. However, about 20% of patients present with a sudden onset of polyarthritis, many accompanied by fever and constitutional symptoms.[60] Joint involvement presents clinically as pain, stiffness, decreased range of motion, and signs of inflammation. Typically, the hands, wrists, knees, and feet are initially and most commonly involved. However, as the disease progresses, the arthritis spreads to the elbows, shoulders, and sternoclavicular joints. In the beginning, there may be any pattern of joint disease; however, the pattern generally is bilateral, symmetric, and polyarticular. Nonetheless, in a small percentage of patients, the process remains monoarticular for months to years.[54]

Upper-extremity involvement is common and therefore after gleaning a questionable history, the physician should search for a few early signs on physical examination. The glenohumeral, acromioclavicular, and scapulothoracic articulations all are at risk, and involvement of the shoulder on the whole is much more common than previously thought. Characteristic physical findings are limitation of motion, tenderness inferior and lateral to the coracoid process, and the absence of swelling and erythema. Infrequently, associated subacromial bursitis can result in prominent soft-tissue swelling. Radiographs are very helpful and reveal joint-space narrowing (destruction of chondral surface), cysts, sclerosis of opposing humerus and glenoid, osteopenia, superolateral cystic changes in the humeral head, and centralization of the glenoid[52] (Fig. 2-9). Occasionally, radiographs may illustrate avascular necrosis of the humeral head secondary to corticosteroid therapy (Fig. 2-10).

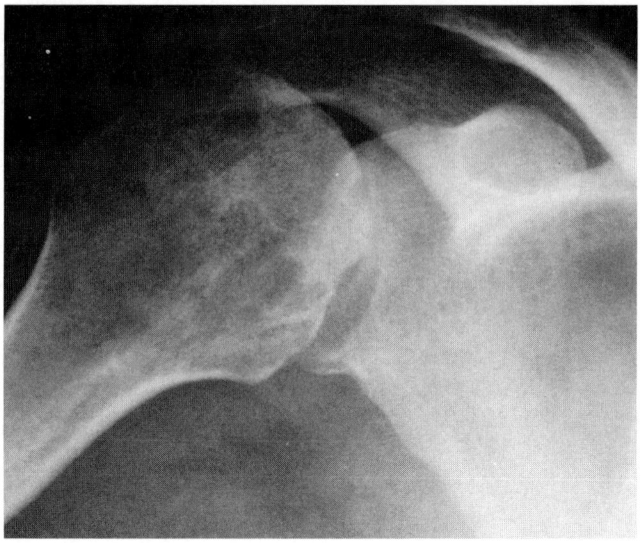

FIGURE 2-9 Rheumatoid arthritis of the glenohumeral joint displaying joint-space narrowing, subchondral cysts, and osteopenia.

Juvenile Rheumatoid Arthritis

Several forms of juvenile rheumatoid arthritis (JRA) commonly involve the upper extremity; however, shoulder involvement is generally late.[39] JRA is included in this chapter because of the common age of onset (any age during childhood) and the symptom complex. Children rarely complain of joint pain but rather limit any motion that causes pain. Rest pain or significant joint pain is rare. Morning or inactivity stiffness, on the other hand, is very common.[48] Physical examination reveals swelling, loss of range of motion, and sometimes tenderness and warmth of the affected upper-extremity joints. The arthritis may be the polyarticular type (40% of children), usually in a symmetric fashion, or the pauciarticular type (40% of children), with asymmetric involvement usually of the large joints.[48] Of children with the pauciarticular type, 10% to 50% develop iridocyclitis (inflammation of anterior uveal tract) that begins simultaneously with the joint complaints. Unfortunately, this inflammation often is insidious and chronic and, if undiagnosed, may cause visual loss or blindness.[48] Generalized growth retardation, epiphyseal undergrowth or overgrowth, and micrognathia also may become apparent. In general, any young athlete complaining of multiple joint pains with a predominant complaint of shoulder or upper-extremity stiffness (especially morning) should not be dismissed as suffering "growth pains" but rather should be evaluated for possible JRA.

Seronegative Spondyloarthropathies

The seronegative spondyloarthropathies are "rheumatoid variants" that can affect the shoulder earlier and to a greater extent than can the seropositive (RA) disease. These maladies include (1) ankylosing spondylitis, (2) psoriatic arthritis, (3) polyarthritis of inflammatory bowel disease, and (4) Reiter's syndrome. Because of their propensity to affect the shoulder, the discussion will focus on ankylosing spondylitis and psoriatic arthritis.

Ankylosing spondylitis (AS) is well known for its devastating effects on the spine and hips. However, shoulder involvement can be significant and can occur early in the disease process. From 10% to 20% of patients initially demonstrate peripheral articular manifestations.[46] The involvement of the peripheral joints in AS typically is noted concurrently or shortly after the involvement of

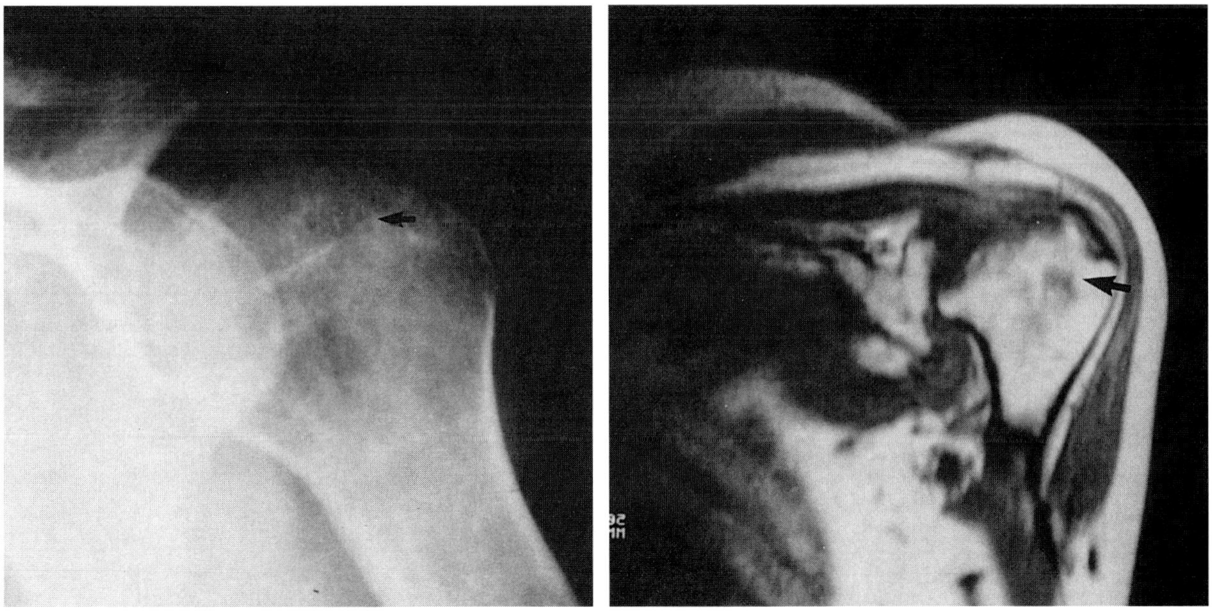

FIGURE 2-10 Shoulder radiograph and corresponding MRI illustrating avascular necrosis of the humeral head.

the spine. Peripheral joint involvement sometimes precedes the findings of central articulations.[46] Unfortunately, many people with AS remain undiagnosed because the symptoms may be mild with minimal, early morning stiffness.[55] Asymmetric involvement of a few joints is common and predominantly found in the shoulders, hips, and knees. Radiographically, patients with AS can show abnormalities of the glenohumeral and acromioclavicular joints or at the site of the coracoclavicular ligaments. The findings in the glenohumeral joint include osteoporosis, diffuse joint-space narrowing, and erosive changes on the superolateral aspect of the humeral head. These findings are similar to rheumatoid arthritis. The acromioclavicular joint demonstrates destructive articular changes identical to those of rheumatoid arthritis. Scalloped clavicular erosion beneath the coracoclavicular ligament also has been noted.[46] Therefore in a patient under 40 years of age with morning stiffness, diffuse tenderness, improvement with exercise, nonanatomic pain distribution, and symmetric decreases in range of motion, a diagnosis of AS should be considered.

Psoriatic Arthritis

In most patients, a history of psoriatic disease is evident, and the articular abnormalities coincide with the skin disease. In as many as 20% of patients with psoriatic arthritis, the appearance of arthritis precedes the skin manifestations.[51] Fortunately, articular disease is much more prevalent in patients with moderate or severe skin abnormalities. The articular disease is variable. Monoarticular, pauciarticular, and polyarticular distribution can be encountered most frequently in the hands and feet and, to a lesser extent, the shoulder[38,51] (Fig. 2-11, *A*). Radiographs of the shoulder can show changes that vary from minor degrees of osseous erosion to extensive osteolysis of the glenohumeral, sternoclavicular, and acromioclavicular joints.[51] Basically, special attention should be given to any skin abnormalities, especially of the hands and feet, when these radiographic findings are observed (Fig. 2-11, *B*).

Miscellaneous Conditions

Cardiac Ischemia

Shoulder and arm pain secondary to cardiac ischemia (CI) is well documented in the literature.[27,56,61] A careful history of the pain, determining location, radiation, timing, and subjective feeling, is the key to the diagnosis. As the population ages and the zest for prolonged athletic competition continues, upper-extremity symptoms related to cardiac ischemia will increase. The typical history is one of exertional chest discomfort for a duration of several minutes that is relieved by rest. The discomfort generally involves the sternal region and secondarily radiates to the shoulders, arm (especially left), neck, jaw, or back.[56] Commonly, the sensation is projected over the left pectoral region, to the left shoulder, and down the medial aspect of the left arm to the elbow.[61] The discomfort sometimes may continue through the forearm along the distribution of the ulnar nerve. Infrequently, the pain may radiate to the right shoulder and arm with or without involvement of the left side. The pain also may present with bilateral shoulder and inferior anterior and posterior neck radiation.[61] Most patients quantify the discomfort as a deep "tightness" or "heaviness" rather than a definite pain. It is never stabbing and is never pre-

A

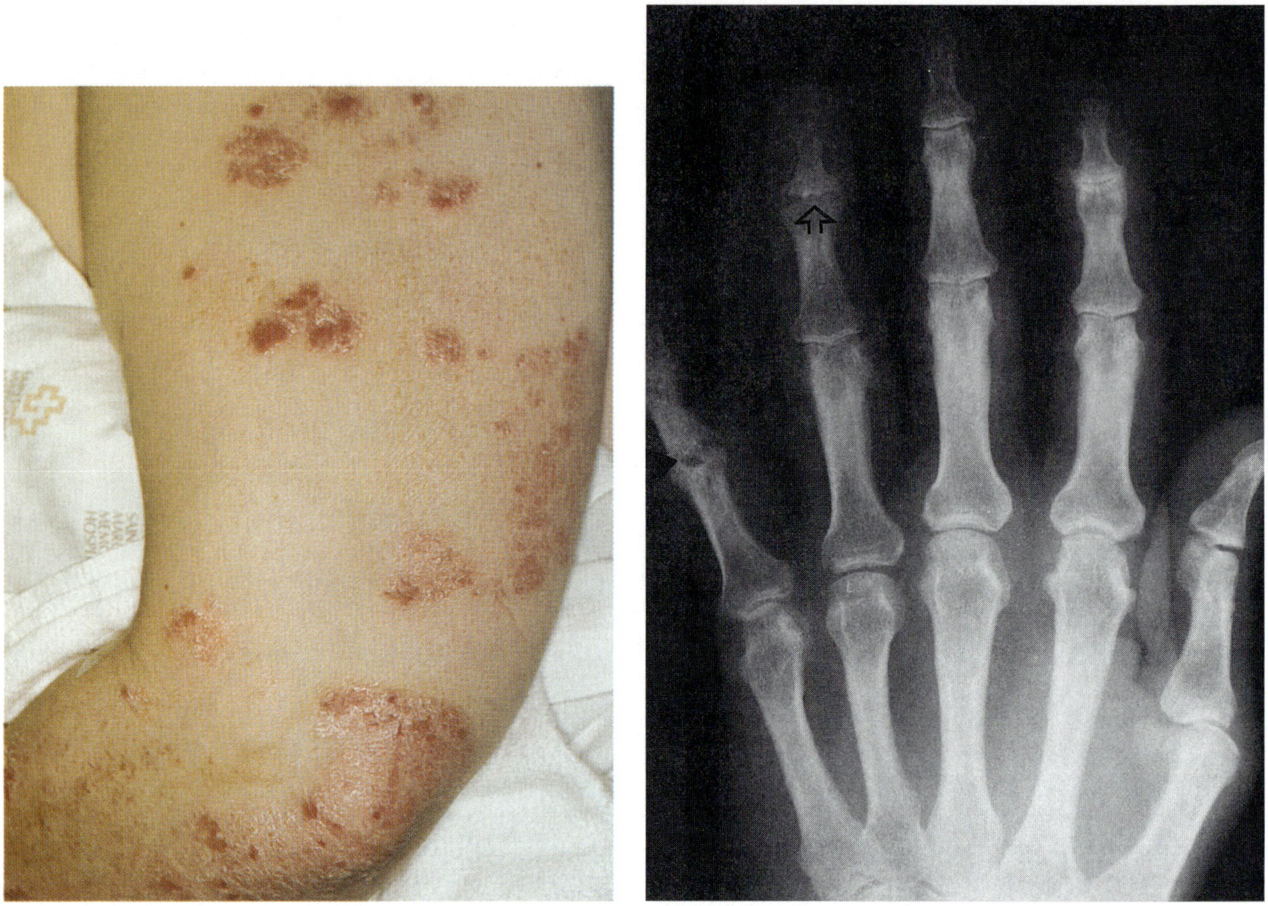

B

FIGURE 2-11 **A,** Typical skin manifestations of psoriasis. **B,** Radiograph of same patient's hand demonstrating destructive changes in the distal and proximal interphalangeal joints.

cipitated by coughing or respiratory movements. The pain lasts several minutes. Pain lasting less than 1 minute is rarely anginal, but pain of constant intensity, lasting longer than 20 minutes, should arouse suspicion of myocardial infarction or pain unrelated to cardiac ischemia. Angina usually is incited by exertion, but pain associated with emotion (fear, anger, anxiety), lying down (angina decubitus), or sleep (nocturnal angina) all have been cited.[56]

Physical examination of the extremities is usually normal. Cardiac examination also can be normal or may uncover one of the following: increased blood pressure, increased heart rate, splitting of the second heart sound, presence of a fourth heart sound (S4), or a diastolic bulge (S3). Pulmonary transient rales or pulmonary venous congestion also may be present.

Cardiac ischemia causing upper-extremity pain in older athletes during exertion may masquerade as a common inflammatory ailment unless a thorough history is available to arouse suspicion.

Phrenic Nerve Irritation

The phrenic nerve arises primarily from C4. It innervates the diaphragm and also sends sensory branches to the pericardium. The diaphragmatic pleural and peritoneal surfaces are supplied by a dual pain innervation through the phrenic and intercostal nerves. Central irritation of the diaphragm refers a sharp pain to the region of the superior ridge of the trapezius muscle, while peripheral irritation causes pain in the distribution of the fifth and sixth intercostal nerves.[23] This anatomic consideration substantiates the common finding of referred posterior shoulder and/or subscapular pain associated with diseases that irritate the diaphragm.

Many disease processes can aggravate the phrenic nerve; some of the more common are subphrenic abscess, pneumonia, pericarditis, rapid hepatic enlargement (viral hepatitis, alcoholism), hepatic abscess, acute pancreatitis, ruptured abdominal viscus, biliary colic, and cholecystitis. One commonly seen process is that of acute cholecystitis with pain referred to the shoulder and/or the posterior angle of the scapula. The history usually reveals the onset of pain several hours after a large meal is ingested. The pain gradually increases in intensity and may wax and wane, but it does not completely disappear until the attack subsides. Physical examination of the right upper quadrant discloses tenderness, muscular rigidity, and occasionally an inflammatory

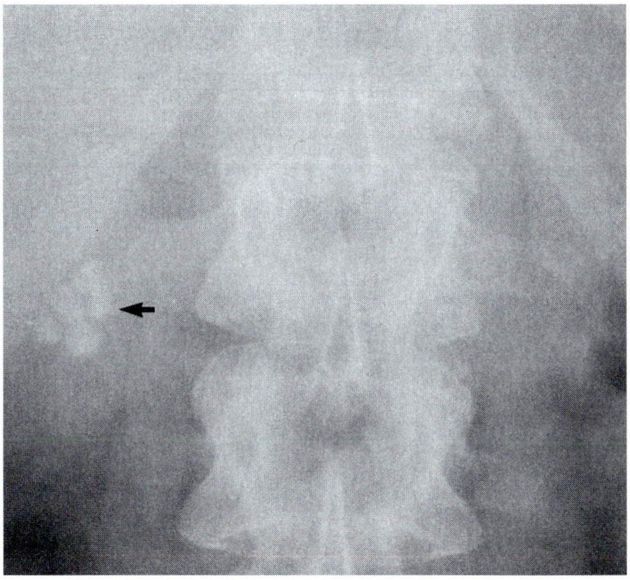

FIGURE 2-12 Abdominal flat plate showing calcified gallstones.

mass or distended gallbladder. Murphy's sign, consisting of inspiratory arrest during deep palpation of the right upper quadrant, is an inconsistent finding but is almost pathognomic when positive.[41] The patient is typically febrile and appears toxic.[1] Two thirds of patients have had a previous history of typical biliary pain with spontaneous subsidence.[36] Anorexia, nausea, and vomiting often are present. Plain x-ray examination may divulge calcified gallstones (Fig. 2-12); however, ultrasound is a more specific method of detecting gallstones in these patients.[36] At present, the most specific test for acute cholecystitis is a technetium-iminodiacetic acid scan with a sensitivity of nearly 100%.[41]

Reflex Sympathetic Dystrophy Syndrome

Reflex sympathetic dystrophy syndrome (RSDS) is caused by a vasomotor dysfunction that produces a significant amount of pain, discoloration, and stiffness. Reported associations are many and include myocardial infarction; cerebrovascular disorders; degenerative disease of the cervical spine; disc herniation; polymyalgia rheumatica; posttraumatic, postsurgical, postinfection, calcific tendinitis; vasculitis; immobilization; and neoplasm.[30,50] The exact etiology of RSDS is still unclear. However, the most credible theory is that three conditions must be present at the same time before a patient develops RSDS: (1) persistent painful lesion, (2) diathesis (predisposition), and (3) abnormal sympathetic reflex.[30] The four principal signs of RSDS are pain, swelling, stiffness, and discoloration. The secondary signs, which are noted in the majority of patients, are osseous demineralization, submotor changes, temperature changes, trophic changes, and vasomotor instability.[30] The symptoms usually greatly outweigh the degree of trauma or disease. The characteristic distribution involves the shoulder and hand, although any site may be involved.[50]

Radiographic manifestations are primarily soft-tissue swelling and regional osteopenia, which can involve both the cancellous and trabecular bone.[50] The best scenario is noted when early diagnosis is followed by early treatment. The goal is to eliminate one or more of the etiologic factors responsible for the pain. Early conservative treatment (physical therapy) has been very helpful; however, sometimes a pharmacologic interruption of the sympathetic activity of the upper extremity (sympathetic block) is needed.

ELBOW

The elbow is involved to some degree in a considerable number of the problems discussed in the prior segments on the shoulder; this section highlights some of the more common but atypical conditions sometimes seen in an athletic population.

Neurovascular Conditions

Cervical Disc Disease/Thoracic Outlet Syndrome

Cubital tunnel syndrome is fairly common in overhand athletes, especially those involved in repetitive, high-velocity motions (e.g., pitchers).[28] The radicular pain and numbness of cervical disc disease may mimic cubital tunnel syndrome, especially if the C7-T1 disc level (C8 nerve root) is the site of the pathology. Pain radiating down the medial aspect of the forearm, terminating in the ring and small fingers and sometimes associated with numbness, is common with C8 nerve root involvement. Weakness of the triceps and small muscles of the hand with no reflex changes also is seen.[59] Cervical foramina encroachment also may present with identical symptoms. Restricted neck motion, positive foramina compression maneuvers (Spurling test), radiographic degenerative changes, and EMG and nerve conduction studies may help differentiate the exact etiology.

The differential diagnosis of cubital tunnel syndrome includes thoracic outlet syndrome (TOS). Because the medial portion of the brachial plexus generally is affected and therefore the neural presentation is along the medial aspect of the arm and into the fourth and fifth fingers, TOS should be investigated. Clinical localizing symptoms and signs, as discussed in the shoulder section, are helpful. Confirmatory EMG and conduction delays across the thoracic outlet help in determining the level of neural involvement.

Neurogenic Arthropathy

Neurogenic arthropathy of the upper extremity is unusual. There are many causes of neuropathic joints, but only tabes dorsalis, syringomyelia, and diabetes mellitus affect the upper extremity with any frequency.[63] Although the pathogenesis of neuropathy remains incompletely understood, the general cascade implicates loss of deep sensation and proprioception; leading to relaxation and hypotonia of supporting structures; leading to recurrent injury; leading to malalignment; leading to erosion of chondral surface, subchondral sclerosis, fracture, and fragmentation; and terminating with joint disorganization.[49] Elbow arthropathy may be the presenting complaint, but neurologic symptoms typically predate the arthropathy. Common features of the history are lack of significant trauma and the absence of appreciable pain. Physical examination usually demonstrates joint swelling with or without deformity. The full-blown radiographic findings of bone destruction, joint debris, resorption of bone ends, reparative callus, gross deformity, and instability are well known.[63] Early findings are similar to osteoarthritis, with bony erosion, subchondral trabecular thickening, osteophytes, and joint-space narrowing. The keys to early detection are the presence of an enlarging and persistent effusion, minimal subluxation, and fracture or fragmentation.[49] Athletes presenting with minimal trauma and pain, a persistent effusion, and early elbow radiographic changes of osteoarthritis should arouse suspicion of arthropathy.

Tumors

Benign and malignant neoplasms of the soft tissue and bone are relatively infrequent, and their appearance in the elbow is rare. The frequency of all bone tumors in the elbow is approximately 1%; of these, the most common benign neoplasms are osteoid osteomas and osteochondromas, whereas lymphomas, Ewing's tumor, and osteogenic sarcoma prevail in the malignant group.[8,34] Lipomas are the most common soft-tissue tumors about the elbow, followed by ganglia and myxomas, whereas in the malignant group, epithelioid and synovial sarcomas appear to predominate.[45]

The clinical presentation is typically pain (night pain) and/or a mass about the elbow. The physical examination varies, depending on the exact etiology of the lesion, but significant findings are restricted motion, swelling, increased warmth, dilated veins, and signs of local compression of one or more of the nerves that traverse the elbow. The symptomatology generally does not indicate the type of lesion but usually calls attention to the underlying pathology. Any soft-tissue mass should be evaluated for consistency (firm or soft), mobility (fixed or free), palpable thrill, bruit, and transillumination characteristics (solid versus cystic). Granted, most neoplasms about the elbow are benign. However, the possibility of malignancy does exist, and the best defense is a careful history, physical examination, and appropriate radiographic studies (Fig. 2-13).

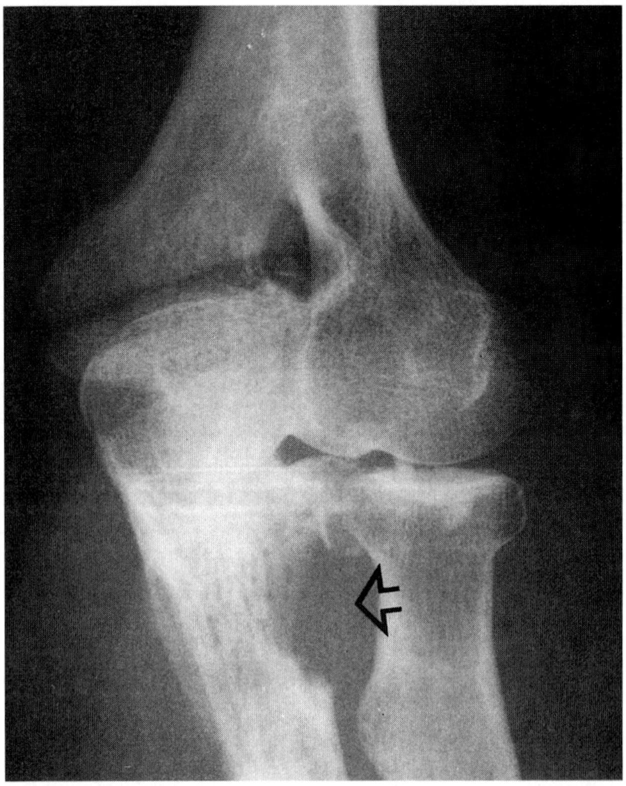

FIGURE 2-13 Malignant hemangioma pericytoma involving the proximal ulna.

Metabolic Problems

No metabolic disease has a specific predilection for the elbow, with the possible exception of tumoral calcinosis.[3] Considering the trend of the long-term participation of athletes, a few of the more common metabolic disorders are discussed. The most common metabolic condition of the immature athlete is rickets (vitamin D deficiency). Although the signs and symptoms of rickets usually present in the weight-bearing joints, the elbow has obvious radiographic findings of the disease common to the larger joints. The predominant radiographic sign in the elbow is profound widening of the radiohumeral joint, whereas the wrist shows the typical cupping of the metaphysis and widening of the physis.[40]

Vitamin D deficiency of the mature adult precipitates the production of uncalcified osteoid secondary to many mechanisms.[37] Again, radiographic findings are most demonstrative, displaying a striking loss of overall bone density associated with a coarsening of the trabecular pattern.[40] Radiolucent lines sometimes can be seen in the cortex perpendicular to the long axis of the bone; they are referred to as *pseudofractures* or *Looser's zones.* They represent cortical stress fractures filled with poorly mineralized callus and fibrous tissue. Looser's zones usually are not evident around the elbow but can be seen in the scapula and ribs on upper-extremity films.[17] Basically, radiographic osteopenia (decreased bone density) in the adult should not always be considered exclusively osteoporosis.

The pathophysiology of tumoral calcinosis is unclear, but it does have a predilection for the elbow and shoulder.[20] There does, however, seem to be a relationship between tumoral calcinosis and hyperphosphatemia, and thus a metabolic etiology is suspected.[3] Calcium salts (calcium phosphate and carbonate) are deposited in the anterior and posterior extraarticular region of the elbow. These extensive periarticular calcifications are readily seen in radiographs.[3,40]

When radiographic findings are consistent with the aforementioned descriptions, a metabolic work-up is useful in determining the diagnosis.

Miscellaneous Conditions

Hemoglobinopathy

The primary hematologic problem about the elbow is sickle cell anemia. In a prospective study, the elbow was involved in 42% of patients, usually in association of other large joints.[13] Nearly 8% of blacks in the United States carry the gene for Hbs, with an incidence of homozygous sickle cell anemia (SS disease) at birth of 1 in 625.[15] Typically, blacks with sickle cell traits (hemoglobin AS) rarely have aseptic necrosis or demonstrable joint disease. However, patients with SS disease experience bone and joint crisis, with the onset usually occurring before the age of 6.

The pathogenesis is an inherited substitution of valine for glutamic acid in position six of the beta chain of hemoglobin. This small change greatly changes the stability and solubility of hemoglobin, causing the classic sickle-shape deformity.[5]

Clinically, there is an acute onset of joint pain, swelling, warmth, erythema, and limitation of function (sickle cell crisis). These crises are caused by the erythrocytes periodically sickling, leading to infarction of the affected areas, usually secondary to capillary stasis induced by the sickle-shaped cells. Multiple joints are involved in more than 80% of cases, and involvement usually is symmetric.[15] This polyarticular involvement is occasionally migratory and may imitate rheumatic fever. Radiographic studies show soft-tissue swelling and possible prior evidence of periostitis, and bone infarction may be seen in adjacent long bones. Nevertheless, degenerative or hypertrophic changes rarely are noted in the elbow unless concomitant infection is present. Dactylitis of the hand with periosteal new bone formation in the metacarpals may help in the diagnosis.[42]

The initial orthopedic manifestation of sickle cell disease may be an acutely swollen joint or joints in the upper extremity with significant pain, limitation of motion, and fever in a young, black athlete.

Hypertrophic Osteoarthropathy

In the adult athlete, complaints of upper-extremity arthralgia and/or aching bone pain usually are secondary to degenerative or inflammatory musculoskeletal problems. However, the clinical presentation of secondary hypertrophic osteoarthropathy, as well as early rheumatoid arthritis, can mimic these typical complaints. Typically, pain and tenderness appear about one or more articulations of the upper extremity. The pain is irritated by motion and is more pronounced at night. The subcutaneous tissue is swollen, and overlying skin may be warm and dusky red. Elbows, wrists, and metacarpophalangeal joints most commonly are affected. Synovial effusions are frequent.[47,58] Articular signs and symptoms are present in approximately 30% to 40% of the cases and, most important, may be the presenting manifestation.[58]

Radiographic findings show periostitis with symmetric periosteal new bone formation in the diaphysis of the bones of the appendicular skeleton. The periostitis is commonly found in the radius and ulna, and less frequently noted in the humerus and metacarpals.[12,47,58]

The causes of secondary hypertrophic osteoarthropathy are many and include pulmonary, pleural, diaphragmatic, abdominal, and cardiac causes. However, pulmonary and hepatic associations seem to be the most prevalent. Pulmonary associations are carcinoma, abscess, bronchiectasis, emphysema, Hodgkin's disease, metastasis, and cystic fibrosis. Hepatic causes are portal or biliary cirrhosis, biliary atresia, bile duct carcinoma, and chronic active hepatitis.[47,58]

In the older athlete with clinical findings of arthrosis associated with diaphyseal periosteal new bone formation, the diagnosis of secondary hypertrophic osteoarthropathy should be entertained.

WRIST

Neurovascular Conditions

Hypothenar Hammer Syndrome

Hypothenar hammer syndrome (HHS) has been reported in association with many sports, including baseball, judo, karate, hockey, and handball.[6,24,44,53] The pathogenesis of HHS is either repeated trauma or a single traumatic episode occurring during a sporting activity and producing ulnar artery spasms, thrombosis, and aneurysms.[53] The extent of arterial damage determines whether arterial spasm (wall contusion), thrombosis (intimal tear), true aneurysm (swelling of all arterial layers), or false aneurysm (rupture and organization of the vessel wall) occurs.

The clinical presentation usually is associated with pain and coolness of the fingers, and occasionally periodic radiation into the forearm. In advanced cases, night pain and rest pain are present. Ulnar nerve symptoms involving the motor branch are rare because vascular compression typically occurs distal to the division of the motor nerve.[53]

Physical findings may be grouped into those of vascular insufficiency and those of ulnar nerve irritation. Guyon's canal can be tender, possibly with an apparent palpable or pulsatile mass. The ulnar palm and digits can be cool. The digits may appear cyanotic or pale, and in progressive cases, ischemic ulcerations may be present. Ulnar motor findings generally are not present because of the neurovascular anatomy of the motor branch. A negative Tinel's sign indicates that there is no compression or irritation of the ulnar nerve and that the numbness is secondary to vascular insufficiency.[44] The Allen test is generally positive.[44,53]

The differential diagnosis includes thoracic outlet syndrome, Raynaud's phenomenon, collagen vascular diseases, subclavian steal syndrome, thromboangiitis obliterans, effort thrombosis syndrome, and proximal arteriovenous malformation.[6,24,44,53]

The definitive diagnostic test is arteriography, which one should perform concomitantly with an axillary block to decrease sympathetic tone. Noninvasive tests such as Doppler flowmeter studies, thermography, and cold intolerance testing are sometimes helpful.[53]

Surgical alternatives include exploration of the thrombosed ulnar artery with excision and ligation or vein graft to reestablish flow.[53]

Pitcher's Hand

Pitchers notoriously have problems with their shoulders and elbows; however, the throwing hand also may be affected, with vascular alterations.[26,53] Several etiologies are possible, but compression of the vascular supply to the index and middle fingers within the lumbrical canal secondary to lumbrical hypertrophy or thickening of the palmar aponeurosis is most probable.[25] Microtrauma and hypertrophy of the intrinsic muscles secondary to repetitive pitching seem to be the pathogenesis.[25,53] A clinical presentation of coolness and aching pain of both the long and index fingers of the throwing hand is common. Coolness and pain are present while pitching and are relieved by rest. During physical examination, the coolness and numbness in the index and middle fingers are aggravated by the intrinsic-plus position (active flexion of the MP joint to 90° with extension of the PIP and DIP joints). Atrophic ulcers over the tops of index and long fingers also may be present.[25]

Digital subtraction angiograms help in the definitive diagnosis, displaying narrowing of the first and second digital arteries.[53] A surgical option is exploration with release of any constricting structure about the arteries (thick vertical septa, superficial transverse fibers, first and second lumbrical canals, and sometimes Cleland's ligaments).[25,53]

Metabolic Conditions

Hyperparathyroidism

Rarely, athletes present with an injury to their wrist and/or hands in which a radiographic assessment is warranted. Although fracture or carpal instability is not apparent, erosion of the tufts of the phalanges and subperiosteal cortical resorption, especially on the radial side of the middle phalanges, are noted. The history may reveal subtle symptoms of headaches, nausea, vomiting, and weakness. A medical history of peptic ulcers and recurrent kidney stones should be sought. In these cases, primary or secondary hyperparathyroidism is the usual cause, and medical work-up should be instituted. Multiple other metabolic diseases have a predilection for the hand and wrist. Serendipitous radiographic pathology may lead to their early detection and treatment. Gout demonstrates articular erosion, with preservation of part of the joint, an overhanging edge of erosion, lack of osteoporosis, and periarticular swelling, whereas hemochromatosis involves the second and third metacarpophalangeal joints, with beaklike osteophytes.[18] Pseudogout is manifested by calcification of the intercarpal ligaments and triangular fibrocartilage complex. Subtle radiographic changes in the small bones of the hand and wrist may be the first clue to an insidious metabolic problem.

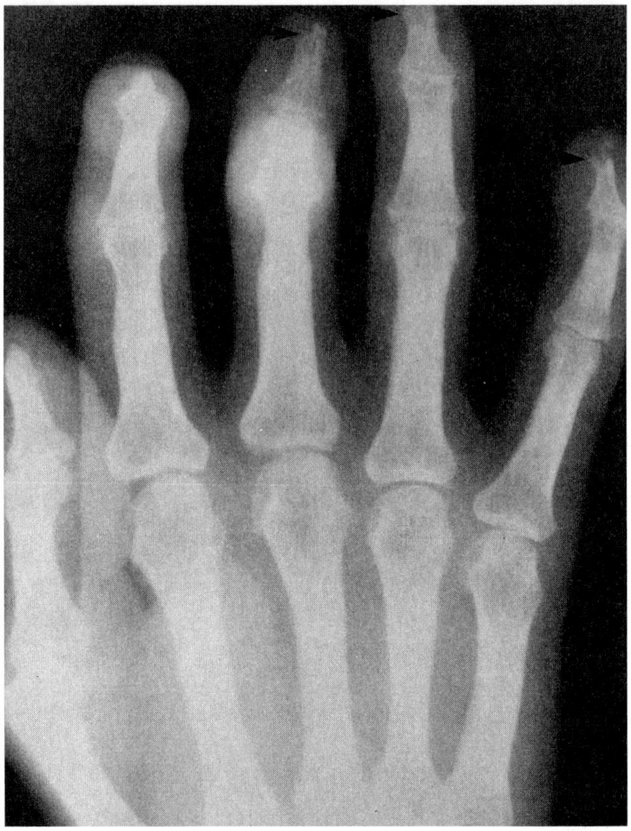

FIGURE 2-14 Hand radiograph with tapering of distal phalanges and interphalangeal destructive changes typical of scleroderma.

Connective-Tissue Disorders

The plethora of connective-tissue disorders and their clinical presentation about the hand and wrist are beyond the scope of this chapter. However, these syndromes exhibit a proclivity for involvement of the hand and wrist. Systemic lupus erythematosus (SLE) demonstrates sclerosis of the distal phalanges and flexible joint contractures. On the other hand, scleroderma shows skin changes (edema, thickening), soft-tissue calcifications, tapering of the distal phalanges, and interphalangeal destructive changes (Fig. 2-14). Mixed connective-tissue disease illustrates overlap of the clinical features of SLE, scleroderma, and rheumatoid arthritis. Radiographically, erosions and destructive changes in the PIPs, MPs, and radiocarpal and midcarpal articulations associated with joint-space narrowing are common.[18] As with metabolic problems, connective-tissue disorders have a predisposition for involvement of the hand and wrist; therefore an understanding of their clinical and radiographic nuances is very helpful.

SUMMARY

This chapter presents uncommon causes of pain and dysfunction in the athlete that may mimic common athletic injuries. Primarily, this chapter is intended to raise the reader's index of suspicion concerning these uncommon maladies and thereby facilitate their diagnosis and treatment. Again the cornerstone to appropriate treatment of upper-extremity injuries in the athlete is an accurate diagnosis. The most important tools in attaining this goal include a thorough history, physical examination, and an awareness of these uncommon problems. Second, this chapter discusses the clinical presentation or serendipitous radiographic findings of these masquerading lesions so that appropriate triage could be instituted early.

References

1. Aach RD: Abdominal pain. In MacBryde CM, Backlow RD, editors: *Signs and symptoms, applied pathologic physiology and clinical interpretation,* ed 5, Philadelphia, 1970, JB Lippincott, p 189.
2. Adams JT, DeWeese JA: "Effort" thrombosis of the axillary and subclavian veins, *J Trauma* 11:923-930, 1971.
3. Baldursson H et al: Tumoral calcinosis with hyperphosphatemia, *J Bone Joint Surg* 51A:913, 1969.
4. Bateman JE: Neurologic painful conditions affecting the shoulder, *Clin Orthop* 173:44-54, 1983.
5. Boone DC: Common musculoskeletal problems and their management. In Boone DC, editor: *Comprehensive management of hemophilia,* Philadelphia, 1976, FA Davis, pp 52-85.
6. Conn J, Bergan JJ, Bell JL: Hypothenar hammer syndrome: posttraumatic digital ischemia, *Surgery* 68(6):1122-1127, 1970.
7. Crowe FW, Schull WJ, Neel JV: *A clinical, pathological and genetic study of multiple neurofibromatosis,* Springfield, Ill, 1956, Charles C Thomas.
8. Dahlin DC: Bone tumors. In *General aspects and data on 6221 cases,* Springfield, Ill, 1978, Charles C Thomas, p 445.
9. Dillin L, Hoaglund FT, Scheck M: Brachial neuritis, *J Bone Joint Surg* 67A(6):878-880, 1985.
10. Ellertsson AB: Syringomyelia and other cystic spinal cord lesions, *Acta Neurol Scand* 45:403, 1969.
11. Enneking WF: *Musculoskeletal tumor surgery,* New York, 1983, Churchill Livingstone, pp 1-60.
12. Epstein D et al: Hypertrophic hepatic osteoarthropathy, *Am J Sports Med* 67:88-97, 1979.
13. Espinoza LP, Spilberg I, Osterland CK: Joint manifestations of sickle cell disease, *Medicine* 53:295, 1974.
14. Feldman F: Tuberous sclerosis, neurofibromatosis, and fibrous dysplasia. In Resnick D, Niwayama G, editors: *Diagnosis of bone and joint disorders,* ed 2, Philadelphia, 1988, WB Saunders, pp 4033-4040.
15. Gilchrist GS: Hematologic arthritis. In Morrey BF: *The elbow and its disorders,* Philadelphia, 1985, WB Saunders, pp 674-681.
16. Grant B, Rowe CR: Motor paralysis of the extremities in herpes zoster, *J Bone Joint Surg* 43A:885, 1961.
17. Greenspan A: *Orthopedic radiology,* New York, 1988, Gower Medical Publishing, p 208.
18. Greenspan A: *Orthopedic radiology, a practical approach,* New York, 1988, Gower Medical Publishing, pp 122-127.
19. Harner RN, Wienir MA: Differential diagnosis of spinal disorders. In Rothman RH, Simeone FA, editors: *The spine,* ed 2, Philadelphia, 1982, WB Saunders, pp 52-57.
20. Hensley DC, Lin JJ: Massive intra-synovial deposition of calcium pyrophosphate in the elbow, *J Bone Joint Surg* 66A:133, 1984.
21. Hershman EB: Brachial plexus injuries, *Clin Sports Med* 9(2):311-329, 1990.
22. Hershman EB, Wilbourn AJ, Bergfeld JA: Acute brachial neuropathy in athletes, *Am J Sports Med* 17(5):655-659, 1989.
23. Hinsey JC, Phillips RA: Observations upon diaphragmatic sensation, *J Neurophysiol* 3:175-181, 1940.
24. Ho PK, Dellon AL, Shaw Wilgis EF: True aneurysms of the hand resulting from athletic injury, *Am J Sports Med* 13(2)136-138, 1985.
25. Itoh Y et al: Circulatory disturbances in the throwing hand of baseball pitchers, *Am J Sports Med* 15:264-269, 1987.
26. Jobe FW, Bradley JP: Rotator cuff injuries in baseball prevention and rehabilitation, *Sports Med* 6:378-387, 1988.
27. Jobe FW, Bradley JP: The diagnosis and nonoperative treatment of shoulder injuries in athletes, *Clin Sports Med* 8(3):419-438, 1989.
28. Jobe FW, Bradley JP: Ulnar neuritis and ulnar collateral ligament instabilities in overarm throwers. In Torg JS, Welsh RP, Shephard RJ, editors: *Current therapy in sports medicine—2,* Philadelphia, 1990, BC Decker, pp 419-421.
29. Karas SE: Thoracic outlet syndrome, *Clin Sports Med* 9(2):297-310, 1990.
30. Lankford LL: Reflex sympathetic dystrophy. In Green DP, editor: *Operative hand surgery,* vol 1, New York, 1982, Churchill Livingstone, pp 539-548.
31. Layzer RB: The phakomatoses. In Wyngaarden JB, Smith LH Jr, Bennett JC, editors: *Cecil textbook of medicine,* ed 19, Philadelphia, 1992, WB Saunders, pp 2143-2144.
32. Leffert RD: Lesions of the brachial plexus, including thoracic syndrome. In *Instructional course lectures,* vol 26, St Louis, 1977, Mosby.
33. Leffert RD: Thoracic outlet syndrome and the shoulder, *Clin Sports Med* 2:439-452, 1983.
34. Malawer MM, Abelson HT, Suit HD: Sarcomas of bone. In DeVita VT Jr, Hellman S, Rosenberg SA, editors: *Cancer, principles and practice of oncology,* ed 2, Philadelphia, JB Lippincott, pp 1293-1294.
35. Malawista SE: Lyme disease. In Wyngaarden JB, Smith LH Jr, Bennett JC, editors: *Cecil textbook of medicine,* ed 19, Philadelphia, 1992, WB Saunders, pp 1772-1774.
36. Malet PF, Soloway RD: Diseases of the gallbladder and bile duct. In Wyngaarden JB, Smith LH Jr, Bennett JC, editors: *Cecil textbook of medicine,* ed 19, Philadelphia, 1992, WB Saunders, pp 804-811.
37. Mankin HJ: Rickets, osteomalacia and renal osteodystrophy, part 1, *J Bone Joint Surg* 56A:101, 1974.
38. McCarty DJ: *Arthritis and allied conditions, a textbook of rheumatology,* ed 11, Philadelphia, 1989, Lea & Febiger, p 957.
39. Mills JA: Arthritis of the shoulder. In Rowe CA, editor: *The shoulder,* New York, 1988, Churchill Livingstone, p 473.
40. Morrey BF: The elbow in metabolic disease. In Morrey BF, editor: *The elbow and its disorders,* Philadelphia, 1985, WB Saunders, pp 752-755.

41. Nahrwold DL: Acute cholecystitis. In Sabiston DC, editor: *Textbook of surgery, the biological basis of modern surgical practice,* ed 14, Philadelphia, 1991, WB Saunders, pp 1050-1051.
42. *Orthopaedic knowledge update 2,* home study syllabus, Park Ridge, Ill, 1987, American Academy of Orthopaedic Surgeons, p 15.
43. Parker F: Skin diseases of general importance. In Wyngaarden JB, Smith LH Jr, Bennett JC, editors: *Cecil textbook of medicine,* ed 19, Philadelphia, 1992, WB Saunders, pp 2296-2309.
44. Porubsky GL, Brown SI, Urbanik JR: Ulnar artery thrombosis: a sports-related injury, *Am J Sports Med* 14(2):170-175, 1986.
45. Pritchard DJ, Cahlin DC: Neoplasms of the elbow. In Morrey BF: *The elbow and its disorders,* Philadelphia, 1985, WB Saunders, pp 713-735.
46. Resnick D, Niwayama G: Ankylosing spondylitis. In Resnick D, Niwayama G, editors: *Diagnosis of bone and joint disorders,* ed 2, vol 2, Philadelphia, 1988, WB Saunders, pp 1103-1144.
47. Resnick D, Niwayama G: Enostosis, hyperostosis, and periostitis. In Resnick D, Niwayama G, editors: *Diagnosis of bone and joint disorders,* ed 2, vol 4, Philadelphia, 1988, WB Saunders, pp 4104-4105.
48. Resnick D, Niwayama G: Juvenile chronic arthritis. In Resnick D, Niwayama G, editors: *Diagnosis of bone and joint disorders,* ed 2, vol 2, Philadelphia, 1988, WB Saunders, pp 1069-1074.
49. Resnick D: Neuroarthropathy. In Resnick D, Niwayama G, editors: *Diagnosis of bone and joint disorders,* ed 2, Philadelphia, 1988, WB Saunders, pp 3154-3185.
50. Resnick D, Niwayama G: Osteoporosis. In Resnick D, Niwayama G, editors: *Diagnosis of bone and joint disorders,* ed 2, vol 4, Philadelphia, 1988, WB Saunders, pp 2023-2037.
51. Resnick D, Niwayama G: Psoriatic arthritis. In Resnick D, Niwayama G, editors: *Diagnosis of bone and joint disorders,* ed 2, Philadelphia, 1988, WB Saunders, pp 1171-1178.
52. Resnick D, Niwayama G: Rheumatoid arthritis. In Resnick D, Niwayama G, editors: *Diagnosis of bone and joint disorders,* ed 2, vol 2, Philadelphia, 1988, WB Saunders, pp 995-996.
53. Rettig AC: Neurovascular injuries in the wrists and hands of athletes, *Clin Sports Med* 9(2):389-417, 1990.
54. Rodnan GP, Schumacher HR, editors, Zvaifler NJ, associate editor: *Primer on the rheumatic diseases,* ed 8, Atlanta, 1983, Arthritis Foundation, p 40.
55. Rodnan GP, Schumacher HR, editors, Zvaifler NJ, associate editor: *Primer on the rheumatic diseases,* ed 8, Atlanta, 1983, Arthritis Foundation, pp 86-87.
56. Rogers WJ: Angina pectoris. In Wyngaarden JB, Smith LH Jr, Bennett JC: *Cecil textbook of medicine,* ed 19, Philadelphia, 1992, WB Saunders, pp 298-299.
57. Sadat-Ali M, Al-Awami SM: Wind-surfing injury to axillary artery, *Br J Sports Med* 19:165-166, 1985.
58. Segal AM, Mackenzie AH: Hypertrophic osteoarthropathy: a 10-year retrospective analysis, *Semin Arthritis Rheum* 12(2):220-232, 1982.
59. Simeone FA, Rothman RH: Cervical disc disease. In Rothman RH, Simeone FA, editors: *The spine,* ed 2, Philadelphia, 1982, WB Saunders, pp 440-456.
60. Short CL, Bauer W, Reynolds WS, editors: *Rheumatoid arthritis,* Cambridge, 1957, Harvard University Press.
61. Smith JR, Paine R: Thoracic pain. In MacBryde CM, Blacklow RD, editors: *Signs and symptoms, applied pathologic physiology and clinical interpretation,* ed 5, Philadelphia, 1970, JB Lippincott, p 172.
62. Sotta RP: Vascular problems in the proximal upper extremity, *Clin Sports Med* 9(2):379-388, 1990.
63. Stevens JC: Neurotrophic arthritis. In Morrey BF, editor: *The elbow and its disorders,* Philadelphia, 1985, WB Saunders, pp 682-690.
64. Swash M: Diagnosis of brachial root and plexus lesions, *J Neurol* 233:131-135, 1986.
65. Tibone J, Bradley JP: Management of resistant subacromial impingement lesions in competitive athletes. In Bigliani, editor: *Complications in shoulder surgery,* Baltimore, 1994, Williams & Wilkins, pp. 258-271.
66. Tullos HS, Erwin WD, Woods GW: Unusual lesions of the pitching arm, *Clin Orthop* 88:169-182, 1972.

CHAPTER 3

Diagnostic Imaging of the Upper Extremity

SCOTT KINGSTON

INTRODUCTION

With today's emphasis on sports and exercise, the potential for bodily injury is increasing. Whether the patient is a professional athlete or amateur, the need for a quick and accurate diagnosis is essential in limiting the time the patient must abstain from the physical activities or athletic endeavors. The extreme ranges and remarkable physical stresses applied to the various joints of the upper extremity place these individuals at considerable risk to injury.

Although a wide variety of diagnostic imaging modalities are available to help the clinician arrive at the proper diagnosis, many of the diagnoses can be made with a good clinical history and physical examination. However, the injured person often is in too much pain or discomfort for a proper physical examination or may be unable to give an accurate account of the injury. The accident may have conflicting aspects, or the patient may have associated injuries that are not routinely discovered by history and examination alone but that, nevertheless, must be treated to ensure recovery.

The ideal appropriate diagnostic imaging test for an injured person is quick, safe, simple to obtain, reproducible, and accurate, with little or no discomfort to the patient. The major tools in the radiologic armamentarium include plain film radiography, ultrasound, computed tomography (CT), contrast studies (arthrography), nuclear scintigraphy (bone scans), and magnetic resonance imaging (MRI). Each of these modalities has its own advantages and limitations. The imaging choice should be complementary to, but not supplant, the history and physical examination. The clinician is always treating the patient and not the scan. However, any additional important information obtained by such tests may not only confirm the suspected diagnosis but also obviate further invasive tests.

IMAGING MODALITIES

Radiography

After a careful history is obtained and the patient is examined, further diagnostic work-up may be indicated. Plain radiographs may be all that is required in many cases but often are necessary for comparison with subsequent diagnostic images. The importance of radiographing the injured area in the proper projection cannot be overemphasized because unique tangential views or radiographic examination with applied stress maneuvers may be necessary when evaluating for ligamentous injury and joint laxity.

Ultrasound

Ultrasound has a limited role in the evaluation of musculoskeletal injuries. Although it can be performed quickly with little stress to the patient, it is very operator dependent and therefore is less consistent and reproducible. Its inability to image and penetrate cortical bone because of acoustic shadowing significantly reduces its use in most instances.[83]

Computed Tomography

CT affords high-spatial-resolution images ideally suited for evaluating fine bony detail. The use of thin slices (2 to 4 mm) minimizes partial volume averaging, thereby allowing proper inspection. Although usually limited to the transverse or axial plane, the area to be examined may be repositioned within the CT gantry to allow orthogonal planar imaging and viewing of the pathology in a different perspective. The CT scan also allows multiplanar reconstruction to be performed in a variety of different planes. This becomes increasingly important when one is evaluating for intraarticular fractures and loose bodies. One major drawback in CT stems from the poor soft-tissue contrast, often making it difficult or impossible to distinguish between normal and abnormal tendons, muscles, and ligaments. Small fluid collections associated with inflammation or posttraumatic edema imperceptibly blend with the adjacent soft tissues.

Arthrography

Not infrequently, intraarticular injections of contrast or air are necessary to provide contrast for a more detailed analysis of the adjacent capsular and ligamentous attachments. Injected iodinated contrast medium or air in arthrography may be used in conjunction with either plain radiography or CT.* However, this technique may give only limited information, such as the presence of a full-thickness or partial synovial surface tear of the rotator cuff of the shoulder. It also does not allow visualization of intratendinous pathology or any additional abnormalities outside of the injected joint capsule. There is also the remote possibility of adverse allergic reactions to the injected contrast material.

*References 11, 20, 41, 49, 60-63, 73, 74, 83.

Radionuclide Scintigraphy

In the presence of acute trauma, a radionuclide bone scan is extremely sensitive in detecting pathology.[37-39,44,74] In patients under 65 years of age, approximately 95% of all fractures may be detected by the first day after the injury, and nearly 100% are detected by the third day. When older patients are taken into account, the sensitivity decreases to 80% by the first day, 95% by the third day, and nearly 100% by the end of the first week.[38] Unfortunately, the bone scan's sensitivity far exceeds its specificity. This reduced specificity in conjunction with poor spatial resolution usually mandates additional correlation with other diagnostic tests. One major advantage of the bone scan is its ability to demonstrate the metabolic or physiologic activity of the injury, thereby revealing the lesion's age. However, even after simple fractures, the scan may remain positive for months while it reflects the dynamic healing and remodeling process.

Magnetic Resonance Imaging

The inherent soft-tissue discrimination, multiplanar imaging capability, noninvasive technique, and high spatial resolution make MRI most attractive when evaluating musculoskeletal injuries.* The ability to distinguish the different soft tissues, such as muscle, fat, bone, tendons, and ligaments, from one another and to distinguish normal from abnormal tissues with unparalleled sensitivity gives MRI a distinct advantage over most other imaging modalities. With more sophisticated technology, including dedicated surface coils and faster imaging sequences, greater anatomic detail can be portrayed in less time, thereby minimizing the motion artifact that often degrades image quality. Although the physics underlying MRI is beyond the scope of this chapter, a basic understanding of them is needed before specific applications in imaging the upper extremity are discussed.

Basics of Magnetic Resonance Imaging

During an MRI study, small amounts of energy are deposited in the body in the form of radiowaves (radiofrequency [RF] pulse) at specific time intervals (time of repetition [TR], measured in milliseconds). This boosts the hydrogen nuclei (protons) to a higher energy level within the body such that, as the protons return to equilibrium (rate of relaxation), they emit weak signals (the MR echo) that are detected by a closely applied surface coil and are then converted into anatomic images. The particular time of echo detection or sampling is referred to as the *echo time* (TE, also measured in milliseconds). The rate of relaxation for each tissue in the body (T_1 and T_2 relaxation rates) is governed by a variety of factors but is essentially fixed for each specific tissue type. Therefore fat appears different from muscle on the MR images due to its distinct T_1 and T_2 relaxation values. A multitude of parameters must be factored into each sequence acquisition; these factors bias the images to be either T_1- or T_2-weighted. The most important of these factors include changing the TR, TE, and flip angle (which in turn varies the amount of RF energy deposited in the tissues). In general, T_1-weighted images (short TR, short TE) have a higher signal-to-noise ratio, resulting in a clearer depiction of the anatomy. In contrast, T_2-weighted images (long TR, long TE) have a lower signal-to-noise ratio, resulting in grainier images, but also highlight pathologic processes by exhibiting fluid (present in effusions, edema, inflammation, and certain neoplasms) as white areas because of their high signal intensity. Proton-density or intermediate-weighted images utilize long TRs with short TEs. Tissue then can be characterized by noting what type of signal is detected on each image. Signal-void (black areas) structures such as cortical bone, tendons, and ligaments appear similar on all pulse sequences (T_1, proton-density, and T_2). Hyaline articular cartilage, fluid, and muscle appear intermediate in signal (gray) on T_1-weighted and proton-density images. Fluid becomes hyperintense or appears white on the more T_2-weighted images. Whether subcutaneous or within bone marrow, ubiquitous fat also appears quite bright or hyperintense in signal on T_1-weighted images, contributing to MR's excellent soft-tissue contrast and discrimination (Fig. 3-1).

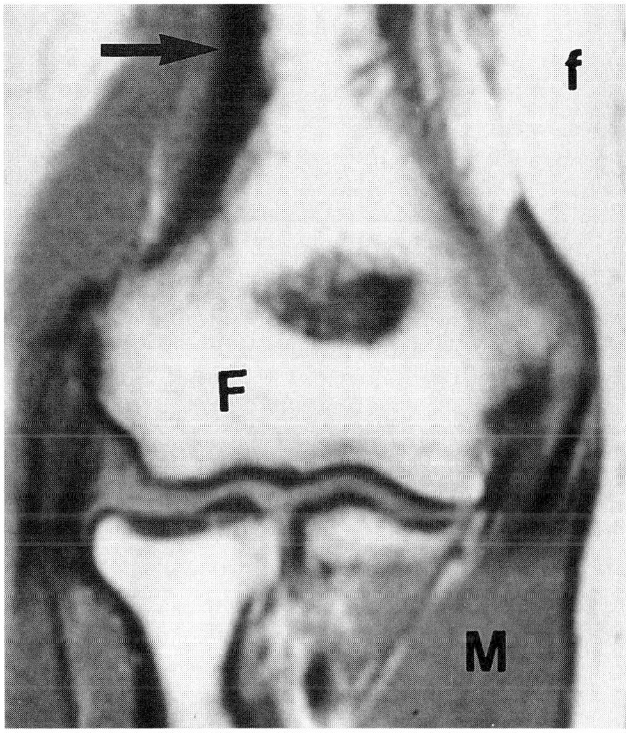

FIGURE 3-1 T_1-weighted coronal MR image of the elbow illustrates bright signal from subcutaneous *(f)* and bone-marrow fat *(F)*. The intermediate signal is from muscle *(M)*, and the signal void *(black arrow)* is from cortical bone.

*References 15, 17-19, 24, 26-28, 30-32, 34, 74.

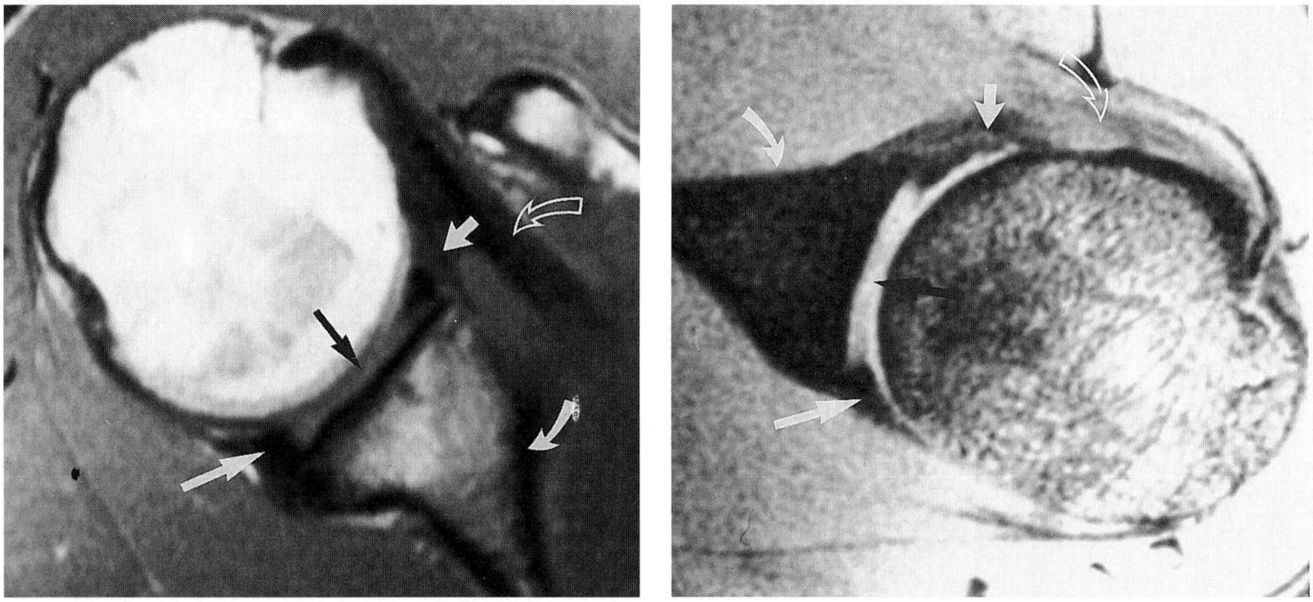

FIGURE 3-2 **A,** Axial T_1-weighted spin-echo and, **B,** gradient-echo images of the shoulder joint. Note the higher signal from fat within the bone marrow in **A** in contrast to the decreased signal in **B** caused by a magnetic susceptibility effect on gradient-echo images. Cortical bone *(curved solid arrows),* tendons *(curved open arrows),* ligaments *(short solid arrows),* and fibrocartilage *(long solid arrows)* demonstrate decreased signal and appear black or dark gray on both sequences. Hyaline cartilage *(black arrow)* appears gray on T_1-weighted spin-echo images and appears white on gradient-echo images.

Gradient-Echo Scanning

Most MR acquisitions or sequences are obtained in the spin-echo mode. However, newer sequences have been developed that alter image appearance and highlight only specific tissues, improving tissue characterization. Faster scans (gradient scanning) may be obtained by reversing the weak-gradient magnetic coils that are built into the main MR scanner. Normally, these gradient coils are used for spatial encoding of the weak MR signals to properly localize and specify where each signal should fit in the particular scan image. This ability to produce such faster gradient scans dramatically reduces the scanning times, thereby reducing motion artifact. Depending on the selected flip angle of the initial RF pulse, gradient images also may be T_1- or T_2-weighted, just like the conventional spin-echo sequence. However, the physician must exercise caution when interpreting gradient and spin-echo MR images because the signal characteristics or image appearances will differ in each sequence (Fig. 3-2).

Fat-Suppression Techniques

Other specialized sequences that suppress the high signal from fat are particularly useful when examining the musculoskeletal system. There are basically two ways of accomplishing this effect. A true fat-suppression technique delivers an additional RF pulse that cancels incoming signals from fat. The second way combines T_1 and T_2 effects while also suppressing the bright appearance of fat. The latter method is called a *STIR sequence* (short T_1 inversion recovery) and frequently is used to enhance soft-tissue edema or inflammation while suppressing the background signal from fat (see Fig. 3-54).

Intraarticular Contrast

Intraarticular injections of contrast medium such as gadolinium-DTPA (Magnevist, Berlex Laboratories, Wayne, NJ) may be used in MRI to highlight subtle cartilaginous defects such as labral tears in the shoulder (Fig. 3-3). This also has been helpful in delineating small undersurface (Fig. 3-4) or synovial abnormalities in the rotator cuff as well as capsular or ligamentous defects.[12,60,74,83] This method is not universally accepted because of the technique's invasiveness and because it requires the approval of each institution's investigational review board because the intraarticular use of such contrast medium is not currently approved by the U.S. Food and Drug Administration.

MRI Variability

Despite the superiority of MRI over most other imaging tests, there are marked differences between MR studies. The different MR scanners, wide array of pulsing sequences, and unique set of selected parameters (e.g., TR, TE, flip angle) result in disparate scan quality and appearance. This is not to imply that many scans are being

A

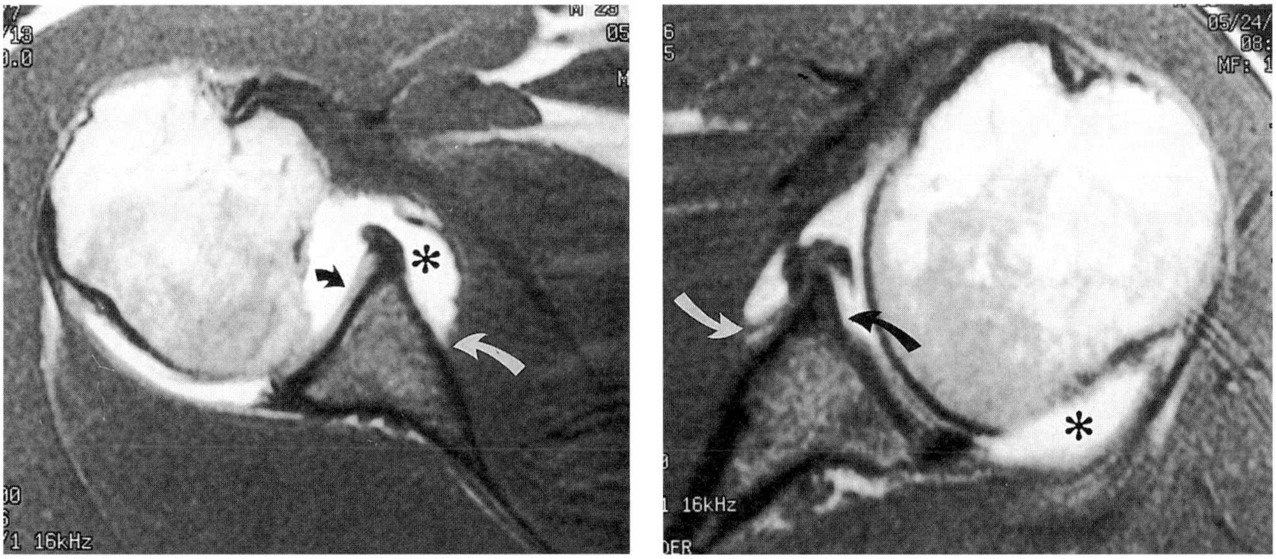

B

FIGURE 3-3 Axial T_1-weighted contrast-enhanced *(asterisk)* images of the shoulder show a normal appearance of the hyaline cartilage and anterior labrum *(curved black arrow)*, **A**, versus a torn cartilage undermining the anterior labrum *(curved black arrow)*, **B.** Anterior capsular insertions *(curved white arrows)* (**A,** type 3; **B,** type 2).

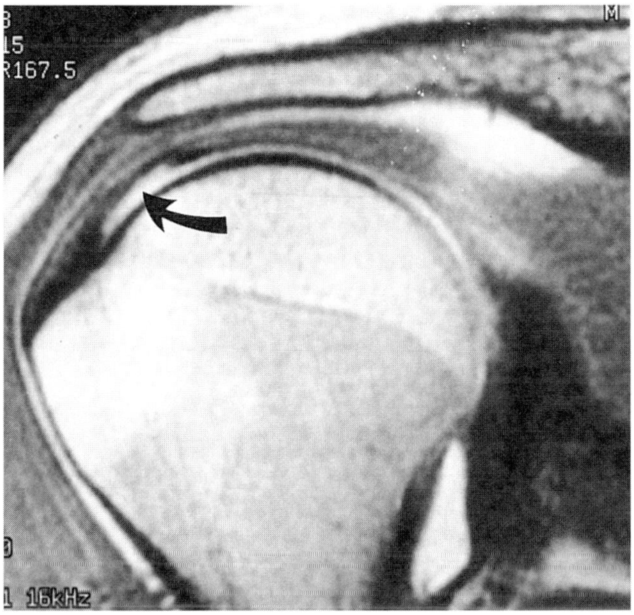

FIGURE 3-4 Oblique coronal T_1-weighted image of the shoulder after the intraarticular injection of gadolinium. A small partial undersurface tear of the rotator cuff *(curved arrow)* is demonstrated.

performed improperly but is simply to emphasize the lack of a universal acquisition technique. Each examination is specifically tailored by the interpreting physician to identify the suspected pathology.

The remainder of this chapter concentrates on the use of imaging modalities in the study of the more common injuries of the upper extremity. The pathogenesis of each offending injury is discussed only briefly; the imaging tests and how they detect and demonstrate particular findings are discussed in more detail.

Angiography

Conventional Angiography and MRA

Subjecting an athlete to an invasive procedure such as an angiogram is a rare practice. However, in the event of a traumatic fracture or dislocation where there is concern about the status of the adjacent vascular structures, the physician may resort to conventional arteriography, venography, and, more recently, magnetic resonance angiography (MRA).

Whether the condition is a vascular occlusion or an

extrinsic compression resulting from adjacent musculoskeletal pathology, conventional angiography or venography depicts the true vessel lumen (Fig. 3-5). MRA, on the other hand, depicts a "flow-map" of the vascular system rather than demonstrating the true anatomic correlate. The MRA images are generated using extremely short TRs, resulting in background soft-tissue suppression. Thus all stationary soft tissues become saturated and contribute no significant signal to the image; however, moving blood within the vessels is not effectively saturated and therefore does emit signal (Fig. 3-6). The MRA images also can be targeted to select out and image only the arteries or veins, depending on the imager's discretion. Because the technique of MRA does not rely on an invasive injection of contrast material but merely the body's natural, flowing blood, any perturbation of normal laminar blood flow will alter the vessel's appearance on the MR images. Areas of vascular stenosis or obstruction will cause either turbulence or lack of flow within the affected segment. This results in areas of little or no detectable signal. Focal areas of signal dropout or altered anatomy that suggest underlying vascular pathology are carefully evaluated. Although the concept of MRA, including its different methods of acquisition (time-of-flight and phase contrast), is quite complex, this relatively new technique may play an increasing role in the injured athlete.

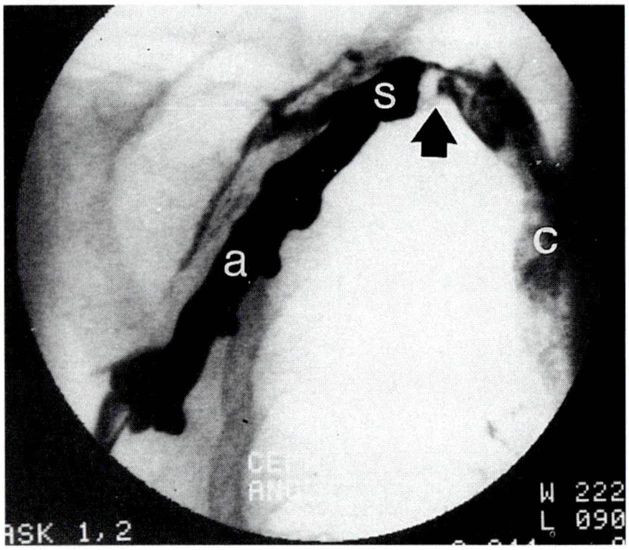

FIGURE 3-5 Right digital subtraction arm venogram after the injection of contrast demonstrates opacification of the axillary *(a)* and subclavian *(s)* veins draining into the superior vena cava *(c)*. There is an area of constriction in the distal subclavian vein *(arrow)* resulting from surrounding hematoma and compression in this weight lifter after an acute injury.

SHOULDER

Acromioclavicular Joint

Separations and Fractures

Direct blunt trauma or falling on an outstretched arm may result in fractures of the clavicle with or without subluxation or dislocation at the acromioclavicular (AC) joint. This area is imaged primarily with plain radiography. Generally, plain x-ray studies, with or without weight-bearing views, suffice in evaluating AC joint injuries. A comparison of both shoulders may reveal subtle malalignment of either joint. Malalignment of more than 2 to 3 mm is highly suggestive of capsular or ligamentous injury[55] (Fig. 3-7). No specific radiographic findings may be present with simple grade I injuries (stretching of the AC joint capsule and adjacent coracoclavicular ligaments). More significant damage occurs in grade II injuries (disruption

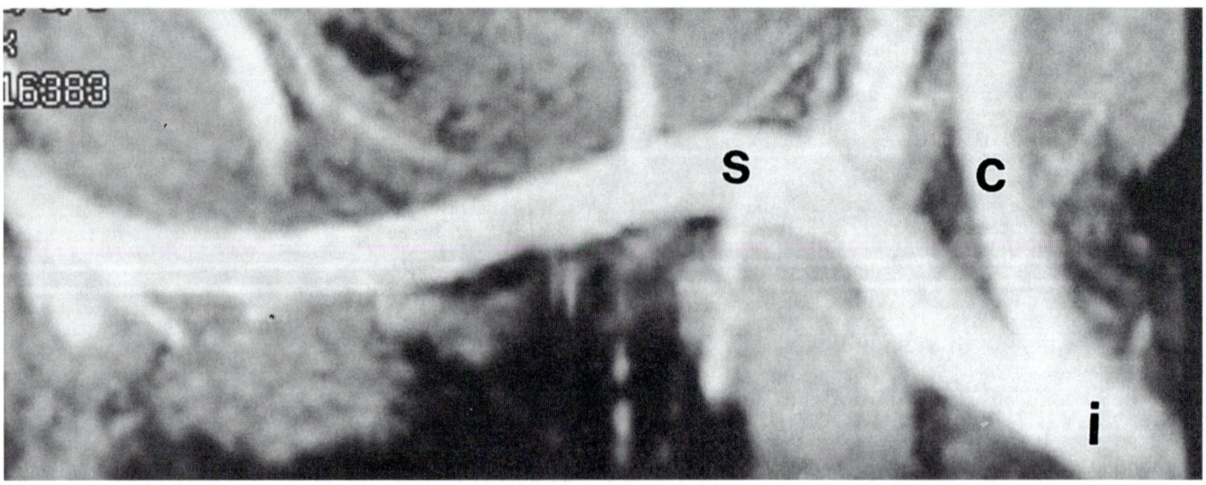

FIGURE 3-6 An MRA (three-dimensional time-of-flight technique) of the right innominate artery *(i)* bifurcating into the right subclavian *(s)* and common carotid *(c)* arteries. The study was performed to rule out injury to the subclavian artery. No intravascular contrast was administered for the examination. Note the background suppression on this MR image and selective visualization of the arteries alone.

of the AC joint capsule with separation). As the severity of the injury progresses to grade III, flagrant cephalad displacement of the distal clavicle results from complete tearing of the coracoclavicular ligaments. Although these soft-tissue injuries may be inferred from plain x-ray tests, the actual damage may be better assessed with MRI in the coronal or sagittal planes (Fig. 3-8). Posttraumatic sequelae with osteolysis of the distal end of the clavicle or dys-

A
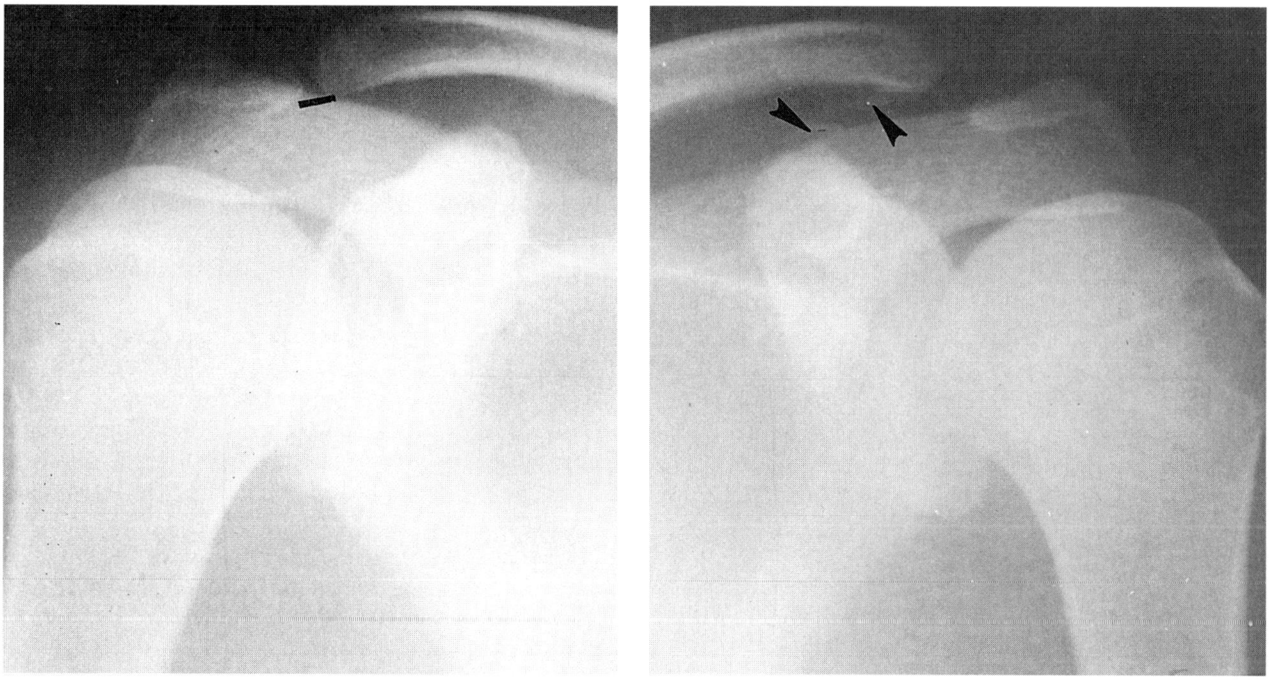
B

FIGURE 3-7 AP radiographs of a normal right AC joint (**A**) with alignment of the undersurfaces of both the acromion and distal clavicle *(short bar)* and separation of the left AC joint (**B**). *Arrows,* Calcification of portions of the injured coracoclavicular ligament.

A
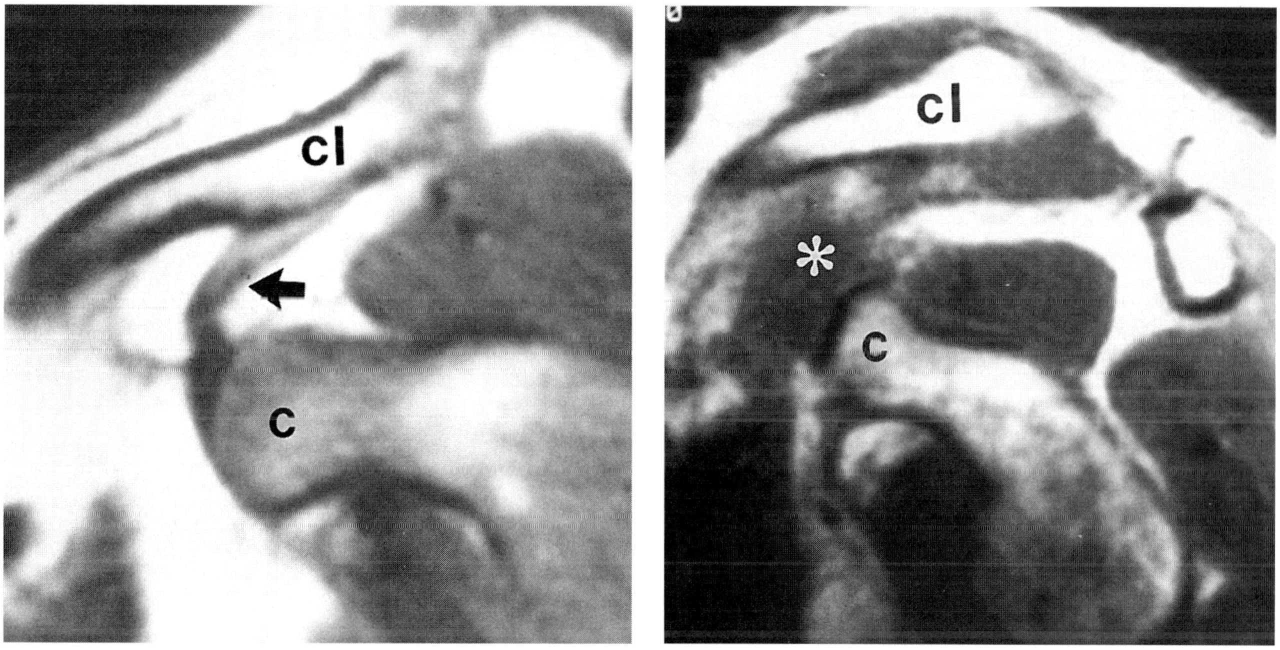

B

FIGURE 3-8 Oblique sagittal T_1-weighted images through the level of the coracoid process *(c)* of the scapula and distal clavicle *(cl)*. **A,** A normal coracoclavicular ligament *(solid black arrow)* surrounded by fat. **B,** Hemorrhage and edema from a torn and disrupted ligament *(asterisk)*.

trophic calcification and ossification of the traumatized coracoclavicular ligaments may be readily apparent on x-ray film[55] (see Fig. 3-7, *B*).

Occult stress or subtle avulsion fractures may be suggested with bone scintigraphy, especially in individuals who have sustained trauma to the shoulder girdle with negative x-ray examination.[74] Assessing relative intensities on the bone scan normally distinguishes an inactive process from a more acute or metabolically active one[37,57,69] (Fig. 3-9). However, more definitive tests, including CT, special radiographic views, and MRI, still may be clinically necessary to further characterize the type and extent of the injury because of the nonspecificity of the bone scan (Fig. 3-10).

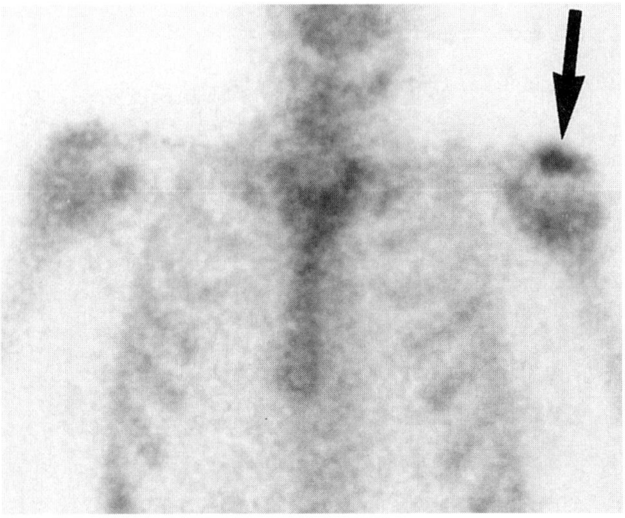

FIGURE 3-9 Bone scan demonstrates increased activity at the acromioclavicular joint *(arrow)*, suggesting an acute injury although the extent of the injury is unknown because of the nonspecific nature of the bone scan.

Glenohumeral Joint

Fractures and Dislocations

The strong physical demands placed on the glenohumeral joint, capsule, and adjacent ligaments during athletics predispose the shoulder to undue stress and subsequent structural alterations leading to a vast array of disorders. Covering only one quarter of the surface area of the humeral head, the glenoid fossa is deepened by the fibrous labra and adjacent capsuloligamentous structures. This serves to prevent the humeral head from dislocating.[40] Approximately 95% of all humeral head dislocations are anterior and inferior.[55,74] This usually results from forces acting on the shoulder with the arm fully abducted and externally rotated. The few remaining dislocations are posterior and rarely superior. Although associated with falling on a somewhat forward flexed, adducted, and internally rotated arm (as occurs in football linemen), the infrequent posterior dislocations are more often encountered in patients with seizure disorders.[55]

A

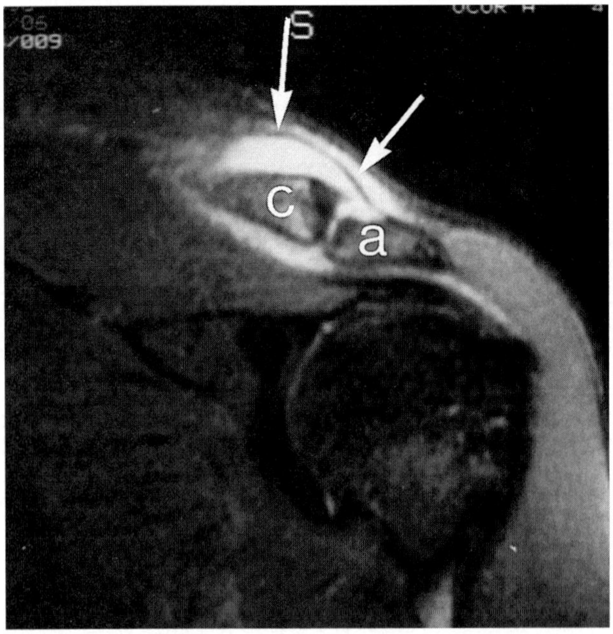

B

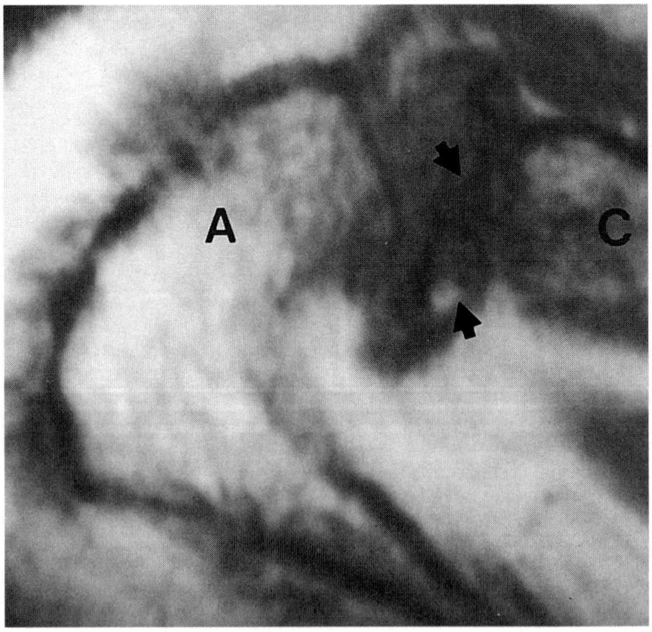

FIGURE 3-10 **A,** Coronal STIR image of the same patient shown in Fig. 3-9 demonstrating stripping of the AC joint capsule *(arrows)* with a large effusion. There is no obvious separation. **B,** Axial MR image in another patient demonstrates an avulsed bony fragment *(arrows)* with surrounding hemorrhagic effusion. *A,* acromion; *C,* clavicle.

Radiographic analysis of the glenohumeral joint demonstrates the humerus overlying the anterior and inferior bony glenoid margin of the scapula with anterior dislocation (Fig. 3-11). This is readily recognizable with simple AP x-ray studies but also may be confirmed with lateral, scapular-Y, or axillary views if necessary. A posteriorly dislocated humerus may be more subtle, with the internally rotated humerus barely overlying the glenohumeral joint on the AP views (Fig. 3-12). Recognizing the various associated impaction or compression fractures of the humeral head and bony glenoid helps in distinguishing the type of dislocation. As the humeral head dislocates anteriorly and inferiorly, typical posterolateral wedge-shaped impaction fractures occur on the posterolateral aspect of the humeral head (Hill-Sachs lesion) with or without associated chip fractures of the anteroinferior bony glenoid (Bankart lesion) (Fig. 3-13). Just as the presence of a Hill-Sachs lesion near the cephalad aspect of the humeral head confirms the suspected diagnosis of a prior anterior dislocation, a reverse Hill-Sachs lesion also may be noted along the anteromedial location of the humeral head with posterior dislocations. Such osseous changes may be apparent on plain radiographs (see Fig. 3-12, *B*) but are exceptionally demonstrated on axial CT and MR images (Fig. 3-14).[86] The last two modalities also allow inspection of any potential bony glenoid fractures unencumbered by overlapping bony shadows on conventional radiographs.

More complex fractures of the scapula, glenoid, or humerus are better evaluated with CT (Fig. 3-15).[74] Identifying the presence and extent of articular surface fractures or displaced fragments and angulation is vitally important in determining the prognosis. According to Neer,[29] the displacement of fragments by more than 1 cm or angulation by more than 45 degrees is considered significant and usually requires surgery. Any loose

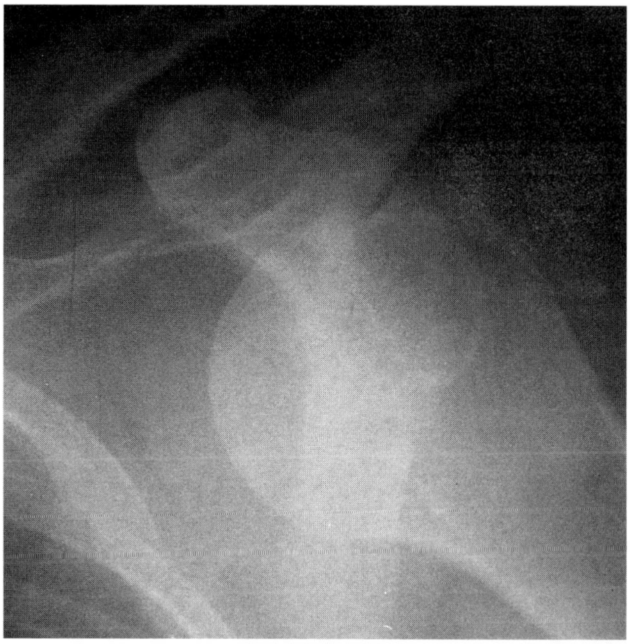

FIGURE 3-11 Humeral head overlies the lower glenoid in this anterior-inferior dislocation.

A

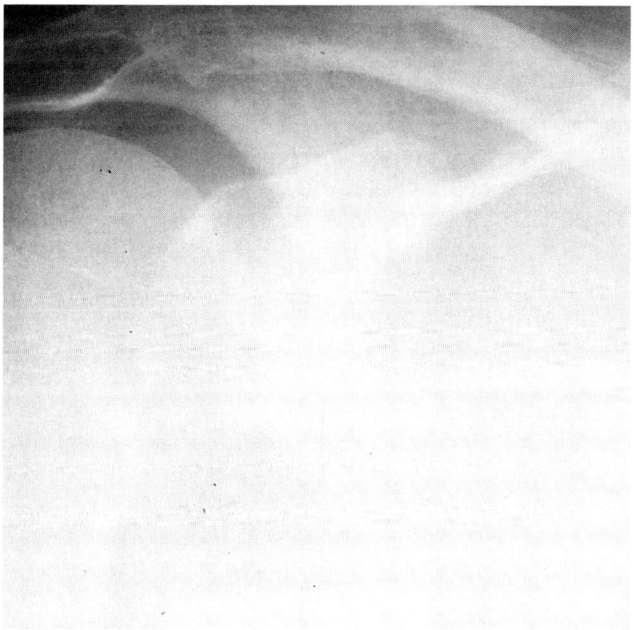

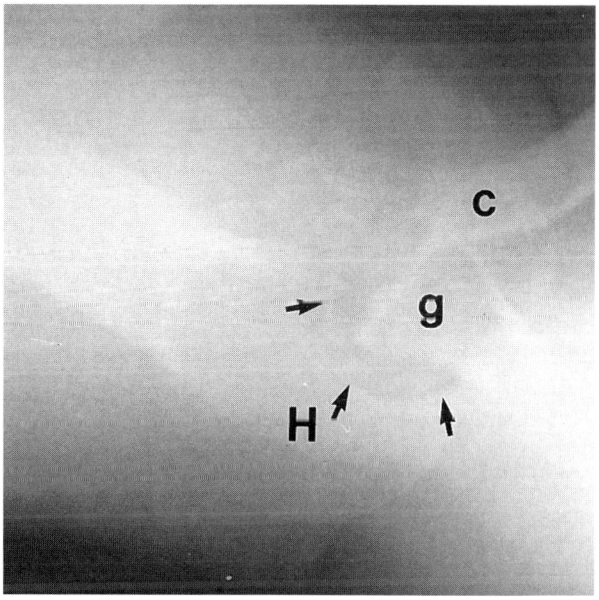

B

FIGURE 3-12 Posterior humeral dislocation is not as evident on the AP radiograph, **A,** but is noticeable on the axillary view, **B,** showing the humerus *(H)* lying posterior to the glenoid *(g)*. A large impaction fracture *(outlined by arrows)* is present. (*c*) represents the distal clavicle.

A

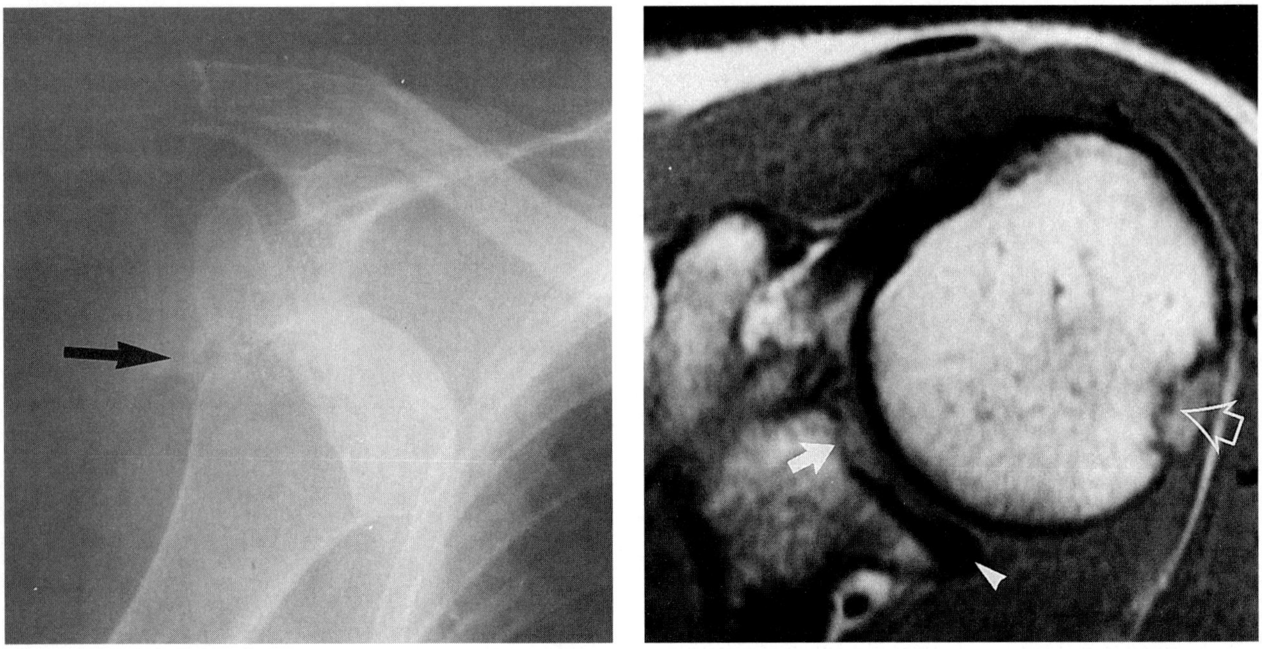

B

FIGURE 3-13 **A,** Bony Bankart lesion *(arrow)* is noted off the inferior glenoid with anterior dislocation of the humerus. **B,** Axial MR image demonstrates the osseous Bankart lesion *(white arrow)* of the anterior glenoid and the associated Hill-Sachs compression fracture *(open white arrow)* of the posterolateral aspect of the humeral head. *White arrowhead,* normal posterior labrum.

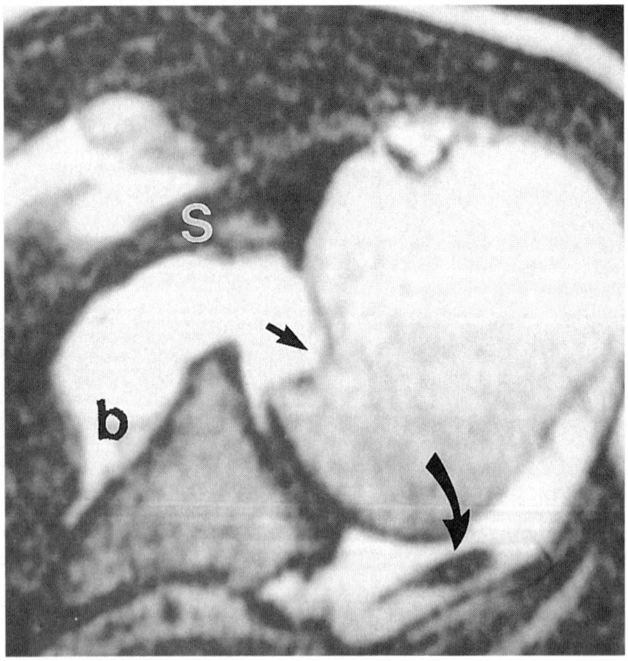

FIGURE 3-14 A reverse Hill-Sachs lesion *(short straight arrow)* is seen in the anteromedial aspect of the humerus, resulting from previous posterior dislocation and impaction on the posterior glenoid in this axial T_2-weighted MR image. *Curved arrow,* osteocartilaginous intraarticular loose body within the posterior glenohumeral joint; *S,* subscapularis tendon; *b,* subscapularis bursa.

intraarticular bone fragments are easily visualized on axial CT images.

Instability

Glenohumeral joint instability may be present in the anterior, posterior, superior, or inferior directions relative to the glenoid fossa or may exhibit a multidirectional instability depending on the underlying pathology. After major trauma, the humerus may become acutely dislocated. However, recurrent glenohumeral subluxations or instability without dislocation usually results from repetitive overuse, particularly in sports of throwers or swimmers, where overhead arm motion is so prevalent.[1,2,22,75] The glenoid labra, glenohumeral ligaments, and capsule provide glenohumeral joint stability throughout a full range of motion.[35,72] With repeated stress applied to the glenohumeral capsuloligamentous structures in overuse activities, the capsule and ligaments may stretch and attenuate, leading to glenohumeral joint instability. Two imaging modalities used to accurately examine these structures are CT arthrography and MRI. The former requires the intraarticular injection of contrast or air, whereas MRI normally does not require such injections. Unfortunately, in the absence of significant joint fluid, the detection of labral and glenohumeral ligament or capsule pathology can be somewhat difficult with MRI.[12] This has prompted the use of contrast-assisted MRI after the intraarticular injection of gadolinium or normal saline in

A

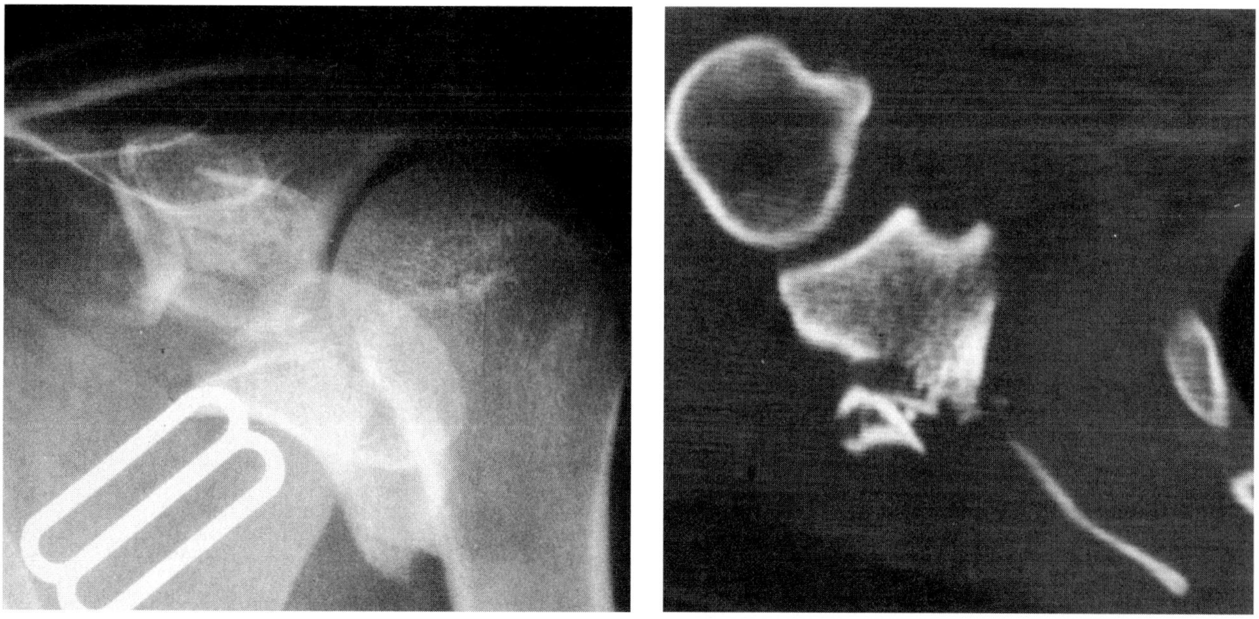

B

C

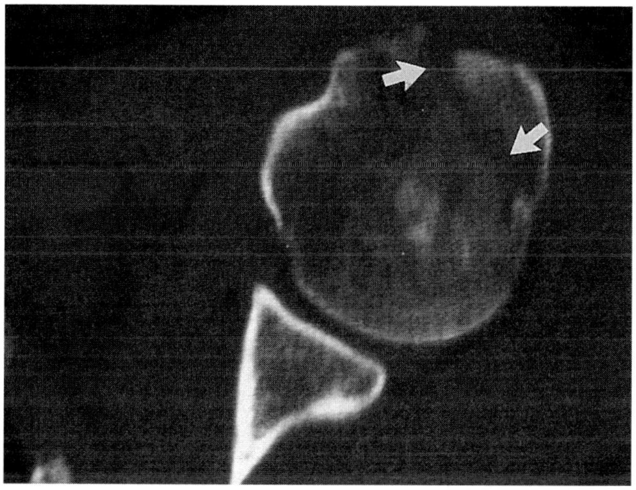

D

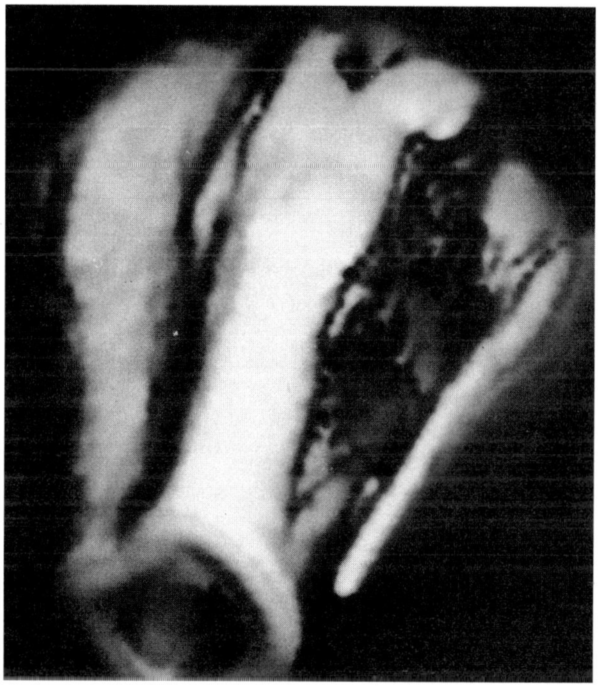

FIGURE 3-15 Scapular and humeral fractures. **A,** Radiograph demonstrating comminuted fracture through the glenoid neck. **B,** Axial CT scan shows the comminution in better detail. **C,** Axial two-dimensional and, **D,** three-dimensional reformatted CT scans show a vertical cleavage fracture of the humeral greater tuberosity.

instances where instability or labral pathology is of primary concern. As previously mentioned, this technique is controversial and not universally accepted. Rather than routinely employing MR arthrography, the physician may reserve this practice for the highly competitive athlete in whom small labral tears or instability is being evaluated.

Glenohumeral Ligaments

One of the most important static stabilizers of the glenohumeral joint against translational instability in the overhead athlete is the inferior glenohumeral ligament.[6,40,75] This ligament is composed of an anterior and posterior band with a redundant intervening axillary pouch. The intimate relationship of the anterior band with the anterior fibrous glenoid labrum acts as the primary structure preventing recurrent anterior glenohumeral subluxation (Figs. 3-16 and 3-17). In overuse syndromes with repetitive overhead motion of the arm in external rotation, chronic stresses are applied to the anterior capsular mechanism and glenohumeral ligaments.[1] If such physical stress exceeds the capacity of the normal reparative response, microtears and possibly rupture of these vital structures may result. Increasing anterior-posterior trans-

A

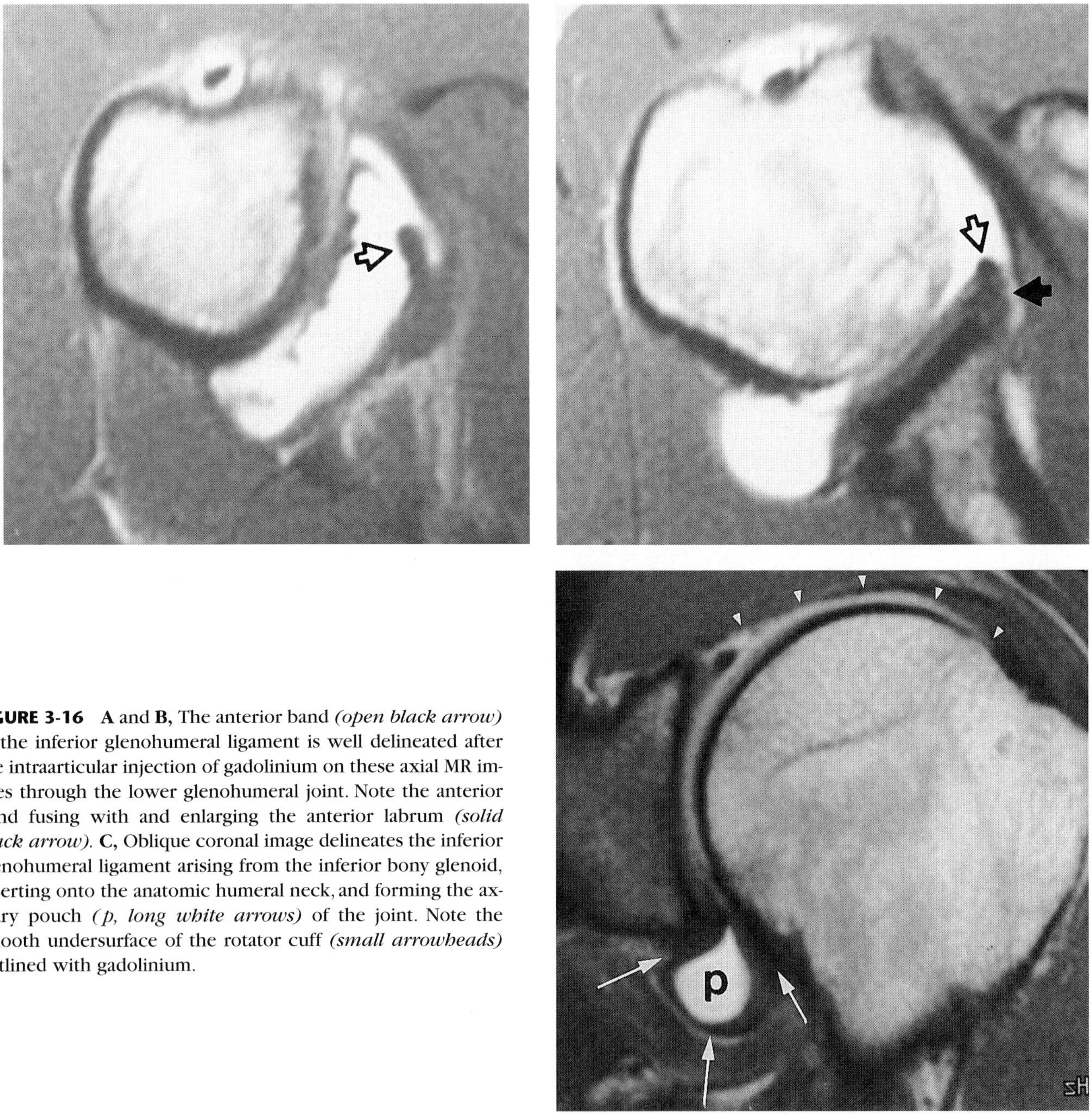

B

C

FIGURE 3-16 **A** and **B,** The anterior band *(open black arrow)* of the inferior glenohumeral ligament is well delineated after the intraarticular injection of gadolinium on these axial MR images through the lower glenohumeral joint. Note the anterior band fusing with and enlarging the anterior labrum *(solid black arrow).* **C,** Oblique coronal image delineates the inferior glenohumeral ligament arising from the inferior bony glenoid, inserting onto the anatomic humeral neck, and forming the axillary pouch *(p, long white arrows)* of the joint. Note the smooth undersurface of the rotator cuff *(small arrowheads)* outlined with gadolinium.

lation of the humeral head ensues, with the development of anterior glenoid erosions, blunting of the labrum with fibrillation, tear formation, and degeneration[2,74] (Figs. 3-18 and 3-19). Abnormalities of the anterior labroligamentous complex, such as Bankart lesions, may be identified.

The middle glenohumeral ligament is the most inconsistent ligament, being absent or atrophic nearly 30% of the time.[6] However, when it is present, it may appear as a linear structure outlined by fluid in the presence of joint effusions. It is easily recognized as lying beneath the anterior capsule or subscapularis tendon on axial CT or MR images. The widely variable appearance of this ligament is important to the examiner because it may resemble a thick, cordlike structure or a thin linear band, usually adjacent to the anterior labrum, and therefore should not be mistaken for a detached anterior labral fragment (Fig. 3-20). Its attachment at or just below the superior labrum anteriorly may simulate a notched appearance of the normal anterior labrum.

The superior glenohumeral ligament is often noted on axial CT or MR images as a small soft-tissue band joining the anterior-superior labrum at the level of the biceps

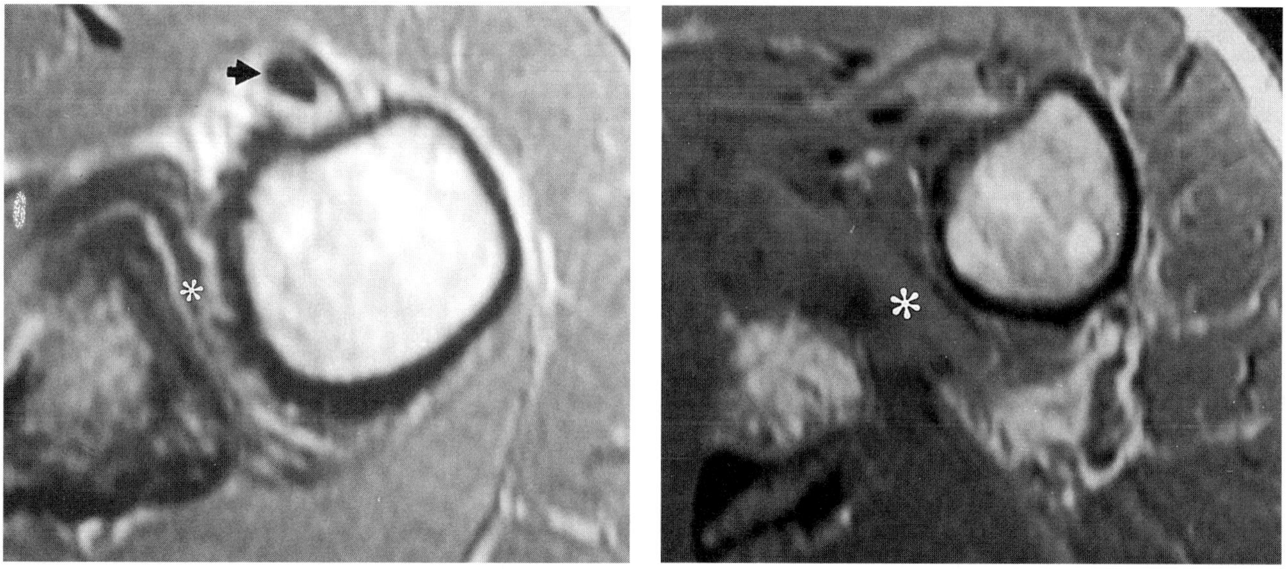

FIGURE 3-17 **A,** A noncontrast axial MR image through the same level as in Fig. 3-16 demonstrates the intact inferior glenohumeral ligament *(asterisk). Black arrow* indicates the biceps tendon. **B,** The inferior glenohumeral ligament *(asterisk)* is disrupted in another patient.

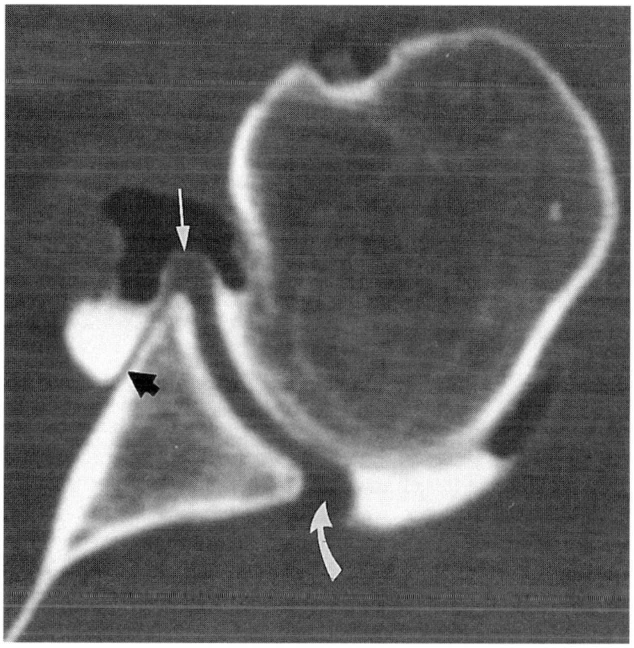

FIGURE 3-18 Normal contrast-enhanced axial CT scan through the glenohumeral joint demonstrating a normal anterior *(straight white arrow)* and posterior *(curved white arrow)* labrum. *Black arrow,* normal anterior capsular insertion onto midglenoid.

tendon (Fig. 3-21). The function of this structure appears to be mainly to provide an inferior restraint of the humerus in adduction.[6,40,75]

Glenohumeral Joint Capsule

The anterior and posterior capsular insertions onto the glenoid also are well displayed with CT arthrography. Soft-tissue swelling with capsular elevation or stripping off scapular cortex is highly suggestive of instability[60,61,72] (see Figs. 3-19, *B*, and 3-22). In throwing athletes, the formation of a crescentic bony spur at the capsular insertion often may be seen on axial images (Fig. 3-23). Presumably, this is caused by chronic traction stress resulting in periosteal reaction, the so-called Bennett lesion frequently noted in baseball pitchers. This lesion is more frequent posteriorly adjacent to the base of the posterior labrum, and may be associated with a posterior labral tear, with the clinical presentation of posterior pain and instability. The metabolic activity of such a lesion may be documented through nuclear scintigraphy,[74] but CT or MRI usually is still needed to further evaluate this area (Fig. 3-24).

A B

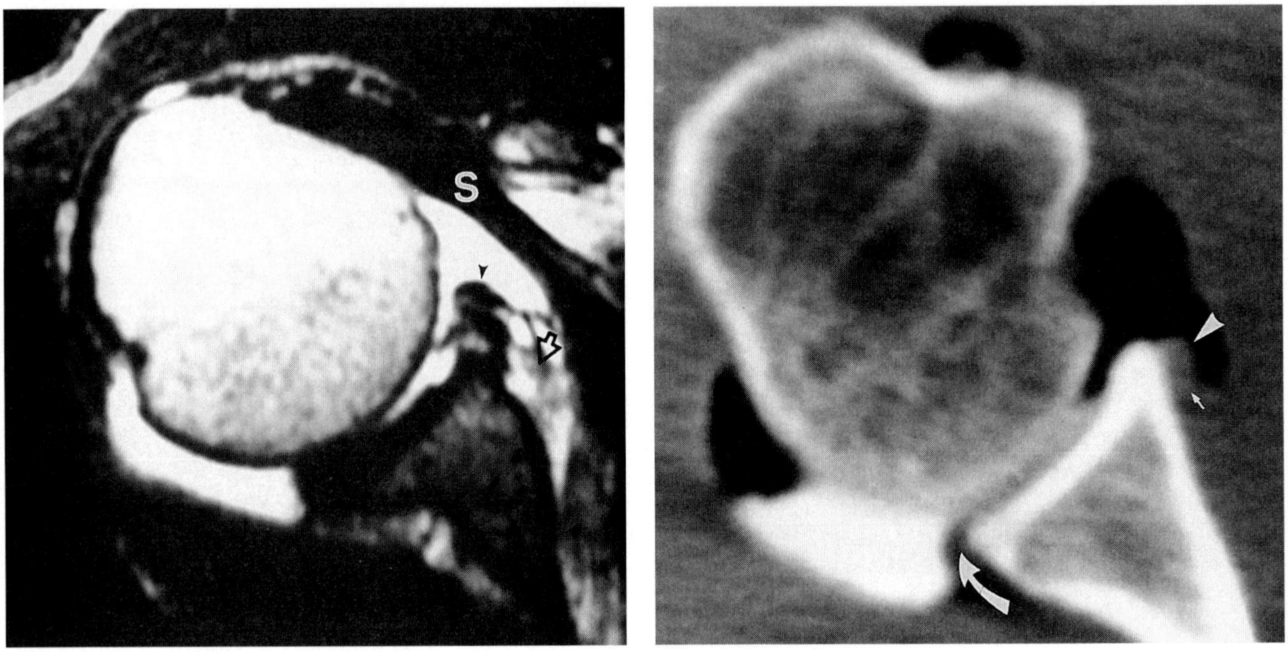

FIGURE 3-19 Torn anterior labral complex. **A,** Axial T_2-weighted MR image shows complete avulsion of the anterior labroligamentous complex *(black arrowhead)* from the underlying glenoid. *Open black arrow,* synovial stranding and debris extending onto the anterior scapular cortex; *S,* subcapularis tendon. Axial contrast-enhanced CT scan, **B,** demonstrates medial displacement of the avulsed anterior labrum and inferior glenohumeral ligament complex *(white arrowhead)* with thickening and scarring at the capsule insertion *(small white arrow). Curved white arrow,* normal posterior labrum.

A B

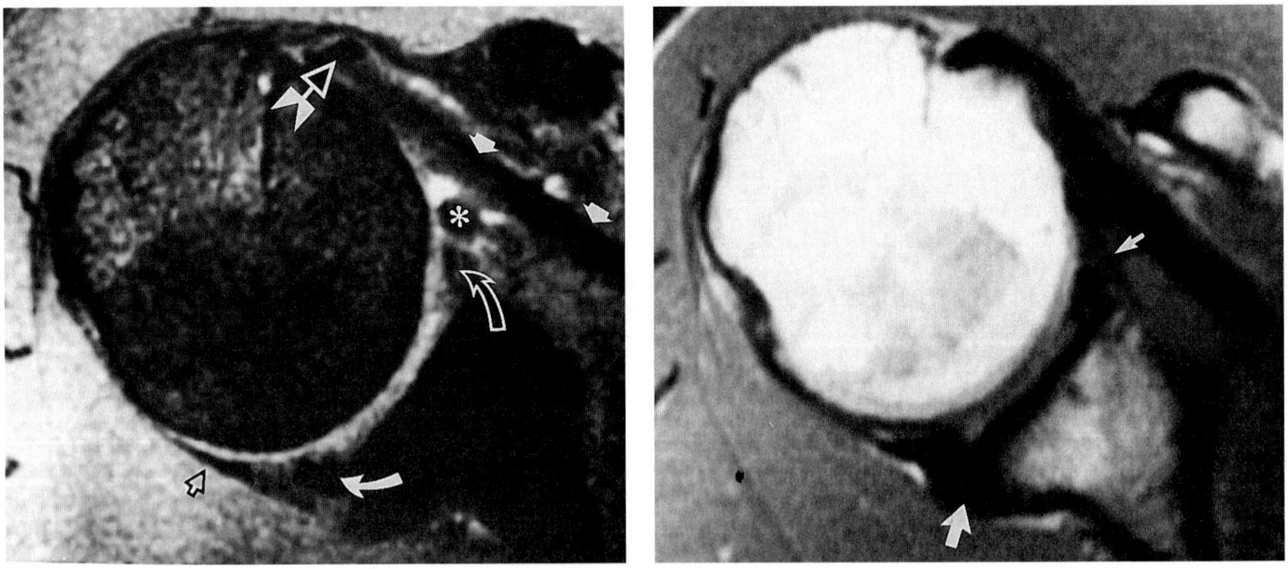

FIGURE 3-20 Middle glenohumeral ligament. **A,** A thick cordlike middle glenohumeral ligament *(asterisk)* is noted on this axial gradient-echo image. This should not be mistaken for an avulsed anterior labrum *(open curved white arrow). White arrowheads,* subscapularis tendon; *flagged arrow,* biceps tendon; *curved solid white arrow,* posterior labrum; *open black arrow,* posterior capsule. **B,** A more common appearance of the middle glenohumeral ligament *(small arrow)* is a linear signal-void area noted anterior to the anterior labrum. *Large arrow,* subcortical sclerosis within the posterior glenoid.

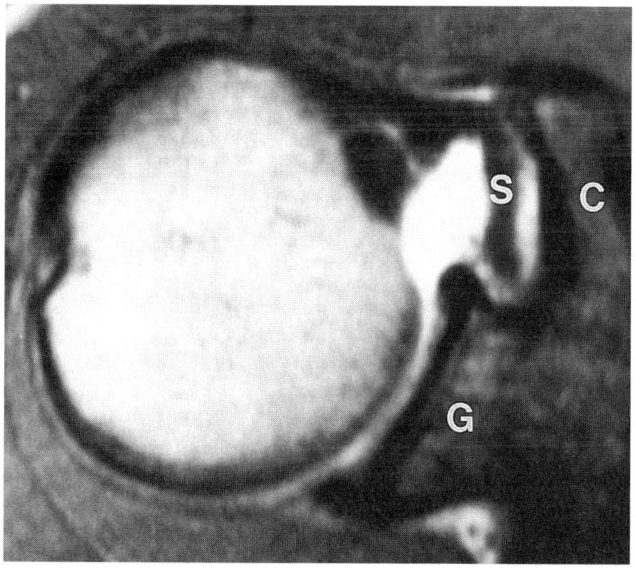

FIGURE 3-21 Superior glenohumeral ligament *(S)* is seen coursing on this high-axial MR image, inserting onto the glenoid neck, adjacent to the anterior labrum. *C,* coracoid process; *G,* glenoid.

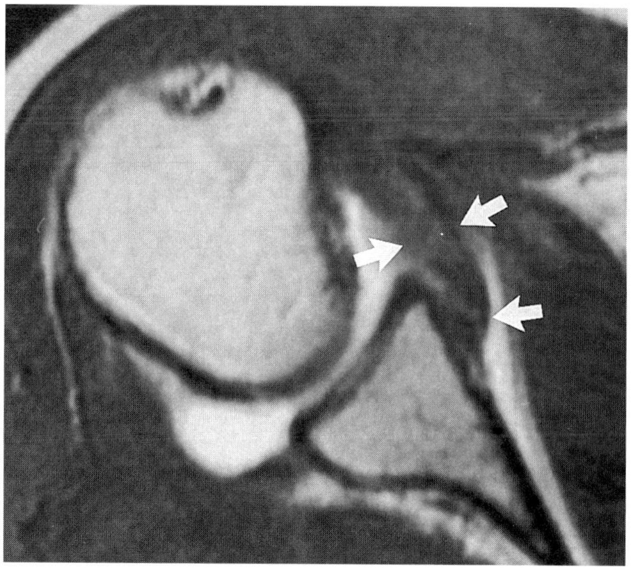

FIGURE 3-22 Axial gadolinium-enhanced MR image demonstrates noticeable thickening of the anterior capsule *(outlined by arrows)* inserting onto the midglenoid.

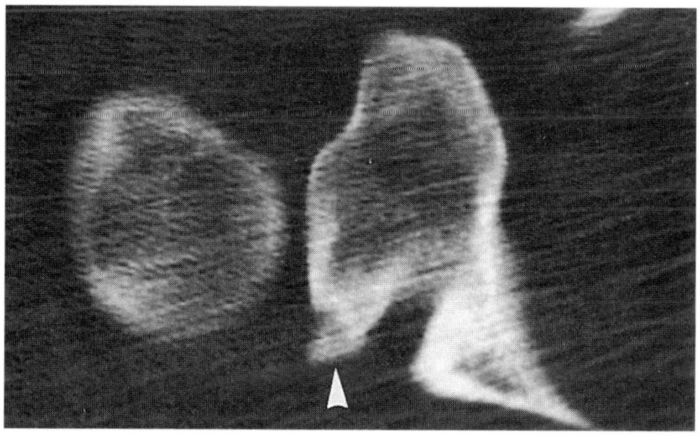

FIGURE 3-23 Axial CT image of crescentic calcific spur *(arrowhead)* at the base of the posterior labrum and the posterior capsular insertion.

A

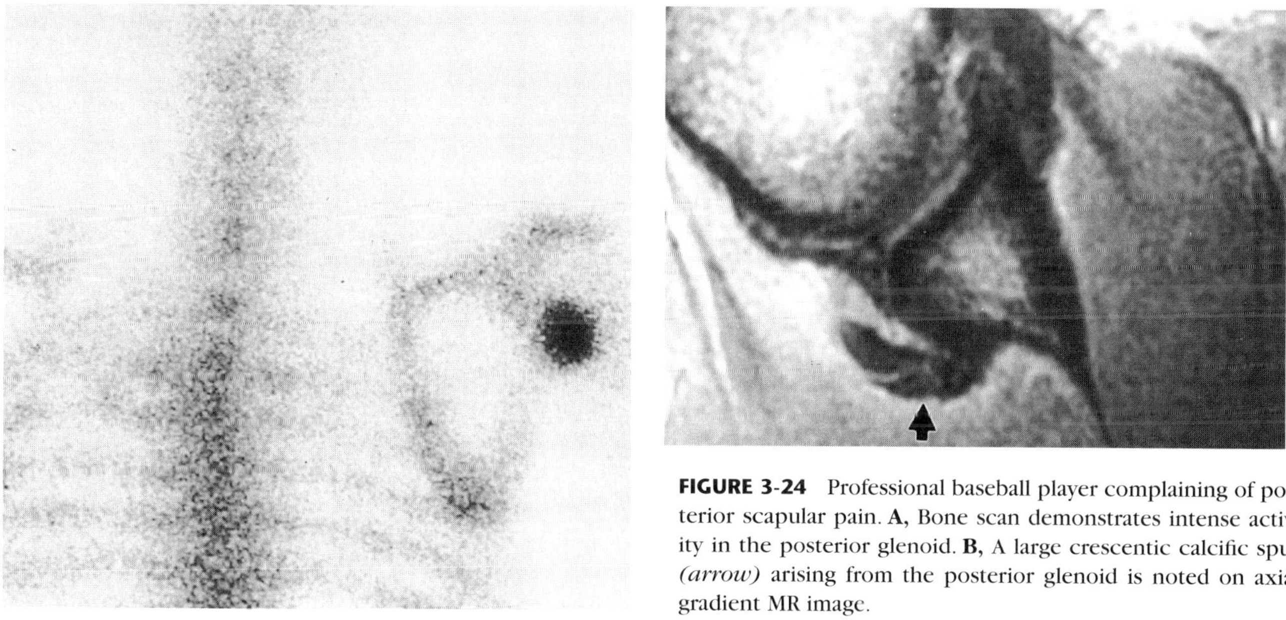

B

FIGURE 3-24 Professional baseball player complaining of posterior scapular pain. **A,** Bone scan demonstrates intense activity in the posterior glenoid. **B,** A large crescentic calcific spur *(arrow)* arising from the posterior glenoid is noted on axial gradient MR image.

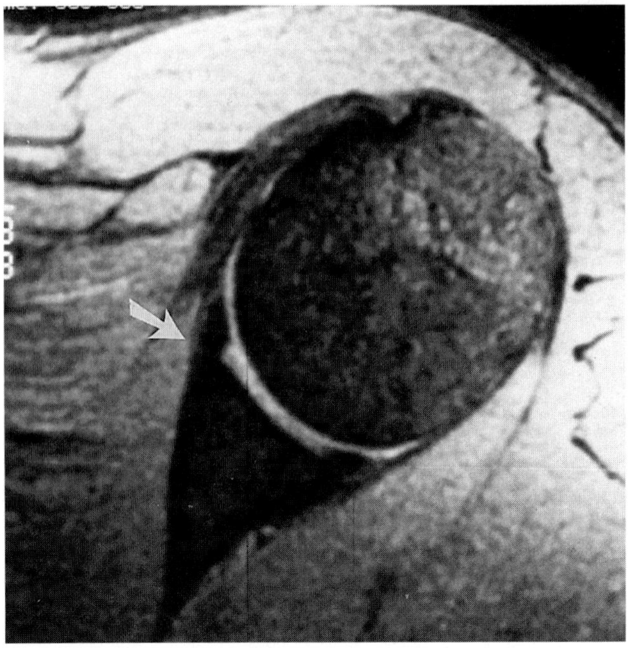

FIGURE 3-25 Axial gradient-echo MR image showing attachment of the anterior capsule *(white arrow)* at the base of the anterior labrum.

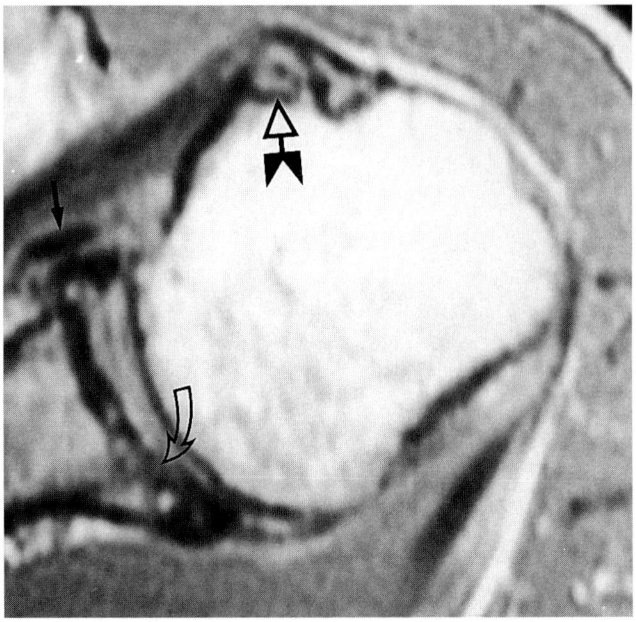

FIGURE 3-26 Posterior humeral shift within the glenohumeral joint demonstrating bony remodeling of the posterior glenoid *(open curved arrow)* from eccentric wearing of the articular surface. *Black arrow,* linear middle glenohumeral ligament; *flagged arrow,* subcortical cyst within the lesser tuberosity.

The site of the anterior capsular insertion onto the scapula has received a lot of attention regarding the presence of anterior instability. Normally the anterior capsule inserts at or near the base of the anterior labrum (type 1 insertion) (Fig. 3-25). Type 2 (see Fig. 3-3, *B*) and type 3 (see Fig. 3-3, *A*) insertions occur at the mid-glenoid level and medial scapular neck, respectively.[61] These insertions are well delineated with CT arthrography but are less reliably seen on MR scans in the absence of any significant joint effusion. Anterior instability has been correlated with the type 3 insertions.[60,74] However, because of the wide normal variation in capsular insertions in asymptomatic patients, any ancillary information must be considered before anterior instability can be diagnosed with certainty.

Bony Glenoid Changes

In addition to capsulolabral abnormalities and heterotopic bone formation at the capsular insertion as signs of instability, additional findings of bony sclerosis or fatty marrow conversion with subcortical cyst formation in the underlying bony glenoid margins also strongly suggest posterior instability resulting from the eccentric wearing of the joint (Fig. 3-26). The abnormal biomechanical forces exerted on the unstable glenohumeral joint result in reactive changes within the underlying cancellous bone marrow of the glenoid as well as of the humeral head. Because of the superiority of MRI over CT in demonstrating cancellous marrow, these structural alterations would be more apparent on MRI and would manifest as areas of decreased signal intensity in areas of sclerosis or areas of high intensity where fatty marrow reconversion has resulted from chronic stress and alteration in the bone marrow's blood supply.

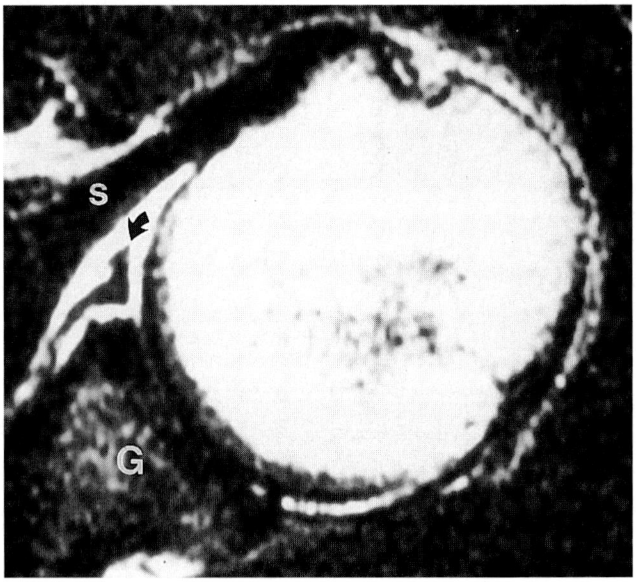

FIGURE 3-27 Axial T_2-weighted MR image with joint fluid demonstrating avulsion of the anterior labrum *(curved black arrow)* with fluid seen dissecting between the glenoid *(G)* and displaced labrum and stripped anterior scapular periosteum. *S,* subscapularis tendon.

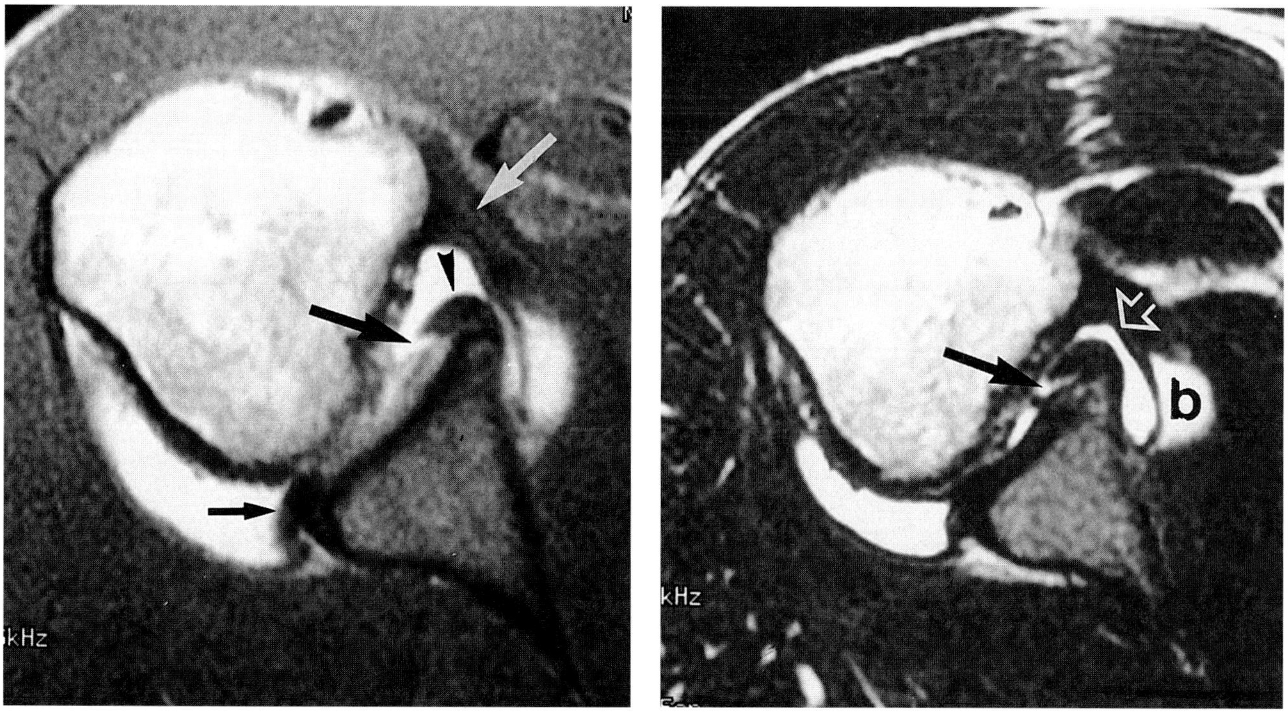

FIGURE 3-28 After the intraarticular injection of gadolinium, axial T_1-weighted, **A,** and T_2-weighted, **B,** images demonstrate an oblique undersurface tear *(large black arrows)* of the anterior labrum *(black arrowhead). Small black arrow,* posterior labrum; *white arrow,* subscapularis tendon; *open white arrow,* middle glenohumeral ligament and anterior capsule; *b,* subscapularis bursa.

Glenoid Labral Tears

In the younger athlete, recurrent subluxations without dislocations often may be explained by the soft-tissue variety of Bankart lesions. This may consist of a tear, partial avulsion, or detachment of the labrum or injury to the capsuloligamentous complex.* Although bony abnormalities are ideally portrayed on plain radiography, CT, and MRI as already mentioned, the recognition of these intraarticular soft-tissue injuries is facilitated by the presence of joint fluid with both MRI and CT.[74] This is accomplished on MRI by the inherent contrast produced on T_1-weighted images when gadolinium is used and on T_2-weighted images when normal saline is injected (Fig. 3-27). Labral tears appear as linear collections of contrast or native fluid within the joint extending into the labral tissue (Fig. 3-28). The labrum also may appear irregular, with blunting of its normal triangular configuration, or may demonstrate complete detachment from the underlying glenoid bony rim with or without associated fracture (Fig. 3-29). Similar findings of the posterior labrum may manifest themselves in cases of posterior dislocations. Tears of the posterior labrum and capsulolabral junction appear as linear areas of contrast within the normally rounded labrum or frank extravasation into the posterior soft tissues, respectively (Figs. 3-30 and 3-31).

*References 2, 11, 15, 18, 32, 41, 49, 52, 60, 63, 73, 74.

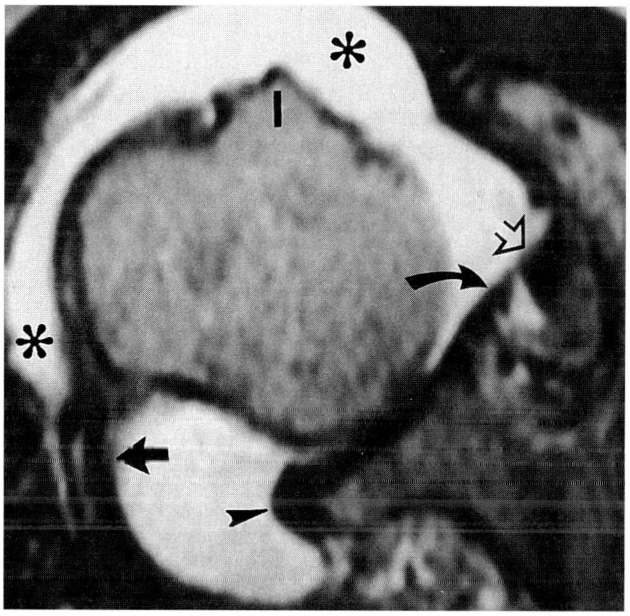

FIGURE 3-29 Axial T_2-weighted MR image with large effusion *(asterisk)* within the subdeltoid bursa attesting to a complete full-thickness rotator cuff tear. The subscapularis tendon is avulsed from the lesser tuberosity *(1),* with medial displacement of the long head of the biceps tendon *(open black arrow).* Detached and displaced anterior labrum *(curved black arrow)* with normal posterior labrum *(black arrowhead)* is noted. *Large black arrow,* infraspinatus tendon insertion.

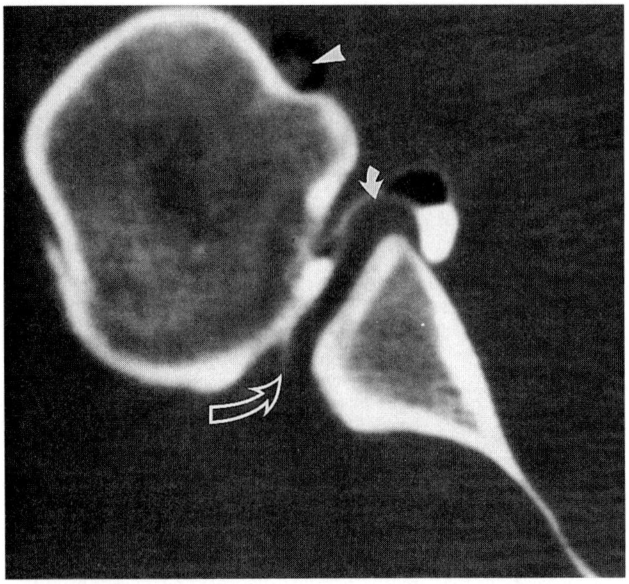

FIGURE 3-30 Axial contrast-enhanced CT scan shows linear posterior labral tear *(open curved white arrow). Small curved white arrow,* normal anterior labrum; *arrowhead,* biceps tendon surrounded by air within its sheath located within the intertubercular groove.

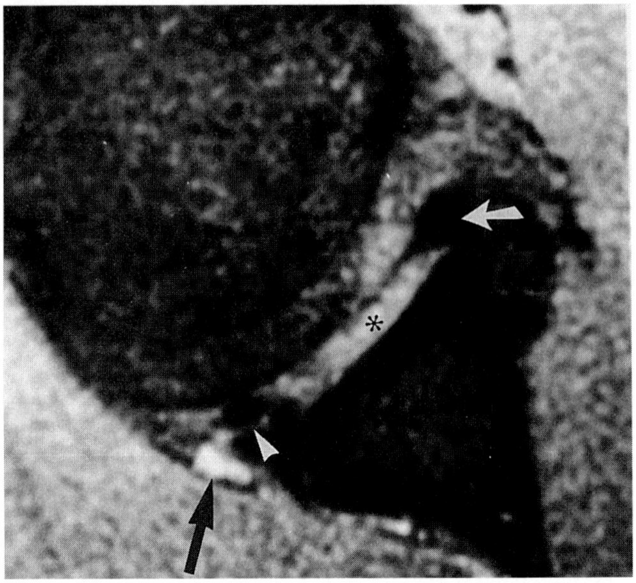

FIGURE 3-31 Axial gradient-echo MR image reveals a linear signal *(white arrowhead)* within the posterior labrum reflecting a tear and injury at the capsulolabral junction *(black arrow). White arrow,* normal anterior labrum; *asterisk,* hyaline articular cartilage.

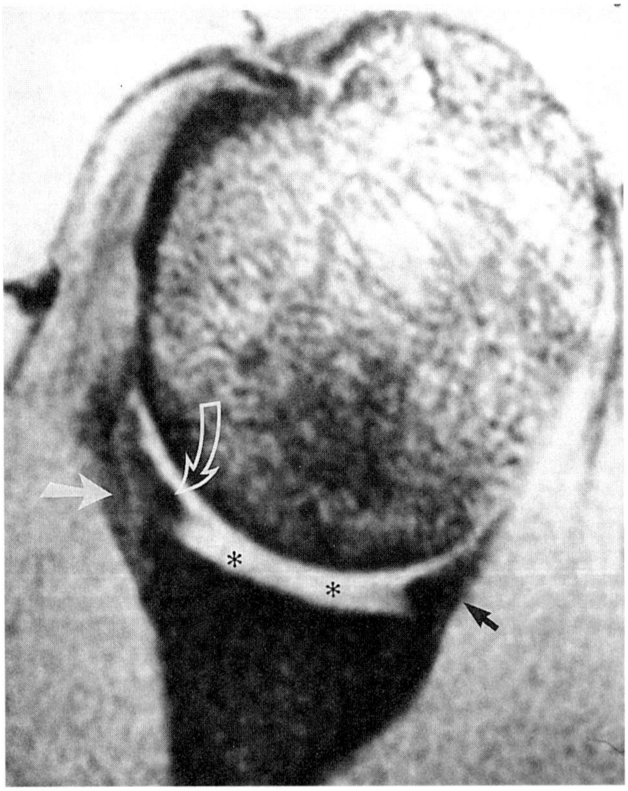

FIGURE 3-32 Normal hyaline articular cartilage *(asterisk)* is seen at the base of both the anterior *(open curved white arrow)* and posterior *(black arrow)* labra and should not be confused with detached or torn labra. *White arrow,* middle glenohumeral ligament.

One pitfall when evaluating labral pathology on MRI is not recognizing the glenoid articular hyaline cartilage that normally undermines the labra (Fig. 3-32). This hyaline cartilage, which appears intermediate in signal intensity on T_1-weighted and proton-density images and high in signal intensity on gradient-echo images, may mimic the appearance of fluid at the labral base.[52] Another potential concern in shoulder MRI is the presence of a normal sublabral foramen that occurs in the anterosuperior quadrant at or above the level of the coracoid process (Fig. 3-33). Neither of these conditions should be mistaken for true labral tears.

A unique labral injury occurs at the insertion of the long head of the biceps onto the superior labrum at the supraglenoid tubercle. This injury often is associated with the overhead-throwing athlete. The violent contraction of the biceps on the superior labrum may result in a central labral tear with subsequent detachment from the underlying glenoid margin in an anterior-to-posterior manner. This has been termed the *SLAP lesion* (superior labrum, anterior to posterior) and has been described as a small central fissure with early detachment progressing all the way to a bucket-handle type tear where the displaced labral fragment may become entrapped between the humeral head and medial glenoid margin.[2,20,24,60,77] Although contrast dissecting within the abnormal superior labrum may be noted on both axial CT and MR images, MRI is particularly suited for this lesion because only MRI can directly image the shoulder in the coronal plane as well (Fig. 3-34).

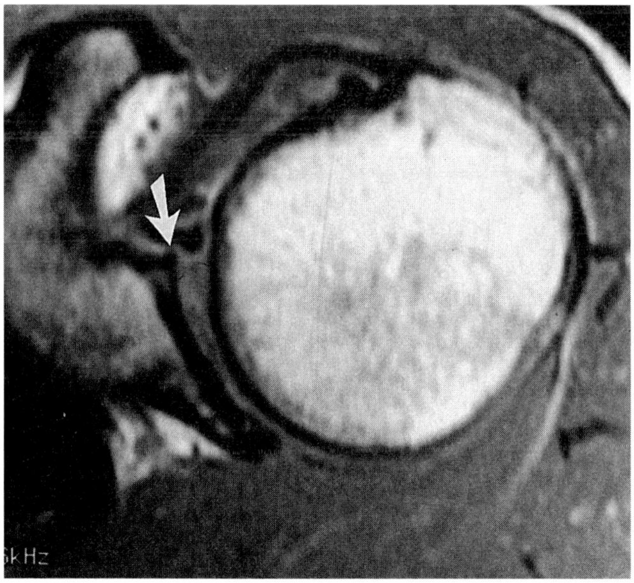

FIGURE 3-33 A small foramen *(arrow)* is present beneath the anterior labrum at the upper coracoid level. This should not be mistaken for a tear at the labral base.

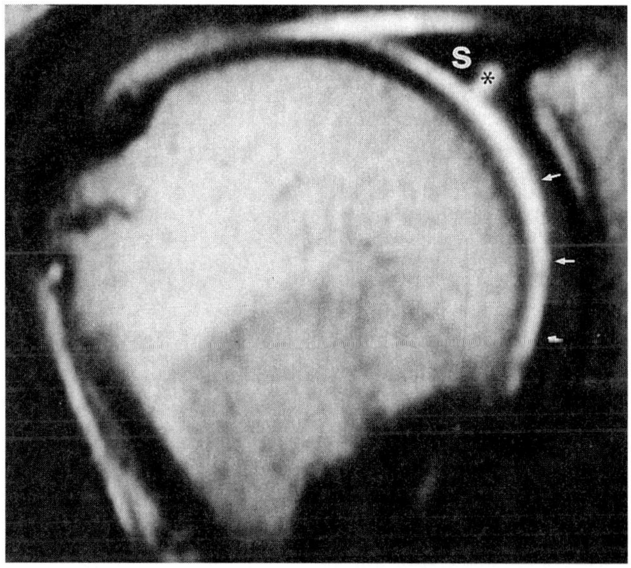

B

A

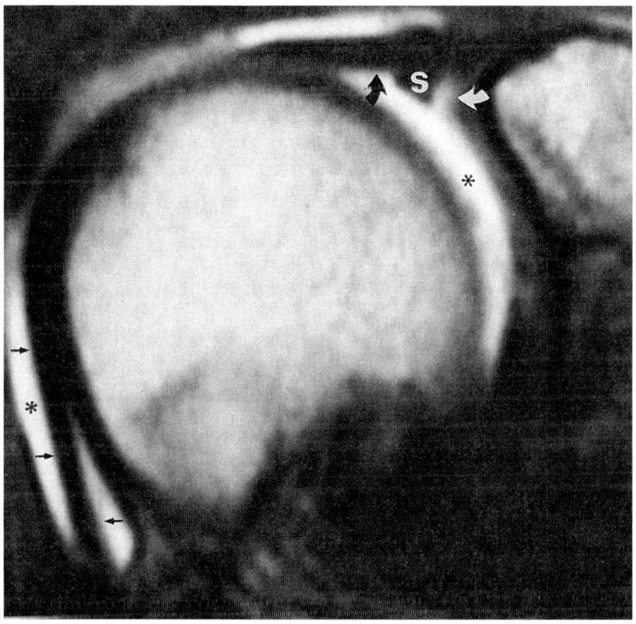

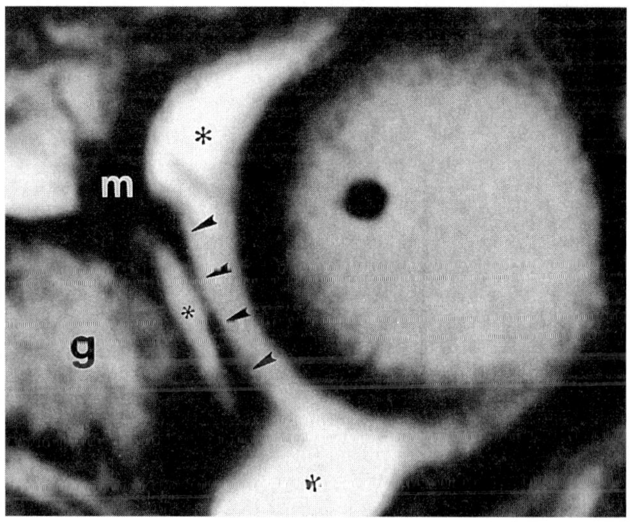

C

FIGURE 3-34 SLAP (superior labrum, anterior to posterior) lesion on oblique coronal (**A** and **B**) and axial (**C**) T_1-weighted MR images after the intraarticular injection of gadolinium *(asterisk).* The torn superior labrum *(S)* is separated (*black arrowheads* in **C**) from the underlying glenoid *(g). Small black arrows,* biceps tendon within the sheath; *black arrow,* intraarticular portion of the biceps tendon; *white arrows,* hyaline articular cartilage; *m,* middle glenohumeral ligament.

Impingement Syndrome and Rotator Cuff Disease

There is a close association between the impingement syndrome and the presence of underlying rotator cuff disease.[21,54,74] The classic form of impingement results in loss of the normal gliding motion between the cephalad aspect of the glenohumeral joint and the coracoacromial arch. This is accomplished by encroachment on the subacromial space with a decrease in the normal humeral-acromial space.[9,54] The etiology and location of impingement in the young athlete are a matter of opinion, and these less-known theories as well as the long-recognized form of impingement are discussed elsewhere in this text.

Acromioclavicular Joint and Humeral Head Changes

Although the diagnosis of impingement should be based on a good history and physical examination, radiographic findings may be obvious on plain x-ray studies. Neer and others have emphasized the importance of the anterior acromion and AC joint with the development of rotator cuff disease leading to rupture through an orderly progression of cuff degeneration beginning with hemorrhage and edema, leading to fibrosis and eventually cuff disruption.[4,53,54] A variety of radiographs of the acromion and AC joint should be obtained and examined for hypertrophic spurs and the development of osteophytes along the undersurface of the anterior acromion and AC joint. Secondary changes of the humeral head consisting of sclerosis and subcortical cystic changes near the greater tuberosity may be noted.[21] With advancing cuff disease and cephalad humeral shift, one can infer marked degeneration or disruption of the rotator cuff with proximal retraction.

Shoulder Arthrography

For a long time, the gold standard in diagnosing rotator cuff tears was shoulder arthrography. This method had an extremely high sensitivity, approaching 100% for acute complete rotator cuff tears[7,48] (Fig. 3-35); however, no information about intratendinous tears, superior bursal side tears, or tendinitis and cuff degeneration could be obtained.[74] Of course, one advantage was that after an arthrogram had been performed, CT arthrography often provided additional information regarding the capsule, glenohumeral ligaments, and glenoid labra.

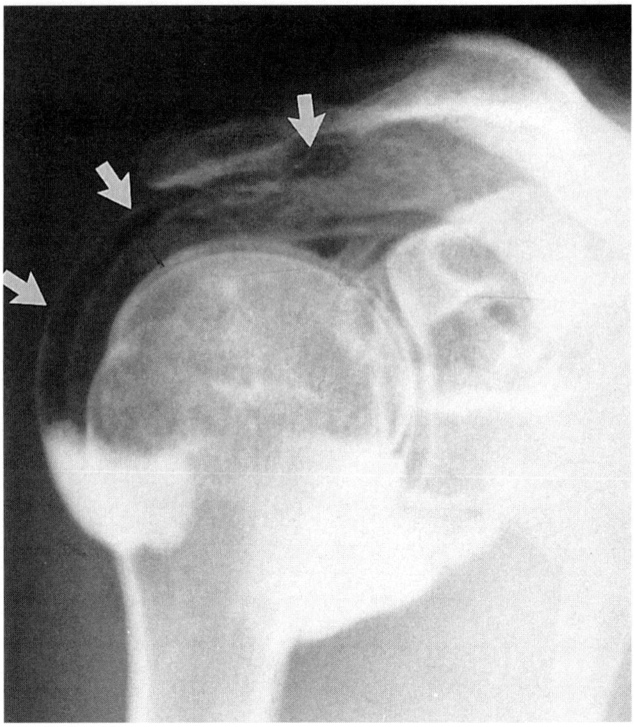

FIGURE 3-35 Air-contrast arthrogram of the shoulder demonstrating communication of the glenohumeral joint with the subacromial-subdeltoid bursa *(arrows)* secondary to a full-thickness tear of the rotator cuff.

Shoulder Sonography

Ultrasound was heralded in the past as a sensitive technique for rotator cuff evaluation.[78] Unfortunately, this technique is extremely operator-dependent, and subsequent studies failed to display the predicted high sensitivity that was previously touted.[7,74] There was difficulty in consistently demonstrating partial or intratendinous tears (Figs. 3-36 and 3-37). Hyperechoic and hypoechoic areas both were noted within the rotator cuff. The examination also was limited by the sonogram's inability to scan beneath the acromion. Examination of the glenoid labra, ligaments, and AC joint is impossible, and this precludes an adequate evaluation of the shoulder.

Shoulder MRI

With the advent of MRI, a new and comprehensive imaging modality for the shoulder came into existence. With the newer scanning sequences, dedicated surface coils resulting in a smaller field of view and high-resolution images, excellent soft-tissue discrimination, and multiplanar capability, MRI easily became the imaging procedure of choice in evaluating impingement and rotator cuff pathology.[26,74]

Acromial Morphology

Direct oblique sagittal imaging with MRI perpendicular to the scapular axis easily demonstrates the relationship of the anterior acromion to the subacromial space and nearby rotator cuff. There is a low correlation between rotator cuff tears caused by impingement and an upward-sloping or straight acromion process (type 1) as depicted on the sagittal images. A higher incidence

A

B

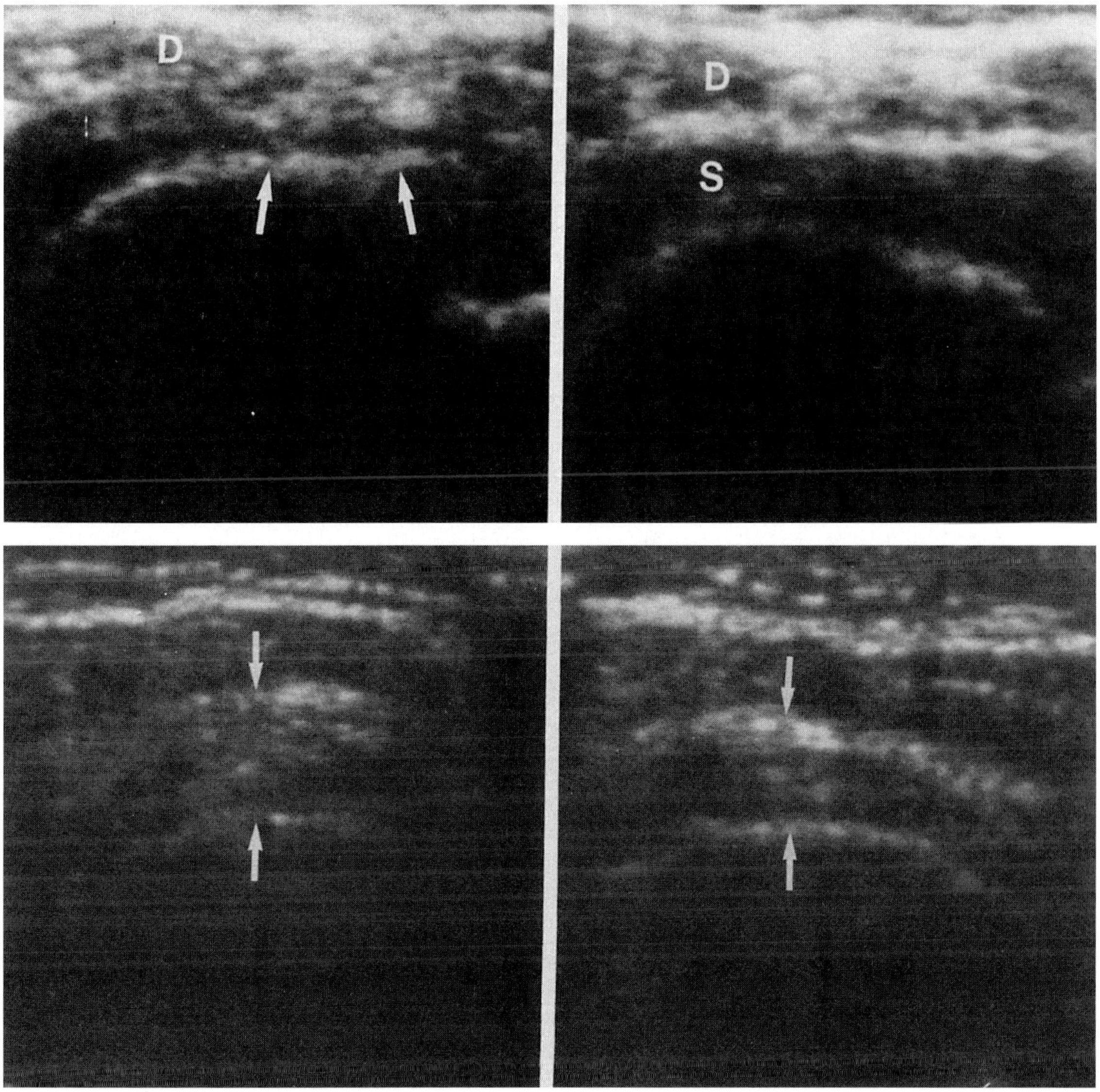

FIGURE 3-36 **A,** Transverse sonograms through the distal supraspinatus tendon *(S)* demonstrate peribursal echogenic fat *(arrows)* and adjacent deltoid muscle *(D)* filling in a tendon gap caused by a full-thickness tear; normal contralateral side is provided for comparison. **B,** Another individual with a false-negative study for partial-thickness tear. Mildly thickened supraspinatus tendon *(outlined by arrows)* is noted on the left with no discernible tear. Normal contralateral side is on the right. (Reprinted with permission from Burk DL et al: *AJR* 153:87, 1989.)

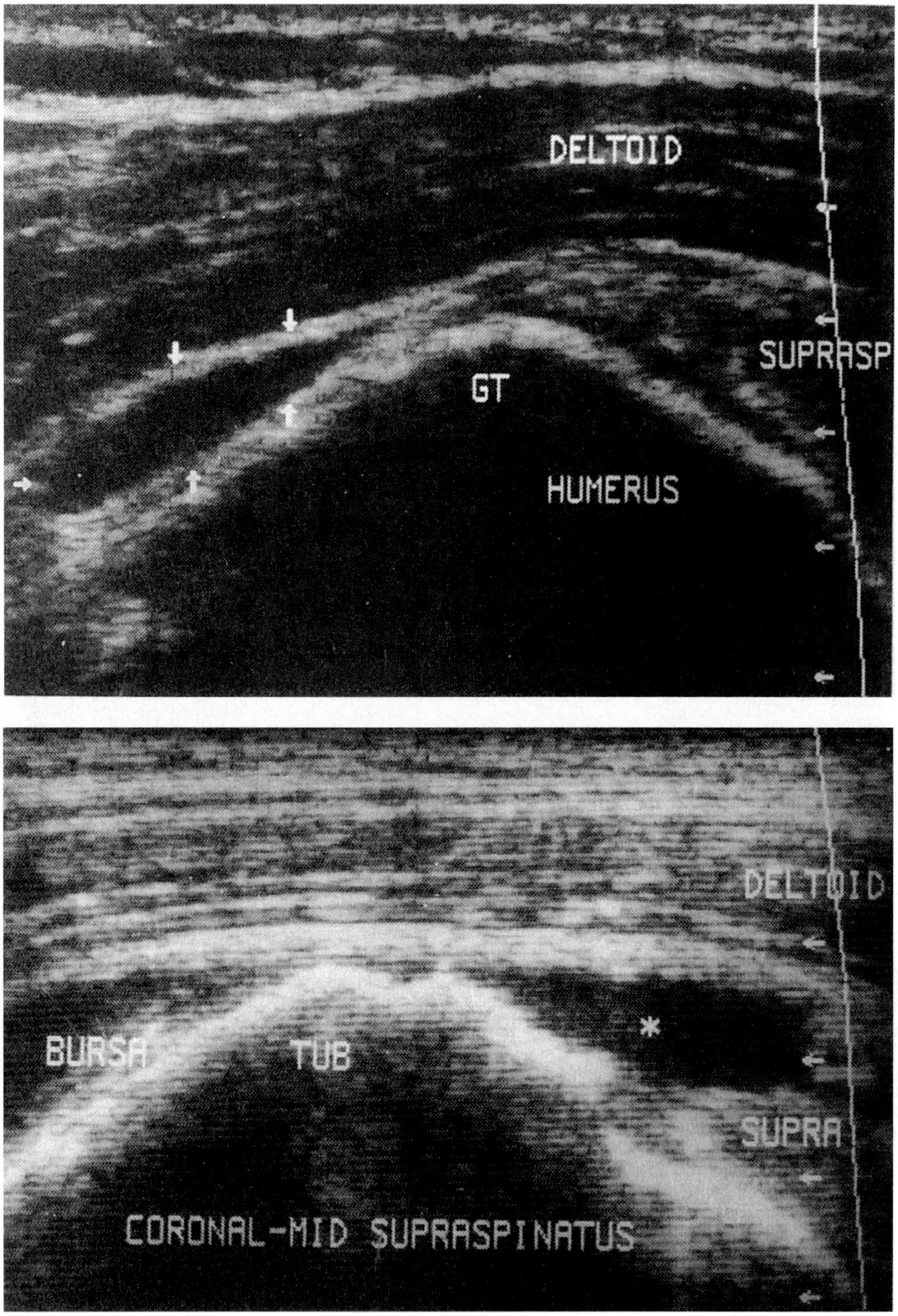

FIGURE 3-37 **A,** Longitudinal sonogram in a normal person with the supraspinatus tendon *(suprasp)* inserting onto the greater tuberosity *(GT)* of the humerus. Fluid is noted in a distended subacromial-subdeltoid bursa *(outlined by arrows)*. **B,** Torn rotator cuff with retracted end of supraspinatus tendon. Fluid *(asterisk)* fills in the cuff defect and communicates with the subacromial-subdeltoid bursa. (Reprinted with permission from Van Holsbeeck M, Strouse PJ: *AJR* 160:561, 1993.)

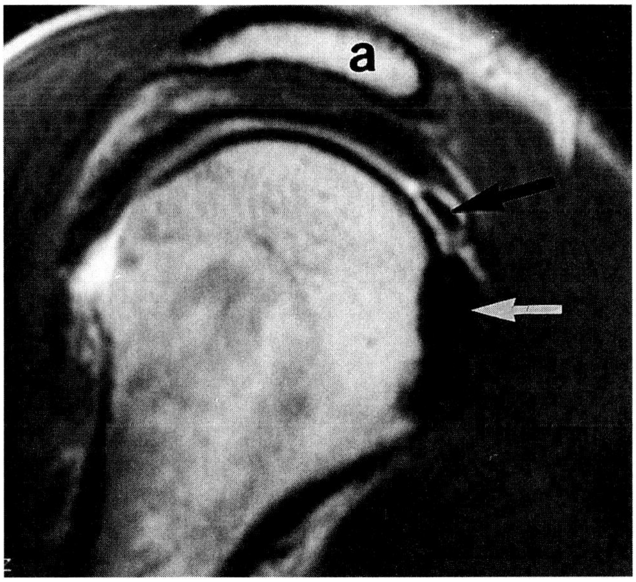

FIGURE 3-38 Oblique sagittal MR image revealing the lateral acromion *(a)* gently curving parallel to the upper humeral cortical surface. *Black arrow,* indicates intraarticular portion of the biceps tendon; *white arrow,* distal subscapularis tendon inserting onto the lesser tuberosity.

A

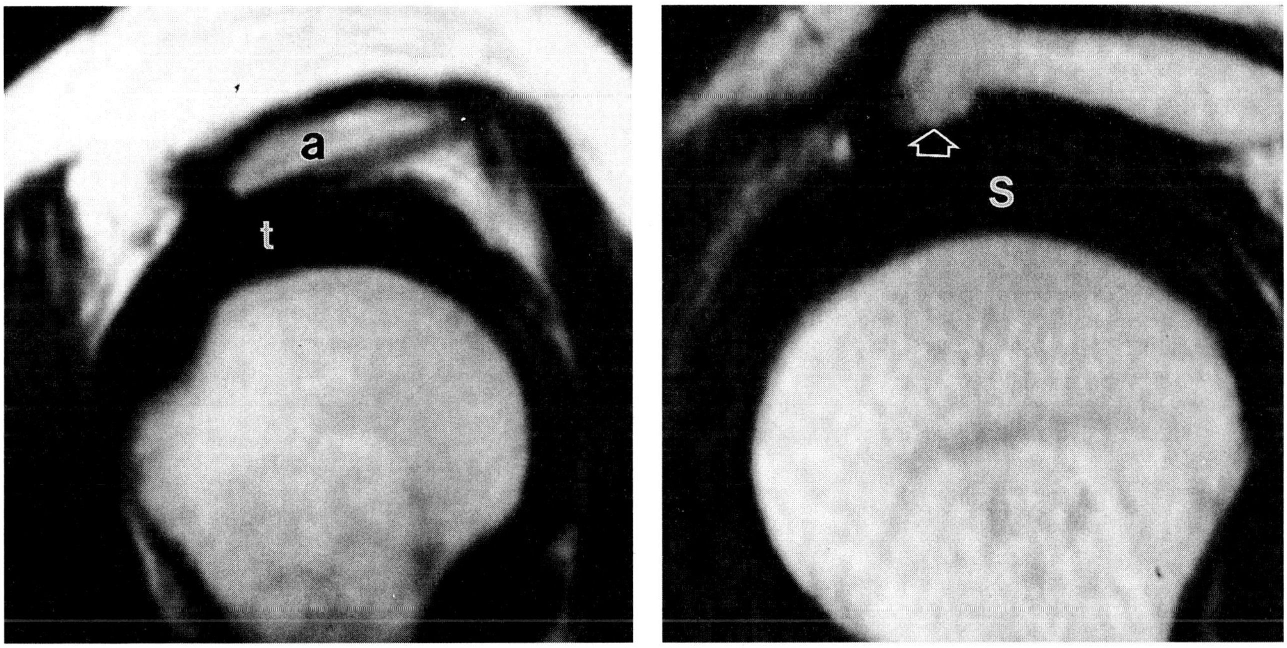

B

FIGURE 3-39 Oblique sagittal MR images reveal downward sloping of the anterior acromion *(a)* abutting the bursal surface of the rotator cuff *(t)* in **A** and a congenital hook *(open arrow)* projecting caudal in **B.** *S,* supraspinatus.

of impingement and underlying cuff pathology has been associated with acromions running parallel to the humeral cortical surface (type 2) (Fig. 3-38). The highest correlation between impingement and cuff tears is found with an acromion that is downward-sloping anteriorly or has a congenital hook (type 3) projecting caudad from its anterior aspect[4] (Fig. 3-39). In addition to the acromial morphology in the sagittal projections, abnormally laterally sloped acromions on the direct oblique coronal MR images also may be apparent and may demonstrate signs of impingement with changes in the peribursal soft tissues and underlying rotator cuff (Fig. 3-40).

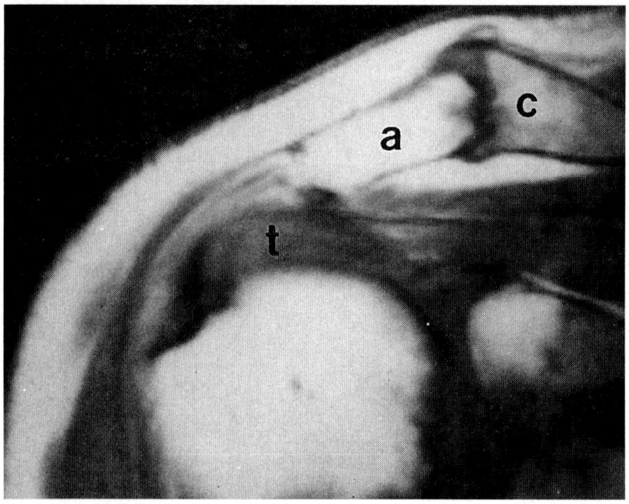

FIGURE 3-40 Laterally sloped acromion *(a)* with obliteration of the normal subacromial fat. Note the markedly thickened rotator cuff *(t)* with heterogeneous internal signal from tendinitis. *c,* clavicle.

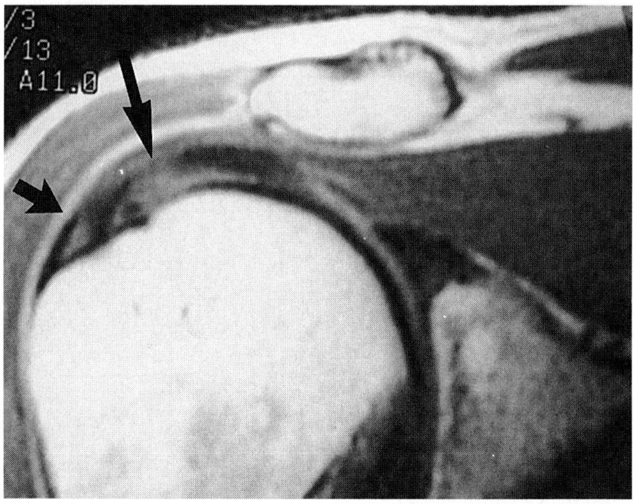

FIGURE 3-41 Coronal oblique T_1-weighted image demonstrating a thickened rotator cuff with focal increased signal indicative of tendinitis or partial tear *(large arrow).* Note the preserved fat planes *(small arrow)* in the subacromial-subdeltoid region.

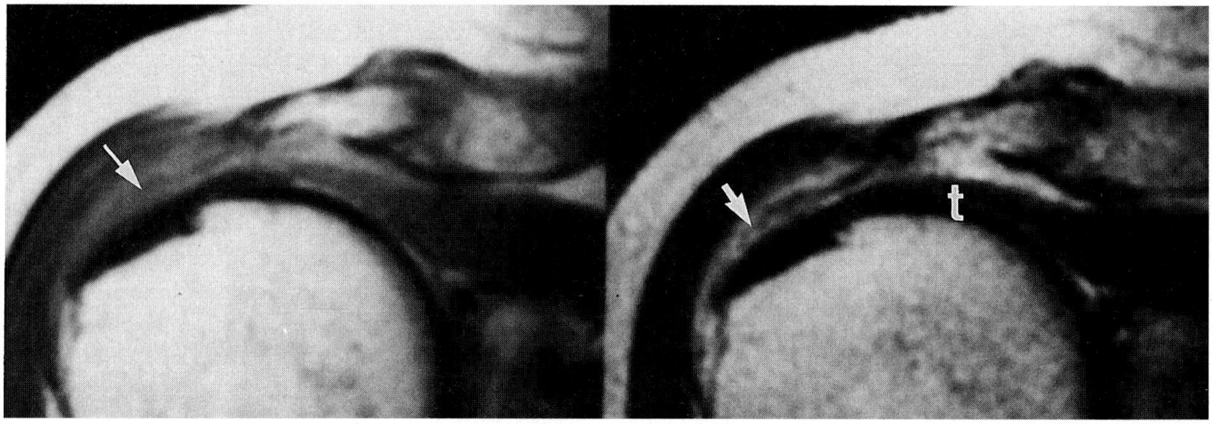

FIGURE 3-42 Chronic peribursal inflammation with synovial hypertrophy *(white arrows)* in a patient who has undergone a previous acromioplasty (note deformity of lateral aspect of acromion). *t,* Normal rotator cuff tendon. Left image, proton-density; right image, T_2-weighted.

Subacromial and Subdeltoid Bursa

The presence of a normal subacromial or subdeltoid space with preservation of the normal fat planes strongly speaks against a full-thickness cuff tear. With the onset of tendinitis, an enlarged rotator cuff with increased signal is expected, although the signal may be focal, linear, or diffuse[59,81] (Fig. 3-41). Ensuing peribursal inflammation with synovial proliferation and effusions will further compromise the subacromial space.[74,82] This may result in the appearance of low- to moderate-signal tissue in the presence of chronic granulation or scar tissue on T_1-weighted images and bright fluid collections on T_2-weighted or gradient-echo sequences when effusions are present (Figs. 3-42 and 3-43). Poor definition of the bursal side of the rotator cuff with fraying may progress to frank partial bursal side tears. These lesions are much less common than underside or synovial tears. As further changes within the cuff and subacromial space develop, the impingement syndrome becomes more apparent, with progressive development of proliferative bony spurs and reactive osteophytes along the undersurface of the anterior acromion and AC joint[1,9,27,28,71,74] (Fig. 3-44). Although small cortical spurs may appear as signal-void structures on MR, larger osteophytes typically have high-signal fat within the marrow space. A pseudospur off the inferior lateral acromion often is encountered on MRI of

A

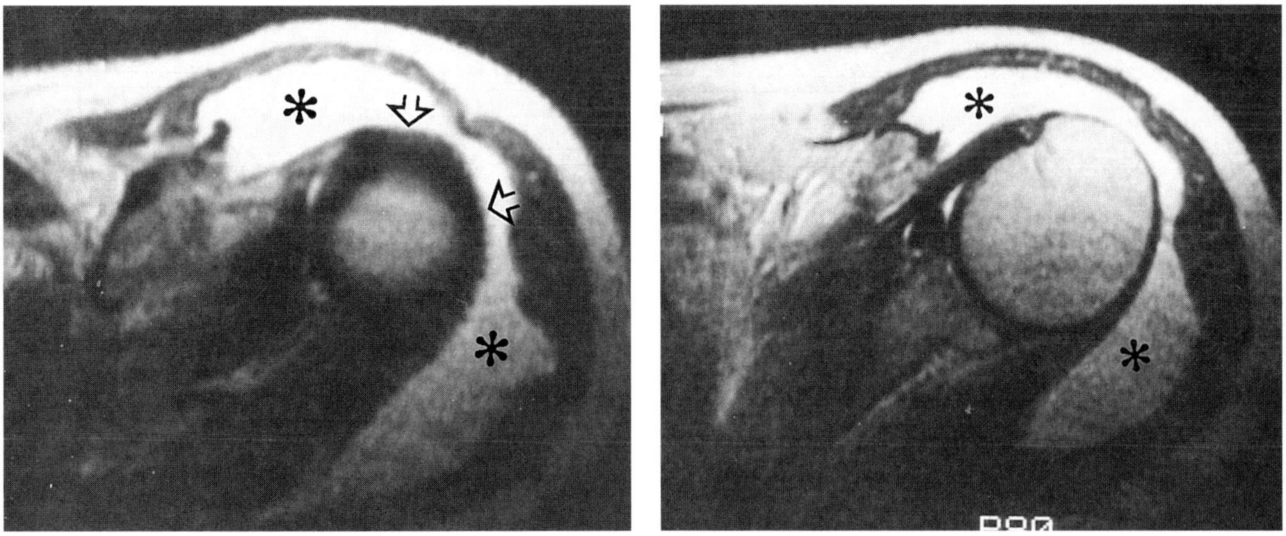

B

FIGURE 3-43 Axial T_2-weighted MR images showing a massive effusion *(asterisk)* within the subdeltoid bursa outlining the normal rotator cuff *(open black arrows)*. Note the uniform thickness of the cuff as it inserts onto the greater tuberosity. Image **A** is more cephalad than image **B.**

A

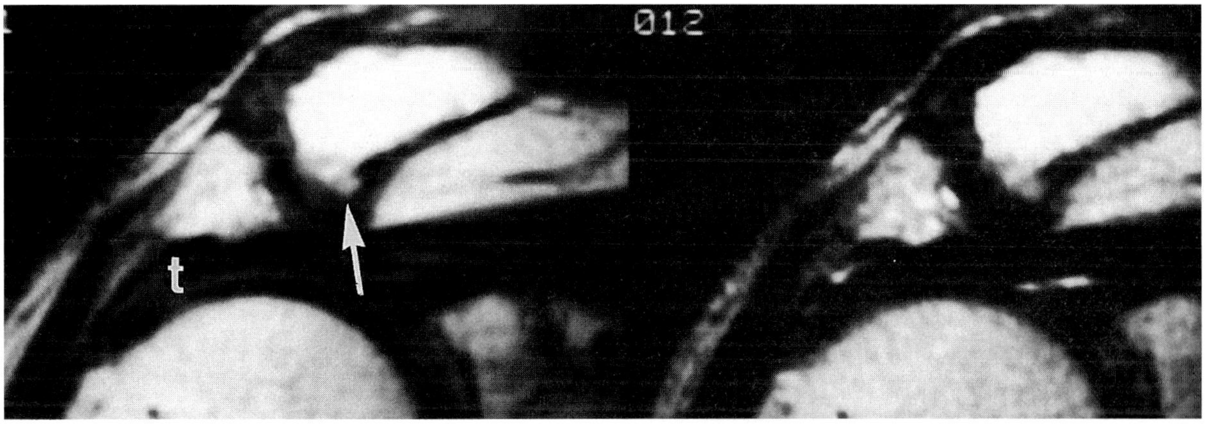

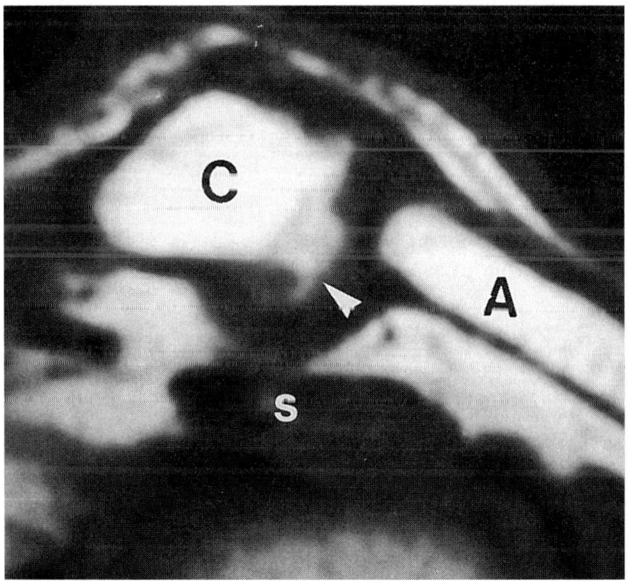

B

FIGURE 3-44 **A,** Oblique coronal and, **B,** sagittal, MR images demonstrate high-signal marrow within distal clavicular osteophytes *(white arrowhead and arrow)* together with hypertrophy of the acromioclavicular joint impinging on the supraspinatus muscle *(S)* and tendon *(t)* below.

the shoulder and is thought to represent a portion of the distal coracoacromial ligament or the origin of some of the deltoid tendon slips[26] (Fig. 3-45, *A*).

Rotator Cuff Pathology

The normal rotator cuff appears as a homogeneous decreased-signal structure of uniform thickness on all MR sequences[3,19,47,89,90] (Fig. 3-45, *B* and *C*). With the repetitive overuse occurring in many sports, the abrasion forces exerted on the rotator cuff result in microtears of the cuff's fibers.[1] Intermediate and then increased signal changes appear within the cuff. As these areas of degeneration coalesce to form actual cuff defects (Fig. 3-46), marked hyperintense or bright areas appear within the cuff until a full-thickness rupture from the synovial surface to the bursal side is encountered* (Fig. 3-47). This can be noticed in all three planes (sagittal, axial, coronal) on MRI. Cuff retraction and chronic atrophy of the muscle will become apparent as the intermediate signal from muscle increases with subsequent fatty replacement.[74] Most cuff tears occur at the so-called critical zone, several centimeters proximal to the insertion of the cuff onto the greater tuberosity.[9,74] This area appears to be a focal zone of relative hypovascularity caused by the anas-

*References 27, 28, 30, 60, 64, 81, 83, 89, 90.

A

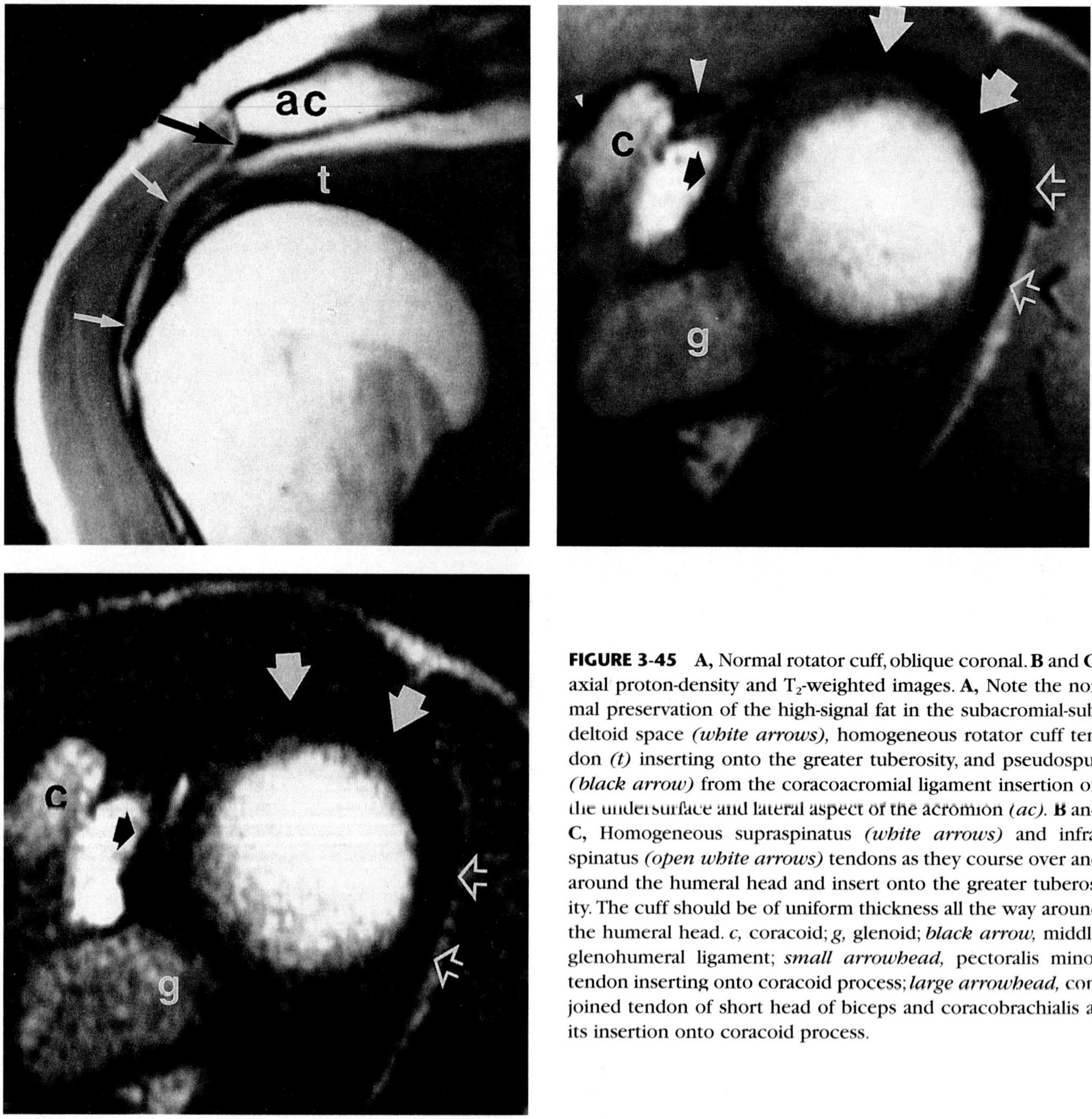

B

C

FIGURE 3-45 **A,** Normal rotator cuff, oblique coronal. **B** and **C,** axial proton-density and T_2-weighted images. **A,** Note the normal preservation of the high-signal fat in the subacromial-subdeltoid space *(white arrows),* homogeneous rotator cuff tendon *(t)* inserting onto the greater tuberosity, and pseudospur *(black arrow)* from the coracoacromial ligament insertion on the undersurface and lateral aspect of the acromion *(ac).* **B** and **C,** Homogeneous supraspinatus *(white arrows)* and infraspinatus *(open white arrows)* tendons as they course over and around the humeral head and insert onto the greater tuberosity. The cuff should be of uniform thickness all the way around the humeral head. *c,* coracoid; *g,* glenoid; *black arrow,* middle glenohumeral ligament; *small arrowhead,* pectoralis minor tendon inserting onto coracoid process; *large arrowhead,* conjoined tendon of short head of biceps and coracobrachialis at its insertion onto coracoid process.

A

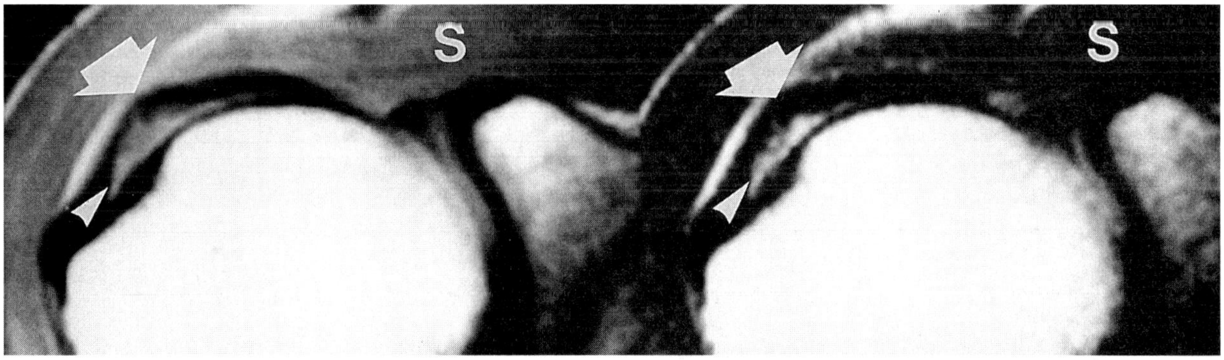

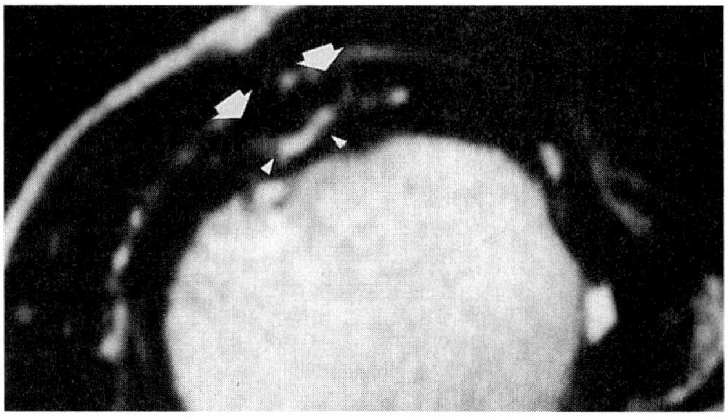

B

FIGURE 3-46 **A,** Proton-density and T_2-weighted oblique coronal and, **B,** axial T_2-weighted MR images demonstrate hyperintensity *(white arrowheads)* along the synovial surface of the rotator cuff indicative of a partial undersurface tear. Note the intact bursal surface *(white arrows)* of the cuff in both planes.

A

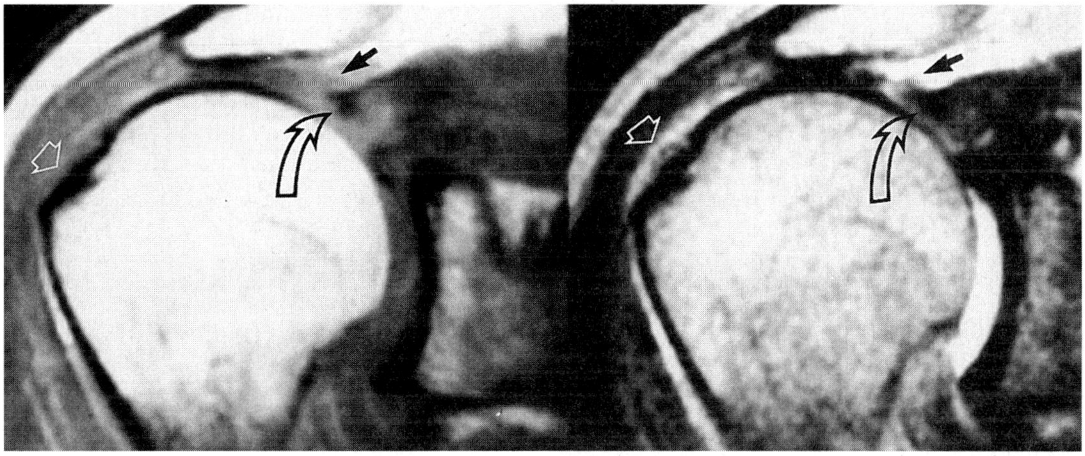

B

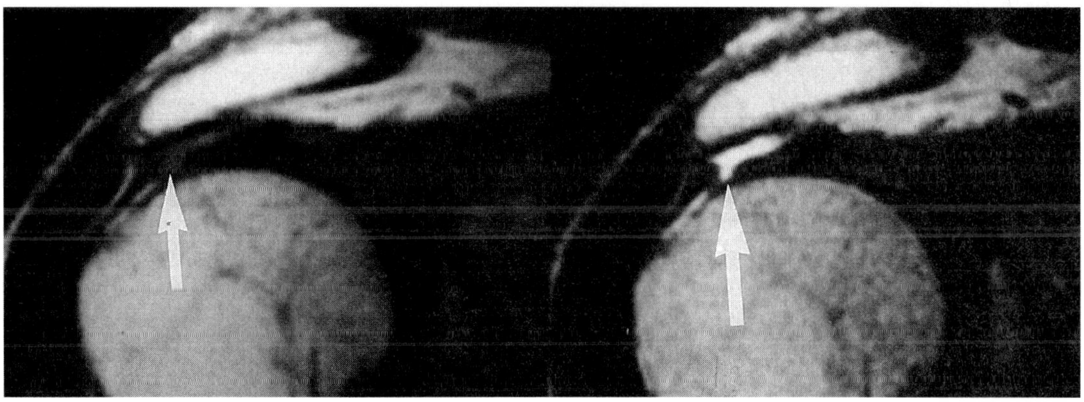

FIGURE 3-47 **A,** Oblique coronal proton-density and T_2-weighted images of a full-thickness cuff tear with retraction of the remaining cuff end *(curved open black arrow)* and fluid in the subacromial *(small black arrow)* and subdeltoid *(open white arrow)* bursa. **B,** Proton-density and T_2-weighted oblique coronal images demonstrating an oblique full-thickness tear *(arrow)* without cuff retraction.

A

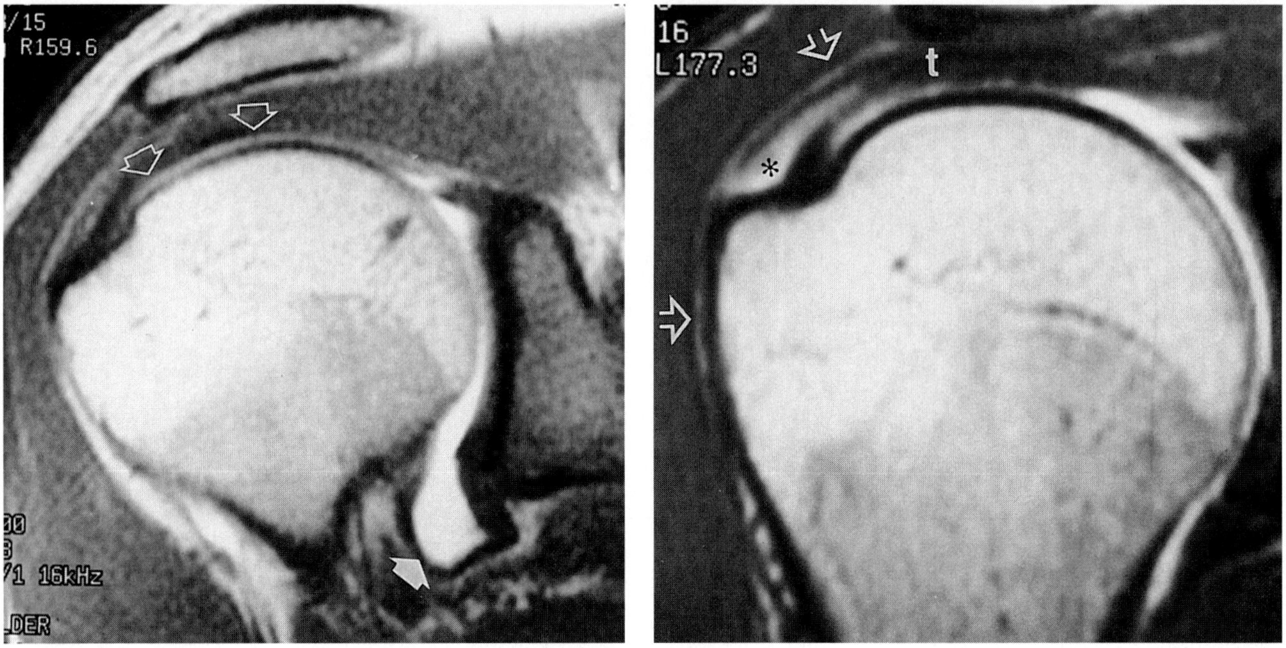

B

FIGURE 3-48 Oblique coronal MR images after the intraarticular injection of gadolinium. Note the smooth undersurface of the intact cuff in **A** *(open white arrows). Solid white arrow,* axillary pouch of the inferior glenohumeral ligament. A collection of gadolinium *(asterisk)* is seen within the substance of the rotator cuff *(t)* in **B,** indicative of a partial undersurface tear, although no definite defect was identified. *Open arrows,* normal subdeltoid fat plane.

tomotic blood vessels originating from the adjacent osseous and muscular arterial branches.[8] This location also may demonstrate an area of increased signal that may be related to the orientation of the imaged cuff fibers (magic angle phenomenon) within the magnetic scanner. Therefore additional findings (e.g., actual interruption of normal cuff fibers, abnormal cuff morphology such as thinning, cuff retraction, or discrete markedly hyperintense fluid collections within the cuff defects entering the subacromial-subdeltoid bursa with obliteration of the normal peribursal fat) should be sought to confirm the diagnosis of a true cuff tear.[60,74]

As can be expected, distinguishing a partial and intratendinous tear from cuff degeneration may be extremely difficult on MRI because of the overlap of similar image findings. The visualized tendinopathy is a continuum of rotator cuff pathology. In some instances, the use of intraarticular gadolinium has improved the detection of subtle undersurface synovial tears (Fig. 3-48) because up to 20% of full-thickness tears may not demonstrate the typical high signal on T_2-weighted images, but instead display a low to intermediate signal caused by the chronic granulation or scar tissue within the cuff defect.[60]

Nevertheless, despite MRI's limitations, it has clearly proven to be superior in its overall accuracy in the detection and analysis of rotator cuff pathology.[89] MRI can aid preoperative planning by revealing such crucial information as the size of the cuff tear, degree of retraction, atrophy of the supraspinatus muscle, and morphology (intact or frayed) of the retracted cuff stump.

Because most rotator cuff tears arise in the anterior portion of the supraspinatus tendon,[9] we have found T_2-weighted axial MR images most useful at this institution (Fig. 3-49). These axial views often demonstrate the tear to the best advantage and usually can distinguish between a partial-thickness and a full-thickness tear. The subdeltoid space also can be evaluated in this plane for bursal fluid that may help to confirm the presence of a full-thickness cuff tear.

Bicipital Tendon Pathology

The remaining muscles and tendons of the rotator cuff, including the subscapularis, infraspinatus, and teres minor, are best inspected with MRI. The normal signal-void tendon of the subscapularis may be avulsed from the lesser tuberosity with medial displacement of the long head of the biceps tendon (Fig. 3-50). In addition to dislocation of the biceps tendon, bicipital tendinitis or degeneration may be diagnosed if there is increased signal within the biceps tendon and surrounding fluid within its synovial sheath.[74] Degeneration or complete rupture of the biceps tendon may present as either severe atrophy or absence of the normal tendon within the intertubercular groove, respectively (Fig. 3-51).

A

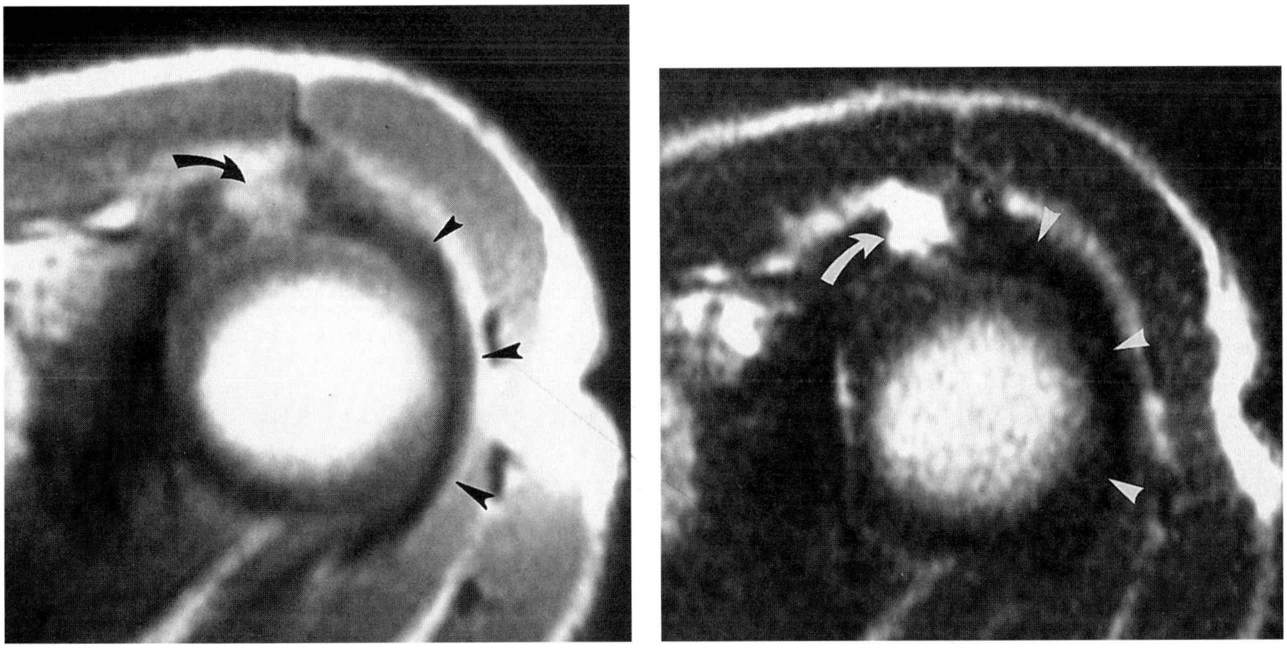

B

FIGURE 3-49 Full-thickness rotator cuff tear (*curved black and white arrows* on proton-density, **A**, and T_2-weighted, **B**, axial images, respectively) involving the smaller anterior band of the supraspinatus tendon. Note the normal infraspinatus tendon *(black and white arrowheads)* surrounding the remainder of the humeral head.

A

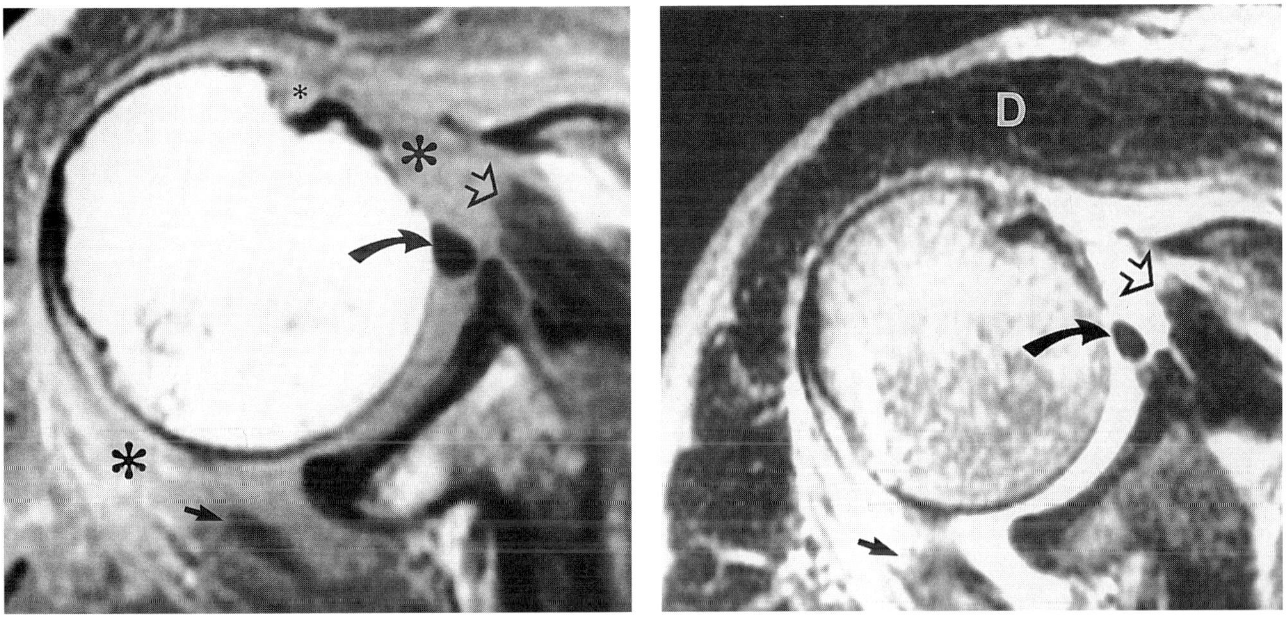

B

FIGURE 3-50 **A,** Axial proton-density and, **B,** T_2-weighted images show a torn distal subscapularis tendon *(open black arrow)* from its insertion onto the lesser tuberosity with medially dislocated biceps tendon *(curved black arrow)* lying adjacent to the anterior labrum. A large effusion *(asterisk)* is noted within the joint and within the subdeltoid bursa anteriorly from the rotator cuff tear. A less common posterior tear of the infraspinatus tendon *(small black arrow)* is also noted.

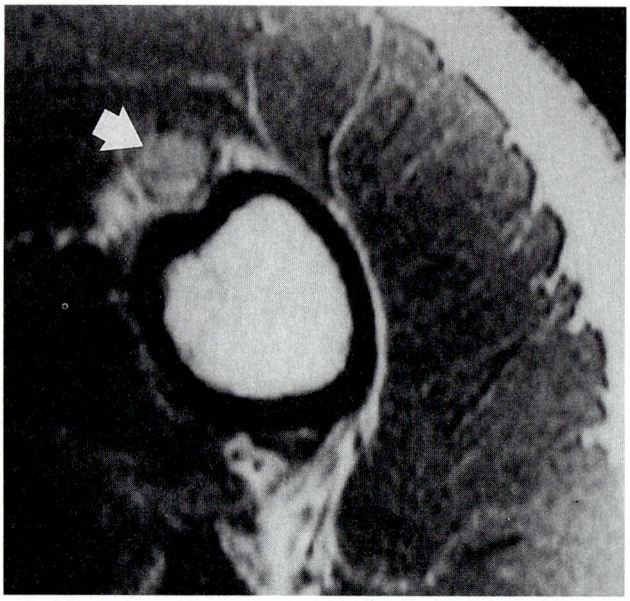

FIGURE 3-51 Axial proton-density MR image demonstrating rupture of the biceps tendon with retraction. Hemorrhage and edema *(white arrow)* instead of the signal-void tendon is noted within the intertubercular groove.

Synovial Cystic Ganglions

Another entity that is ideally suited for MR imaging is the periarticular synovial cyst. Usually connected with the glenohumeral joint via a narrow neck, these cysts can dissect superiorly, posteriorly, and medially over the scapula near the base of the scapular spine (Fig. 3-52). As fluid preferentially flows into the cyst, the cyst may reach a substantial size, and patients may present clinically with pain, atrophy, and weakness about the shoulder girdle caused by pressure effects on the adjacent suprascapular nerve. Because this nerve has both sensory and motor components supplying the supraspinatus and infraspinatus muscles, selective symptoms related to that particular muscle group will be present, depending on the precise location of the cyst.[14] MRI can clearly demonstrate the size and exact location of the cyst, thereby facilitating surgical extirpation.[14,60]

ELBOW

The elbow is a hinged joint that provides primarily flexion and extension but also pronation and supination of the forearm with no significant lateral or medial motion. This motion is afforded by the anatomic configuration of the radiohumeral, ulnohumeral, and proximal radioulnar joints and by the redundant anterior and posterior capsular reflections with the more taut radial and ulnar collateral ligaments (lateral and medial collateral ligaments, respectively). The two major intracapsular but extrasynovial anterior and posterior fat pads are helpful indicators of hemarthrosis or synovitis with secondary joint effusions.

The elbow has traditionally been imaged by a number of modalities, including plain radiography, arthrography, nuclear scintigraphy, and CT; however, MRI has been gaining increasing popularity and, as elsewhere in the body, often has replaced the more conventional diagnostic tests because of its more comprehensive look at the surrounding paraarticular soft tissues, including the muscles, ligaments, and tendons.[54]

Magnetic Resonance Imaging of the Elbow

Specific imaging techniques will be discussed in each of the following sections, beginning with our MR protocol. We currently obtain spin-echo sequences (proton-density or intermediate-weighted as well as T_2-weighted images) in the axial, coronal, and sagittal planes using a field of view of 12 to 14 cm, one excitation, and a 256 × 192 matrix, with slice thicknesses of 3 mm and an interslice gap of 1 mm. The patient is placed in the prone position, with the arm extended over the head and elbow centrally placed within the bore of the magnet. Using an extremity or flexible wraparound surface coil allows small field-of-view imaging, resulting in high-resolution images with a good signal-to-noise ratio and uniformity of signal across the anatomic region. The prone position may be physically demanding for the patient, resulting in motion artifact, therefore placing the arm in the neutral position comfortably by the patient's side while scanning is optimal. If the magnet bore can accommodate the patient with the surface coil in this position, then lateral off-centering is necessary. The addition of STIR imaging in the coronal or axial planes has helped in delineating the presence and location of areas involved with inflammation or edema associated with ligamentous or tendinous tears. When these additional sequences are performed, a 256 × 128 matrix is sufficient (thereby reducing scanning time) because of the inherent exquisite sensitivity of STIR imaging.

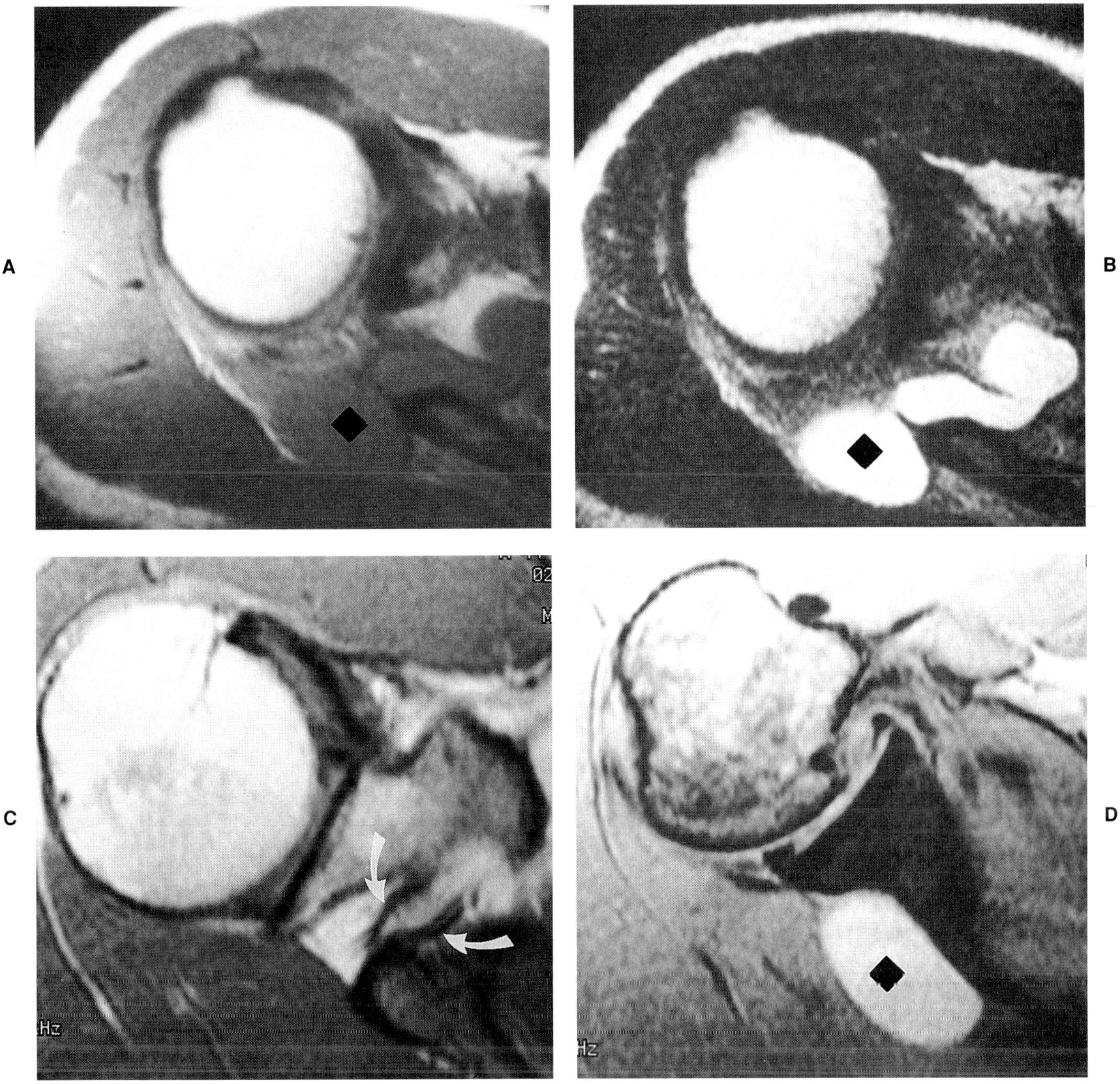

FIGURE 3-52 Synovial cystic ganglion *(black diamond)* dissecting through the scapular notch into the supraspinatus fossa on T_1-weighted **(A)** and T_2-weighted **(B)** axial MR images. **C,** Pressure effects on the underlying suprascapular nerve and vessels *(curved white arrows)* may occur with larger cysts. **D,** Isolated ganglion *(black diamond)* in the infraspinatus fossa is noted on this gradient-echo axial image in another patient.

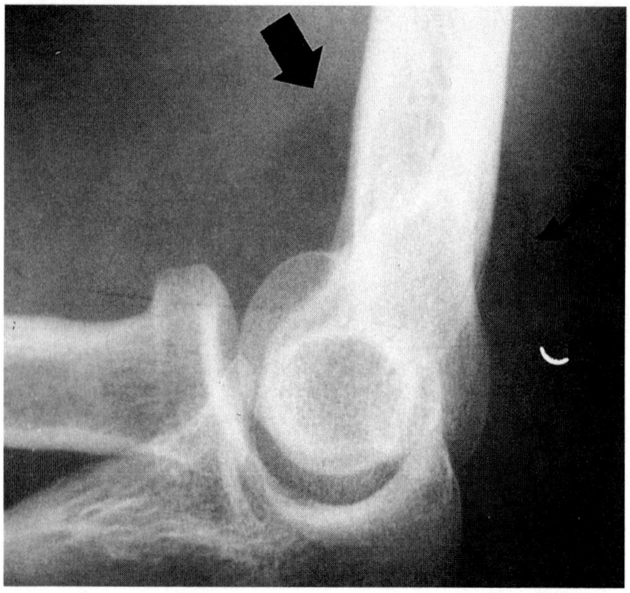

FIGURE 3-53 Lateral radiograph of the elbow demonstrates a "sail" sign from the displaced anterior fat pad *(thick black arrow)* and a posterior fat pad *(curved arrow)* displaced by fluid in the joint space.

Synovitis

Synovial fluid often is encountered after trauma, especially in the setting of acute intraarticular fractures. Such effusions are easily detected with plain radiographs obtained in the lateral projection with the elbow in 90° of flexion. Typically, the anterior and posterior fat pads are tucked within the coronoid and olecranon fossae of the distal humerus, respectively, and are barely visible on normal elbow films. In the presence of joint fluid, a positive fat-pad sign results when the anterior and posterior fat pads are elevated out of their respective fossae from the distended synovial capsule (Fig. 3-53). Resembling a ship's sail, the elevated anterior fat-pad sign has been referred to as the *sail sign.*[55] The exquisite soft-tissue contrast of MR allows direct visualization of both fat pads and their relationship to fluid within the joint (Fig. 3-54).

Fractures and Dislocations

The identity of the fracture or dislocation usually is confirmed by obtaining x-ray films in the anterior-posterior, lateral, or oblique projections, if necessary (Fig. 3-55). In the adolescent with skeletal immaturity, a thorough knowledge of the various ossification centers of the distal humerus is important to avoid mistaking the nonunited ossification centers for fractures. Comparison views of the contralateral elbow often resolve any question. Before these ossification centers fuse with the humeral shaft in the late teen years, traction forces applied to them from the flexor or extensor tendons may result in displacement away from the humeral shaft, with the onset of pain or joint immobility and locking.[55,56]

A

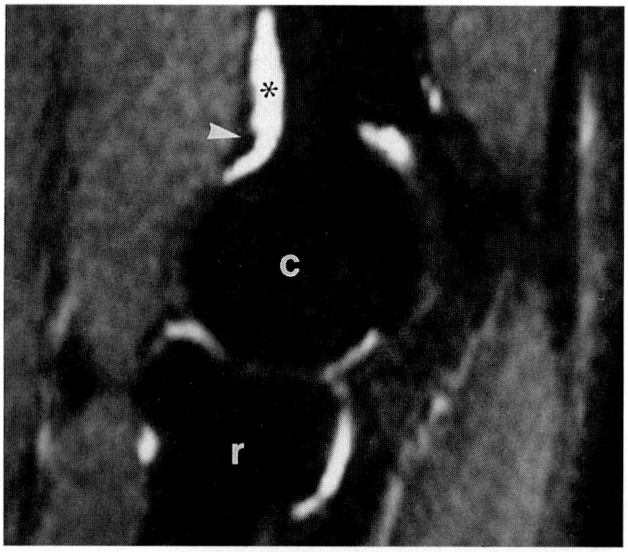

B

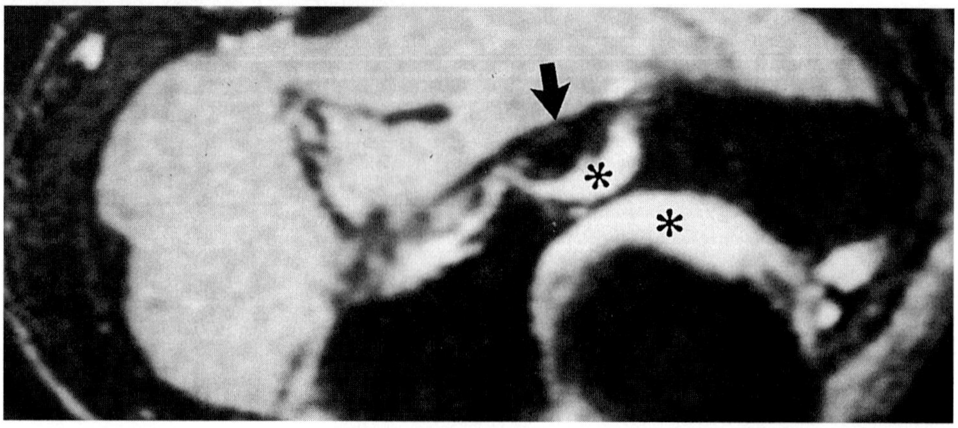

FIGURE 3-54 **A,** Sagittal and, **B,** axial STIR MR images of the elbow demonstrate synovial fluid *(asterisk)* in the anterior and posterior joint compartments. Signal from fat is suppressed on STIR sequences, and fluid becomes hyperintense. The extrasynovial anterior fat pad *(white arrowhead and black arrow)* is contrasted against the fluid within the coronoid fossa. There is no significant fat pad displacement because of the extended position of the elbow while being scanned. *c,* Capitellum of humerus; *r,* radius.

Occasionally, a follow-up radiograph in 1 week may be necessary to visualize a healing occult fracture as bone resorption occurs around the fracture. A radionuclide bone scan may be helpful in identifying a fracture (Fig. 3-56) when there are no radiographic abnormalities other than the presence of an effusion;[56] however, little additional information is obtained from the bone scan about any potential surrounding soft-tissue trauma that may be more devastating than the fracture itself.

CT scanning with the arm fully extended or held in flexion and using 2- to 3-mm cuts often delineates the extent and location of intraarticular fractures (Fig. 3-57) that may be obscured by overlapping bony shadows, considerably helping the orthopedist in presurgical planning. CT is unsurpassed in its ability to detect and localize small intraarticular loose bodies that might dictate whether an anterior or posterior arthroscopic or open surgical approach should be employed (Fig. 3-58).

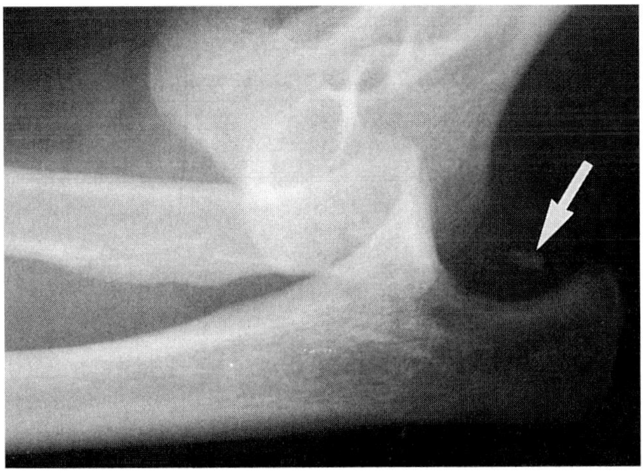

FIGURE 3-55 Lateral radiograph shows posterior dislocation of the proximal radius and ulna with small avulsion chip fracture *(arrow)*.

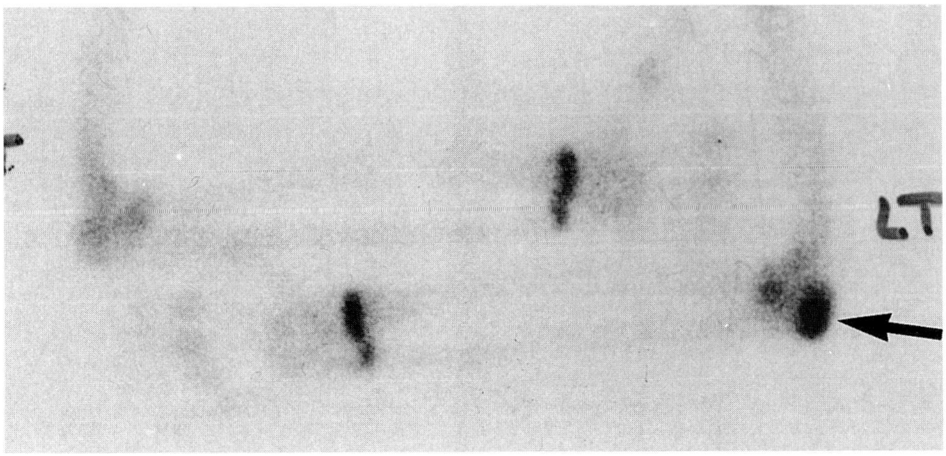

FIGURE 3-56 Radionuclide bone scan reveals intense uptake *(arrow)* within the olecranon of the left elbow. This is a nonspecific finding but is correlated clinically with a fracture. Other foci of activity reflect active epiphyseal growth plates in a young adolescent.

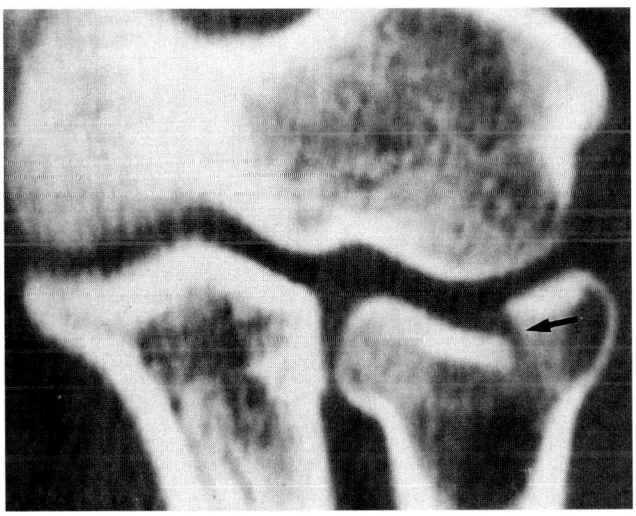

FIGURE 3-57 High-resolution CT scan demonstrating mildly depressed articular surface fracture of the radial head.

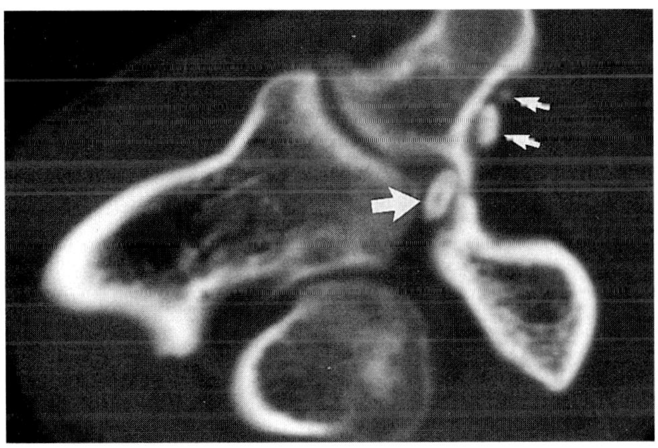

FIGURE 3-58 Multiple intraarticular loose bodies are noted within the anterior coronoid *(single arrow)* and posterior olecranon fossae *(double arrows)* on axial CT.

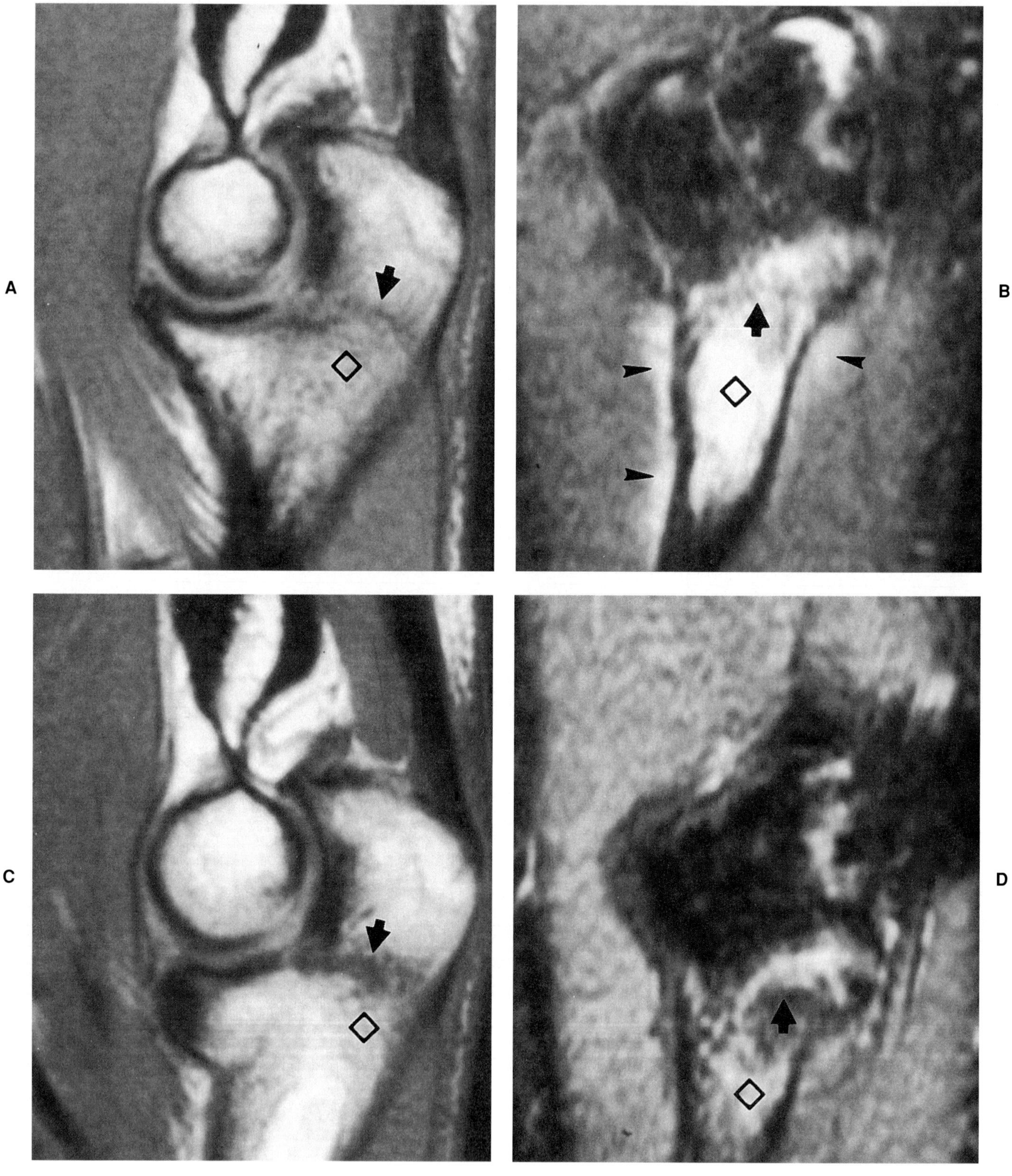

FIGURE 3-59 Sagittal proton-density (**A** and **C**) and coronal STIR (**B** and **D**) MR images of a healing olecranon fracture. With healing, the fracture line *(black arrow)* becomes more apparent with a reduction in the intraosseous *(black diamond)* and periosteal *(black arrowheads)* edema.

A

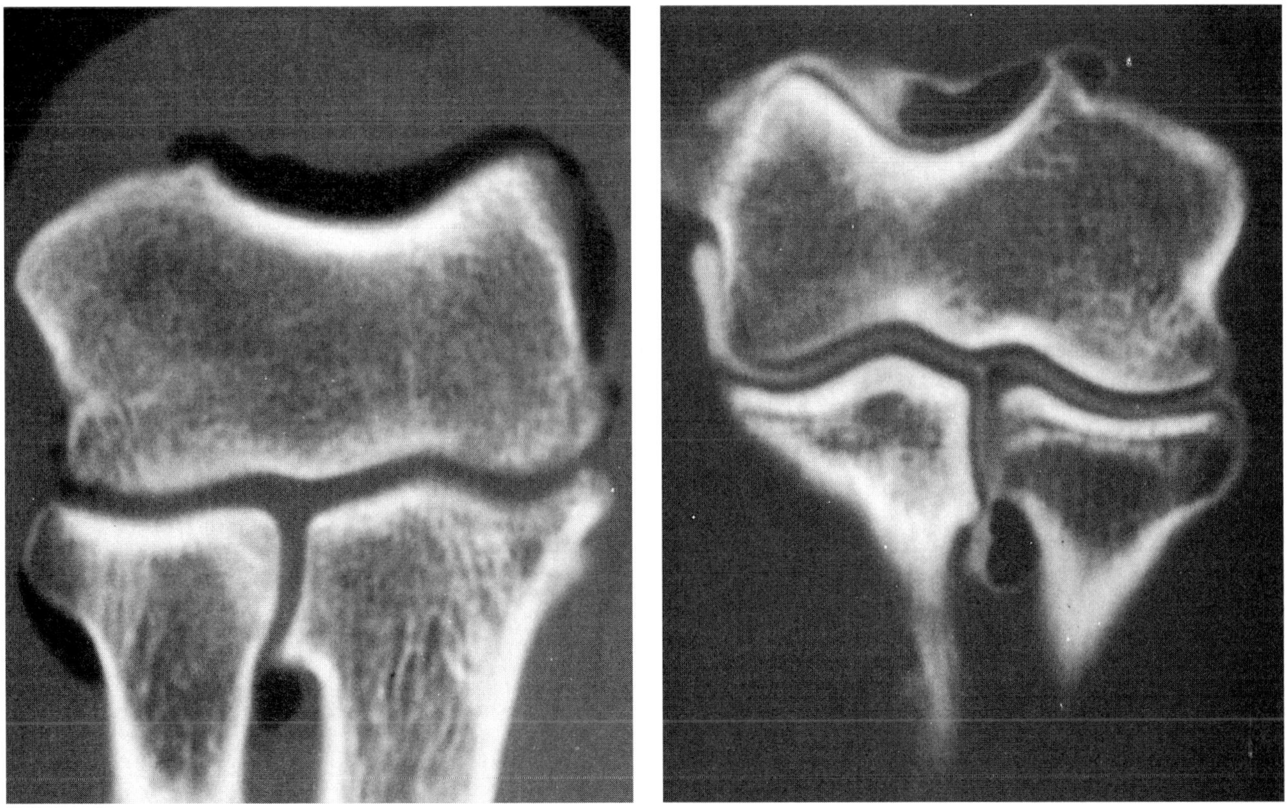

B

FIGURE 3-60 Coronal CT scans of the elbow after the intraarticular injection of air, **A,** and both air and contrast, **B,** portray the cortical and cartilaginous surfaces with clarity.

MRI has demonstrated sensitivity comparable to CT in displaying acute bone fractures and is unsurpassed in delineating any associated paraarticular soft-tissue injury.[17,46] Intraosseous hemorrhage or edema associated with fractures is easily identified by its low- to intermediate-signal intensity on T_1-weighted or proton-density images and by its high signal on T_2-weighted or STIR images, in contrast to the high signal from normal cancellous marrow on T_1-weighted images and extreme loss of signal on the STIR images. As the fracture continues to heal with sclerosis, the low-signal fracture line is noted on all pulse sequences, with a reduction in the surrounding edema on follow-up scans (Fig. 3-59).

Loose Bodies

The detection of intraarticular loose bodies always should begin with plain radiography; however, because of their small size, radiographic detection may prove difficult. Conventional tomography in the AP and lateral projections after the intraarticular injection of air or contrast material has helped considerably in identifying small osteochondral fragments.[56,76] However, CT-arthrography demonstrates the integrity of the cartilaginous and cortical surfaces of the elbow with unsurpassed quality (Figs. 3-60 and 3-61).

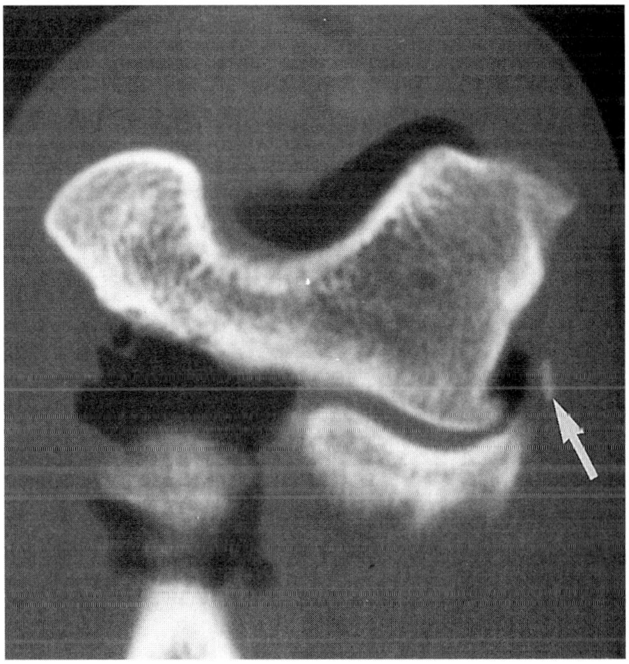

FIGURE 3-61 A small ossicle at the medial joint line on a conventional radiograph is noted to lie within the capsule or ulnar collateral ligament after the installation of air into the joint. The ossicle *(arrow)* is not surrounded by air, thus confirming its extraarticular location.

Pure cartilaginous fragments have a density on CT similar to fluid or synovium but may be distinguished if coated by contrast and completely surrounded by air (Fig. 3-62).[76] The physician should exercise caution to avoid mistaking any small projecting synovial strands or buds for noncalcified loose bodies. Although MRI also may demonstrate large intraarticular loose bodies (Fig. 3-63) noncontrast CT is preferable when searching for small intraarticular bony chips or calcified cartilaginous fragments because of CT's superb ability to detect subtle calcifications.

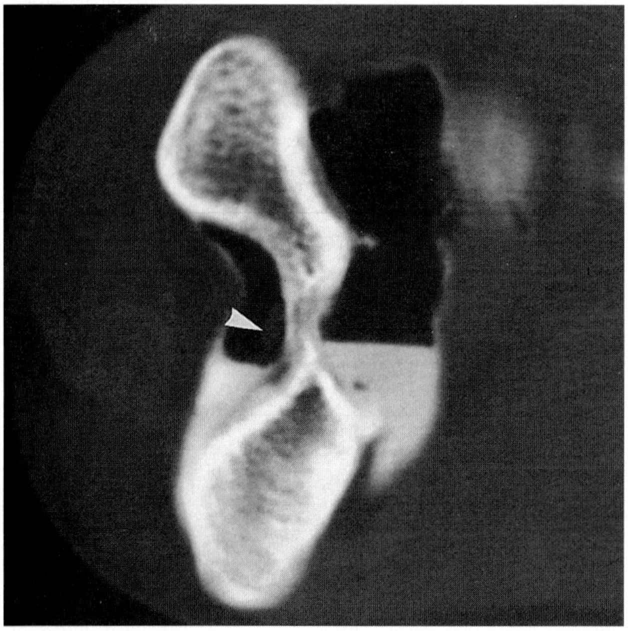

FIGURE 3-62 A small cartilaginous loose body *(arrowhead)* is totally surrounded by air and therefore lies within the posterior joint compartment on this CT arthrogram.

Hypertrophic Osseous Changes

In the highly competitive athlete, repetitive stresses are routinely applied to the elbow resulting in characteristic bony changes. These changes may manifest as traction spurs on the medial aspect of the coronoid tubercle at the insertion of the ulnar collateral ligament (UCL) resulting from valgus forces in throwing athletes.[56] Small spurs or osteophytes with fragmentation at the tip of the olecranon with possible intraarticular loose body formation as well as spurring at the proximal radioulnar articulation and tip of the coronoid process may be observed (Fig. 3-64). In the face of UCL insufficiency, laterally applied compressive forces may result in subcortical bone marrow signal changes on MRI. Although the aforementioned traction spurs and osteophytes may be observed with routine radiography, tomography, and CT, the cancellous bone marrow changes are best demonstrated with MRI[17] (Fig. 3-65). In the setting of an ulnar nerve neuropathy, CT is excellent in delineating stress-related spurs in the medial posterior ulnohumeral compartment, where the ulnar nerve courses posterior to the medial epicondyle (Fig. 3-66). The bone scan, on the other hand, is used to evaluate metabolic activity and to distinguish between an acute and a chronic inactive process[37,39] (Fig. 3-67).

Osteochondritis Dissecans

Areas of devitalized bone in the capitellum may occur in the idiopathic form or may result from the excessive cumulative compressive forces applied to this area from the radial head. Radiographic evaluation may demonstrate findings ranging from vague lucencies to gross morphologic changes in advanced cases, with irregular cortical margins and bony fragmentation with displaced intraarticular loose bodies. The diagnostic work-up in

A

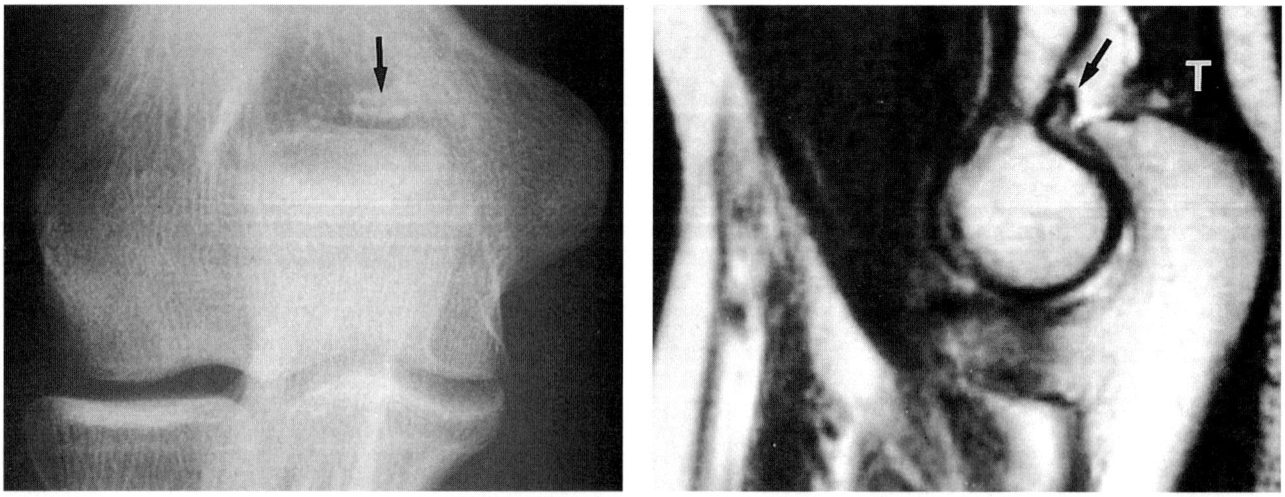

B

FIGURE 3-63 An ossific intraarticular loose body within the olecranon fossa *(arrow)* is better delineated on the radiograph **(A)** than on the sagittal MR image **(B).** Note the signal-void of the loose body on MR resulting from cortical bone. *T,* triceps tendon.

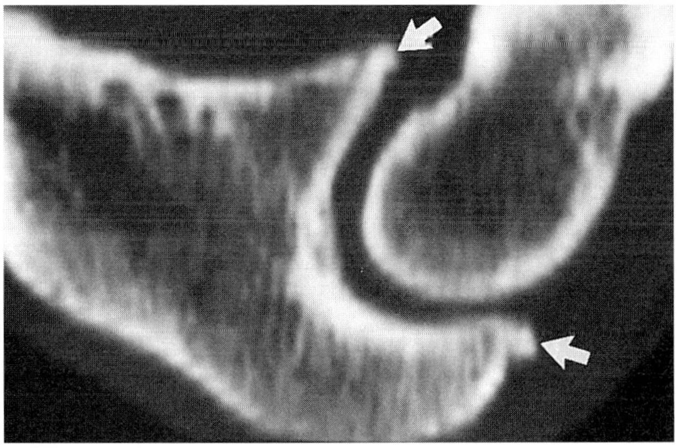

FIGURE 3-64 Sagittal reformatted CT image demonstrates small spurs at the tips of the coronoid and olecranon processes.

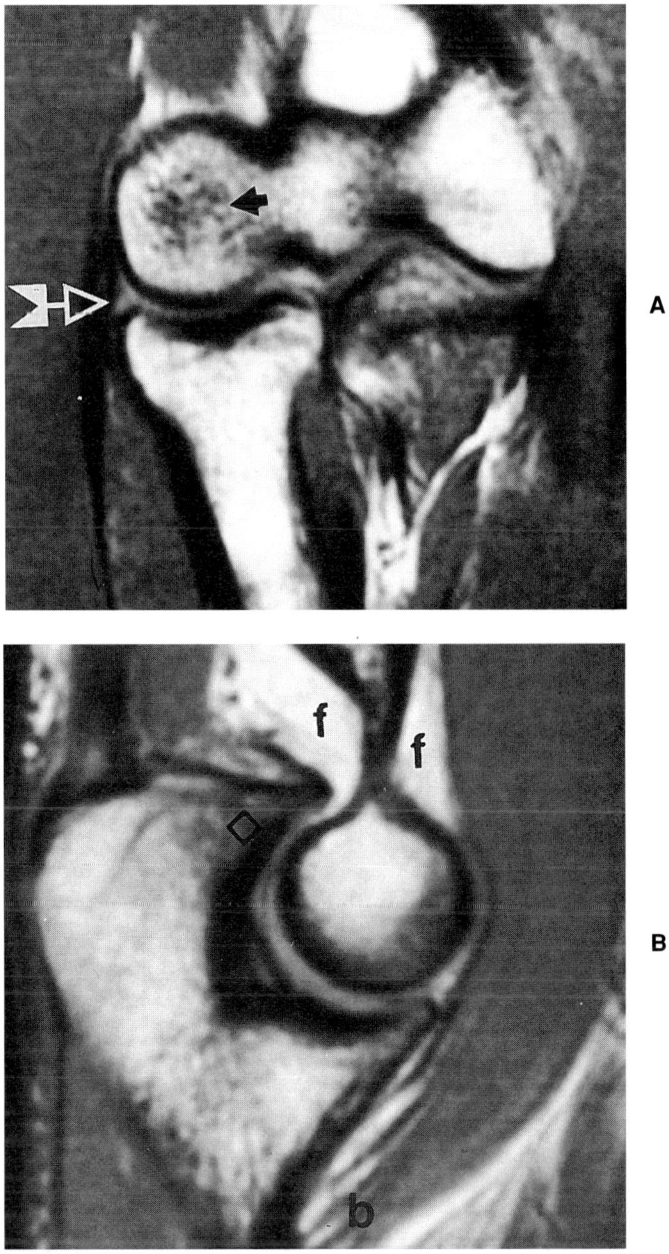

FIGURE 3-65 Decreased marrow signal is noted within the capitellum (*black arrow in* **A**) and olecranon tip (*black diamond in* **B**) and is caused by reactive changes within the bone marrow resulting from repetitive stress in two different baseball players. The changes in **A** probably reflect abnormally transmitted forces during valgus stress in conjunction with ulnar collateral ligament insufficiency. Olecranon marrow changes are most likely due to chronic abutment with the posterior humerus. Note the clear anterior and posterior fat pads (*f*) in **B.** *Flagged arrow,* intact radial collateral ligament; *b,* distal brachialis tendon inserting onto the proximal ulna.

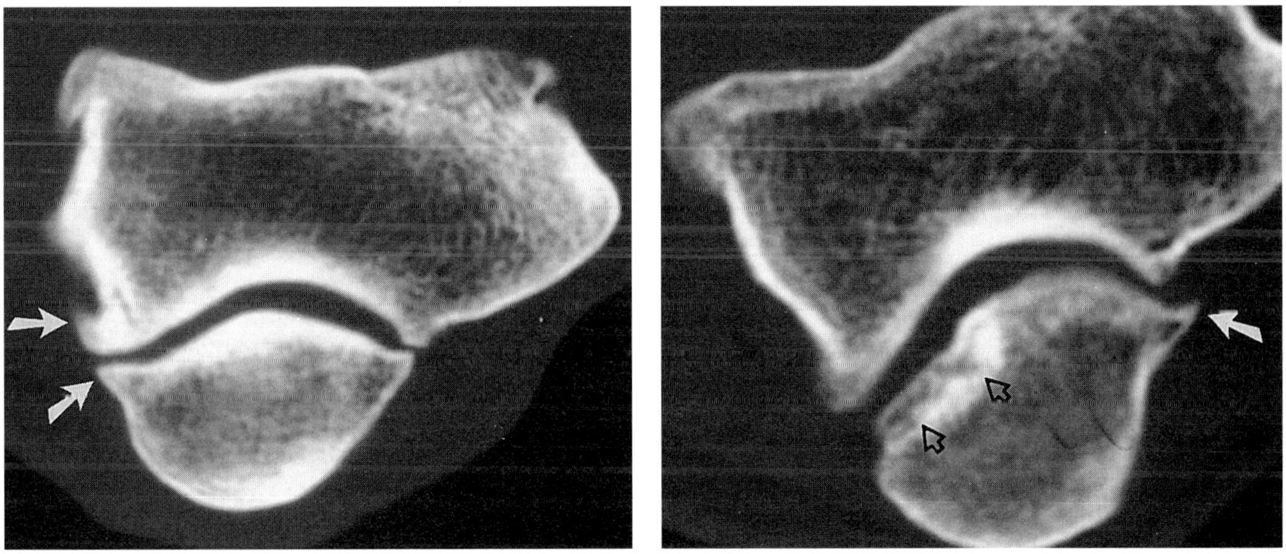

FIGURE 3-66 Axial CT scans through the posterior ulnohumeral compartments demonstrate spurs *(white arrows)* and posttraumatic and degenerative sclerosis with subcortical irregularity *(open black arrows).*

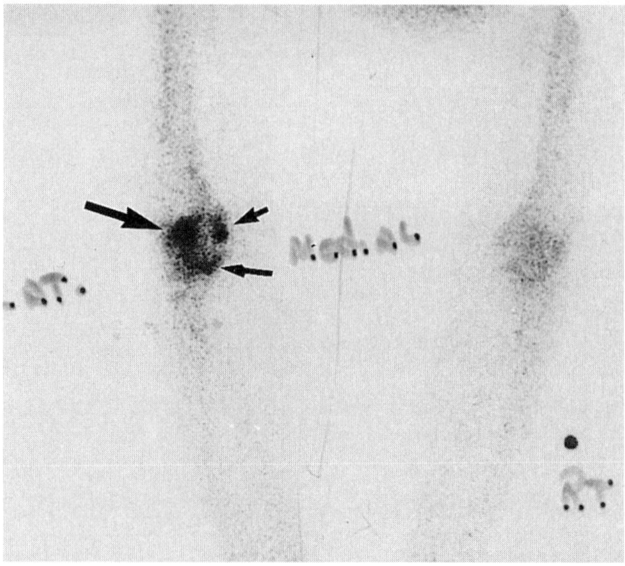

FIGURE 3-67 Radionuclide bone scan of both elbows in a professional baseball pitcher. Note the active uptake within the posterior olecranon *(largest arrow)* and at the insertion sites of the ulnar collateral ligament *(small and medium-size arrows)* along the medial aspect.

evaluating for loose bodies already has been discussed; however, early detection may be established with MRI by portraying decreased bone marrow signal within the capitellum before any cortical or articular cartilage disruption ensues (Fig. 3-68). Proper conservative therapy at such an early stage may avert the development of osteochondritis dissecans and its later complications.

In MRI of the elbow, a small field of view is necessary to obtain high-resolution images to visualize the hyaline articular surfaces. However, the signal intensities of both synovial fluid and hyaline cartilage are similar on gradient-echo images, and therefore non-gradient-echo sequences (T_1- or T_2-weighted) are obtained in a variety of planes when evaluating the integrity of the overlying cartilage. After the integrity of the overlying cortex and articular cartilage is interrupted, intraosseous high signal from synovial fluid intravasation or loose fibrovascular granulation tissue formation may be seen at the lesion's base, indicative of fragment instability (Fig. 3-69). Another potential problem in MR interpretation of the elbow is in mistaking the normally flattened and cartilage-void area of the posterior capitellum on sagittal images as being pathologic (Fig. 3-70).

Tendon Tears

MRI is clearly the preferred imaging modality and is unsurpassed when evaluating tendon injuries.[3,46] It can characterize the condition and degree of retraction of the tendon stump similar to rotator cuff imaging, thereby altering the surgical approach or management. The normal signal-void of dense collagen within the tendon is either poorly defined with intratendinous areas of increased signal in the case of partial tears or discontinuous in instances of complete ruptures with intervening hemorrhage and edema between the torn tendon and its bony insertion (Fig. 3-71).

One common tendinous injury of the elbow occurs when the distal biceps tendon avulses from its insertion onto the radial tuberosity either with or without retraction of the tendon stump. In the presence of complete or near-complete rupture, posttraumatic changes consisting of hematoma and developing granulating scar tissue may be palpable at surgery via an anterior surgical approach; however, on direct visual examination through a posterior approach, the true nature of the tear may become more obvious (Fig. 3-72). The distal bicipital aponeurosis or lacertus fibrosus is easily evaluated with axial MR scanning because of the normal contrast of adjacent fat and the signal-void curvilinear aponeurosis as it courses over the brachial artery and blends with the fascial covering of the pronator teres muscle (Fig. 3-73).

Epicondylitis

Medial or lateral epicondylar pain (golfer's elbow and tennis elbow, respectively) is frequent in athletes. The proposed mechanism in lateral tennis elbow is repetitive stress from vigorous extension and rotation of the forearm.[56] This results in partial or complete tear of the origin of the common extensor tendon. Similar actions on the medial epicondyle account for the tearing of the origin of the common flexor tendon medially.[17]

MRI is ideally suited in evaluating both of these conditions with spin-echo (T_2-weighting) and STIR imaging in the coronal and axial planes (Figs. 3-74 and 3-75). Localizing the edematous and inflammatory changes to the injured tendon on MR and distinguishing them from the adjacent collateral ligament or other soft tissues helps in assessing the patient with medial or lateral joint pain.

A

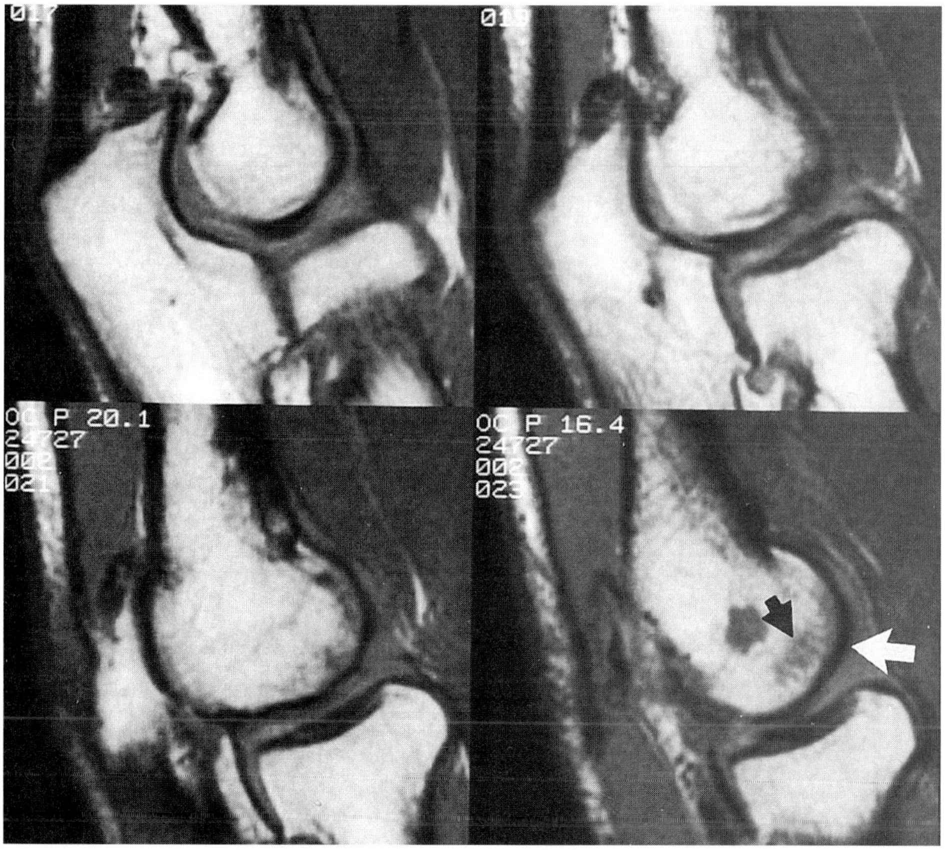

B

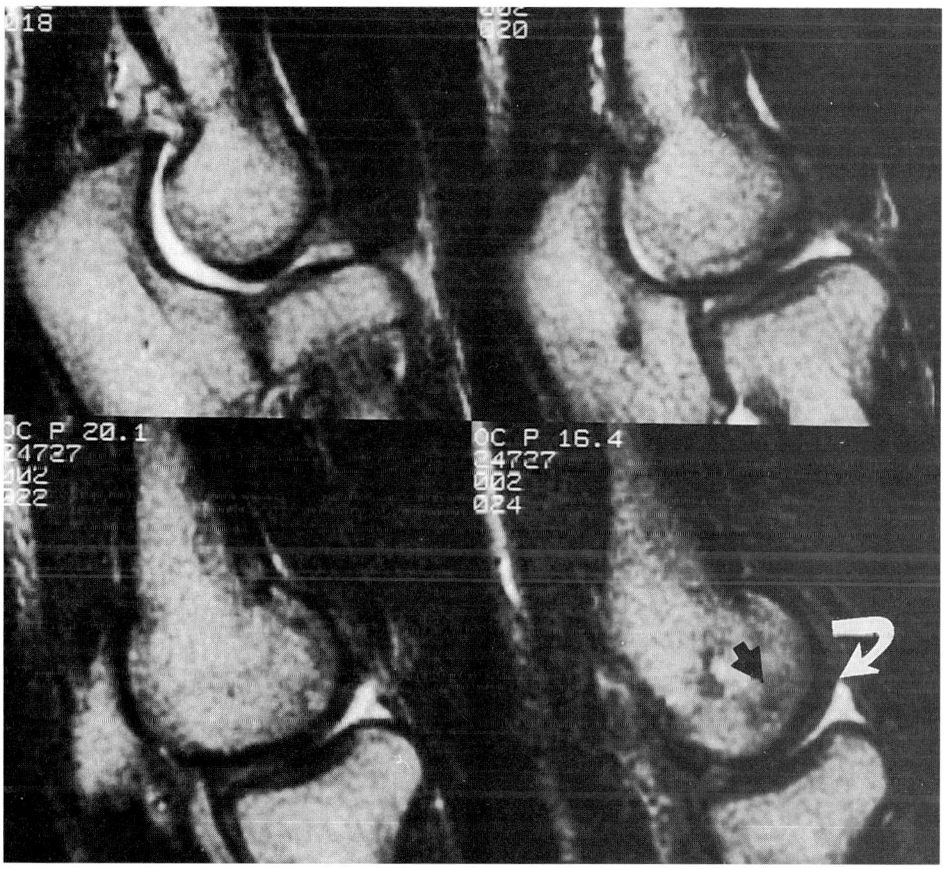

FIGURE 3-68 **A,** Sagittal proton-density and, **B,** T_2-weighted images show early marrow changes *(black arrow)* in the capitellum with an intact overlying cortex and articular hyaline cartilage *(straight and curved white arrows, respectively).*

A

B

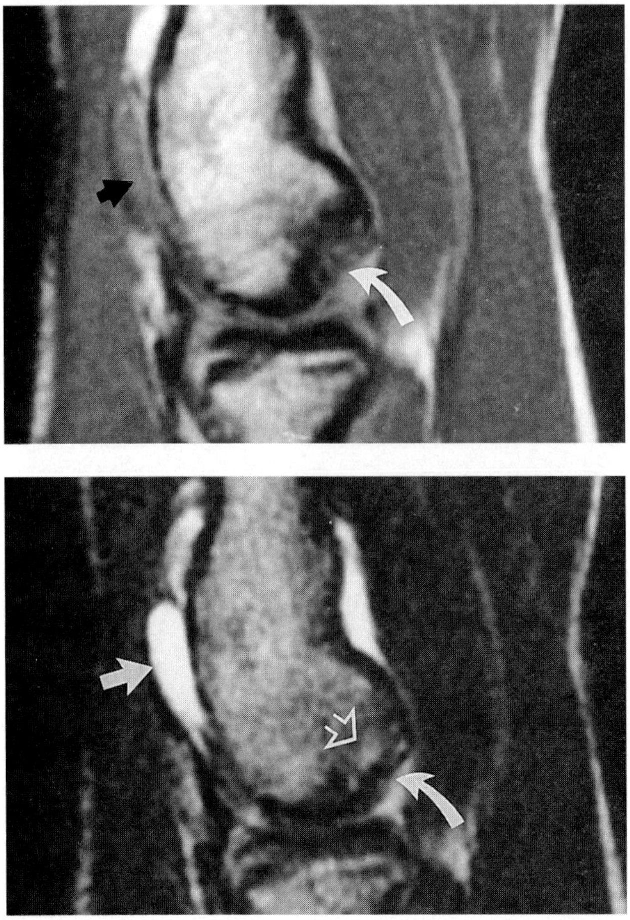

FIGURE 3-69 **A,** Sagittal proton-density and, **B,** T_2-weighted MR images demonstrating osteochondritis dissecans of the capitellum with disruption of the overlying cortex and cartilage *(curved white arrow)* with intravasation of joint fluid into the underlying bone resulting in hyperintensity *(open white arrow). Solid black and white arrows,* synovial fluid.

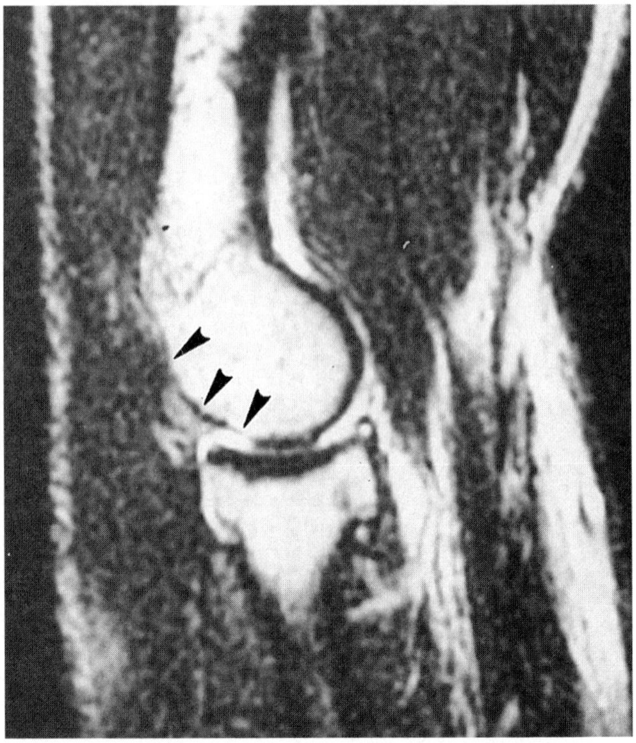

FIGURE 3-70 Sagittal T_2-weighted MR image shows the normal flattened posterior aspect of the capitellum that is not covered with a thick cartilaginous lining and may demonstrate normal cortical thinning.

A

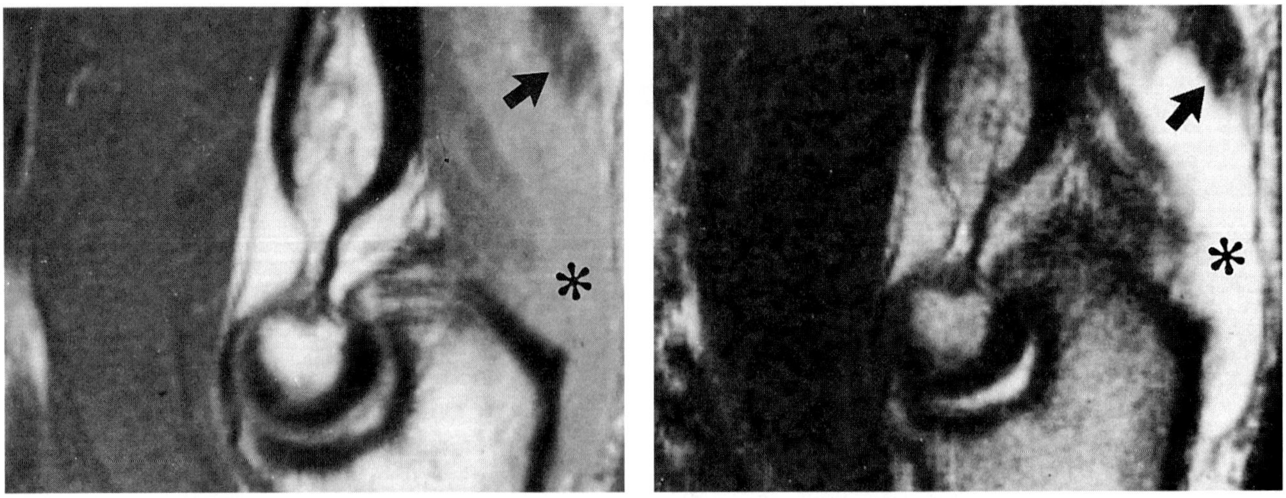

B

FIGURE 3-71 Acute rupture of the distal triceps tendon with retraction of the tendon stump *(black arrow)* and surrounding hemorrhage and edema *(asterisk)* extending to the olecranon is portrayed on both T_1-weighted **(A)** and T_2-weighted **(B)** sagittal images.

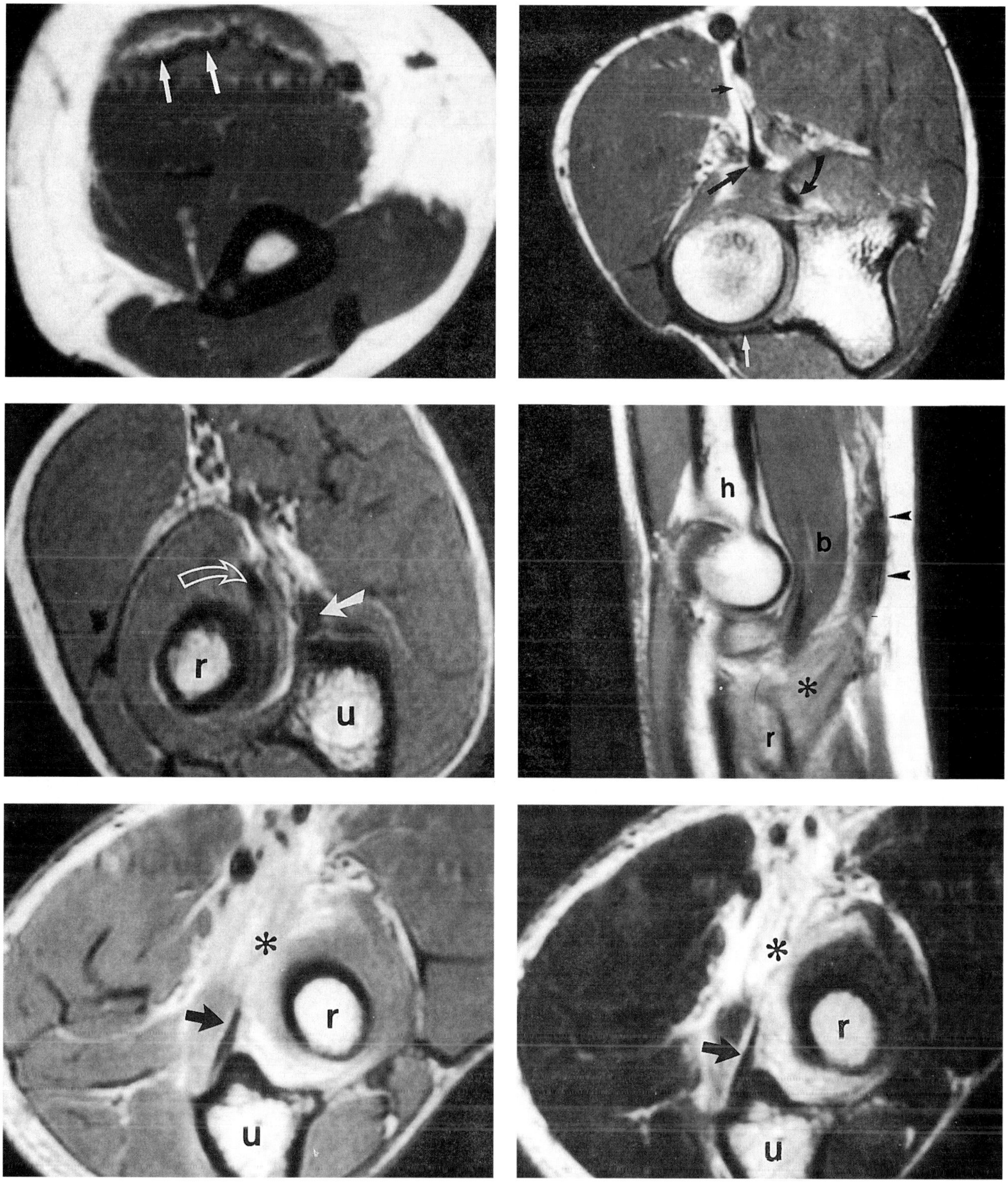

FIGURE 3-72 Normal and ruptured distal biceps tendon. **A,** Musculotendinous junction of biceps tendon with linear signal-void tendon *(white arrows)*. **B,** Biceps tendon *(large straight black arrow)*, coursing within the antecubital fossa with the adjacent brachialis tendon *(curved black arrow)*, is noted. *White arrow,* annular ligament of the radioulnar joint; *short black arrow,* lacertus fibrosus. **C,** Distal biceps *(open white arrow)* and brachialis *(solid white arrow)* tendons are noted at their insertions on the radius and proximal ulna, respectively. **D** to **F,** Distal biceps tendon ruptured from its insertion. There is absence of the normal tendon with hemorrhage and edema *(asterisk)* on T_1-weighted **(D),** proton-density **(E),** and T_2-weighted **(F)** images. *Black arrowheads,* frayed and retracted biceps tendon; *straight black arrow,* **E,** inserting brachialis tendon; *h,* humerus; *r,* radius; *u,* ulna.

FIGURE 3-73 Axial proton-density image demonstrates biceps tendon *(curved black arrow)* and its associated aponeurosis *(black arrowhead)* ventral to the brachial artery *(open black arrow)* at the antecubital fossa. *Small black arrow,* brachialis tendon.

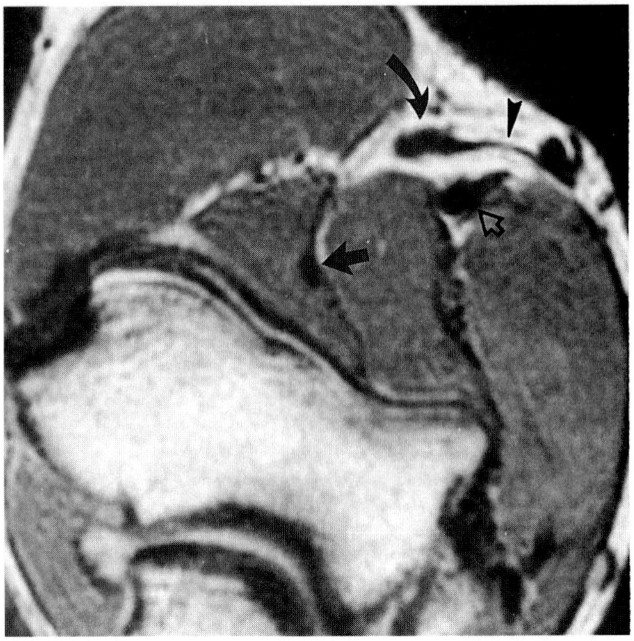

A

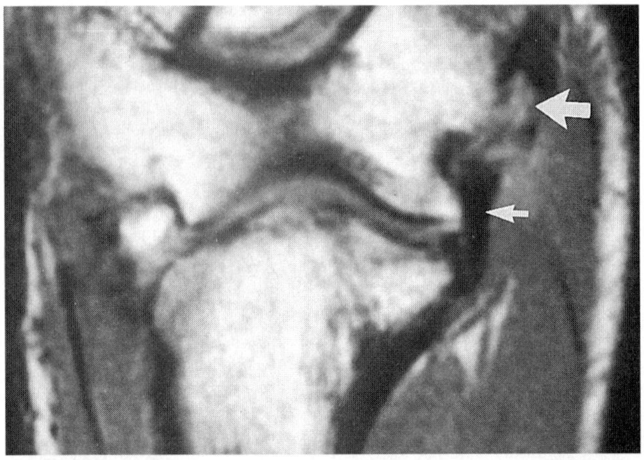

B

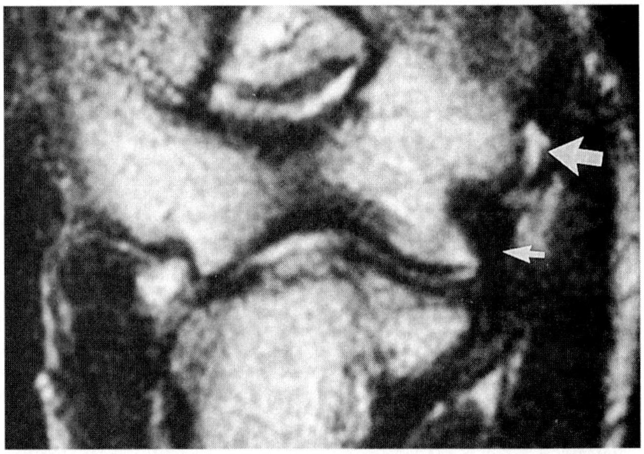

C

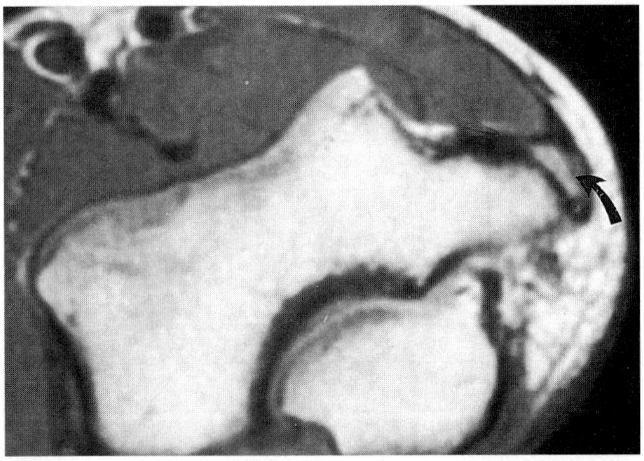

D

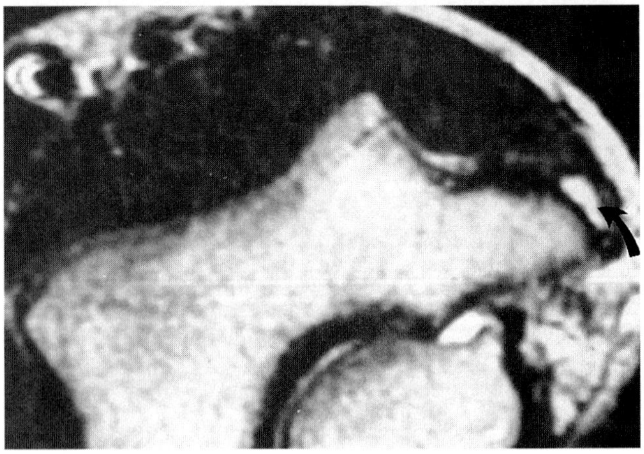

E

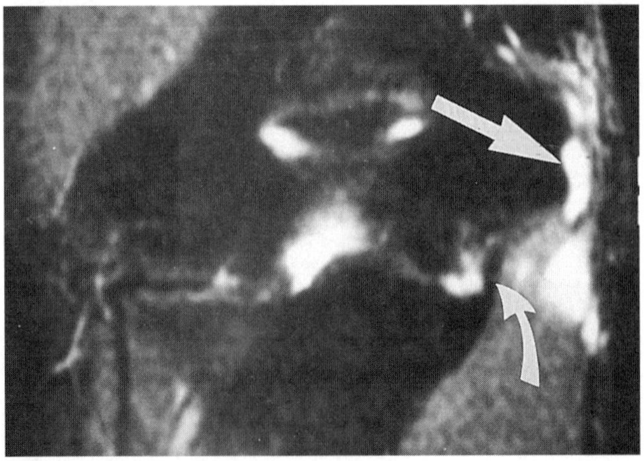

FIGURE 3-74 Partial tear of the common flexor tendon *(large white arrows)* appearing as focal fluid collections within the common tendon on both coronal (**A** and **B**) and axial (*curved black arrows on* **C** *and* **D**) intermediate and T_2-weighted images. Small white arrow, distal ulnar collateral ligament. **E,** STIR coronal image also demonstrates the focal tear *(straight white arrow)* with an intact ulnar collateral ligament *(curved white arrow).*

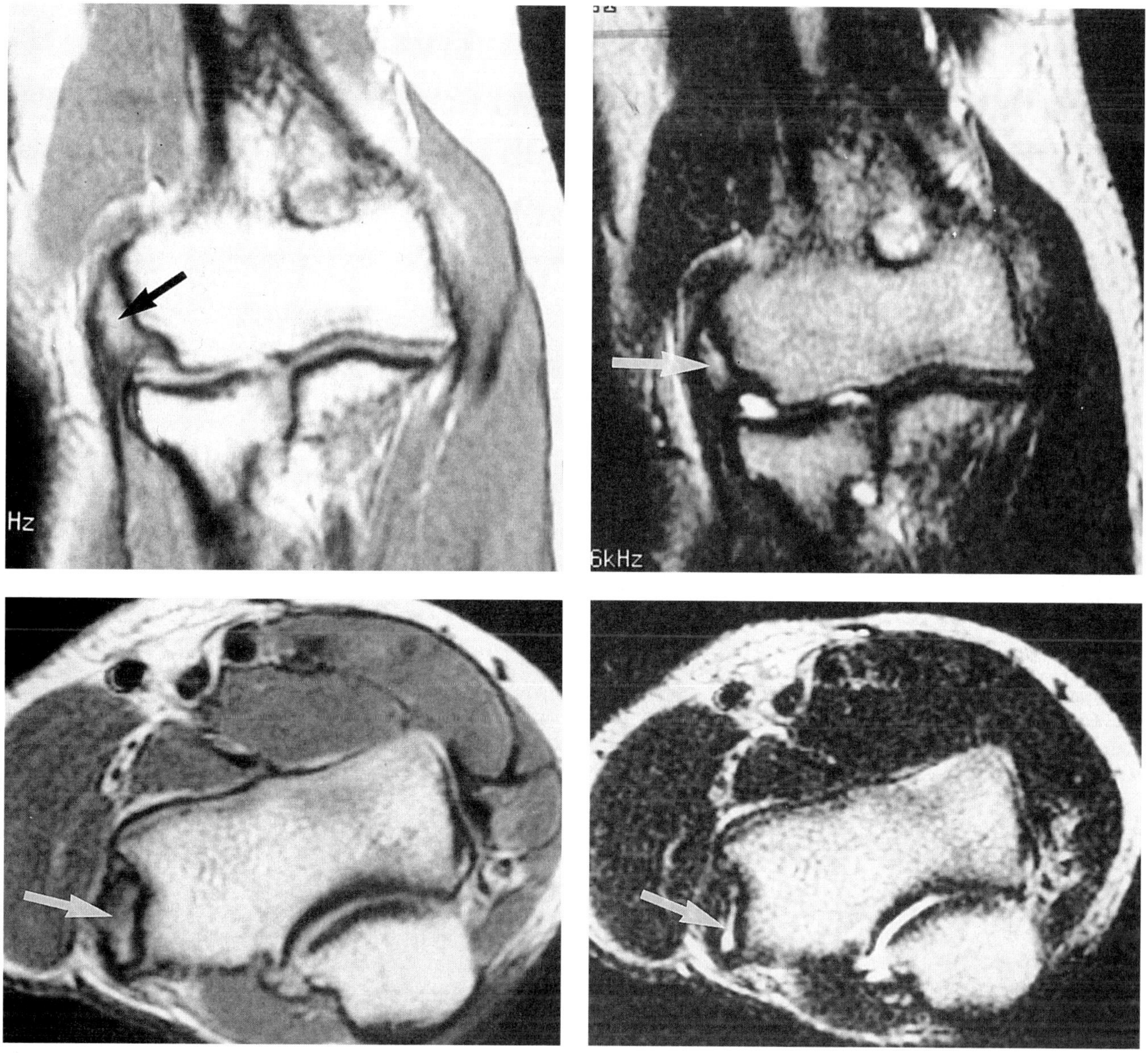

FIGURE 3-75 Coronal (**A** and **B**) and axial (**C** and **D**) proton-density and T_2-weighted images of a partial tear of the common extensor tendon.

Collateral Ligament Injuries

Ulnar Collateral Ligament

The ulnar collateral ligament (UCL) is considered the most important stabilizer of the elbow in resisting valgus stress. This structure is critical in maintaining elbow stability and is responsible for major disability in throwing athletes, primarily baseball players (pitchers).[50] Although contrast arthrography was used in the past as a test for imaging the ligament's and capsule's integrity, this technique has been largely abandoned and replaced with MRI.

The strong anterior band of the UCL is directly visualized on both the coronal and axial MR images as a discrete, thin, signal-void band stretching from the undersurface of the medial epicondyle to the medial aspect of the coronoid process (Fig. 3-76). The thinner and less functional posterior and transverse bands are not as well delineated. A small area of fibrofatty tissue is consistently located between the UCL and the trochlea in the normal setting.

Radiographic stress views of the elbow resulting in valgus angulation, coupled with instability on physical examination, is strong evidence for a tear of the UCL[23] (Fig. 3-77); however, only MRI allows direct visualization of the injured ligament. Increased signal within and surrounding the ligament or discontinuity of the ligament

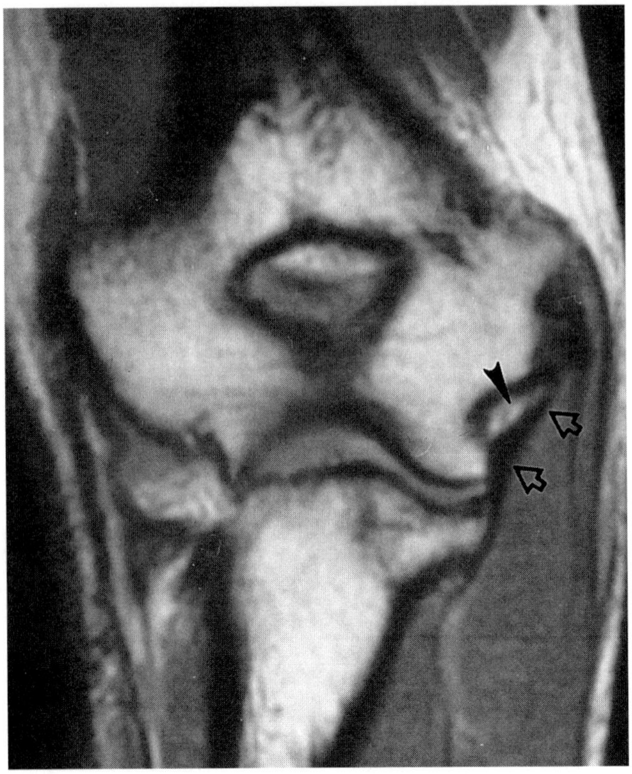

A

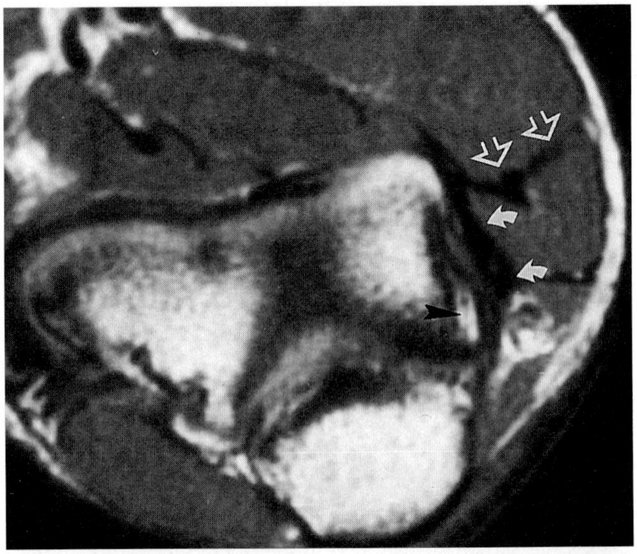

B

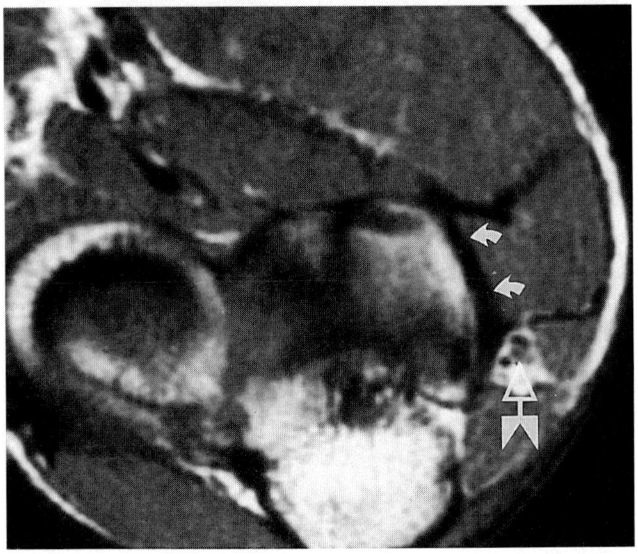

C

FIGURE 3-76 Normal ulnar collateral ligament on coronal **(A)** and axial (**B** and **C**) MR. **A,** Note the well-defined straight anterior band *(open black arrows)* as it bridges the medial aspect of the coronoid process with the undersurface of the medial epicondyle of the distal humerus. *Black arrowhead,* normal fibrofatty tissue between the ligament and humeral cortex. **B** and **C,** The distal insertion of the ulnar collateral ligament still appears as a discrete signal-void structure *(curved small white arrows)* inserting onto the medial side of the coronoid process. *Black arrowhead,* normal fibrofatty tissue; *open white arrows,* common flexor tendons; *flagged arrow,* ulnar artery and nerve.

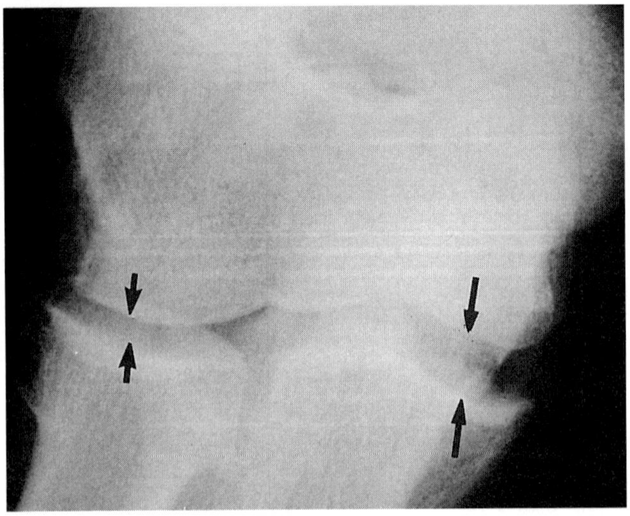

FIGURE 3-77 Elbow radiograph with manual valgus stress demonstrates asymmetric widening of the medial joint compartment suggesting ligamentous insufficiency of the ulnar collateral ligament.

with obliteration of the normal adjacent fat pad suggests an acute partial or complete tear with associated edema and hemorrhage[50] (Fig. 3-78). Over long periods of time, ligamentous stretching from overuse may result in chronic microtears during the course of the athlete's career, resulting in the development of loose granulation or scar tissue. The MR appearance of these chronic injuries may mimic a normal UCL at first glance, but on further inspection, a broader band of inhomogeneous signal with poorly defined margins usually is present in the absence of any adjacent edema (Fig. 3-79). This should be regarded as highly suggestive of a chronically torn and scarred ligament and should be correlated with the physical examination and accompanying radiographic stress views in cases of instability and medial elbow pain.

Radial Collateral Ligament

Tearing of the radial collateral ligament is less common but may present with similar MR findings (Fig. 3-80).

A B

C D

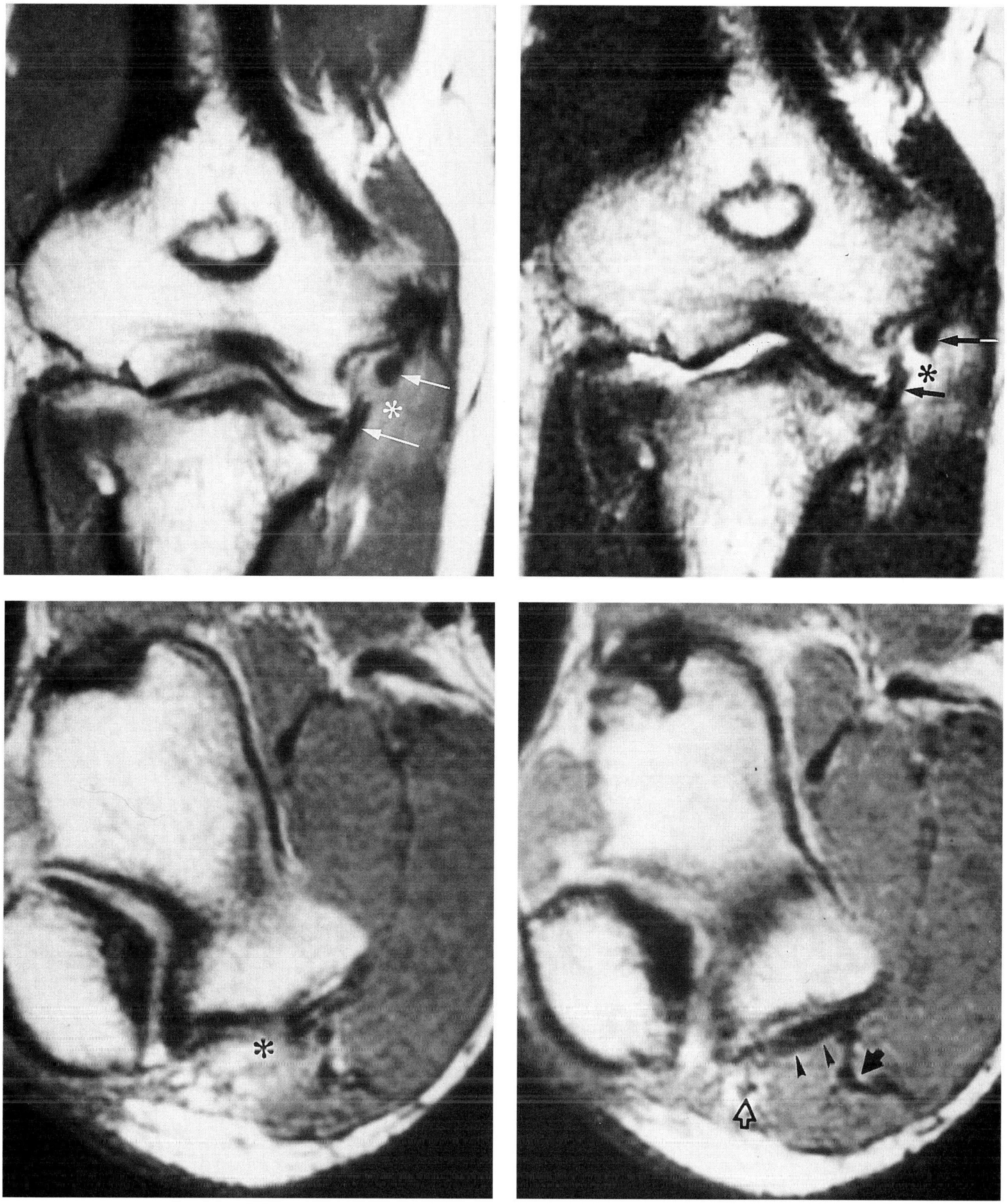

FIGURE 3-78 Acute rupture of the ulnar collateral ligament. Proton-density (**A, C,** and **D**) and T_2-weighted **(B)** MR images reveal a midligament rupture with intervening hemorrhage and edema *(asterisk)* between the proximal and distal ends *(white and black arrows)*. Note the absence of any normal ligament on image **C** with a normal distal segment *(black arrowheads)* on image **D. D,** *Open arrow*, ulnar artery and nerve; *black arrow,* flexor tendons.

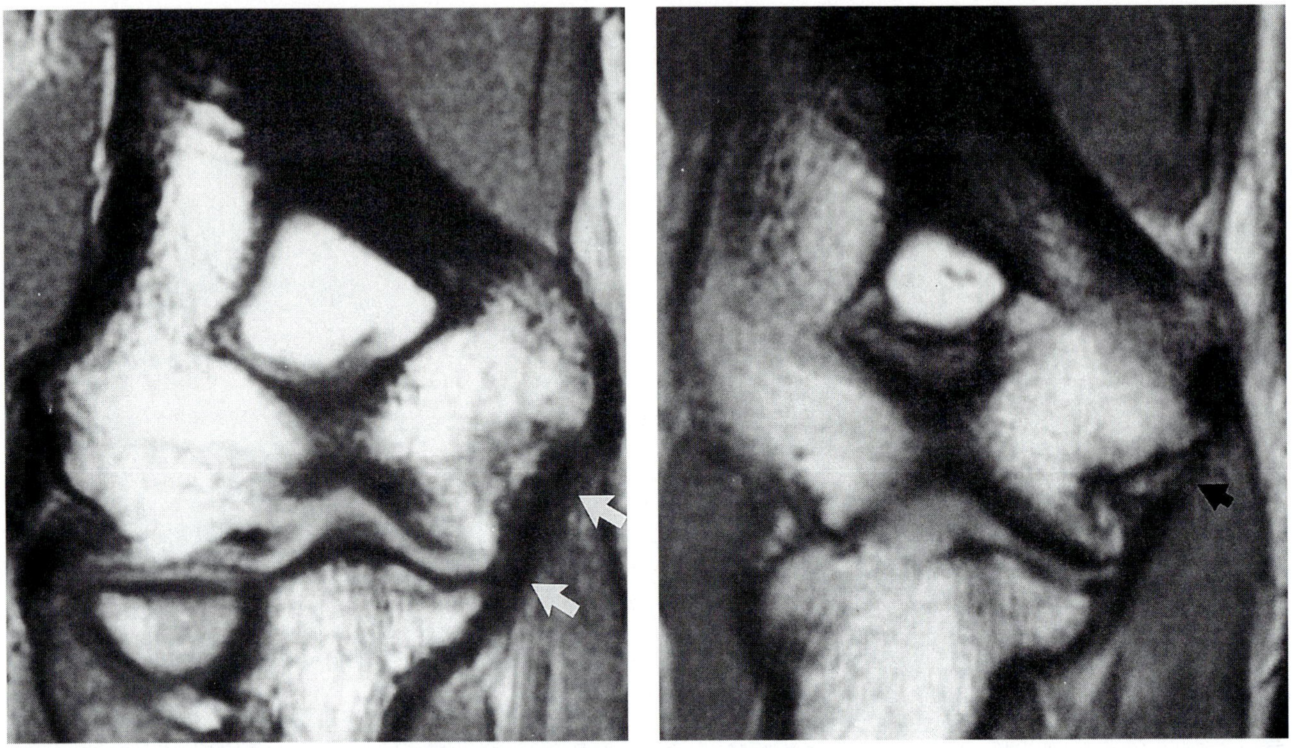

FIGURE 3-79 Surgically proven chronic ruptures of ulnar collateral ligaments. Chronic tearing with subsequent fibrosis results in a decreased signal, simulating normal ligaments. Closer inspection reveals hazy margins with a thickened and slightly heterogeneous structure with poor definition and obliteration of normal fibrofatty tissue lateral to the ligament.

There may be posterior-lateral rotational instability in the case of a torn collateral ligament, posterior capsule, or adjacent radial slip of the UCL that normally passes posterolateral to the radial head and inserts onto the proximal ulna (Fig. 3-81).

WRIST AND HAND

The precise anatomic and functional relationships between the various osseous and ligamentous structures of the wrist allow its complexity and wide range of motion. Therefore it is frequently injured during sports. A simple "sprain" must be differentiated from a more serious injury that might lead to functional impairment, deformity, and permanent disability. The various imaging techniques currently available are extremely helpful in making an early, accurate diagnosis, which is critical for a successful treatment and outcome.

Fractures and Dislocations

Radiography

After an acute traumatic episode, plain radiographs should be obtained after an appropriate clinical assessment and physical examination is performed. The radiographs usually are sufficient to determine a diagnosis. However, a fracture line often is not initially apparent and may require repeat radiographs 10 to 14 days later after sufficient bone resorption occurs at the fracture site or periosteal reaction becomes radiographically evident[34,56,65] (Fig. 3-82). The injured person may complain of localized pain over the traumatized area where soft-tissue swelling is present. This may manifest itself on the radiograph as obliteration or displacement of the normal fat planes. In the case of scaphoid fractures, there usually is displacement or loss of the normal navicular fat stripe situated between the radial collateral ligament and tendon sheaths of the abductor pollicis longus and extensor pollicis brevis muscles (Fig. 3-83). Such soft-tissue findings are not specific for scaphoid fractures or any other particular fracture, and a careful search should be made to exclude other neighboring pathology.[65]

Common hand injuries usually are diagnosed with routine radiography. Direct trauma to the metacarpals and phalanges may result in fractures that are readily noted on the radiographs (Fig. 3-84). Smaller avulsion fractures of the phalanges with contractual deformities suggest underlying tendon or ligament ruptures. A typical example is the flexion deformity of the distal interphalangeal (DIP) joint with avulsion of the dorsal lip of the base of the distal phalanx (mallet finger), which should be distinguished from avulsion of the terminal extensor tendon. This type of injury is commonly seen in

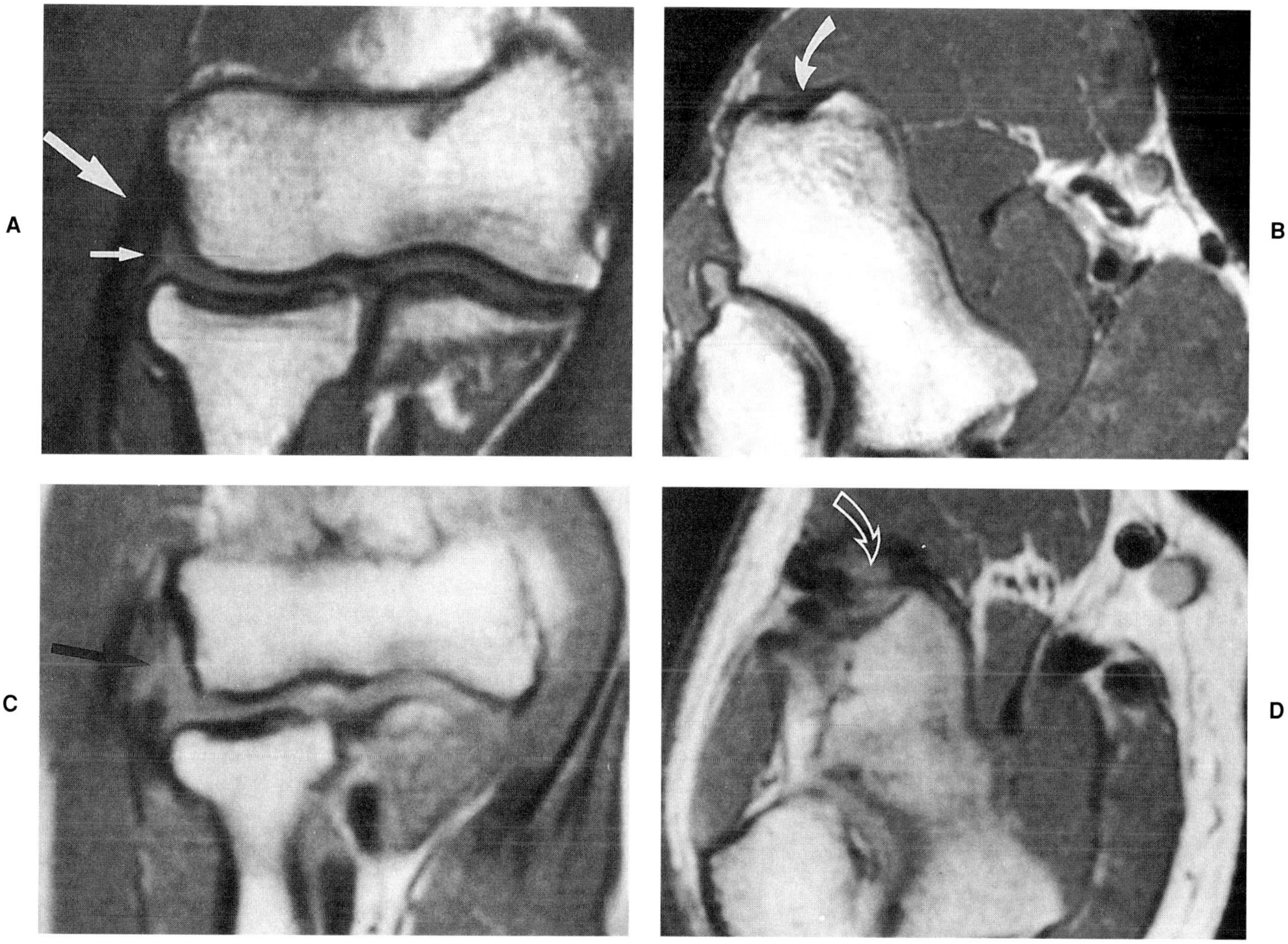

FIGURE 3-80 **A** and **B**, Normal radial collateral ligament *(small straight and curved white arrows)*. Note the thin discrete signal-void continuous linear structures arising from the lateral aspect of the capitellum and inserting onto the radial head. The thicker common extensor tendon *(large white arrow)* is immediately adjacent to the ligament. **C** and **D**, Subacute rupture of both the common extensor tendon and radial collateral ligament *(arrows)* with focal fluid filling in the discontinuous segment on coronal and axial intermediate-weighted images.

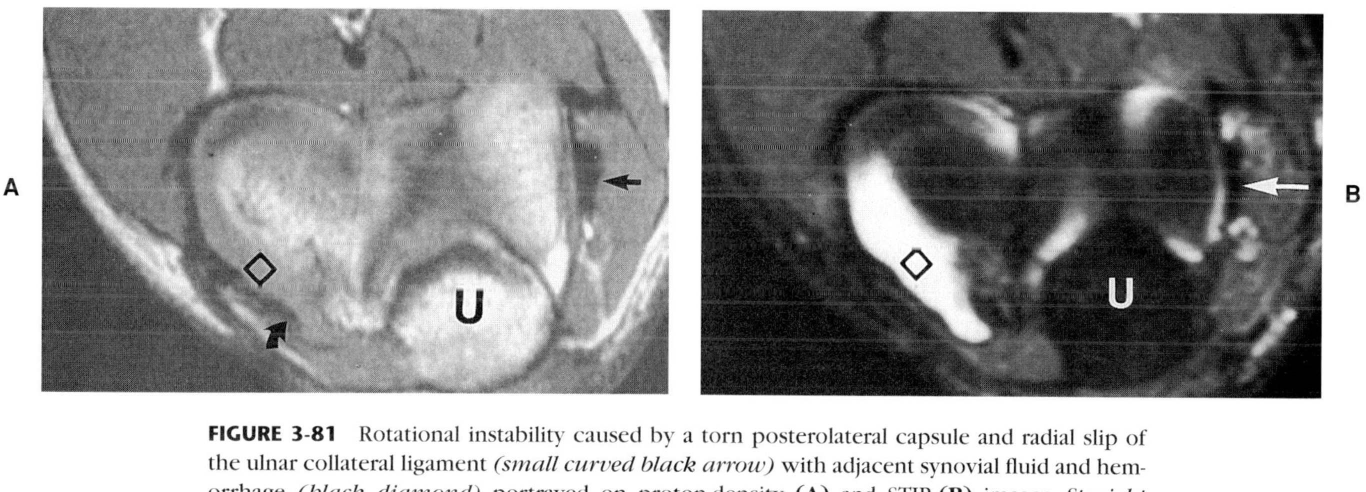

FIGURE 3-81 Rotational instability caused by a torn posterolateral capsule and radial slip of the ulnar collateral ligament *(small curved black arrow)* with adjacent synovial fluid and hemorrhage *(black diamond)* portrayed on proton-density **(A)** and STIR **(B)** images. *Straight black and white arrows,* distal ulnar collateral ligament insertion onto coronoid; *U,* ulna.

A

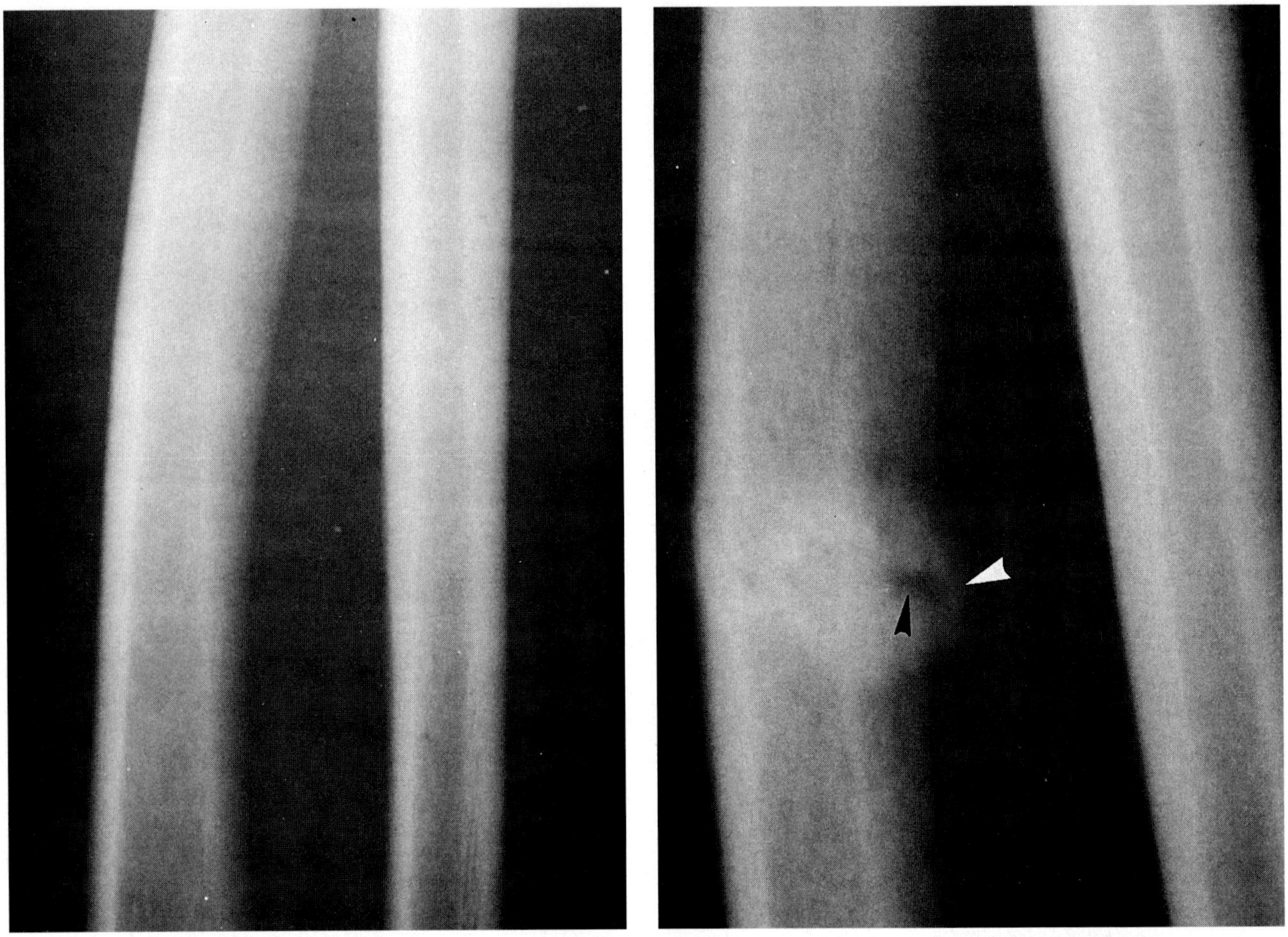

B

FIGURE 3-82 Professional athlete who had an acute injury to the distal forearm with localized tenderness. Initial radiograph **(A)** was normal. A follow-up radiograph **(B)** 14 days later showed bone resorption at the fracture site *(black arrowhead)* with developing periosteal callus formation *(white arrowhead).*

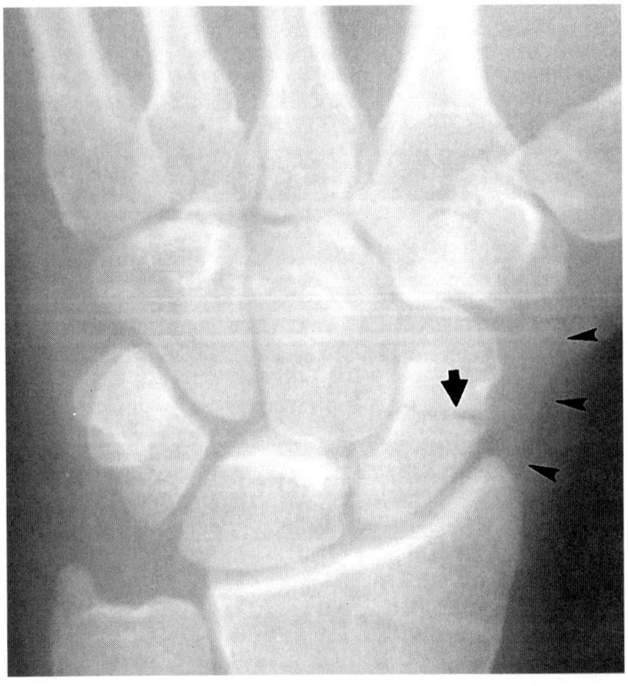

FIGURE 3-83 Marked bowing with indistinctness of the navicular fat stripe *(black arrowheads)* caused by hemorrhage from the adjacent midscaphoid fracture *(arrow).*

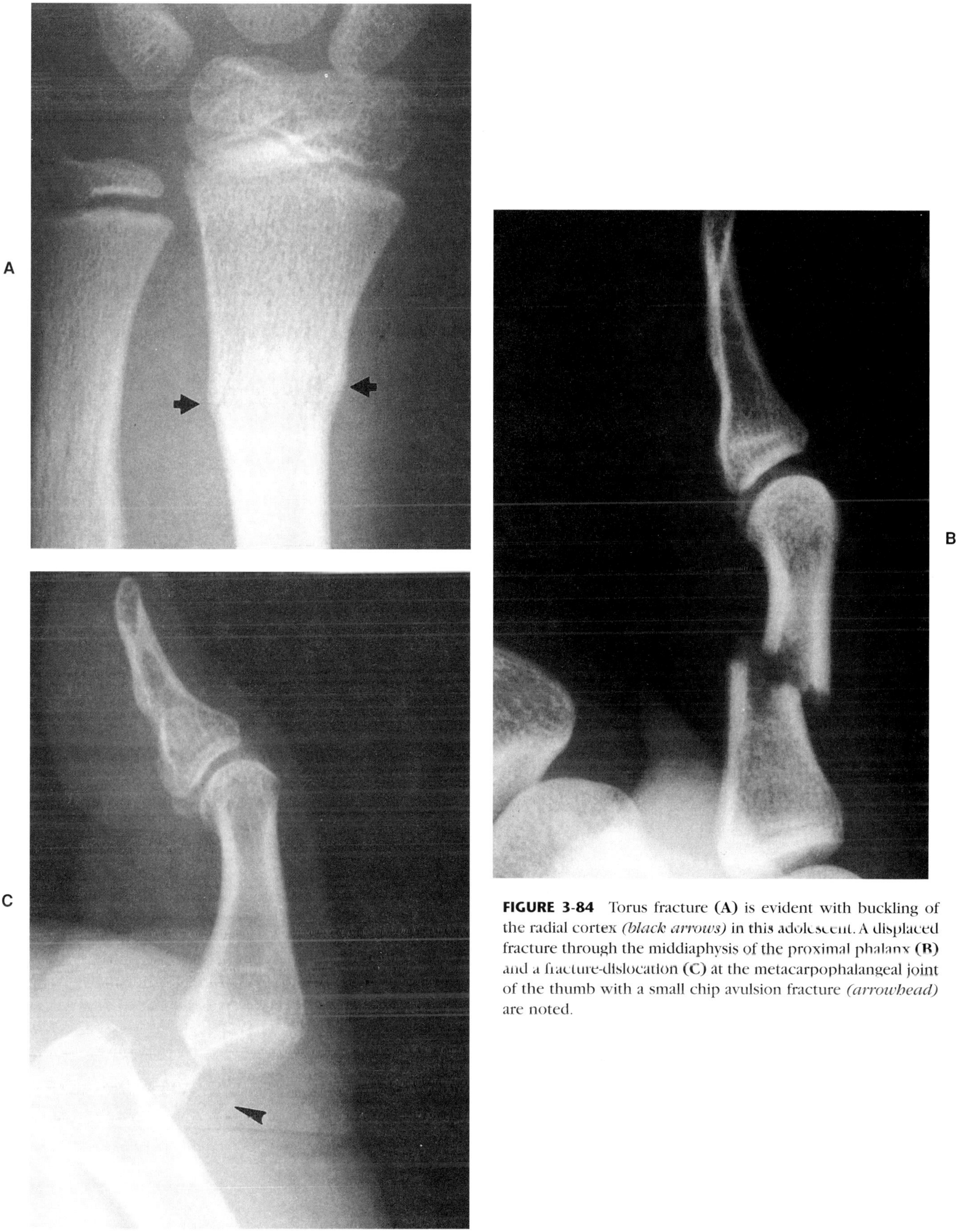

FIGURE 3-84 Torus fracture **(A)** is evident with buckling of the radial cortex *(black arrows)* in this adolescent. A displaced fracture through the middiaphysis of the proximal phalanx **(B)** and a fracture-dislocation **(C)** at the metacarpophalangeal joint of the thumb with a small chip avulsion fracture *(arrowhead)* are noted.

baseball, basketball, and football players. Volar fractures of the fingers may be seen with ruptures of the flexor profundus tendon, avulsing a small bony fragment off the base of the distal phalanx, with volar plate fractures off the base of the middle phalanx in hyperextension injuries (Fig. 3-85), or with ulnar collateral ligament avulsions from the proximal phalangeal base of the thumb[25,36] (Fig. 3-86).

Alignment deformities resulting from ligamentous injuries, such as the boutonnière deformity secondary to disruption of the central slip of the extensor tendon and interphalangeal joint dislocations, may be evident on plain radiographs. These deformities may be aggravated after the application of stress, as in the aforementioned "gamekeeper's thumb" caused by a ruptured ulnar collateral ligament.[36]

Routine radiography of the wrist should include at least PA, oblique, and lateral views. Additional supplemental views can be obtained with the hand in a fist and the wrist in ulnar deviation, thereby elongating the proximal carpal row and facilitating detection of subtle scaphoid fractures. Other special views, such as a carpal tunnel view, might help disclose occult fractures at the base of the hook of the hamate (a common injury in golfers and baseball players), or fractures in individuals in whom a direct blow to the hamate from the butt of a bat, club, or tennis racquet produced the fracture.[56,79] CT is useful in identifying these fractures about the wrist (Fig. 3-87).

Radionuclide Scintigraphy

Triple-phase bone scanning has been shown to be very sensitive in detecting acute fractures after the first 24 hours.[37-39,56,69] Immediately after the fracture there is a generalized increase in soft-tissue activity in the vascular phase secondary to hyperemia; this is followed by diffuse background activity on the blood pool images. The delayed static images obtained 2 to 4 hours later depict a "hot spot" at the fracture site, indicating the physiologically active bony metabolism or turnover. The bone scan's poor spatial resolution is offset by the fact that the scintigraphic findings may precede positive radiographic findings by days to weeks, thus allowing prompt immobilization and treatment.

Computed Tomography

Because intraarticular fractures may predispose the joint to premature degenerative arthritis as a late sequela to healing, knowing the exact nature and extent of the fracture is critical for successful management of the injury. Therefore high-resolution thin-slice CT scanning using 1.5- to 2-mm cuts through the area of concern is most helpful[5,34,58] (Fig. 3-88).

Direct scanning performed in orthogonal planes or multiplanar reconstructions often delineates the fracture from the articular surface (Fig. 3-89). Intraarticular loose bodies restricting full motion of the joint as well as small chip avulsion fractures from underlying ligamentous injuries are easily demonstrated on CT.

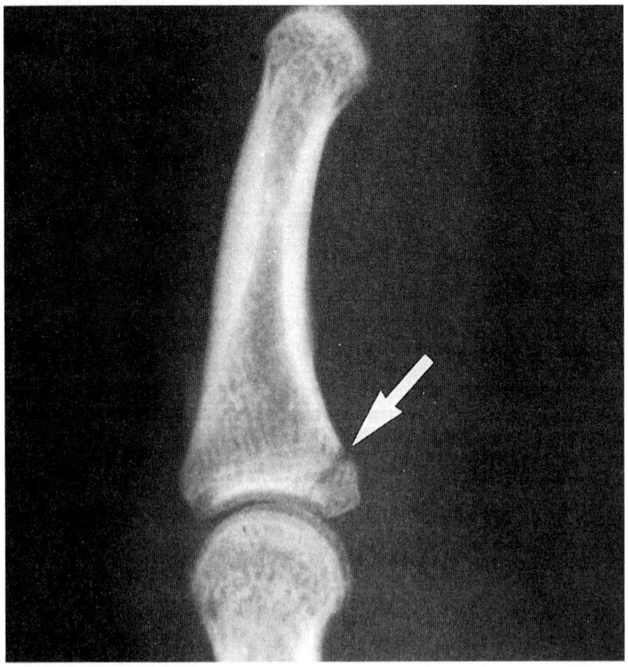

FIGURE 3-85 Lateral radiograph demonstrates a nondisplaced fracture *(arrow)* of the volar plate off the base of the middle phalanx resulting from a hyperextension injury.

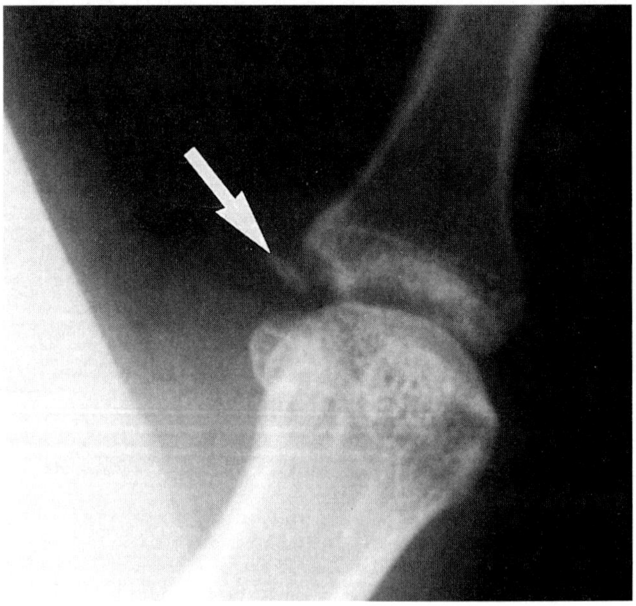

FIGURE 3-86 Gamekeeper's thumb fracture *(arrow)* with avulsion of the base of the proximal phalanx of the thumb, resulting from rupture of the ulnar collateral ligament. This is a common injury in skiers who fall with their hands holding onto their ski poles, resulting in forced abduction.

A 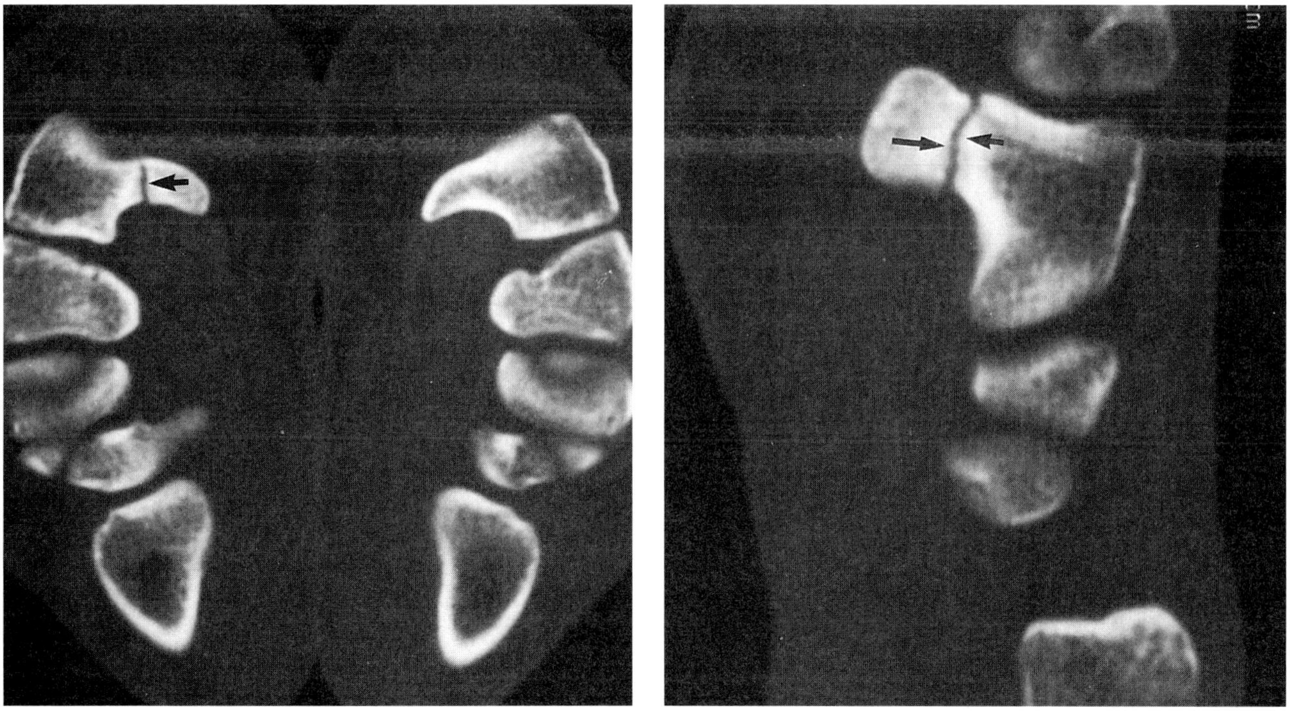 B

FIGURE 3-87 CT scans of the wrist in the axial **(A)** and sagittal **(B)** planes demonstrating bony nonunion of a fracture through the hook of the hamate in this baseball player. Note the sclerosis *(arrows)* with healing despite the lack of bridging trabeculae.

A 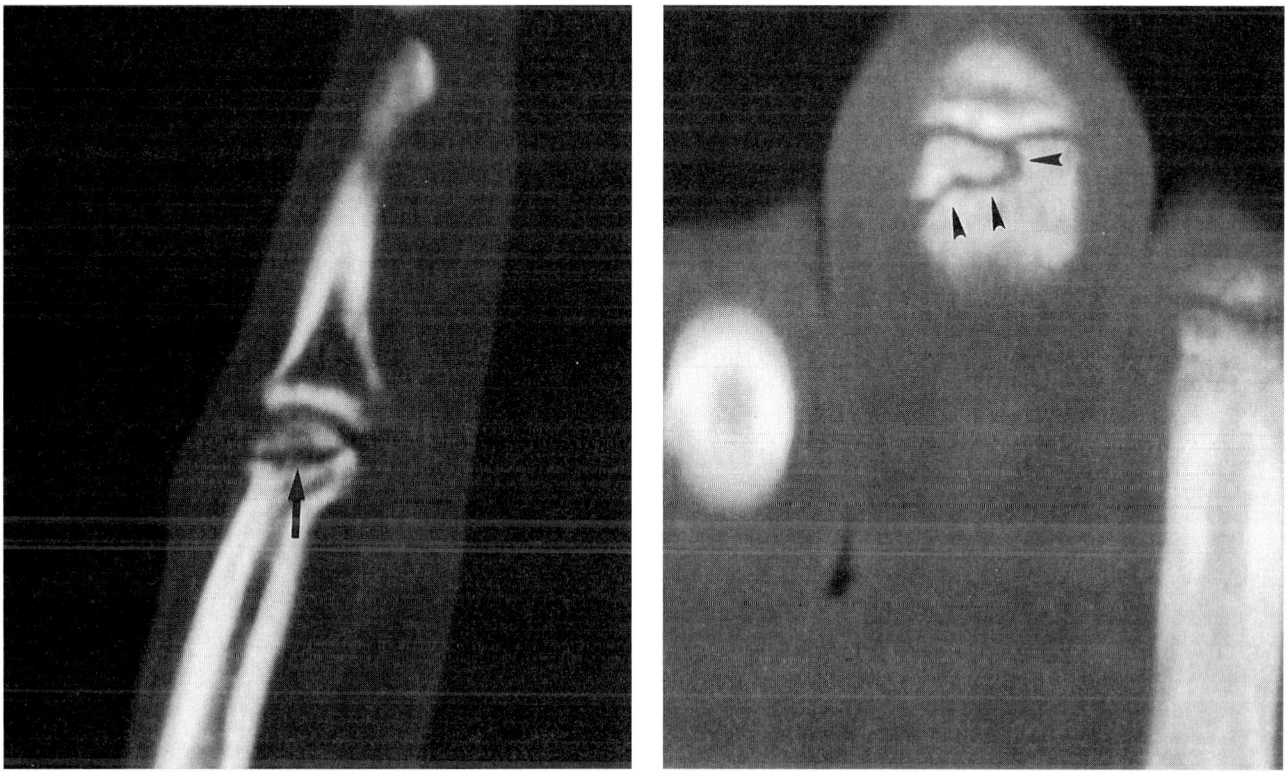 B

FIGURE 3-88 An unusual fracture involving the head of the proximal phalanx of the middle finger extends into the joint and bisects the articular surface. The CT scans demonstrate smooth sclerotic margins *(arrowheads)* of the fracture with no evidence of bridging bone.

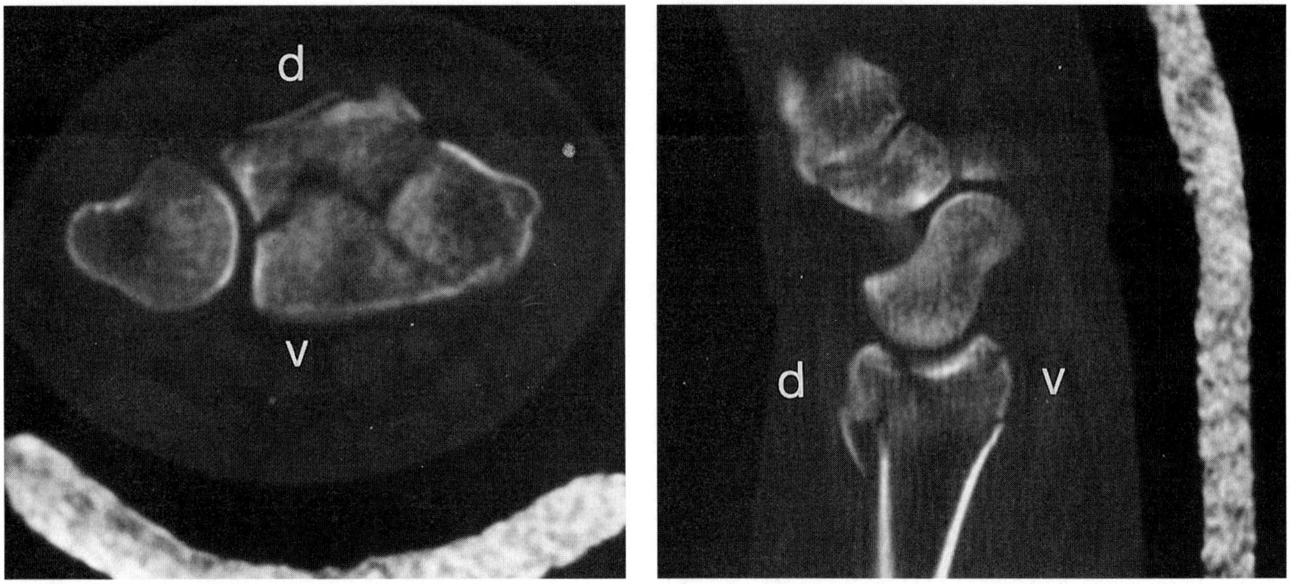

FIGURE 3-89 High-resolution CT scans through the wrist in the axial **(A)** and sagittal **(B)** planes with the forearm and wrist in plaster show the extent of the comminuted fracture of the distal radial articular surface. There is buckling of the dorsal *(d)* radial cortex, resulting in the loss of the normal palmar tilt (normal angle is 10° to 14°). The normal tilt must be restored to prevent limited range of motion resulting from abnormal mechanics at the radioscaphoid articulation. *V,* volar.

Delayed bony union or nonunion is a late complication of fractures; often the physician can detect this on serial follow-up radiographs by noting the lack of bridging bony trabeculae across the fracture as well as the development of sclerosis about the fracture margins.[5,17,34,56,58] These findings are best appreciated with CT because of the lack of overlapping bony shadows and artifacts that normally would arise with union even if the part were immobilized in plaster (see Figs. 3-87 and 3-88).

MRI

MRI has been shown to be extremely sensitive and is comparable to the bone scan in detecting fractures because of the associated intraosseous hemorrhage and edema that contrast against the normal high signal of fat (Fig. 3-90). In such cases as acute trauma, decreased or intermediate signal is noted on T_1-weighted images, but increased signal is present on the T_2-weighted, STIR, or gradient-echo images. The fracture line itself appears as a linear signal-void band on all imaging sequences; however, nonunion may be difficult to diagnose unless high-signal fluid is visualized within the fracture. Most osseous pathology is examined with thin-slice spin-echo imaging rather than gradient-echo imaging, where emphasis is on the extrinsic and intrinsic carpal ligaments. A dedicated surface coil (wrist coil, flexible wraparound coils, or properly positioned 3-inch round coil) allows small field-of-view (8 to 10 cm), high-resolution images, which are needed when imaging the wrist.[84,85]

Avascular Necrosis

When a bone's normal blood supply is interrupted, aseptic necrosis can occur, leading to fragmentation and subsequent bony collapse. This is most frequently encountered within the lunate and the proximal end of the scaphoid, although no bone is absolutely immune to this disorder.

AVN of Scaphoid

Branches of the radial artery pierce the distal pole of the scaphoid and travel proximally, eventually supplying the proximal pole. Because 70% to 80% of scaphoid fractures occur at the wrist and 20% at the proximal pole, avascular necrosis (AVN) of the proximal scaphoid fragment is common after an untreated nonunion or displaced fracture.[56,65] The more proximal the fracture, the more likely the proximal pole will undergo AVN.[17]

Although this AVN may manifest on follow-up radiographs as increased bone density of the proximal fragment, the devitalized bone eventually may suffer structural collapse, which, if left untreated, may lead to a degenerative arthritis. The bone scan frequently was used to demonstrate the photopenic or "cold" area resulting from the regional lack of blood supply, while subsequent scans demonstrated areas of increased activity during the reparative or healing phase.[56,57,69]

In cases of suspected AVN, MRI now is considered the imaging procedure of choice and not only can detect marrow viability, but also may be used in postoperative patients in assessing the success of bone grafts

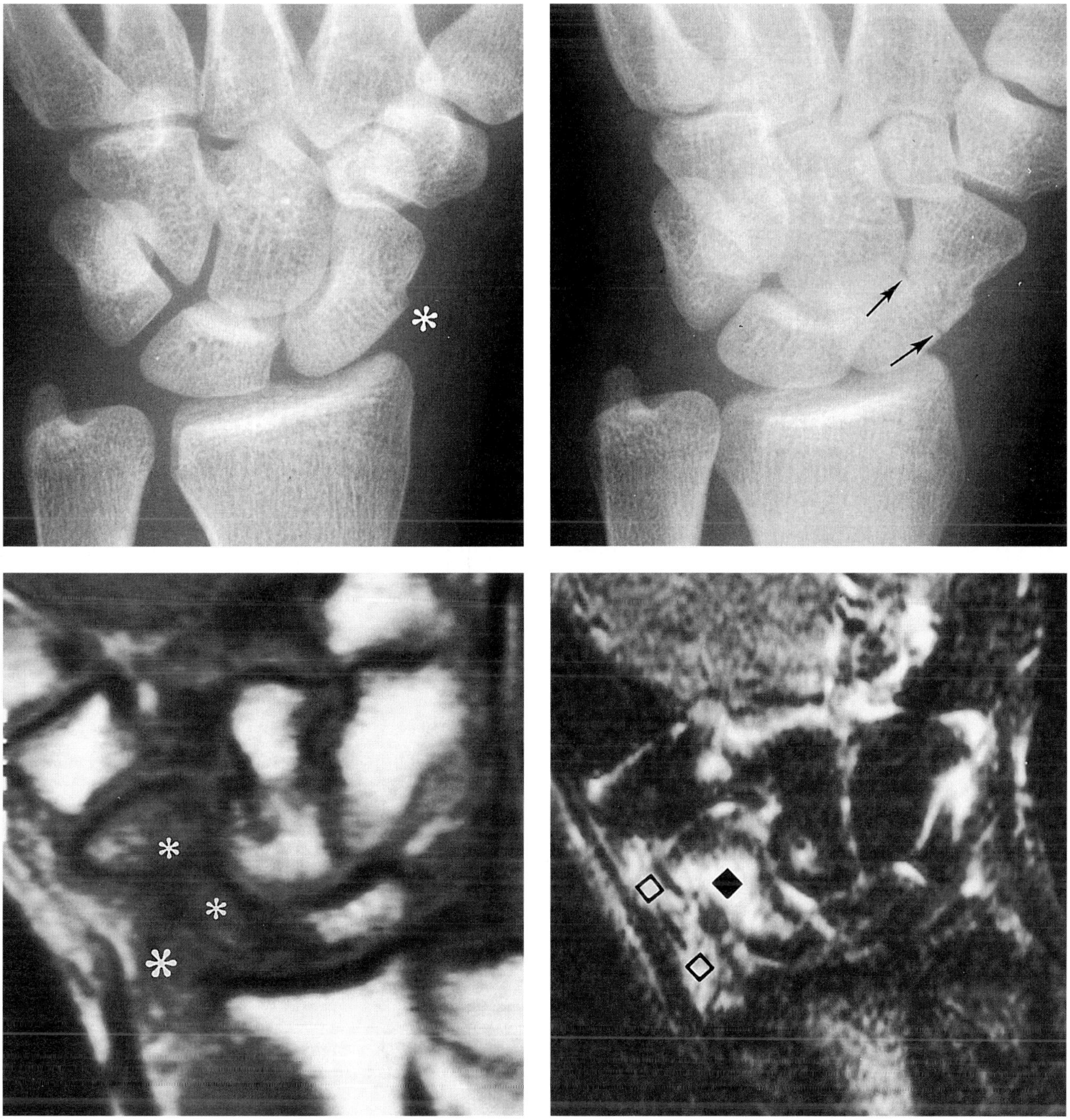

FIGURE 3-90 AP radiograph, **A,** demonstrates obliteration of the normal navicular fat stripe *(asterisk)* and no detectable fracture in this patient with localized pain in the anatomic snuff-box after trauma. **B,** The scaphoid fracture *(arrows)* becomes evident on the oblique projection. **C,** Coronal T_1-weighted and, **D,** STIR MR images demonstrate the intraosseous hemorrhage and edema *(small asterisks, solid black diamond)* resulting from the scaphoid fracture. Note replacement of the adjacent extraosseous fat with hemorrhage and edema *(large asterisk, open black diamonds),* accounting for the obliterated navicular fat stripe on the radiograph.

A 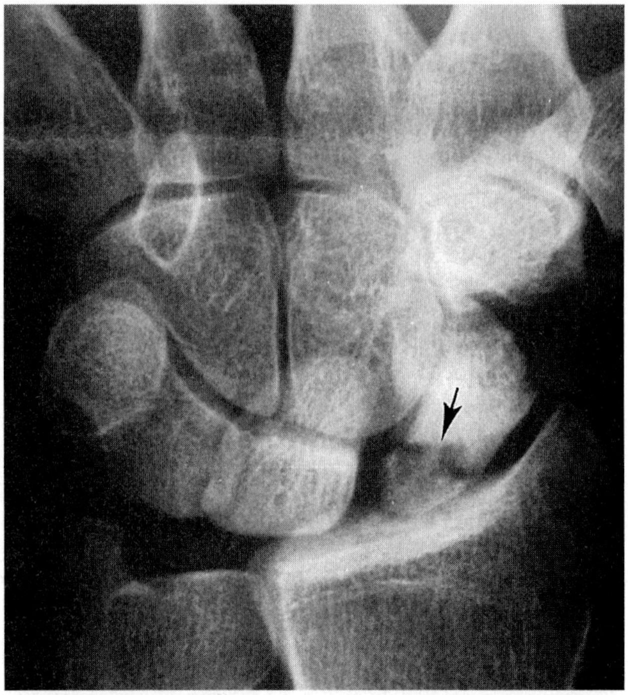

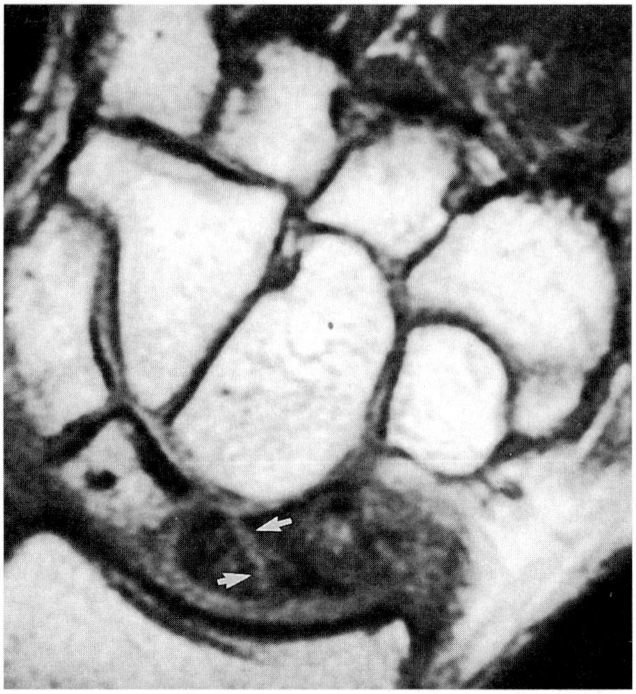 B

C 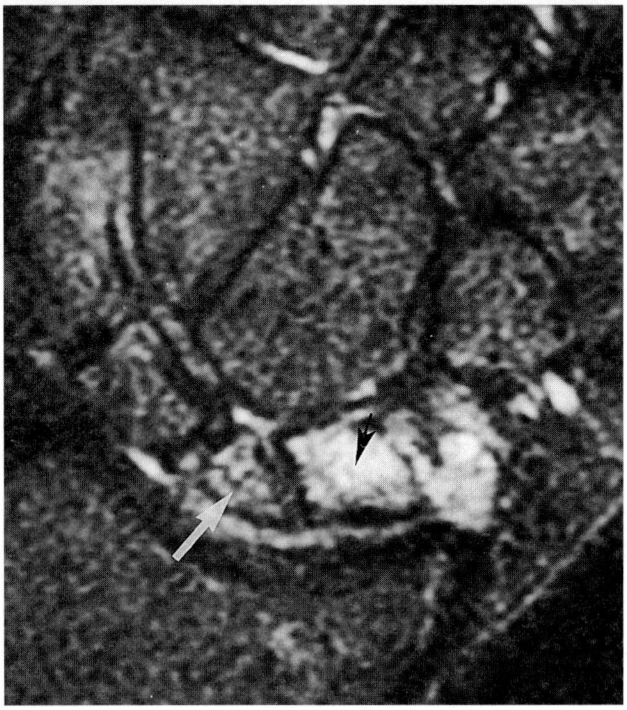

FIGURE 3-91 Developing avascular necrosis of the scaphoid. **A,** Transcaphoid fracture *(black arrow),* with bony nonunion. **B,** Coronal T_1-weighted and, **C,** STIR MR images demonstrate the fracture line *(small white arrows in* **B***)* with decreased signal from the bone marrow. **C,** Hyperintensity within the marrow of the distal scaphoid pole *(black arrowhead)* is due to vascular congestion and hyperemia. Less pronounced effects are seen within the proximal pole *(white arrow)* caused by interruption of the normal blood supply to the proximal scaphoid.

used to avoid the long-term complications of AVN.* In advanced cases of AVN, the involved bone marrow appears dark on both T_1- and T_2-weighted sequences, corresponding to the osteosclerosis depicted on plain radiography. However, in the early stages of AVN, one may observe increased signal within the marrow, presumably resulting from hyperemia. MRI therefore can demonstrate the changes occurring within the marrow long before the occurrence of any deformity and collapse of bone (Fig. 3-91).

AVN of Lunate

Similar to imaging of the scaphoid, MRI is extremely valuable in diagnosing avascular necrosis of the carpal lunate (Kienböck's disease). Although its etiology is still controversial, chronic repetitive stress leading to microfractures in the lunate and resulting in disturbance to the lunate's blood supply has been postulated as one cause.[17] This is in keeping with the association of lunate ischemic necrosis with a negative ulnar variance (shorter ulnar length than radial) (Fig. 3-92). This variance results in an increase in the normal biomechanical stress forces applied directly to the lunate from the radius alone. Normally, applied stress is distributed between the radius and ulna together, and the interposed triangular fibrocartilage complex (TFCC) acts as a cushion between the lunate and ulnar head. Just as with AVN of the scaphoid, sclerosis, fragmentation, and structural collapse of the lunate eventually occur, with the capitate migrating proximally.[17,66,91]

*References 17, 66, 70, 84, 85, 91.

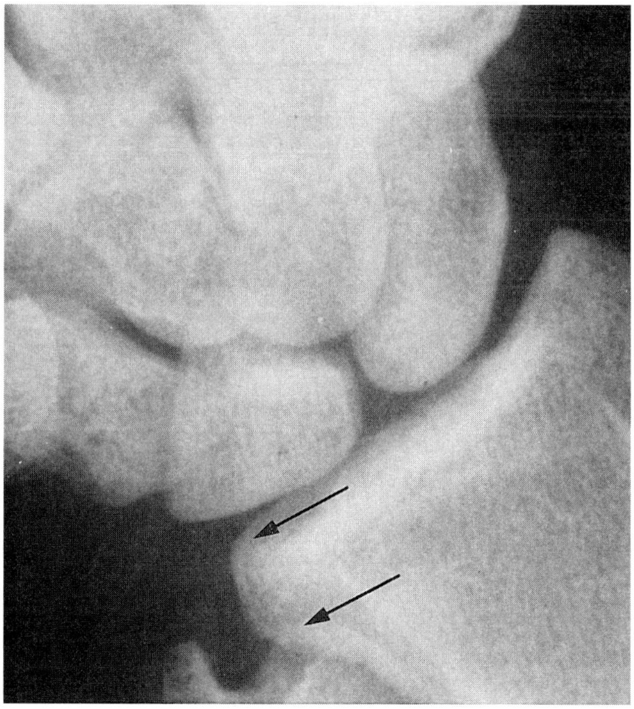

FIGURE 3-92 AP radiograph depicting negative ulnar variance, the distance between arrows, measured between midarticular surface of distal radius and articular surface of distal ulna. Ulnar variance may be misinterpreted when either the distal or proximal cortical surfaces of the radius are used because these correspond to the dorsal and volar lips, respectively, because of the normal palmar tilt of the radial articular surface.

Disorders of the Radioulnar Joint

The radioulnar joint consists of the shallow sigmoid notch of the medial aspect of the distal radius and the head of the distal ulna, and is stabilized by the TFCC.

Acting as a single functional unit, the TFCC actually is composed of several structures, including the triangular fibrocartilage (articular disc or TFC), volar and dorsal radioulnar ligaments, meniscus homolog, ulnar collateral ligament, and sheath of the extensor carpi ulnaris tendon. It is intimately related to the triquetrum and lunotriquetral ligament along its volar aspect.

In the patient with ulnar-sided wrist pain, disorders of the TFCC may consist of traumatic ruptures or degenerative perforations of the articular disc, chronic ulnolunate impingement, or subluxation and inflammation of the extensor carpi ulnaris tendon.[10,17,34,91]

Arthrography

Traumatic tears of the TFC were radiographically evaluated primarily with wrist arthrography before the advent of MRI. Injecting contrast material into the radiocarpal joint will demonstrate leakage of contrast with subsequent opacification of the distal radioulnar joint in the presence of a torn TFC[33,67] (Fig. 3-93). Complete disrup-

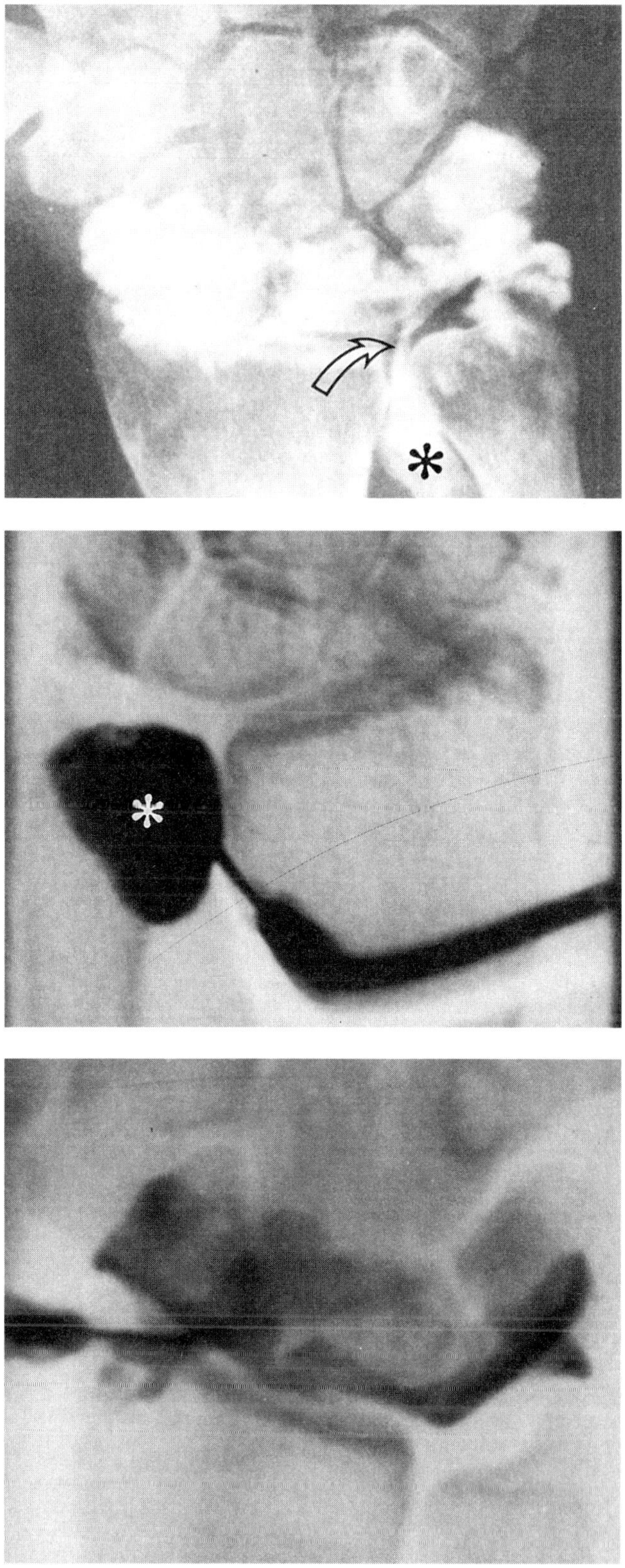

A

B

C

FIGURE 3-93 **A,** Wrist arthrogram demonstrating a tear within the triangular firbrocartilage *(open curved black arrow),* allowing communication between the radiocarpal compartment and the distal radioulnar joint *(asterisk).* Normal appearance of the distal radioulnar joint, **B,** labeled with an asterisk, and the radiocarpal joint, **C,** after contrast injection.

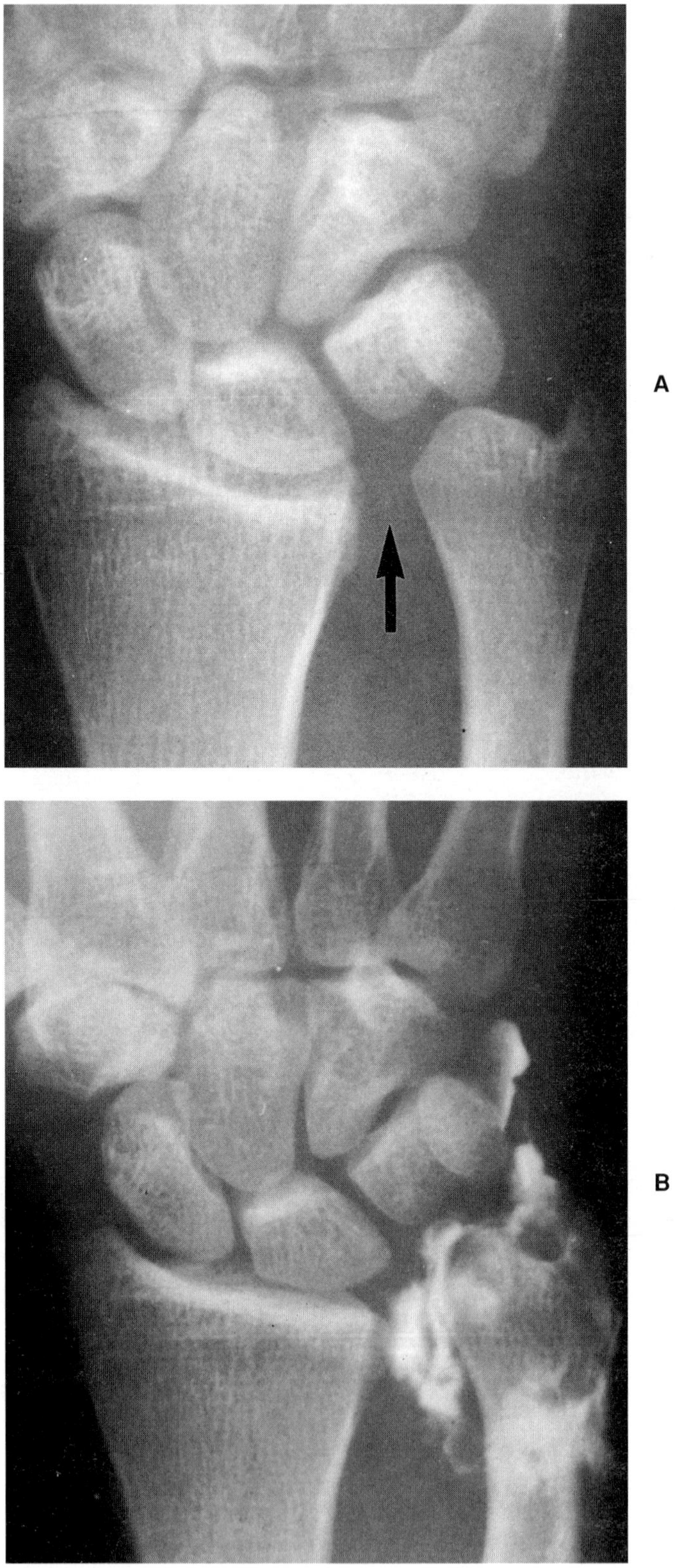

FIGURE 3-94 **A,** Complete disruption of the distal radioulnar joint *(black arrow)* with extravasation into the periarticular soft tissues on the arthrogram **(B).**

A
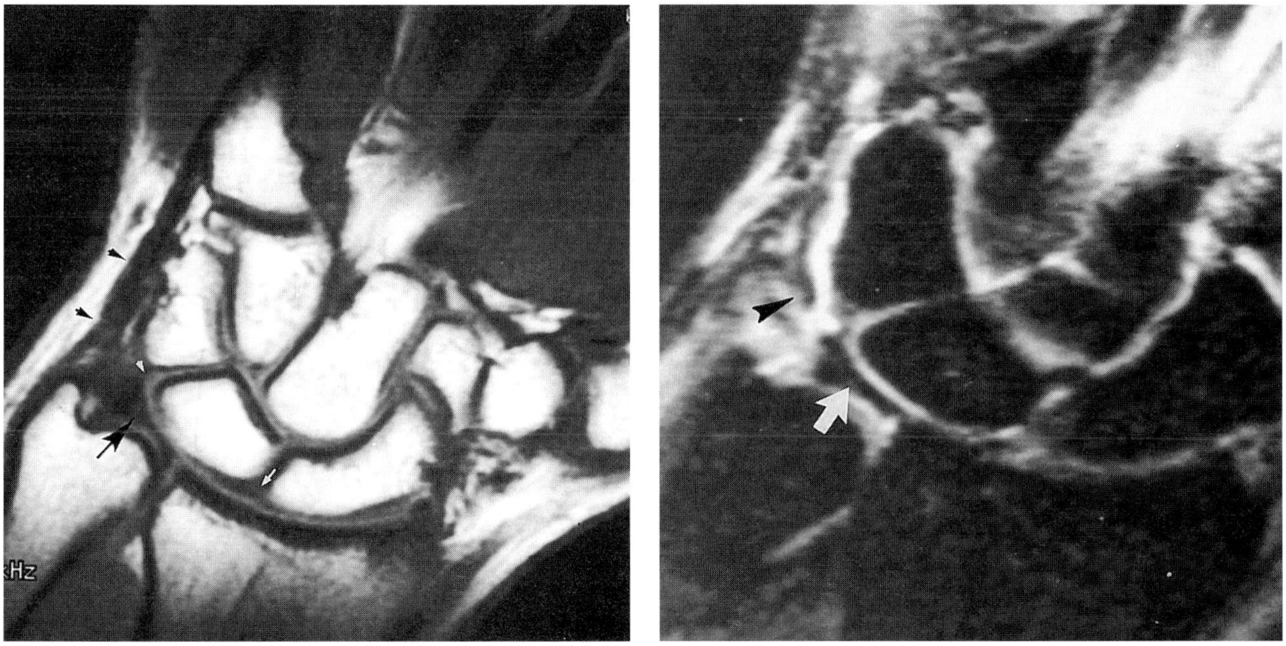
B

C
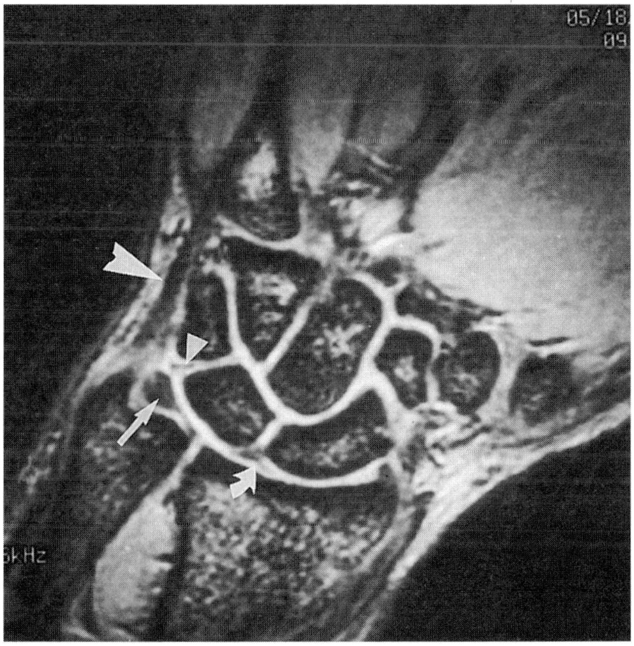

FIGURE 3-95 The articular disc, or triangular fibrocartilage (TFC), is demonstrated on coronal T_1-weighted **(A)**, routine gradient-echo **(B)**, and 1.5-mm-thick high-resolution three-dimensional gradient-echo **(C)** MR images. Note the signal-void appearance of the TFC (**A**, *large black arrow;* **B** and **C**, *white arrow*) on all pulse sequences. The extensor carpi ulnaris tendon (**A**, *small black arrowheads;* **C**, *large white arrowhead*), meniscus homolog (**B**, *black arrowhead*), lunotriquetral ligament (**A** and **C**, *small white arrowheads*), and scapholunate ligament (**A**, *white arrow;* **C**, *curved white arrow*) are well delineated.

tion of the distal radioulnar joint also may demonstrate extravasation of contrast in the surrounding soft tissues as well as within the adjacent tendon sheath (Fig. 3-94). Unidirectional flow patterns on arthrography have prompted injections of the radiocarpal and midcarpal compartments as well as the radioulnar joint.[88] Digital subtraction has obviated the need to wait for the contrast to be absorbed between wrist compartment injections.[68]

MRI

MRI is the only imaging modality to date that allows direct visualization of the TFC. Through coronal and sagittal imaging, the articular disc is well seen as a biconcave triangular band of low signal on all sequences (Fig. 3-95). It is thinner in its center, where chronic degenerative perforations are common in the elderly. An increased signal of the TFC on MRI is presumed to result from internal mucoid degeneration, similar to meniscal pathology of the knee. Increased lunate loading in patients with positive ulnar variance can result in chronic ulnolunate impingement caused by attritional degenerative perforations of the TFC, which may manifest as erosive changes of the proximal lunate and distal ulna with chondromalacia and the development of subcortical sclerosis, cyst formation, and remodeling[17] (Fig. 3-96). In contrast, younger individuals with normal ulnar length or negative ulnar variance more often acutely tear the TFC after an injury. This tear usually occurs several millimeters from the TFC's radial attachment. A tear should not be diagnosed, how-

A
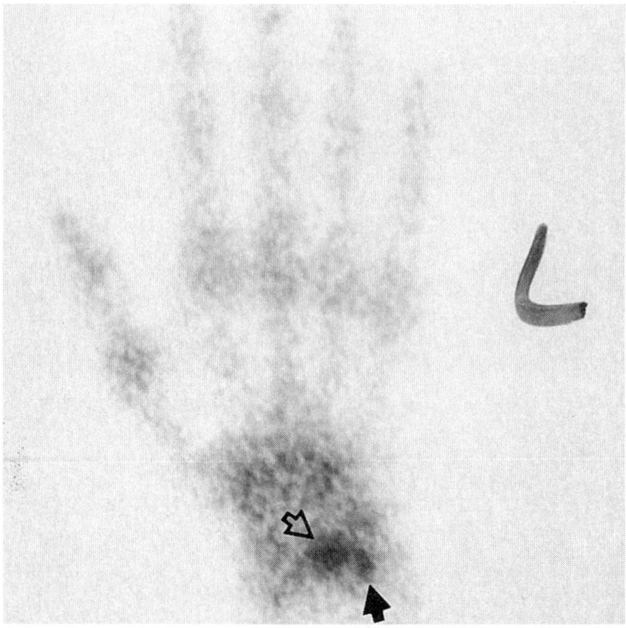

B
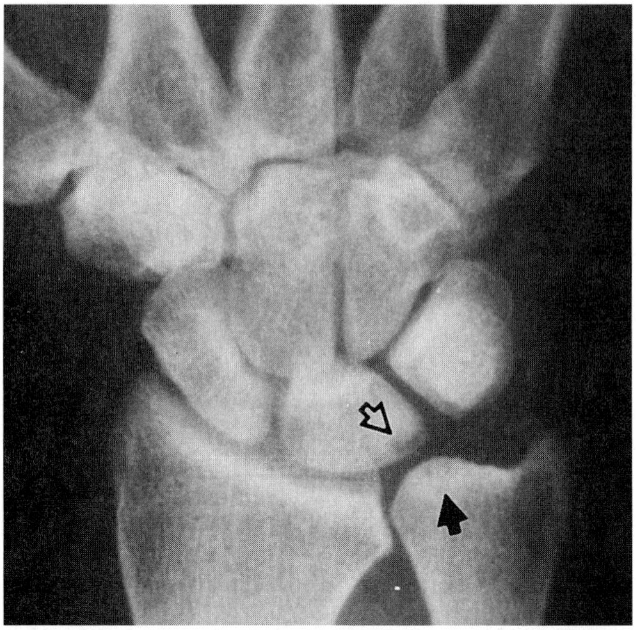

C
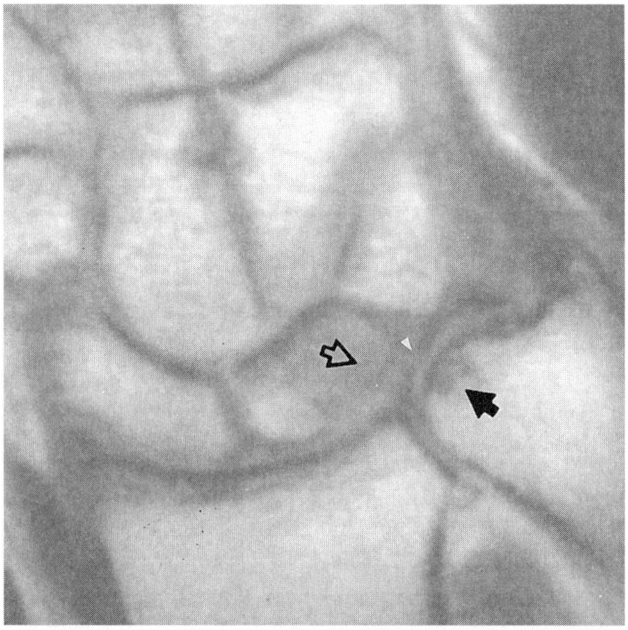

D
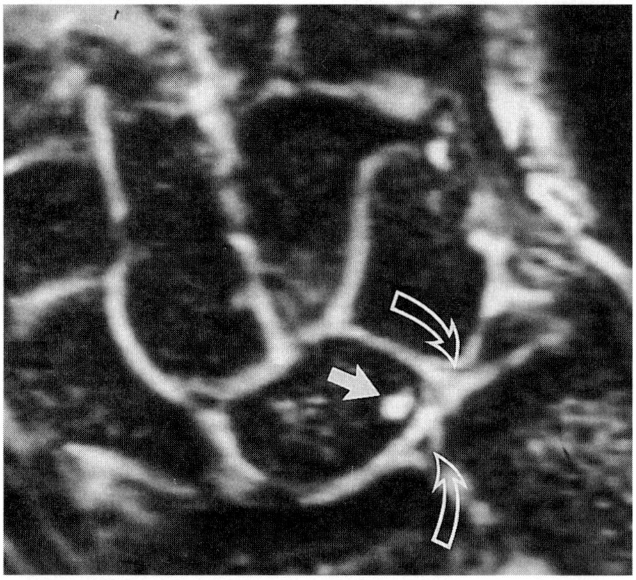

E
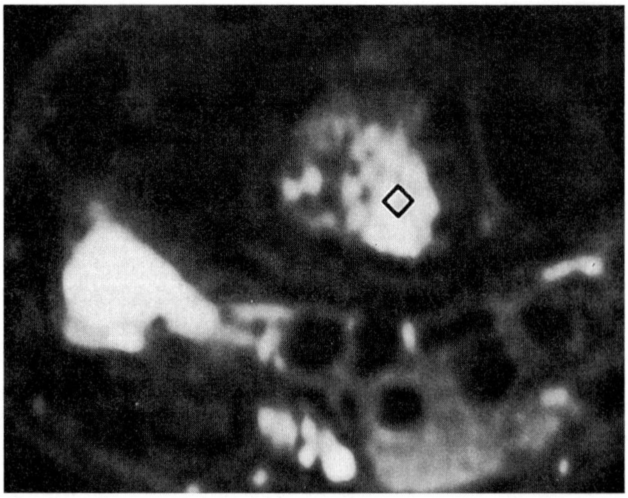

FIGURE 3-96 Ulnolunate impingement. **A,** Positive bone scan demonstrates increased activity within the lunate bone *(open black arrow)* and radial aspect of the distal ulnar articular surface *(black arrow).* **B,** Subcortical sclerosis and cyst formation are noted in the same areas on the radiograph. **C,** Generalized decreased signal within the lunate bone is evident on the coronal T_1-weighted MR image as is a more focal subcortical cyst *(open black arrow).* The adjacent ulna displays a similar finding *(solid black arrow).* Note the small central perforation *(white arrowhead)* of the TFC. A gradient-echo image **(D)** demonstrates the small fluid-filled lunate cyst *(solid straight arrow),* as well as the torn TFC with its distal radial attachment and free edge of the remainder of the disk *(open white curved arrows).* **E,** An axial STIR image is more sensitive in demonstrating the chronic hyperemic changes occurring within the lunate *(open black diamond)* than the corresponding gradient-echo image **(C).** These changes within the bone marrow account for the bone-scan findings and the decreased marrow signal seen in image **C.**

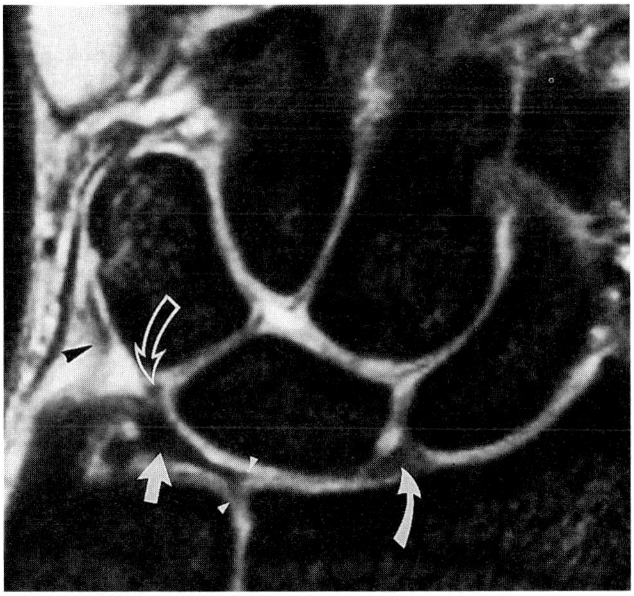

FIGURE 3-97 Gradient-echo MR image demonstrating the normal triangular configuration of the TFC *(large straight white arrow)* with its radial attachments *(small white arrowheads).* Note the normal radial hyaline articular cartilage undermining the radial attachments. This should not be confused with a detachment from the adjacent radius. The proximal attachment of the TFC can be seen at the base of the ulnar styloid process (fovea). *Black arrowhead,* meniscus homolog; *open curved white arrow,* lunotriquetral ligament; *solid curved white arrow,* scapholunate ligament.

A

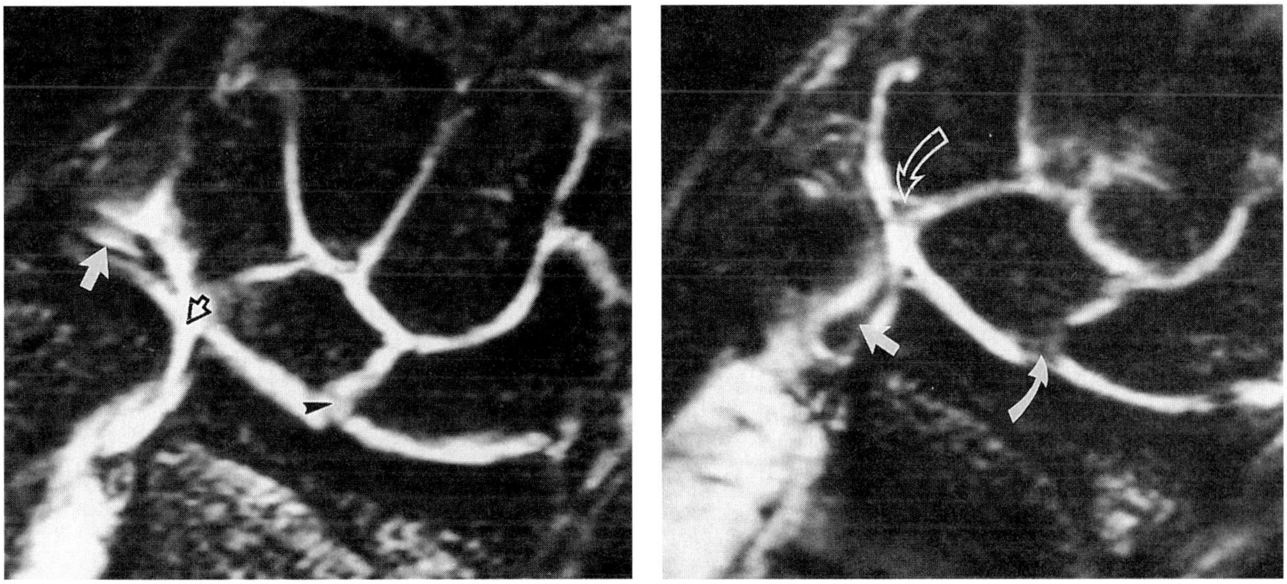

B

FIGURE 3-98 Torn TFC. **A,** Internal degenerative tears of the TFC *(solid white arrow)* and a torn radial attachment *(open black arrow).* A high signal within the scapholunate ligament *(black arrowhead)* is consistent with a tear. **B,** Deformed and detached TFC *(solid straight white arrow)* has prolapsed into the distal radioulnar joint. Note the normal lunotriquetral *(open curved white arrow)* and scapholunate *(solid curved white arrow)* ligaments.

ever, when the normal hyaline articular cartilage of the distal radius appears to undermine the insertion site of the TFC on the coronal MR images (Fig. 3-97). Rather, torn TFC is diagnosed when disruption or a discontinuous disc is noted with fluid in the distal radioulnar joint* (Fig. 3-98).

*References 10, 16, 31, 70, 85, 91.

Subluxations

Subluxations of the distal radioulnar joint are best observed with either axial CT or MRI scanning because obtaining a true lateral radiograph often is difficult (Fig. 3-99).[56] Localizing the distal ulna within the sigmoid notch virtually excludes this entity; however, scanning should be performed in both pronation and supination, in addition to the neutral position, to rule out dynamic instability that might go undetected if the wrist were scanned in

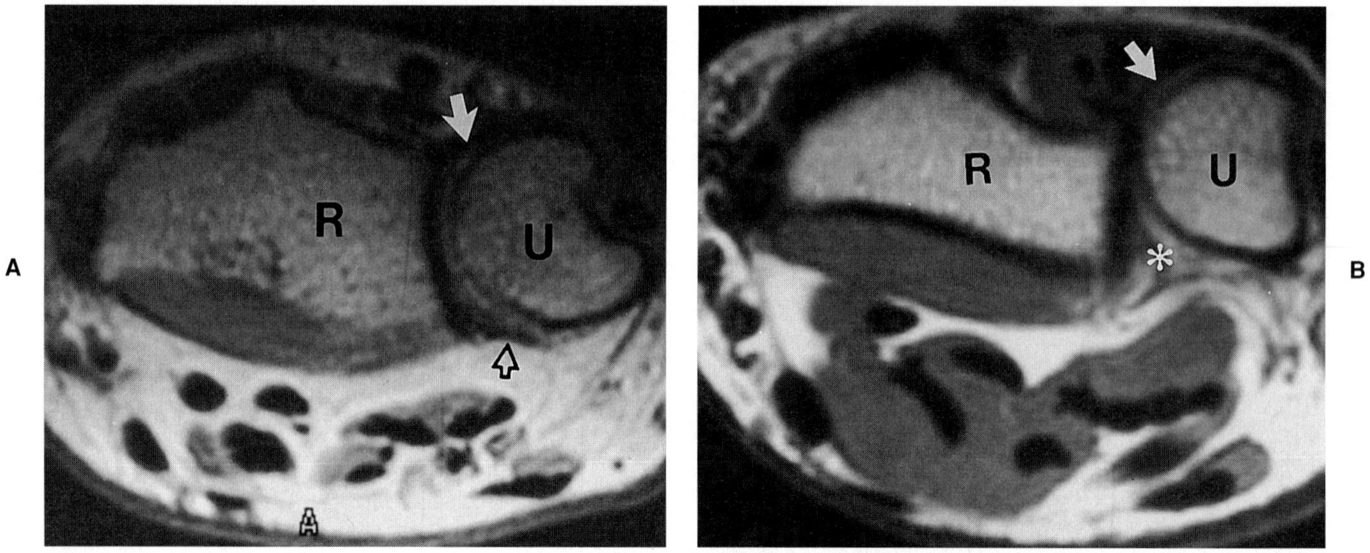

FIGURE 3-99 **A,** Axial T_1-weighted MR image through the distal radioulnar joint demonstrate the normal dorsal *(solid straight white arrow)* and volar *(open black arrow)* radioulnar ligaments, with the ulna *(U)* centrally located within the sigmoid notch of the radius *(R)*. **B,** The volar radioulnar ligament is ruptured *(asterisk)* with dorsal displacement of the ulna. The dorsal radioulnar ligament *(white arrow)* is still intact.

just one position.[56] Minor volar and dorsal translation of the distal ulna can be seen with forceful supination and pronation, respectively, and should not be confused with true subluxation.[91]

Ligamentous Injuries and Instability

A number of lines and angles are derived from plain radiographs of the wrist through a variety of projections to evaluate for ligamentous disruptions[34] (Fig. 3-100). A detailed analysis of these measurements is beyond the scope of this section; however, these lines and parallel arcs must be maintained for carpal stability.

Extrinsic and Intrinsic Ligaments

Wrist stability is maintained primarily through a complex arrangement of extrinsic dorsal and volar ligaments. The extrinsic ligaments can be further classified into various radiocarpal and ulnocarpal ligaments, with the stronger volar radiocarpal ligaments acting as the primary stabilizer of the radiocarpal joint. These are named according to their origins and insertions on the various bones as they traverse the carpus. The intrinsic or interosseous ligaments also are named accordingly and are subject to disruptions, leading to various instability patterns.[51]

Not infrequently, the radioscapholunate (extrinsic) and scapholunate (intrinsic) ligaments are ruptured after a fall on the outstretched hand, resulting in rotatory subluxation of the scaphoid. As the distal pole is volarly tilted, the proximal pole tilts dorsally, and the normal scapholunate space (up to 3 mm) widens (Terry Thomas sign), with foreshortening of the scaphoid on the PA radiograph[34,65] (Fig. 3-101). Stress views of the wrist sometimes are needed to enhance the dissociation of these two carpal bones.[56]

With additional force loading on the wrist, the supporting ligaments of the lunate rupture further, and either perilunate (Fig. 3-102) or lunate (Fig. 3-103) dislocations may occur. This rupture is easily recognized on the lateral radiograph when the long axes of the radius, lunate, and capitate are no longer colinear. In perilunate dislocations, the lunate maintains its normal relationship with the radius, but the lunate becomes volarly displaced with true lunate dislocations.

Intercalated Instability

Dorsal and volar intercalated segmental instability (DISI, VISI) patterns of carpal instability are diagnosed when there is either dorsal or volar tilting of the lunate distal concave articular surface on lateral projections without frank dislocation (Fig. 3-104). DISI and VISI are associated with scapholunate and lunotriquetral ligament disruptions, respectively. Although this instability pattern is recognizable on plain radiography, sagittal reformatted CT images, and direct sagittal MRI, the associated interosseous ligamentous pathology is best evaluated with wrist arthrography. High-resolution MRI also has proved sensitive in detecting interosseous ligamentous pathol-

A

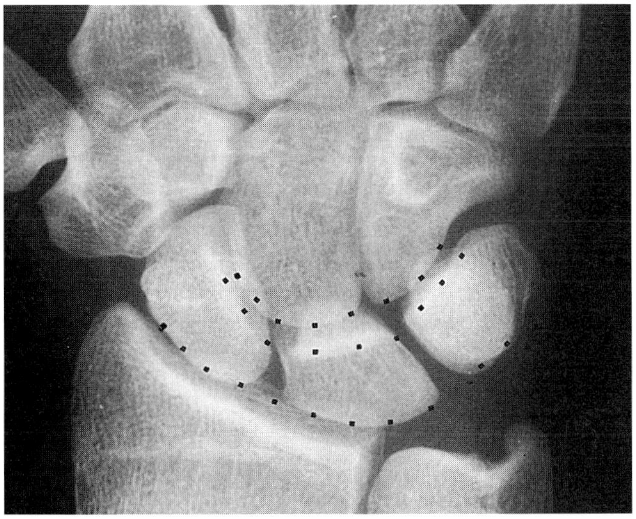

B

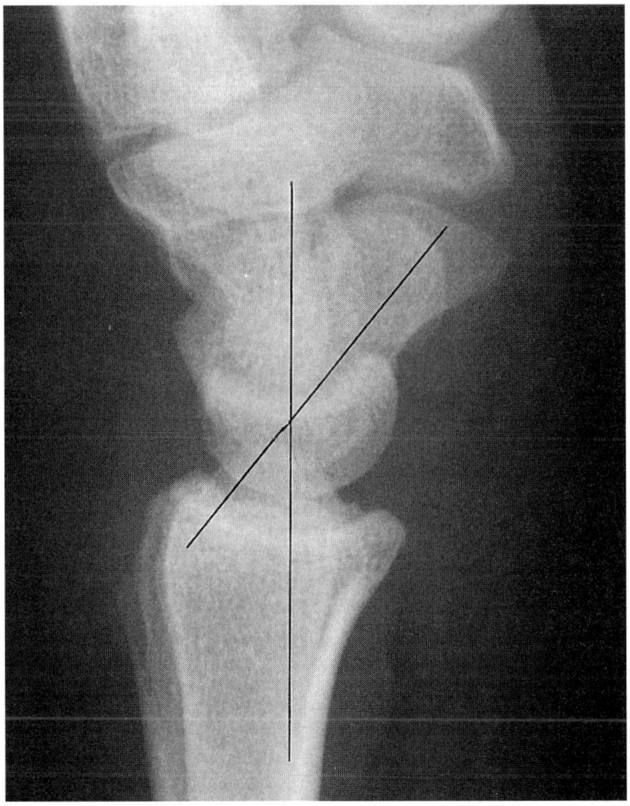

FIGURE 3-100 Anteroposterior **(A)** and lateral **(B)** radiographs of the wrist demonstrate the normal anatomic relationships of the carpus. Three parallel arcs *(dotted lines)* are formed by the proximal and distal articular cortical surfaces of the proximal carpal row and by the proximal articular cortical surface of the distal carpal row. The lateral radiograph demonstrates the normal colinear relationship of the capitate, lunate, and radius, with a normal scapholunate angle (normal angle is 30° to 60°).

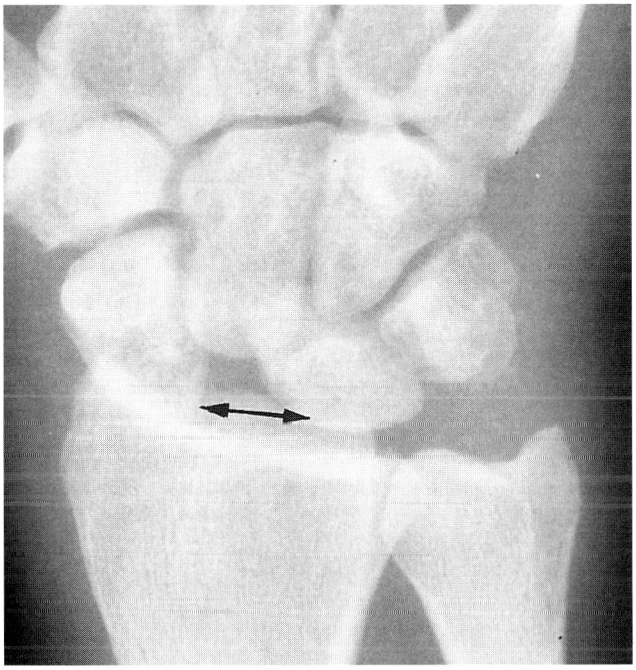

FIGURE 3-101 Widening of the scapholunate space caused by disruption of the scapholunate and radioscapholunate ligaments with subsequent instability and rotational subluxation of the scaphoid, causing foreshortening on the AP radiograph.

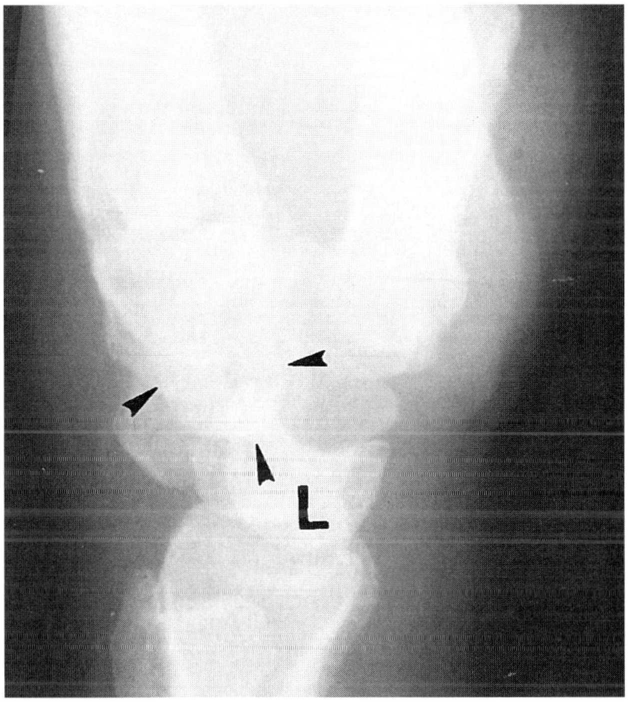

FIGURE 3-102 Perilunate dislocation of the distal carpal row with dorsal displacement relative to the proximal carpal row. The lunate *(L)* maintains its relationship with the radius. Black arrowheads outline the displaced capitate.

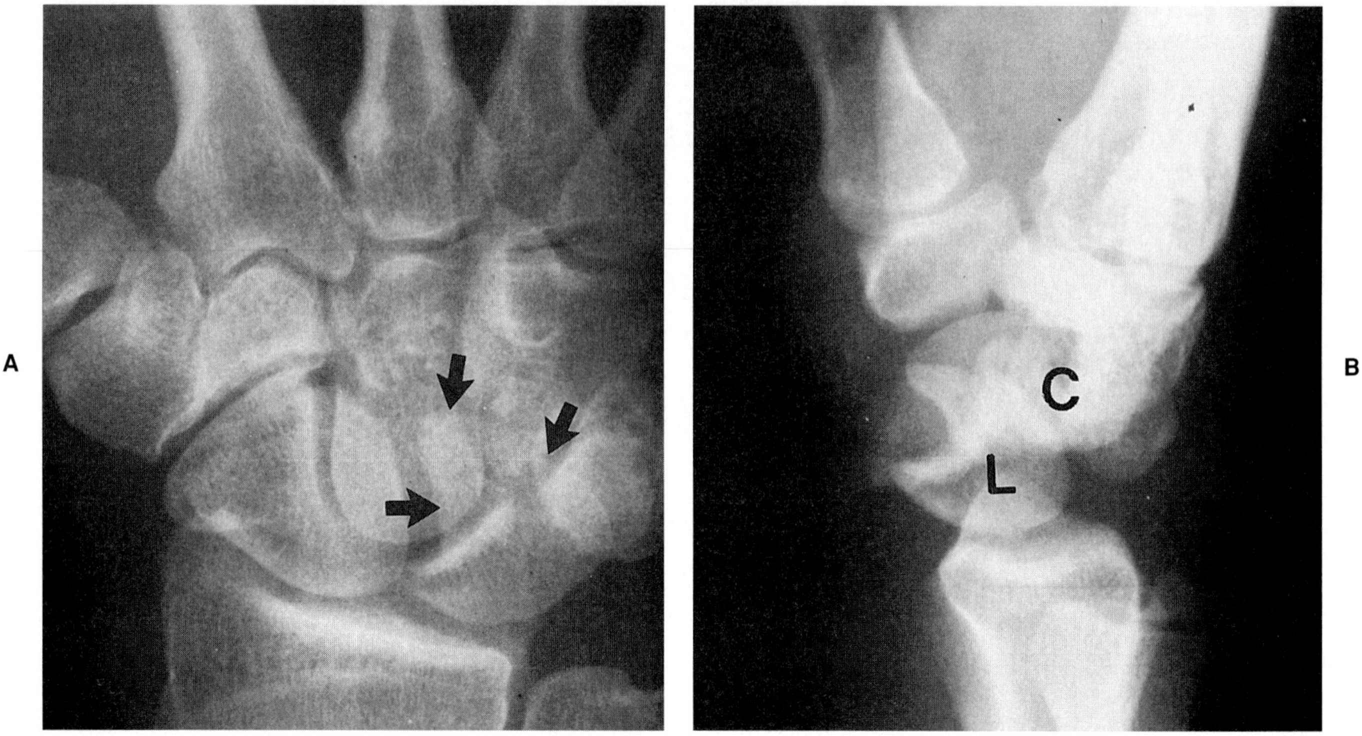

FIGURE 3-103 **A,** Loss of the normal carpal arcs with triangular configuration of the lunate *(outlined with arrows).* **B,** A lunate dislocation accounts for the abnormal appearance on the AP radiograph. There is also dorsal subluxation of the distal carpal row. *L,* lunate; *C,* capitate.

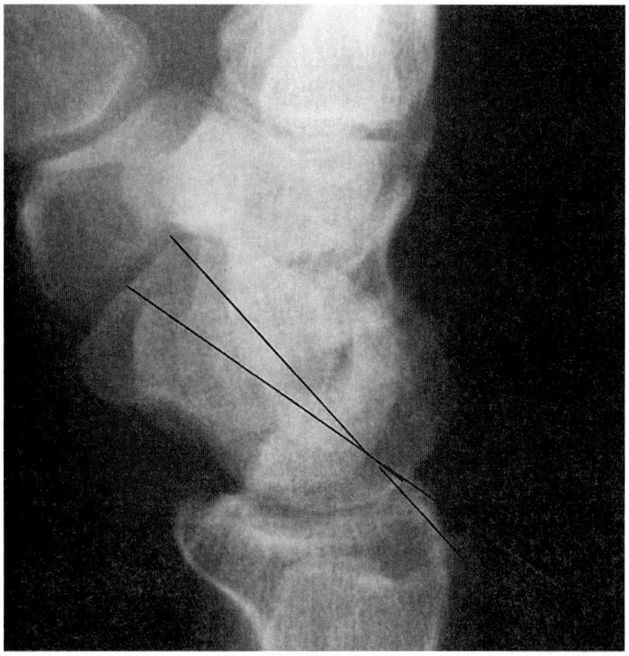

FIGURE 3-104 Volar intercalated segmental instability (VISI) pattern on a lateral radiograph of the wrist. There is volar tilting of the distal concave articular lunate surface with a reduction of the normal scapholunate angle (normal angle is 30° to 60°). The capitate and radius still have a normal relationship without evidence of frank dislocation. This instability pattern is accompanied by a torn lunotriquetral ligament.

ogy. Videofluoroscopy is reserved for evaluating dynamic instability of the wrist in patients with intermittent pain, clicking, and functional instability.

Magnetic Resonance Evaluation

As previously mentioned, triple-compartment wrist arthrography has demonstrated a high sensitivity and accuracy, and is still considered the gold standard in the detection of interosseous ligament tears, especially tears of the scapholunate and lunotriquetral ligaments as well as the TFC.[13,33,67,68,88] With further refinements, MRI has shown comparable results in detecting abnormality of the scapholunate ligament but is not as sensitive in detecting tears of the lunotriquetral ligament, presumably because the latter is smaller, thinner, and curvilinear, making the lunotriquetral more difficult to consistently image.[17,31,84,85,91] Despite this flaw, conventional MR imaging in the coronal plane using T_1-weighted and gradient-echo imaging demonstrates the signal-void bands of these small intrinsic intercarpal ligaments with marked clarity. Volumetric or three-dimensional gradient-echo MRI acquisitions allow 1 mm thick slices, resulting in near-textbook detail (see Figs. 3-95 and 3-97). Discontinuity with localized fluid collection is strong evidence for ligamentous tears (see Figs. 3-96, *D,* and 3-98). MRI has the additional benefit of imaging the extrinsic volar and dorsal radiocarpal ligaments in the axial and sagittal

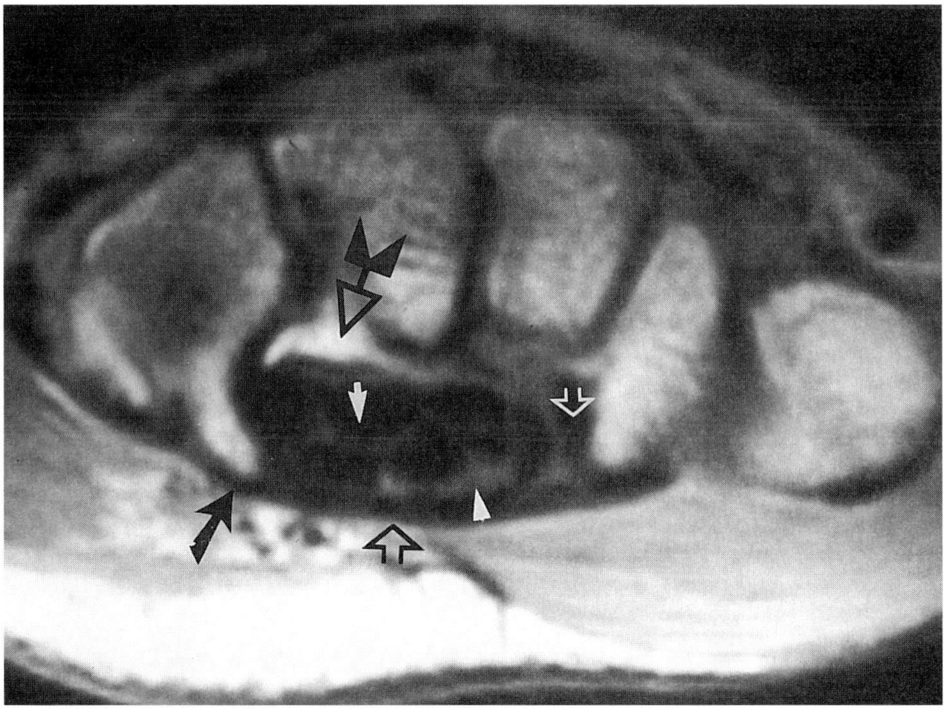

FIGURE 3-105 Normal carpal tunnel demonstrated on an axial T_1-weighted MR image. Signal-void flexor tendons *(small solid white arrow)* traverse the carpal tunnel and are bounded ventrally by the straight or minimally bowed carpal ligament *(open black arrow)*. Note the oval intermediate-signal median nerve *(white arrowhead)* just dorsal to the ligament. *Flagged arrow*, normal fat within the roof of the carpal tunnel; *solid black arrow*, insertion of the carpal ligament onto the hook of the hamate; *open white arrow*, flexor carpi radialis tendon lying adjacent to the scaphoid.

planes, although the accuracy of these assessments remains to be seen.

Carpal Tunnel Syndrome

In patients with median nerve entrapment at the wrist, the classic physical findings of pain and paresthesias confined to the sensory distribution of the median nerve (positive Phelan's test) and thenar muscular atrophy may not be apparent or may conflict with the electromyographic (EMG) study. This clinical condition results from encroachment on the median nerve within the carpal tunnel. Regardless of the etiology of encroachment, the anatomic structures within the carpal tunnel are beautifully demonstrated with axial MRI, affording identification of the enlarged and hyperintense median nerve on T_2-weighted images[42,43,45,84,85] (Figs. 3-105 to 3-107). Synovial hypertrophy of the individual flexor tendon sheaths often is responsible for this condition and has been documented to cause compression of the normal median nerve with wrist flexion.[87] Other rare causes, including osseous fractures, cysts, and anomalous muscles and arteries within the confines of the carpal tunnel, also may be investigated with MRI. Evaluation of the flexor retinaculum after surgical decompression may reveal subtotal resection or subsequent scar formation, accounting for the absence of pain relief in the postoperative patient.

Tendon Injuries

Ruptures and Tenosynovitis

Tendon ruptures or inflammation of their synovial sheaths (tenosynovitis) are best illustrated with MRI. Sagittal scanning will portray the tendon in its length, allowing recognition of focal ruptures and retraction or scarring at the site of injury. Axial images reveal the normal signal-void of tendons and the surrounding fluid from their synovial effusions that occurs with tenosynovitis[84,85] (Fig. 3-108). These images can be obtained through a variety of MRI sequences (T_2, STIR, gradient-echo), but they necessitate small-field-of-view, high-resolution images with a properly selected surface coil (dedicated wrist coil or 3-inch circular coil) appropriately positioned.

Soft-Tissue Masses

Solid Masses

With a soft-tissue mass of the hand or wrist, plain radiography plays a minor role unless there are secondary osseous changes immediately adjacent to the mass or characteristic calcifications specific to certain disorders (Fig.

A
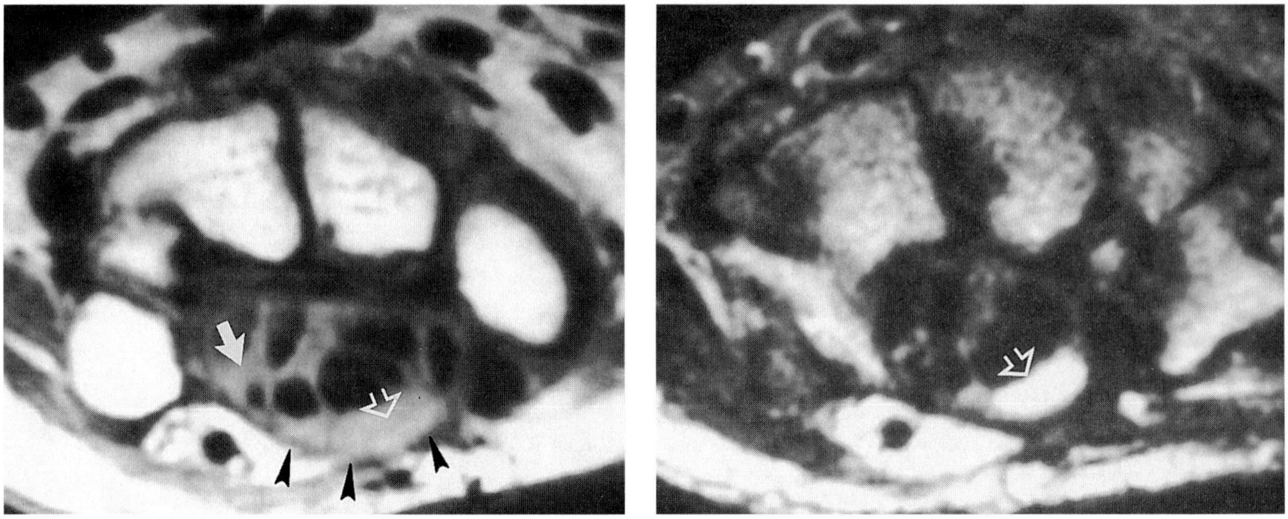
B

FIGURE 3-106 Intermediate-weighted **(A)** and T_2-weighted **(B)** MR images demonstrating typical features in carpal tunnel syndrome. Synovial proliferation of the flexor tendon sheaths *(large white arrow)* results in increased volume of the carpal tunnel, with separation of the individual superficial and deep flexor tendons (in contrast to Fig. 3-105) and bowing of the flexor retinaculum or carpal ligament *(black arrowheads)*. The median nerve *(open white arrow)* is enlarged by edema, which is reflected by its hyperintensity on the T_2-weighted image. Note the obliteration of the normally high-signal-intensity fat stripe normally present dorsal to the flexor tendons.

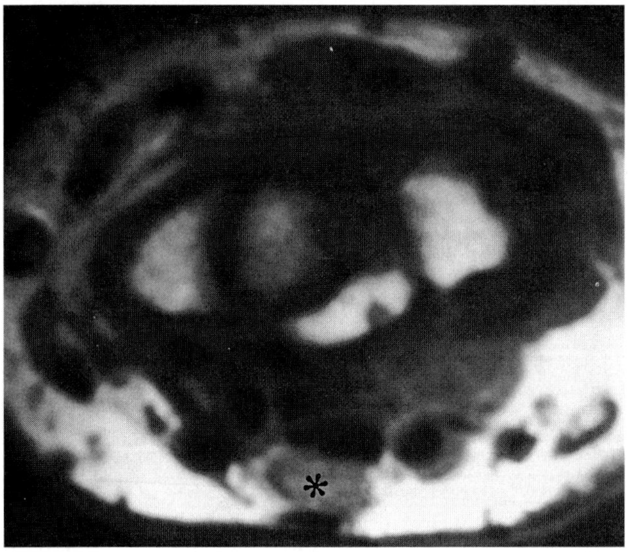

FIGURE 3-107 A pseudotumor of the median nerve *(asterisk)* is present just proximal to the entrance to the carpal tunnel in the same patient as in Fig. 3-106. The enlarged and edematous median nerve simulates a neural tumor.

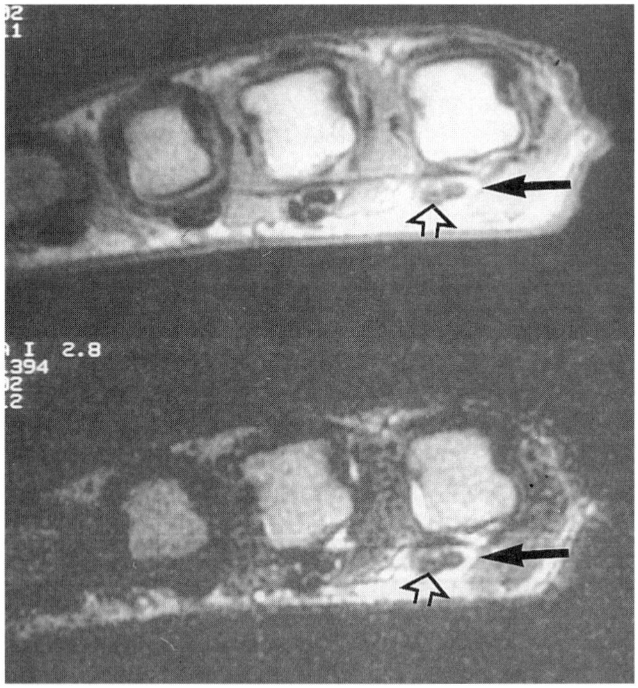

FIGURE 3-108 Tenosynovitis of the index finger. Axial T_1-weighted *(top)* and T_2 weighted *(bottom)* MR images through the distal metacarpals demonstrate fluid *(solid black arrow)* within the common tendon sheath surrounding both the superficial and deep flexor tendons *(open black arrows)*.

3-109). Limited by its inability to discriminate between normal and abnormal tissues in the absence of calcifications, CT also is of limited value.[80] Rather, MRI is preferable in the vast majority of cases. Although MRI may be able to demonstrate soft-tissue neoplasms, hematomas, ligamentous tears, and tendon tears with associated edema, caution should be exercised when evaluating soft-tissue neoplasms because of the overlap of MR findings seen in both benign and malignant tumors.[80] Identifying and staging the tumor rather than determining its malignant potential and histology always should be the prime objective with MRI.

Cystic Ganglion

Ganglion cysts of the wrist and hand, as in the shoulder, are filled with mucinous fluid and are easily detected on

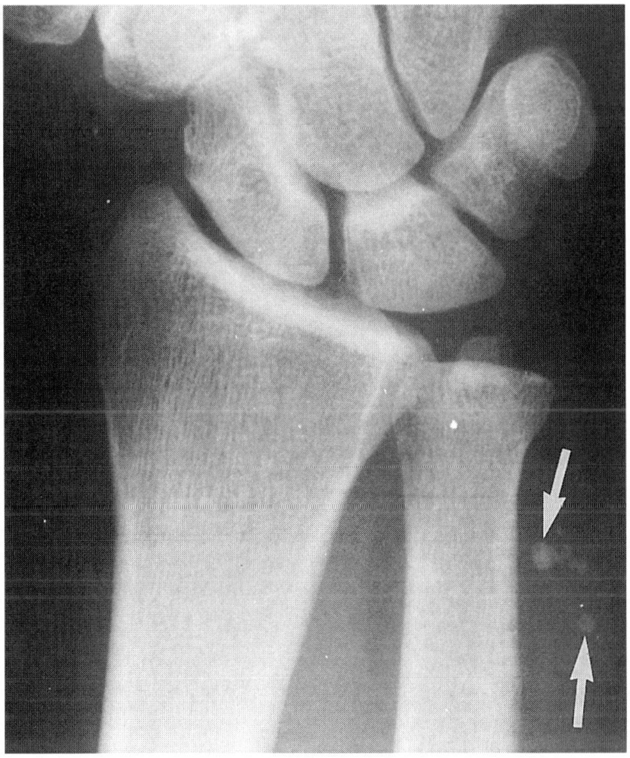

A

FIGURE 3-109 Intermuscular hemangioma of distal forearm. **A,** Radiograph shows typical calcified phleboliths *(arrows)* associated with hemangiomas. **B,** Axial T_1-weighted MR images demonstrate a mass *(black diamond)* with interspersed areas of high signal (fat). The combination of radiographic and MR findings allows a specific diagnosis to be concluded with confidence. Normally, histologic diagnoses should not be inferred based on scan findings alone.

B

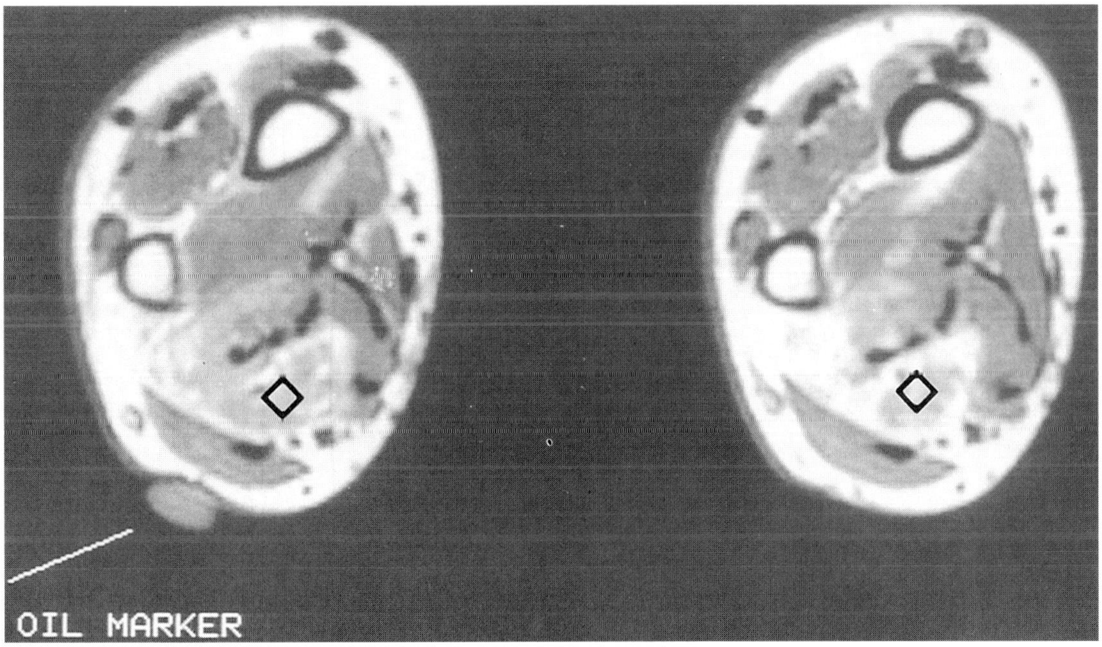

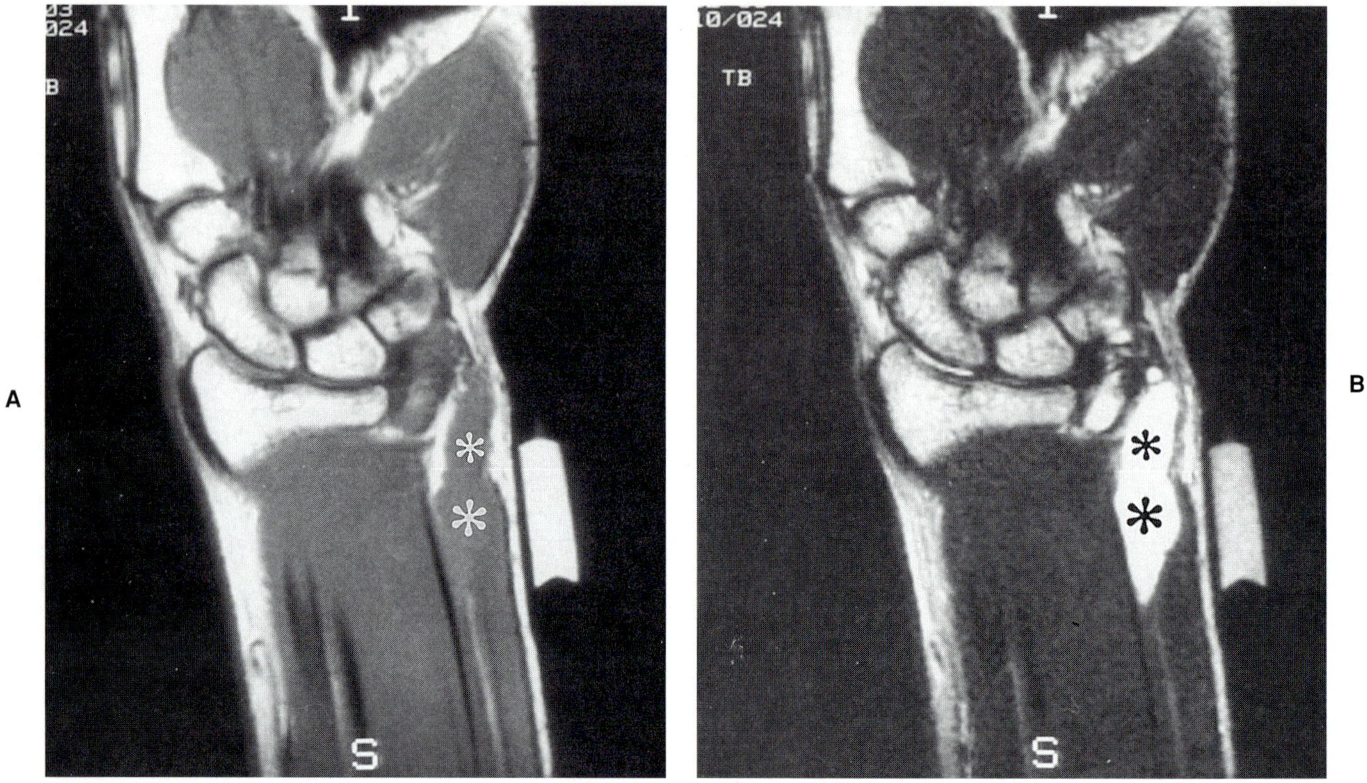

FIGURE 3-110 Proton-density **(A)** and T_2-weighted **(B)** MR images of the distal forearm and wrist show typical features of a ganglion cyst. The cystic fluid (asterisk) has intermediate signal in image **A,** appearing hyperintense in image **B.** Note the proximal dissection of the cyst originating from the distal radioulnar joint.

MRI.[17] They appear as low to intermediate signal on T_1-weighted images and as hyperintense signal on T_2-weighted images (Fig. 3-110). Their stalk connecting to a nearby joint or tendon sheath often is too small to be detected, but determining its precise location and its relationship to the neurovascular structures and other soft tissues is invaluable to the surgeon.[56]

SUMMARY

With the increasing popularity of sports and health-related activities, sports- and exercise-related injuries are becoming more common. A wide variety of imaging modalities are currently available to the physician and should be used only after the physician obtains a good clinical history and performs a proper physical examination. The additional information provided by these imaging techniques has proven invaluable in diagnosis, treatment, and prognosis.

REFERENCES

1. Abrams JS: Special shoulder problems in the throwing athlete: pathology, diagnosis, and nonoperative management, *Clin Sports Med* 10(4):839, 861, 1991.
2. Andrews JR, Kupferman SP, Dillman CJ: Labral tears in throwing and racquet sports, *Clin Sports Med* 19(4):901, 911, 1991.
3. Beltran J et al: Tendons: high field-strength surface coil MR imaging, *Radiology* 162:735-740, 1987.
4. Bigliani LU et al: The relationship of acromial architecture to rotator cuff disease, *Clin Sports Med* 10(4):823-838, 1991.
5. Biondetti PR et al: Wrist: coronal and transaxial CT scanning, *Radiology* 163:149-151, 1987.
6. Bowen MK, Warren RF: Ligamentous control of shoulder stability based on selective cutting and static translation experiments, *Clin Sports Med* 10(4):757-782, 1991.
7. Burk DL et al: Rotator cuff tears: prospective comparison of MR imaging with arthrography, sonography, and surgery, *AJR* 153:87-92, 1989.
8. Chansky HA, Iannotti JP: The vascularity of the rotator cuff, *Clin Sports Med* 10(4):807-821, 1991.
9. Cofield RH: Rotator cuff disease of the shoulder, *J Bone Joint Surg* 67(A):974-979, 1985.
10. Dell PC: Traumatic disorders of the distal radioulnar joint, *Clin Sports Med* 11(1):141-159, 1992.
11. Deutsch AL et al: Computed and conventional arthrotomography of the glenohumeral joint: normal anatomy and clinical experience, *Radiology* 153:603-609, 1984.
12. Flannigan B et al: MR arthrography of the shoulder: comparison with conventional MR imaging, *AJR* 155:829-832, 1990.
13. Freiberger RH, Kay JJ: *Arthrography,* New York, 1979, Appleton-Century-Crofts.
14. Fritz RC et al: Suprascapular nerve entrapment: evaluation with MR imaging, *Radiology* 182:437-444, 1992.

15. Garneau RA et al: Glenoid labrum: evaluation with MR imaging, *Radiology* 179:519-522, 1991.
16. Golimbu CN et al: Tears of the triangular fibrocartilage of the wrist: MR imaging, *Radiology* 173:731-733, 1989.
17. Golimbu CN: Elbow and wrist. In Firooznia H et al, editors: *MRI and CT of the musculoskeletal system,* St Louis, 1992, Mosby, pp 564-633.
18. Gross ML et al: Magnetic resonance imaging of the glenoid labrum, *Am J Sports Med* 18(3):229-234, 1990.
19. Huber DJ et al: MR imaging of the normal shoulder, *Radiology* 158:405-408, 1986.
20. Hunter JC, Blatz DJ, Escobedo EM: SLAP lesions of the glenoid labrum: CT arthrographic and arthroscopic correlation, *Radiology* 184(2):513-518, 1992.
21. Jobe FW, Bradley JP: The diagnosis and nonoperative treatment of shoulder injuries in athletes, *Clin Sports Med* 8:419-438, 1989.
22. Jobe FW, Kvitne RS: Shoulder pain in the overhand or throwing athlete, *Orthop Rev* 18:963-975, 1989.
23. Jobe FW, Nuber G: Throwing injuries of the elbow, *Clin Sports Med* 5:621-636, 1986.
24. Hodler J et al: Injuries of the superior portion of the glenoid labrum involving the insertion of the biceps tendon: MR imaging findings in nine cases, *AJR* 159:565-568, 1992.
25. Kahler DM, McCue III FC: Metacarpophalangeal and proximal interphalangeal joint injuries of the hand, including the thumb, *Clin Sports Med* 11(1):57-76, 1992.
26. Kaplan PA et al: MR imaging of the normal shoulder: variants and pitfall, *Radiology* 184:519-524, 1992.
27. Kieft GJ et al: Rotator cuff impingement syndrome: MR imaging, *Radiology* 166:211-214, 1988.
28. Kilcoyne RF: Imaging choices in the shoulder impingement syndrome, *Appl Radiol* 59-62, 1993.
29. Kilcoyne RF et al: The Neer classification of displaced proximal humeral fractures: spectrum of findings on plain radiographs and CT scans, *AJR* 154:1029-1033, 1990.
30. Kneeland JB et al: MR imaging of the shoulder: diagnosis of rotator cuff tears, *AJR* 149:333-337, 1987.
31. Kong HS et al: Triangular fibrocartilage and intercarpal ligaments of the wrist: MR imaging cadaveric study with gross pathologic and histologic correlation, *Radiology* 181:401-404, 1991.
32. Legan JM et al: Tears of the glenoid labrum: MR imaging of 88 arthroscopically confirmed cases, *Radiology* 179:241-246, 1991.
33. Levinsohn EM, Palmer AK: Arthrography of the traumatized wrist: correlation with radiography and the carpal instability series, *Radiology* 146:647-651, 1983.
34. Linn MR, Mann FA, Gilula LA: Imaging the symptomatic wrist, *Orthop Clin North Am* 21(3):515-543, 1990.
35. Maki NJ: Cineradiographic studies with shoulder instabilities, *Am J Sports Med* 16(4):362-364, 1988.
36. Markiewitz AD, Andrish JT: Hand and wrist injuries in the preadolescent and adolescent athlete, *Clin Sports Med* 11(1):203-225, 1992.
37. Martire JR: The role of nuclear medicine bone scans in evaluating pain in athletic injuries, *Clin Sports Med* 6(4):713-737, 1987.
38. Matin PM: The appearance of bone scans following fractures, including immediate and long term studies, *J Nucl Med* 20:1227, 1979.
39. Matin PM: Bone scintigraphy in the diagnosis and management of traumatic injury, *Semin Nucl Med* 12:104-122, 1983.
40. Matsen III FA, Harryman II DT, Sidles JA: Mechanics of glenohumeral instability, *Clin Sports Med* 10(4):783-788, 1991.
41. McNiesh LM, Callaghan JJ: CT arthrography of the shoulder: variations of the glenoid labrum, *AJR* 149:963-966, 1987.
42. Mesgarzadeh M et al: Carpal tunnel: MR imaging part II, carpal tunnel syndrome, *Radiology* 171:749-754, 1989.
43. Mesgarzadeh M, Schneck CD, Bonakdarpour A: Carpal tunnel: MR imaging. I. Normal anatomy, *Radiology* 171:743-748, 1989.
44. Mettler FA, Guiberteau MJ: *Essentials in nuclear medicine imaging,* New York, 1983, Grune & Stratton.
45. Middleton WD et al: MR imaging of the carpal tunnel: normal anatomy and preliminary findings in the carpal tunnel syndrome, *AJR* 14:307-316, 1987.
46. Middleton WD et al: MR imaging of the normal elbow: anatomic correlation, *AJR* 149:543-547, 1987.
47. Middleton WD et al: High resolution MR imaging of the normal rotator cuff, *AJR* 148:559-564, 1987.
48. Mink JH, Harris E, Rappaport M: Rotator cuff tears: evaluation using double-contrast shoulder arthrography, *Radiology* 157:621-623, 1985.
49. Mink JH, Richardson A, Grant TT: Evaluation of the glenoid labrum by double contrast shoulder arthrography, *AJR* 133:883-887, 1979.
50. Mirowitz SA, London SL: Ulnar collateral ligament injury in baseball pitchers: MR imaging evaluation, *Radiology* 185:573-576, 1992.
51. Mooney JF, Siegel DB, Koman LA: Ligamentous injuries of the wrist in athletes, *Clin Sports Med* 11(1):129-139, 1992.
52. Munk PL et al: Glenoid labrum: preliminary work with use of radial-sequence MR imaging, *Radiology* 73:751-753, 1989.
53. Neer CS: Anterior acromioplasty for chronic impingement syndrome in the shoulder: a preliminary report, *J Bone Joint Surg* 54(A):41, 1972.
54. Neer CS: Impingement lesions, *Clin Orthop* 173:70-77, 1973.
55. Newberg AH: The radiographic evaluation of shoulder and elbow pain in the athlete, *Clin Sports Med* (4):785-809, 1987.
56. Palmer AK: Hand, wrist, forearm, and elbow. In Martire JR, Levinsohn EM, editors: *Imaging of athletic injuries: a multidisciplinary approach,* New York, 1992, McGraw-Hill, pp 229-280.
57. Papanicolaou N et al: Bone scintigraphy and radiology in young athletes with bone pain, *AJR* 145:1039-1044, 1985.
58. Pennes DR, Jonsson K, Buckwalter KA: Direct coronal CT of the scaphoid bone, *Radiology* 171:870-871, 1989.
59. Pope CF: Radiologic evaluation of tendon injuries, *Clin Sports Med* 11(3):579-599, 1992.
60. Rafii M: Shoulder. In Firooznia H, Golimbu CN, Rafii M, Rauschning W, Weinrob JC, editors: *MRI and CT of the musculoskeletal system,* St Louis, 1992, Mosby, pp 464-549.
61. Rafii M et al: CT arthrography of capsular structures of the shoulder, *AJR* 146:361-367, 1986.
62. Rafii M et al: Athlete shoulder injuries: CT arthrographic findings, *Radiology* 162:559-564, 1987.
63. Rafii M et al: Computed tomography (CT) arthrography of shoulder instabilities in athletes, *Am J Sports Med* 16(4):352-361, 1988.
64. Rafii M et al: Rotator cuff lesions: signal patterns at MR imaging, *Radiology* 177:817-823, 1990.
65. Recht MP, Burk DL, Dalinka MK: Radiology of wrist and hand injuries in athletes, *Clin Sports Med* 6(4):811-828, 1987.
66. Reinus WR et al: Carpal avascular necrosis: MR imaging, *Radiology* 160:689-693, 1986.
67. Reinus WR et al: Arthrographic evaluation of the carpal triangular fibrocartilage complex, *J Hand Surg* 12(A):495, 503, 1987.
68. Resnick D et al: Digital arthrography of the wrist: a radiographic-pathologic investigation, *AJR* 142:1187-1190, 1984.
69. Rupani HD et al: Three phase radionuclide bone imaging in sports medicine, *Radiology* 156:187-196, 1985.
70. Schweitzer ME et al: Chronic wrist pain: spin-echo and short tau inversion recovery MR imaging and conventional and MR arthrography, *Radiology* 182:205-211, 1992.
71. Seeger LL et al: Shoulder impingement syndrome: MR findings in 53 shoulders, *AJR* 150:343-347, 1988.
72. Seeger LL, Gold RH, Bassett LW: Shoulder instability: evaluation with MR imaging, *Radiology* 168:695, 1988.

73. Shuman WP et al: Double contrast CT of the glenoid labrum, *AJR* 141:581-584, 1983.
74. Silberstein CE: Shoulder and humerus. In Martire JR, Levinsohn EM, editors: *Imaging of athletic injuries: a multimodality approach,* New York, 1992, McGraw-Hill, pp 181-228.
75. Silliman JF, Hawkins RJ: Current concepts and recent advances in the athlete's shoulder, *Clin Sports Med* 10(4):693-705, 1991.
76. Singson RD, Feldman F, Rosenberg ZS: Elbow joint: assessment with double contrast CT arthrography, *Radiology* 160:167-173, 1986.
77. Snyder SJ et al: SLAP lesions of the shoulder, *Arthroscopy* 6:274-279, 1990.
78. Soble MG, Kaye AD, Guay RC: Rotator cuff tear: clinical experience with sonographic detection, *Radiology* 173:319-321, 1989.
79. Stark HH et al: Fractures of the hook of the hamate in athletes, *J Bone Joint Surg* 59(A):575-582, 1976.
80. Totty WG, Murphy WA, Lee JK: Soft tissue tumors: MR imaging, *Radiology* 160:135-141, 1986.
81. Uhthoff HK, Sarkar K: Classification and definition of tendinopathies, *Clin Sports Med* 10(4):707-720, 1991.
82. Van Holsbeeck M, Strouse PJ: Sonography of the shoulder: evaluation of the subacromial-subdeltoid bursa, *AJR* 160:561-564, 1993.
83. Vellet AD, Munk PL, Marks P: Imaging techniques of the shoulder: present perspectives, *Clin Sports Med* 10(4):721-756, 1991.
84. Weiss KL et al: High-field MR surface-coil imaging of the hand and wrist. I. Normal anatomy, *Radiology* 160:143-146, 1986.
85. Weiss KL, Beltran J, Lubbers LM: High-field MR surface coil imaging of the hand and wrist. II. Pathologic correlations and clinical relevance, *Radiology* 160:147-152, 1986.
86. Workman TL et al: Hill-Sachs lesion: comparison of detection with MR imaging, radiography, and arthroscopy, *Radiology* 185:847-852, 1992.
87. Zeiss J et al: Anatomic relations between the median nerve and flexor tendons in the carpal tunnel: MR evaluation in normal volunteers, *AJR* 153:533-536, 1989.
88. Zinberg EM et al: The triple-injection wrist arthrogram, *J Hand Surg* 13(A):803-809, 1988.
89. Zlatkin MB et al: The painful shoulder: MR imaging of the glenohumeral joint, *J Comput Assist Tomogr* 12:995, 1988.
90. Zlatkin MB et al: Rotator cuff tears: diagnostic performance of MR imaging, *Radiology* 172:223-229, 1989.
91. Zlatkin MB et al: Chronic wrist pain: evaluation with high-resolution MR imaging, *Radiology* 173:723-729, 1989.

CHAPTER 4

Psychology of the Athlete

HERNDON P. HARDING, JR.
ROBERT K. KERLAN

I bandaged them, but God healeth them
Ambroise Paré

The French playwright Molière observed that humor is potent because it touches truth. The old joke that, "The operation was a success, but the patient died," underscores the fact that after surgery the physician's role is not complete. During rehabilitation the treatment can fail even though the operation was successful.

This chapter deals with the psychologic and emotional concomitants of physical injury and rehabilitation, their etiologies and expression, and some approaches to their treatment. Although follow-up care is important for all patients, there are additional concerns for athletes that complicate treatment. There are further special concerns for injured children and other special populations that are beyond the scope of this chapter.

INJURY AND THE ATHLETE

There are many benefits to being an athletic individual. In addition to the increasing evidence of improved longevity[17] and reduced rates of certain diseases,[12] there is the subjective improved sense of well-being and increased sexual satisfaction[10] experienced by those who are physically active. Intellectually and emotionally, these factors provide a basis for a positive sense of identity and a foundation for a sense of self-esteem. For professional or accomplished amateur athletes, many of these benefits are increased by the great investment of time and effort in perfecting their skills, often to the exclusion of other aspects of personality development. This single focus on athletic skill can compress the normal stages of growth and ultimately compromise the full, adult development of the athlete.[15]

A sense of being in control of life is part of being emotionally healthy. It is partially determined by the ability to control bodily functions. Especially for athletes, anything that threatens that control or ability can also threaten their sense of wholeness.

An injury to an athlete may feel like a loss of the only thing that makes the athlete attractive and worthwhile. This is especially true when the patient has few other areas of self-esteem, so that the athlete's esteem "investment portfolio" does not have the diversity that allows loss of esteem in one area to be buffered by esteem in another area. This precarious self-esteem is the result of more than just the patient's very focused life. As far back as 5 BC, Euripides observed that society's overvaluing of athletics had a negative effect on athletes' behavior.[6] Society often gives athletes opportunities for self-gratification beyond the norm. In return for this special treatment, society expects much from athletes, including an increase in society's own sense of worth. When a city has the winning team, then somehow the citizens who live in that city must be more valuable beings: "We're number one!" Consequently, if athletes can no longer fulfill their end of the tacit bargain, the athletes may suffer a loss of those privileges and a loss of partial identity.

Equally threatening is the potential loss of income for the injured professional and the possible change in relationships with family and friends. If the patient's family and friends are overly invested in the patient's ability to perform, regardless of the patient's age, there may be a loss in those relationships when the ability is jeopardized by injury. This is especially so if the patient's family or friends have been living vicariously through the patient's fame and glory. The threat of loss is more than physical; it may mean a loss of connectedness to others and a loss of self. It adds insult to injury.

Despite the personality pitfalls of athleticism, an athlete's mental health is often better before injury than the average person. After injury, however, the athlete may tend to experience psychologic distress in somatic symptomatology more frequently than nonathletes,[11] thereby complicating rehabilitation.

Athletic injury can result in various emotional reactions. A loss of self-esteem, depression, emotional tension, and confusion are some of the most common initial experiences.[2] The process of grieving may be an expected reaction, especially with severe or prolonged injury. This may entail the well-known, nonsequential stages of grieving described by E. Kubler-Ross[9] and associates: denial, anger, bargaining, depression, and finally acceptance.

Denial occurs when the patient minimizes or treats as insignificant what is commonly viewed as a significant threat or loss. Although some individuals will have a remarkable ability to adapt to the threatening situation, beware of those who take injury too much in stride. Although denial is a major problem if it lasts too long, it is often a normal component of grieving and should not be too worrisome as an initial reaction. It may be viewed as a way by which the mind gives itself time to assimilate the ramifications of the injury. Until the timing is right, the mind must hold the notion in abeyance by pretending that the injury does not exist or is not severe enough to warrant much adjustment.

Anger, like denial, is not pathologic, even if it does not seem entirely logical in the way it is displayed. Anger may be directed at God or the universe or be expressed by blaming others either for causing the injury or for not providing proper care. This latter charge is often leveled at the physician and is not always vocalized. Although anger should be accepted, the physician should never allow it to be expressed in a way that might physically or seriously emotionally harm patients or others. It is a temporary stage of adjustment, if it appears at all, and the physician does not want the patient to suffer remorse for harm inflicted during a time when the patient may not have had all of his or her mature personality in gear.

Depression is a common reaction to serious athletic loss or threat of loss. Some components of depression, like anger, are frequently experienced with a major injury[18] and are pathologic only if they do not resolve as treatment progresses or if the symptoms are so overwhelming that they interfere significantly with the healing process. Some symptoms of depression are listed in Box 4-1 and can be usefully cataloged by the mnemonic A SAD CAGE. If depression seems prolonged, longer than 2 to 3 weeks, if the possibility of suicide enters the picture, or if any of the symptoms seem overwhelming, a psychiatric consultation may help determine the best approach to treatment.

The Patient's Personality

In addition to the emotional reaction to injury, an individual's personality, including specific weaknesses and strengths, is an important factor in the reaction to injury. Psychologic testing reveals that some personality factors may even predict the likelihood of a surgery's success.[20] A patient with mature defense mechanisms[19] (Fig. 4-1)—mental approaches for coping—may experience even the regressive stages of anxiety and grief but steadily proceed toward healthy adjustment. A less-mature defense structure, such as one using displacement and projection, may result in the patient getting stuck in thoughts and behaviors that undermine the therapeutic process.

Humor

Mature mechanisms facilitate not only the psychologic process of healing but perhaps also the physical process. Humor, if used to help cope with the situation, can be an extremely useful defense mechanism.[3] However, as with all strong treatments, its power is a two-edged sword and

BOX 4-1
SYMPTOMS OF DEPRESSION: A S-A-D C-A-G-E

A - Activity level is reduced. The patient may speak and think as though moving through molasses.
S - Sleeping patterns are disturbed with either much more sleep than usual or insomnia. Depression's insomnia is usually characterized by little trouble falling asleep (unless there is also concomitant anxiety) and rather periodic awakening throughout the night and early morning.
A - Appetite and/or weight changes are observed with either increases or decreases.
D - Death may become a preoccupation. This may be thoughts of suicide or a fear of dying during sleep for almost any reason. This may be any preoccupation with death.
C - Concentration is dramatically reduced. The patient may find it difficult to maintain focus.
A - Anhedonia, the loss of the sense of pleasure in activities that usually bring pleasure; frequently is elicited by inquiring about the patient's current interest in sexual behavior.
G - Guilt or remorse to an unrealistic degree in the given situation is observed.
E - Energy is decreased. In addition to an actual decrease of activity, the patient may have a profound sense of lacking energy, called anergia.

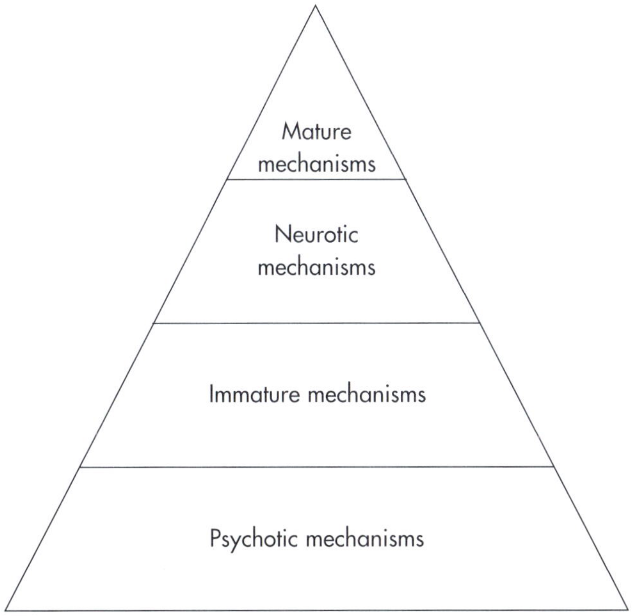

FIGURE 4-1 A hierarchy of adaptive psychological mechanisms.

can be used destructively and beneficially. Playful joking by the patient may be a positive way of dealing with a difficult situation, or it may reveal a hidden belief that they are now valuable only as the butt of jokes.

Humor is also a powerful, two-edged tool in the physician's hands. It can be used to help make the unbearable a bit easier to bear, or it can be used to erode the spirit. Knowing when and how to use humor is the key. Timing is important, but even more so is the type of humor used. Some forms of humor, like sarcasm, are less likely to have a helpful effect, even in skilled and caring hands. Just as different defense mechanisms can be seen as being more useful or more mature than others, so can different kinds of humor be more valuable than others.

Binding the Wound

Physicians must observe and listen carefully so that they understand and respond to not only what patients say, but also what they mean.

Patients may be unable to clearly communicate their true concerns about their injury and treatment, since patients may not be aware of their concerns. This may be because the concerns arise from the unconscious mind. Because a concern is not conscious, it is reflected indirectly through behavior that may be confusing to both patients and caregivers. Accurately interpreting these behaviors by carefully observing and listening is the first goal, just as accurate data-gathering is the first step in any diagnostic and treatment approach. Listening to patients not only is useful as a tool to understanding, but also has a therapeutic effect. The act of listening to patients' stories helps bind the psychologic wound. Listening or binding assembles the scattered pieces of psyche, a process as important as juxtaposing the edges of a physical wound to promote healing.

The true measure of a big man is the way he treats little men.

A useful practice is to put aside defensive reactions when patients say or do something provocative. Instead, try to identify the message behind the behavior. One way to do this without allowing emotions to interfere is to realize that patients are the ones under the most stress in this situation, and that they are not operating at their highest level. Because physicians really care for their patients, the physician must recognize their patients' temporary inadequacy and not take the provocation personally. Instead, physicians must compassionately and dispassionately listen to the hidden message with what therapists sometimes call the *third ear*. The message may be something as simple as "I'm afraid I won't make it through the operation," or "I'm too embarrassed to ask, but will this affect my sex life?" Or it may be as complex as, "I feel so alone and the only way I think I can really connect with you is to fight with you. I desperately need to feel connected," or "Since I feel out of control physically, and therefore less valuable, I have to feel as though I can have some effect on people even if it's just proving my ability to get a negative response. If I can get others to be out of control, they will be with me in a way. By being out of control emotionally, they are helpless, just as I feel helpless because of my injury."

This last meaning is a good example of the defense mechanism, "killing two birds with one stone," where one defense deals with two intolerable and ineffable internal reactions simultaneously. Wise and caring physicians realize that patients are doing the best they can to communicate and, even though patients are doing so ineffectively, does not hold that against them. Instead, physicians listen beyond what is said to hear what patients are unable to say and respond to their patients' needs with reassurance, rather than retaliation.

Although there are different approaches to organizing this search for the hidden message,[14] the one presented here is useful, in part, because it is easy to remember. It fits the mnemonic EAR, which stands for empathy, appreciation, and repetition.

Empathy

Empathy first.
Robert Kenersen

Although the physician's goal is to hear the patient's story and discover the meaning of the injury to the patient, the physician may not accomplish this as quickly as desired. The physician should establish an empathic connection first and keep it a high priority,[13] even if it means that the first interview reveals very little specific information about the person. No matter how thorough a physician is, how brilliant the assessment is, and how skillfully the work in the operating room is done, if the physician fails to get the patient to return after the initial examination, the physician will not succeed.

We only know what we love.
Goethe

Although talking about love may seem strange in a chapter about sports injuries, it is a vital ingredient in the healing process. This is especially true when trying to understand hidden meanings. This need to "love" the patient does not mean romantic love, rather the Greek love of agape, in which one person considers another's needs to be of equal importance. This does not mean physicians must like every patient; this will not happen. It means wanting the best for their patients.[16] When physicians emphatically sense their patients' perspectives and care about their patients' needs, then these physicians are loving their patients within the boundary of the medical profession. That kind of love leads to real knowledge of their patients.

It is much easier to comprehend the totality of another's experience by walking a mile in the other person's moccasins. Everyone has a story to tell; hearing that story tells a lot about the person. Imagining what the patient is experiencing provides a more complete picture of that patient's situation than probably any other tool. Not everyone is naturally empathic, but the skills can be learned.

By hearing from the physicians that they are there to understand, not to judge, the patients know their physicians are trying to be supportive. This helps provide a setting wherein patients are less worried about saying the "right things." Physicians are often seen as authority figures, as well as just having expertise in their specializations. Because of this aura, patients often try to make a good impression on their physicians and, consequently, may not easily reveal things that might not please the physicians such as problems with the rehabilitation process. Physicians must listen for what is *not* being said. This does not mean just words; acts of omission may reveal as much as acts of commission.

One way to determine whether physicians are understanding their patients is if the physicians can anticipate their patients' thoughts. Physicians should keep these guesses to themselves, however, because jumping ahead of a patient's story is an infraction of the common courtesy of not interrupting. One of the most common means by which people determine whether another is listening to them is whether they think they are being interrupted. In addition, physicians who show patience in listening to their patients encourage these patients to think about what they are saying. This may lead to less superficial information being provided.

Some patients tend to ramble and test their physician's best efforts at listening patiently. Sometimes these patients ramble in any situation, or they may not know what kind of information the doctor needs, thereby leading them to be overly inclusive. One way to help such a patient is for the physician to tell the patient that there may be times during this talk when the physician will need to interrupt with questions. These questions are to better clarify and understand what the patient is saying. The physician tells the patient this ahead of time so the patient will not think the physician is being rude. Then, even if the physician must direct the discussion, the patient knows that the physician was not intending to slight the patient.

Appreciation

Empathy is the ability to care about the patient. Appreciation is the tangible expression of caring that is shown by being interested in the patient's story. Genuinely wanting to listen is half the battle. It demonstrates the physician's interest in the patient as a person and not as just a case; this interest usually helps patients talk more easily about what matters to them.

To know that the doctor is interested in "who I am" provides reassurance and fosters trust. Too often physicians talk about "care providers" who are really only "service providers." The difference is easily sensed. Physicians who keep one hand on the doorknob and convey a sense of insouciance, or those who call their patients by the wrong names, are viewed as uncaring when compared to physicians who pull up a chair, sit close, and show animated responses to what their patients say. Although both physicians are busy, the latter takes the time to be attentive. Physicians can help patients understand time constraints during a visit by telling patients at the beginning of their visit how much time the visit can take. Then full attention should be given during that time. To a degree, quality can make up for a lack of quantity.

Eye contact is also a means of showing interest in and appreciation of who the patient is. Eyes may or may not be the windows to the soul, but looking into someone's eyes always carries some kind of meaning. Interest, understanding, and caring may be better expressed to the patient by good eye contact than by most verbal approaches. Uncertainty, shame, and boredom may be revealed in poor eye contact. Physicians should be aware of the quality of their own eye contact, as well as that of their patients. Eye contact is one of the many nonverbal clues that reveals a patient's level of connectedness to the physician.

Repetition

By restating what the patient said, the physician not only makes sure that the information has been heard correctly, but also lets the patient know the physician was listening. If the patient often corrects the clarifying comment, then perhaps the physician was not listening as well as believed.

Bearing

Just as the cast on a fracture at some point may assist in weight-bearing in addition to providing its function of binding the wound, the aforementioned approach of active listening not only helps put the pieces together but also helps the patient bear the difficult situation of injury. Beyond listening techniques, other techniques help make the injury bearable, as a crutch may be of use in addition to the cast.

Patient Stories

One method for encouraging patients is to tell patients about similar situations that the physician has seen in the past in which another patient was successful. This is especially useful if the previous patient is someone with whom the patient can relate or identify, and whom the patient would want to emulate. This technique is useful not only because it provides some emotional removal from the immediate situation, but also because it provides a history of hope. Positive examples should always be used rather than ones that imply a threat of failure with noncompliance. These examples may help patients get in touch with their own feelings because they may no longer feel alone with the experience.

Informed Consent

Physicians often view informed consent as a necessary evil that impedes their efficiency in alleviating the suffering caused by illness. Why do we include it as a means of support to the patient? One of the most elegant arts in life is turning apparent liabilities into assets. Instead of considering the informed consent process an onerous duty, physicians can use it as a process for gathering information and as a forum for sharing the uncertainties inherent in medical care.[7]

In addition to minimizing malpractice liability, informed consent helps the patient face the reality that no outcome can be guaranteed and that there is risk in life. By sharing the reality of uncertainty, physicians not only help their patients deal with reality, but also serve as a model in coping with that situation. Most important, even though the outcome cannot be guaranteed, physicians can promise to be with their patients through any outcome. Patients need to be reassured that they will not be abandoned and that they are in this thing together.

Being with a patient throughout a poor outcome is part of being responsible to that patient; it has nothing to do with blame. Unfortunately, the legal forums often see blame and responsibility as synonyms, but caring physicians see responsibility as part of their role and separate from the issue of blame. Even though a physician may not be to blame for a bad outcome, that physician is still responsible for making the best of the situation with the patient. This is part of the difference between providing care and providing only a service.

Related to the area of informed consent is the issue of who makes treatment decisions. Patients must make their own decisions as long as they are competent. Struggling with patients about treatment decisions is usually a waste of time and frustrating for both patients and physicians. Making the options clear, even to the point of recommending an option, is reasonable. However, patients hold the ultimate authority. A patient may have issues of which the physician has no knowledge. Because this may occur, physicians should treat their patients as if patients are the bosses from the beginning. By doing so patients believe they are regarded as people of power and control. This also makes it easier for physicians to accept their patients' decisions and not feel insulted when patients choose to go against the advice given by their physicians.

Education

One way to approach healing is to educate patients in techniques that will help psychologically in the rehabilitation process. For example, a rehabilitating athlete often obsesses about the injury and its current stage of healing. This athlete also experiences an acute awareness of any sensation associated with the injury. This preoccupation is understandable but may interfere with the healing process. The patient may worry excessively and be hypersensitive to any sensation near the injured area. The patient needs to understand the difference between the pain of damage and the normal discomfort associated with the return to use. Being overly focused on the injured spot, constantly going through the range of motion to see how it feels, and being unable to focus on other things indicate that the injury is taking up too much of the patient's mental life and does not benefit the healing process. The physician should help the patient find ways to put aside the worrying and go on with the other aspects of daily life. Finding analogies in the patient's experience will help do this.

Case Example

When a pitcher obsessed about the surgical repair and rehabilitation of his shoulder, he found himself preoccupied with the situation in a way that intruded on his life. The analogy that worked for him was that of the "lock box," which is a personal safe for a baseball player to put a wallet, watch, ring, or other valuables into when coming into the clubhouse before a game. The box enables the baseball player to be free from concern about those valuables while out on the field. This patient understood that thinking about the injury should not be treated as unimportant; rather the injury should be treated by the patient as an important assessment, but not *all* of the time. The patient visualized a mental lock box into which he placed his worries and assessment. This athlete realized that, even though the thinking was an important process, it did not need to be done all the time.

Trying to eradicate the worrying does not work. Indeed, physicians want their patients to play an active part in assessing their progress. Finding familiar analogies, like telling stories, is a way to help patients deal with the healing process and emphasize that the patients already have methods of coping in their repertoire. This technique makes use of a preexisting strength.

Another common problem in the rehabilitation process is the athlete's belief that it is taking too long to mend and the fear that the athlete might never return to competitive form.

Case Example

A rehabilitating relief pitcher was experiencing dysphoria and anger after shoulder surgery. His coach referred him to the team psychiatrist. During discussions, the player discovered a new level of maturity when he found that he could be satisfied with small steps in the right direction and did not need to have his arm functioning at 100% immediately. Helping him realize that healing is a step-by-step process encouraged him and helped him realize that not everything in life is immediately gratifying, yet may eventually work out. An analogy of his many years spent achieving major-league proficiency in the first place was helpful. He did not achieve his success overnight. Too often athletes believe that they are either injured and on the disabled list or 100% healthy. Rather than view the situation as black or white, athletes need to see the situation in colors of reality.

Supporters of Injured Athletes

As busy practitioners, physicians cannot spend as much time with their patients as they might wish. A sensitive staff that relates well with patients can take the place of physicians and provide continuity of care from the operating room through the rehabilitation process. Physical therapists, who not only know their business but can serve as a communications link, are invaluable assets. In many cases, even though physicians set the approach, therapists are responsible for the implementation. Thinking in terms of a team approach is helpful, where the strengths of each team member are different and complementary. The entire team is dedicated to the patient's benefit. Remembering this goal can help the team deal with the inevitable turf issues that arise when the team's priorities are forgotten because of concern for individual team members or departments. A good model for personnel management has a team leader who worries about meeting the needs of the immediate subordinates. This helps each management level focus on the tasks for that group.[8]

In addition to the support provided by the treatment team, there are other kinds of support for rehabilitating athletes. Support groups made up of people experiencing similar types of rehabilitation can provide a forum to explore fears about the process. It is easier to bear any difficulty when people can bear it together. The Athletic Counseling and Treatment Institute,[1] a nonprofit organization, fosters the development of such groups nationwide and publishes a journal for rehabilitating athletes. Articles focus on various injuries, treatments, and the rehabilitation process. These articles are intended to inform athletes about what to expect and to decrease the sense of isolation athletes may be experiencing.

Medication

Occasionally psychotropic medications are needed in the treatment of rehabilitating athletes. For a professional or collegiate athlete, physicians must avoid prescribing a substance banned by that athlete's sport organizations. Each organization has a different list, and physicians should consult the organization if there is any doubt. Most organizations allow the use of antidepressants, when needed, and many permit the use of benzodiazepines. A knowledgeable psychiatrist should be consulted before using psychoactive medications to ensure that other therapeutic issues are not being overlooked, to ensure that issues of tolerance and addiction are addressed, and to determine which medications may be less sedating and less likely to interfere with the athlete's performance.

Confidentiality

A unique situation occurs when a professional athletic organization hires a physician to care for its athletes. The athletes and management often presume that the physician must report all information to the organization's management. In this situation, athletes may not reveal how much pain they are experiencing, especially during the rehabilitation process, because of its effect on contract negotiations. The physician should clearly explain the reporting relationship and the bounds of confidentiality so the patient can decide how much to confide in the physician. Professional athletes may hesitate to be totally honest because of the effect that a seemingly trivial comment might have on future negotiations.

Believing

> *The reasonable man adapts himself to the world. The unreasonable man persists in trying to adapt the world to himself. Therefore, all progress depends on the unreasonable man.*
>
> George Bernard Shaw

In the old question of whether a glass is half empty or half full, patients benefit by viewing the glass as half full. Optimism may actually lead to a greater probability of success in the treatment process.

The specialty of sports psychiatry gives us a psychologic illustration of this mind-body interaction. In golfing, the golfer can choose either to hit toward a target or to hit away from an obstacle. With the latter choice, the unconscious tends to view the area to be avoided as a negative target and perversely directs the action toward that target. The body tends to move action toward the mind's focus, regardless of the command. This conflict between the conscious and unconscious turns a simple command process into a psychologic battle that reduces the chance of success. The remedy is simple. Keep the messages to the conscious and unconscious the same by self-talking in positive languages[5] and hitting toward, not away from, targets.

This does not mean that just thinking positive thoughts always achieves positive results. It does illustrate, however, that positive thinking can improve probability. A hopeful patient has a better chance at success than a despondent one. Giving the patient the statistical odds of recovery is usually enough reality for the patient to assimilate over time. Some people's responses do, in fact, fall outside of the statistical norm; this is part of how norms are derived. Patients are not statistics, and helping them to be positive gives them the best opportunity to beat the bell-shaped curve. Physicians should foster hope, rather than denial. There is no such thing as false hope.[4] Hope is what propels people toward health.

SUMMARY

In all injuries there are psychologic components that can either help or hinder the healing process. Athletes have unique social and psychologic elements that require special attention, especially personality traits and aspects of grieving.

This chapter focuses on the physician's ability to observe and listen in ways that enable the physician to help patients through empathy, appreciation, and repetition. Approaches to informed consent, education about the healing process, other health professionals, medication use, and confidentiality also play a role in the rehabilitation process. Finally, promoting optimism and hope helps in healing and in sport.

References

1. Athletic Counseling and Treatment Institute, 134 N Payne Street, Alexandria, VA 22314.
2. Chan CS, Grossman HY: Psychological effects of running loss on consistent runners, *Percept Motor Skills* 66:875, 1988.
3. Cousins N: *Anatomy of an illness as perceived by the patient,* Toronto, 1979, Bantam Books.
4. Cousins N: Denial. Are sharper definitions needed? *JAMA* 248(2): 210, 1982.
5. Dorfman HA, Kuehl K: *The mental game of baseball,* South Bend, Indiana, 1989, Diamond Communications.
6. Euripides A: In Olyvova V: *Sports and games in the ancient world,* London, 1984, Orbis.
7. Gutheil T: Malpractice through the sharing of uncertainty, *N Engl J Med* 311(1):49, 1984.
8. Hawken P: *Growing a business,* New York, 1987, Fireside, Simon & Schuster.
9. Kubler-Ross E: *On death and dying,* New York, 1969, Macmillan.
10. Levin S: Does exercise enhance sexuality? *Phys Sports Med* 21(3):199, 1993.
11. Little JC: The athlete's neurosis—a deprivation crisis, *Acta Psychiatr Scand* 45:187, 1969.
12. Manson JE et al: A prospective study of exercise and incidence of diabetes among US male physicians, *JAMA* 268(1):63, 1992.
13. Margulies A, Havens L: The initial encounter: what to do first? *Am J Psychiatry* 138(4):421, 1981.
14. Moss N: The psychology of the aging athlete, *Clin Sports Med* 10(2):431, 1991.
15. Nicholi AM: Psychiatric consultations in professional football, *N Engl J Med* 316(17):1095, 1987.
16. Orr R: Personal and professional integrity in clinical medicine, *Update* 8(4):1, 1992.
17. Paffenbarger RS et al: The association of changes in physical-activity level and other lifestyle characteristics with mortality among men, *N Engl J Med* 328(8):538, 1993.
18. Scott SC: Current concepts in the rehabilitation of the injured athlete, *Mayo Clin Proc* 59:83, 1984.
19. Vaillant G: *Adaptation to life,* Boston, 1977, Little, Brown.
20. Wise A, Jackson DW, Rocchio P: Preoperative psychologic testing as a predictor of success in knee surgery, *Am J Sports Med* 7(5):287, 1979.

PART TWO

The Shoulder

CHAPTER 5

Biomechanics

MARILYN M. PINK
JACQUELIN PERRY

The shoulder is a highly mobile joint, with an estimated 16,000 positions of planar motions that can be differentiated by less than 1°.[9,43] This mobility comes from an absence of skeletal constraints, as well as from the versatility of the muscles that position the arm in space (the deltoids) and the muscles that contribute power to the overhead athletic maneuver (the pectoralis major and the latissimus dorsi). Balancing this mobility are components of stability. The stability is afforded by both static components (labrum, capsule, ligaments, and negative intraarticular pressure) and dynamic components of the muscles that protect the glenohumeral joint (the rotator cuff muscles) and the muscles that pivot the scapula (the scapular muscles).

To produce the high velocities, accelerations, moments, torques, and precise timing required in sports, all of these mobility and stability components must work together. An analogy is the synchronous motion of gears meshing to drive a motor (Fig. 5-1). If any one of the gears fails, all of the antecedent and subsequent gears become jammed, and injury ensues.

An understanding of the component gears during overhead athletic activities offers keys to optimal injury prevention, rehabilitation, and surgical procedures. Thus the purpose of this chapter is to discuss the static and dynamic components of mobility and stability in the shoulder. Baseball pitching and swimming will be used as paradigms to describe in three dimensions the uniqueness of the components in overhead athletes with normal and injured shoulders.

MOBILITY

The extreme mobility characteristics of the shoulder result from the skeletal configuration and from the muscular contributions. The shallow, dish-shaped glenoid af-

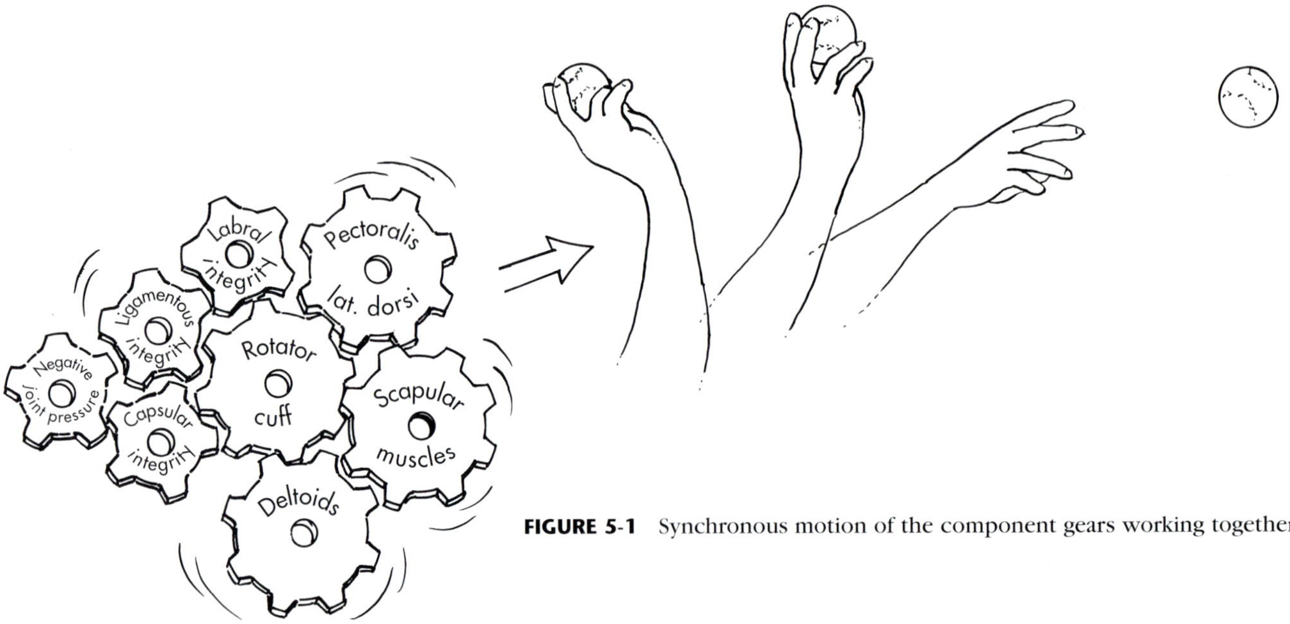

FIGURE 5-1 Synchronous motion of the component gears working together.

fords a surface on which the humeral head can pivot. The alignment of the glenoid (i.e., its tilt relative to the scapular axis) has been debated. Various authors have identified different upward/downward and retroversion/anteversion tilts.* Upon scrutiny, it is evident that the differences in opinion of the glenoid tilt are the result of differences in the method of measurement. Rather than discuss the technical differences in instrumentation at this point, note that the studies stand united in the opinion that the glenoid tilt varies widely among individuals, and thus the clinical implications vary widely. If an individual's glenoid faces upward or is retroverted, the glenoid then contributes a factor of stability as the fossa inhibits the humeral head subluxation inferiorly or anteriorly respectively. However, if an individual's glenoid faces downward or is anteverted, it allows for more vulnerability to inferior or anterior subluxation.

Three muscles contribute to gross glenohumeral mobility—the deltoids, pectoralis major, and latissimus dorsi. Because of their insertion distal to the axis of rotation, the deltoids clearly do not precisely center the humeral head in the glenoid but rather grossly place the arm in space. The rotator cuff muscles create a force couple with the deltoids to do the fine-tuning of humeral head placement. For this reason, the deltoids have been called the drivers; they get the humerus where it needs to go. The rotator cuff muscles have been called the steerers[51]; they ensure accurate positioning of the head in the glenoid. The pectoralis major and latissimus dorsi may be the only muscles that add power to overhead athletic activities. A study by Bartlett and associates[3] demonstrated that these muscles are the only two upper-extremity muscles that have a positive correlation between peak torque and pitching velocity. As will be seen later in this chapter, these muscles also demonstrate a phasic peak during the freestyle swim stroke.[45]

*References 4, 18, 31, 34, 46, 49-51, 55.

STABILITY

Static Component

The labrum has been described as both a consistent fibrocartilaginous structure[6,22] and a redundant fold of the capsular tissue.[36] Generally, the labrum is more meniscal superiorly and is more solidly attached to the bone inferiorly. There is a large degree of individual variation of the labrum, as there is of the glenoid, and there is no significant correlation between the size of the labrum and that of the glenoid (i.e., if the glenoid is large, the labrum is not always correspondingly large).[26] The additive result is numerous and unpredictable combinations of sizes. There are two relative consistencies in glenolabral anatomy. The first is that the anterior and inferior portions of the labrum are the largest within an individual, thus affording extra stability in these two critical directions.[26] The second is that the combination of the labrum and the glenoid approximately doubles the depth of the socket both anteroposteriorly and superoinferiorly.[29]

The depth of the glenohumeral socket in normal shoulders not only increases the surface area of contact with the humeral head, but also keeps it centered. Some investigators have described the head as rolling across the glenoid face from one margin to another.[15,51] Yet, such an intraarticular displacement does not occur.[55] Roentgenologic studies have only demonstrated a 3-mm upward shift during the first 30° of arm elevation, and only 1-mm shift thereafter.[46] In a separate study the humeral head was found to be relatively centered in the glenoid cavity throughout the horizontal plane of motion.[29] The maximum deviation was only 4 mm posterior to the center of the glenoid cavity during maximal horizontal humeral extension and external rotation. So, instead of allowing a rolling motion, the labrum forms a sufficiently deep socket to keep the humeral head centered. This supports the thought that a normal shoulder acts as a ball-and-socket joint.

People with dysfunctional shoulders exhibit variable and greater excursions of the humeral head on the glenoid. Poppen and Walker first reported this in the arcs of humeral planar motion.[46] Howell and associates also noted an increased anterior translation in the majority of patients with anterior instability when abducting the humerus to 90° and during horizontal extension.[28] Likewise, people with inferior and multidirectional instability demonstrated excessive excursion and sliding motions.[41] Obviously, people with dysfunctional shoulders are demonstrating glenohumeral instability, and their joints are not functioning as a ball seated within its socket.

The glenohumeral ligaments are also static stabilizers of the shoulder. The coracohumeral ligament bounds the superior aspect of the joint between the subscapularis and the supraspinatus, and reinforces the superior stability afforded by the cuff muscles.[11] The superior, middle, anteroinferior, and posteroinferior glenohumeral ligaments are of most interest when considering anterior instability. The general consensus from multiple researchers with different methodologies is that the superior glenohumeral ligament is the primary restraint when the humerus is adducted. As the arm abducts to 45°, the middle glenohumeral ligament becomes the main stabilizer. When the humerus reaches 90° of abduction, the inferior glenohumeral ligament plays the role of primary restraint.[12,17,38,54,56]

The joint capsule is the next layer of stability in the normal shoulder. The thickest portion of the capsule is the inferior portion.[40,54] When the arm is held in neutral rotation, this reinforces the thickened inferior portion of the labrum. When the arm is abducted and externally rotated, the inferior aspect of the capsule tightens to provide additional anterior support.

As overhead athletic activities require repetitive motions at 90° of humeral elevation, the anteroinferior glenohumeral ligament appears to be a critical provider of stability and also is at risk of injury. Intraoperative observations support this deduction, since the anteroinferior glenohumeral ligament is typically found to be lax. Likewise intraoperatively, anterior and inferior capsular laxity is noted. During positions of exaggerated humeral extension or abduction with external rotation (such as during the baseball pitch and the freestyle swim stroke), the humeral head can be angled to press against the anterior capsule and inferior glenohumeral ligament. With enough repetitions, this motion can stretch out the capsule and ligament. The best defense against the pathology of stretched anterior structures is to strengthen the anterior wall muscles (subscapularis, latissimus dorsi, pectoralis major, teres major), which reinforces the capsule and strengthens the muscles that afford posterior restraint in the vulnerable abducted/rotated position (infraspinatus, teres minor, supraspinatus).

Negative intraarticular pressure has recently been discussed as a means of static stability. Cadaver studies have shown that a vented capsule (thus a loss of negative intraarticular pressure) has an effect on superoinferior humeral translation.[7,20,25,32,56] Conceptually, if there is undersurface fraying of the rotator cuff caused by instability and impingement of the cuff between the superior glenoid rim and the humeral head, there is likely to be a loss of capsular integrity. The loss of integrity could mean a loss of capsular negative intraarticular pressure. This would result in additional instability. However, in the living human, the whole body is under negative intraarticular pressure. Thus the effect of loss of capsular integrity (i.e., a vented capsule and the presumable loss of negative intraarticular pressure) in patients may not be as dramatic as that evidenced in cadavers.

All of the static components of glenohumeral stability are noncontractile tissue but can be stretched. If damage has been done to any of these components, the options are either to compensate by strengthening the dynamic stabilizers through a carefully planned rehabilitation program and rest from the offending activity for 6 weeks, or to undergo a surgical repair. By understanding these static stabilizers, optimal surgical procedures can be developed. Ideally, however, the risk to these static structures is minimized through an exercise program. Following an exercise program requires an understanding of the dynamic stabilizers.

Dynamic Component

The scapular muscles and the rotator cuff muscles are the dynamic stabilizers. The scapular muscles position the glenoid for optimal alignment with the humeral head, and the rotator cuff muscles precisely position the head within the glenoid.

Multiple force couples are formed by the scapular muscles throughout the range of motion. The force couples are dynamic and change as the degree of scapular elevation, rotation, and protraction changes. By forming force couples, the muscles tether the scapula from every corner. If one corner were not controlled, scapular lag or scapular winging could occur. For example, to upwardly rotate the scapula, there are three complementary forces: upward rotation, medial contraction, and an anterolateral force from the inferior angle. The upper trapezius, lower trapezius, and upper three digitations of the serratus anterior work together for scapular upward rotation. The middle trapezius, levator scapulae, and rhomboids supply the medial force, and the last four digitations of the serratus anterior afford the anterolateral force at the inferior angle.[30,37] If any one of these muscles diminishes its contribution, the rest of the force couple would have to compensate, asynchronous scapular motion would occur, and the propensity toward injury would be enhanced. (In this example, please note the different functions of the upper and lower portions of the serratus anterior. Because of the relatively wide span of origin of the fibers on the ribs and the narrow area of insertion on the scapula, there are several different angles of pull.)

The rotator cuff muscles surround approximately one half of the glenohumeral joint as they approximate the humeral head into the glenoid and stabilize the joint throughout elevation.[5,50,53,54] The supraspinatus compresses the humeral head from the superior aspect of the joint. The subscapularis is just outside the capsule and thus it is the next layer of the anterior wall and the first contractile tissue barrier. The infraspinatus and teres minor help to center the axis of humeral rotation by depressing and retracting the head during elevation.[44,53]

The rotator cuff muscles are quite vulnerable to injury. One of the first muscles of the glenohumeral joint to fatigue is the supraspinatus.[24,27] The subscapularis also can easily become stretched in the case of recurrent dislocation and then becomes unable to function as an anterior wall muscle.[13] If any one of the rotator cuff muscles develops pain, a reflexive inhibition or premature fatigue may occur,[2,27] and the other muscles begin to compensate.[35] Thus when adding together fatigue, stretch, pain, and compensation, it is easy to see how the synchronous motion may break down.

The complexities of the gears of motion are multiplied when considering the scapular muscles and the rotator cuff muscles together. Not only must each muscle work synchronously within the group, but the groups must work together to optimally position the glenoid and to approximate the glenohumeral joint. When the scapular muscles and the rotator cuff muscles work with the deltoids and the pectoralis major and latissimus dorsi, the much-discussed scapulohumeral rhythm[1,8,46] and dynamic stability[5] are attained.

Thus the rotator cuff tendons, capsule, and ligaments are imbricated and surround the glenohumeral joint to provide stability.[10] Because of the interwoven nature of these structures, a lesion will most likely involve more than one isolated component. The scapular muscles, although not directly surrounding the glenohumeral joint, also provide stability by positioning the glenoid for optimal congruency with the humeral head. Therefore the aggregate effect of these tissues must be considered in understanding stability of the glenohumeral joint.

Now that the groundwork has been laid in understanding the static and dynamic components of mobility and of stability, the next level of understanding is the three-dimensional paradigms of the overhead athlete. The basic arm mechanics are similar in the baseball pitch,[14] tennis serve,[48] volleyball serve, and the javelin throw.[23] Because the most extensive biomechanical studies have examined the baseball pitch, the pitching motion is used for the first paradigm for overhead activity. Freestyle swimming is also a common overhead activity, but has slightly different mechanics. Thus the freestyle swimming stroke serves as the second model of overhead activity.

BASEBALL PITCHING

The six consecutive phases of the baseball pitch are as follows:

1. Wind-up: begins with the start of motion and ends when the nondominant hand leaves the ball.
2. Early cocking: continues until the front foot comes into contact with the ground.
3. Late cocking: ends with maximal humeral external rotation.
4. Acceleration: terminates at the point of ball release.
5. Deceleration: is the first one third of the time from ball release to the end of arm motion.
6. Follow-through: is the last two thirds of the time from ball release to the end of arm motion (Fig. 5-2).

Wind-up

The wind-up phase is relatively nonchallenging for the shoulder. Both hands are in contact with the ball, and the muscles demonstrate relatively low activity in both the normal and unstable shoulders.[14,21] There are no known differences in the mechanics of normal and unstable shoulders during this phase.[21]

Early Cocking

In early cocking the shoulder is abducted to 104° and externally rotated to 46°.[16] Two force couples are formed during early cocking—one for the scapular motion and one for glenohumeral motion. The goal of the scapular muscles is to position the glenoid for the humeral head as the arm moves into abduction. The scapula is then a stable platform on which the humeral head can move. The upper and lower trapezius muscles upwardly rotate the scapula as they pull on the spine of the scapula. At the same time, the serratus anterior pulls the inferior angle upward, and the middle trapezius, rhomboids, and levator scapulae retract the superior, medial border of the scapula.[14] Each scapular muscle is active to ensure smooth movement of this relatively large, smooth, and free-floating bone (Fig. 5-3).

The three heads of the deltoid and the supraspinatus are synergistically working during early cocking to elevate the humerus.[14] The supraspinatus, which inserts closer to the joint axis than does the deltoid, helps to keep the humeral head congruent with the glenoid and

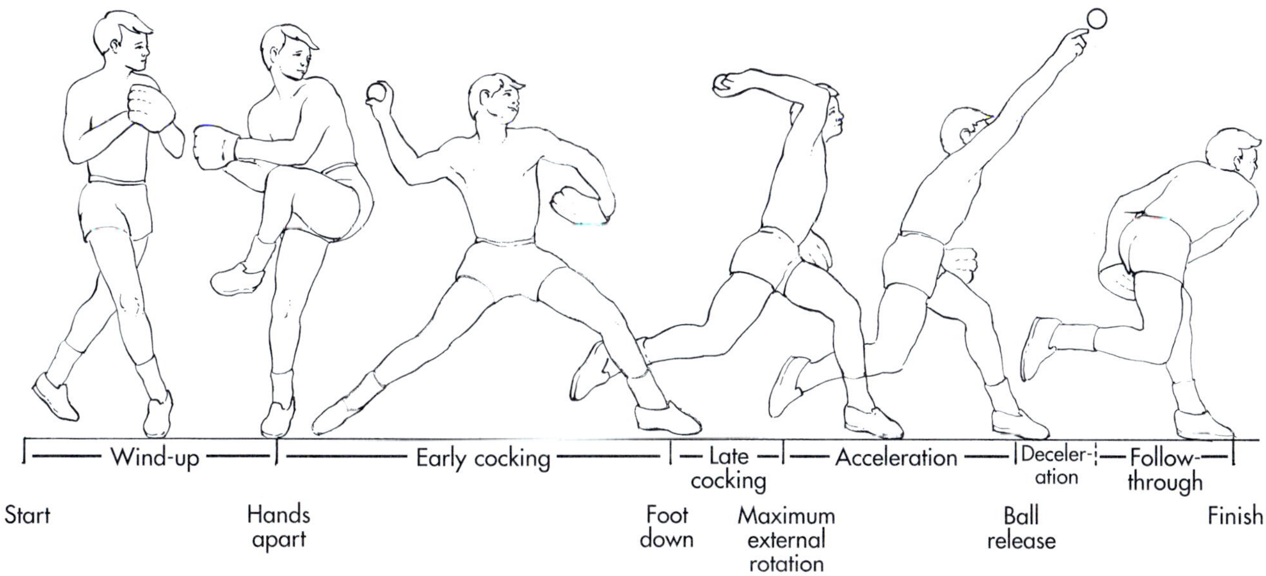

FIGURE 5-2 Phases of the baseball pitch.

prevents the head from riding up the glenoid rim (Fig. 5-4). If the deltoids were to abduct the humerus without the supraspinatus, they would be able to mechanically displace the humeral head. The deltoids position the arm in space, and the supraspinatus stabilizes the head within the glenoid. The relationship of the deltoid and supraspinatus has been noted during planar motions as well.[30] This separates the supraspinatus from the rotators of the rotator cuff and functionally aligns it with the deltoids for humeral elevation.

There are no significant differences during early cocking in the normal and unstable shoulders during the baseball pitch.[21]

Late Cocking

During late cocking the humerus maintains its level of abduction and moves into the scapular plane while externally rotating from 46° to 170°.[16] In this position the head of the humerus is angled so that it can stretch the anterior structures. This creates the potential for anterior instability and the resultant impingement. If the muscles of the anterior wall are fatigued, the propensity toward overstretching is intensified. In that the anterior structures are functionally stretched (and actually stretched beyond the desired balance of stability and mobility) during the pitching motion, there is no need to further stretch the anterior structures with pregame stretches. The additional pregame stretching would only increase the risk for injury.

Because the humerus maintains, rather than increases, its elevation during late cocking, the scapula does not need additional elevation. However, it does need to provide a stable base for the external rotation of the

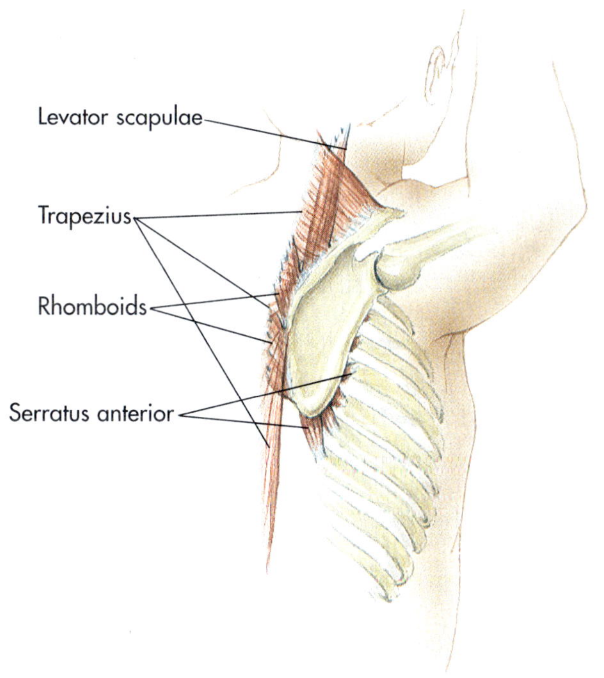

FIGURE 5-3 Force couple of the upper, middle, and lower trapezius, serratus anterior, rhomboids, and levator scapulae during the early cocking phase of the baseball pitch.

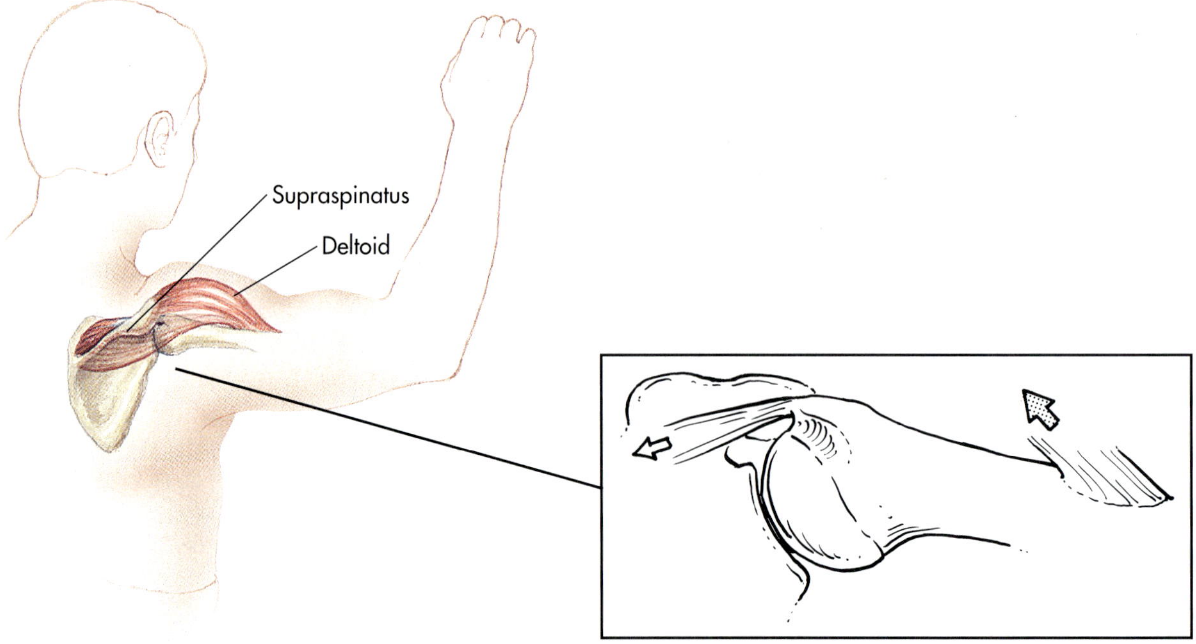

FIGURE 5-4 Supraspinatus and deltoids function together during the early cocking phase of the baseball pitch.

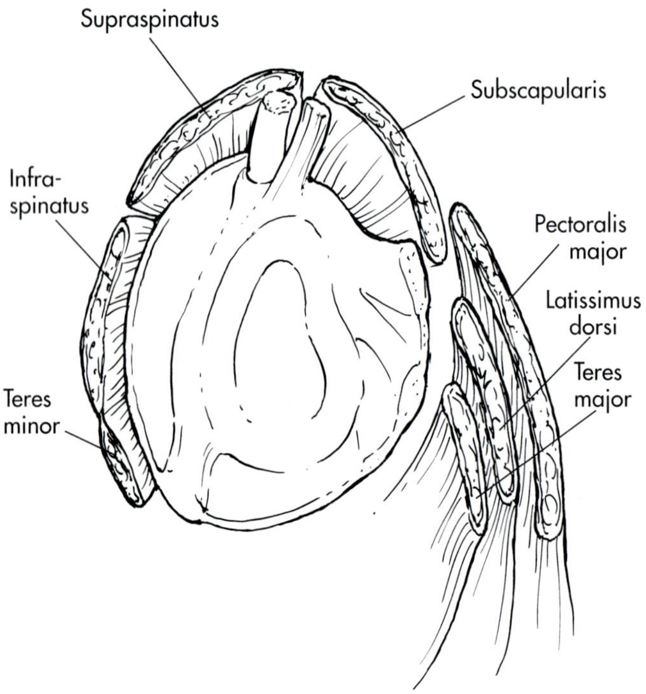

FIGURE 5-5 Position of the tendons and ligaments around the glenohumeral joint in the position of 90° abduction and 90° external rotation. (Modified from Turkel et al.[54])

humerus. The middle trapezius, rhomboids, and levator scapulae have all been shown to be scapular retractors that function isometrically at the end of the range.[37] These are key muscles in providing scapular stabilization. The serratus anterior is the key muscle opposing the retractors while stabilizing and protracting the scapula.[14] In addition to forming a force couple for stabilization, these muscles may help to "tip" the scapula so that the glenoid offers maximum congruency for the humeral head.

At this time the subscapularis, pectoralis major, and latissimus dorsi are all anterior to the glenohumeral joint. Turkel and associates[54] described the relative position of the tendons and ligaments around the glenohumeral joint in a position of 90° abduction and 90° external rotation (Fig. 5-5). Although this is not exactly the humeral position during late cocking, it is a similar example of the dynamics of positioning and demonstrates the position of the muscles that form the anterior wall along with the capsule and the ligaments. The anterior wall provides stability to the anterior aspect of the joint.

The posterior rotator cuff muscles are also quite active during late cocking.[14] The infraspinatus and teres minor are externally rotating the humerus. In addition, their posterior placement offers a posterior restraint to the anterior subluxation as they hold the humeral head back (Fig. 5-6).

In the position of extreme external rotation the supraspinatus is rotated posteriorly. At this point the supraspinatus is relatively ineffective as a superior compressive force. In part, this force may be provided by the

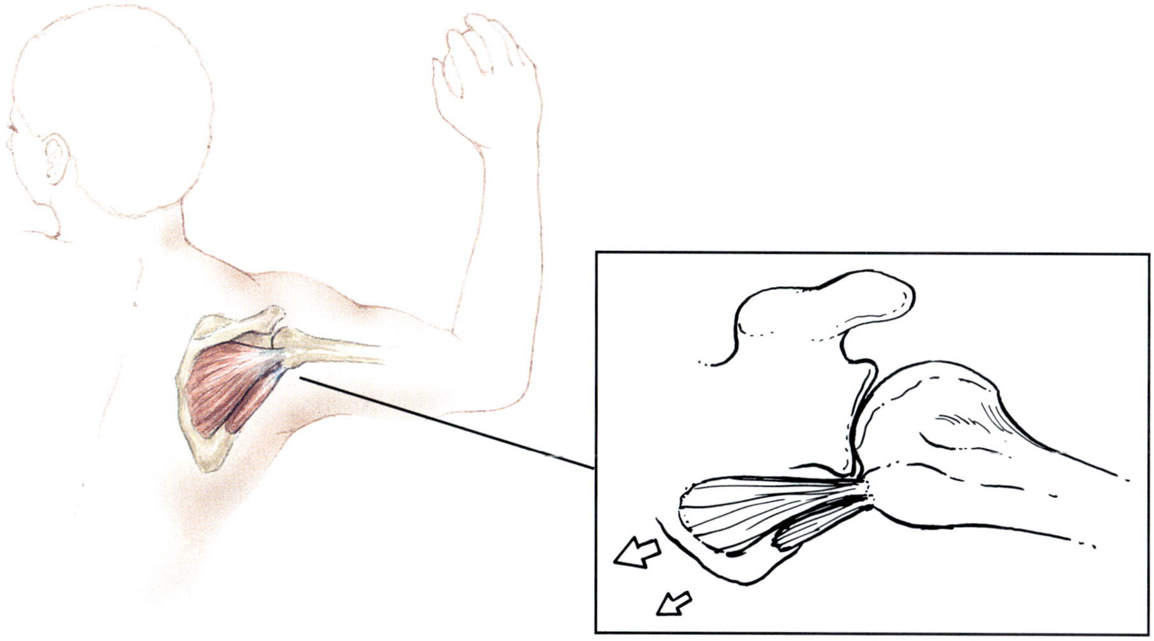

FIGURE 5-6 Posterior restraint of the infraspinatus and teres minor during the late cocking phase of the baseball pitch.

subscapularis, which is now positioned superiorly. The electromyographic firing pattern supports this, because the upper portion of the subscapularis is more active than the lower portion, and it is more active than the supraspinatus.[14] This shows that the subscapularis has different functions when it is in different positions. Also, the angle of pull differs within the broad origin of fibers.

Baseball pitchers with unstable shoulders demonstrated several significant differences from pitchers with normal shoulders during the late cocking phase. First, the serratus anterior was significantly less active.[21] This can be related to the clinical world because one of the most subtle signs of impending injury is scapular lag, winging, or asymmetry. When the serratus anterior is no longer able to perform adequately, no other muscles can effectively substitute. In this subtle stage, the astute eye of the coach or medical practitioner notes that the player tends to drop the elbow. The "dropped elbow" is really decreasing the degree of necessary scapular elevation. In the next level of pathology, the player may begin with some compensatory mechanics, such as moving the humerus into the coronal plane (Fig. 5-7). When the humerus moves into the coronal plane, the head of the humerus angles even further anteriorly. The player also loses some external rotation.

Experience has shown that if the scapular asynchrony can be identified at the earliest stage, even before the athlete complains of pain or before there is a tangible consistent drop in performance, then he can be pulled off the field and put on a specific strengthening program to prevent anatomic damage to the static stabilizers.

Chronically unstable shoulders have also demonstrated significantly less activity in the subscapularis and pectoralis major.[21] The result of this is obviously a lack of support to the anterior wall.

As the subscapularis becomes less active in pitchers with unstable shoulders, the supraspinatus becomes more active.[21] This could be partially related to a decrease in humeral external rotation. If the humerus is not rotated to quite the degree of the normal shoulder, the supraspinatus moves back into position to offer the superior compression to the humeral head.

Acceleration

During acceleration the humerus internally rotates about 100° in 0.05 second. Very high angular velocities, torques, and joint compressive forces are reported at this time.[16,19,42] A stable scapula is needed as a fulcrum for the high angular velocities and torques. In keeping with this, the scapular muscles all demonstrate relatively high activity during the acceleration phase.[14]

As the humerus internally rotates, the posterior deltoid is optimally positioned to restrain the humerus with horizontal abduction (Fig. 5-8), as noted by its extremely high electrical activity. The supraspinatus also is highly active as it again demonstrates its relationship to the deltoid.[14]

The teres minor demonstrates much higher activity than the infraspinatus during acceleration.[14] This may have clinical relevance, because posterior cuff tenderness in baseball pitchers can frequently be isolated to the teres minor. In addition, during electromyographic manual muscle testing, there were higher levels of activity in

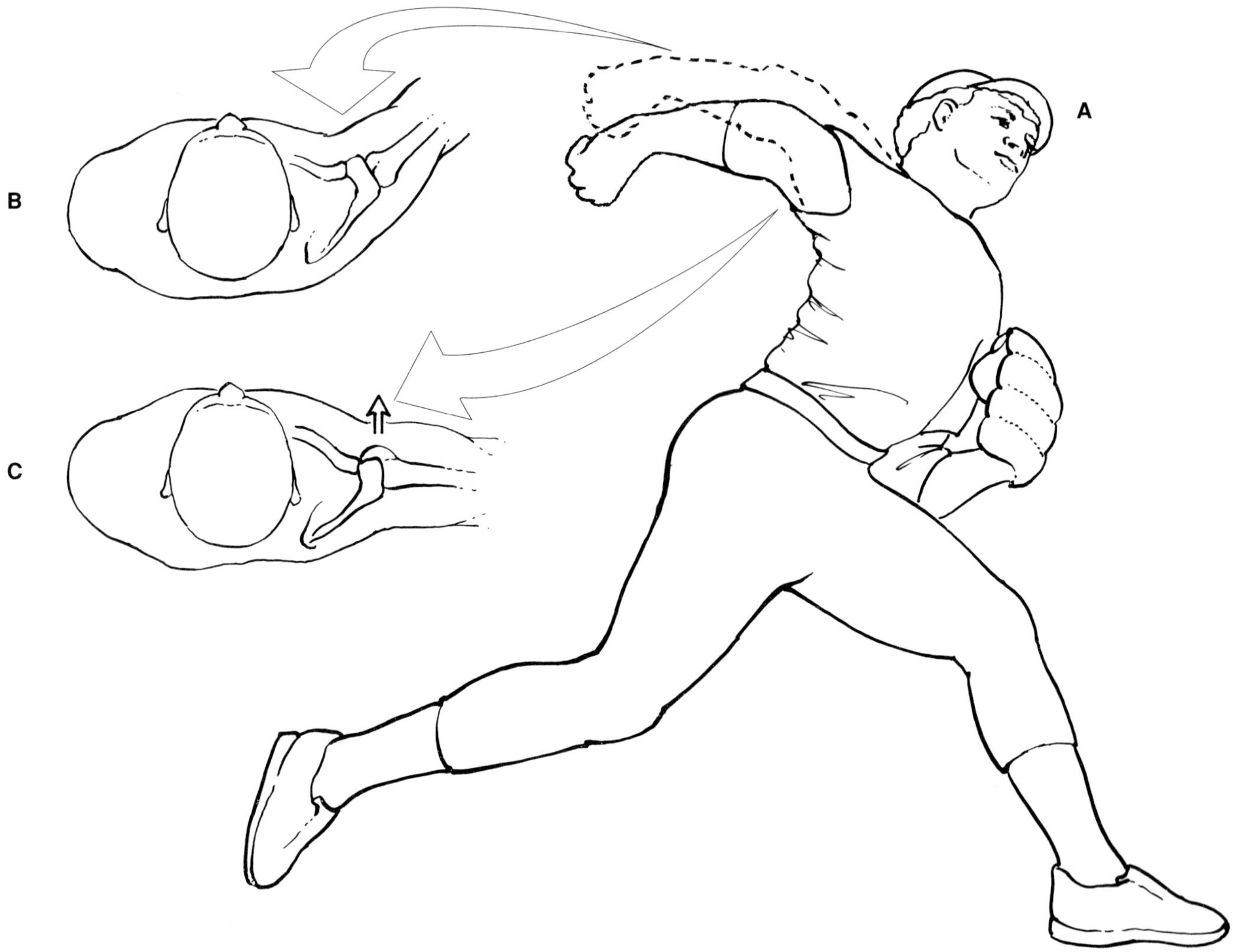

FIGURE 5-7 **A,** Baseball pitching mechanics with humerus moving from the scapular plane to the coronal plane. **B** and **C,** Overhead view of humerus moving from scapular plane (normal mechanics) to the coronal plane (poor mechanics).

the teres minor than in the infraspinatus when the humerus was abducted or extended. A subtle but important point exemplified here is that the teres minor and infraspinatus function differently from each other.

The pectoralis major and teres minor form a force couple during acceleration. As the pectoralis major forcefully contracts at high elevation[14] for adduction and internal rotation, the teres minor holds the head back and controls the humeral internal rotation. The direction of fibers of the teres minor gives it an extension component, which may be the reason it outperforms the infraspinatus in this position.

The subscapularis, especially the upper portion, also exhibits very high activity during this phase and functions with the latissimus dorsi and the pectoralis major.[14] The insertion of the subscapularis is closer to the joint axis of rotation than is the insertion of the pectoralis major and latissimus dorsi. This allows the subscapularis to function as a steering muscle as it precisely positions the humeral head in the glenoid. This is similar to the relationship of the supraspinatus with the deltoid.

The large angular velocity during acceleration is the result of energy that is transferred from the ground reaction force, through the trunk, and up to the arms. As previously mentioned, the latissimus dorsi and pectoralis major may be the only upper-extremity muscles to augment that force.[3] During this time, these muscles exhibit a peak of muscle activity.[21]

Pitchers with unstable shoulders demonstrate several significant differences from pitchers with normal shoulders.[21] First, the serratus anterior is less active. This is a carryover from the late cocking phase with the same clinical implications. Additionally, the latissimus dorsi and subscapularis are less active. The force couple they form in the pitchers with normal shoulders is not in effect. The support for the anterior wall is also diminished.

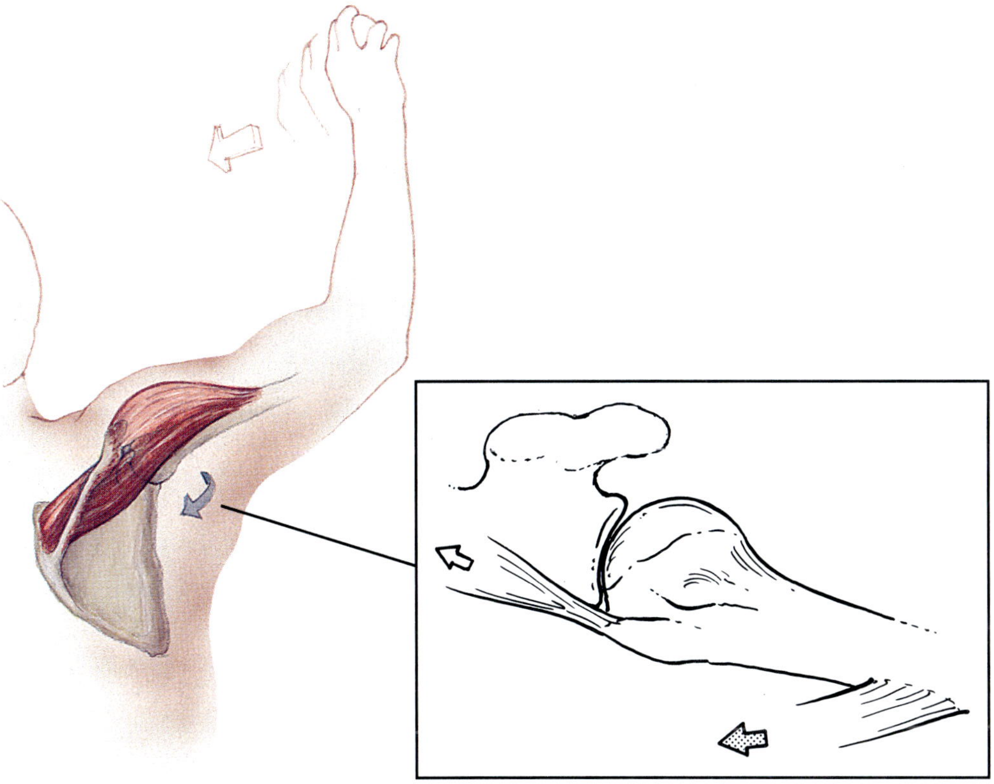

FIGURE 5-8 Posterior restraint of the posterior deltoid and supraspinatus during the acceleration phase of the baseball pitch.

Furthermore, the augmentation of power supplied by the latissimus dorsi is no longer present. All of these factors demonstrate the compound effect of the loss of the smooth gear functioning and, as a result, asynchronous motion.

Deceleration

The deceleration phase is the first one third of the time from ball release to the end of arm motion. During this phase the excess kinetic energy that was not transferred to the ball is dissipated. As in the acceleration phase, there are high calculated forces and torques.[7,17] In general, all posterior muscles of the shoulder are active to control the deceleration. The teres minor demonstrates the highest level of activity of all the glenohumeral muscles. This is a carryover of its activity in the acceleration phase and is clinically substantiated by the posterior rotator cuff pain, which can be isolated to the teres minor in baseball pitchers and can be reproduced in a motion mimicking the deceleration phase. The teres minor pain is frequently noted during spring training; it is because of the intensity of throwing when this muscle has been deconditioned during the off-season.

The latissimus dorsi is more active than the pectoralis major during deceleration.[14] This is logical because the pectoralis major loses its mechanical advantage when the humerus drops below 90° elevation. The subscapularis also has high activity.[14] In its role as a companion muscle to the latissimus dorsi, it creates an anterior compressive force to stabilize the humeral head as the joint rapidly rotates inward.

Unstable shoulders exhibit the same patterns of muscle firing as that seen in the normal shoulders during the deceleration phase.

Follow-through

Follow-through appears to be a fairly inconsequential motion for the shoulder. The serratus anterior is the only muscle in the normal pitcher that demonstrates activity above 35% of the maximum.[14] It is active as it protracts the scapula when the arm finishes its movement across the body.

In a comparison of pitchers with unstable shoulders and those with normal shoulders, the only significant differences in muscle activity were a decrease of both the latissimus dorsi and serratus anterior in the pitchers with unstable shoulders. These two large muscles obviously diminish their functions for scapular protraction, humeral adduction, and internal rotation.

In pitching there are multiple force couples that ensure optimal scapular and humeral motion. The dynamic concept of force couples communicates the complexities of muscles working together, as opposed to muscles working in isolation. These force couples combine and trade-off with one another for smooth functioning in the normal shoulder. Pitchers with unstable shoulders demonstrate a logical diminution of specific muscles, and the result is asynchronous motion.

FREESTYLE SWIMMING

The four consecutive phases of the freestyle stroke are as follows:

1. Early pull-through: begins with the hand entering the water and ends when the humerus is perpendicular to the axis of the torso.
2. Late pull-through: continues until the point that the hand exits the water.
3. Early recovery: terminates at the point when the humerus is perpendicular to the water's surface.
4. Late recovery: ends at the point when the hand enters the water again (Fig. 5-9).

Although hand entry into the water is used to designate the beginning of pull-through, the first underwater action is still a forward reach. Only after the maximum arm length is attained is the motion reversed to a pull.

The hand enters forward of and lateral to the head, and just medial to the shoulder. The flexed elbow is above the hand, so that the fingers are the first to enter the water with the palm facing out.[33] This is similar to clinical tests for impingement (Fig. 5-10). Current research on cadavers demonstrates that the impingement is of the anterior rotator cuff on the anterosuperior glenolabral rim (Fig. 5-11).

At the time of hand entry, there is a peak of muscle action in the upper trapezius, rhomboids, supraspinatus, anterior and middle deltoids, and serratus anterior.[45] The two force couples at work here are similar to those discussed during the baseball pitch. The serratus anterior is upwardly rotating the scapula and protracting the inferior border while the rhomboids are retracting the medial superior border and the upper trapezius is upwardly rotating the scapula. This muscle action positions the glenoid fossa for the humeral head as the arm is abducted and flexed by the supraspinatus and anterior and middle deltoids.

The hand follows an S-shaped curve during the pull-through phase[47] (Fig. 5-12). The pectoralis major and the teres minor fire initially.[45] This is another force couple not unlike that found in pitching. The pectoralis major, one of the two upper-extremity power muscles, fires while the arm is elevated above 90°. As the pectoralis major propels the body over the arm by adducting, extending, and internally rotating the humerus, the teres minor counterbalances the strong internal rotation force.

Swimmers with painful shoulders have a different pattern of hand entry than do those with normal shoulders. The hand enters further away from midline, and the humerus is lower to the water. Coaches note this position as a dropped-elbow position and remark that they can tell when swimmers are hurt, tired, or lazy because they fail to hold the elbow up. Actually, the dropped elbow is a result of decreased humeral elevation and internal rotation. This is consistent with the significant decrease in activity in the anterior and middle deltoids. In addition, the scapula does not need to be upwardly rotated or retracted as much in this position. Accordingly, there is significantly less activity in the upper trapezius and rhomboids. This position of hand entry avoids the

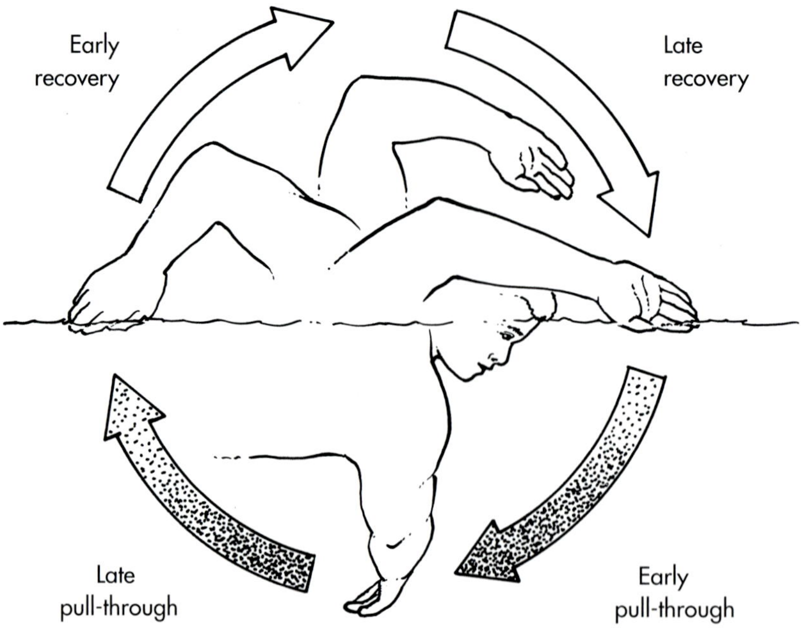

FIGURE 5-9 Four phases of the freestyle swim stroke.

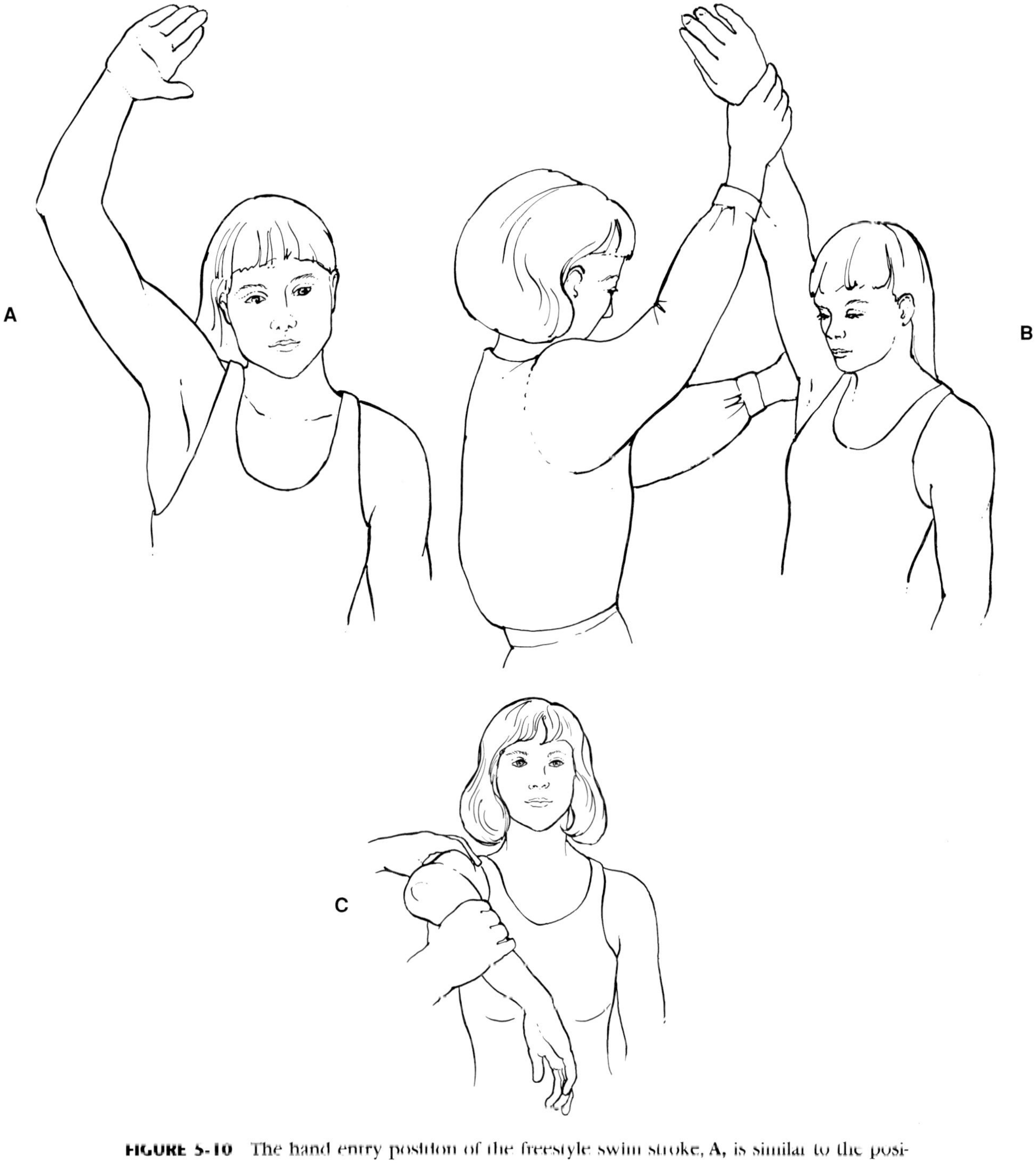

FIGURE 5-10 The hand entry position of the freestyle swim stroke, **A,** is similar to the positions of the Neer and Hawkins clinical tests for impingement, **B** and **C.**

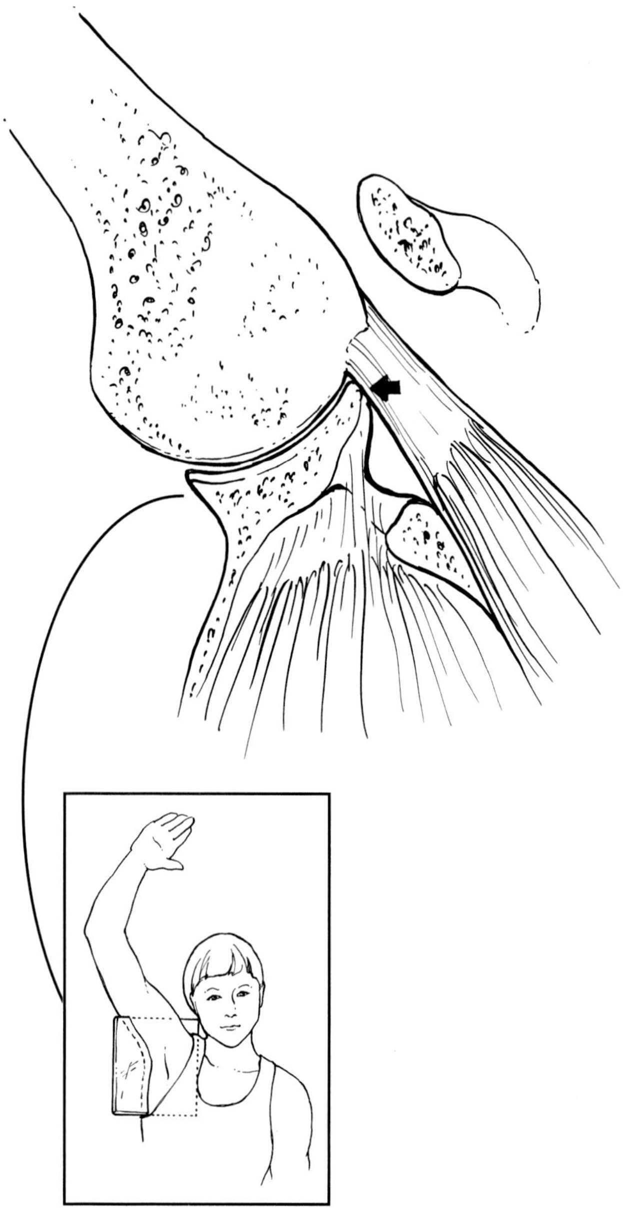

FIGURE 5-11 Impingement at hand entry is on the anterosuperior glenoid rim.

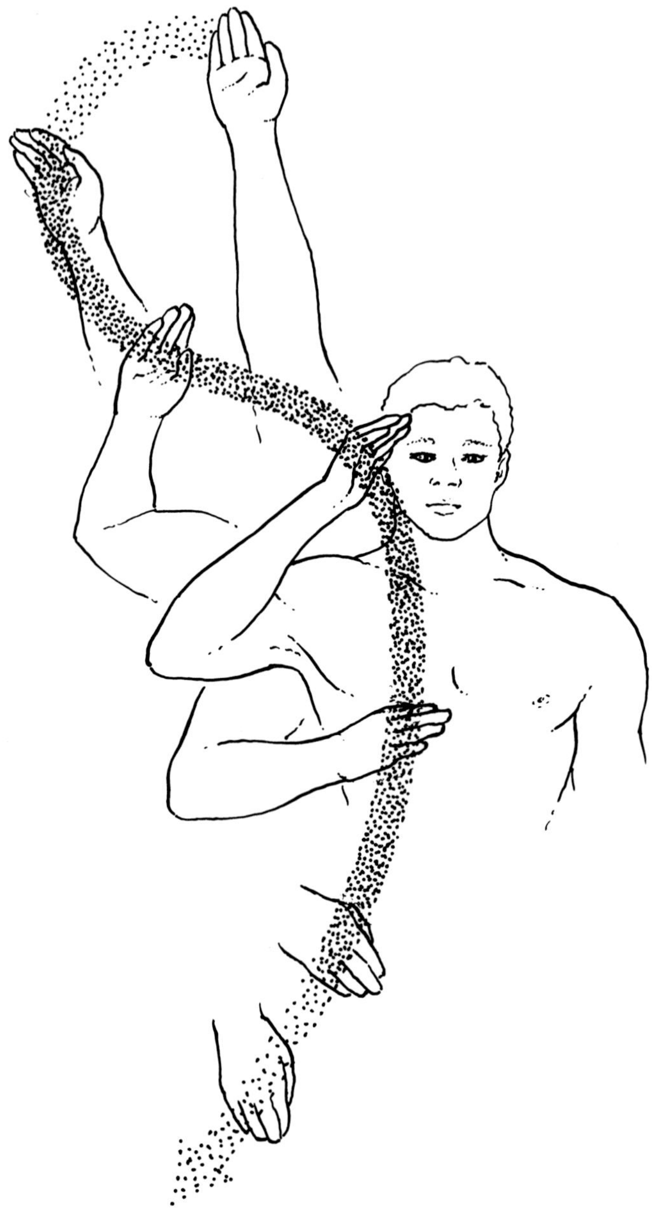

FIGURE 5-12 S-shaped curve during the freestyle swim stroke.

classic impingement position of humeral forward flexion described by Neer and Welsh,[39] which is now known to be an impingement of the supraspinatus on the glenoid.

After the humerus crosses the point where it is perpendicular to the body, the latissimus dorsi becomes the propulsive force in swimmers with normal shoulders as the latissimus dorsi now has the mechanical advantage. The trade-off of the pectoralis major firing at elevations above 90° and the latissimus dorsi firing at levels below 90° was also seen in pitching. The subscapularis fires with the latissimus dorsi to protect the glenohumeral joint as the humerus internally rotates. The serratus anterior is also active throughout pull-through as it stabilizes the scapula and pulls the body over the arm. At the end of the pull-through phase, the deltoids and supraspinatus become active to lift the extended humerus out of the water.[45]

Swimmers with painful shoulders demonstrated several differences from swimmers with normal shoulders during the pull-through phase. The most dramatic difference is the significantly depressed action of the serratus anterior and the significantly increased action of

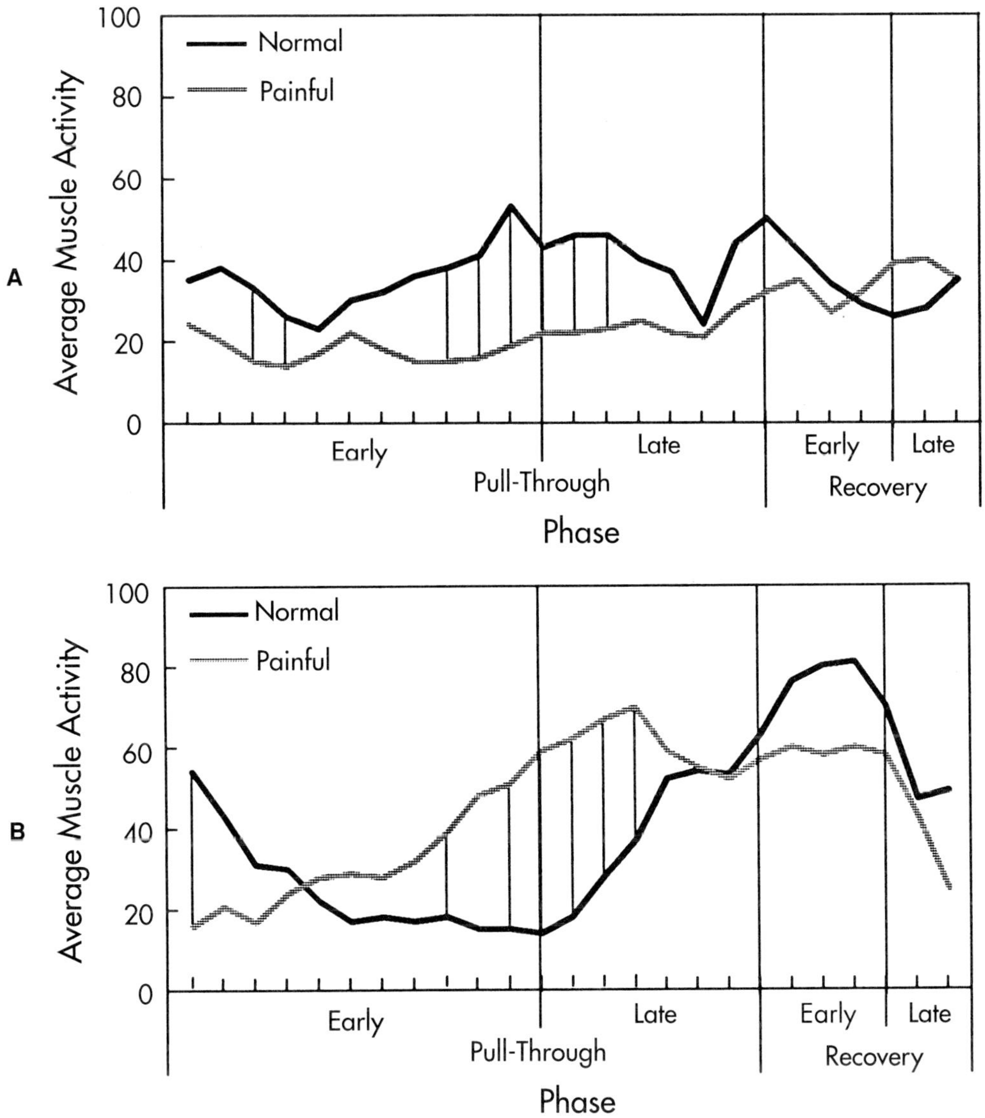

FIGURE 5-13 **A,** Muscle activity of the serratus anterior in swimmers with normal and painful shoulders. Vertical lines show periods of significant differences. **B,** Muscle activity of the rhomboids in swimmers with normal and painful shoulders. Vertical lines show periods of significant differences.

the rhomboids[52] (Fig. 5-13). The serratus anterior may well fatigue in swimmers with painful shoulders. As a result the scapula would not be a stable base for humeral motion. Fatigue is highly probable in that the serratus anterior is consistently active throughout the stroke. Competitive swimmers frequently undergo high-mileage workouts, and the potential of fatigue is multiplied. To compensate for an unstable scapula, the rhomboids fire. The rhomboids may be able to stabilize the scapula, but oddly enough the function of the rhomboids is directly opposite that of the serratus anterior. Thus the compensatory action could not possibly lead to smooth functioning.

At the end of pull-through, the infraspinatus in swimmers with painful shoulders increases its activity while the anterior deltoid action is reduced.[52] The infraspinatus is probably increasing the humeral external rotation to avoid the painful extreme in internal rotation with the humerus in hyperextension. In addition, the position of extreme internal rotation with humeral hyperextension can cause the humeral head to stretch the anterior structures. This could lead to anterior instability. At this time, coaches note a blunting of humeral lift (i.e., a dropped elbow); thus the decreased action of the anterior deltoid is reasonable.

Recovery is a much shorter phase than pull-through. The purpose of recovery is simply to bring the arm into position to pull once again. The sequence of muscle action in the normal shoulder is to lift and abduct the humerus (middle deltoids and supraspinatus), retract the scapula (rhomboids), internally rotate the humerus (subscapularis), and finally externally rotate the humerus to swing the forearm and hand forward (infraspinatus).[45] The hand is then in position to enter the water again.

Swimmers with painful shoulders continue with their lower arc of motion and dropped elbow during recovery. Thus the anterior deltoid in these swimmers continues to demonstrate depressed action. The subscapularis also has decreased activity.[52] Like the serratus anterior in the normal population, this muscle is constantly firing. As a result, there is potential for fatigue. The decreased action of the subscapularis also may allow more humeral external rotation rather than the extreme, and painful, internal rotation.

To summarize freestyle swimming, the two muscles that appear most likely to fatigue are the serratus anterior and the subscapularis. If they were to fatigue, the smooth interactive gear motion undoubtedly would be upset. This information is clinically applied by placing freestyle swimmers with painful shoulders on a specific strengthening program for the serratus anterior and subscapularis. These swimmers are frequently able to return to their prior level of competition without surgical intervention.

SUMMARY

The extreme mobility of the glenohumeral joint is the result of the lack of skeletal restraint and the muscle action around the joint. The mobility is balanced by the stability afforded by the labrum, capsule, ligaments, negative intraarticular pressure, and muscles of the rotator cuff and the scapula. By understanding the tissues that are at risk in specific sports and by understanding muscle mechanics, an effective and efficient exercise program can be designed to prevent and rehabilitate injury. Severe damage of the noncontractile tissue may result from the high velocities, great forces, extreme ranges of motion, and repetition of the motion. If rehabilitation fails, surgery may be necessary. This process for understanding sport mechanics and muscle mechanics demonstrates the inextricable union of function, injury prevention, rehabilitation, and surgery. This knowledge also allows a dynamic problem-solving approach when problems occur in the athlete. Furthermore, it helps to identify the core of the problem rather than focusing on the symptomatology.

References

1. Bagg S, Forrest W: A biomechanical analysis of scapular rotation during arm abduction in the scapular plane, *Am J Phys Med Rehabil* p 238, 1988.
2. Bain AM: Supraspinatus tendinitis, *Physiotherapy* 57:17, 1971.
3. Bartlett LR, Storey MD, Simons BD: Measurement of upper extremity torque production and its relationship to throwing speed in the competitive athlete, *Am J Sports Med* 17:89, 1989.
4. Basmajian JV, Bazant FJ: Factors preventing downward dislocation of the adducted shoulder joints: an electromyographic and morphological study, *J Bone Joint Surg* 41A:1182, 1959.
5. Blasier R, Guldberg R, Rothman E: Anterior shoulder stability: contributions of rotator cuff forces and the capsular ligaments in the cadaver model, *J Shoulder Elbow Surg* 1(3):140, 1992.
6. Bost FC, Inman VT: The pathological changes in recurrent dislocation of the shoulder, *J Bone Joint Surg* 24(3):595, 1942.
7. Browne AO et al: Glenohumeral elevation studied in three dimensions, *J Bone Joint Surg* 72B:843, 1990.
8. Calliet R: *Shoulder pain,* ed 2, Philadelphia, 1981, Davis.
9. Carpenter JL, Blasier RB, Pellizon GG: The effect of muscular fatigue on shoulder proprioception, 19th Annual Meeting of the Orthopedic Research Society, San Francisco, Calif, Feb 1993, p 311.
10. Clark M, Harryman DT: Tendons, ligaments, and capsule of the rotator cuff: gross and microscopic anatomy, *J Bone Joint Surg* 74A (5):713, 1992.
11. Clark J, Sidles JA, Matsen FA: The relationship of the glenohumeral joint capsule to the rotator cuff, *Clin Orthop* 254:29, 1990.
12. Connell P et al: The contribution of the glenohumeral ligaments to anterior stability of the shoulder joint, *Am J Sports Med* 18(6): 579, 1990.
13. DePalma AF, Cooke AJ, Prabhakar M: The role of the subscapularis in recurrent anterior dislocation of the shoulder, *Clin Orthop* 54:35, 1967.
14. DiGiovine N et al: An electromyographic analysis of the upper extremity in pitching, *J Shoulder Elbow Surg* 1(1):15, 1992.
15. Dvir Z, Berme N: The shoulder complex in elevation of the arm: a mechanism approach, *Biomechanics* 11:219, 1978.
16. Feltner M, Dapena J: Dynamics of the shoulder and elbow joints of the throwing arm during a baseball pitch, *Int J Sports Biomech* 2:235, 1986.
17. Ferrari D: Capsular ligaments of the shoulder anatomical and functional study to the anterior superior capsule, *Am J Sports Med* 18(1):20, 1990.
18. Freedman L, Munro RR: Abduction of the arm in the scapular plane: scapular and glenohumeral movements, *J Bone Joint Surg* 48A: 1503, 1966.
19. Gainor BJ et al: The throw: biomechanics and acute injury, *Am J Sports Med* 8:114, 1980.
20. Gibb TD et al: The effect of capsular venting on glenohumeral laxity, *Clin Orthop* 268:120, 1991.
21. Glousman R et al: Dynamic electromyographic analysis of the throwing shoulder with glenohumeral instability, *J Bone Joint Surg* 70A(2):220, 1988.
22. Gray H: *Gray's anatomy: anatomy of the human body,* Philadelphia, 1973, Lea & Febiger.
23. Gregor R, Pink M: Biomechanics analysis of a world record javelin throw: a case study, *Int J Sports Biomech,* 1985.
24. Hagberg M: Electromyographic signs of shoulder muscular fatigue in two elevated arm positions, *Am J Phys Med* 60(3):111, 1981.
25. Harryman D et al: Laxity of the normal glenohumeral joint: a quantitative in vivo assessment, *J Shoulder Elbow Surg* 2:66, 1992.
26. Hata Y et al: Anatomic study of the glenoid labrum, *J Shoulder Elbow Surg* p 207, 1992.
27. Herberts P, Kadefors R: A study of painful shoulder in welders, *Acta Orthop Scand* 47:381, 1976.
28. Howell S, Galinat BJ: The glenoid-labral socket, *Clin Orthop* 243: 122, 1989.

29. Howell SM et al: Normal and abnormal mechanics of the glenohumeral joint in the horizontal plane, *J Bone Joint Surg* 70A:227, 1988.
30. Inman VT, Saunders DM, Abbott CL: Observations of the functions of the shoulder joint, *J Bone Joint Surg* 26A:1, 1944.
31. Itoi E et al: Scapular inclination and inferior stability of the shoulder, *J Shoulder Elbow Surg* 1(3):131, 1992.
32. Kumar VP, Balsubrananian P: The role of atmospheric pressure in stabilizing the shoulder: an experimental study, *J Bone Joint Surg* 67B(5):719, 1985.
33. Maglischo EW: *Swimming faster,* Mountain View, CA, 1982, Mayfield Publishing.
34. Maki S, Gruen T: Anthropometric study of the glenohumeral joint. Transactions, 22nd Annual Meeting of the American Orthopedic Research Society, 1:173, 1976.
35. Michaud M et al: Muscular compensatory mechanism in the presence of a tendinitis of the supraspinatus, *Am J Phys Med* 66(3): 109, 1987.
36. Moseley HF, Overgaard B: The anterior capsular mechanism in recurrent anterior dislocation of the shoulder, *J Bone Joint Surg* 44B:913, 1962.
37. Moseley JB et al: EMG analysis of the scapular muscles during a shoulder rehabilitation program, *Am J Sports Med* 20(2):128, 1992.
38. Motzkin N et al: Role of capsular structures in inferior shoulder stability (abstract), *J Shoulder Elbow Surg* 2(1):517, 1993.
39. Neer CS, Welsh RP: The shoulder in sports, *Orthop Clin North Am* 8:583, 1977.
40. O'Brien SJ et al: The anatomy and histology of the inferior glenohumeral ligament complex of the shoulder, *Am J Sports Med* 18(5):449, 1990.
41. Ozaki J: Glenohumeral movements of the involuntary inferior and multidirectional instability, *Clin Orthop* 238:107, 1989.
42. Pappas AM, Zawacki RM, Sullivan TJ: Biomechanics of baseball pitching: a preliminary report, *Am J Sports Med* 13:216, 1985.
43. Perry J: Normal upper extremity kinesiology, *Phys Ther* 58(3): 265, 1978.
44. Pink M, Jobe FW: Shoulder injuries in athletes, *Clin Manage* 11(6):39, 1991.
45. Pink M et al: The normal shoulder during freestyle swimming: an electromyographic and cinematographic analysis of twelve muscles, *Am J Sports Med* 19(6):569, 1991.
46. Poppen N, Walker P: Normal and abnormal motion of the shoulder, *J Bone Joint Surg* 58A(2):195, 1976.
47. Richardson AB: The biomechanics of swimming: the shoulder and knee, *Clin Sports Med* 5:103, 1986.
48. Ryu R et al: An electromyographic analysis of shoulder function in tennis players, *Am J Sports Med* 16(5):481, 1988.
49. Saha AK: Anterior recurrent dislocation of shoulder, *Acta Orthop Scand* 68:479, 1967.
50. Saha AK: Dynamic stability of the glenohumeral joint, *Acta Orthop Scand* 42:491, 1971.
51. Saha AK: Mechanics of elevation of glenohumeral joint: its application in rehabilitation of flail shoulder in upper prachial plexus injuries and poliomyelitis and in replacement of the upper humerus by prosthesis, *Acta Orthop Scand* 44:668, 1973.
52. Scovazzo ML et al: The painful shoulder during freestyle swimming: an electromyographic and cinematographic analysis of twelve muscles, *Am J Sports Med* 19(6):577, 1991.
53. Townsend H et al: Electromyographic analysis of the glenohumeral muscles during a baseball rehabilitation program, *Am J Sports Med* 19(3):264, 1991.
54. Turkel SJ: Stabilizing mechanisms preventing anterior dislocation of the glenohumeral joint, *J Bone Joint Surg* 63A(8):1208, 1981.
55. Walker P: *Human joints and their artificial replacements,* Springfield, Ill, 1977, Charles C Thomas.
56. Warner J: Static capsuloligamentous restraints to superior-inferior translation of the glenohumeral joint, *Am J Sports Med* 20(6):675, 1992.

CHAPTER 6

Anatomy and Surgical Approaches

CHRISTOPHER M. JOBE

All art is but imitation of nature.
Seneca[71]

My philosophy is—as near normal anatomy as possible.
C.S. Neer letter to Reinhard Kölbel

The aim of the shoulder surgeon is to recreate the structure and function provided by nature. Nowhere is this truer than in sports medicine because of the highly involved and intricate mechanics of athletic endeavors. Procedures that substitute rather than restore normal anatomy seldom succeed in athletes.

This chapter describes the anatomy that the surgeon who treats athletic patients tries to restore by operative or nonoperative means. This purpose focuses our attention on those structures most likely to be affected by athletic injuries.

This chapter also describes the surgical approaches that are least disruptive to the functional anatomy of the shoulder. Because of the focus, and in the interest of brevity, information generally available in reference texts is abbreviated. In addition, discussion of congenital variations and nonphysiologic surgical approaches (e.g., tumor resection) is omitted.

This chapter is organized to show first the functional anatomy of the region from the skeleton outward, placing emphasis on structures affected by sports injuries. The discussion of these structures should aid in the surgical handling of these structures. The final portion of the chapter discusses arthroscopic and open surgical approaches to the shoulder most useful to the sports medicine physician.

ANATOMY

Bones and Joints

The shoulder region is a combination of joints, the purpose of which is to position the extremity in space. The shoulder is made up of the scapulothoracic joint and three diarthrodial joints—the sternoclavicular, the acromioclavicular, and the glenohumeral. The shoulder joint is comparable to the wrist joint, which is also made up of multiple articulations. Like the wrist, these joints function as one. There is a varying rhythm among the motions of the three shoulder joints and an interrelation among the joints. Like the joints at the wrist and other combination joints, it is difficult for someone to voluntarily move only one diarthrodial joint.

Motion of the shoulder as a whole is described in terms of the position or motion of the shaft of the humerus relative to the longitudinal axis of the body and rotation about the axis of the shaft (i.e., flexion-extension, abduction-adduction, and internal rotation–external rotation).

Sternoclavicular Joint

The most proximal diarthrodial joint connecting the upper limb with the axial skeleton is the sternoclavicular joint. This is the joint that suspends the clavicle from the manubrium of the sternum and the first rib. In the coronal plane, the orientation of the joint is from superomedial to inferolateral, and in the axial plane from anterolateral to posteromedial.[20] The joint is divided by a disc that is complete in 97% of specimens.

There are many ligaments supporting this joint, the most important of which is the posterior sternoclavicular ligament. There is an interior sternoclavicular ligament that assists in the stabilization of the joint. The anterior ligament is not quite as strong as the posterior ligament, which may account in part for the fact that anterior dislocations are more frequent than posterior dislocations. The interclavicular ligaments assist in this suspension of the clavicle, and the intraarticular disc contributes to stability.[6] The costoclavicular ligaments control displacement along the longitudinal axis of the clavicle: The anterior costoclavicular ligament resists lateral displacement, and the posterior ligament resists medial displacement.[15] The range of motion of this joint is 35° of anterior posterior angulation in the axial plane, 30° to 35° of elevation in the coronal plane, and 44° to 50° of upward rotation in the sagittal plane.[39] Almost all motions are a combination of these.

The coronal elevation of the scapula through the sternoclavicular joint contributes to the ability of the glenohumeral joint to be elevated as it positions the glenoid beneath the humeral head. This motion provides bony support to the weight of the arm. In addition, the upward rotation of the clavicle in the sagittal plane creates some of the apparent elevation of the glenohumeral joint, as will be shown in the description of the glenohumeral joint. Because of these two effects, sternoclavicular fusion is debilitating for an overhand athlete. In addition, because of the presence of the trachea and great vessels immediately behind the sternoclavicular joint, reconstruction (except to decompress these structures) is rarely indicated.[42]

Clavicle

The clavicle is an S-shaped bone that suspends the shoulder. The clavicle is the site of multiple muscle and ligament attachments and serves as a bony protection for the brachial plexus (Fig. 6-1). In addition to suspending the shoulder, it maintains the length-tension curves of some of the larger muscles, especially the pectoralis major and trapezius. Some have reported that removal of portions of the central clavicle has little consequence. There are, on the other hand, many patients for whom a clavicle resection would be disabling, especially those individuals who are involved in vigorous activities.[2,48]

The medial epiphysis of the clavicle is the last physis of the body to fuse. In males younger than 25 years old, an apparent sternoclavicular dislocation may, in fact, be a growth plate injury.

Acromioclavicular Joint

The acromioclavicular (AC) joint has very little motion but much pathology.[39] It is a joint separated by a meniscus that is usually perforated[22] (Fig. 6-2). The acromioclavicular joint routinely degenerates, showing considerable changes by the fourth decade in almost all individuals. Only occasionally is the joint itself painful, usually secondary to acute or chronic trauma. Recent studies have shown that the acromioclavicular ligaments main-

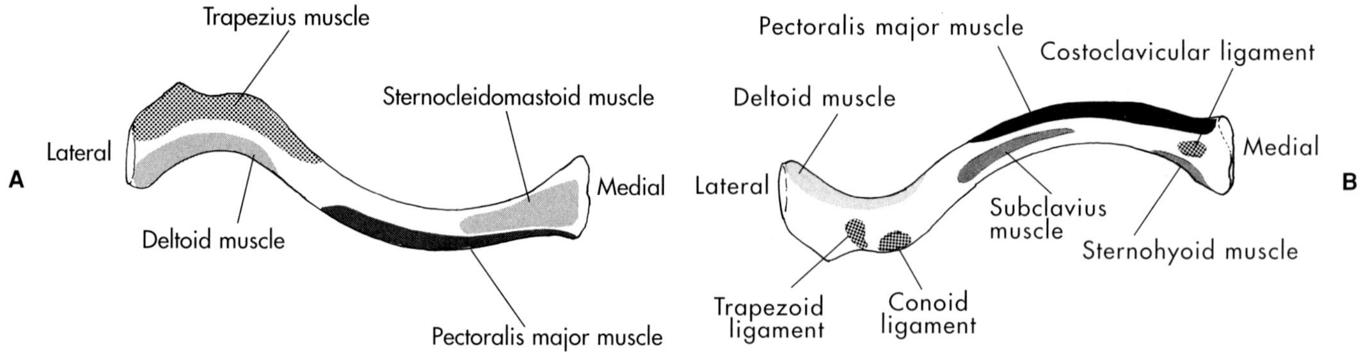

FIGURE 6-1 **A,** The superior view of the right clavicle with muscle attachments. **B,** The inferior view of the clavicle with muscle and ligament attachments.

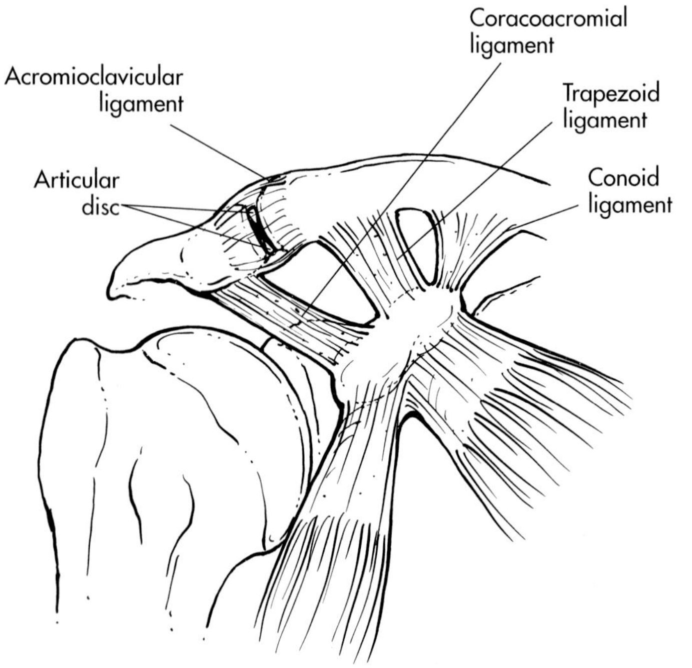

FIGURE 6-2 Anterior view of the acromioclavicular joint showing the relationship of the acromioclavicular joint to the two coracoclavicular ligaments, the conoid and trapezoid ligaments, and the coracoacromial ligament.

tain the alignment of this joint for low-level forces.[25] For high loads, the coracoclavicular ligaments resist the vertical and compressive loads. The posterior coracoclavicular ligament, the conoid ligament, is the strongest ligament resisting downward movement of the scapula relative to the clavicle. The conoid ligament probably also functions to rotate the clavicle upward as the scapula is pulled forward and up. The trapezoid ligament, the anterior portion of the coracoclavicular ligaments, resists downward motion and compression of the AC joint. Anterior posterior displacement of the acromion on the clavicle is most strongly resisted by the acromioclavicular ligaments.[25,78]

Scapula

The scapula functions mainly as a thin sheet of bone for muscle attachments (Fig. 6-3). Almost all of the surfaces of the scapula are covered by muscle. Scapular bone is metaphyseal in type, in that it has a thin cortex with frequent vascular perforations.[82] This means that there is considerably more bleeding with subperiosteal dissection than there is over diaphyseal bone. In addition, the muscle insertions on the scapula tend to be indirect insertions (see section on muscles), which also predisposes the scapula to bleeding when ligaments and tendons are detached.

Bony Anatomy

The scapula has four important processes—the spine, the acromion, the coracoid, and the glenoid.

The spine, an extension off the back of the scapula, functions as a muscle insertion site for the trapezius muscle and origin for the posterior third of the deltoid muscle. The scapular spine adds to the lever arm of these muscles.

The acromion also functions as a site of muscle attachment for the trapezius above and the deltoid below, and acts to extend the muscle lever arm, particularly that of the deltoid. The acromion is essential for athletic function. Despite reports in the literature of satisfactory strength after excision of the acromion,[9] these patients were not professional athletes.

Failure of fusion of ossification centers of the acromion occurs in about 1% to 2% of the population and is frequently bilateral. If present, it can be a source of shoulder pain.

The third important process is the coracoid. This is an anterior projection to which muscles and ligaments are attached. The base of the coracoid is the attachment site of the coracoclavicular ligaments. The tip serves as an important palpation landmark, especially for arthroscopy. It also serves as the origin of the short head of the biceps and the coracobrachialis, as well as serving as the insertion of the pectoralis minor. The arm of the cora-

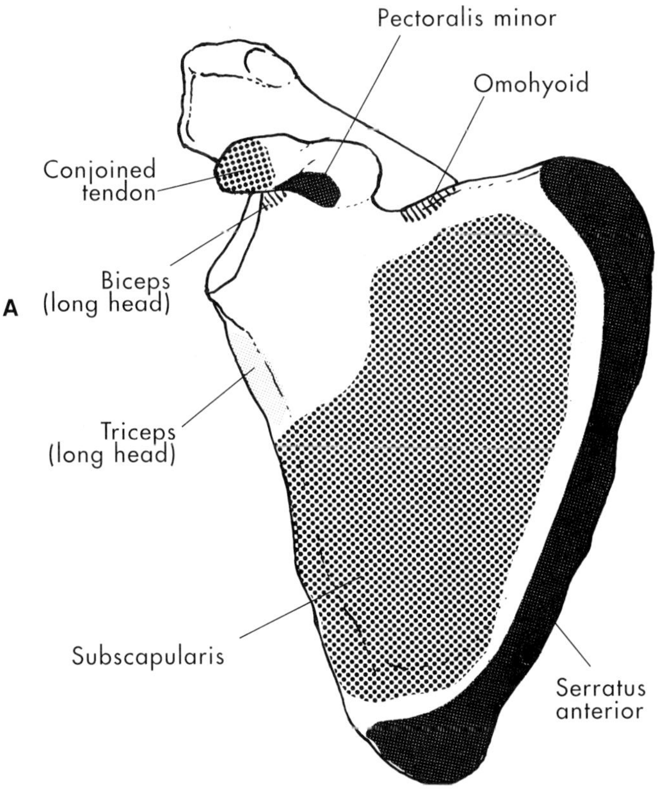

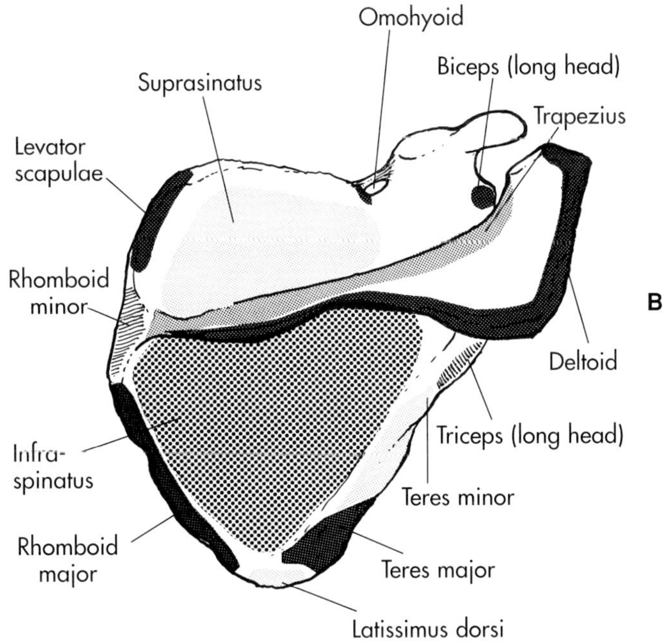

FIGURE 6-3 **A,** Anterior view of the scapula showing the sites of muscle attachment. **B,** A posterosuperior view of the scapula with its muscle attachments.

coid behind the tip forms the anterior limit of the coracoacromial arch or supraspinatus outlet. The inside of the arm of the coracoid also is the origin of the coracohumeral ligament. The coracoid is also the roof of the axillary space.

The glenoid will be discussed with the glenohumeral articulation.

Supraspinatus Outlet

The acromion, the coracoid process, and the coracoacromial ligament make up the roof of the supraspinatus tendon (Fig. 6-4). The coracoacromial ligament inserts on the inferior tip and the lateral portion of the undersurface of the acromion for a distance of up to 2 cm. On the medial side of the acromion lies the acromioclavicular joint. Compromise of this outlet has been blamed on several things: curvature of the undersurface of the acromion,[7,52,53] mobility of an unfused ossification center,[53] thickening of the coracoacromial ligament,[53] and decreased angle of the acromion orientation with respect to the horizontal.[3] Osteophytes located along the anteroinferior margin of the acromion on each side of the acromioclavicular joint may also compromise this outlet. However, compromise of the outlet is not always secondary to distortions of the rigid outer boundary or "roof." The outlet may often be compromised by dynamic motion of the humeral head toward the roof.

Nerve Entrapment

There are two potential sites of nerve entrapment on the scapula.[17,61,62] The suprascapular notch through

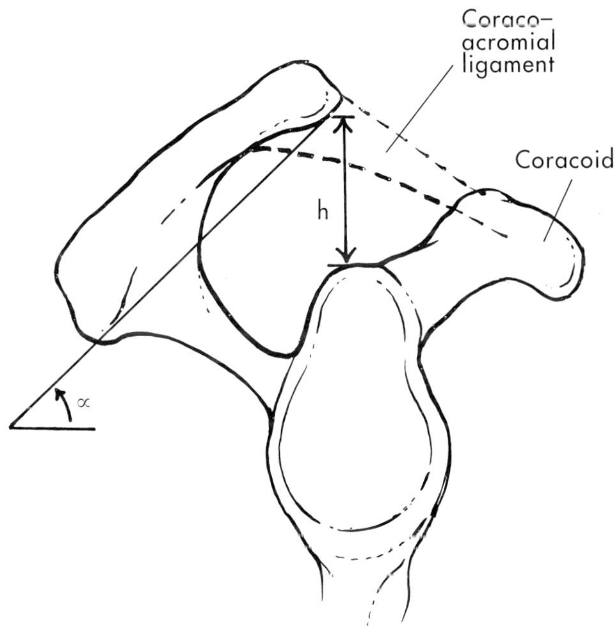

FIGURE 6-4 The roof of the supraspinatus outlet and some of the factors that affect it. Compromise of this outlet has been attributed to a decreased angle of the acromion, as indicated by the Greek letter α, decreased height as indicated by the letter *h*, a primary curve or hook shape to the undersurface of the acromion, and secondary changes such as a bone spur projecting into the ligament or thickening of the coracoacromial ligament itself. The ligament inserts onto the inferior portion of the anterior acromion and then along the lateral edge of the inferior acromial surface.

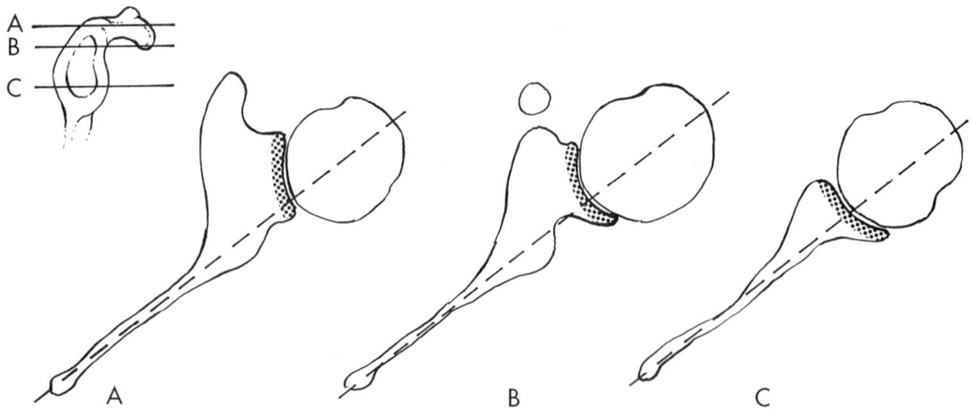

FIGURE 6-5 Three cross-sectional drawings that will illustrate the relationship of the glenoid to the humerus and to the remaining scapula. *(A)* The superior portion of the glenoid is set off anteriorly relative to the blade of the scapula and is retroverted about 7°. *(B)* Moving inferiorly, the glenoid begins to align with the scapula. *(C)* In a more inferior cross-section, the glenoid lines up with the blade of the scapula and is more perpendicular or perhaps even slightly anteverted.

which the suprascapular nerve passes is bordered superiorly by the transverse scapular ligament and is a site of entrapment.[17] The artery accompanying the nerve (suprascapular artery) usually passes over this ligament. After innervating the supraspinatus muscle, the suprascapular nerve passes around the base of the glenoid and scapular spine in what is referred to as the spinoglenoid notch. This may be bounded superiorly by collagenous material, allowing the nerve to become entrapped by space-occupying lesions, such as a ganglion cyst extending from the glenohumeral joint, or by fibrous tissue bands or other structures in athletes who perform repetitive overhand activities, such as throwers or volleyball players.

Glenohumeral Joint

The glenohumeral joint has features that make it different by comparison with many of the other joints about the body. This discussion begins with a description of the bony and articular structures, including articular cartilage and the labrum, and then describes the passive restraints of the shoulder capsule and tendons, both as a gross description and with some of the more salient histologic features. The true motion of the glenohumeral joint is then mentioned, as are implications for capsule tensioning and a description of the function of the capsule joint. The conclusions describe how the paths of stabilizers aid in resisting translation and angulation.

Bone and Articular Anatomy

The glenoid, the articular process of the scapula, lines up almost perpendicular to the blade of the scapula with approximately 7° of retroversion.[20] At the upper end, it is formed with the base of the coracoid. The glenoid is offset anterior to the blade of the scapula and is somewhat more retroverted (Fig. 6-5). The lower end of the glenoid is less retroverted. As the entire scapula curves around the thorax, the scapula is angled anteriorly about 30° from the axial plane so that the glenoid is anteverted 20° to 30° relative to the body. In the sagittal plane, the scapula is tilted forward (about 20°) at rest at its upper end. The glenoid is about 40 mm long and 30 mm wide at its widest point, which is located in the inferior portion[38,79] (Fig. 6-6). There is an easily identifiable indentation along the anterior rim of the glenoid that is sometimes called the equator. This notch can serve as a reference point to divide the glenoid roughly in half.

The articular surface of the glenoid is covered with hyaline cartilage and is rimmed around its edge by the labrum, which is almost entirely fibrous.[19] In the lower half of the glenoid, the labrum appears to be a fibrous continuation of the articular cartilage. In this lower area, the labrum does not perform a meniscus-like function. In the upper half of the joint, the labrum has a more variable form and may appear to be somewhat meniscal in its appearance and function because it may overlap the articular cartilage. Also in the upper half, the labrum is less tightly adherent to the glenoid. The anterosuperior portion of the labrum often has a normal fenestration, or "sublabral recess." In 9% of cases, it is complete and communicates with the subscapularis recess.[29]

The function of the labrum is the subject of some debate. The current thinking is influenced by "Wolff's law" and proposes that the labrum does have a function (i.e.,

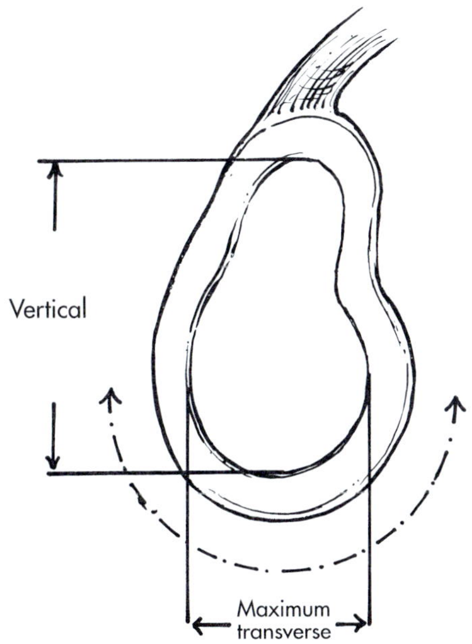

FIGURE 6-6 An en face view of the glenoid labrum. The widest portion of the glenoid is in its lower half, and it averages about 30 mm. The vertical dimension of the bony glenoid is approximately 40 mm. The upper portion of the labrum often appears to be almost meniscal in its shape in that its attachment is peripheral but much of the glenoid labrum may overhang the articular cartilage, much in the same way the meniscus overhangs the articular cartilage of the knee. In the lower half of the glenoid, the labrum does not overhang the glenoid, and in fact it is difficult arthroscopically to demarcate where the articular cartilage ends and labrum begins. The notch in the anterior glenoid is sometimes called the "equator" and is a convenient arthroscopic landmark.

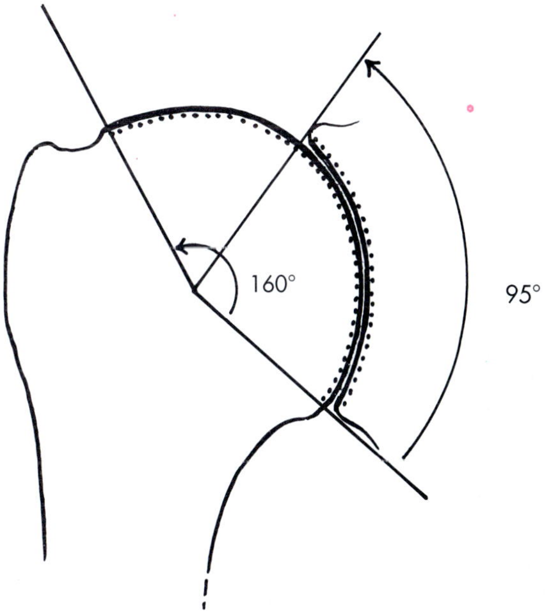

FIGURE 6-7 An anterior view of the glenohumeral joint in the coronal plane. The articular cartilage of the humeral head covers an arc of approximately 160°, and this cartilage is opposed by a vertical glenoid that covers 95°. In pure coronal abduction, there would be only 65° of motion before contact occurs between the greater tuberosity and the superior labrum.

it exists, therefore it has a function). The following are functions proposed: (1) the labrum acts as part of the ligaments or capsule reinforcing their attachment to bone[51,75]; (2) the labrum acts as an extension of the glenoid to deepen the "cup"[36]; (3) the labrum acts as a washer, maintaining the negative pressure within the area of cartilage contact, allowing stabilization by atmospheric pressure[28]; and (4) the labrum acts to restrict angulation toward itself (i.e., as a bumper against soft tissues adjacent to the humeral articular cartilage). These mechanisms are not mutually exclusive, and the roles may change with the amount and direction of force applied. The author's opinion is that, as in most positions of the shoulder, the passive stabilizers are not in a condition of tension, and the labrum functions to deepen the cup of the glenoid into which the forces generated by the rotator cuff muscles compress the head of the humerus. This is probably most important in resisting a first-time dislocation, which often does not occur in a position of tension on the ligamentous structures. In positions of extreme angulation, the labrum probably functions to reinforce the insertion of the capsule, thereby assisting the capsule to resist dislocation. This function helps the shoulder resist recurrent dislocations. The contribution of the labrum to stability by controlling negative intraarticular pressure is, at best, negligible.[4,10]

There are two bony tubercles at the superior and inferior poles of the glenoid. The superior tubercle, known as the bicipital tubercle, serves as part of the origin of the long head of the biceps, although most of the tendon inserts through the superior labrum. The inferior tubercle lies outside the joint and serves as an attachment of the long head of the triceps.

Although there is not much conformity of bone between the glenoid and humerus, the actual glenoid articular surface and the adjacent labrum conform nicely to the articular cartilage surface of the humeral head. As to bony constraint, the glenoid covers only 25% to 33% of the humeral head surface area. In any one plane, the linear arc of the glenoid covers 50% to 60% of the arc of the head[38,40,79] (Fig. 6-7). This is a more significant limitation on joint motion than containment (an area function) because joint angulation occurs in planes. The vertical arc of the humeral head is about 155° to 160°.[40,79] Thus a line of glenoid articular surface that covers 50% to 60% of the humeral surface would leave about 65° of angulation before the labrum makes contact with the rotator cuff or biceps tendon.

In shape, the articular surface of the humerus is largely spherical, with an average 24-mm radius of curvature.[38] The central axis of the articular cartilage is offset from the axis of the shaft by about 130° to 150°, similar to the neck shaft angle found at the hip (Fig. 6-8). In addition, the articular position of the head is retroverted approximately 20° to 40° in the axial plane relative to the axis of the epicondyles of the elbow (Fig. 6-9).

The diameter of the humeral head averages about 48 mm compared with the glenoid, which averages 35 mm

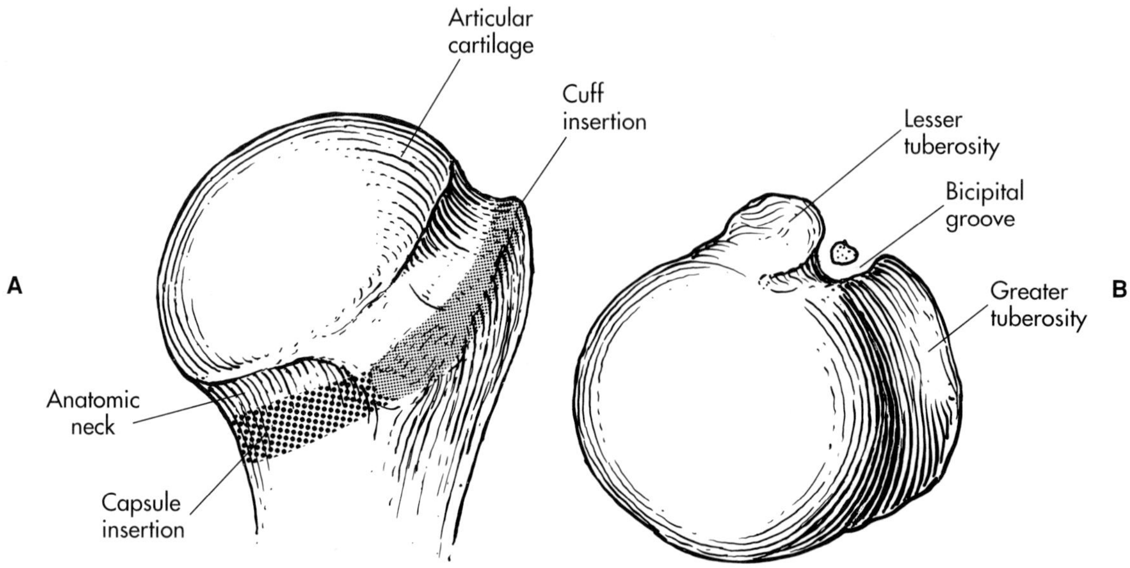

FIGURE 6-8 **A,** A posterior view of the proximal humerus demonstrating the articular cartilage, the insertion of the capsule and rotator cuff and the intervening anatomic neck, referred to as the bare area by arthroscopists. **B,** A superior view of the right humerus showing the tuberosities with their cuff attachments and the intervening bicipital groove.

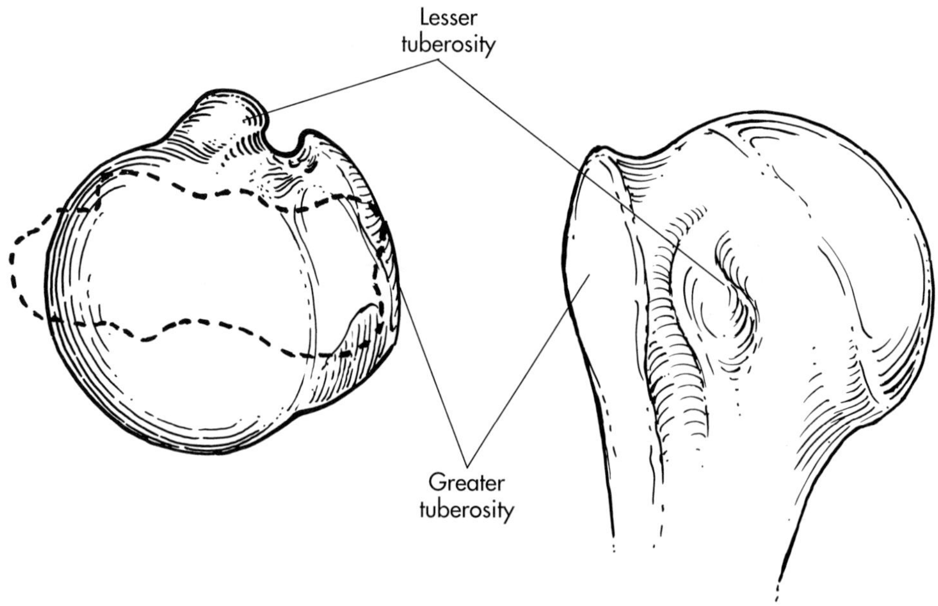

FIGURE 6-9 A superior view of the proximal humerus showing the retrotorsion of the humeral head relative to the shaft of the humerus. (The dotted line demonstrates the configuration at the level of the epicondyles.) When the forearm is held straight anterior, the humeral head is somewhat (20° to 40°) retroverted relative to the shaft of the humerus. The bicipital groove lies approximately 1 cm lateral to the midline of the arm.

at its greatest diameter. Therefore at all times a portion or portions of the humeral head overhang the edges of the glenoid.[5,24,50,67] The humeral head is also prominent with respect to the ring of cuff muscles and ligament attachments on the anatomic neck of the humerus. In various positions of the shoulder, the ligaments and tendons aid in stability by contouring this prominence of the humeral head.[52]

Capsule and Ligaments

An understanding of the glenohumeral joint capsule and its ligaments is essential to understanding shoulder function. The innervation of the capsule, as with all joints, is via nerves that are passing by and innervating adjacent structures. These are the suprascapular nerve above and the axillary nerve below.[27] As will be seen in later discussion, the shoulder capsule functions in a manner that is different from the usual ligaments.

If the orientation of collagen fascicles in the capsule is an indication of internal tensile stresses, the stresses on the shoulder capsule are different from those of other ligaments.[57] In general, the glenohumeral capsule has two layers of fascicles that run perpendicular to each other (Figs. 6-10 and 6-11). In the inner layer, the collagen fascicles run proximally in a radial direction, that is, from glenoid to the humerus. In the outer layer, the collagen fascicles run circumferentially rather than from bone to bone. This basic arrangement is more complex in various regions of the capsule, particularly in areas adjacent to the individual glenohumeral ligaments (Fig. 6-12).

The uppermost thickening of the capsule, the superior glenohumeral ligament, takes its origin from the upper labrum, often in continuity with the origin of the long head of the biceps. Alternative sites of origin are either in common with the middle glenohumeral ligament or by a solitary origin between the biceps and middle glenohumeral ligament. The superior glenohumeral ligament is almost universally present (97%), although it may be obscured by synovial tissue, and inserts just medial to the upper end of the lesser tuberosity.

Inferiorly, the next ligament is the middle glenohumeral ligament. This is the most variable region of the capsule in its appearance, not only in the recesses, which will be discussed, but also in the actual presence of this ligament. The middle glenohumeral ligament may be entirely absent (10%) or extremely poorly developed (20%).[22] Conversely, the middle glenohumeral ligament may be very well developed and thickened. When the ligament is present, it originates from the anterior-superior labrum or adjacent bony glenoid, runs obliquely and inferiorly across the inner surface of the subscapularis, and then reascends to the humerus just medial to the upper end of the lesser tuberosity and just below the insertion of the superior glenohumeral ligament.[22,29] The lower

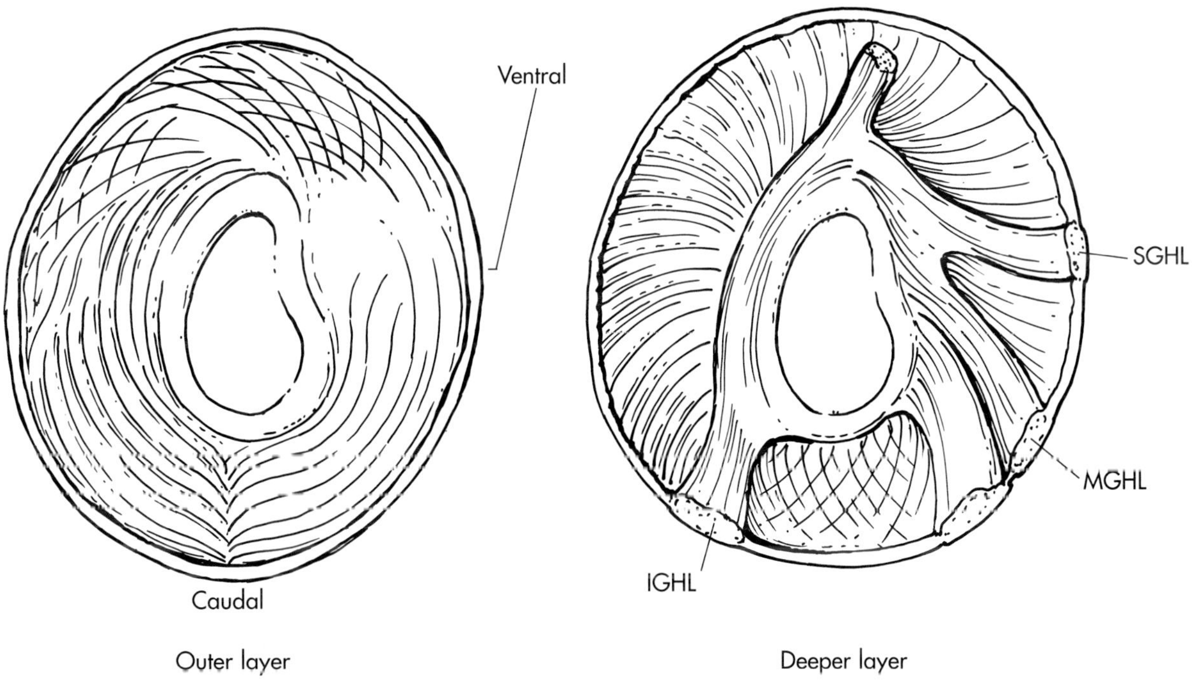

FIGURE 6-10 The orientation of the collagen fascicles in the capsule of the glenohumeral joint. The outer layer consists of circularly running fascicles, and the deeper running layer consists of longitudinal fascicles, including the specialized areas of the glenohumeral joint, such as the superior glenohumeral ligament, the middle glenohumeral ligament, and the inferior glenohumeral ligament with its anterior and posterior bands. (Modified from Gohlke F, Essigkrug B, Schmitz F: The pattern of the collagen fiber bundles of the capsule of the glenohumeral joint, *J Shoulder Elbow Surgery* 3[3]:111, 1994.)

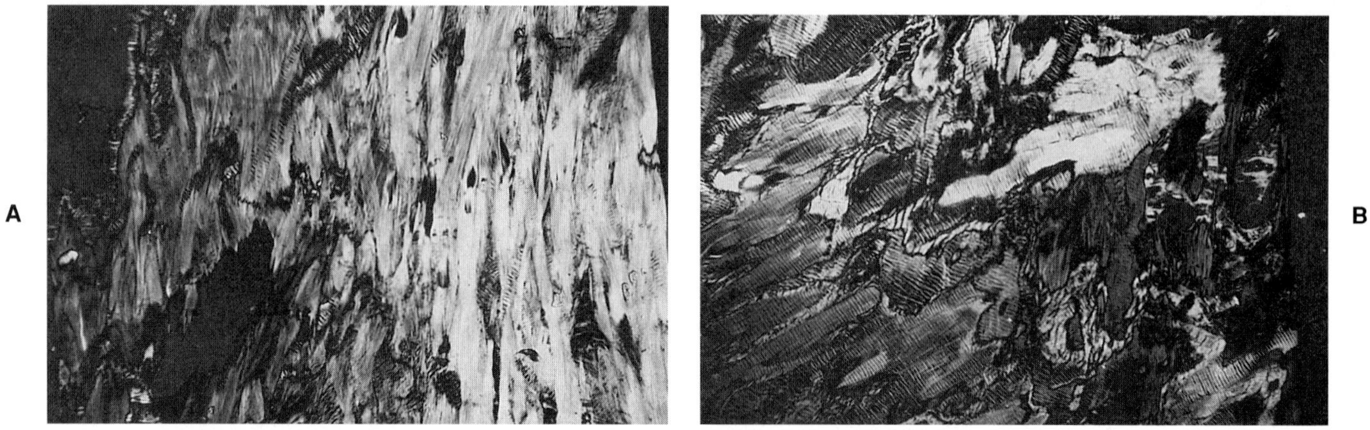

FIGURE 6-11 A, View under a polarizing microscope of a histologic section of the inferior glenohumeral ligament showing the inner collagen fascicles running radially (from inferior to superior here). B, A more peripheral section through the same ligament as in A showing the appearance of the circular fibers running transversely.

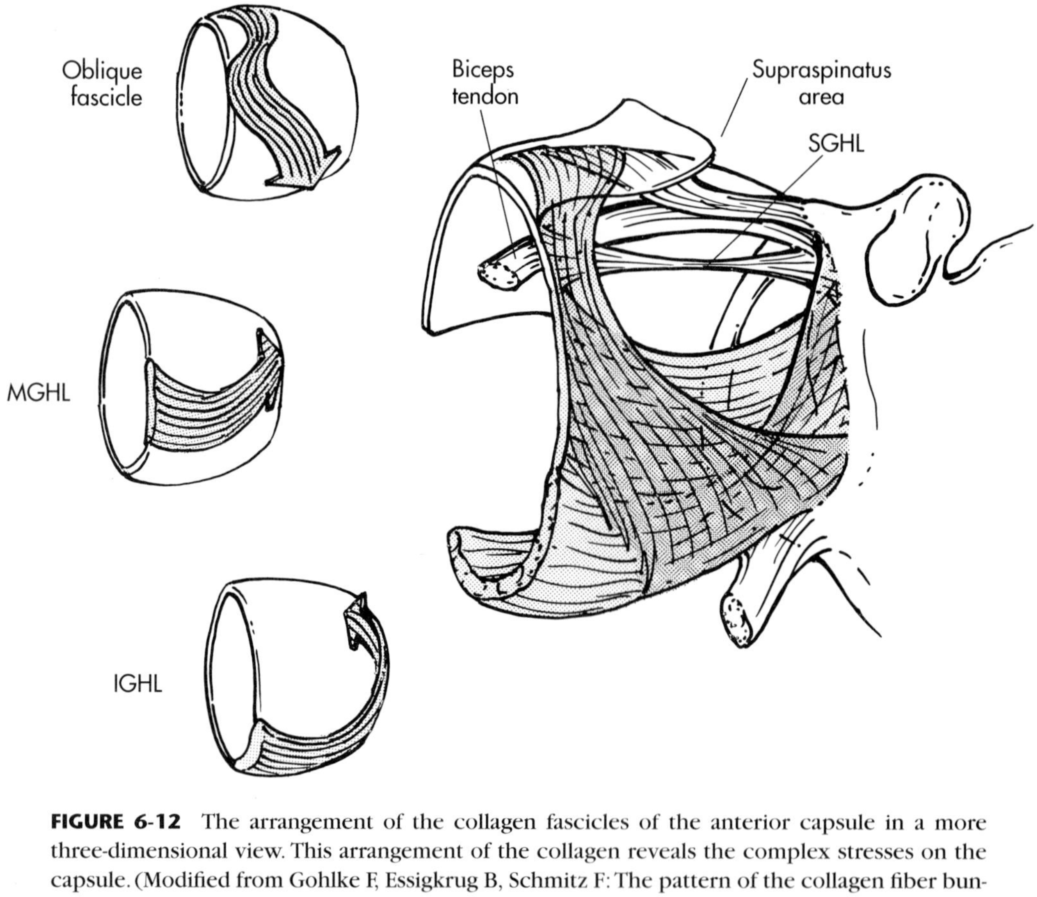

FIGURE 6-12 The arrangement of the collagen fascicles of the anterior capsule in a more three-dimensional view. This arrangement of the collagen reveals the complex stresses on the capsule. (Modified from Gohlke F, Essigkrug B, Schmitz F: The pattern of the collagen fiber bundles of the capsule of the glenohumeral joint, *J Shoulder Elbow Surgery* 3[3]:11, 1994.)

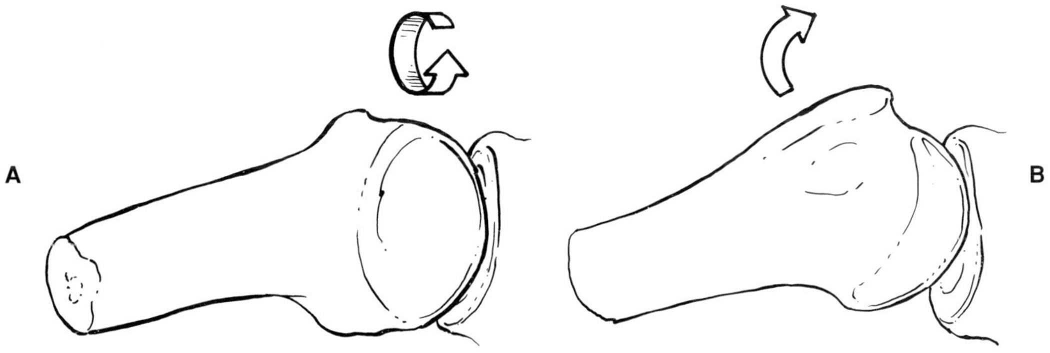

FIGURE 6-13 **A,** Rotation occurs at the glenohumeral joint when the orientation of the humeral head remains unchanged and the bone rotates about the axis. **B,** Angulation occurs at the glenohumeral joint when the orientation of the axis of the humeral head changes relative to the glenoid.

portion of the middle glenohumeral ligament originates outside the anterior band of the inferior glenohumeral ligament.

The inferior glenohumeral ligament is the most substantial region of the capsule.[29,57] The inferior glenohumeral ligament takes origin from the lower half of the glenoid, usually through the labrum, and has additional indirect fibers of origin from the neck of the glenoid. The anterior limit of this glenoid origin is usually in the area of the equator of the glenoid. The posterior limit of the origin of the inferior glenohumeral ligament is somewhere in the posterior inferior quadrant of the glenoid and varies more widely than does the anterior limit.[56,57]

The inferior glenohumeral ligament is bordered anteriorly by a thick band of collagen called the anterior band. Below the anterior band lies the anterior region of the ligament, and further posteriorly lies the posterior region of the ligament. There is often a demarcation between the anterior and posterior regions in the form of a V-shaped humeral insertion. The two regions function together but have a different orientation to the glenoid surface, as will be discussed later under ligament function. Most posteriorly, the inferior glenohumeral ligament may or may not have an arthroscopically visible posterior band.

The posterior capsule above the inferior glenohumeral ligament conforms in its histology to the simple description of the capsule discussed previously (i.e., an inner layer of radially running fibers and an outer layer of circumferentially running fibers).

There are often recesses or defects within the capsule. In the majority of glenohumeral joints (85%), there is a recess through which the subscapularis tendon can be visualized. This recess is variable in size and most often lies between the superior and middle glenohumeral ligaments (35%). In 40% of cases, there will be two recesses, one above and one below the middle glenohumeral ligament, and in 2.4% there will be a recess below the middle glenohumeral ligament only. Finally, there is a group of patients in whom the middle glenohumeral ligament is impossible to detect, either because it is absent (9%) or because there is no recess above or below it, creating a confluence of the middle and inferior glenohumeral ligaments (5%).[22,55]

There are two tendons that are usually visible from within the glenohumeral joint, the tendon of the long head of the biceps and the upper edge of the subscapularis tendon. The tendon of the long head of the biceps takes origin from the superior glenoid labrum and tubercle and passes through the joint to the bicipital groove, which is another defect in the capsule and lies on the humeral head between the greater and lesser tuberosities. The tendon is retained in this groove by an extension of the coracohumeral ligament.[59,72]

Glenohumeral Motion and Implications for Capsule Tensioning

To better understand the function of these ligaments, a more exact and simplified description of shoulder motion is needed. The purpose of the shoulder region as a whole is to provide motion of the arm in relation to the axial skeleton. This description of shoulder motion has been used to describe the motion of the glenohumeral joint alone. This has been done in spite of the fact that the two axes used, those of the axial skeleton and the humeral shaft, do not correspond to the axes of the articular cartilages involved. This motion description is easier for clinicians to follow because the two axes involved have a bony representation. However, to understand the motion of the glenohumeral joint alone, it is more accurate to use the axes of the articular cartilages.

In a ball-and-socket joint such as the glenohumeral joint, there are two basic motions, rotation and angulation. Pure rotation is motion about a selected axis of the humerus without changing the orientation of the axis relative to the glenoid (Fig. 6-13, *A*). Pure angulation is a change in the orientation of that axis without rotation about it. As will be seen, there are very few motions that are pure angulation or pure rotation (Fig. 6-13, *B*).

There are three inaccuracies inherent in using the axis of the humeral shaft as a descriptor of glenohumeral joint motion. First, a comparison of the angulation ranges of the two axes demonstrates more angulation of the glenohumeral joint when using the shaft axis as a reference than occurs when using the axis of the humeral head. The 135° angle of the articular cartilage from the shaft allows rotation about the axis of the humeral head to appear as increased angulation of the shaft.

The second issue is that motion of the head axis (Figs. 6-14 and 6-15) is smoother because it does not have discontinuity at the top of the circle of motion. This "notch" in the motion is necessitated by a reversal in humeral rotation, which must occur in moving from superior angulation anterior to the plane of the scapula to superior angulation posterior to the plane of the scapula.

The third inaccuracy is that there is little correlation between the direction of humeral head axis angulation and the direction of humeral shaft angulation. For the purposes of the model, the humeral head axis will be used to describe glenohumeral motion.

To simplify the discussion, the humeral head will be considered spherically convex, articulating with the glenoid, which will be considered spherically concave. Although this is not strictly true given the bony anatomy, it is more nearly true when considering the articular cartilage and soft tissue, such as the labrum. With these two tissues attached, the articular surfaces are more nearly spherical and congruent.

An additional simplification is needed, because within a particular broad ligament, such as the inferior glenohumeral ligament, different regions of the ligament may be oriented differently. Therefore the discussion will focus on a single fascicle or small group of fascicles within the capsule, such as a small region of the inferior glenohumeral ligament.

For most shoulder positions, there is little passive tensioning in the fascicle under discussion. There are two basic types of passive tensioning and a continuum of positions between the two, where tension arises as a combination of the two basic types.

The first basic position of passive tensioning is that of pure angulation (Fig. 6-16). This is angulation of the joint away from the glenoid origin of the fascicle. Other fascicles of the joint will not be in pure angulation at this time. To achieve this position of angulation, the head must rotate about its axis to a position where the humeral insertion of the fascicle is directly opposite its

A

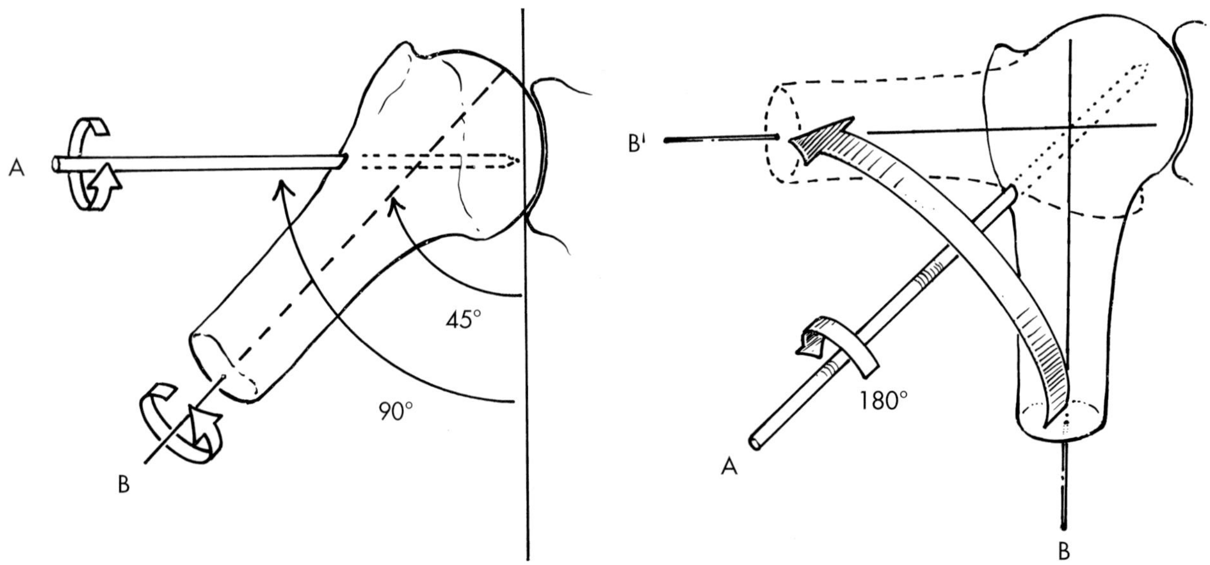

B

FIGURE 6-14 **A,** The two axes by which the motion of the glenohumeral joint can be determined. Axis *A* is that of the anatomic neck and articular cartilage. This axis, identified by what appears to be a rigid pin, would pass through the center of rotation and the center of articular cartilage. At roughly 45° of coronal abduction, this axis should be perpendicular to the glenoid. Axis *B* is the axis of the humeral shaft. It is the most convenient axis to use clinically and is therefore the more commonly used. At 90° of glenohumeral abduction, this axis becomes perpendicular to the glenoid. **B,** This is a schematic drawing showing a glenohumeral joint held in the anatomic position, *B,* and a rotating bearing, *A,* passed through the axis of the humeral head, into the glenoid. If the axis of the bearing rotated 180°, this rotation would appear as 90° of abduction, *B′* if one is measuring the motion of the shaft of the humerus. However, the joint has not changed in angulation but only in rotation. The angulation only appears to have changed. In this way, the glenohumeral joint can produce a wider range of angulation of the humeral shaft relative to the glenoid without sacrificing additional bony stability.

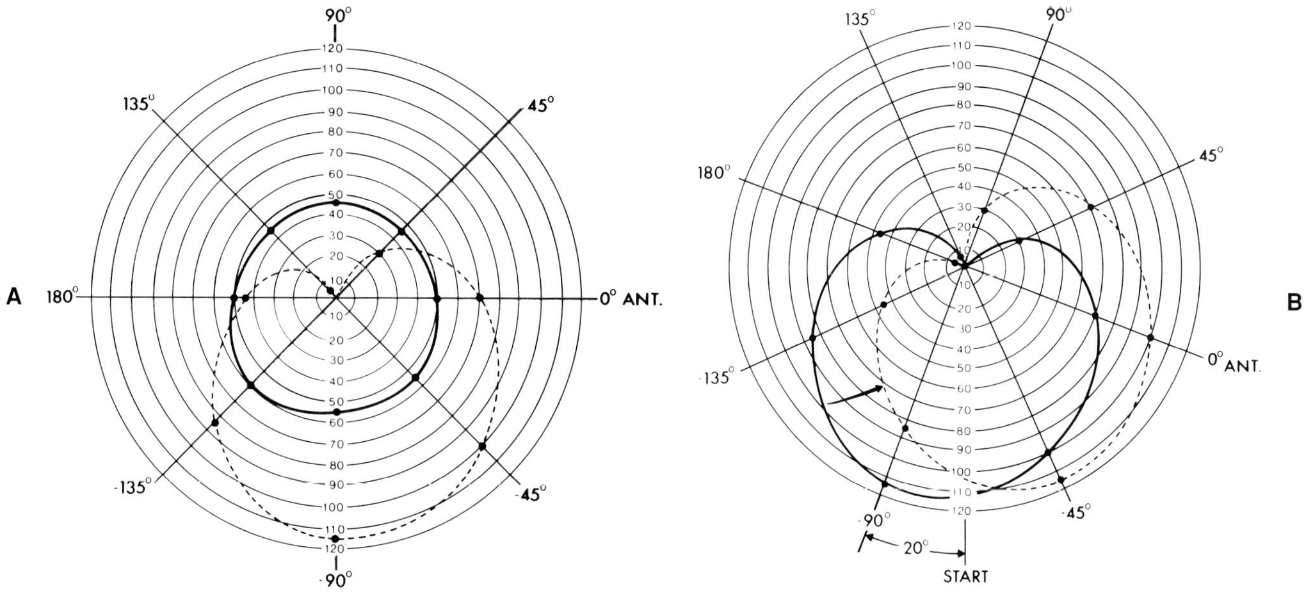

FIGURE 6-15 **A,** The range of angulations from a perpendicular to the center of the glenoid in various directions. The solid line demonstrates the path described by the axis of the articular cartilage, which is roughly a circle. (Zero degrees is directly anterior, 90° is directly superior, and 180° is directly posterior.) The path followed by the humeral shaft *(broken line)* demonstrates a much wider but irregular path. This reveals that rotation of the glenohumeral articular cartilage produces an apparently wider range of angulation of the joint. **B,** The contribution of the 135° offset in the humerus is amplified by upward rotation of the scapula in the sagittal plane. The solid line is the motion of the humeral shaft relative to the scapula plotted on the diagram with the scapula in its position of rest (i.e., angulated 20° forward on the thoracic cage). The broken line is a diagram of the range of angulations of the humeral shaft relative to the scapula at the end of the scapula's 45° upward rotation in the sagittal plane. This illustrates how the angular offset of the humerus allows rotation of the scapula in the sagittal plane to increase the apparent range of glenohumeral angulation.

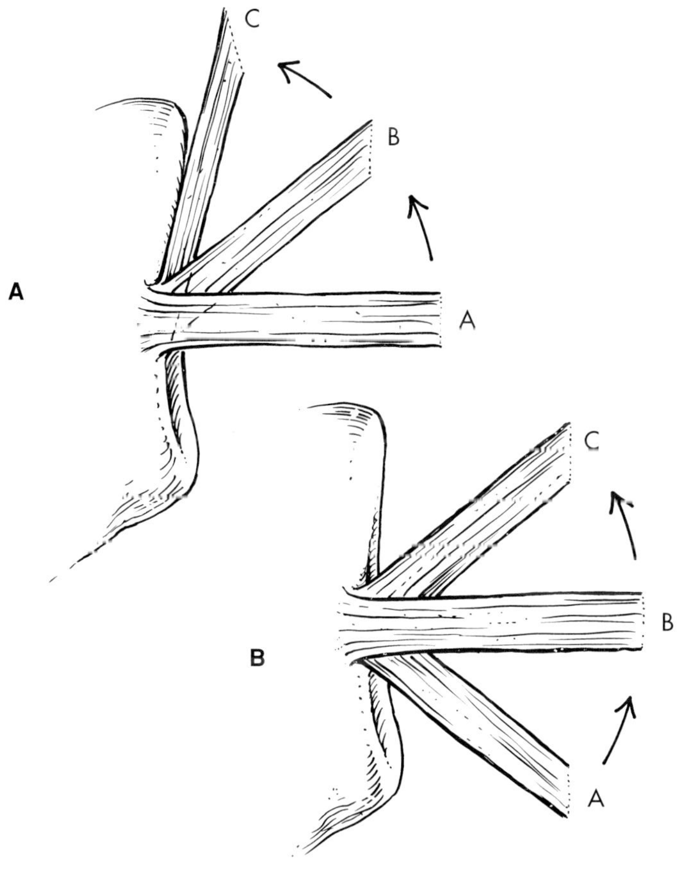

FIGURE 6-16 **A,** Three positions in which a fascicle may be held in passive tension and contribute to the stability of the glenohumeral joint. The positions are named according to the motion of the humeral head axis that produced the tension. In position *A,* the axis of the humeral head has been angulated maximally away from the glenoid origin of the fascicle or group of fascicles. In this position, the humeral insertion of this group of fascicles lies directly opposite the glenoid origin. In this way, angulation determines a specific rotation. In position *C,* the humeral insertion of the group of fascicles has been rotated maximally away from the glenoid insertion. The humeral insertion must be drawn toward the rim of the glenoid. In this fashion, an extreme position of rotation determines a specific angulation. Position *B* is one of the many intervening positions in which the group of fascicles is tensioned by a combination of angulation and rotation. When the humeral insertion lies closer to the glenoid origin than the arc described by *A, B,* and *C,* there is no passive tensioning of this group of fascicles. **B,** The range of positions that are available for most fascicles. All fascicles can achieve their positions of maximum angulation, but only a few have a range that includes maximum rotation. Most have a range between two intermediate ranges of rotation, as denoted by the letters *A* and *C.*

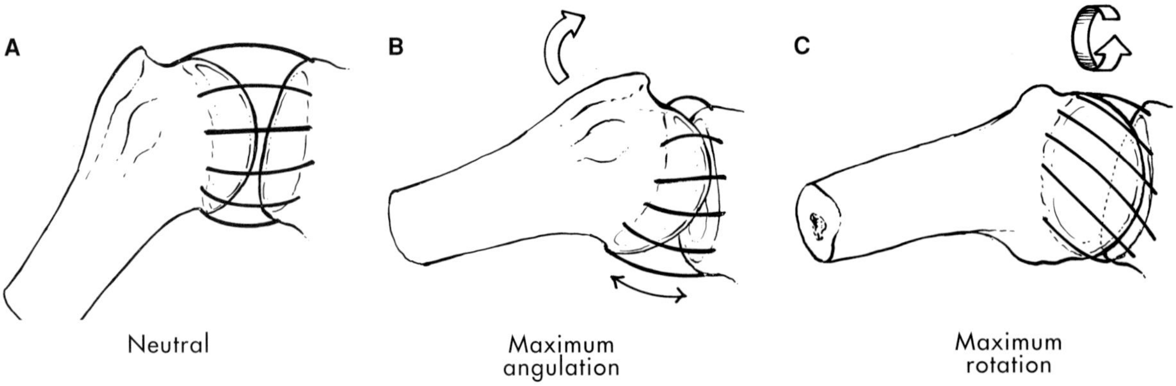

FIGURE 6-17 **A,** The neutral position of the fascicles. **B** and **C,** The effect of maximum angulation and rotation on passive tensioning. In maximum angulation, **B,** the group of fascicles acts as a tension band to compress the glenohumeral joint and thereby increase stability. Because the humeral head overhangs the glenoid, the capsule contours the prominent humeral head, which creates a force that resists translation in the direction of the group of fascicles. In the position of maximum rotation, **C,** the passive tensioning of the group of fascicles creates an internal rotation moment that resists further rotation. This moment also creates a force that resists some translation of the joint. The intervening positions have a combination of these two mechanisms for stabilizing the joint.

glenoid insertion. Because of this, it can be said that joint angulation determines a certain position of glenohumeral rotation about the axis of the head.

The other basic passive-tensioning position is that in which the head is rotated about its axis so that the humeral insertion of the coracohumeral ligament is rotated maximally away from the glenoid insertion.[26] In this position of rotation, the ligament acts as a tether and draws its humeral insertion toward the rim of the glenoid. Thus extreme rotation determines a particular position of angulation. As a rule, by choosing a position of maximum angulation, a position of rotation is determined, and by choosing a maximum rotation, a particular angulation is determined.[60] Because there are many directions of maximal angulation but only two of rotation, most fascicles can achieve maximal angulation, but only two areas of capsule reach maximal angulation in a position of rotation.

Between these two basic positions of passive tensioning, there is a continuous arc of positions in which the fascicle will be passively tensioned. These intermediate positions represent combinations of angulation and rotation (see Fig. 6-16). The large triangle underneath this arc represents the positions of the glenohumeral joint in which there is no passive tensioning of the fascicle. This is consistent with the finding that in most positions of the shoulder, the capsule is lax.

Resistance to Translation

What are the stabilizing effects of the fascicle in the two basic positions (Fig. 6-17)? In maximum angulation of the joint, the fascicle acts as a tension band that produces compression of the joint.[10] This helps stabilize the joint against translation in any direction. In addition, this fascicle resists further angulation away from its origin. Because of the prominence of the humeral head, this region of the ligament (by contouring of the head) provides force in a direction away from its glenoid origin.[30,32,35,50]

In the second basic passive-tensioning position, that of rotation, the passive tensioning within the fascicle resists further rotation. Because of the orientation of the fascicles, this position also develops internal forces that limit translation in the direction of its humeral insertion. The tense positions between rotation and angulation have a combination of the above effects.[31]

To amplify this discussion, the positions of various capsule regions and the mechanisms resisting the standard translations will be described. Recurrent anterior dislocation of the shoulder occurs in an abducted–externally rotated position. In fact, the standard clinical test is the apprehension test performed in 90° of shoulder abduction. This is approximately 60° of glenohumeral abduction and maximum external rotation about the axis of the humeral shaft. To the anterior band of the inferior glenohumeral ligament and the adjacent anterior portion of the inferior glenohumeral ligament, this represents the position of maximum angulation. This region of the capsule is stretched over the prominence of the humeral head, which it may be said to "contain."* There is some additional contribution from the middle glenohumeral ligament, which is mainly angulated but partially rotated in this position.[23] The posterior portion of the inferior

*References 50, 51, 57, 69, 70, 75, 77

glenohumeral ligament is partially rotated forward and partially angulated, creating a combination effect that further resists anterior translation of the humeral head.

The opposite instability, the recurrent posterior instability, occurs with the arm in forward flexion to 90 degrees and internal rotation. In this position, the axis of the humeral head is maximally angulated in the anterosuperior direction, creating a posteroinferior bulge of the humeral head that is contained by the posterior portion of the inferior glenohumeral ligament.[58] In this position, this area of the capsule may be seen to be mainly in its angulated position, where it also "contains" a volume of humeral head. In the position of posterior instability, the superior structures, the coracohumeral ligament and the superior glenohumeral ligament, have their humeral insertion rotated posteriorly so that they act in a rotated position to resist posterior translation of the humeral head on the glenoid.[31,57,58,70,81] A comparison of these two instabilities reveals how an area of ligament, particularly the inferior glenohumeral ligament, can be effective in resisting translation in two directions, and how two regions of the same inferior ligament may be functioning in a slightly different fashion to resist the same translation or opposing translatory forces. Thus a shoulder with anterior instability would have increased posterior laxity, and vice versa.

With the arm at the side, the superior portion of the capsule, especially the superior glenohumeral ligament and the anterior band of the inferior glenohumeral ligament, resists inferior translation of the humeral head on the glenoid. With the arm in 90° of abduction, it is the inferior glenohumeral ligament that resists inferior translation.[11] Thus we can see that positive resistance to translation also depends on the starting position of the glenohumeral joint.

Rotation, Angulation, and Motion

In addition to excessive translation, angulation occurs to a degree that may be pathologic at the shoulder. The two structures that may possibly resist angulation are the ligament that is at the apex of the deformity covering the normal protrusion of the humeral head over the edge of the glenoid and the labrum and humeral bone on the opposite side of the joint (Fig. 6-18). The ligament functions in tension; the latter two structures would function by compressing each other.

In abduction and external rotation the structure resisting further angulation is the anterior portion of the inferior glenohumeral ligament. The area of compression is where the rotator cuff contacts the posterosuperior labrum.

The ligament at the apex of the angulation (i.e., the inferior glenohumeral ligament) is probably the primary resistance to increased angulation (Fig. 6-19). In angulation, as opposed to translation, there is little overlap of function between ligaments. The stress applied to the capsule by angulation tends to be concentrated in one

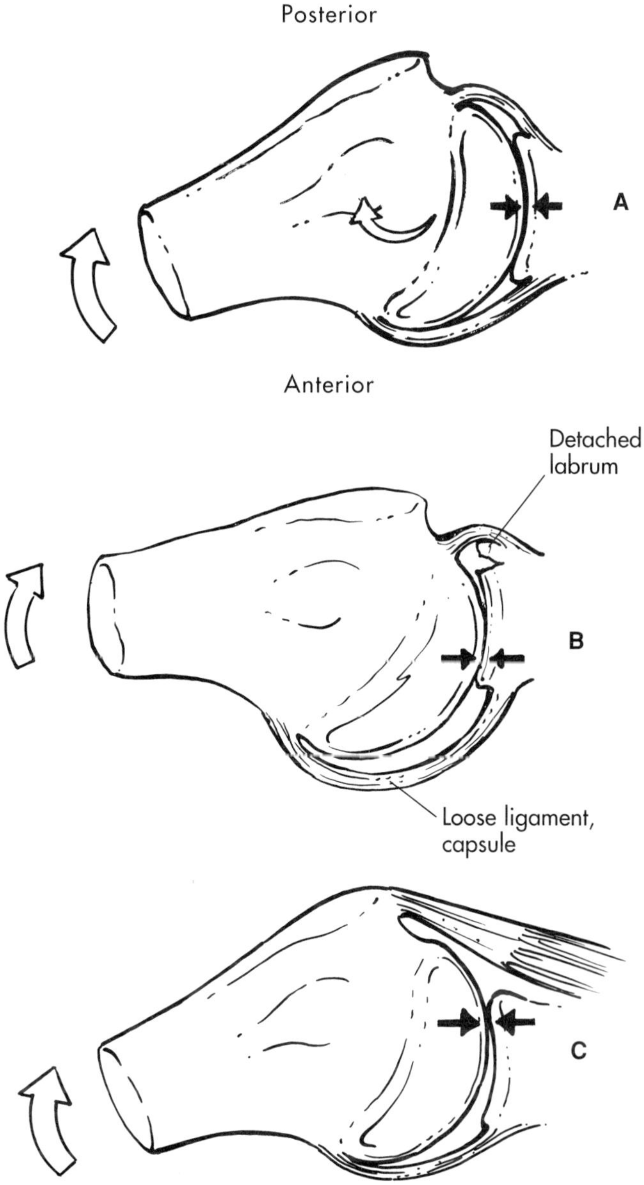

FIGURE 6-18 Illustration of the concept of "capacity" of the glenohumeral capsule. Because the humeral head overhangs the glenoid, there is a normal volume of humeral head that must be contained within a volume of capsule. **A,** The area of the inferior capsule that is distended in abduction and external rotation. **B,** A necessary condition for instability to occur is increased capacity. Because of labral detachment and stretching and ligament stretching, the anterior soft tissues can accept a larger volume of humeral head. **C,** The opposite pathology, in which a surgeon or a pathologic condition has decreased the capacity of this area of the joint to less than normal. Not only is the patient's range of motion reduced, but the decreased capacity causes a posterior subluxation of the humeral head, causing the humeral head to rest in a noncongruous fashion against the posterior glenoid, which often leads to later arthritic changes.[96]

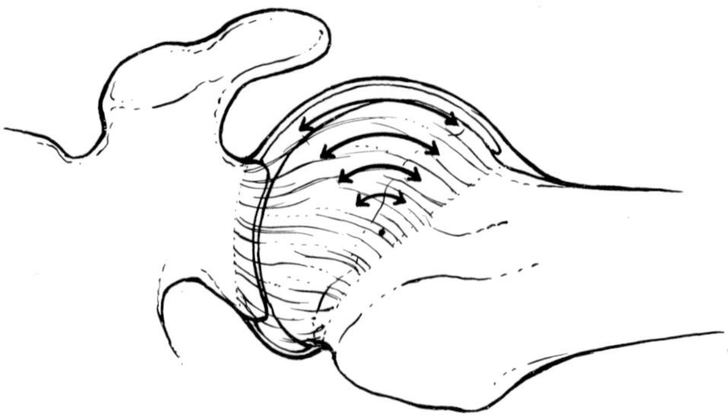

FIGURE 6-19 The effect of hyperangulation, as opposed to translation, on the capsule. Earlier illustrations in this chapter showed that several areas of the capsule can act together to restrain translation. In angulation, an uneven distribution of stress reaches a maximum at the apex of the angulation and decreases as one moves away from the apex fascicle until the center of rotation is achieved. Beyond the center of rotation there is no passive tensioning of the capsule. This mechanism, similar to tearing a phone book in half one page at a time, explains how young athletes can develop instability over an extended period of time.

A

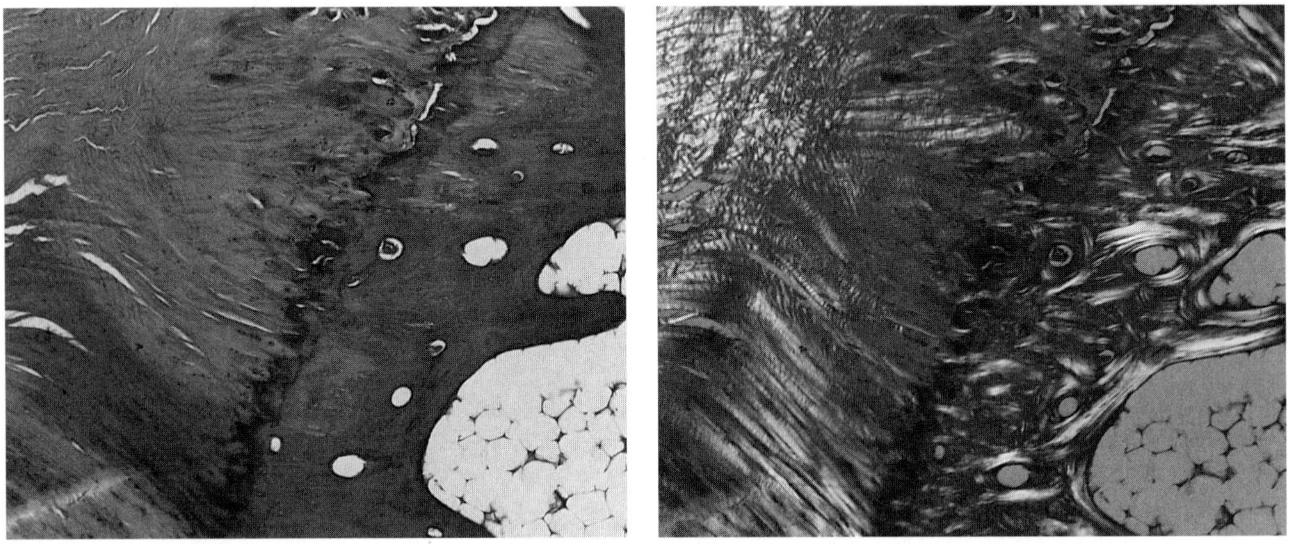

B

FIGURE 6-20 The direct insertion of the supraspinatus into the greater tuberosity of the humerus. **A,** The typical direct insertion with the four layers, and, **B,** the same section under polarized light. The four layers are the flexible supraspinatus tendon, the less flexible unmineralized fibrocartilage, the mineralized fibrocartilage, and then finally the bone of the greater tuberosity.

small area of the capsule. In translation, loads are spread throughout a larger portion of the capsule.

Extraarticular Humerus

The proximal humerus outside of the joint consists of the two tuberosities, greater and lesser, the bicipital groove, and the surgical neck of the humerus. The normal position of the humeral head is 20° to 30° of retroversion (see Fig. 6-10). With the axis of the elbow in the coronal plane, the bicipital groove lies about 1 cm lateral to the midline of the humerus. The groove is bound anteriorly by the transverse humeral ligament, but the strongest restraint to dislocation of the bicipital tendon is the coracohumeral liagment, with its insertion on both tuberosities.[72]

The blood supply to the humeral head enters through the upper portion of the bicipital groove in the form of the arcuate artery, which is a branch of the anterior humeral circumflex artery. This artery receives many collaterals before it enters into the bone but has few, if any, collaterals after entering the bone. The arteries with which it may communicate are branches from the posterior humeral circumflex that enter the inferior portion of the head posteriorly. Damage to the end branches of the anterior humeral circumflex and the posterior humeral circumflex arteries invariably leads to avascular necrosis.

Muscles

Muscles are the producers of force and therefore the producers of action in athletes. The sports medicine surgeon wants to recreate or preserve the normal muscle connections to bone so that the actions of the muscle are correct. They also want to preserve the innervations and the circulation.

If it is necessary to detach the muscular insertion from bone, the type of insertion is the factor that determines how that is done. Direct insertions (Fig. 6-20) are very thick collagenous structures in which the fibers of the tendons seem to insert directly into bone through a

A

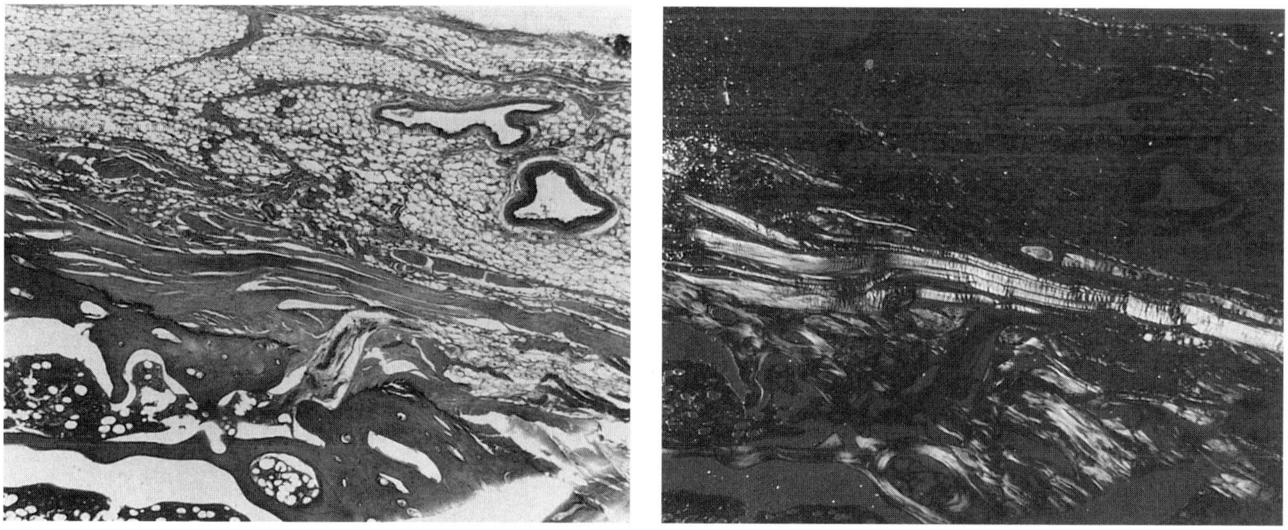

B

FIGURE 6-21 **A** and **B,** The indirect insertion of the deltoid on the acromion under polarized light. Note that the layer of collagen is less abundant. The muscle does not insert directly into bone but seems to pass over the bone into the periosteum, with only a few collagen fascicles inserting into bone. A blood vessel in the center of the illustration supplies both the muscle and the bone. Blood vessels are not shared in direct insertions.

four-layer transition zone that eases the transition of mechanical properties.[82] This type of insertion would be seen at the insertion of the supraspinatus onto the greater tuberosity.

Indirect insertions (Fig. 6-21) are usually broad, muscular insertions or origins, and because the force is thereby spread out, there is usually a broad thin collection of collagen.[82] Little of this collagen seems to pass directly into bone. Most of the collagen goes into periosteum. The surgical handling of indirect insertions is problematic because of the lack of collagen. Surgeons try to split these insertions and leave the collagen in continuity over the bone so that there is little interruption of these collagen fibers. When it is necessary to interrupt the collagen fibers, a portion of periosteum is taken with the muscle so that there will be some collagenous tissue with which to reattach the muscle.

Muscles often have a different insertion at each end. For example, the supraspinatus is fleshy at its origin and direct at its insertion. A single insertion also may vary. For example, the upper subscapularis insertion is direct, and the lower insertion is indirect.[44]

The insertions of the rotator cuff muscles on the humerus are somewhat more complicated. There are connecting fascicles between adjacent tendons (Fig. 6-22). There are also connections to the adjacent capsule.[16,29] The subscapularis muscle is very collagenous toward its upper half and acts in some ways as a passive stabilizer for anterior stability.[73,77]

With respect to function, muscles are divided into three groups: glenohumeral muscles (Table 6-1), scapulothoracic muscles (Table 6-2), and multiarticulation

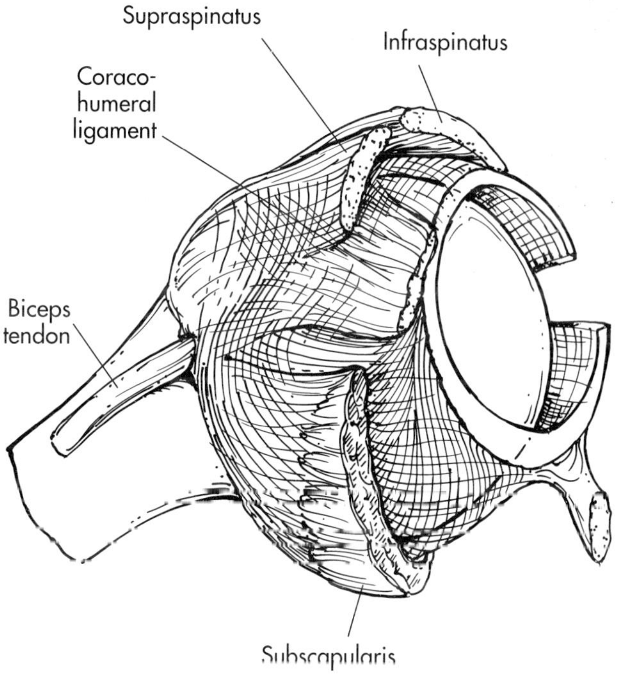

FIGURE 6-22 The complex interconnection between the rotator cuff insertions with each other and with the underlying capsule. This is a glenohumeral joint with the capsule divided posteriorly from glenoid to humerus and the labrum divided from the glenoid. (Modified from Gohlke F, Essigkrug B, Schmitz F: The pattern of the collagen fiber bundles of the capsule of the glenohumeral joint, *J Shoulder Elbow Surgery* 3(3):111, 1994.)

TABLE 6-1
Glenohumeral Muscles

Name	Origin	Insertion	Nerve (C-spinal Level)	Artery	Function
Deltoid					
Anterior third	Lateral third of clavicle, anterior acromion	Deltoid tubercle	Axillary (C5, C6) anterior branch	Posterior humeral circumflex	Elevation in anterior sagittal plane (e.g., flexion)
Middle third	Lateral acromion	Deltoid tubercle	Axillary (C5, C6) anterior branch	Posterior humeral circumflex	All elevations
Posterior third	Posterior acromion and spine of scapula	Deltoid tubercle	Axillary (C5, C6) anterior branch	Posterior humeral circumflex	Posterior elevations
Rotator Cuff	Scapula	Humerus	C5, C6	Multiple	Glenohumeral joint compress
Supraspinatus	Supraspinatus fossa	Uppermost facet of the greater tuberosity	Suprascapular nerve (C5, C6)	Suprascapular artery	Abduction especially in the plane of scapula with internal rotation of the humerus
Infraspinatus	Infraspinatus fossa	Middle facet of the greater tuberosity	Suprascapular nerve (C5, C6)	Suprascapular artery and/or circumflex scapular artery	External rotation in abduction
Teres minor	Middle half of lateral scapula	Lower facet of the greater tuberosity	Axillary nerve posterior branch	Circumflex scapular artery	External rotation in abduction
Subscapularis upper portion	Subscapularis fossa	Lower tuberosity	Upper subscapular nerve (C5)	Subscapular artery	Internal rotation in abduction
Subscapularis lower portion	Subscapularis fossa and lateral scapula	Humerus below lesser tuberosity	Lower subscapular nerve (C5, C6; see text)	Subscapular artery	Internal rotation in abduction
Teres major	Inferior lateral scapula	Medial lip and floor of bicipital groove	Lower subscapular nerve (C5, C6)	Subscapular artery	Adduction and internal rotation against resistance[12]
Coracobrachialis	Coracoid process	Anteromedial humeral diaphysis	Musculotaneous nerve	Branch of brachial nerve	Flexion adduction

muscles (Table 6-3). The tables list the action of the muscle and its innervation and vessel supply.[5,18,68] The drawings of the bones demonstrate the origin and insertion sites (see Figs. 6-1 and 6-3).

Nerve fibers generally travel parallel to the muscle fibers. This makes muscle-splitting incisions convenient in those areas where the muscles cannot be adequately retracted. However, the major nerve to the muscle may in fact be traveling perpendicular to the muscle fibers and can be endangered by muscle-splitting incisions. The following are six areas where the relationship of nerve to muscle is critical: (1) the deltoid muscle and axillary nerve, (2) the trapezius muscle and spinal accessory nerve, (3) the conjoined muscle and tendon and musculocutaneous nerve, (4) the subscapularis muscle and upper and lower subscapular nerves and the axillary nerve, (5) the infraspinatus muscle and the suprascapular nerve, and (6) the quadrilateral space.

TABLE 6-2
Scapulothoracic Muscles

Name	Origin	Insertion	Nerve (C-spinal Level)	Artery	Function
Trapezius					
Upper	Occiput nuchal ligament C7	Distal third of clavicle	Spinal accessory	Transverse cervical and/or dorsal scapula	Upward rotation and elevation (of scapula)[66]
Middle	T1-T6 spinous process	Acromion and distal scapular spine	Spinal accessory (cranial nerve XI)	Transverse cervical and/or dorsal scapula	Scapula retraction
Lower	T7-T12	Base of spine of scapula	Spinal accessory (cranial nerve XI)	Transverse cervical and/or dorsal	Upward rotation and retraction
Rhomboids					
Major	T2-T5	Medial border of scapula below base of spine of scapula to inferior angle	Dorsal scapular nerve (C5)	Dorsal scapular artery	Retraction
Minor	C7-T1	Base of spine of scapula			
Levator Scapulae	C1-C3 Transverse process	Upper angle of scapula	C3, C4 Dorsal scapular nerve	Adjacent vessels	Elevation
Pectoralis Minor	Ribs 3 to 5	Coracoid process	Medial pectoral (C8-T1)	Pectoral artery	Protraction
Subclavius	Ribs (first rib)	Clavicle (lower surface of clavicle)	Nerve to subclavius (C5)	Clavicular artery	Sternoclavicular stabilization
Serratus Anterior					
Upper slip	Ribs 1 and 2	Upper vertebral border of scapula	Long thoracic (C5-C7)	Supreme thoracic	Protraction
Middle slips 2 to 4	Ribs 2 to 4	Vertebral border of scapula	Long thoracic	Lateral thoracic (thoracodorsal)	Protraction
Slips 5 to 9	Ribs 5 to 9	Inferior angle of scapula	Long thoracic	Lateral thoracic (thoracodorsal)	Upward rotation

The axillary nerve is the sole innervation of the deltoid muscle (Fig. 6-23).[1] The nerve exits the quadrilateral space posteriorly and splits into two branches: a smaller posterior branch that ascends along the posterior inferior border of the muscle innervating the posterior fibers of the muscle, and a larger anterior branch that ascends to a level approximately 5 cm below the rim of the acromion. The anterior branch travels anteriorly at this level, innervating the anterior two thirds of the muscle. It is important to remember that this distance from the acromion varies from individual to individual based on patient size, and that the position varies with arm position. Since muscle is a structure with an inconstant length, abduction of the shoulder will bring the nerve closer to the rim of the acromion.[13]

The trapezius muscle has a similar relationship to the spinal accessory nerve (Fig. 6-24). This nerve is well known to be endangered by dissection in the posterior

TABLE 6-3
Multiple Joint Muscles

Name	Origin	Insertion	Nerve (Spinal Nerve)	Vessel	Function
Pectoralis major Upper third	Medial clavicle	Lateral lip of bicipital groove	Lateral pectoral (C5-C7)	Deltoid branch of thoracoacromion	Flexion, adduction
Pectoralis major Middle third	Manubrium, upper two thirds, body of sternum	Lateral lip of bicipital groove	Medial pectoral (C7, C8, T1)	Pectoral	Internal rotation, adduction
Pectoralis major Lower third	Lower body of ribs 5 and 6	Lateral lip of bicipital groove (inverted orientation angle to fiber rotation)	Medial pectoral (C8, T1)	Pectoral	Internal rotation, adduction
Latissimus dorsi	Spinous process of T7-L5 posterior of iliac crest	Crest of the lesser tubercle, the floor of bicipital groove of the humerus	Thoracodorsal (C6, C7)	Thoracodorsal	Adduction against resistance (internal rotation, extension)
Biceps brachii	Glenoid and coracoid	Lacertus fibrosus and radius (tuberosity of radius)	Musculocutaneous	Branch(es) of brachial	Supination and elbow flexion
Triceps brachii long head	Inferior glenoid (other heads from humerus	Olecranon	Radial	Profunda brachii	Elbow extension (shoulder compression)

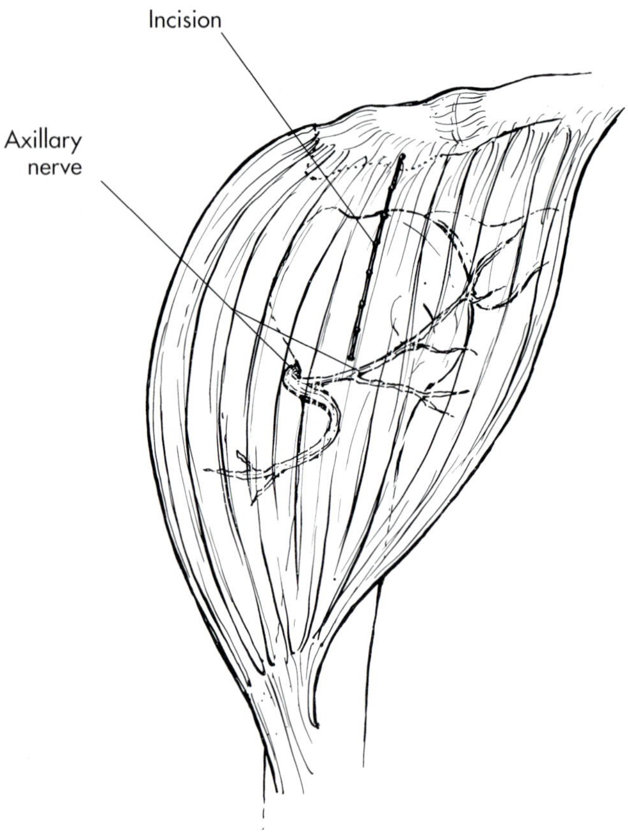

FIGURE 6-23 An anterolateral view of the deltoid and possible position of a muscle-splitting incision. Note the anterior branch of the axillary nerve as it passes forward beneath the deltoid and lies approximately 4 to 5 cm below the edge of the acromion. If the arm is passively abducted or if the deltoid actively contracts, this nerve will be brought closer to the acromion.

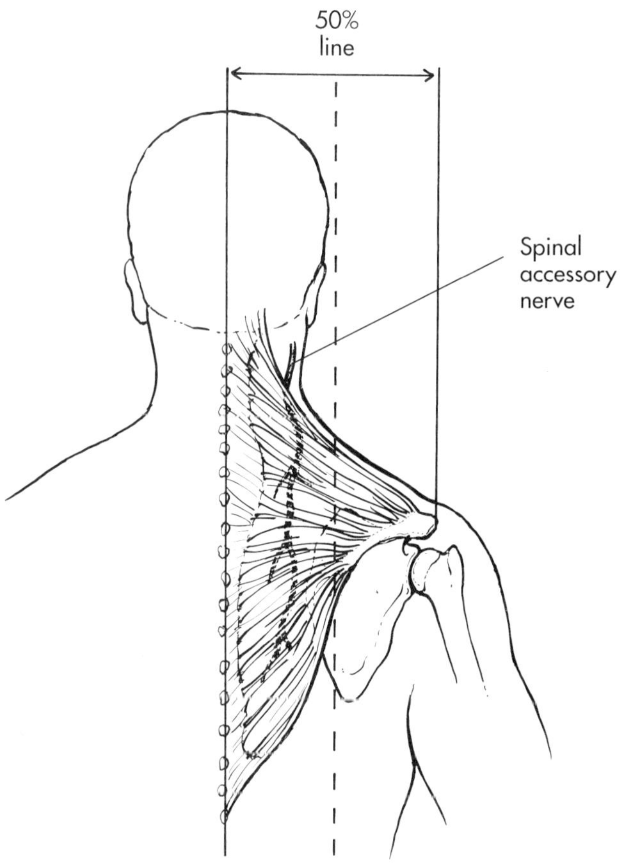

FIGURE 6-24 The trapezius and its relationship to its nerve on the deep surface. The nerve enters the muscle approximately 2 to 3 cm superior and medial to the insertion of the trapezius onto the clavicle. If one considers muscle length to be the distance from the origin on the spinous processes to the insertion on the acromion, the branches of the spinal accessory nerve (three to six in number) always lie medial to the 50% line.

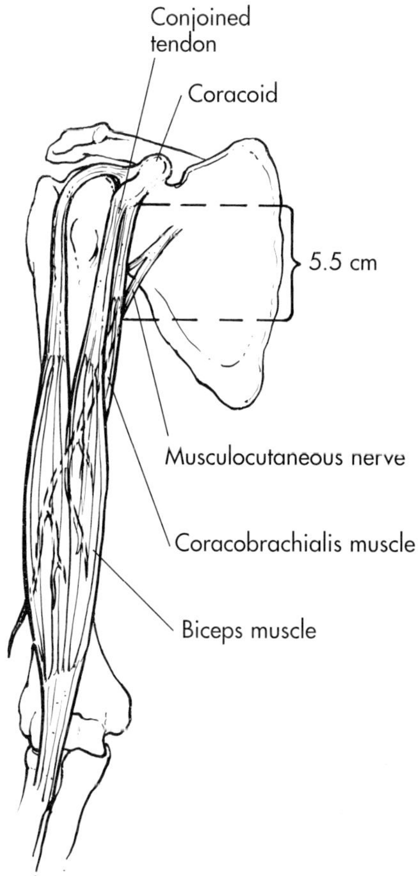

FIGURE 6-25 The conjoined tendon of the coracobrachialis and biceps brachialis (short head) muscles is penetrated by the musculocutaneous nerve 5.5 cm below the tip of the coracoid. Because of the frequent appearance of accessory nerves and the variability in the point of penetration by the musculocutaneous nerve, 75% of cadavers have nerve tissue entering the conjoined tendon and muscle above this 5.5-cm limit.

triangle of the neck. The nerve exits the sternocleidomastoid muscle, travels across this posterior triangle, enters the trapezius about 2 cm above the clavicle, and travels to the deep surface of the trapezius. The trapezius, like the deltoid, varies in length.

The position of the spinal accessory nerve was measured as a percentage of the muscle length taken as the distance from the spinous processes of the vertebrae to the tip of the acromion. The spinal accessory nerve travels slightly medial to a line midway between the spinous processes and the acromion. This path lies at about the level of the vertebral border of the scapula. There appear to be about five (three to six) major branches lying medial to this 50% line.[41] Thus the nerve would be endangered if the trapezius muscle were split medially from the scapula.

The conjoined tendon and muscle represent the origins of the coracobrachialis and short head of the biceps muscles. The musculocutaneous nerve penetrates these muscles about 5.5 cm below the tip of the coracoid (Fig. 6-25). Because there are accessory nerves to these two muscles coming off the lateral cord, and because the position of the main musculocutaneous nerve itself is highly variable, 75% of specimens have nerve material within the 5.5-cm supposed "safe zone."[24] Therefore dissection in this area must be performed carefully to avoid damage to the main musculocutaneous nerve or these auxiliary branches.

The subscapularis muscle entirely covers the anterior glenohumeral joint. To approach the joint and yet avoid transecting muscle and taking down its insertions, it is often convenient to perform a muscle-splitting approach. The upper half of the muscle is innervated by the upper subscapular nerve or nerves, and the lower 20% is innervated by the lower subscapular nerve or nerves[44] (Fig. 6-26). The intervening 30% of the muscle has a variable innervation. Although there have not been any documented cases of denervation of this muscle resulting

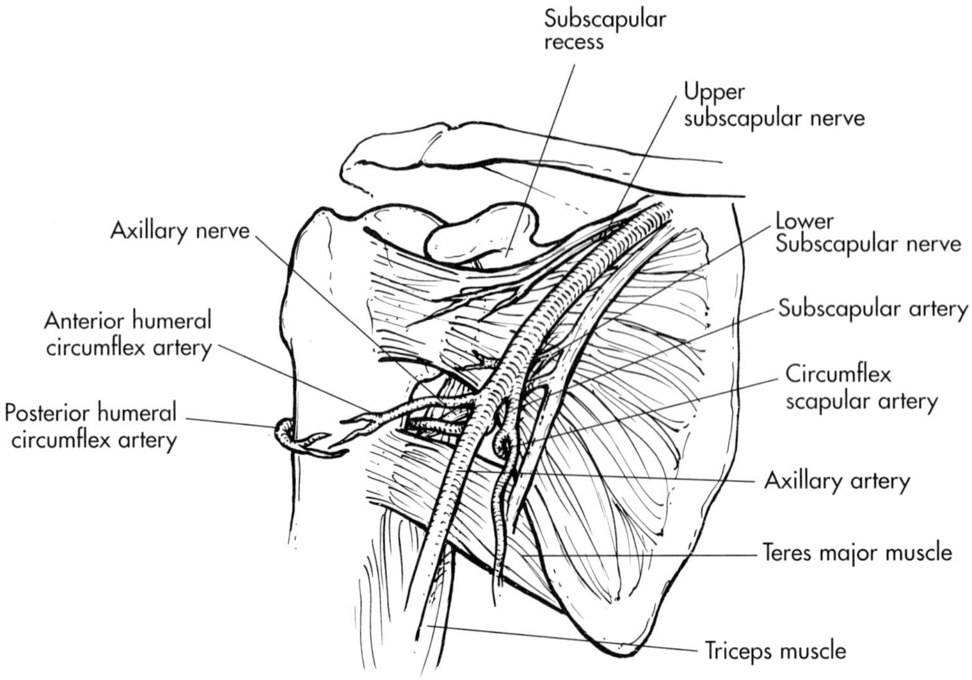

FIGURE 6-26 An anterior view of the subscapularis and the quadrilateral space. The subscapularis muscle forms the posterior wall of the axillary space and therefore has a close association with the nerves of the brachial plexus and the axillary artery and veins. In addition, the muscle itself has a dual innervation. The upper 50% of the muscle is penetrated by the superior subscapular nerves, and the lower 30% of the muscle is innervated by the lower subscapular nerves. The intervening 20% of the muscle is variable in its innervation. These subscapular nerves frequently are multiple. The inferior border of the subscapularis anteriorly is indicated by the anterior humeral circumflex artery, but a portion of the muscle inserts even more inferiorly on the humeral head than shown. This portion of the subscapularis is obscured anteriorly by the tendon of the latissimus dorsi. The axillary nerve and the posterior humeral circumflex artery pass through the quadrilateral space, of which the subscapularis muscle forms the superior border.

from a muscle-splitting procedure, it is a possibility. In addition, immediately anterior to the subscapularis muscle lies the axillary nerve en route to the inferior border of the subscapularis, where it enters the quadrilateral space. Because of this position of the axillary nerve, all muscle-splitting incisions of the subscapularis must be performed under direct vision to avoid injuring the nerve.

The internal structure of the subscapularis muscle is worthy of note. The upper muscle lies above the center of glenohumeral motion and is therefore almost at its maximum excursion at rest. This portion of the muscle shortens as the arm is elevated. This upper area has more collagen and a direct insertion into the lesser tuberosity and acts almost as a passive stabilizer.[73] The lower portion of the subscapularis rests near its shortest length and has greater need for excursion. This region has longer, more parallel fibers and a fleshy indirect insertion. This lower indirect insertion is difficult to repair.

The infraspinatus muscle (Fig. 6-27) overlies what would be the most desirable place to enter the glenohumeral joint posteriorly. Because it is largely a fleshy muscle with not as much tendon as the subscapularis, it is a more desirable location for muscle-splitting incisions rather than to take down the distal insertion. The suprascapular nerve lies immediately deep to the muscle. At the upper portion of the muscle, where the nerve is in the spinoglenoid notch, it may lie as close as 1.7 cm medial to the glenoid rim. This dictates a limit to muscle-splitting incisions of the infraspinatus and submuscular dissection.

The teres minor muscle resembles the lower portion of the subscapularis. It is most active with the arm in abduction and has a fleshier insertion compared with the infraspinatus muscle. This muscle is the posterior roof of the quadrilateral space.

The quadrilateral space (Figs. 6-28 and 6-29) represents the inferior portion of the glenohumeral joint. Here the axillary nerve is adjacent to the muscles and capsule. As these are soft-tissue structures, there is not a lot of fat

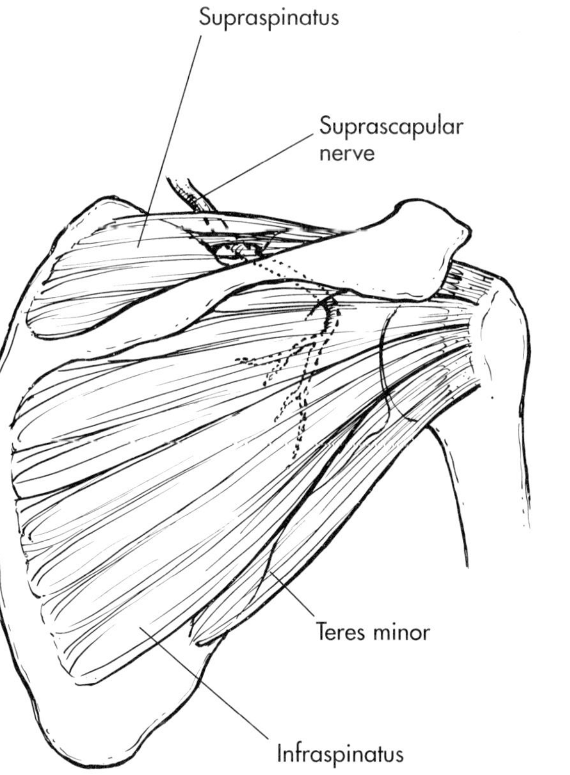

FIGURE 6-27 The supraspinatus and infraspinatus muscles have an intimate relationship with the suprascapular nerve. This nerve lies on the deep surface of the muscles, making muscle-splitting incisions hazardous. Although muscle-splitting incisions of the supraspinatus are used rarely to never, those of the infraspinatus are not as rare, and at the upper portion of the glenoid this nerve may lie only about 2 cm medial to the rim of the glenoid. Thus muscle-splitting incisions of the infraspinatus are not taken very far medially.

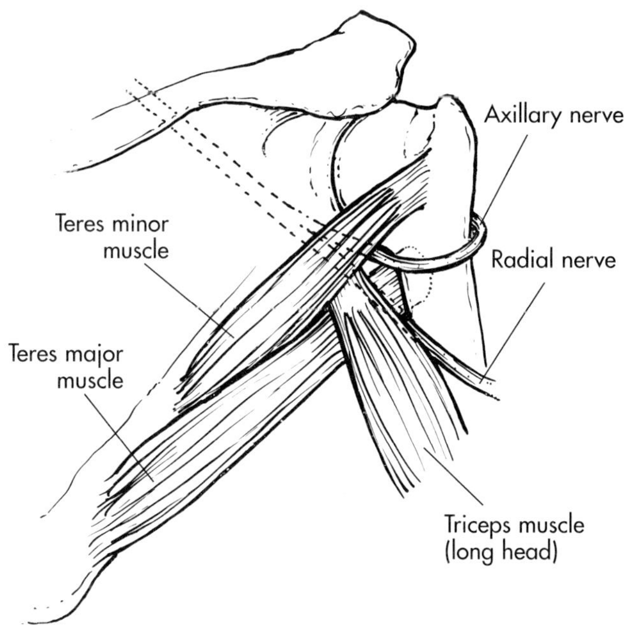

FIGURE 6-28 The boundaries of the quadrilateral space as seen from behind. This space is never as large as is represented in textbooks because it is really only a potential space. It is filled with very little perineural fat. The nerve lies very close to the fascia of the muscles, if not directly on it.

in this area to protect the nerve and to signal the nerve's presence to the surgeon. Anteriorly, the quadrilateral space is bounded by the subscapularis above and teres major and latissimus dorsi below. The shaft of the humerus lies lateral and the long head of the triceps lies medial to the space. Posteriorly, the space has the same medial and lateral borders but is bounded by the teres minor above and teres major below. Adhesions and additional collagenous tissue can develop in this space, leading to an entrapment of the nerve and the posterior humeral circumflex artery when the arm is in an abducted externally rotated position.[14]

Nerves

Nerves have a relatively constant arrangement in terms of their paths to various important structures.[33,74] Nerves poorly tolerate changes in length.[49] There is obstruction of venous outflow from the nerves with only an 8% change in length.[49] With this in mind, it is easy to understand why nerves tend to be arranged near centers of rotation so that their changes in length are less for each change in angulation of the joint. In addition, the nerves travel in the soft tissues and avoid crossing planes of motion. Where it is necessary to cross a plane of motion, they do so obliquely and at the edges of the motion so there is less absolute and relative motion. Nerves receive blood supply throughout their length and tolerate only 8 cm of dissection from their blood supply.[49]

The brachial plexus consists of spinal nerves, trunks, anterior and posterior divisions, lateral, medial, and posterior cords, and peripheral nerves.[33,43] Histologically, all of these structures are peripheral nerves. Table 6-1 lists the peripheral nerves, their nerve of origin, their division, their trunk, and their spinal nerves for reference.

In the shoulder region, as in other parts of the body, there are areas where the nerves have a special relationship with adjacent structures that may endanger the nerves. In the shoulder there are, in addition to the muscle relations and quadrilateral space mentioned in the muscle section, the suprascapular notch and the

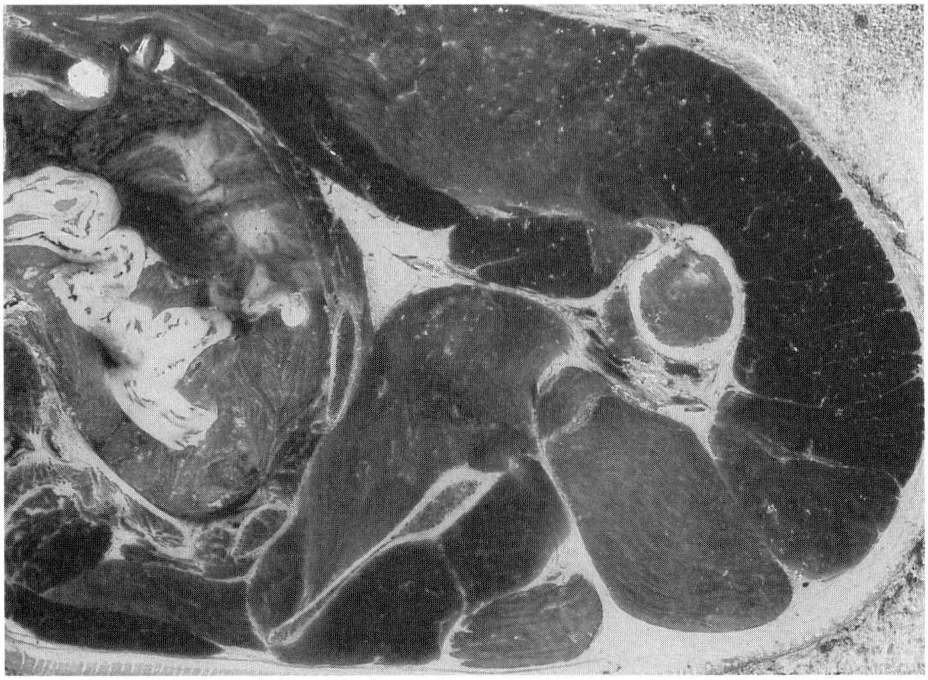

A

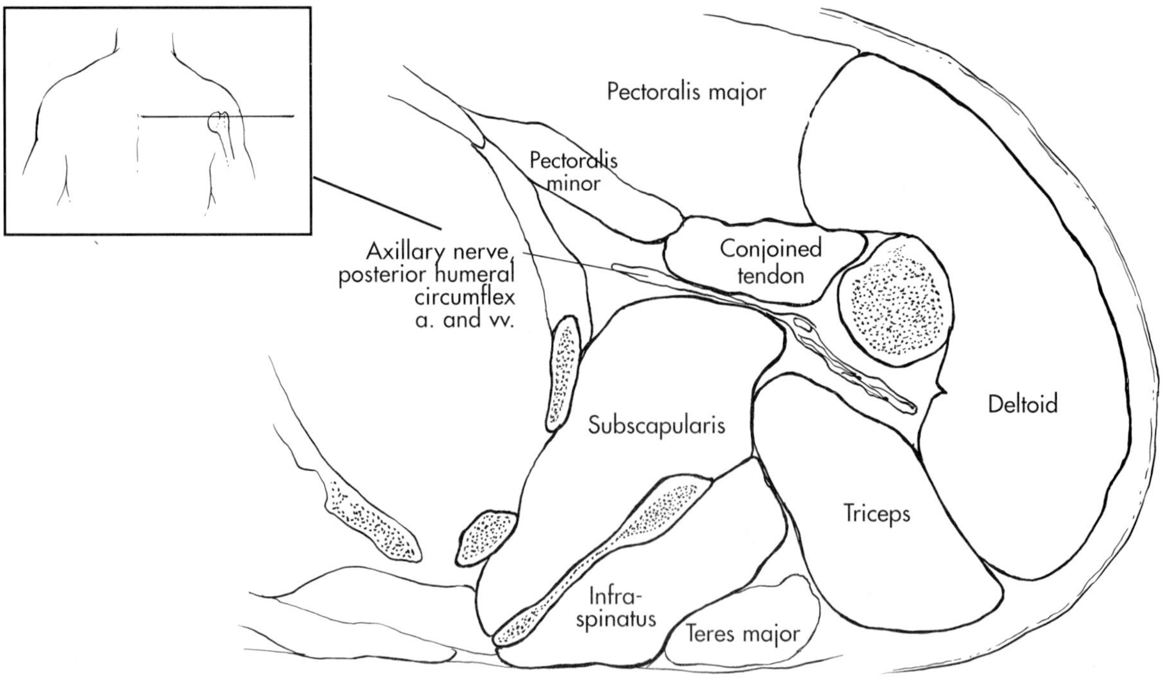

B

FIGURE 6-29 **A** and **B,** An axial cross-section of the quadrilateral space. The axillary nerve and its accompanying posterior humeral circumflex artery are seen exiting the axilla between the subscapularis muscle and the conjoined tendon. Medial to the humerus, they lie on top of the teres major and then pass between the triceps and humerus to the deltoid muscle.

TABLE 6-4
Nerves of the Shoulder

Name	Parent Nerve	Cord Representation	Muscle	Skin
Dorsal scapular	C5	C5 (C4 also)	Rhomboid minor Rhomboid major Levator (occasionally)	
Long thoracic	C5, C6, C7	C5, C6, C7	Serratus anterior	
Suprascapular	Superior trunk	C5, C6	Supraspinatus Infraspinatus	Upper lateral arm
Axillary	Posterior cord	C5, C6	Deltoid, teres minor	
Lateral pectoral	Lateral cord	C5, C6, C7	Pectoralis major Pectoralis minor	
Medial pectoral	Medial cord	C8, T1 (C7 from lateral pectoral nerve)	Pectoralis major	
Upper subscapularis	Posterior cord	C5	Subscapularis (upper)	
Lower subscapularis	Posterior cord	C5, C6	Subscapularis (lower) and teres major	
Thoracodorsal	Posterior cord	C7, C8	Latissimus dorsi	
Musculocutaneous	Lateral cord	C5-C7	Biceps, coracobrachialis Brachialis	Forearm
Radial	Posterior cord	C5-C8	Triceps brachii (and distal muscles)	Posterior arm
Medial brachial cutaneous	Medial cord	C8, T1		Medial arm
Intercostal brachial	Intercostal nerves 2 and 3	T2, T3		Axilla
Supraclavicular	C3, C4	C3, C4		Skin of upper shoulder and chest

spinoglenoid notch, both of which can be areas of entrapment of the suprascapular nerve.

The supraclavicular nerves are often cut during dissection over the clavicle. Anterior and superior shoulder incisions also regularly leave areas of numbness by sectioning supraclavicular nerves. Fortunately, this usually leaves little effect on the patient.

The intercostal brachial (second intercostal space) nerve is endangered in approaches to the axilla, as seen in breast surgery and thoracic outlet surgery. Transecting the intercostal brachial nerve can produce symptoms.

The long thoracic nerve is endangered where it is draped over the second rib and can be injured indirectly by positioning the patient improperly at surgery or by the patient's own lifting activities.[34]

The thoracic outlet is a similar area of potential nerve entrapment[66] (Fig. 6-30). The area of entrapment is a triangle above the first rib that is bordered anteriorly by the scalenus anterior muscle and posteriorly by the middle scalene. The subclavian vein enters the chest anterior to the scalenus anticus, but the subclavian artery and all of the nerves of the brachial plexus travel within the triangle, where they may be entrapped and become symptomatic, particularly the lower trunk, which is draped over the first rib.

An additional important facet of innervation of the shoulder is the autonomic nerve supply. There is a rich sympathetic innervation in the shoulder that comes from the cervical sympathetic ganglia and travels within the peripheral nerves. The highest spinal cord representation of the sympathetic nervous system is usually reported as T2 but may be T1 or C8 in some individuals. The upper portion of the brachial plexus seems to carry fewer sympathetic nerve axons than the lower portion.

Vessels

In general, blood vessels follow the same pattern of distribution as the nerves.[71] There are more variations of the vessels than of the nerves because the vessels act as high-pressure conduits, and their efficiency of function is not directly related to their distance from the heart. Their embryology is also not one continuous path. This leads to a greater variation in the arterial tree than is seen in the arrangement of the brachial plexus. Each of the arteries is accompanied by two veins, the venae comitantes.

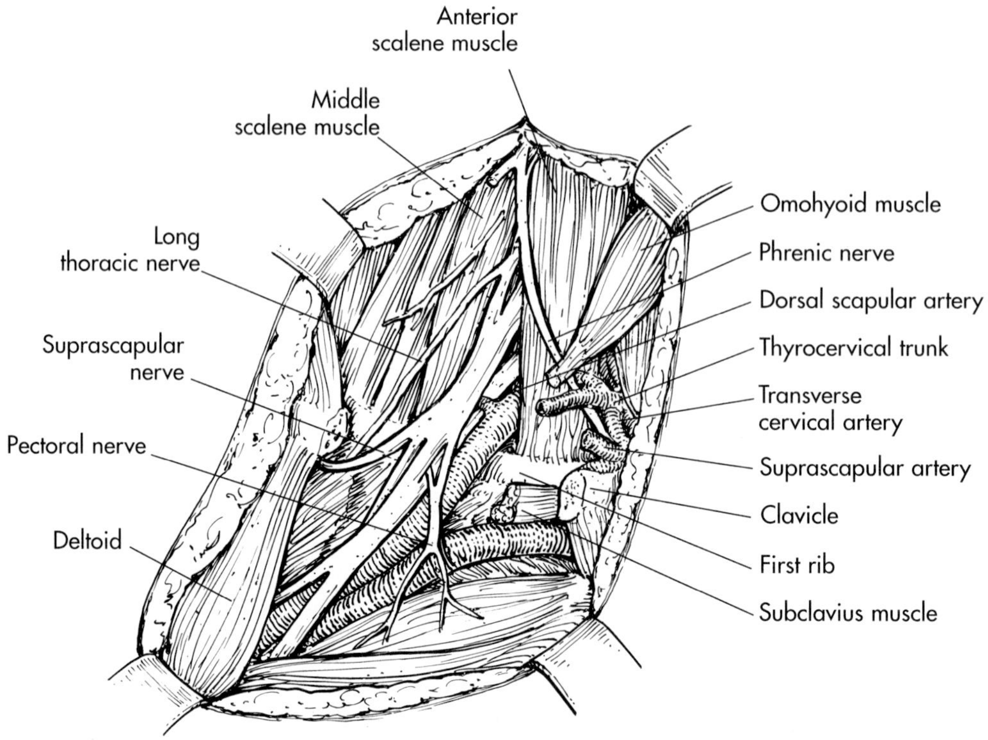

FIGURE 6-30 The thoracic outlet and its boundaries. This also illustrates the brachial plexus as it would appear at dissection.

Fig. 6-31 illustrates the statistically average distribution of vessels in the shoulder and their relationship to the pectoralis minor muscle. Because of the great variability in vessel distribution, almost no individuals actually have the so-called normal distribution.[21,37,76] This is the major reason that vascular surgeons frequently rely on arteriography to accurately visualize the vascular anatomy.

The collateral vessels are affected by the same tendencies that govern the distribution of vessels in general. In the areas where there are dense collagenous structures, there are planes of motion and therefore not many crossing vessels.[61] Most of these large collateral vessels travel in areas of muscle.

The cephalic vein is an important solitary structure. In the shoulder it travels within the deltopectoral groove, sometimes adjacent to the deltoid artery, which is a branch of the thyrocervical trunk. The cephalic vein drains the deltoid muscle in addition to the superficial arm and forearm, and in most patients, this relationship should be maintained. If the vein is injured and ligated, the resultant congestion in the arm and deltoid leads to a more painful postoperative course.

Bursae and Planes of Motion

There are various ways by which the body accommodates motion. The best known of these is the diarthrodial joint. There are other accommodations by which relatively dense soft tissues move past each other. For very dense collagenous structures, these are called bursae (Fig. 6-32). These are synovially lined structures whose histology and ultrastructure vary from site to site depending on what structure is deep to the bursal surface. These bursae accommodate motion of skin past bone and bone or tendon past bone. The most important of these in the shoulder are the subacromial and the coracobrachialis bursae. The first facilitates motion between the acromion and the underlying supraspinatus tendon; the second between subscapularis and the overlying conjoint tendon and coracoid process. These two bursae are often connected.

The most abundant motion-facilitating structure in the shoulder is the loose alveolar tissue, which is most often seen where muscles move past each other. These planes of motion are convenient not only for the motion of the athletic patient but also to facilitate the dissection by the surgeon. As mentioned previously, nerves and vessels do not cross these planes of motion. Therefore the plane at which motion occurs tends to provide a relatively safe and bloodless area for dissection.

The cross-sectional drawings in Figs. 6-33 to 6-38 show not only the relationship of the shoulder structures, but by bold lines also demonstrate the planes where one can attain relatively bloodless dissection.

Text continues on p. 156.

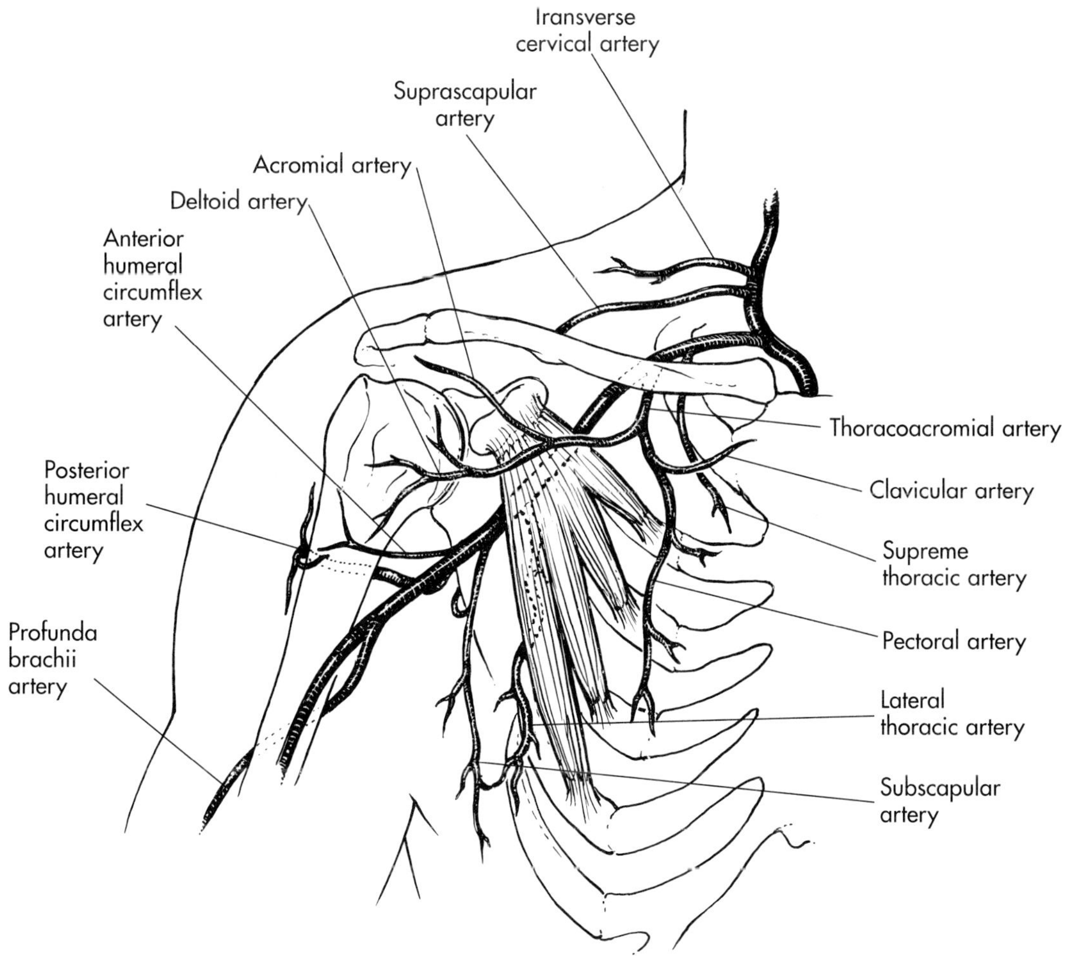

FIGURE 6-31 The named arteries of the shoulder region and their branching from the axillary artery relative to the pectoralis minor muscle. The thoracoacromial artery is shown originating above the pectoralis minor. It usually is shown originating deep to the pectoralis minor.

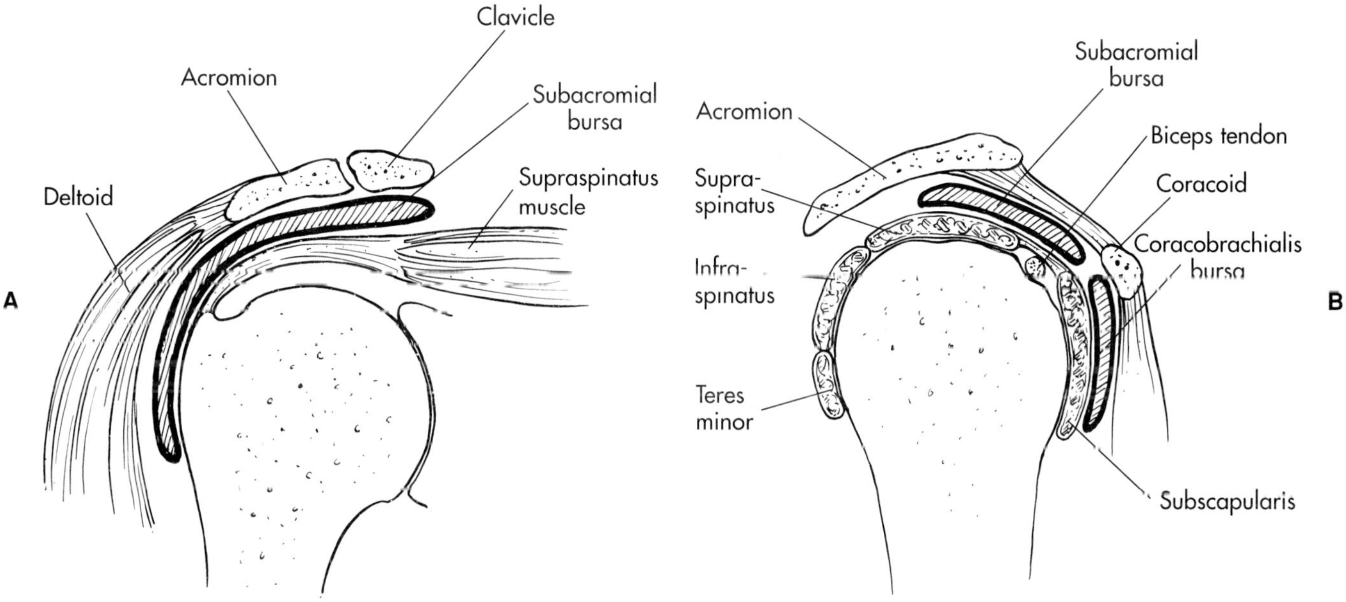

FIGURE 6-32 **A** and **B**, Anterior view and sagittal view of the major bursae of the shoulder. The coracobrachialis bursa here is shown as a separate structure; however, in 80% of specimens it connects with the subacromial bursa. The subacromial bursa is present only in the anterior one half to two thirds of the subacromial space. The posterior portion of that space is occupied by fat.

A

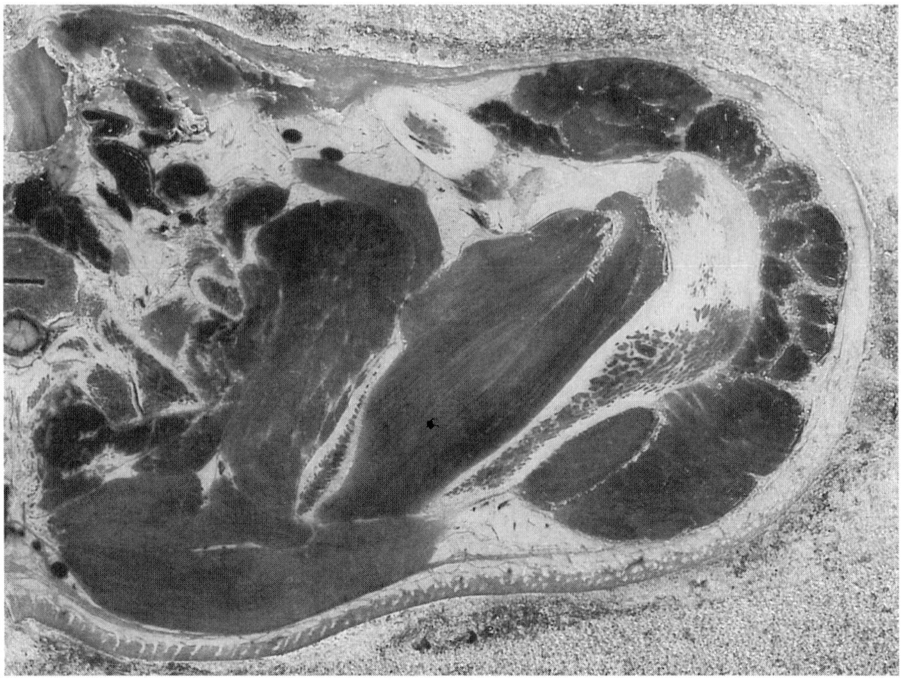

B

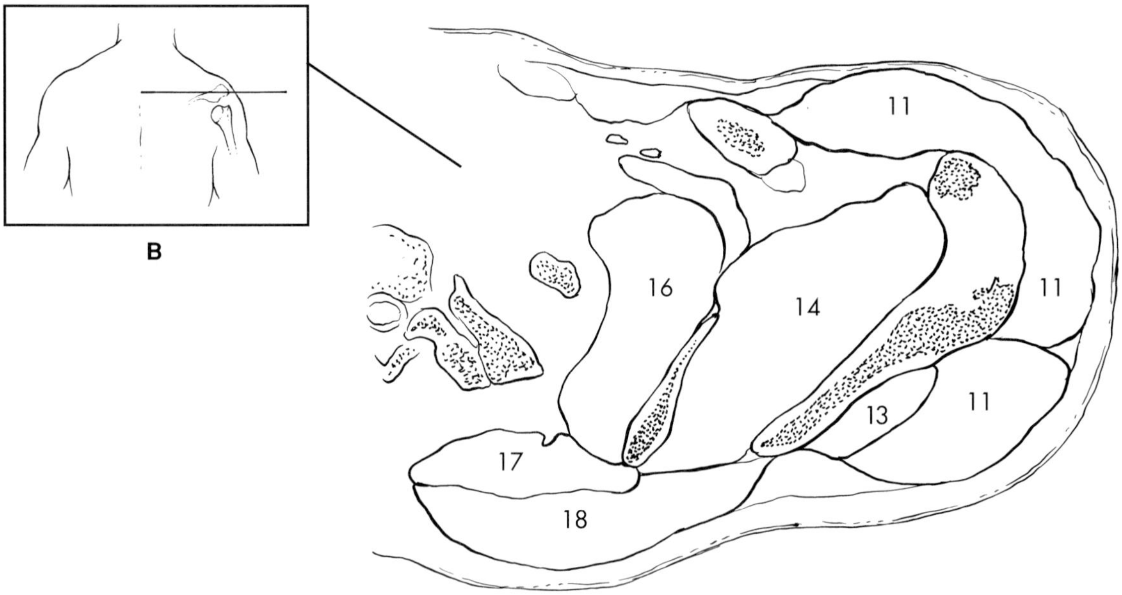

FIGURES 6-33 and 6-34 Serial axial cross-sections moving from cephalad to caudad. These illustrations demonstrate relationships in the axial plane. They also demonstrate the thinness or complete closure of the potential spaces. Note that in figures 6-33 to 6-38 the lines demarcating the potential spaces on the photograph (the *A* figures) are thinner than the artist's line (the *B* figures) in the drawing. The heavier line in the drawings indicates potential spaces that are useful in surgical approaches. The structures are numbered 1 through 25 to indicate the bones and muscles. Bones are: (1) scapula, (2) humerus, (3) clavicle, (4) rib 1, (5) rib 2, (6) rib 3, (7) rib 4, (8) rib 5, and (9) rib 6. Muscles are: (10) pectoralis major, (11) deltoid, (12) supraspinatus, (13) infraspinatus, (14) subscapularis, (15) teres minor, (16) serratus anterior, (17) pectoralis minor, (18) trapezius, (19) rhomboid, (20) coracobrachialis, (21) biceps (short), (22) biceps (long), (23) teres major and latissimus dorsi, (24) subclavius, and (25) triceps.

A

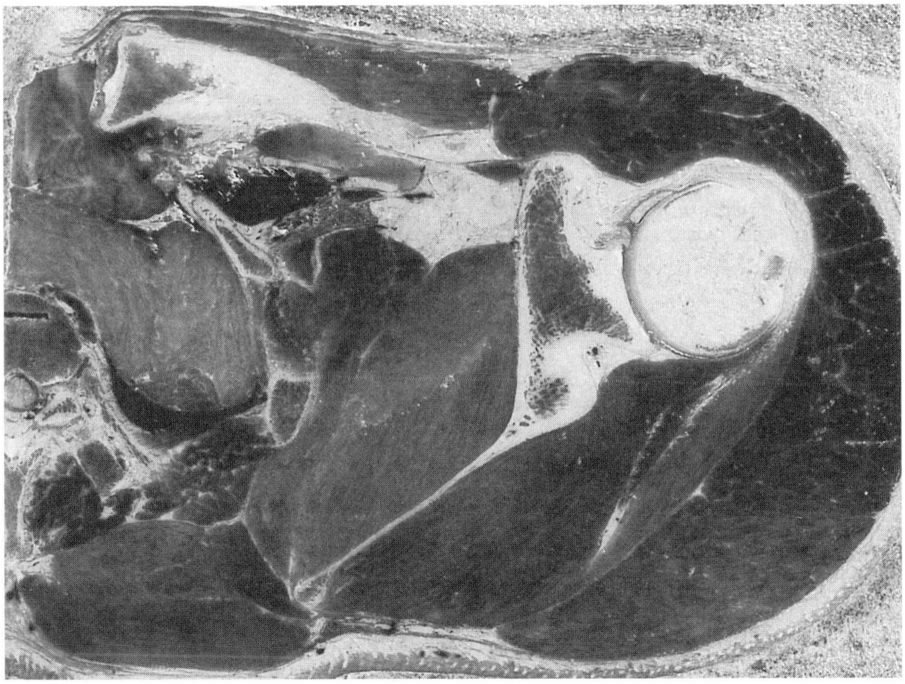

B

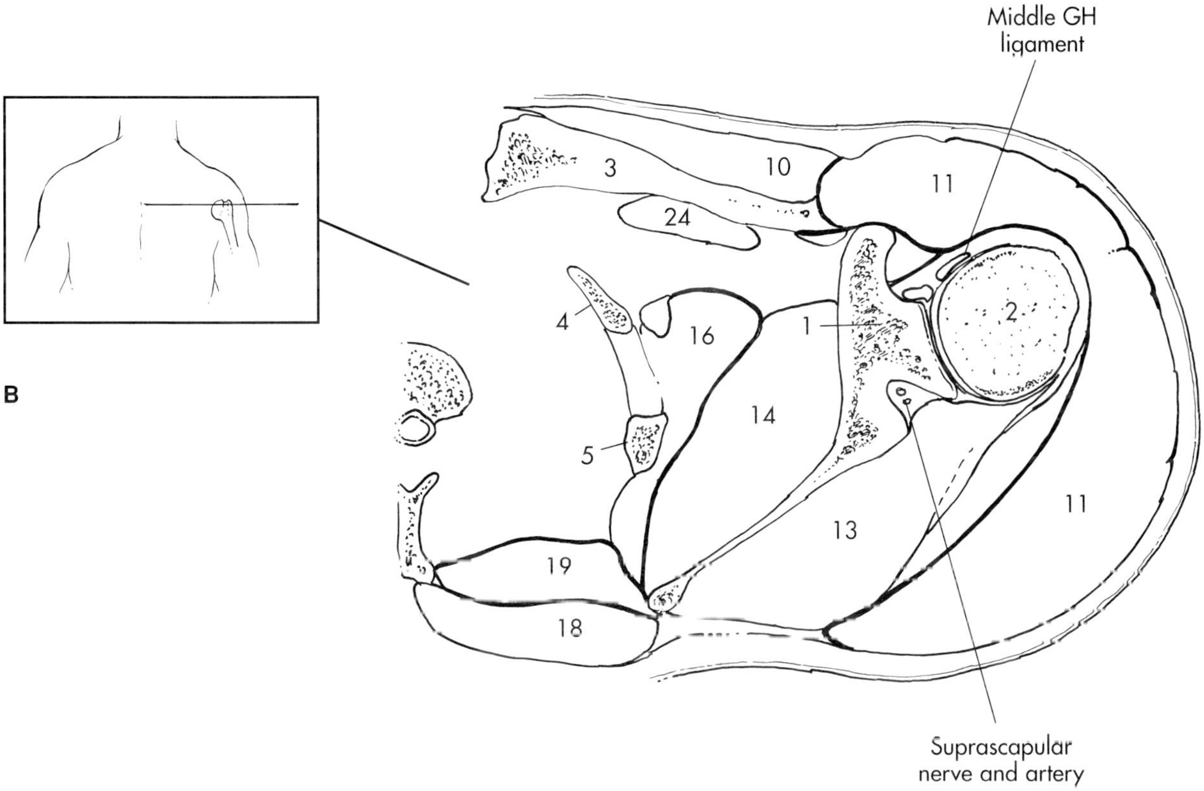

FIGURE 6-34, A and B. For legend see opposite page.

A

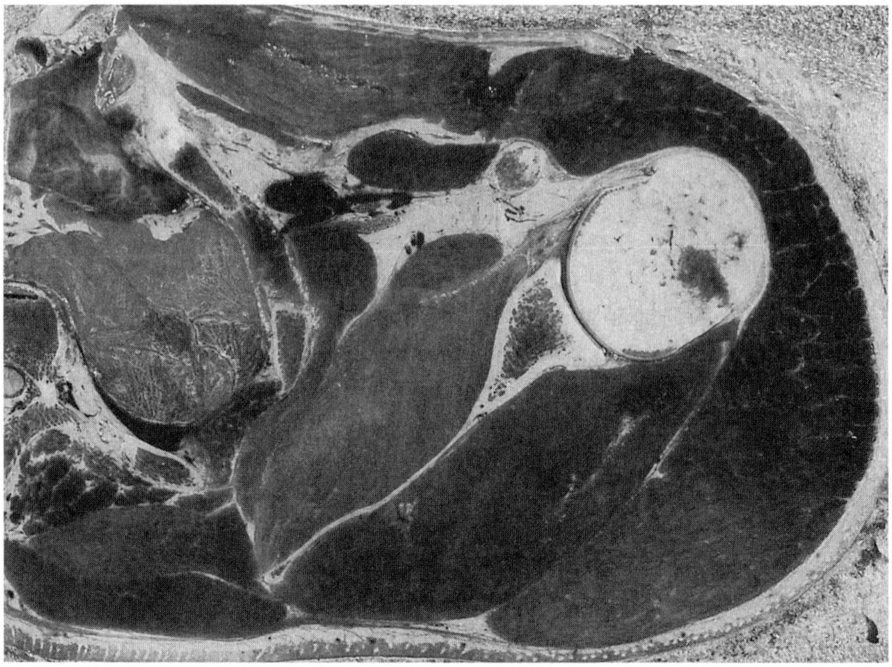

B

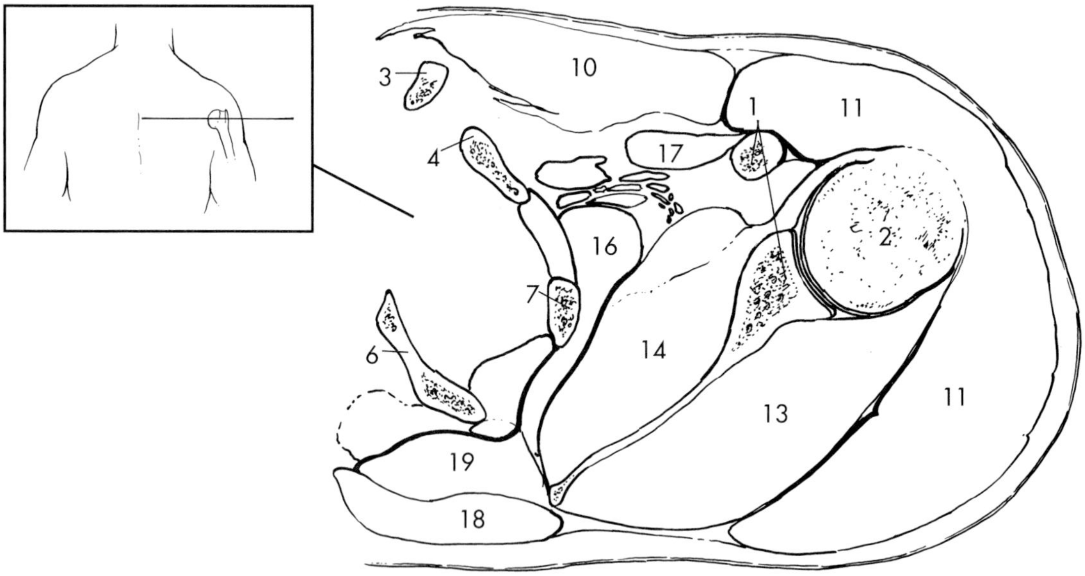

FIGURES 6-35 and 6-36 Serial axial cross-sections moving from cephalad to caudad. These illustrations demonstrate relationships in the axial plane. They also demonstrate the thinness or complete closure of the potential spaces. Note that in figures 6-33 to 6-38 the lines demarcating the potential spaces on the photograph (the *A* figures) are thinner than the artist's line (the *B* figures) in the drawing. The heavier line in the drawings indicates potential spaces that are useful in surgical approaches. The structures are numbered 1 through 25 to indicate the bones and muscles. Bones are: (1) scapula, (2) humerus, (3) clavicle, (4) rib 1, (5) rib 2, (6) rib 3, (7) rib 4, (8) rib 5, and (9) rib 6. Muscles are: (10) pectoralis major, (11) deltoid, (12) supraspinatus, (13) infraspinatus, (14) subscapularis, (15) teres minor, (16) serratus anterior, (17) pectoralis minor, (18) trapezius, (19) rhomboid, (20) coracobrachialis, (21) biceps (short), (22) biceps (long), (23) teres major and latissimus dorsi, (24) subclavius, and (25) triceps.

A

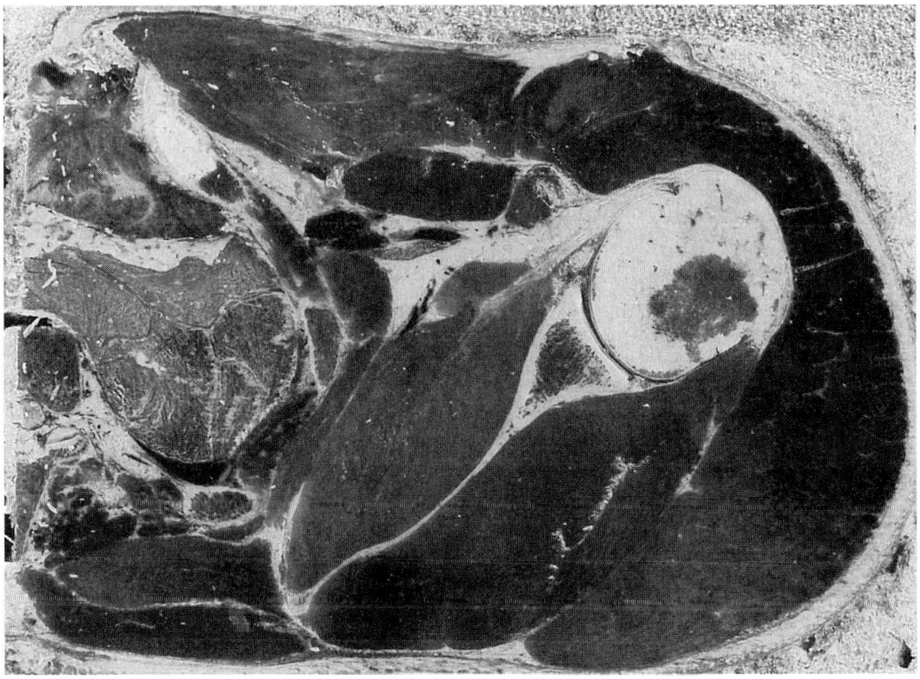

B

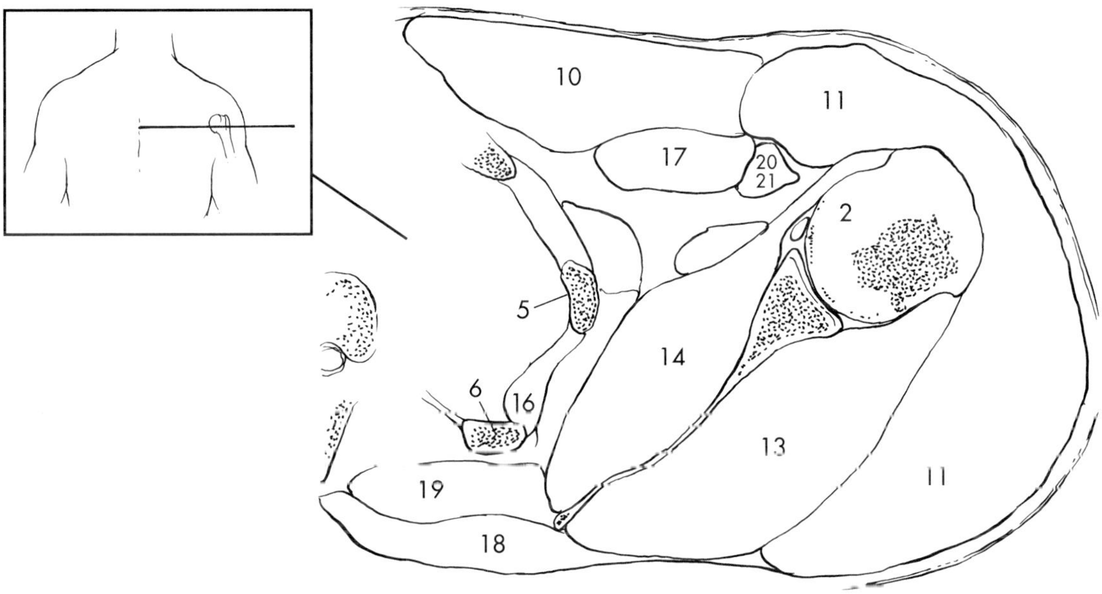

FIGURE 6-36, A and B. For legend see opposite page.

A

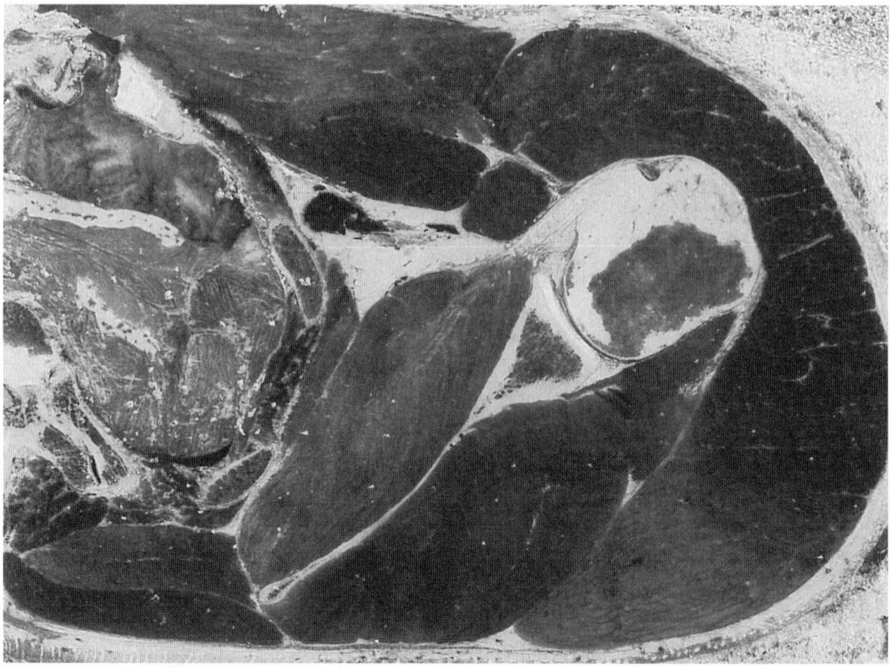

B

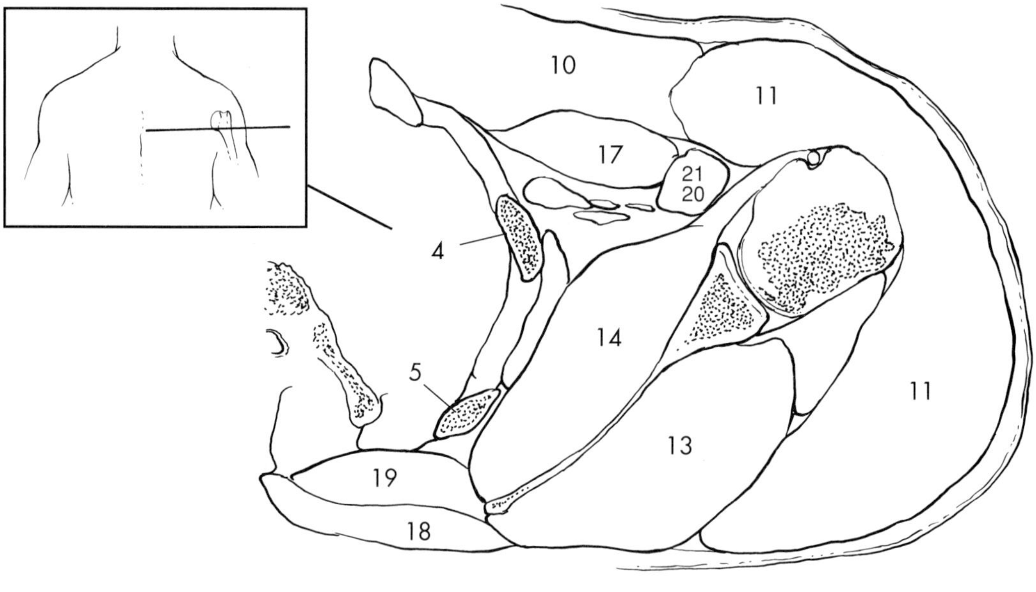

FIGURES 6-37 and 6-38 Serial axial cross-sections moving from cephalad to caudad. These illustrations demonstrate relationships in the axial plane. They also demonstrate the thinness or complete closure of the potential spaces. Note that in figures 6-33 to 6-38 the lines demarcating the potential spaces on the photograph (the *A* figures) are thinner than the artist's line (the *B* figures) in the drawing. The heavier line in the drawings indicates potential spaces that are useful in surgical approaches. The structures are numbered 1 through 25 to indicate the bones and muscles. Bones are: (1) scapula, (2) humerus, (3) clavicle, (4) rib 1, (5) rib 2, (6) rib 3 (7) rib 4, (8) rib 5, and (9) rib 6. Muscles are: (10) pectoralis major, (11) deltoid, (12) supraspinatus, (13) infraspinatus, (14) subscapularis, (15) teres minor, (16) serratus anterior, (17) pectoralis minor, (18) trapezius, (19) rhomboid, (20) coracobrachialis, (21) biceps (short), (22) biceps (long), (23) teres major and latissimus dorsi, (24) subclavius, and (25) triceps.

A

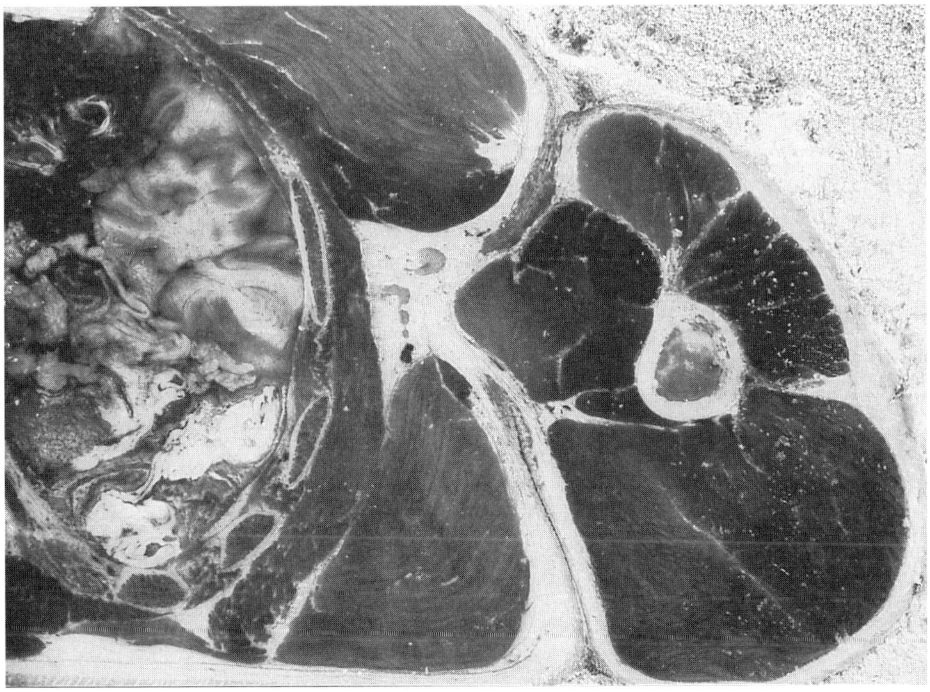

B

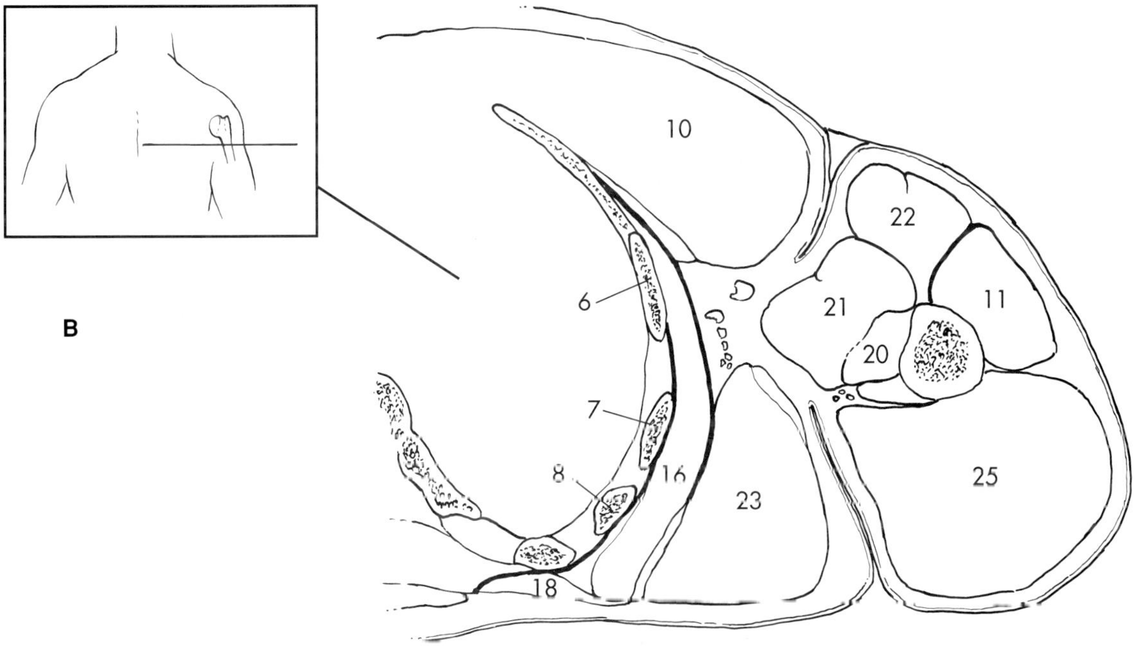

FIGURE 6-38, A and B. For legend see opposite page.

Skin

The skin overlying the shoulder is frequently exposed to view. The important general considerations are the vascular supply to the skin, cosmesis, and sensation. Cosmesis often becomes the primary consideration. This occurs because sensation in the area of the skin of the shoulder is less important to function, and numbness infrequently arises as a complaint from the patient. In addition, there is an abundant blood supply to the skin of the shoulder so that there is rarely wound necrosis.

The auxiliary blood to the skin (i.e., those vessels that supplement supply to the dermis) of the anterior shoulder reaches the skin from the axilla and at the edges of the sternum from the internal mammary arteries (Fig. 6-39). The auxiliary vessels travel in the subcutaneous fascia. This leaves a large bloodless plane anteriorly where skin and fat can be elevated off the deep fascia of the pectoralis major without loss of blood supply. This freedom allows the surgeon to pick more cosmetic incisions. Posteriorly, there is a similar auxiliary blood supply to the skin coming from the circumflex scapular artery; this is frequently used by our colleagues in microvascular surgery.[79,80]

With cosmesis being the usual overwhelming consideration, it is important to place incisions in the skin in such a way that they line up with the usual stresses on the skin. In more recent history, plastic surgeons have referred to these as the lines of relaxed skin tension[8,46,47,54] (Fig. 6-40). In the past, Langer referred to them as the lines of "splitability" of the skin.[45] These lines are made more apparent by pinching the skin in different directions, looking for a smooth and parallel pattern. They rep-

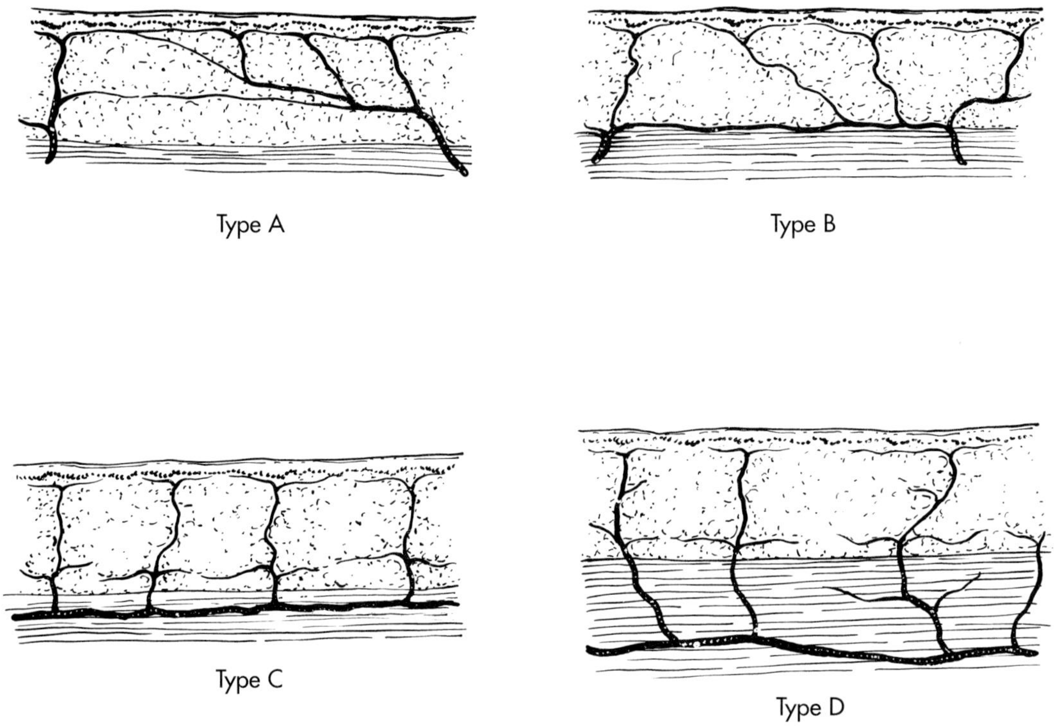

FIGURE 6-39 The four potential relationships of the direct circulation to the skin. There is always a plexus of vessels in the dermis and a direct circulation connecting the dermis with a deeper layer. This layer of deeper circulation provides the direct circulation to the dermal plexus and always is located just superficial to the plane of motion between skin and the deeper structures. Over the pectoralis major, the plane of motion is between muscle fascia and skin, as in type A. In the type A circulation, the auxiliary blood supply lies in the subcutaneous fascia and thereby moves with the skin. Over the biceps and the arm, the plane of motion is between the circumferential fascia of the forearm and the fascia of the individual muscles. In this area, the auxiliary blood supply lies directly on the deep fascia, as shown in type B. The circulation shown in type B lends itself to fasciotendinous flaps. The circulation shown in type C is found on the plantar and palmar surfaces of the body, where the auxiliary blood supply lies deep to a thick fascial structure that adheres very tightly to the skin. In these areas, raising skin flaps could be detrimental to the skin circulation. Type D is the type of circulation that is common in an area such as over the gluteus maximus. In this type of circulation, the auxiliary blood supply lies deep to the muscle and then supplies the skin directly. In these areas, a myocutaneous flap often proves to be the best strategy. (Modified from Taylor GI, Palmer JH: The vascular territories [angiosomes] of the body: experimental study and clinical applications, *Br J Plast Surg* 40:113, 1987.)

resent the overwhelming collagen orientation of the skin. The current theory regarding their origin is the same as Langer's. The orientation of these lines are determined by the shape of the structure underlying the skin and the motion of that underlying structure.

SURGICAL APPROACHES

The surgical approaches mentioned here are the ones most important to sports medicine. A few others are mentioned for the sake of comparison. They are listed by the body surface through which the approach is made.

Open Procedures

Anterior or Deltopectoral Approaches

The anterior or deltopectoral approaches can be either short or long.[65] In sports medicine, the short, more cosmetic incision is used. This incision is made anteriorly in the vertical lines of relaxed skin tension. In most female patients (because of the smaller muscle mass) the incision can actually be placed even more inferiorly into the axilla. In either case this is a cosmetic incision. The long oblique deltopectoral incision is made to allow extensibility of the incision. It has a poorer cosmetic result and is rarely needed in sports medicine.

The skin and subcutaneous fat are elevated off the deep fascia in a usually bloodless dissection. The one exception to this is that the crossing vessels are present as they come from the deltoid artery as it lies in the deltopectoral groove. In such cases the small bleeding vessels are an additional clue in localizing the deltopectoral groove.

The deltopectoral groove also signals its location by a fat stripe, or occasionally the cephalic vein is visible immediately beneath the deep fascia. In any case the fascia is split over the deltopectoral groove, taking care not to injure the vein, and leaving the vein attached to the deltoid muscle from which it receives several tributaries. Finger dissection easily splits the deltopectoral groove deep to the vein. Then the fascia of the deep surface of the groove is split with scissors. In some patients the surgeon may elect to release the superior 1 cm of the pectoralis major insertion from the humerus to gain additional exposure. Care is taken to release the deep fascia on the deep surface of the deltoid to enable placement of a Goelet retractor beneath the deltoid. An additional Goelet retractor is placed medially to retract the pectoralis major muscle.

The conjoint tendon and muscle are retracted medially with a long, thin Richardson retractor to expose the subscapularis muscle. Shoulder adduction and external rotation brings the subscapularis muscle into the wound from beneath the conjoint tendon. This is because the upper subscapularis muscle is above the center of glenohumeral rotation, and abduction hides the upper subscapularis under the coracoid and conjoint tendon. The subscapularis muscle is split in line with its fibers in most sports medicine procedures described in this text. The subscapularis may occasionally need to be divided for more extensive procedures. When dividing the subscapularis, it is best to remember that the lower subscapularis has little internal collagen with which to hold sutures. The lower subscapularis should be retracted and

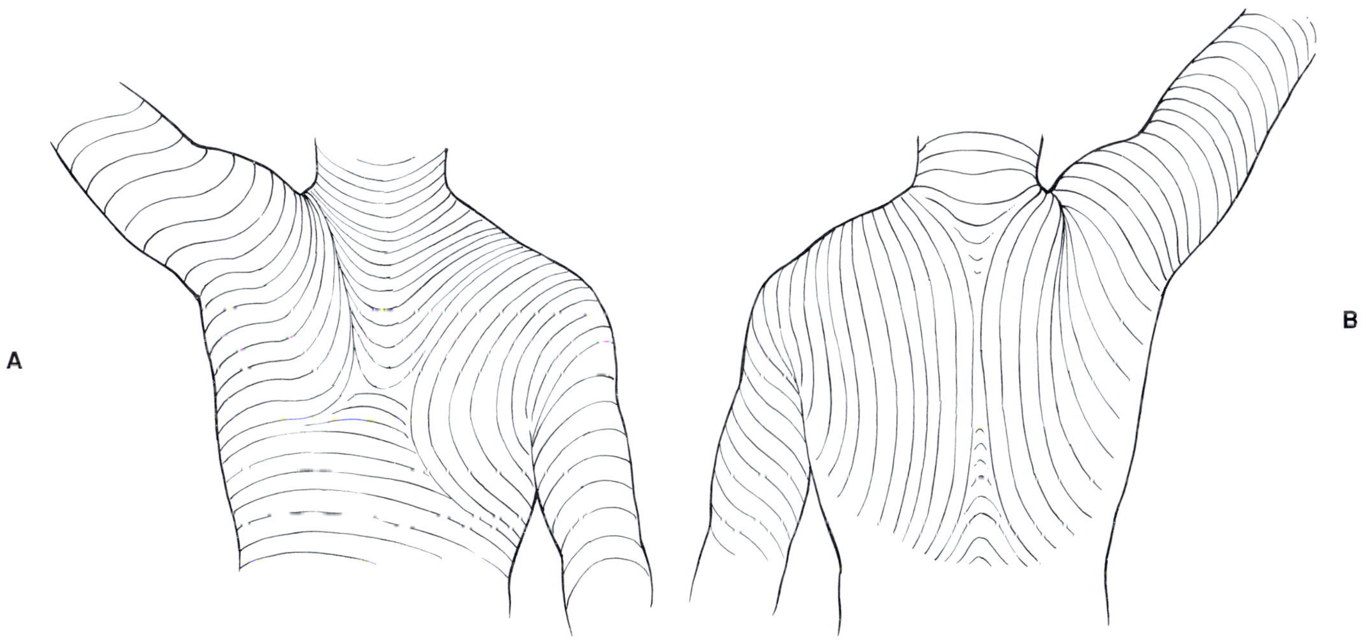

FIGURE 6-40 **A** and **B,** The usual location of the lines of relaxed skin tension in the adult male. Incisions placed in these lines lie parallel to the usual tension in the skin and therefore are less prone to stretching. (Modified from Kraissel CJ: Selection of appropriate lines for elective surgical incisions, *Plast Reconstr Surg* 8:1, 1951.)

not divided. If release of the lower subscapularis is necessary, subperiosteal release on the bone is more desirable than division.

The split in the subscapularis lies between its upper two thirds and lower one third. Cautery is usually needed to coagulate branches of the anterior humeral circumflex artery along the anterior surface of the muscle. Care is taken to work under direct vision to avoid dividing the axillary nerve that crosses the subscapularis muscle on its anterior surface. The split is initiated along the entire length that the surgeon has selected, but the deeper work is begun medially, where it is easier to separate muscle from the underlying capsule. When an appropriate plane between muscle and capsule has been reached, the dissection is continued laterally to the lesser tuberosity and then superiorly and inferiorly. Sharp dissection, generally in the form of a #15 blade, is required to initiate the dissection in the inferior and superior directions. A periosteal elevator is then used. In the inferior direction, care is taken to stay directly on capsule and bone to avoid injuring the axillary nerve. A Gelpi retractor and a glenoid neck retractor are used to retract the split subscapularis muscle. The Gelpi is placed laterally in the tendinous portion of the muscle because this retractor tends to tear through muscle tissue.

When the capsule has been cleanly exposed, it can then be split in line with its radially directed fibers. The arm is placed at about 45° of abduction and external rotation. In this position the fibers of the capsule lie in a roughly horizontal orientation in relation to the torso. The level of the split should be selected so that the medial exit of the split is within the surgeon's area of vision so that the surgeon is able to work. When the capsule has been split, the arm can be placed in a partially abducted neutral-rotation position to put the capsule in maximum relaxation. In this position the humeral head retractor often can be placed without scratching the glenoid cartilage by sliding it in on the interior surface of the inferior glenohumeral ligament until the teeth are beyond the glenoid. Then the teeth are slid superiorly behind the glenoid. Using this retractor, the head can be levered laterally so that the remaining medial capsulolabral work can be performed under direct vision. Occasionally the inferior capsule needs to be released from the glenoid to place the humeral head retractor.

Posterior Approaches[65]

The posterior transdeltoid approach to the glenohumeral joint is carried out through a vertical incision in the lines of relaxed skin tension. Here again, it is fairly easy and safe to mobilize skin flaps by carrying out the dissection just superficial to or at the level of the deep fascia. The skin is retracted with Goelet retractors. The medial-lateral positioning of this vertical incision is usually at the level that one would use for performing an arthroscopy, roughly 1 to 2 cm medial to the posterior lateral corner of the acromion.

After elevating the skin, the deltoid is split in line with its fibers. The line of the deltoid split is also centered over the posterior arthroscopy portal, roughly 1 to 2 cm below the level of the spine. The lower portion of the split is carried out more carefully because the axillary nerve exits from the quadrilateral space just below the teres minor. Work here is performed under direct vision after one has split the upper deltoid and obtained direct vision of the deep layer of the fascia of the deltoid.[65]

If more exposure is required, the deltoid can be elevated off the spine and acromion of the scapula in the required direction. Because this deltoid origin is an indirect insertion, care is taken to maintain considerable periosteum with the deltoid muscle to facilitate reattachment. An alternative extension is to carry the superior split into the trapezius so that the external collagen of both muscles can be left in continuity even though they have been detached from the spine of the scapula. In this way a side-to-side repair can be effected at the end of a surgery. Because of the spinal accessory nerve, the trapezius split is not continued more than 2 cm. The deltoid is retracted with Goelet retractors.

After the infraspinatus has been exposed, it is split at its median raphe. This is directly over the midportion of the joint and is where the arthroscopic portal occurs posteriorly. The surgeon must remember that there is a medial limit to dissection here of about 2 cm from the glenoid rim because of the presence of the suprascapular nerve. The neck retractor is placed medially and the Gelpi laterally as in the anterior approach. The capsule can then be visualized and split. Again, it may be necessary to release some capsule before replacing the humeral head retractor, but usually this is not necessary.

The posteroinferior incision is also made in the skin vertically in the same medial-lateral position but more inferiorly. Skin flaps are elevated and retracted with Goelet retractors. Through this wound the quadrilateral space can be approached by gently rolling the deltoid muscle superiorly and following the muscle's deep surface to the quadrilateral space and the axillary nerve. In this way the quadrilateral space can be approached without the discomfort caused by muscle detachment.

The posterior midline approach is rarely, if ever, used in sports medicine and is mentioned here for completeness. This approach is usually used by pediatric orthopedic surgeons (i.e., in correcting a Sprengel's deformity). The deep surface of the trapezius and the deep surface of the rhomboids are relatively avascular and provide nice bloodless planes for dissection, the shortcoming being that the surgeon has to divide the collagen connecting the proximal tendons of these muscles to the spinous processes of the vertebra.

Superior Approaches

The transdeltoid superior approach to the shoulder is used most often for subacromial disease, such as rotator cuff tears, impingement syndrome, and bicipital tendinitis. Skin incisions are made in the lines of relaxed skin tension. The deltoid is usually split between the anterior and middle thirds or slightly into the middle third. The deltoid incision extends medially into the periosteum over the acromion to carry some periosteum with the anterior muscle and to avoid dividing the longitudinal collagen fibers of the deltoid muscle. This split is performed over the anterior acromion for ease of surgical exposure and because the periosteum is thickest at this location. This incision can be continued with the collagen fibers of the acromioclavicular ligaments and into the trapezius, creating two relatively solid structures for side-to-side repair. The split is carried only 2 to 3 cm into the deltoid muscle to prevent injury to the axillary nerve.

The anterior third of the deltoid is then elevated off the bone. There is often abundant bleeding here, first because this is a metaphyseal-type bone and there is abundant sharing of circulation between the medullary blood supply and the vessels of the muscle, and second because of the proximity of the acromial artery. Sponges are packed underneath the deltoid as a technique of stripping the soft tissues off the coracoacromial ligament while simultaneously creating a tamponade of the acromial artery. Through this approach, the coracoacromial ligament spurs, the acromion, the rotator cuff, and the acromioclavicular joint can be reached as needed. The deltoid repair at the end of the case is probably the most crucial part of this approach. By using this technique, abundant periosteum has been left on the anterior third of the deltoid for use with a transosseous mattress repair.

The transtrapezius approach can be used to approach several areas because this rather large muscle covers a significant portion of the shoulder girdle. We again use lines of relaxed skin tension, which are more desirable cosmetically and more convenient. The trapezius muscle can be split with relative safety only in its lateral 40%. The lateral 40% is determined by measuring the distance from the spinous process of the vertebrae to the tip of the acromion. Branches of the spinal accessory nerve (cranial nerve XI) are rarely, if ever, found lateral to a vertical line representing 50% of the distance from vertebra to acromial tip.[41]

A similar technique in the posterior approach is dissection from the deltoid superiorly or posteriorly into the trapezius to avoid making a flap of deltoid and detaching the longitudinal fibers of the insertion. This trapezius-splitting incision can be conveniently used to approach the suprascapular nerve. Traditionally, the suprascapular nerve has been approached through a horizontal noncosmetic incision through which the trapezius insertion onto the spine of the scapula is elevated and the muscle retracted. The suprascapular nerve is then released from its entrapment in the scapular notch. This incision is a little more extensible in that it allows both the suprascapular and spinoglenoid notches to be approached by allowing a split that can be continued into the deltoid if the spinoglenoid notch needs to be approached. The traditional horizontal incision, although cosmetically poor, still affords a reasonable quick recovery. In a more medial superior approach, such as over the upper angle of the scapula, it is better to elevate the insertion of the trapezius from the scapula rather than splitting the muscle because of the immediate proximity of the eleventh cranial nerve.

Inferior or Axillary Approaches

This incision is on the axillary wall rather than the axillary extension of the anterior incision described previously. It is most often used as an approach to the first rib in thoracic outlet syndrome.[66]

The major structures at risk in this approach include the long thoracic nerve on the lateral surface of the serratus anterior muscle and the intercostal brachial nerve, which comes through the second intercostal space and provides sensation down the medial surface of the arm. With the patient in the lateral decubitus position, the incision is made in the lines of relaxed skin tension within the axilla. This approach is very traction-dependent, and the arm here is held in abduction. Upon locating the deep surface of the subcutaneous fat and the serratus anterior muscle, care is taken to preserve the long thoracic nerve. The lateral thoracic artery and its accompanying vein may be sacrificed. The axillary fat is then gently dissected from the underlying muscle until the intercostal brachial nerve is encountered in the second intercostal space. Care is taken to maintain the intercostal brachial nerve. The supreme thoracic artery is sacrificed. In this way a relatively bloodless plane can be followed to the root of the neck. Less frequently, the thoracic outlet area can also be approached anteriorly and posteriorly.

Arthroscopic Procedures

The considerations in the placement of arthroscopic portals are similar to, yet somewhat different from, those that determine the open surgical approaches. Our primary objective after accessibility is the maintenance of tissue viability and the preservation of nerve function. In general, there is a trade-off in arthroscopy. The surgeon gives up the advantages of open surgery, which are the ability to recognize and retract the vital structures and the ease of movement and placement of instruments. In return, the surgeon gains greater intraarticular visibility, although this is only two-dimensional and somewhat distorted. In addition, the arthroscopic surgeon hopes to achieve smaller incisions and to shorten the patient's rehabilitation (although shoulder arthroscopy patients often are immobilized for a longer period than patients with open procedures). To compensate for the inability to see and retract sensitive structures, the arthroscopist selects portals in safe areas.

The plane of the glenoid is the operative area that is best to achieve because it provides the greatest visibility and the greatest mobility of the operative instruments.

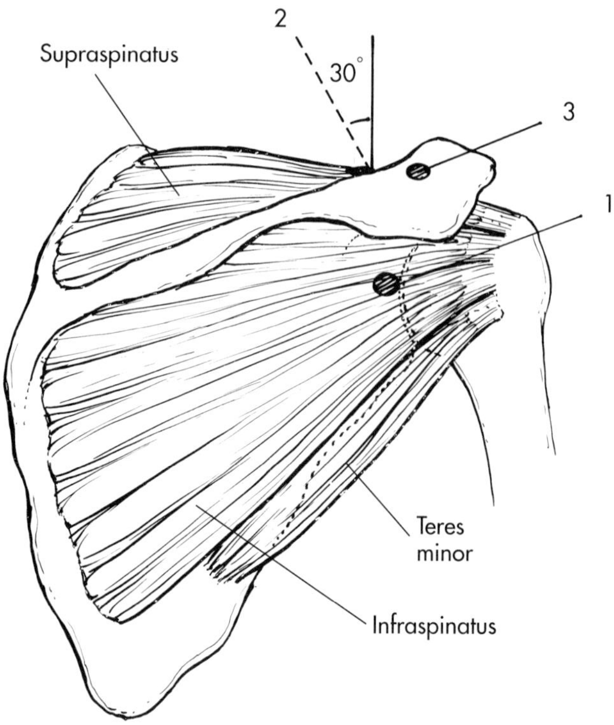

FIGURE 6-41 The usual location of the posterior and superior portals. Portal #1 is the usual posterior portal for arthroscopic surgery. If it is placed in the usual fashion, it lies roughly at the median raphe of the infraspinatus and enters the joint at that point. Portal #2 is directed 30° lateral and slightly posterior. It penetrates the muscular portion of the supraspinatus rather than the tendinous portion, as one might fear. This portal is useful as a point of exit for cannulae or as a source of superior visualization. Portal #3 is a transacromial portal and is used only rarely for repair of a superior labral lesion.

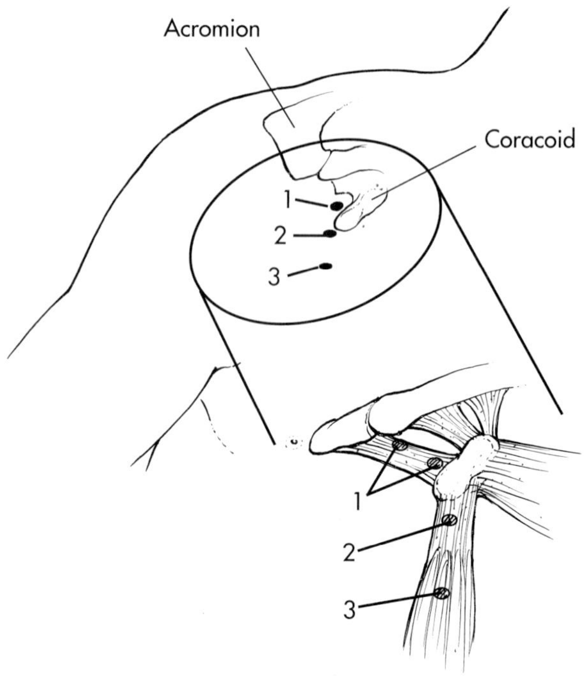

FIGURE 6-42 The anterior structures and the positions of the portals. Portal #1 is the anterosuperior portal and is safe. Portal #2 is the anterior middle portal, is directly under the tip of the coracoid, and carries a moderate amount of risk. Portal #3 is the anteroinferior portal, is a useful portal if one is attempting arthroscopic repair of the labrum, but carries a large risk, necessitating a special technique to reduce that risk.

This plane runs from posterolateral to anteromedial, approximately 30° from the sagittal plane.

Posterior Portal

The posterior portal is created about 1 to 2 cm medial and 1 to 2 cm inferior to the posterolateral corner of the acromion (Fig. 6-41). These distances may increase or decrease as the shape of the acromion varies and the thickness of the soft tissue of the patient varies. This position indicates the entry point of the posterior portal. The line of insertion is completed by placing a fingertip anteriorly on the tip of the coracoid. In this position, the arthroscope traverses skin, fat, and the posterior third of the deltoid, where there is no danger of contacting the axillary nerve, and runs through the midportion of the infraspinatus. A cannula misplaced too far medially could endanger the suprascapular nerve and artery, and too far inferior might damage the axillary nerve. The internal entry point is within the posterior superior glenohumeral capsule.

Anterior Portals

There are several anterior portals[63] (Fig. 6-42). One approach is made from "outside in" through the deltoid above to the level of the coracoid, possibly through the coracoacromial ligament and through the rotator interval or coracohumeral ligament. A needle first is used to develop the desired path through the skin and the point of entry within the glenohumeral joint. The skin is then incised and the cannula passed in the same direction as the needle had passed.

Further inferiorly, a path may be located from "inside out" by replacing the arthroscope with a long blunt tipped trocar and then passing that trocar through the anterior tissues. The point of exiting the joint selected by arthroscopy lies just above the subscapularis tendon. One hopes to pass superior and lateral to the coracoid, through the deltoid muscle (above the axillary nerve), and then through skin. If the rod is passed just above the subscapularis tendon and somewhat inferiorly, this portal is actually immediately inferior to the coracoid, a

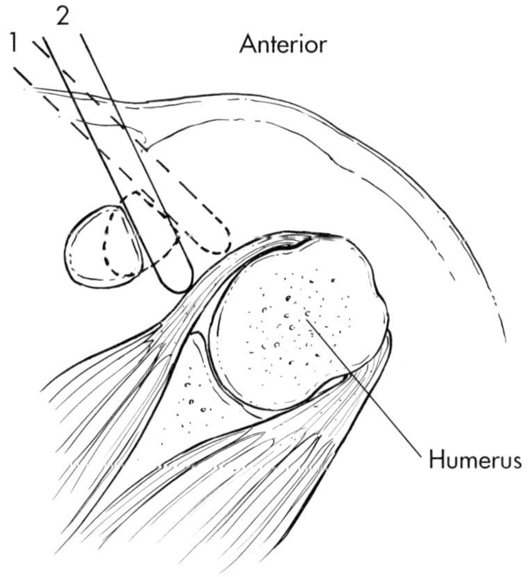

FIGURE 6-43 The creation of the anteroinferior portal in three steps: the surgeon makes the incision about 3 cm below the tip of the coracoid and advances the cannula in the plane of the glenoid, aiming for the anteroinferior quadrant of the shoulder. The surgeon advances the cannula until the conjoined tendon is encountered. In the second step, the surgeon advances the cannula laterally off the conjoined tendon until the humeral head and its adjacent structures are encountered. Then the surgeon angulates the cannula back medially, causing the cannula to retract the conjoined tendon medially. The cannula then penetrates the inferior, more muscular portion of the subscapularis for use in this anteroinferior quadrant of the joint.

riskier position because of the proximity of the musculocutaneous nerve and its branches. Some surgeons consciously accept this risk when they want to work on the inferior glenohumeral joint.

Most inferiorly, there are rare instances in which an anteroinferior portal is made by incising the skin 2 or 3 cm below the tip of the coracoid and passing an arthroscopic instrument cannula with a blunt obturator until the conjoint tendon is palpated (Fig. 6-43). At this point the cannula and obturator are directed posterolaterally until the head of the humerus, with its overlying subscapularis muscle, is encountered. Then the cannula is angled medially. The surgeon hopes by this maneuver to sweep the conjoint tendon and the musculocutaneous nerve out of the way, as is done in open procedures. The obturator then can be used to penetrate the lower muscular portion of the subscapularis.[63]

Superior Portals

There are two basic superior portals. If the surgeon passes an arthroscopic cannula with a sharp trocar through a skin incision made just medial to the angle created by the clavicle and spine of the scapula, and directs this cannula 30° laterally and slightly posterior, the cannula can be brought into the glenohumeral joint. This is especially useful for egress of fluid from the joint.

If arthroscopic work needs to be done in the area of the superior labrum, particularly if suture anchors or absorbable tacks are being attached to the upper glenoid, a cannula directed from superior lateral to inferior medial would be necessary. To achieve this arthroscopically, the superior portal must lie immediately adjacent to the anterior edge of the acromion, or rarely it must actually pass through the acromion.[64] Some surgeons have drilled a small hole in the acromion and then confirmed the utility of this position by passing a long spinal needle into the glenohumeral joint. The hole is then widened to accept an arthroscopic instrument cannula, through which the necessary procedures are performed.

Lateral Portals

Posterolateral, straight lateral, and anterolateral portals can be made about 2 to 3 cm below the lateral margin of the acromion with relative safety of the axillary nerve. These portals are selected as necessary in performing subacromial surgery.

Acromioclavicular Joint Portal

This joint may be approached anterosuperiorly or posterosuperiorly in the plane of the acromioclavicular joint. From either position, a smaller arthroscope can be placed to visualize the acromioclavicular joint, and instruments can be used to perform any necessary procedures. When the acromioclavicular joint is entered without going through the subacromial bursa, the small scope is used initially until there is enough room for the 4-mm scope.

Posteromedial Portals

Finally, some authors have proposed arthroscopy of the scapulothoracic bursae. A portal at the superior angle of the scapula may endanger the spinal accessory nerve (cranial nerve XI). Granted, this nerve is a small nerve lying in a rather large target of the trapezius, but it does lie in the area where these portals are made.

References

1. Abbott LS, Lucas DB: The tripartite deltoid and its surgical significance in exposure of the scapulohumeral joint, *Ann Surg* 136:392, 1952.
2. Abbott LS, Lucas DB: The function of the clavicle: its surgical significance, *Ann Surg* 140:583, 1954.
3. Aoki M, Ishii S, Usui M: The slope of the acromion in the rotator cuff impingement, *Orthop Trans* 10(2):228, 1986.
4. Bankart ASB: The pathology and treatment of recurrent dislocation of the shoulder joint, *Br J Surg* 26:23, 1938.
5. Basmajian JV: *Muscles alive: their functions revealed by electromyography*, ed 4, Baltimore, 1979, Williams & Wilkins.
6. Bearn JG: Direct observations on the function of the capsule of the sternoclavicular joint in clavicular support, *J Anat* 101:159, 1967.
7. Bigliani LU, Morrison DS, April EW: The morphology of the acromion in its relationship to rotator cuff tears, *Orthop Trans* 10(2):228, 1986.

8. Borges AF: The relaxed skin tension lines (RSTL) vs other skin lines, *Plast Reconstr Surg* 73:144, 1984.
9. Bosley RC: Total acromionectomy: a twenty year review, *J Bone Joint Surg* 73A:961, 1991.
10. Bowen M et al: The effect of joint compression on stability of the glenohumeral joint, *Trans Orthop Res Soc* 17:289, 1992.
11. Bowen M et al: Role of the inferior glenohumeral ligament complex in limiting inferior translation of the glenohumeral joint, *Trans Orthop Res Soc* 17:497, 1992.
12. Broome HL, Basmajian JV: The function of the teres major muscle: an electromyographic study, *Anat Rec* 170:309, 1971.
13. Burkhead WZ, Scheinberg RR, Box G: Surgical anatomy of the axillary nerve, *J Shoulder Elbow Surg* 1:31, 1992.
14. Cahill BR, Palmer RE: Quadrilateral space syndrome, *J Hand Surg* 8:65, 1983.
15. Cave AJE: The nature and morphology of the costoclavicular ligament, *J Anat* 95:170, 1961.
16. Clark J, Sidles JA, Matsen FA: The relationship of the glenohumeral joint capsule to the rotator cuff, *Clin Orthop* 254:29, 1990.
17. Clein LJ: Suprascapular entrapment neuropathy, *J Neurosurg* 43:337, 1975.
18. Colachis SC Jr, Strohm BR: Effects of suprascapular and axillary nerve block on muscle forces in the upper extremity, *Arch Phys Med Rehabil* 52:22, 1971.
19. Cooper DE et al: Anatomy, histology, and vascularity of the glenoid labrum—an anatomical study, *J Bone Joint Surg* 74A:46, 1992.
20. Cyprien JM et al: Humeral retrotorsion and glenohumeral relationship in the normal shoulder and in recurrent anterior dislocation (scapulometry), *Clin Orthop* 175:8, 1983.
21. De Garis CF, Swartley WB: The axillary artery in white and Negro stocks, *Am J Anat* 41:353, 1928.
22. DePalma AF, Callery G, Bennett GA: Variational anatomy and degenerative lesions of the shoulder joint, *Am Acad Orthop Surgeons Instr Course Lect* 6:255, 1949.
23. Ferrari DA: Capsular ligaments of the shoulder—anatomical and functional study of the anterior-superior capsule, *Am J Sports Med* 18:20, 1990.
24. Flatow EL, Bigliani LU, April EW: An anatomical study of the musculocutaneous nerve and its relationship to the coracoid, *Clin Orthop Rel Res* p 244, 1989.
25. Fukuda K et al: Biomechanical study of the ligamentous system of the acromioclavicular joint, *J Bone Joint Surg* 68A:434, 1986.
26. Gagey O, Bonfait H, Gillot C: Anatomic basis of ligamentous control of elevation, *Surg Radiol Anat* 9:19, 1987.
27. Gardner E: The innervation of the shoulder joint, *Anat Rec* 102:1, 1948.
28. Gibb T et al: The effect of capsular venting on glenohumeral laxity, *Clin Orthop Rel Res* 268:120, 1991.
29. Gohlke F, Essigkrug B, Schmitz F: The pattern of the collagen fiber bundles of the capsule of the glenohumeral joint, *J Shoulder Elbow Surgery* 3(3):111-128, 1994.
30. Harryman D et al: Translation of the humeral head on the glenoid with passive glenohumeral motion, *J Bone Joint Surg* 72A:1334, 1990.
31. Harryman DT et al: The role of the rotator interval capsule in passive motion and stability of the shoulder, *J Bone Joint Surg* 74A:53, 1992.
32. Hawkins RJ, Angelo RL: Glenohumeral osteoarthritis—a late complication of the Putti-Platt repair, *J Bone Joint Surg* 72A:1193, 1990.
33. Hollinshead WH: *Anatomy for surgeons,* vol 3, ed 3, Philadelphia, 1982, Harper & Row.
34. Horwitz MT, Tocantins LM: An anatomical study of the role of the long thoracic nerve and the related scapular bursae in the pathogenesis of local paralysis of the serratus anterior muscle, *Anat Rec* 71:375, 1938a.
35. Howell S et al: Normal and abnormal mechanics of the glenohumeral joint in the horizontal plane, *J Bone Joint Surg* 70A:227, 1988.
36. Howell SM, Galinat BJ: The glenoid-labral socket—a constrained articular surface, *Clin Orthop* 243:122, 1989.
37. Huelke DF: Variation in the origins of the branches of the axillary artery, *Anat Rec* 135:33, 1959.
38. Iannotti JP et al: The normal glenohumeral relationships: an anatomic study of one hundred and forty shoulders, *J Bone Joint Surg* 74A:491, 1992.
39. Inman VT, Saunders M, Abbott LC: Observations on the function of the shoulder joint, *J Bone Joint Surg* 26:1, 1944.
40. Jobe CM, Iannoti JP: Limits on glenohumeral motion-joint biometry, accepted by *J Shoulder Elbow Surg,* 1994.
41. Jobe CM, Kropp WP, Wood V: The spinal accessory nerve in trapezius splitting approaches, accepted by *J Shoulder Elbow Surg,* 1994.
42. Kennedy JC: Retrosternal dislocation of the clavicle, *J Bone Joint Surg* 31B:74, 1949.
43. Kerr AT: The brachial plexus of nerves in man: the variations in its formation and branches, *Am J Anat* 23:285, 1918.
44. King WD et al: Anatomic and electromyographic studies of the subscapularis muscle following longitudinal splitting, presented at the AAOS Specialty Day, American Orthopaedic Society of Sports Medicine, Feb 27, 1994, New Orleans.
45. Kraissel CJ: Selection of appropriate lines for elective surgical incisions, *Plast Reconstr Surg* 8:1, 1951.
46. Langer K: On the anatomy and physiology of the skin. I. The cleavability of the skin, *Br J Plast Surg* 31:3, 1978.
47. Langer K: On the anatomy and physiology of the skin. II. Skin tension, *Br J Plast Surg* 31:93, 1978.
48. Lewis MM et al: En bloc clavicular resection: operative procedure and postoperative testing of function: case reports, *Clin Orthop* 193:214, 1985.
49. Lundborg G: Ischemic nerve injury. Experimental studies on intraneural microvascular pathophysiology and nerve function in a limb subjected to temporary circulatory arrest, *Scand J Plast Reconstr Surg (Suppl)* 6:1, 1970.
50. Matsen FA: Biomechanics of the shoulder. In Frankel VH, Nordin M, editors: *Basic biomechanics of the skeletal system,* Philadelphia, 1980, Lea & Febiger.
51. Moseley H, Overgaard B: The anterior capsular mechanism in recurrent anterior dislocation of the shoulder, *J Bone Joint Surg* 44B:913, 1962.
52. Neer CJ: Anterior acromioplasty for chronic impingement syndrome of the shoulder, *J Bone Joint Surg* 54A:41, 1972.
53. Neer CS: Impingement lesions, *Clin Orthop* 173:70, 1983.
54. Neer CS, Poppen NK: Supraspinatus outlet, *Orthop Trans* 11:234, 1987.
55. O'Brien S: The shoulder. In Rockwood CA, Matsen FA, editors: *The shoulder,* Philadelphia, 1990, WB Saunders.
56. O'Brien SJ et al: The anatomy of the inferior glenohumeral ligament complex of the shoulder, *Am J Sports Med* 18:449, 1990.
57. O'Brien S et al: Capsular restraints to anterior/posterior motion of the shoulder, *Orthop Trans* 12:143, 1988.
58. Ovesen J, Nielsen S: Posterior instability of the shoulder, *Acta Orthop Scand* 57:436, 1986.
59. Petersson CJ: Spontaneous medial dislocation of the tendon of the long biceps brachii: an anatomic study of prevalence and pathomechanics, *Clin Orthop* 211:224, 1986.
60. Radke HM: Arterial circulation of the upper extremity. In Strandness DE Jr, editor: *Collateral circulation in clinical surgery,* Philadelphia, 1969, WB Saunders.
61. Rengachary SS et al: Suprascapular entrapment neuropathy: a clinical, anatomic and comparative study (part 1), *Neurosurgery* 5: 441-446, 1979.

62. Rengachary SS et al: Suprascapular entrapment neuropathy: a clinical, anatomical, and comparative study (part 2, anatomical study), *Neurosurgery* 5:447, 1979.
63. Resch H, Bech E: *Arthroscopy of the shoulder,* Vienna, 1992, Springer-Verlag.
64. Resch H et al: Arthroscopic repair of superior glenoid labral detachment (the SLAP lesion), *J Shoulder Elbow Surg* 2(3):147, 1993.
65. Rockwood CA: Surgical approaches to the shoulder. Keynote address to American Academy of Orthopaedic Surgeons Summer Institute, San Diego, Sept, 1984.
66. Roos DB: New concepts of thoracic outlet syndrome that explain etiology, symptoms, diagnosis and treatment, *Vasc Surg* 13:313, 1979.
67. Saha AK: *Theory of shoulder mechanism: descriptive and applied,* Springfield, IL, 1961, Charles C Thomas.
68. Salmon M, Dor J: *Les arteres des muscles des membres et du tronc,* Paris, 1993, Masson et Cie.
69. Samilson RL, Prieto V: Dislocation arthropathy of the shoulder, *J Bone Joint Surg* 65A:456, 1983.
70. Schwartz RE, Torzilli PA, Warren RF: Capsular restraints to anterior-posterior motion of the shoulder, Transcript of 33rd Orthopaedic Research Society 12:78, 1987.
71. Seneca LA. In Stevenson B, editor: *Epistulae ad lucillium epis. lxv, sec 3. The home book of quotations,* New York, 1949, Dodd Mead.
72. Slatis P, Aalto K: Medial dislocation of the tendon of the long head of the biceps brachii, *Acta Orthop Scand* 50:73, 1979.
73. Symeonides P: The significance of the subscapularis muscle in the pathogenesis of recurrent anterior dislocation of the shoulder, *J Bone Joint Surg* 54B:476, 1972.
74. Taylor GI, Palmer JH: The vascular territories (angiosomes) of the body: experimental study and clinical applications, *Br J Plast Surg* 40:113, 1987.
75. Townley CO: The capsular mechanism in recurrent dislocation of the shoulder, *J Bone Joint Surg* 32A:370, 1950.
76. Trotter M et al: The origins of the branches of the axillary artery in whites and American Negroes, *Anat Rec* 46:133, 1930.
77. Turkel SJ et al: Stabilizing mechanisms preventing anterior dislocation of the glenohumeral joint, *J Bone Joint Surg* 63A:1208, 1981.
78. Urist MR: Follow-up notes on articles previously published in the journal: complete dislocation of the acromioclavicular joint, *J Bone Joint Surg* 45A:1750, 1963.
79. Walker PS: *Human joints and their artificial replacements,* Springfield, Ill, 1977, Charles C Thomas.
80. Watterson PA, Taylor GI, Crock JG: The venous territories of muscles: anatomical study and clinical implications, *Br J Plast Surg* 41:569, 1988.
81. Weber SC, Caspari RB: A biomechanical evaluation of the restraint to posterior shoulder dislocation, *J Arth Rel Surg* 5:115, 1989.
82. Woo S et al: Ligament, tendon, and joint capsule insertions to bone. In *Injury and repair of the musculoskeletal soft tissues,* Park Ridge, Ill, 1988, American Academy of Orthopaedic Surgeons.

CHAPTER 7

Anterior Shoulder Instability, Impingement, and Rotator Cuff Tear

SECTION A
CHRISTOPHER M. JOBE
MARILYN M. PINK
FRANK W. JOBE
BENJAMIN SHAFFER

SECTION B
EDWARD G. MCFARLAND
BENJAMIN SHAFFER
RONALD E. GLOUSMAN
JOHN E. CONWAY
FRANK W. JOBE

SECTION C
RONALD E. GLOUSMAN
FRANK W. JOBE

SECTION D
BENJAMIN SHAFFER
FRANK W. JOBE

SECTION E
LEWIS A. YOCUM
JOHN E. CONWAY

SECTION F
CLIVE E. BREWSTER
DIANE R. MOYNES SCHWAB
JUDY L. SETO

SECTION A Theories and Concepts

Theories of the relationships among anterior shoulder instability, impingement, and rotator cuff tears are currently in a state of flux. The traditional understanding of impingement was based on an older nonathletic population, with impingement occurring as a consequence of mechanical wear of the cuff beneath the coracoacromial arch. However, in the younger athletic population, this mechanism has not been confirmed. Over the past decade it has been determined that anterior instability may be the primary cause of shoulder dysfunction in the young, overhead athlete, and that impingement and rotator cuff tears are secondary conditions. Arthroscopic examination also has failed to demonstrate the expected bursal side cuff pathology, and acromioplasties have failed to return these younger, overhead-throwing athletes to their preinjury level of activity. Therefore researchers have looked for more than one mechanism that would produce impingement in these different groups of patients.

The purpose of this chapter is to examine and review the classic and the more recently understood mechanisms of shoulder function and dysfunction to create a unifying theory by which the continuum of instability and impingement can be understood. This chapter will first review those observations, then suggest a unifying proposition that can be explained in terms of a classification system (see Fig. 7-1).

HISTORICAL OBSERVATIONS

In 1972 Charles Neer introduced a theory of impingement based on cadaveric, surgical, and clinical findings in an older, nonathletic population.[29] In his theory, Neer synthesized a seemingly diverse set of clinical conditions, such as rotator cuff tendinitis, rotator cuff tears, bursitis, and biceps tendinitis, into a comprehensive theory of impingement. He further classified the causes as either *outlet* or *nonoutlet,* thereby suggesting treatment of the specific underlying pathology.[26]

Outlet impingement was thought to be more common than nonoutlet impingement, with encroachment of the cuff by the constricting structures of the coracoacromial arch (anterior acromion, coracoacromial ligament) or acromioclavicular (AC) joint. Compressive cuff wear by this mechanism was thought to be responsible for the majority of rotator cuff tears.[26] The specific causes of outlet impingement reported include abnormal acromial tilt, slope, morphology,[6,24,29,43] and AC joint arthritis.[17,22]

Nonoutlet impingement demonstrates cuff pathology as a consequence of abnormal cuff proximity to an otherwise normal supraspinatus outlet. This is thought to be less common than outlet impingement. Many causes of nonoutlet impingement have been proposed.[17,26] These include abnormal scapular motion (such as with serratus anterior palsy), prominence of the greater tuberosity (malunion or nonunion), loss of humeral head depressors (rotator cuff tear or biceps rupture), loss of the glenohumeral fulcrum (such as occurs in patients with ligamentous laxity or instability), loss of the normal suspensory mechanism of the shoulder (old AC separation), defects of the acromion (unfused acromial epiphysis—os acromiale),[6,23,28] or thickened bursa or cuff (calcium deposits or bursitis).[26] Additionally, atypical use of the upper extremity, such as propelling a wheelchair or ambulating with crutches, may cause nonoutlet impingement.

Although biceps tendinitis has been described as a distinct clinical entity, it has been most commonly implicated in the spectrum of rotator cuff disease.[8,26,27] Primary pathology of the biceps long head was thought to be distinctly uncommon, but fraying, synovitis, and wear and tear of the long head were well-recognized stages in the progression of pathology accompanying the impingement process, primarily because of the biceps tendon's role as a humeral-head depressor functioning in conjunction with the rotator cuff.

Neer and Welsh described the impingement sign as forced elevation of the arm in forward flexion while fixing the scapula.[30] This was thought to result in impingement of the greater tuberosity and cuff against the unyielding acromion and coracoacromial ligament. Reproduction of the patient's pain was considered a positive impingement sign. Hawkins and Kennedy have described an alternative method to demonstrate impingement, in which the arm is flexed foward 90° and forcibly internally rotated against the fixed scapula, eliciting pain in the affected shoulder.[16]

UNIFYING PROPOSITION

Most of Neer's theory was developed based on observations of an older, nonathletic patient population. The proposition to be described here is based on differences between younger and older populations. Specific differences will be described, and a means to group patients with instability will be explained. Related questions about the impingement mechanism will be summarized, as will the current research, which has begun to better define the concept of impingement in the overhead athlete. The unifying proposition will then be discussed in relation to the clinical examination and the biomechanics of sports.

Older vs. Younger Populations

Impingement-type pain in the shoulder can be put into two general categories: pain that tends to occur in people who are over the age of 35 years and pain that tends to occur in people who are 35 years of age and younger. This is the first branch of the classification system of shoulder dysfunction (Fig. 7-1). As with most classification systems, however, overlap between the two groups

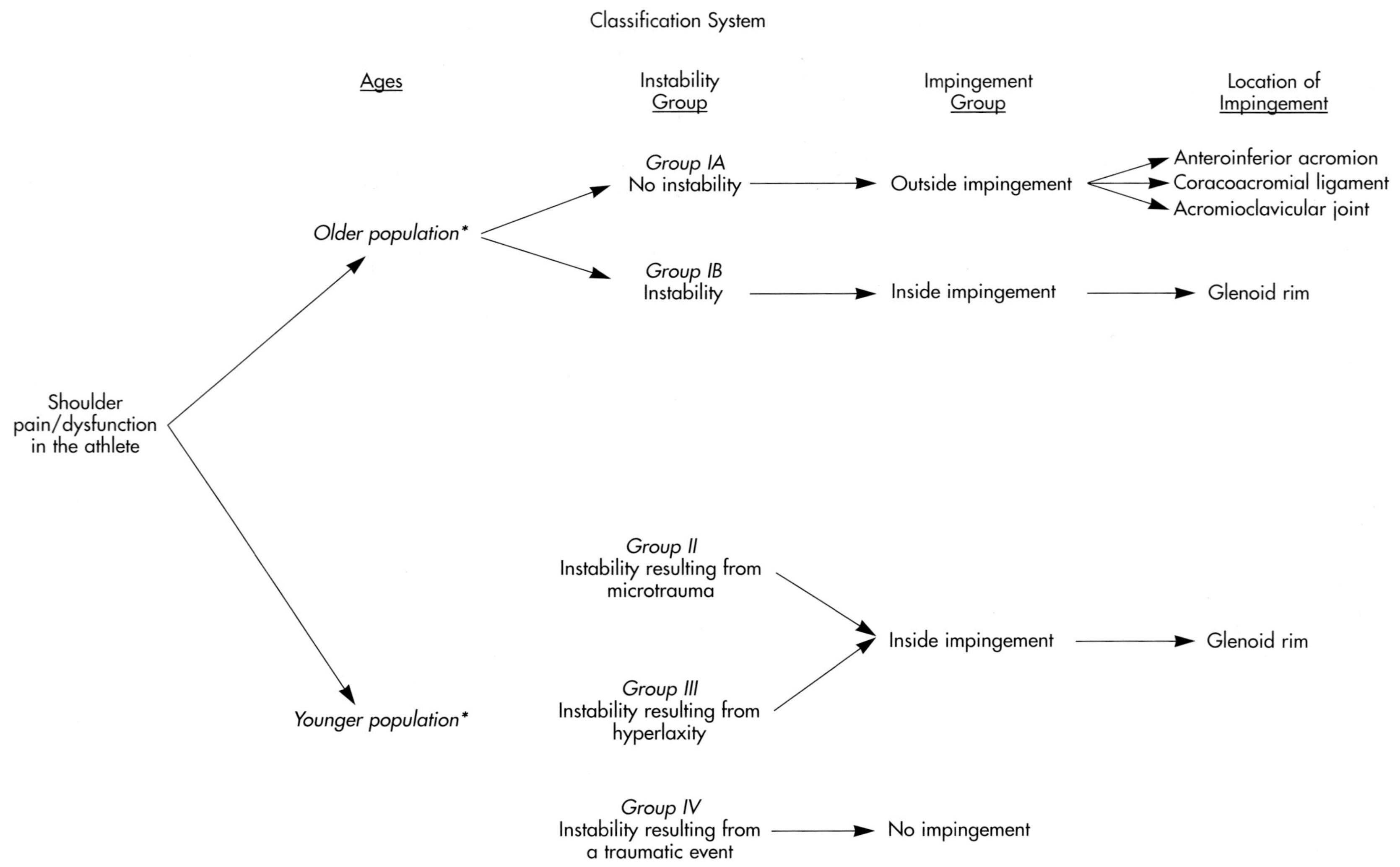

* There is some overlap between the two age groups.

FIGURE 7-1 Classification system for shoulder pain and dysfunction in the overhead athlete.

exists; thus the examiner needs to remain aware of the total picture.

In the older population, shoulder disorders usually are a consequence of the degenerative aging process. Typically, there is compromise of the subacromial space, spur formation, cuff thinning, and a decreased vascular supply*; this is in keeping with outlet impingement. Some of the older patients exhibit weakness of the rotator cuff or scapular muscles; this is in keeping with nonoutlet impingement.

*References 7, 10, 19, 20, 31, 40.

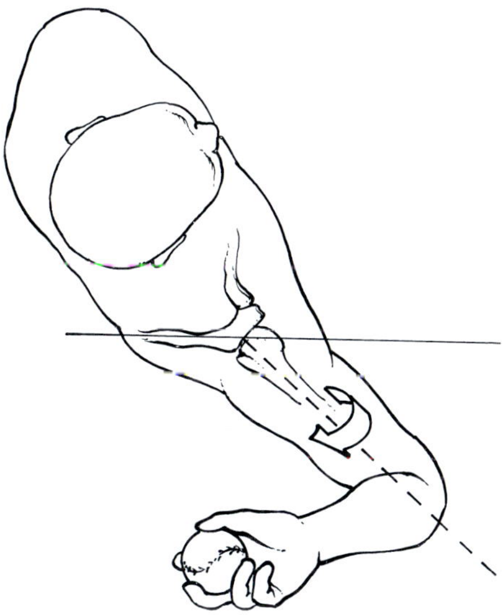

FIGURE 7-2 Hyperangulation.

In the younger population (18 to 35 years) the patient most commonly is an overhead athlete involved in sports such as swimming, tennis, baseball, football, or javelin throwing. These sports subject the shoulder to extremely large ranges of motion (ROM), forces, and accelerations as well as repetitive movement.[3,4,12,14]

When the humerus is abducted into the coronal plane and maximally externally rotated, the humerus *angulates* such that it abuts against the posterosuperior glenoid labrum (Fig. 7-2). This is called *hyperangulation*. The hyperangulation can cause stretching of the anterior structures, and a vicious circle may be set in motion, thereby creating increased angulation and further stretching. During this cycle, microtrauma to the capsular and ligamentous tissues occurs. If the anterior wall muscles (the muscles that provide support for the anterior capsule: the subscapularis, pectoralis major, latissimus dorsi, and teres major; Fig. 7-3) are weak, fatigued, or injured, even more angulation and stretching occur. Thus specific strengthening exercises and periods of rest are obviously important.

Eventually enough capsule may be stretched to allow for anterior subluxation. Anterior subluxation was seen in 100% of a group of patients undergoing capsular reconstruction. Hyperangulation and subluxation deny maximal congruency of the glenoid and humeral head, resulting in the ensuing encroachment of soft tissues. The encroaching, pinching, rubbing, or impingement can damage the undersurface of the rotator cuff. Thus the continuum of instability leads to fraying of the undersurface of the rotator cuff as it impinges on the posterior rim of the glenoid (Fig. 7-4).

It is then evident that impingement and rotator cuff tears cannot be treated as separate and distinct disorders

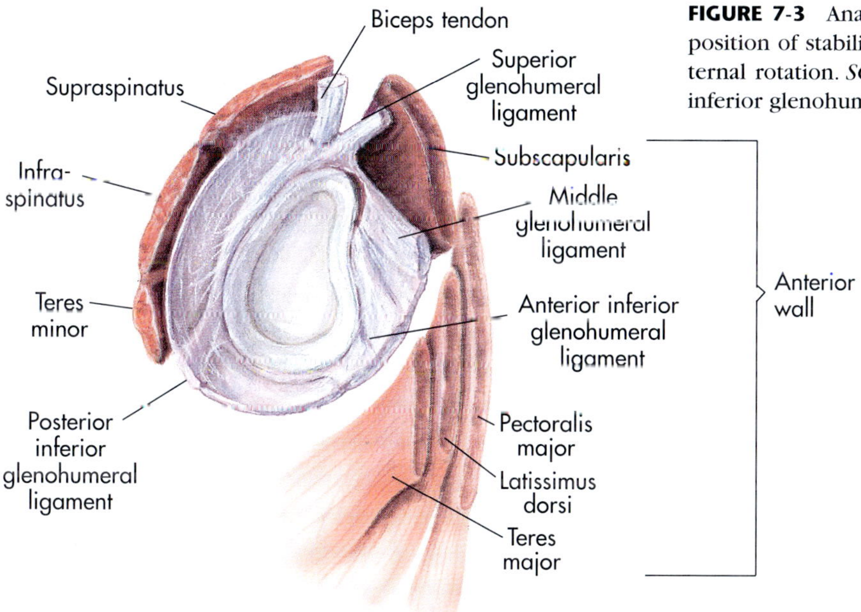

FIGURE 7-3 Anatomy of the glenohumeral joint and relative position of stabilizing structures of 90° abduction and 90° external rotation. *SGHL,* superior glenohumeral ligament; *IGHL,* inferior glenohumeral ligament. (Adapted from Turkel.[38])

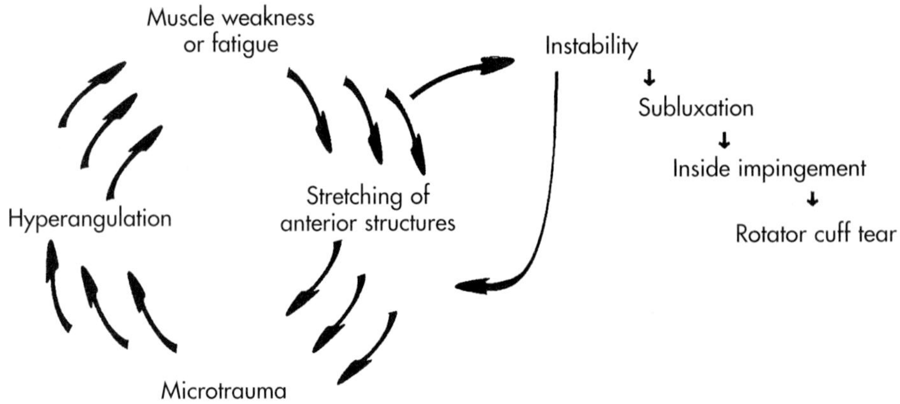

FIGURE 7-4 Instability continuum.

in the young, overhead athlete. The instability may be subtle in its clinical presentation. As a matter of fact, the subluxation may be clinically "silent" in the presence of the more easily diagnosed symptoms of impingement and rotator cuff tear. These "louder" symptoms should be seen as part of a continuum of pathology where increased joint angulation and instability are the core of the problem. The treatment needs to focus on that problem.

The initial treatment consists of a very specific preventive and rehabilitative program to build up the anterior wall muscles, rotator cuff, and scapular rotator muscles. With such a strengthening program, the cycle of damage can be prevented or at least minimized. If the rehabilitation fails, the second option is surgery. Because of the slow, chronic capsuloligamentous overstretching that initially caused the problem, it is believed that correcting this problem arthroscopically is not only difficult, but frequently impossible. The capsule and ligaments have been overstretched to the degree that they no longer fit the rim of the glenoid, and often a large anteroinferior capsular pouch or pocket has been created. Thus the capsule must be taken down and tightened through an open surgical repair. If this mechanism of injury is acknowledged and treated appropriately with rehabilitation or, if necessary, with surgery, more than 95% of competitive, overhead athletes will be able to return to sport.[23]

Grouping of Instability

With this as the background for the two separate pathologies in the older and younger population, along with the instability continuum, the second branch of the shoulder dysfunction classification system is developed (see Fig. 7-1). This second branch includes the four groups described below.

Group I: Group I instability is typically found in the older (i.e., older than 35 years of age) professional or recreational athlete; or the older, nonathletic individual. It is rarely found in the younger population but should be kept in mind. This group is subdivided into group IA and IB. Group IA encompasses patients with pure and isolated impingement on the acromial process or on the coracoacromial ligament. No instability is present. These patients demonstrate positive Hawkins' or Neer's impingement sign. An arthroscopic examination is likely to reveal lesions on the bursal surface of the rotator cuff and may reveal additional pathologic factors such as subacromial spurs. The glenohumeral joint may or may not have evidence of arthritis but does not show signs of instability. This group is analogous to outlet impingement. Group IB demonstrates instability and impingement of the undersurface of the rotator cuff and/or scapular muscles. This group is analogous to the impingement described in Fig. 7-4 (inside impingement), and may include patients identical to group II, except for the age of the patient.

Group II: Group II patients demonstrate instability with impingement secondary to repetitive trauma. This group frequently includes young, overhead athletes. The clinical examination frequently elicits the impingement sign, and the relocation test is positive (Fig. 7-5). When under anesthesia, members of this group may also demonstrate excessive anterior translation of the humeral head. There is a pass-through sign in which the arthroscope is easily passed beneath the head of the humerus along the anterior glenoid rim. The lesions of repetitive trauma are clearly evident along the posterosuperior labrum and/or the anteroinferior capsule. An enlarged bare spot on the posterior humeral head is also common. The glenohumeral ligaments, especially the inferior glenohumeral ligament, are lax or noticeably attenuated when the humerus is externally rotated. In addition, tears on the undersurface of the supraspinatus and infraspinatus are commonly encountered.

Group III: The group III category of shoulder dysfunction also commonly includes young, overhead athletes. The clinical examination demonstrates generalized ligamentous laxity (i.e., elbow and knee recurvation, hyperextensibility of the fingers and thumb), which is the differentiating factor between groups II and III. Shoulder instability is evident, as demonstrated by a positive relocation test.

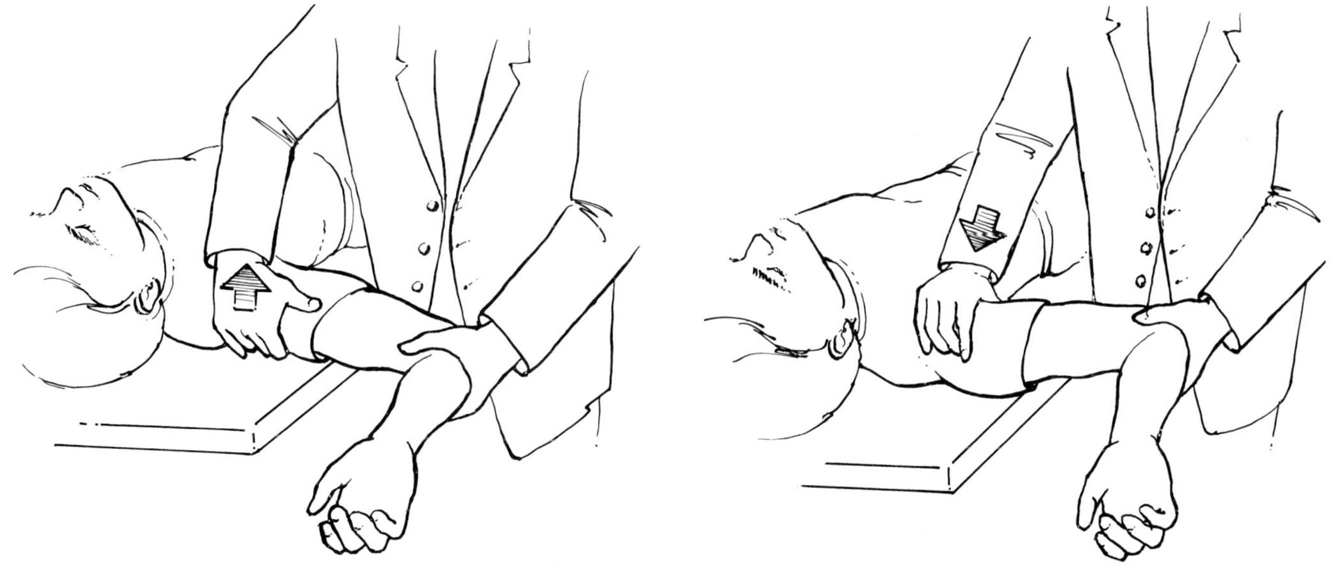

FIGURE 7-5 Relocation test: The patient is supine with the arm off the table at 90° abduction and maximum external rotation. **A,** The examiner grasps the humeral head posteriorly and pushes anteriorly. Sometimes the examiner feels sliding (subluxation) of the humeral head, and this sliding typically elicits pain located at the posterior joint line. **B,** The examiner grasps the humeral head anteriorly and pushes posteriorly to relocate the head and lift the rotator cuff off the posterior labrum. If the patient feels pain in the first half of the test, **A,** it is usually relieved in the second half of the test.

Arthroscopically, the humeral head can easily be displaced, sometimes by merely palpating it with the probe. Because of the ligamentous laxity, the arthroscope can be easily passed between the humeral head and anterior glenoid labrum in the pass-through test. There may be humeral head lesions, such as that seen in group II patients, but they are less severe.

Group IV: The patients in group IV have experienced a traumatic event, such as a fall onto the outstretched arm, or direct trauma, such as sliding into a base under a tag with the arm forcibly hyperabducted and externally rotated. That singular traumatic event renders the shoulder unstable but without impingement. This group may also include patients who have had only partial dislocations. These patients have not developed an apprehension sign but do sometimes have a positive relocation test. Arthroscopically, these patients show evidence of a Bankart lesion from the traumatic event and sometimes erosion of the posterior humeral head caused by the instability.

Impingement Mechanism

Questions arose when trying to relate the historical observations of impingement to rotator cuff tears in the young athletic population. The primary question related to the area of fraying of the rotator cuff muscles. As early as 1934, Codman wrote of undersurface tears and called them "rim rents."[9] If the impingement was indeed between the anterior one third of the acromion or the coracoacromial ligament and the greater tuberosity of the humerus, the fraying should be on the superior surface of the rotator cuff, but this typically is not the case in young, overhand athletes.* Undersurface cuff pathology occurs far more frequently than would be expected based on the traditional subacromial theory of impingement.

If the impingement were on the superior surface, it would be expected to find the pathologic processes of abrasion, inflammation, fibrosis, and adhesions within the subacromial space through arthroscopy. In the throwing population, arthroscopy usually reveals a pristine appearance of the subacromial space.[23] What is actually found arthroscopically is posterosuperior labral tearing, undersurface rotator cuff injury, and posterior humeral head lesions. In arthroscopic evaluations of 66 young, overhead athletes with shoulder dysfunction the following was found: 56% demonstrated anterior, inferior labral fraying; 63% revealed posterior labral fraying; 47% showed posterior humeral head chondromalacia; and 37% had a "Kiss"† lesion.

If the impingement were on the superior or bursal surface of the rotator cuff, positive results from acromioplasty in the younger, athletically inclined population would also be expected. Yet, with this procedure, there are disappointing results with an infrequent return to similar preinjury level of activity.[2,15,21,37,38] The surgical procedure that successfully eliminates impingement symptoms, allowing the majority of young athletes to return to their prior competitive level, is the anterior cap-

*References 10, 13, 20, 33, 35, 40, 42.

†A Kiss lesion is an articulation between an undersurface lesion of the rotator cuff or chondromalacic lesion of the posterior humeral head with the glenoid rim surface when the arm is abducted and externally rotated.

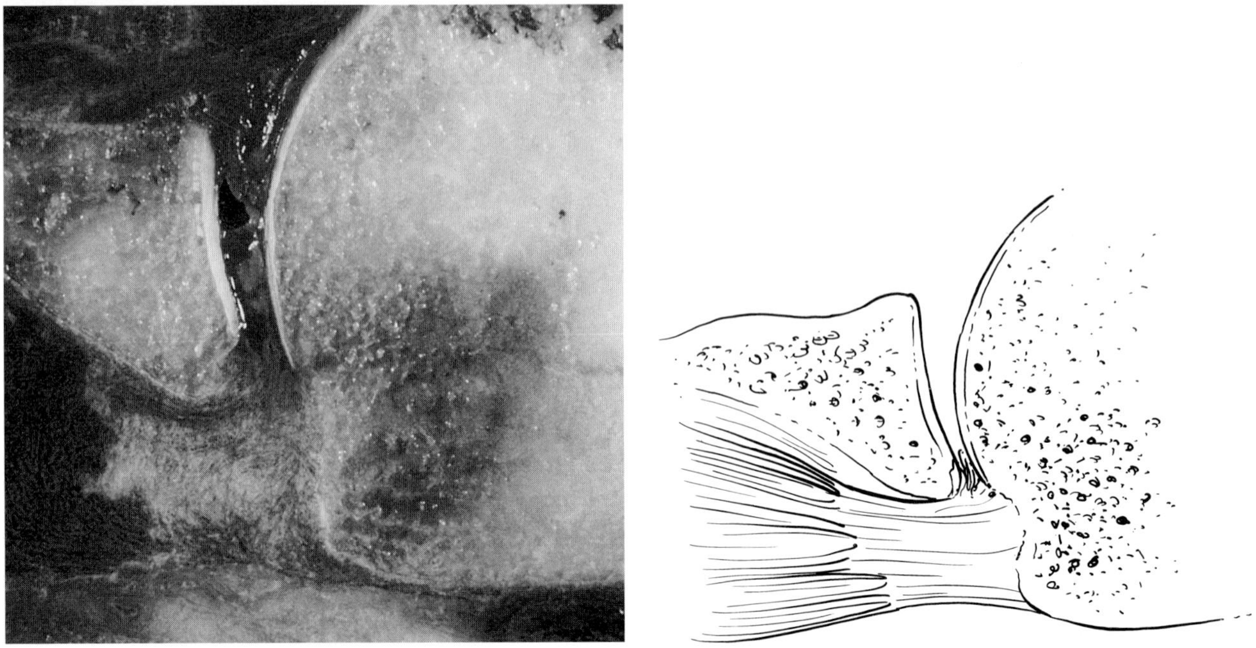

FIGURE 7-6 Impingement of the rotator cuff on the posterosuperior glenoid labrum during humeral abduction and maximal external rotation. **A,** Cross-section from a cadaver. **B,** Schematic of **A.**

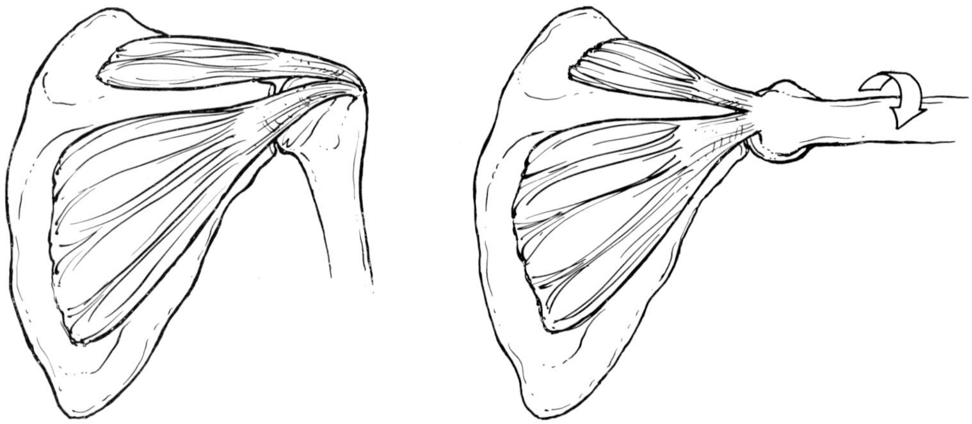

FIGURE 7-7 Reversal of orientation of the rotator cuff fibers with the humerus adducted **A,** abducted to 90° and externally rotated at 90°, **B.**

sulolabral reconstruction,[23,34,36] which does not alter or affect the subacromial space.

The first step of the relocation test, which is used to determine instability rather than impingement (see Fig. 7-5, *A*), has a positive test finding of pain at the posterior joint line. What causes this pain? The humeral position in the relocation test is one of abduction to 90° with hyperangulation and maximal humeral external rotation. This position of the muscles and ligaments can be approximated to the anatomic work of Turkel[39] (see Fig. 7-3). In this position the rotator cuff muscles are rotated too far posteriorly to be impinged beneath the anterior acromion or the coracoacromial ligament. However, something is definitely causing the pain when the humeral head is pushed anteriorly (i.e., subluxed), and something relieves the pain when the head is subsequently pushed posteriorly (i.e., relocated).

Clinically, competitive baseball pitchers may have pain in the posterior cuff. Some have suggested that tension overload causes this pain.[1,33,35] Little scientific information exists to support this hypothesis. Both the infraspinatus and supraspinatus muscles demonstrate relatively less EMG activity at the time this "tension overload" is supposed to occur.[11] In addition, if tension overload were the culprit, why is the tear not more typically through-and-through as opposed to just on the undersurface?

Amid all of this rebuttal of rationales, the posterior shoulder pain is real, and the cause of this pain seems to be a black box that is only now beginning to be opened with new research.

In an anatomic study 10 cadaver joints were fixed at 60° of abduction (which is equivalent to 90° of shoulder abduction if the scapula were allowed to move) and maximum external rotation. A deformity of the posterosuperior labrum was demonstrated that was caused by impingement against the greater tuberosity. In addition, the undersurfaces of the rotator cuff tendons that were positioned posteriorly and superiorly were impinged by rubbing or pounding on the posterosuperior labrum with a deformation of the fibers on the undersurfaces[18] (Fig. 7-6). Cross-sectional cuts of two additional glenohumeral joints frozen in this position confirmed this.

A kinesiologic study was performed on subjects who agreed to have tracking devices attached to their scapula and humerus with Steinmann pins. During the end range of abduction, the greater tuberosity approximated the posterosuperior labrum, and on the computer reconstruction it appeared to move onto the glenoid surface.[18]

An imaging study was performed on two volunteers who were able to fit into the MRI gantry with the arm in the position of the relocation test (i.e., abducted to 90° and externally rotated to 90°). From this a reversal of orientation of the undersurface of the supraspinatus and infraspinatus was evident[18] (Fig. 7-7).

In a separate arthroscopy study the arms of 17 athletes with shoulder pain were placed in 90° of abduction and maximal external rotation. Impingement was found between the posterosuperior border of the glenoid and the undersurface of the tendon insertions of the supraspinatus and infraspinatus. In all cases either a partial capsulotendinous rupture or partial cuff tear was present. In addition, 70% of these cases exhibited lesions of the posterosuperior labrum.[41]

Relationship of Theory to Practice

Relationship of theory to clinical exam: Arthroscopically, humeral motion has qualitatively been evaluated during the relocation test. Because of the anterior capsule laxity, the humeral head can easily be displaced anteriorly when in 90° abduction and maximal external rotation (Fig. 7-8). At this point, the supraspinatus, infraspinatus, and teres minor (which are rotated posteriorly) rub along the glenoid lip and are pinched between the humeral head and the posterosuperior glenoid rim with resultant fraying. Rather than tension overload, it is evident that the lesion results from an anatomic abutment of the humeral head on the posterosuperior glenoid labrum along with pinching of the rotator cuff tendon.

During the second part of the relocation test (Fig. 7-5, *B*), the supraspinatus, infraspinatus, and teres minor are pushed off the rim posteriorly, and the pain is relieved.

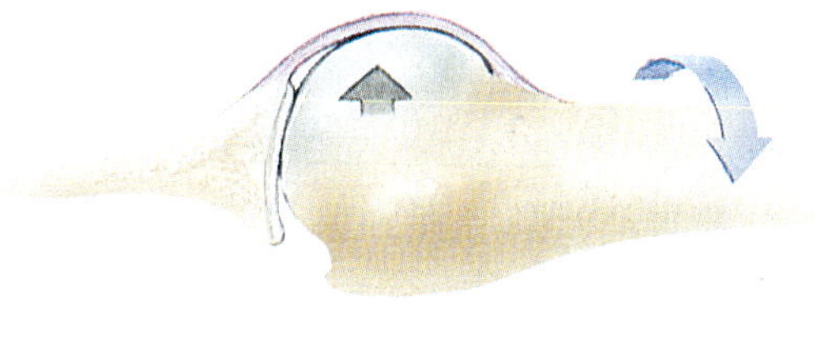

FIGURE 7-8 Anterior displacement of the humeral head with a lax capsule when abducted to 90° and externally rotated.

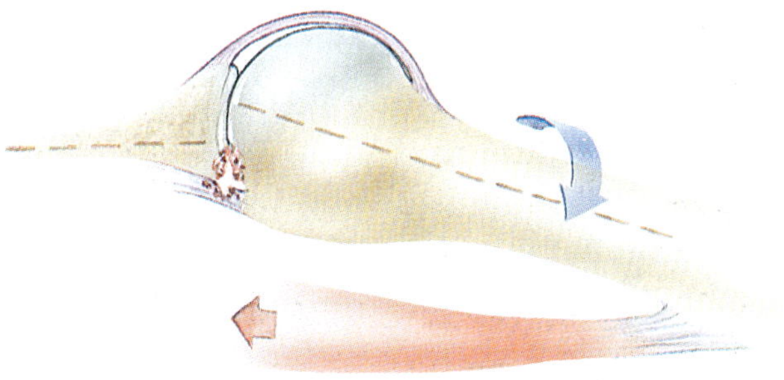

FIGURE 7-9 The angle of pull from the posterior deltoid pushes the humeral head against the glenoid, contributing to hyperangulation and thus accentuating the skeletal, tendon, and labral lesions.

The posterior deltoid muscle plays a role in the impingement during active humeral abduction. If the rotator cuff muscles are not functioning, the posterior deltoid continues to pull on the humerus. The angle of pull from the posterior deltoid pushes the humeral head against the glenoid, contributing to hyperangulation, and thus accentuating the skeletal, tendon, and labral lesions (Fig. 7-9).

The forceful humeral internal rotation during elevation likewise can pinch the anterior rotator cuff on the superior glenoid rim (Fig. 7-10).

Clearly there is potential for impingement of the rotator cuff undersurface with the anterosuperior and posterosuperior glenoid labrum. Taking this concept to the playing field, it can also be seen how the biomechanics of sports that use these extreme positions of the glenohumeral joints contribute to this internal mechanism.

Relationship of theory to the biomechanics of sport: During the late cocking phase of the baseball pitch, the arm is in 104° abduction and moves into the scapular plane[14] with maximal external rotation (Figs. 7-11, *A*, and 7-12, *A* and *B*). This is similar to the humeral position during the relocation test. If the subscapularis, pectoralis major, latissimus dorsi, and teres minor fatigue, the athlete loses the support of the anterior wall, which would

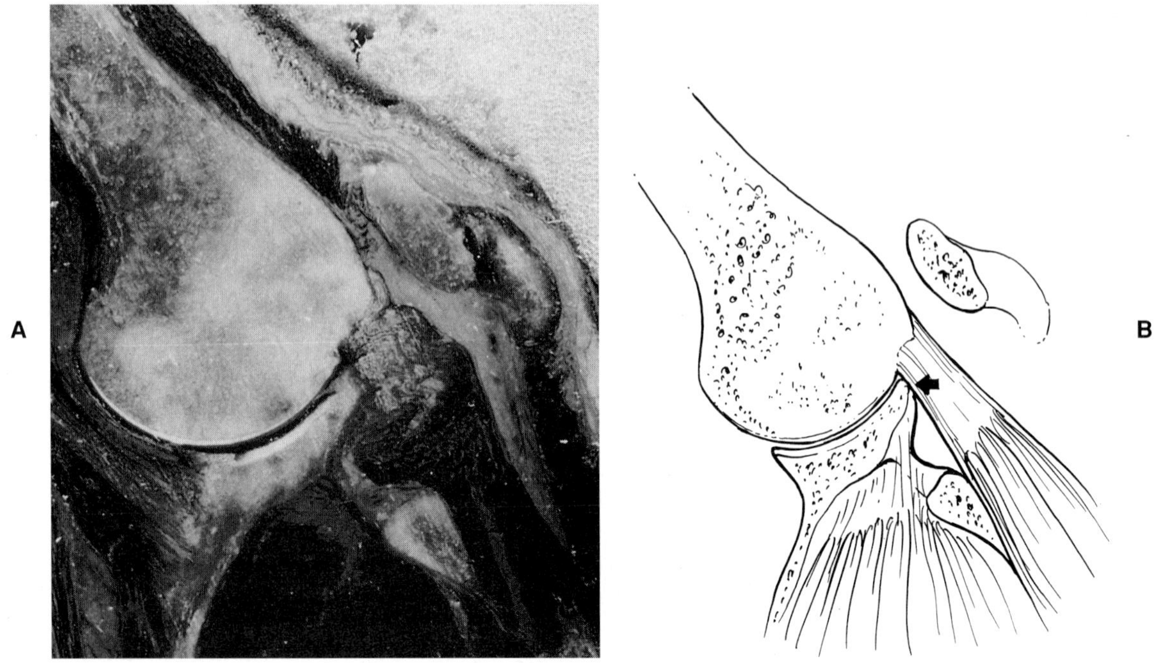

FIGURE 7-10 Impingement of the rotator cuff on the anterosuperior glenoid labrum during maximal humeral flexion and forceful internal rotation. **A,** Cross-section of a cadaver. **B,** Schematic of **A.**

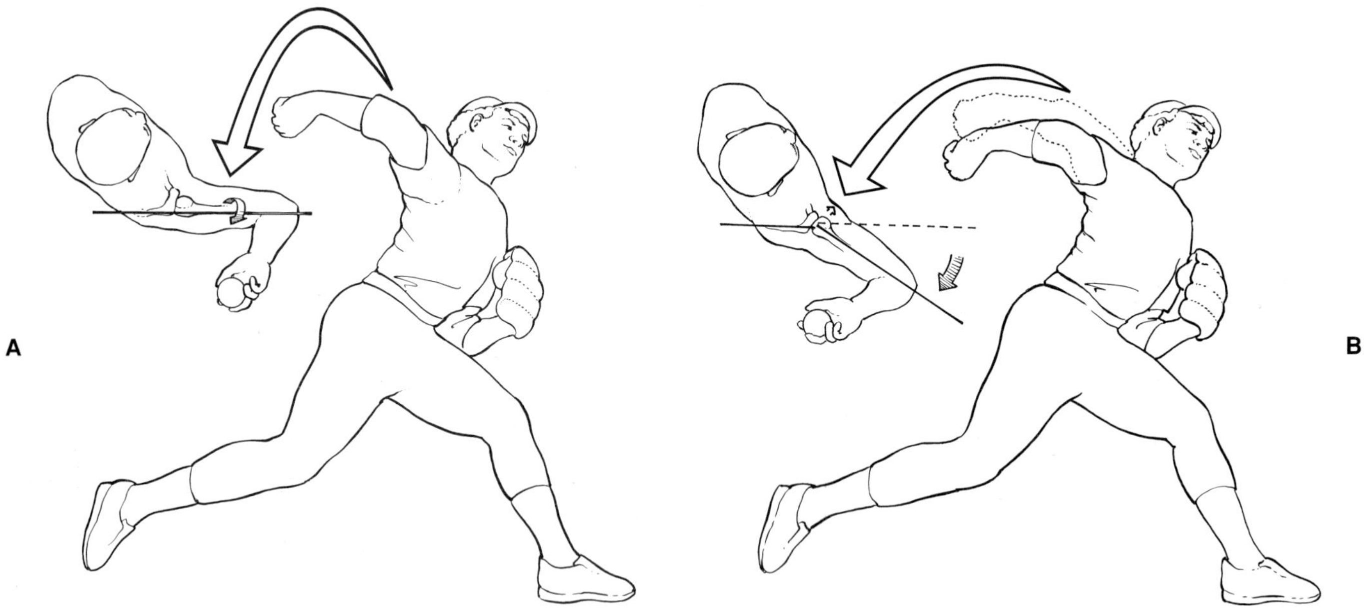

FIGURE 7-11 Pitching mechanics. **A,** Normal pitching mechanics from a side view and an overhead view. **B,** Pathologic pitching mechanics from a side view and an overhead view.

have held the humerus in position (see Fig. 7-3). If the muscles no longer offer support, the capsule and ligaments are challenged in an attempt to restrain the humeral head.[11] As these muscles fatigue, the pitcher begins to alter the mechanics. The humerus moves from abduction in the scapular plane to abduction in the coronal plane, which pathologically further hyperangulates the humerus and allows the humeral head and rotator cuff to come in contact with the posterosuperior labrum (Figs. 7-11, *B,* and 7-12, *C*). The athlete begins trying to "power" the arm by excessive trunk motion and by leaving the arm behind a bit longer, which actually causes even more humeral external rotation and hyperangulation, to "whip" the arm. The result increases stretching of the anterior capsule with the resultant instability and the pinching of the rotator cuff tendons (primarily at the

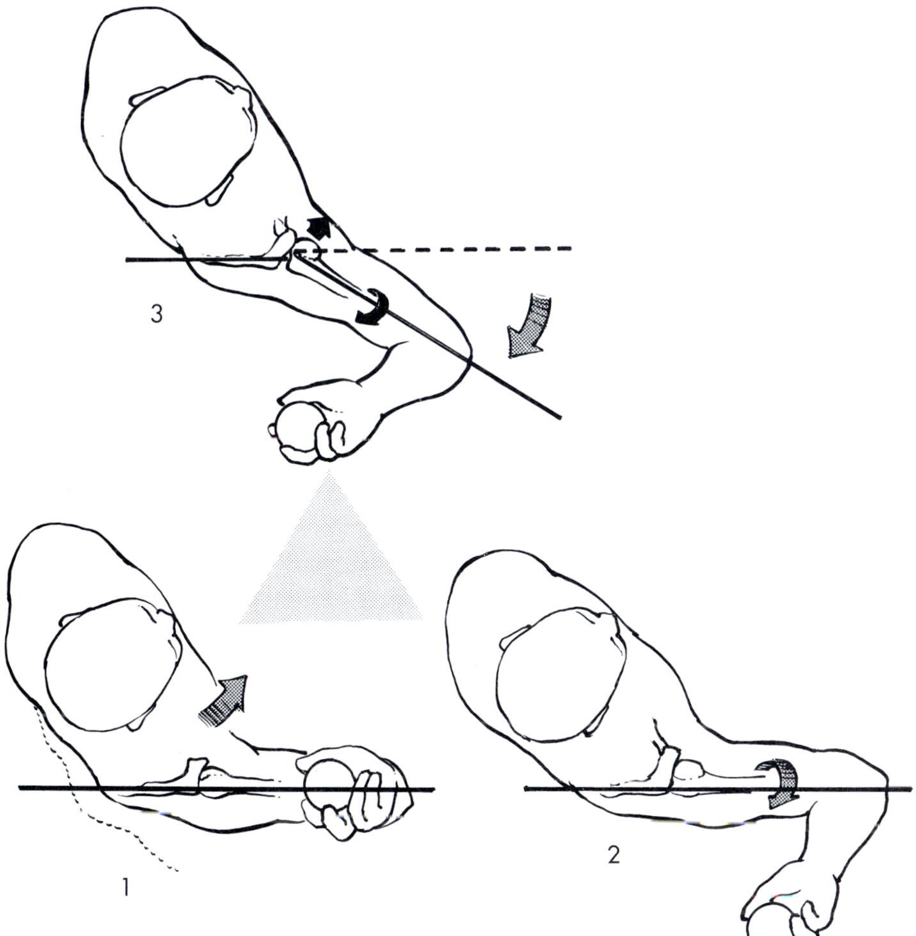

FIGURE 7-12 Triangle of hyperangulation. Hyperangulation has three components in the baseball pitcher. *1* and *2* are considered normal for a pitcher, but *2* places the pitcher in an at-risk posture. Component *3* places the pitcher in a position that can cause rotator cuff undersurface fraying. *1,* Scapula moves forward with the trunk. *2,* Maximal humeral external rotation. *3,* Humerus moves into the coronal plane.

junction of the supraspinatus, infraspinatus, and teres minor tendon) on the glenoid rim.

In swimmers, the pain is frequently found at the point of hand entry (unpublished data, Stocker D and Pink M). The humeral position of hand entry is between that of the Neer and Hawkins impingement tests (Fig. 7-13), for which the mechanics of internal impingement have already been described (see Fig. 7-10). The impingement in this position is of the rotator cuff and occurs along the anterosuperior glenoid labrum or on the coracoacromial ligament.

OUTSIDE AND INSIDE IMPINGEMENT

It now seems apparent there are two types of impingement. Bernard Morrey called these types *outside* and *inside impingement.* They are identified in the third branch of the shoulder dysfunction classification (see Fig. 7-1). The previous discussion delineates the mechanics of undersurface rotator cuff tears, or *inside impingement.* The progression of injury is translation of the humeral head and hyperangulation of the humerus, which leads to skeletal, labral, and tendinous lesions as the undersurface of the cuff impinges along the posterosuperior glenoid labrum. There is also potential for *outside impingement,* which was described by Neer[25] and more recently by Bigliani.[5] In a small percentage of cases fraying of the superior surface is seen. These patients, who are usually in the older population, may have contact of the rotator cuff with the acromion or coracoacromial ligament. As mentioned earlier in this chapter, the older patient is subject to the degenerative process, which includes decreased joint space, spurring, and decreased vascularity. These factors would predispose the older population to fraying of the superior surface. In addition, these people are less apt to undergo repetitive, high-velocity, overhead activities with an excess of 90° abduction and 90° external rotation. More than likely, they assume functional positions where the rotator cuff would be in contact with the acromion, especially since the joint space is predisposed to compromise. Additionally, this is a population that does well with acromioplasties. Those patients who do well with acromioplasties most likely have outside impingement.

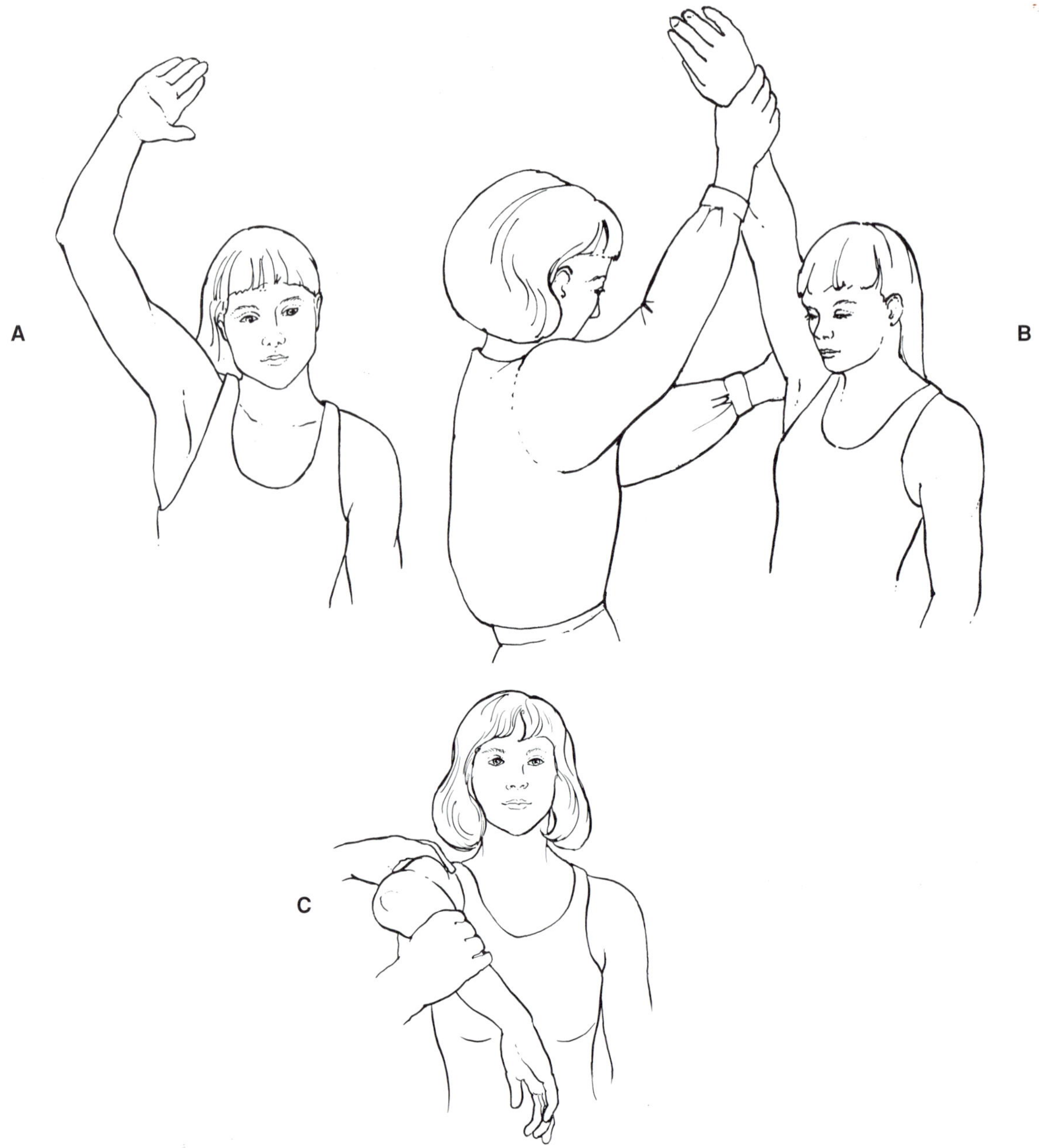

FIGURE 7-13 Hand entry during the freestyle swim stroke is between that of the Neer and Hawkins impingement test. **A,** Hand entry position during freestyle swimming. **B,** Neer impingement test. **C,** Hawkins impingement test.

SUMMARY

The first step in defining the shoulder dysfunction in the overhead athlete is to note the patient's age. An older population (i.e., people over the age of 35 years) can have either outside or inside impingement. The outside-impingement group (group IA) does not have accompanying instability. The impingement involves a compromise of the supraspinatus outlet by the overlying structures or the coracoacromial ligament and is considered outlet impingement. This group responds well to surgical removal of hard tissue constraints, acromioplasty being the best example. The inside-impingement group within the older population (group IB) does have accompanying instability. The impingement appears in patients with poor strength of the rotator cuff and scapular muscles, and it is considered nonoutlet impingement. The impingement is usually of the rotator cuff tendons on the superior or posterior glenoid rim. This group responds well to rehabilitation and may not respond to acromioplasty.

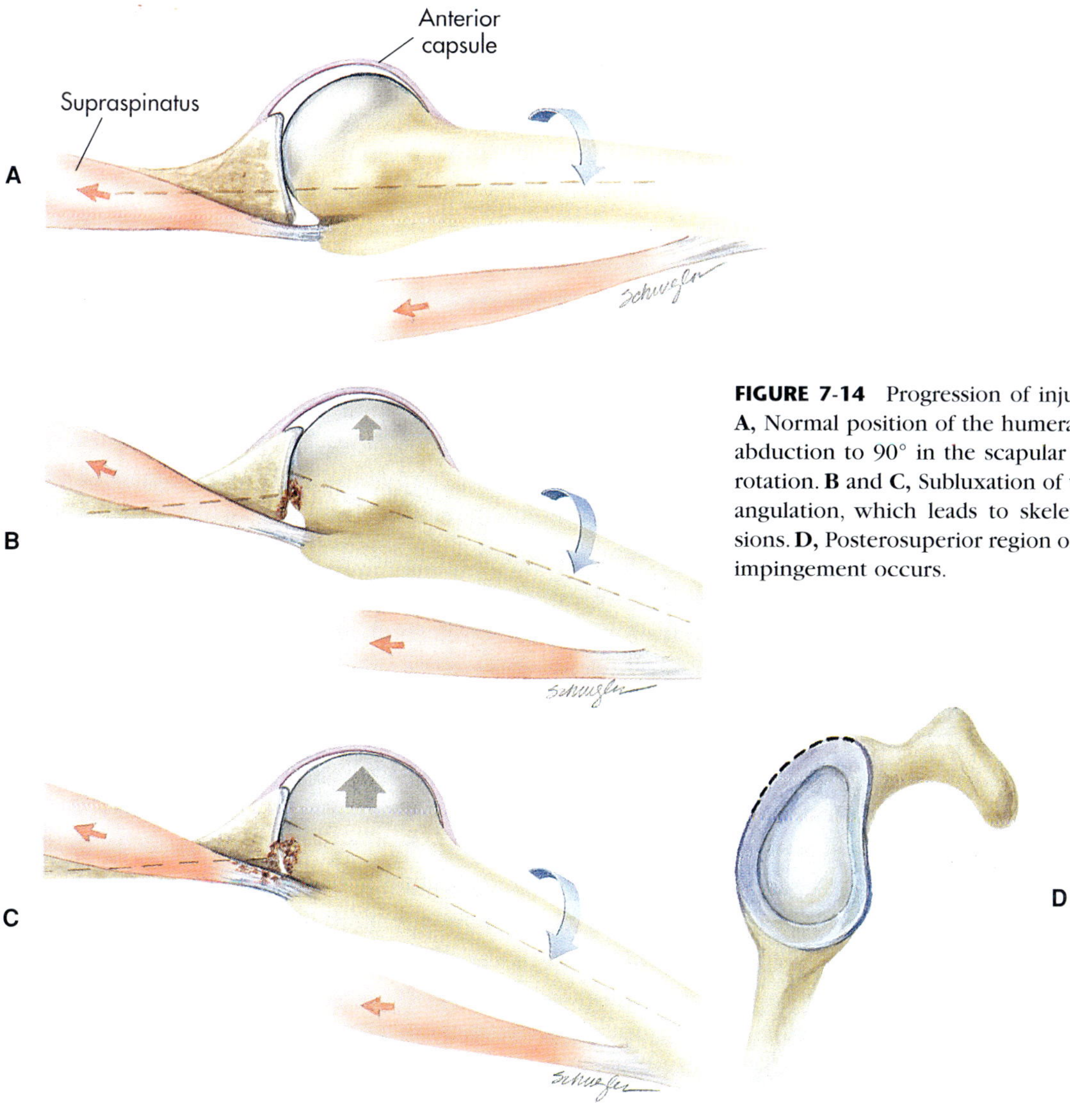

FIGURE 7-14 Progression of injury in internal impingement. **A,** Normal position of the humeral head in the glenoid during abduction to 90° in the scapular plane and maximal external rotation. **B** and **C,** Subluxation of the humeral head and hyperangulation, which leads to skeletal, labral, and tendinous lesions. **D,** Posterosuperior region of the glenoid, which is where impingement occurs.

The younger population is an athletic group whose repetitive overhead sports cause hyperangulation of the humerus. The shoulder dysfunction emanates from a vicious circle of hyperangulation of the humerus; muscle fatigue or weakness; overstretching of the anterior structures; and microtrauma to these tendinous, capsular, and ligamentous tissues. This vicious circle leads to anterior instability, subluxation, impingement, and rotator cuff tears (see Figs. 7-4 and 7-14). Patients in group II demonstrate instability caused by microtrauma; patients in group III reveal instability caused by hyperlaxity. In both cases the instability results from the aforementioned vicious circle. If the instability is not corrected, undersurface tears of the rotator cuff will result from an impingement of the tendons on the glenoid labrum. The impingement is an actual mechanical pinching of the tendon and is in contradistinction to the proposed mechanism of tension overload on the tendon. The patients who have experienced inside impingement have been throwers, and the rotator cuff impingement has been between the posterosuperior glenoid labrum and the humeral head. Other sports, such as swimming, are also at risk for inside impingement. For swimmers, the point of contact appears to be the supraspinatus against the anterosuperior labrum. Both throwers and swimmers may respond to rehabilitation to correct the instability that leads to inside impingement. When continued stress to the capsule has progressed to subluxation and anatomic damage, surgical correction of the capsule may be necessary. Group IV instability is seen in young athletic patients who have had a traumatic event that led to the instability, and who have not, at least in the early stages, demonstrated any impingement.

The classification scheme and unifying proposition suggested in this chapter are a turning point on which to ask many more questions. The answers that come will help refine treatment of shoulder dysfunction in the overhead athlete.

References

1. Abrams JS: Special shoulder problems in the throwing athlete: pathology, diagnosis, and nonoperative management, *Clin Sports Med* 10(4):839, 1991.
2. Altchek DW et al: Arthroscopic acromioplasty, *J Bone Joint Surg* 72A:1198, 1990.
3. Atwater AE: Biomechanics of overarm throwing movements and of throwing injuries, *Exerc Sports Sci Rev* 7:43, 1979.
4. Bassett RW et al: Glenohumeral muscle force and moment mechanics in a position of shoulder instability, *J Biomech* 23: 405, 1990.
5. Bigliani LU et al: *Arthroscopic coracoacromial ligament resection for impingement in the overhead athlete.* Paper presented at the Annual Meeting of the American Shoulder and Elbow Surgeons, Sept 26-28, 1994.
6. Bigliani LU, Morrison DS, April EW: The morphology of the acromion and its relationship to rotator cuff tears, *Orthop Trans* 10:228, 1986.
7. Brewer BJ: Aging of the rotator cuff, *Am J Sports Med* 7:102, 1979.
8. Burkhead WZ: The biceps tendon. In Rockwood CA, Matsen FA, editors: *The shoulder,* vol 2, Philadelphia, 1990, WB Saunders.
9. Codman EA: *The shoulder,* Boston, 1934, Thomas Todd.
10. DePalma AF: Injuries of the shoulder in sports. In *Surgery of the shoulder,* ed 3, Philadelphia, 1983, JB Lippincott.
11. DiGiovine NM et al: An electromyographic analysis of the upper extremity in pitching, *J Shoulder Elbow Surg* 1:15, 1992.
12. Elliott B et al: A three-dimensional cinematographic analysis of the fastball and curveball pitches in baseball, *Int J Sports Biomech* 2:20, 1986.
13. Ellman H: Arthroscopic subacromial decompression: analysis of one-three year results, *Arthroscopy* 3:173, 1987.
14. Feltner M, Dapena J: Dynamics of the shoulder and elbow joints of the throwing arm during a baseball pitch, *Int J Sports Biomech* 2:235, 1986.
15. Hawkins RJ, Brock RM: Anterior acromioplasty: early results for impingement with intact rotator cuffs, *Orthop Trans* 3:274, 1979.
16. Hawkins RJ, Kennedy JC: Impingement syndrome in athletes, *Am J Sports Med* 8:151, 1980.
17. Ianotti JP: Rotator cuff disorders: evaluation and treatment, *American Academy of Orthopaedic Surgeons Monograph Series,* 1991.
18. Jobe CM, Sidles J: Evidence for a superior glenoid impingement upon the rotator cuff: anatomic, kinesiologic, MRI and arthroscopic findings. Presented at the 5th International Conference on Surgery of the Shoulder, Paris, France, July, 1992.
19. Kessel L: *Clinical disorders of the shoulder,* Edinburgh, 1982, Churchill Livingstone.
20. Loehr JF, Uhthoff HK: The pathogenesis of degenerative rotator cuff tears, *Orthop Trans* 11(2):237, 1987.
21. Lowe WR, Tibone JE: Arthroscopic acromioplasty: long term results, Unpublished manuscript, 1992.
22. Matsen FW, Arntz CT: Subacromial impingement. In Rockwood CA, Matsen FA, editors: *The shoulder,* Philadelphia, 1990, WB Saunders.
23. Montgomery WH III, Jobe FW: Functional outcomes in athletes following a modified anterior capsulolabral reconstruction, *Am J Sports Med* 22(3):352, 1994.
24. Morrison DS, Bigliani LU: The clinical significance of variations in acromial morphology, *Orthop Trans* 11:234, 1987.
25. Mudge MK, Wood VE, Frykman GK: Rotator cuff tears associated with os acromiale, *J Bone Joint Surg* 66A:427, 1984.
26. Neer CS II: *Shoulder reconstruction,* Philadelphia, 1990, WB Saunders.
27. Neer CS II: Impingement lesions, *Clin Orthop* 173:70, 1983.
28. Neer CS II: The relationship between the unfused acromial epiphysis and subacromial impingement lesions, *Orthop Trans* 7:138, 1983.
29. Neer CS II: Anterior acromioplasty for the chronic impingement syndrome in the shoulder: a preliminary report, *J Bone Joint Surg* 54A:41, 1972.
30. Neer CS II, Welsh RP: The shoulder in sports, *Orthop Clin North Am* 8(3):583, 1977.
31. Ogata S, Uhthoff HK: Acromial enthesopathy and rotator cuff tear: a radiologic and histologic postmortem investigation of the coracoacromial arch, *Clin Orthop* 254:39, 1990.
32. Ozaki J et al: Tears of the rotator cuff of the shoulder associated with pathological changes in the acromion, *J Bone Joint Surg* 70A:1224, 1988.
33. Paulos LE, Franklin JL: Arthroscopic shoulder decompression development and application: a five year experience, *Am J Sports Med* 18:235, 1990.
34. Rubenstein DL et al: Anterior capsulolabral reconstruction of the shoulder in athletes, *J Shoulder Elbow Surg* 1:229, 1992.
35. Scarpinato DF, Bramhall JP, Andrews JR: Arthroscopic management of the throwing athlete's shoulder: indication, techniques, and results, *Clin Sports Med* 10(4):913, 1991.
36. Seitz WH: Shoulder impingement: instability overlap syndrome, *Orthop Trans* 14(3):685, 1990.
37. Stuart MJ, Azevedo AJ, and Cofield RH: Anterior acromioplasty for treatment of the shoulder impingement syndrome, *Clin Orthop* 260:195, 1990.
38. Tibone JE et al: Shoulder impingement syndrome in athletes treated by an anterior acromioplasty, *Clin Orthop* 188:134, 1985.
39. Turkel SJ: Stabilizing mechanisms preventing anterior dislocation of the glenohumeral joint, *J Bone Joint Surg* 63A:1208, 1981.
40. Uhthoff HK, Sarkar K: Classification and definition of tendinopathies, *Clin Sports Med* 10(4):707, 1991.
41. Walch G et al: Impingement of the deep surface of the supraspinatus tendon on the posterosuperior glenoid rim: an arthroscopic study, *J Shoulder Elbow Surg* 1(5):238, 1992.
42. Yamanaka K, Fukuda H: Pathological studies of the supraspinatus tendon with reference to incomplete thickness tears. Proceedings of the Third International Conference on Shoulder Surgery, Fukuoka, Japan, Oct 28-30, 1986.
43. Zuckerman JD et al: The influence of coracoacromial arch anatomy on rotator cuff tears, *J Shoulder Elbow Surg* 1:4, 1992.

SECTION B Clinical and Diagnostic Evaluation

The athlete with shoulder pain remains a diagnostic and therapeutic challenge for many reasons. The past few decades have seen a significant increase in interest and knowledge about the shoulder complex. The normal shoulder anatomy, biomechanics, and functional capabilities have begun to be reexamined, with continuing appreciation of the wide range of normal variations. Additionally, the pathologic processes have been given more critical attention, and basic assumptions about the pathophysiology have begun to be challenged. The sensitivity and specificity of many findings on physical examination remain untested or are now in question. The shoulder complex remains an enigma where the relationships between pathology, symptoms, and physical examination continue to baffle both the novice and the experienced physician.

The athletic shoulder presents unique challenges in diagnosis. Athletic shoulders are exposed to extremes of motion, strain, and repetition. Adaptations by the shoulder girdle over time can be helpful for the athlete, but there is disagreement over whether and when these changes are pathologic. For example, increased external rotation of the dominant throwing arm is a common finding, but at what point does it contribute to pathologic instability and pain? When an athletic shoulder crosses the line from normal to pathologic function, these adaptations and physical findings may either contribute to or even prevent an accurate diagnosis.

This chapter reviews the diagnostic process for the athletic shoulder, particularly as it relates to the clinical spectrum of instability, impingement, and rotator cuff disease. This chapter will discuss the pathway to a diagnosis through the history, physical examination, imaging, and arthroscopic evaluation. Specifically, the use of these diagnostic tools to distinguish the four groups of patients will be discussed later. Subsequent chapters address the task of successful treatment in these challenging subgroups of patients.

HISTORY

The accurate and thorough history is important for a successful diagnosis in this challenging group of athletes, particularly because the physical examination may not provide consistently helpful information. The symptoms and circumstances in which the injury occurs provide the clinician with hints about the underlying pathology. Familiarity with the athlete's sport and discussions with the athlete and trainer often help the physician determine the precipitating or exacerbating activity, establish a diagnosis, and facilitate treatment strategy. Obtaining information from trainers and coaches sometimes is very helpful in determining whether other factors, such as overuse or poor mechanics, are contributing to the patient's problem.

The history should not be viewed in isolation; an accurate diagnosis is based on a constellation of historical factors or details and findings at the time of the physical examination or arthroscopy. A 20-year-old swimmer with shoulder pain could have a variety of etiologies for that pain, and it should not be presumed that the etiology is instability without a complete and thorough history and physical examination.

Although age is not a definitive criterion for cataloging patients, the athlete with a painful or dysfunctional shoulder tends to have different pathologic problems depending on age. This is especially true for the impingement-instability spectrum. As noted by Neer, impingement and cuff pathology increase in patients in their thirties.[37] In the authors' experience, patients in the late thirties or older are more likely to have classic outside impingement (group IA) unless they are very high-caliber athletes in overhead sports. Some of these older patients do develop inside impingement (group IB). Impingement symptoms in the adolescent and younger overhead sport athlete tend to reflect some underlying instability, and the diagnosis is more likely internal impingement (group II or III).

Dominance of the extremity is a factor in the evaluation of athletes with shoulder pain. Throwers tend to have symptoms in their dominant extremity, whereas in other sports such as swimming and weight-lifting, athletes may have problems in either shoulder. The type, intensity, and level of competition of the sport also influence injury patterns. Athletes should be asked about their cross-training activities and what effect these activities have on symptoms, because cross-training can contribute to injury.[34] The number of years of participation or competition help to determine the possibility of overuse or injury caused by repetition.

The two most common complaints of the athlete with shoulder symptoms are pain and/or instability. The circumstances surrounding the initial symptoms are important to ascertain, especially with a history of trauma. Trauma can cause rotator cuff injury and should be considered in the differential diagnosis of patients involved in contact sports or in older patients. Although unusual, full-thickness rotator cuff tears can occur in younger athletes.[27] Blevins et al reported 12 full-thickness rotator cuff tears in contact-sport athletes with an average age of 23.[4]

Arm position at the time of injury is likewise important. If the patient had a dislocation (group IV), the arm position after it is dislocated may provide sufficient evidence to indicate whether it was anterior (arm would be abducted slightly), posterior (arm would be adducted, internally rotated), or inferior (luxatio position with the arm abducted around 90°) (Fig. 7-15). Athletes should be asked whether they feel their arm sliding or whether it feels loose. Patients who experience subluxations with minor or no trauma typically are in group III, with congenital or developmental hyperlaxity. In these groups, a history of instability in other joints may be an indication of underlying connective-tissue disorders.

Pain is the most common shoulder complaint for most athletes. The "how, what, when, and where" of the pain may give some assistance in diagnosis. In the instability-impingement spectrum, the pain can be anterior, lateral, or posterior. Radiation of the pain down the shoulder into the deltoid is common for impingement symptoms caused by either internal or external impingement. However, patients with internal impingement tend to have more symptoms in the posterosuperior joint line. There is often a vague, poorly localized ache or discomfort felt in the shoulder during nonspecific activity.

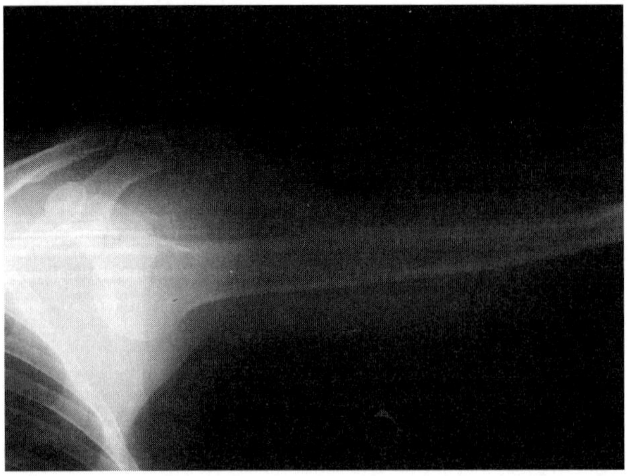

FIGURE 7-15 In traumatic inferior dislocation of the shoulder (luxatio erecta), the arm is in an abducted position, as shown in this radiograph. Associated fractures and neurovascular injuries are common with this type of instability.

Anterior shoulder pain in the region of the biceps tendon may radiate down the arm, but biceps pain does not correlate well with any one pathologic process or type of impingement. The relationship of biceps pain to superior labral pathology (SLAP lesions) is inconsistent.

Impingement pain is most commonly insidious in onset, although it may be dated to one particular throw, swing, or other kind of event. The pain is predictably associated with activity and may persist after the athletic event for varying time intervals. Patients may have pain with activities of daily living and when using the arm overhead. The pain may keep them from sleeping on that shoulder at night. Severe night pain is more common with full-thickness rotator cuff tears but can occur with other shoulder pathologies. However, pain waking the patient from sleep should be evaluated carefully because tumor pain can produce similar symptoms.

Severity of symptoms does not always correlate with the degree of pathology. However, as the stage of impingement progresses from tendinitis to partial and full-thickness rotator cuff tears, the symptoms usually worsen in severity.[52] With persistent or progressive symptoms, the athlete may note weakness, with decreased speed in serving, pitching, or swimming. In tennis, the patient may have difficulty serving and may also have trouble hitting a backhand or reaching for a forehand ground stroke.

The athlete should be questioned about neck pain and any neurologic symptoms such as paresthesias. Radiation of pain proximally from the shoulder to the neck is atypical, although there may be associated trapezius stiffness or periscapular muscle soreness. Symptoms of tingling or numbness caused by instability can be seen, but they are usually transient. The dead-arm syndrome described by Rowe usually presents as a "heaviness" of the arm without true neurologic deficits.[44,45] Persistent paresthesia should alert the examiner to other possible etiologies, such as cervical spine or brachial plexus abnormalities.

Particularly in the throwing athlete, the relationship of the pain to the phases of the pitch should be evaluated. Posterior shoulder pain in follow-through may indicate posterior rotator cuff muscle strain and fatigue, whereas posterior shoulder pain in late cocking may indicate internal impingement.[20,28,31] Classic impingement pain anterolaterally over the shoulder frequently is not associated with any specific phase of the throwing motion. In the young athlete, it is probably caused by a SLAP lesion rather than impingement under the acromion.[28,47]

Particularly in the throwing act, forceful delivery is based on the sequential transmission of energy, relying on the integrity and coordination of the entire body. Pain or dysfunction in the lower extremities, trunk, elbow, or forearm may result in abnormal stress transmission to the shoulder, with symptoms of pain.[40]

Crepitus also is a frequent complaint, but it is neither a sensitive nor a specific finding. Crepitus often is accompanied by no symptoms, but it also can be seen in conjunction with degenerative arthritis, the entire spectrum of impingement pathology from tendinitis to full-thickness tears, acromioclavicular joint problems, and fractures. Throwers often will feel or hear a pop in the shoulder, with increased symptoms. Although the athlete should be examined carefully for rotator cuff pathology or occult instability, in the authors' experience, this complaint alone does not indicate any one pathologic entity but is sometimes associated with SLAP lesions.

Swelling is an uncommon complaint and, if present, vascular etiologies of swelling should be considered. Localized swelling may indicate a ganglion cyst or other tumor. In patients with significant rotator cuff disease, a ruptured biceps tendon gives patients a typical and characteristic arm mass, but this injury can occur in younger patients as well.

The way a patient's perception of pain has responded to previous treatments and modalities may indicate the source of an athlete's pain. Has the patient taken any medications or been given any injections? Has the patient received an adequate rehabilitative and preventive strengthening program? How long has the patient rested from the offending activity in an effort to eliminate symptoms? Has the patient changed pitching rotation or swimming mileage? The success or failure of previous operative procedures complicates the evaluation. In the athlete who has failed previous surgery, a thorough history has increased significance. The examiner needs to consider whether the prior diagnosis was accurate and whether the appropriate surgery was performed.

It is also important to consider the patient's overall health. Does the patient have a history of medical illness such as diabetes, gout, or other systemic disease? Does the patient have a history of cardiac or gastrointestinal disorders, any unintentional weight loss, fatigue, or malaise? Does the patient have pain or swelling in other joints or have any symptoms of inflammatory arthritis? Although shoulder pain in the athlete is usually due to some component of the impingement-instability spectrum, the examiner must keep in mind the variety of other potential causes, such as arthritis, neoplasm, metabolic disease, infection, congenital anomaly, and psychiatric factors.

PHYSICAL EXAMINATION

The physical examination of the athletic shoulder should help confirm the diagnosis and also should rule out other pathologic processes. A thorough physical examination is possible in 5 to 10 minutes. Each examiner should develop a system, but generally the evaluation should include a screening neurologic test, visual inspection, range of motion, palpation, strength testing, and, finally, provocative tests such as impingement and laxity, apprehension, and relocation tests.[23,25,46]

Cervical Spine and Neurologic Testing

Because referred cervical spine pathology can present as shoulder pain, every shoulder evaluation should include a brief cervical spine examination, especially when there are complaints of paresthesia or weakness. Palpate for tenderness and examine for the reproduction of shoulder symptoms during an active range of motion of the neck. Axial loading in various positions of flexion, extension, or lateral bending may reproduce shoulder symptoms in cases of cervical-nerve-root pathology. Rarely, patients with upper extremity complaints will have symptoms in the lower extremities as well, such as in cervical spondylolysis or stenosis. A thorough examination of the upper and lower extremities should include sensation, motor, and reflex testing.

Visual Inspection

Complete visualization of the patient's neck as well as both shoulders and upper extremities is optimal for comparison. This will allow the examiner to find subtle changes in symmetry, swelling, or atrophy around the shoulder girdle. Static inspection both from the front and from the back, with the patient seated or standing, usually reveals no gross asymmetry or atrophy. However, mild asymmetry in the position of the scapula, hypertrophy of the muscles of the dominant arm, and slight drooping of the dominant shoulder are common and are known as "tennis shoulder"[30,42] (Fig. 7-16). These changes also can be found in the dominant arm of throwers.[25]

Prominence of the scapular spine may indicate atrophy of the supraspinatus and/or infraspinatus (Fig. 7-17). In the older group, atrophy is more common in long-standing full-thickness rotator cuff tears. Atrophy in athletes is uncommon, and neurologic causes, such as suprascapular nerve entrapment, should be considered.[15,32,41,43]

Range of Motion

The motion of both shoulders should be evaluated both actively and passively. Motions that are clinically important are elevation in the scapular and forward frontal planes, internal and external rotation at 90° of abduction, external rotation with the arm at the side, and internal rotation with the thumb up the spine.[1] The patient should be observed for any asynchrony of motion, both anteriorly and posteriorly. Asymmetry of scapulohumeral rhythm may indicate compensation for pain or other abnormalities.[7] A painful arc between 70° and 120° of elevation indicates impingement but fails to distinguish between outlet and nonoutlet impingement or between in-

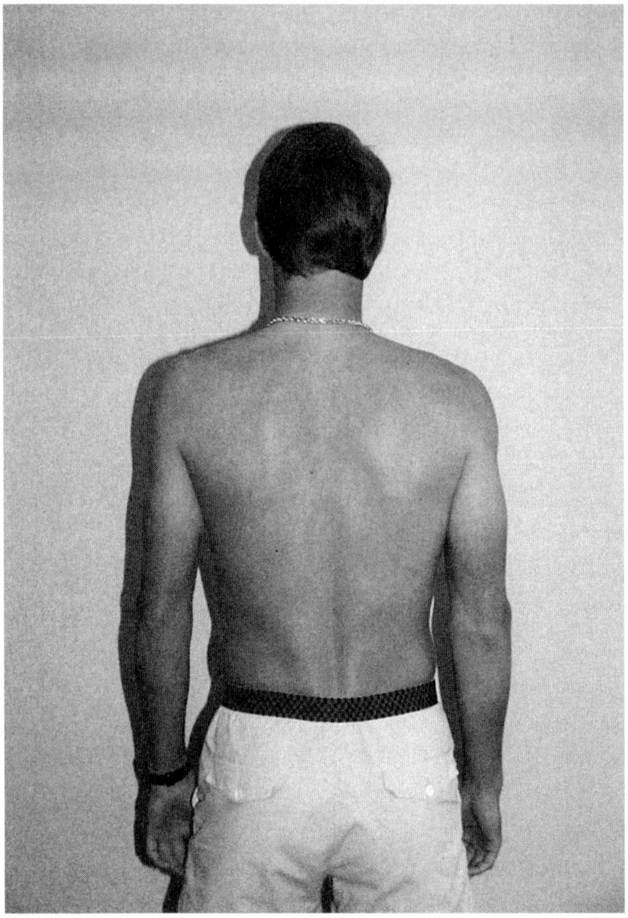

FIGURE 7-16 A tennis player demonstrating findings in the dominant arm that are seen in many athletes. The carrying level of the dominant arm is lower than the nondominant arm.

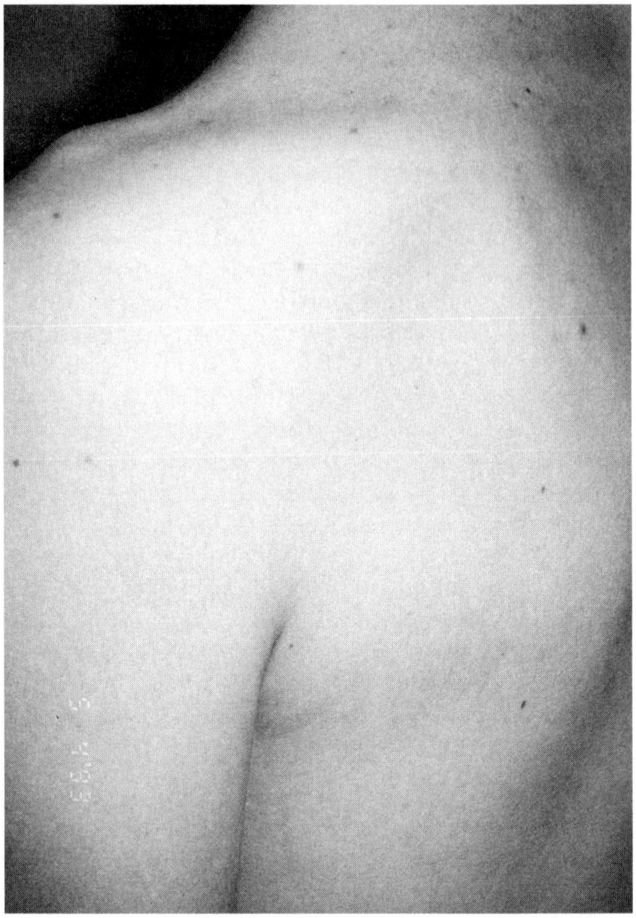

FIGURE 7-17 Suprascapular nerve palsy with a lesion at the scapular notch produces wasting of the supraspinatus and infraspinatus in this "Ultimate Frisbee" player. Most overhead athletes have a lesion at the spine of the scapula, thus causing wasting to the infraspinatus only.

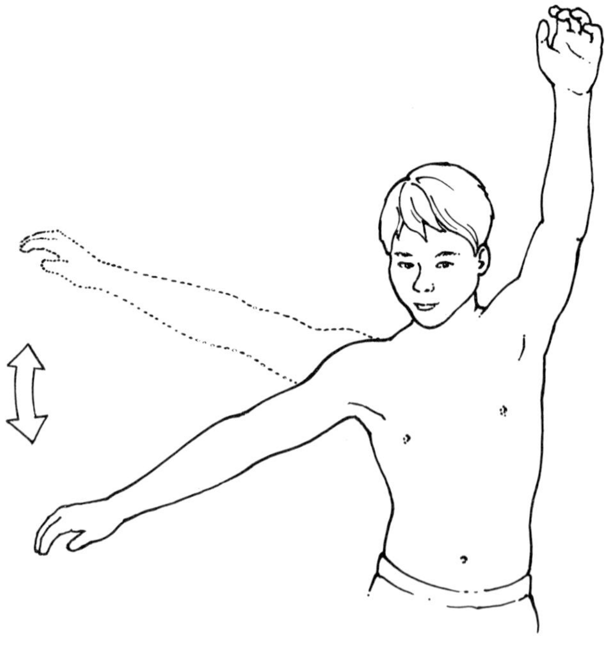

FIGURE 7-18 The arc becomes painful at about 70° to 120° of elevation.

ternal and external impingement[8,29] (Fig. 7-18). If the patient reports pain or symptoms with a certain motion, the examiner should ask the patient to perform such maneuvers. Patients with voluntary or involuntary instability will demonstrate a motion that causes their symptoms that is different from the inciting motion of the patient with subacromial impingement. A "shrug sign" with arm elevation indicates abnormal mechanics resulting from pain, paralysis, weakness, or capsular tightness (Fig. 7-19).

Loss of active forward elevation or abduction is uncommon in athletes except after an acute injury and can have a variety of causes. Loss of elevation or abduction is more common in older patients with chronic or large rotator cuff tears. Adhesive capsulitis is distinctly uncommon in younger athletes, although it may occur in older athletes. The authors have seen several senior-level tennis players with loss of elevation caused by degenerative arthritis of the shoulder, but most of these patients had loss of other shoulder motions as well.

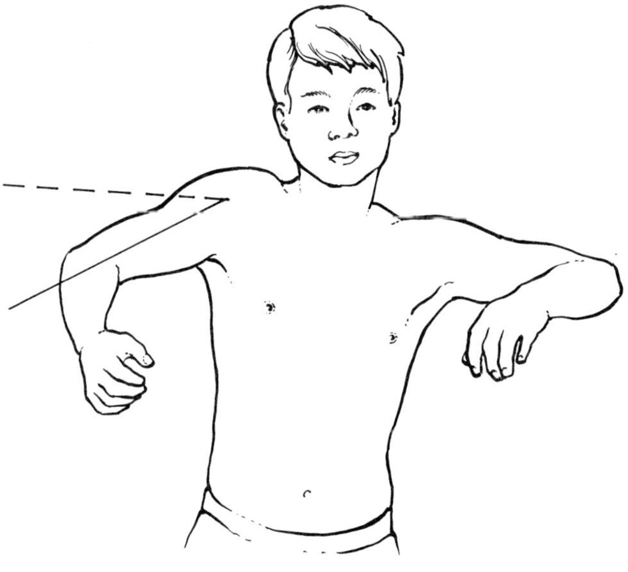

FIGURE 7-19 Patients with a painful, weak, or frozen shoulder may show a "shrug sign," in which they elevate the shoulder complex to compensate for decreased glenohumeral motion.

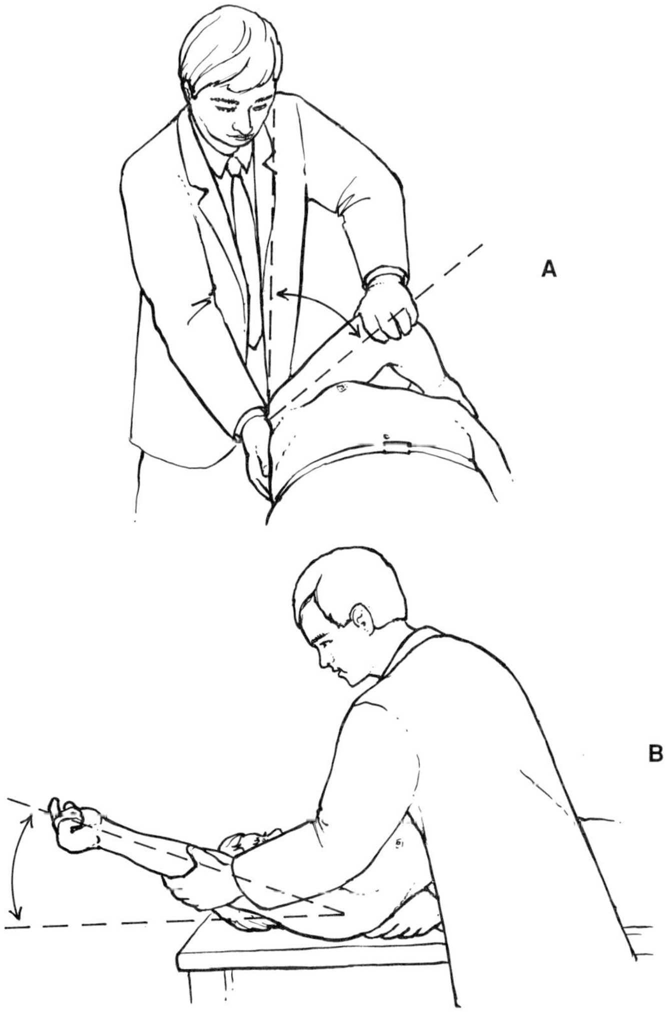

FIGURE 7-20 **A,** The examiner tests for horizontal flexion by stabilizing the scapula. Flexion may indicate shoulder tightness in throwing athletes. **B,** The examiner tests for tightness in forward elevation by stabilizing the scapula and elevating the arm. Both of these tests are used often, but the clinical significance is not well established.

Shoulder internal and external rotation is measured with the patient either standing or sitting. The dominant arm of throwing athletes typically shows increased active and passive external rotation compared with the nondominant arm.[6,25] Swimmers will commonly have increased external rotation of both shoulders. This is not always associated with concomitant loss of internal rotation, nor does it appear to necessarily correlate with symptoms. Kibler et al found loss of internal rotation in tennis players. They postulated that this was due to posterior capsule tightness and that it might contribute to stretching of the anterior structures.[6,30] This is commonly seen in the dominant arm of baseball pitchers.

Passive motion of the shoulder to evaluate scapular and glenohumeral mobility has been recommended by many authors.[6,40,46] With the patient supine, the posterior capsule tightness can be tested by forced horizontal adduction with the arm abducted 90° (Fig. 7-20). Combined abduction also gives a relative measure of the athlete's overhead flexibility (Fig. 7-6). Unfortunately, neither standard measurements for age, gender, or sport nor the reproducibility of this test is known. These tests therefore are not of significant benefit in distinguishing patient subgroups in the instability-impingement spectrum.

Palpation

The location of tenderness to palpation, when present, can give important clues about the source of the pain in the athletic shoulder. Unfortunately, not all patients have pain at the time of the examination, and accurate palpation of the deeper structures often is prevented by large overlying muscles. When indicated, the examination should include the following: the sternoclavicular joint; the clavicle; the acromioclavicular joint; the anterior, lateral, and posterior acromion; the anterior joint line; the posterior joint line; and the biceps tendon. Codman has advocated slight extension of the arm to palpate the supraspinatus insertion.[7] Patients with posterior pain may have a strain of the posterior cuff, posterior capsulitis, or posterior internal impingement (group IB, II, or III). Tenderness along the coracoid may indicate retrocoracoid impingement, but tenderness is not specific for that condition alone.[14,19]

Direct palpation of the biceps tendon is not possible, but tenderness in the region of the bicipital groove is best identified by externally rotating the arm, thereby bringing the biceps tendon away from the anterior joint line. Hawkins et al recommend internal rotation of 10° to bring the biceps straight anteriorly.[23] However, the authors have found that external rotation of 20° to 30°

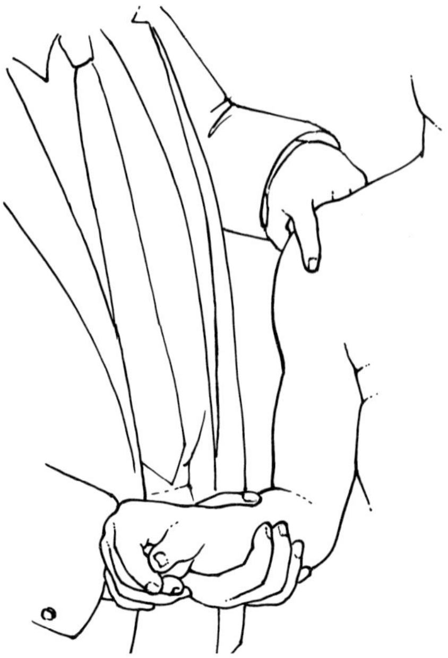

FIGURE 7-21 The examiner palpates the biceps tendon by externally rotating the arm 20° to 30°, flexing and extending the elbow, and feeling for the tendon excursion anteriorly.

with palpation for the tendon of the shoulder, either supine or standing, tends to make the biceps easier to palpate (Fig. 7-21).

Crepitus can be palpated by passively moving the arm at the side or by having the patient reproduce the arm position that produces the crepitus. Crepitation can be due to a variety of causes and may be radiating from sources distant from the shoulder. The "crank test" is considered positive for labral pathology when there is crepitus with the arm in an abducted, externally rotated position.[26] However, localizing the pathology or judging its extent using palpable crepitus or cracking sounds is difficult. There is currently no accurate, reproducible test for labral pathology, although, rarely, larger labral tears may produce painful catching.

Strength Testing

Strength testing of the upper extremity can be used as an integral part of the neurologic examination and to reveal any functional deficits in the athlete's shoulder. In those patients with a suggestion of vascular injury, other tests are recommended (Chapter 14). Muscle testing should be performed according to standard texts, but when in-

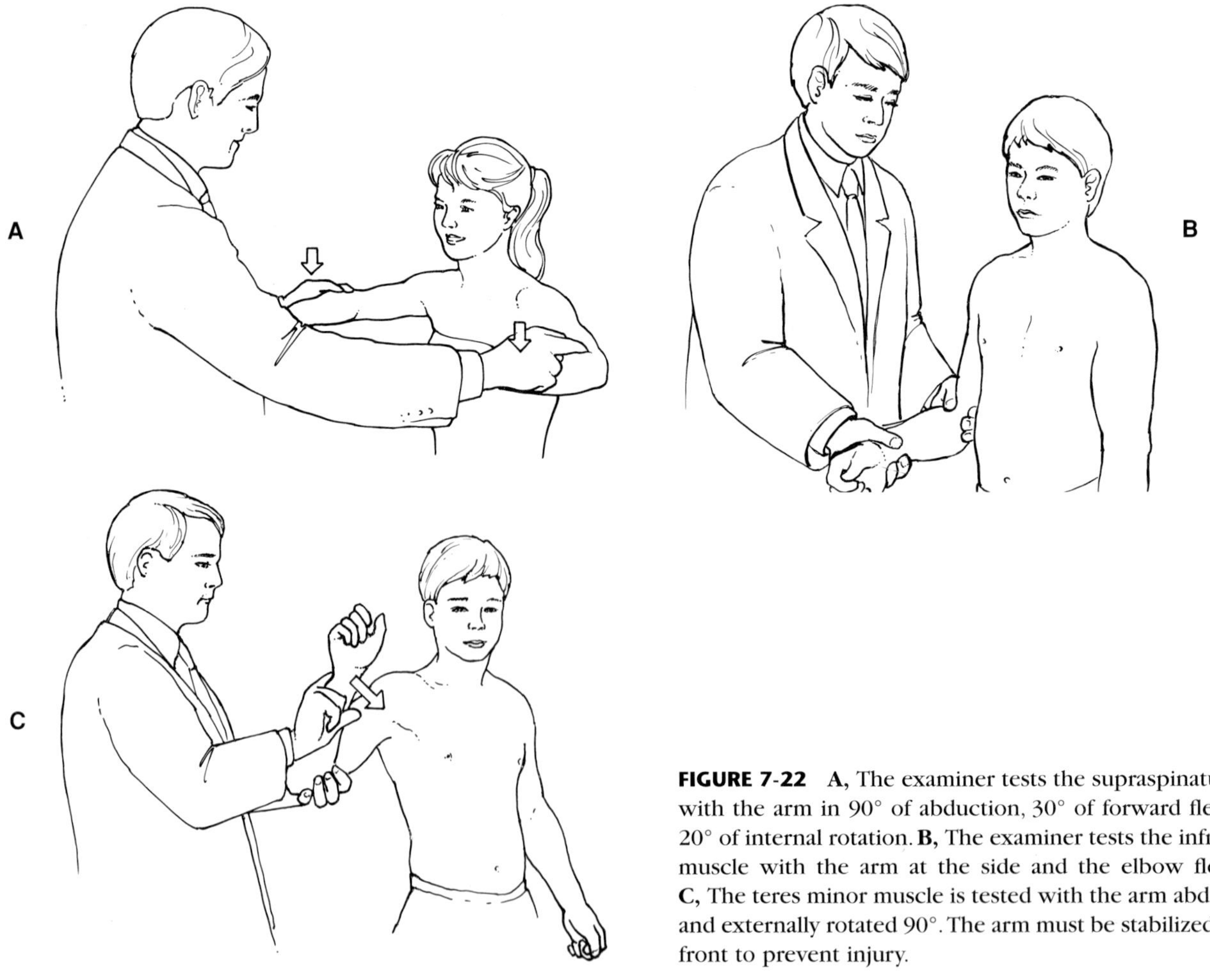

FIGURE 7-22 **A,** The examiner tests the supraspinatus muscle with the arm in 90° of abduction, 30° of forward flexion, and 20° of internal rotation. **B,** The examiner tests the infraspinatus muscle with the arm at the side and the elbow flexed 90°. **C,** The teres minor muscle is tested with the arm abducted 90° and externally rotated 90°. The arm must be stabilized from the front to prevent injury.

dicated a comprehensive examination will include muscles innervated by all peripheral nerves and spinal root levels. In the throwing athlete, testing of the scapular stabilizers or "pivoters" is important as well.

The supraspinatus is best tested in the scapular plane with the arm abducted 90° and internally rotated 20° (Fig. 7-22). Because pain may result in relative weakness or "giving way" during testing, such findings are not necessarily indicative of the severity of structural damage. Loss of strength is not a reliable sign of rotator cuff tear in the earlier stages, particularly in the young athlete.[28,31]

The infraspinatus is tested with the arm at the side. Weakness in external rotation may be because of chronic disuse, pain, or other causes. It is considered to be the sine qua non of rotator cuff tears by some authors, based on studies showing loss of external rotator strength in most full-thickness rotator cuff tears.[7,38] Testing external rotation with the arm abducted above 45° tests primarily the teres minor (see Fig. 7-22). However, strength testing with the arm in this position must be performed carefully to prevent provoking symptoms or subluxations.

Internal rotation strength is best tested with the elbow at the side. Weakness is uncommon but when present may be due to pain. Avulsion of the subscapularis after dislocation or previous surgery also is uncommon but may be the most serious complication after a Bankart procedure. Gerber recommends a "lift-off" test where the patient attempts to push away from the back with the arm in internal rotation. The test also is considered positive if the patient cannot hold the hand away from the back in this position[46] (Fig. 7-23).

Serratus anterior weakness can result in scapular winging, which can be illustrated best by having the patient flex the shoulder forward 90° (Fig. 7-24). More subtle serratus anterior weakness can be detected by having the patient do a "wall push-up." Rhomboid testing can be performed prone with the arms horizontally extended while abducted 90°. Trapezius function can be tested with a shoulder shrug. Weakness and atrophy of this muscle caused by spinal accessory nerve palsy has been described in athletes as well as appearing as a complication after neck surgery.[12,32]

Large rotator cuff tears are unusual in athletic patients, but when present they result in a loss of active motion and significant strength deficits. A positive "drop-arm" test shows an inability to maintain the arm at 90° of abduction, but the test is nonspecific.

Provocative Tests

Impingement Tests

Traditionally, the most widely recognized sign of impingement is described by Neer.[33,37] While fixing the scapula with one hand, the examiner elevates the affected shoulder, which in theory compresses the rotator cuff against the unyielding coracoacromial arch and causes pain (Fig. 7-25). This sign may actually result from impingement of the rotator cuff against the superior glenoid labrum. This test usually will be positive in patients with pure impingement (group I), but it also may be positive when rotator cuff inflammation is seen in other patients with internal impingement (group IB, II, and III). A positive impingement sign may occur in other

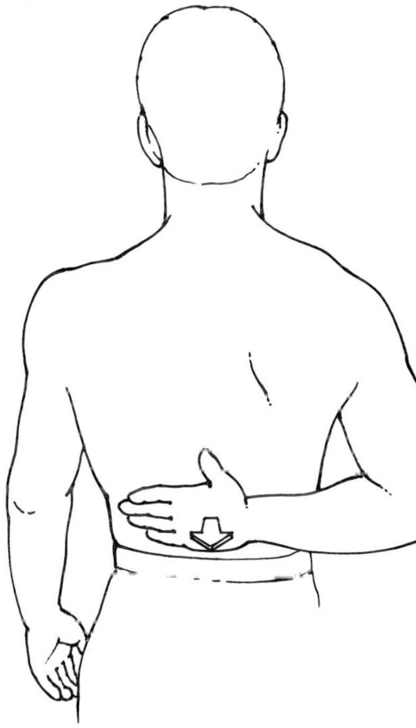

FIGURE 7-23 The test of subscapularis function evaluates the patient's ability to push the hand away from the low back. An inability to perform this maneuver indicates subscapularis pathology.

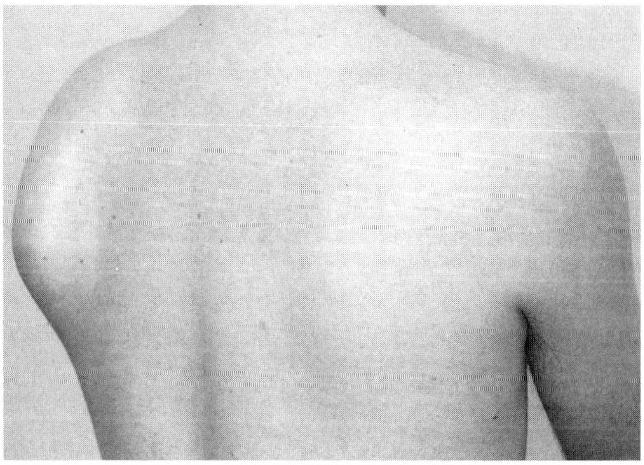

FIGURE 7-24 Winging of the scapula can be due to long-thoracic-nerve palsy or serratus weakness. In this patient, winging was due to pain produced by prominent staples used in a anterior shoulder reconstruction.

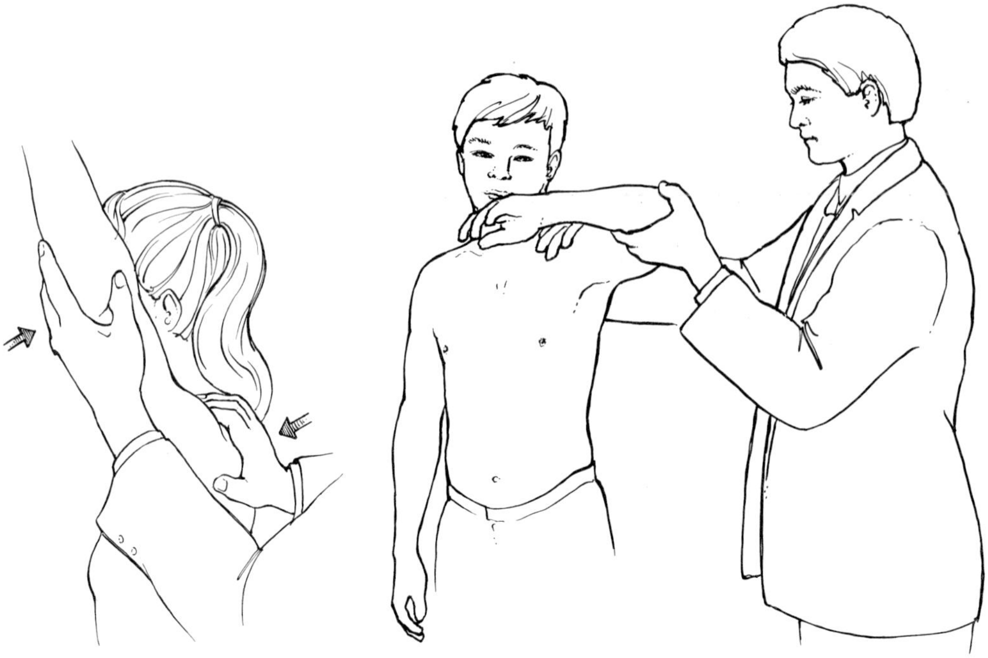

FIGURE 7-25 Two impingement signs are commonly used. **A,** The Neer impingement sign is produced by stabilizing the shoulder and elevating the arm in the frontal plane. **B,** The Hawkins impingement sign is produced by abducting the arm 90° and internally rotating the shoulder. Further abduction may be necessary to reproduce the impingement pain.

conditions, including adhesive capsulitis, acromioclavicular or glenohumeral joint arthritis, calcific tendinitis, or tendinitis from any cause.[17] According to Neer, "there are an infinite number of local and systemic problems that could cause a positive impingement sign."[38]

Hawkins has described a modification of this impingement sign that may more accurately test for subacromial impingement: The arm, elevated forward 90°, is adducted and then forcibly internally rotated against the fixed scapula (see Fig. 7-25). Reproduction of symptoms with anterior shoulder pain under the arch indicates impingement.[24]

Biceps tendinitis frequently coexists in the impingement-instability spectrum. There are no definitive criteria for making this diagnosis either with examination or arthroscopically because many patients with isolated biceps pain have no intraarticular pathology at the time of arthroscopy. The relationship of biceps tendinitis or dysfunction to SLAP lesions is not yet completely understood. The most commonly used provocative tests that presumably indicate biceps tendinitis include Speed's test and Yerguson's test. Speed's test is performed with the arm abducted 90° and forward-flexed 45° with the forearm supinated and the elbow extended (Fig. 7-26). Pain with resistance indicates a positive result, but this test can be positive with impingement resulting from other causes.[11] Yerguson's test (pain with resisted supination of the flexed elbow) is neither sensitive nor specific.[53]

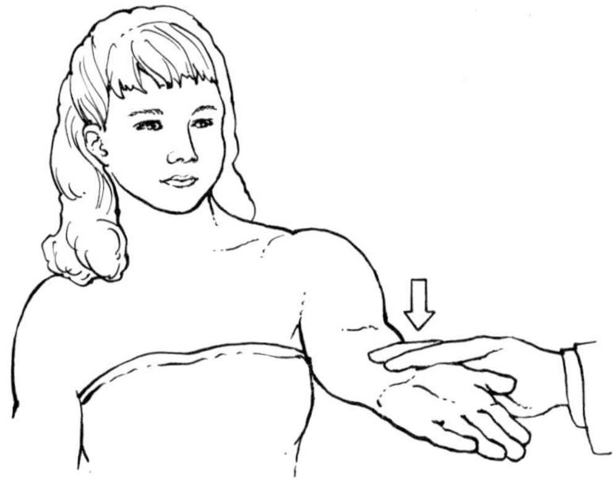

FIGURE 7-26 Speed's test for biceps tendinitis is performed by elevating the arm 90° in a plane 45° in front of the body with the palm up. This test may not distinguish biceps pain from impingement pain.

Acromioclavicular (AC) pathology can both mimic and contribute to internal or external impingement. The AC joint rarely becomes symptomatic in patients with instability alone, but it may be symptomatic in athletes with impingement. Tenderness at the AC joint that reproduces the patient's pain is strong evidence of AC pathology. The other test of the AC joint includes forced passive cross-arm testing (Fig. 7-27), and although sensitive for AC joint pathology, it is not specific.[5,46] To test the AC joint, O'Brien et al recommended a Speed's test with the arm adducted 10° across the body and with the arm

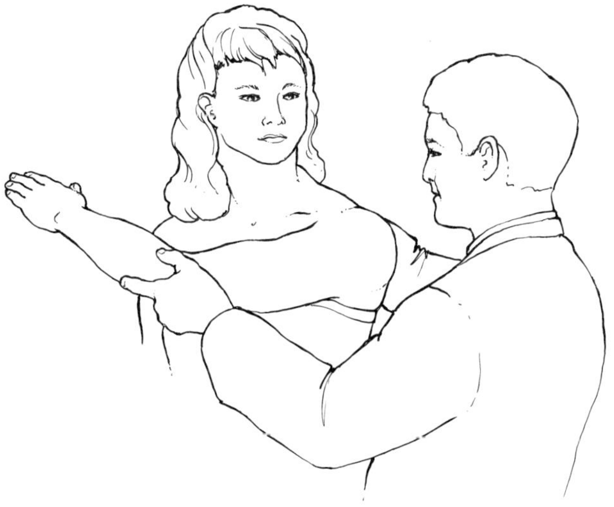

FIGURE 7-27 Forceful horizontal adduction is used to evaluate acromioclavicular joint pathology.

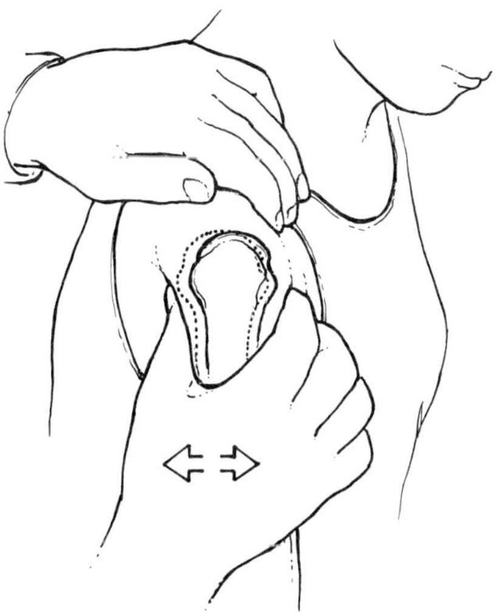

FIGURE 7-28 Shoulder laxity can be evaluated with the "load and shift" test. With the patient sitting, the scapula is stabilized with one hand, a compressive force is applied to the glenohumeral joint, and anteroposterior excursion is measured.

internally rotated. They report a false-positive rate of 8%, with no false-negative responses.[39]

The impingement test of Neer uses injection of an anesthetic into the subacromial space primarily to distinguish shoulder pain from pain originating from other sources.[37,38] The test does not distinguish outlet from nonoutlet causes of impingement, and a positive test (where the pain is relieved by rejection) also can be seen in groups IB, II, and III. Therefore this test will not distinguish inside impingement from outside impingement (group IA). Injection of the acromioclavicular joint usually will determine whether acromioclavicular pathology is contributing to the athlete's pain, but it may not eliminate the pain caused by osteolysis of the distal clavicle.[5] Injection of the posterior joint line in patients with inside impingement at the posterosuperior glenoid has been neither accurate nor beneficial in our experience.

Laxity and Apprehension Tests

Although many of the aforementioned examinations provide useful information about the etiology of shoulder pain in athletes, examination of the shoulder for laxity and instability provides critical information to distinguish the various groups of athletes who present with shoulder pain and dysfunction. There is increasing appreciation that in the shoulder, as in the knee, laxity and instability are not synonymous. The shoulder demonstrates a wide range of normal laxity, and care must be taken not to mistake normal laxity for instability.[16,21,35] Another difficulty with laxity and instability testing is that the examination requires experience and practice. In addition, because there is currently no objective means by which shoulder laxity can be measured, the examination remains subjective, with possible differences between observers. Examination of shoulders in patients with no shoulder complaints both in the office and under anesthesia is recommended to gain experience with these techniques.

Laxity testing can be performed with the patient sitting or supine. Both shoulders must be examined, and the patient must be relaxed. With the patient sitting and the arm at the side, the examiner slides the humeral head anteriorly and posteriorly, feeling for subluxation of the humeral head over the anterior and posterior glenoid rims. Hawkins terms this the "load and shift" test[23] (Fig. 7-28). Gerber recommends performing a "posterior drawer" test with the patient supine[18] (Fig. 7-29). Posterior excursion is measured by flexing the arm forward while directing a posterior force with the other hand. An anterior drawer test is performed by stabilizing the scapula and attempting to subluxate the shoulder anteriorly[18] (see Fig. 7-29). Other authors call this examination of supine anterior and posterior laxity a "push-pull" test.[23] If the shoulder can be subluxated on physical examination, the patient should be asked whether the subluxation is similar to the sensation felt when symptoms occur.

There are three reported methods of classifying the anteroposterior excursion of the humeral head. Some authors have reported the laxity in terms of millimeters, but this method probably is not accurate or reproducible. Another technique is to estimate the percentage of humeral head subluxation during the maneuver, but this entails some guess about the humeral head's size. Hawkins recommends a classification based on whether the humeral head translates minimally (trace), translates to the glenoid rim (type I), translates over the glenoid rim (type II), or locks out (type III). In our experience,

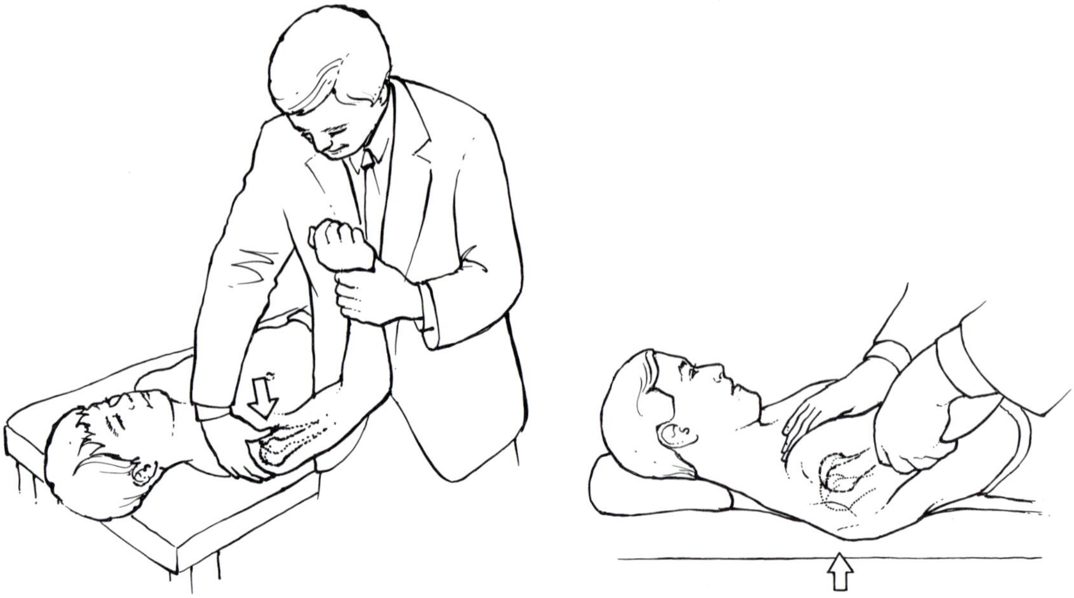

FIGURE 7-29 The anterior and posterior drawer tests described by Gerber are performed with the patient supine and placed near the edge of the table so that the shoulder is unsupported. **A,** To perform the posterior drawer test, the examiner holds the arm at the wrist and applies a posteriorly directed force to the humeral head lateral to the shoulder joint. It is important to forward flex the shoulder as the force is directed posteriorly to evaluate posterior shoulder laxity. **B,** To perform the anterior drawer, the examiner must stabilize the scapula with one hand. The other hand holds the humerus to apply an axial load to the joint. The hand on the humerus then attempts to translate the humeral head anteriorly over the glenoid rim.

type IVs are very rare, and it is difficult to distinguish type I from type II in most patients.[23,33] Until an instrumental device or technique for measuring anteroposterior excursion is created, these classifications will be disputed. The authors have not found fluoroscopy or radiographs helpful in measuring laxity.

Large, asymmetric laxity with subluxation may indicate pathologic laxity, but without symptoms the laxity is probably normal. Two studies of laxity in normal, asymptomatic adolescent athletes have demonstrated asymmetric shoulder laxities in 10% to 25% of those examined.[16,33] Subluxations that reproduce the symptoms of pain or instability are significant, providing important information about the etiology of the patient's dysfunction. When these examinations do not provide helpful information, then other evidence must be obtained to aid in diagnosis, either radiographically or upon arthroscopic evaluation.

Patients with traumatic instability (group IV) typically do not have a positive anterior apprehension test for anterior instability because they have not been dislocated. A shoulder must have been completely out to develop the apprehension sign. Anterior apprehension testing can be performed with the patient sitting or supine. When the patient is tested in a supine position, anterior pressure on the abducted, externally rotated shoulder produces apprehension; this is called the "fulcrum test" by some authors.[23] A relocation maneuver can be performed by stabilizing the humeral head with a posteriorly directed force applied to the anterior proximal humerus. This should eliminate the apprehension in most patients. As has been shown by Speer et al., the relocation test, when used for instability, is both accurate and sensitive.[49]

Relocation Test

An important test on physical examination is the relocation test for pain. The patient is put in a supine position and moved in the abducted externally rotated position until pain is experienced. This position is usually in abduction above 90° and in the extreme of external rotation and hyperextension. Kinematic studies have shown that this reproduces the position of the arm in the late cocking stage of the pitching motion.[20,28] In this position, the humeral head subluxes anteriorly, and hyperangulation of the humerus posteriorly allows the rotator cuff to be captured between the greater tuberosity and the posterosuperior glenoid labrum. A posteriorly directed force at this point will eliminate the impingement pain. Patients with external impingement will not have pain in this position; if they do have pain, they usually will not experience relief with posterior stabilization of the humeral head.

ARTHROSCOPIC EVALUATION

Diagnostic arthroscopy and examination under anesthesia are valuable in the evaluation and treatment of athletes with shoulder problems, especially when the diagnosis is in doubt. Routine diagnostic arthroscopy frequently is not necessary in complete-dislocation group IV with pure instability when the history, physical examination, and supportive radiographs document the instability pattern. Similarly, some patients with obvious rotator cuff tears (group I) do not need arthroscopy to confirm the diagnosis. However, examination under anesthesia and arthroscopy can provide supportive data in cases where the presence or absence of intraarticular pathology or instability is in question.

With the patient under anesthesia, both shoulders should be examined for range of motion, crepitus, and laxity-instability. This is best accomplished with the patient supine and with muscle paralysis. Although shoulder arthroscopy and surgery can be performed successfully with scalene blocks, asymmetry is more difficult to ascertain in the shoulder examination with this technique. A detailed examination as recommended by Cofield can be performed. Although this technique is comprehensive, it is also time-consuming.[8]

Excellent reviews of diagnostic and surgical arthroscopy of the shoulder are available.[35] Salient points of the arthroscopic evaluation as they relate to these patient populations will be discussed here.

The arthroscopy can be performed with the patient sitting or in a lateral decubitus position with equal success. Regardless of the patient position, the shoulder should be capable of being removed from the holding device to allow range of motion and manipulation. This facilitates observation of any internal impingements with the arthroscope through either the posterior or anterior portals.

Arthroscopic evaluation of the shoulder is initially performed through standard anterior and posterior portals. The intraarticular examination should be thorough and should systematically evaluate all of the structures that provide diagnostic information.

Lesions of the biceps tendon can be seen throughout the spectrum of impingement-instability. Flattening and hypertrophy of the tendon can be seen in patients with long-standing rotator cuff disease. Inflammation and scarring are commonly seen at the base of the tendon in patients with impingement. SLAP lesions may reflect some degree of instability and superior impingement. SLAP lesions are frequently seen in patients with instability and internal impingement (group II).

Tears and fraying of the supraspinatus especially can be seen in patients with internal impingement and in patients with instability-impingement (groups IB, II, and III). Rotator cuff tears in patients with traumatic instability increase in incidence in patients over the age of 40.[22,50] Partial tears should be evaluated with bursoscopy to verify that they are partial-thickness tears and should not be converted to full-thickness tears by zealous débridement. The technique of Snyder, using a suture placed through the partial tear, is recommended.[48] Bursal-side tears are more common in patients with outside or classic Neer impingements (group IA).

Fraying and tears of the infraspinatus are less common but may be seen at the posterosuperior border of the glenoid.[13] In the abducted, externally rotated position, the upper and superior infraspinatus can impinge internally between the humeral head, the greater tuberosity, and the labrum. This same mechanism may be responsible for the posterior labrum tears and fraying seen in a high percentage of group II patients.

Examination of the humeral head should include the entire head surface by internal and external rotation of the arm. Special attention should be directed to the posterior and superior surfaces, where chondromalacia or impression fractures (Hill-Sachs lesions) may be detected. Posterior head defects of the Hill-Sachs type are more common in patients with traumatic instability and dislocations, whereas those with subluxation tend to have varying degrees of posterior humeral head chondromalacia. This chondromalacia enlarges the normal bare spot and represents the contact area with the posterior glenoid rim in anterior subluxation. Hill-Sachs lesions are usually a little more anterior and represent the contact area with the anterior glenoid at complete dislocation. Posterosuperior humeral head chondromalacia and impression fractures suggest inferior instability and may be confluent with posterior humeral head lesions (Fig. 7-30). Patients with external impingement (group I) may have diffuse humeral head chondromalacia, but the chondromalacia should not have the appearance of a Hill-Sachs lesion.

The glenoid should be examined for chondromalacia and degenerative changes. The bare spot on the central area is normal and corresponds to the area of high contact between the humeral head and the glenoid. This is a normal variant and does not contribute to symptoms. The anterior glenoid rim should be visualized for wear indicative of instability. This wear is typically at or inferior to the glenoid equator. Glenoid-rim fractures can be difficult to visualize arthroscopically because many heal beneath the glenoid and are covered by soft tissue. However, when glenoid-rim fractures are present, they confirm traumatic instability. The anterior and inferior labrum is typically confluent with the articular cartilage, although in a minority of shoulders it is meniscoid in nature.[9,51] These areas should be examined carefully for detachments (Bankart lesions) and tears. Labrum flap tears that are large enough to be symptomatic are unusual, but débridement of these symptomatic tears can relieve symptoms.[7,10] Débridement of labrum lesions alone in an unstable shoulder does not address the primary pathology. Studies have demonstrated that the débridement alone in this situation produces less-than-satisfactory results.[2,10] Patients with pure external impingement and rotator cuff disease frequently have fraying of the labrum rim, which probably represents a degenerative process. Patients in groups IB, II, and III may not have labrum detachments or tears, but they may have atrophic labra. Superior labrum detachments without biceps involve-

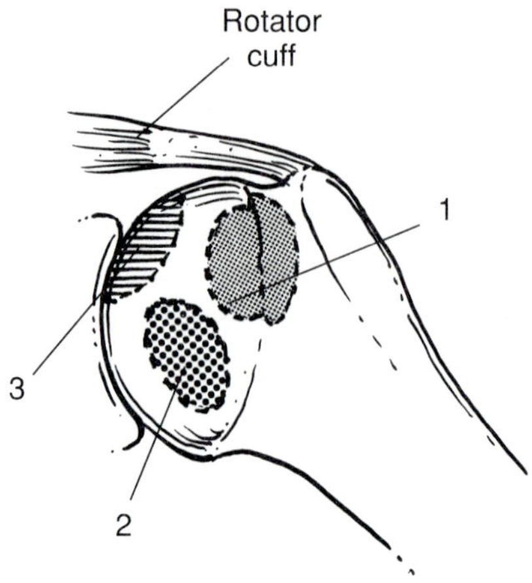

FIGURE 7-30 Chrondromalacia of the humeral head may give evidence of the direction of the instability. Enlargement of the bald spot frequently is seen with occult subluxations *(1)*. Hill-Sachs lesion usually are posteriorly in the humeral head and indicate traumatic instability *(2)*. Superior head chondromalacia may indicate inferior instability *(3)*.

ment may be normal variants (e.g., Buford variant) and are not believed to be of significance for instability or impingement.

Although visualization of the glenohumeral ligaments can provide some information, grading systems are subjective and of unknown accuracy. At least one study suggests that an atrophic inferior glenohumeral ligament is associated with atraumatic instability. Occasionally, rents in the capsule resulting from traumatic dislocations may be visible in the acute situation.[3]

Visualization of the position of the humeral head in reference to the glenoid with light traction can suggest instability if the head perches on the anteroinferior rim of the glenoid. A positive push-through test is a consistent finding in group II and especially group III patients: The arthroscope in the posterior portal can be pushed easily between the glenoid and the humeral head into the anterior axillary recess in the region of the anterior bundle of the inferior glenohumeral ligament. This finding is typical of patients with instability but usually is not seen in patients with pure outside impingement.

Inside impingement is best demonstrated arthroscopically by manipulating the arm while viewing the superoposterior glenoid from either the anterior or the posterior portal. The arm is abducted maximally and externally rotated until contact is observed between the cuff and the labrum. The corresponding frayed cuff and glenoid regions often "kiss."[13] Posterosuperior labrum lesions often will be visualized in this area of impingement.

DIAGNOSTIC GUIDELINES

The preceding discussion demonstrates the necessity of a thorough and comprehensive approach to the athlete with a painful shoulder. No single criterion can establish the diagnosis, because these processes represent a continuum ranging from apparently isolated rotator cuff disease to pure, unidirectional, and traumatic instability. As more is learned about the shoulder through advances in imaging and both clinical and basic research, the distinctions between groups may become either more blurred or more definite. The complexity of the shoulder and progression of the disease process currently make specific classification of the individual athlete difficult.

Athletes with a painful, dysfunctional shoulder who have been determined to be in the impingement-instability spectrum can be basically divided into four groups. Although tremendously oversimplified, a description will be given of a typical patient in each group of the impingement-instability spectrum (assuming a typical patient can exist).

Group I patients are typically older and have a history of classic impingement, as described by Neer. They are involved in overhead sports as a hobby or were more competitive when they were younger. They have pain over the anterolateral acromion or along the biceps tendon. The pain may occur if they roll on the shoulder in their sleep. They may have weakness in abduction and, less commonly, in external rotation because of pain. Their symptoms may worsen as they become more chronic. They will improve at least temporarily with ice, rest, and antiinflammatories. Subacromial injections will relieve their pain. On examination, they may have an element of adhesive capsulitis and possibly a shrug sign. They will be tender over the anterolateral acromion and biceps tendon but usually not over the posterior joint line. They will have pain and may have weakness with resisted abduction and external rotation. Neer and Hawkins impingement signs often will be positive. These patients will have a negative apprehension test. Although they may have increased shoulder laxity with manual testing, they will not show instability on examination that reproduces their symptoms. Radiographs will show greater tuberosity and acromial sclerosis, as well as other typical findings discussed in Chapter 3. The MRI may show partial or complete cuff tearing but no labral pathology. An arthrogram may or may not show a tear. Examination under anesthesia usually will show no pathologic laxity. The arthroscopy will demonstrate either cuff pathology or a thickened, inflamed subacromial bursa. There will not be a Hill-Sachs or a Bankart lesion, although there may be some fraying off the labral rim. Surprisingly, a very small subgroup of these patients will show arthroscopic findings and examination typical of instability (group IB), although this is very uncommon in patients over the age of 35 years.

On the other end of the spectrum are patients with

traumatic unidirectional instability. These patients typically will have had several dislocations and seek treatment because of instability rather than pain. Between dislocations, they usually are asymptomatic, although they may experience subluxations. They generally will have no connective-tissue disorder other than multiple-joint dislocations. On examination, they will have full range of motion, no weakness, and no tenderness. They usually have negative impingement tests but positive anterior apprehension signs. With supine testing, the relocation maneuver will eliminate their apprehension. They may have normal or increased laxity with demonstrable subluxations that are *not* symptomatic in directions other than that of their primary instability. However, they are typically not ligamentously lax upon examination. Plain radiographs may substantiate their instability with glenoid-rim fractures or Hill-Sachs lesions. CT after arthrogram or MRI will demonstrate these lesions along with a Bankart lesion. If necessary, arthroscopy will confirm a Bankart lesion and a Hill-Sachs lesion on the posterior humeral head. Less commonly, there may be a superior Hill-Sachs lesion, indicating an element of multidirectional instability.

Groups II and III are distinguished primarily by the presence of hyperlaxity in group III. Group III patients may not be athletes at all but experinece subluxation or dislocations with minimal or no trauma. They will have congenital hyperlaxity or a connective-tissue disorder. Consequently, they may have several other joint subluxations or dislocations. They will show signs of hyperlaxity on examination, and they may have apprehension in several directions. They easily have a type III sulcus sign and may subluxate palpably with testing. Radiographs will be negative, although they may have glenoid hyperplasia. MRI and CT arthrography are consistently negative. Arthroscopy reveals this hyperlaxity, with a subluxed humeral head and a positive push-through test. Commonly these patients demonstrate an attenuated inferior glenohumeral ligament and a patulous axillary pouch. There is rarely a Bankart lesion, SLAP lesion, cuff tear, or Hill-Sachs lesion. Internal impingement may be demonstrable with shoulder rotation.

Athletes who perform overhead sports and who develop painful dysfunction frequently represent painful instability secondary to microtrauma (group II). This group includes higher-caliber athletes who are throwers, tennis players or, occasionally, swimmers. They develop pain insidiously, often during periods of intense exercise. This pain presents similarly to the impingement pain of group I patients. The pain may be anterolateral or along the posterior joint line. They have no history of dislocation, although the arm may feel loose. Dead-arm symptoms may occur acutely in certain positions or after the athlete's sport activity. Symptoms are relieved initially with rest, ice, antiinflammatories, rehabilitation, and occasionally injections. On physical examination, there is no atrophy with increased external rotation on the affected side. The patient may or may not have a positive Neer and/or Hawkins impingement sign. There is often tenderness over the anterolateral acromion, biceps, or posterior joint line. Laxity testing may show normal or increased laxity. The supine apprehension test reproduces the pain, and a relocation maneuver eliminates it. Plain radiographs may show signs of impingement or a Bennett lesion. MRIs and CT arthrography may show blunting of the anterior labrum but usually are normal. Examination under anesthesia typically demonstrates subluxation anteriorly. Arthroscopic findings are variable but support the diagnosis of occult instability with impingement. Internal impingement is likely with the arm in the position of extreme abduction and external rotation.

SUMMARY

Athletes with painful shoulders present a diagnostic challenge for the sports-medicine physician. The overlapping histories, symptoms, signs on physical examination, and arthroscopic findings make the distinct classification of patients difficult. The spectrum of patient symptoms within the impingement-instability continuum tends to eliminate distinctions among patients. Physical examination remains an inexact science, and the accuracy, sensitivity, and specificity of the findings and tests await further investigation. Although radiographic evaluation provides clues to the diagnosis, it frequently falls short of providing definitive information. The science of arthroscopy of the shoulder is in relative infancy. Arthroscopic normal and pathologic anatomy continues to be delineated, and correlation of these findings with symptoms awaits further studies. A comprehensive framework for the evaluation and understanding of the painful shoulder in the athlete remains a significant challenge. The current schema provides a background for the chapters on treatment that follow.

References

1. Green WB, Heckman JD, editors: *The clinical measurement of joint motion,* Rosemont, Ill, 1994, The Academy.
2. Altchek DW et al: Arthroscopic labral debridement: a three year follow-up study, *Am J Sports Med* 20:702-706, 1992.
3. Baker CL, Uribe JM, Whitman C: Arthroscopic evaluation of acute initial anterior shoulder dislocations, *Am J Sports Med* 18:25-28, 1990.
4. Blevins FT, Pagnani MJ, Warren RF: *Rotator cuff injury in contact athletes.* Fellows research program, American Orthopaedic Society Sports Medicine, Sun Valley, Idaho, July, 1993.
5. Cahill BR: Osteolysis of the distal part of the clavicle in male athletes, *J Bone Joint Surg* 64A:1053-1058, 1982.
6. Chandler TJ et al: Flexibility comparisons of junior elite tennis players to other athletes, *Am J Sports Med* 18:134-136.
7. Codman EA: *The shoulder,* Malabar, Fla, 1934, Robert Kreiger Publishing, reprint 1984.

8. Cofield RH, Irving JF: Evaluation and classification of shoulder instability with special reference to anterior and posterior drawer tests, *Clin Orthop* 223:32, 1987.
9. Cooper DE et al: Anatomy, histology and vascularity of the glenoid labrum: an anatomical study, *J Bone Joint Surg* 74A:46-52, 1992.
10. Cordasco FA et al: Arthroscopic treatment of glenoid labrum tears, *Am J Sports Med* 12:425-431, 1993.
11. Crenshaw AH, Kilgore WE: Surgical treatment of bicipital tenosynovitis, *J Bone Joint Surg* 48A:1496-1502, 1966.
12. Crohn BT, Brahms MA, Cohn M: Injury to the eleventh cranial nerve in a high school wrestler, *Orthop Rev* 15:59-64, 1986.
13. Davidson PA et al: Rotator cuff injury associated with increased glenohumeral motion: a new site of impingement, submitted to *J Shoulder Elbow Surg,* 1994.
14. Dines DM et al: The coracoid impingement syndrome, *J Bone Joint Surg* 72B:314-316, 1990.
15. Drez D: Suprascapular neuropathy in the differential diagnosis of rotator cuff injuries, *Am J Sports Med* 4:43-45, 1976.
16. Emery RJH, Mullaji AB: Glenohumeral joint instability in normal adolescents, *J Bone Joint Surg* 73B:406-408.
17. Fu FH, Harner CD, Klein AH: Shoulder impingement: a critical review, *Clin Orthop* 269:162-173, 1991.
18. Gerber C, Ganz R: Clinical assessment of instability of the shoulder: with special reference to anterior and posterior drawer tests, *J Bone Joint Surg* 66B:551-556, 1984.
19. Gerber C, Terrier F, Ganz R: The role of the coracoid process in the chronic impingement syndrome, *J Bone Joint Surg* 67B:703-708, 1985.
20. Glousman RE et al: Dynamic EMG analysis of the throwing shoulder with glenohumeral instability, *J Bone Joint Surg* 70A:220-226, 1988.
21. Harryman DT et al: Laxity of the normal glenohumeral joint: a quantitative assessment, *J Shoulder Elbow Surg* 1:66-76, 1992.
22. Hawkins RJ et al: Anterior dislocation of the shoulder in the older patient, *Clin Orthop* 206:192-195, 1986.
23. Hawkins RJ, Bokor DJ: Clinical evaluation of shoulder problems. In Rockwood CA, Matsen FA, editors: *The shoulder,* Philadelphia, 1990, WB Saunders.
24. Hawkins RJ, Hobeika PE: Physical examination of the shoulder, *Orthopedics* 6:1270-1278, 1983.
25. Hawkins RJ, Mohtadi N: Rotator cuff problems in athletes. In DeLee JC, Drez D, editors: *Orthopaedic sports medicine, principles and practice,* Philadelphia, 1994, WB Saunders.
26. Hurley JA, Anderson TE: Shoulder arthroscopy: its role in evaluating shoulder disorders in the athlete, *Am J Sports Med* 18:480, 1990.
27. Itoi E, Tabata S: Rotator cuff tears in the adolescent, *Orthopedics* 16:78-81, 1993.
28. Jobe FW, Glousman RE: Rotator cuff dysfunction and associated glenohumeral instability in the throwing athlete. In Paulos LE, Tibone JE, editors: *Operative techniques in shoulder surgery,* Gaithersburg, Md, 1991, Aspen Publications.
29. Kessel L, Watson M: The painful arc syndrome, *J Bone Joint Surg* 59B:166-172, 1977.
30. Kibler WB: Role of the scapula in the overhead throwing motion, *Contemp Orthop* 22:525-532.
31. Kvitne RS, Jobe FW: Diagnosis and treatment of anterior instability in the throwing athlete, *Clin Orthop* 291:107-123, 1993.
32. Lefferts RD: Neurological problems. In Rockwood CA, Matsen FA, editors: *The shoulder,* Philadelphia, 1990, WB Saunders.
33. McFarland EG, Campbell G, McDowell J: Posterior shoulder laxity in asymptomatic adolescent athletes, *Med Sci Sports Exerc* 26:5 (supplement), 1994.
34. McFarland EG, Wasik M: Injuries to competitive female swimmers due to cross-training, *Med Sci Sports Exerc* 24:S125 (supplement), 1992.
35. McGinty JB: *Operative arthroscopy,* New York, 1991, Raven Press.
36. Neer CS II: Anterior acromioplasty for the chronic impingement syndrome of the shoulder: a preliminary report, *J Bone Joint Surg* 54A:41-50, 1972.
37. Neer CS II: Impingement lesions, *Clin Orthop* 173:70-77, 1983.
38. Neer CS II: *Shoulder reconstruction,* Philadelphia, 1990, WB Saunders.
39. Pagnani MJ, O'Brien SJ: *A new diagnostic test for acromioclavicular disease.* Fellows research program, American Orthopaedic Society Sports Medicine, Sun Valley, Idaho, July, 1993.
40. Pappas AM, Zawacki RM, McCarthy CF: Rehabilitation of the pitching shoulder, *Am J Sports Med* 13:223-235, 1985.
41. Post M, Mayer J: Suprascapular nerve entrapment, *Clin Orthop* 223:126-136, 1987.
42. Priest JD, Nagel DA: Tennis shoulder, *Am J Sports Med* 4:28-42, 1976.
43. Ringel SP et al: Suprascapular neuropathy in pitchers, *Am J Sports Med* 18:80-86, 1990.
44. Rowe CR: Recurrent transient anterior subluxation of the shoulder: the "dead-arm syndrome," *Clin Orthop* 223:11, 1987.
45. Rowe CR, Zarins B: Recurrent transient subluxation of the shoulder, *J Bone Joint Surg* 63A:863-872, 1981.
46. Silliman JF, Hawkins RJ: Clinical examination of the shoulder complex. In Andrews JR, Wilk KE, editors: *The athlete's shoulder,* New York, 1994, Churchill Livingstone.
47. Snyder SJ et al: SLAP lesions of the shoulder, *Arthroscopy* 6:274-279, 1990.
48. Snyder SJ et al: Partial thickness rotator cuff tears: results of arthroscopic treatment, *Arthroscopy* 7:1-7, 1991.
49. Speer KP et al: An evaluation of the shoulder relocation test, *Am J Sports Med* 22(2):177-183, 1994.
50. Timjes J, Loyd HM, Tullos HS: Arthrography in acute shoulder dislocations, *South Med J* 72:564-567, 1979.
51. Vlasek R, McFarland EM: *Anatomic variants of the glenoid labrum,* American Academy Orthopaedic Surgeons, New Orleans, La, Feb, 1994.
52. Watson M: Rotator cuff function in the impingement syndrome, *J Bone Joint Surg* 71B:361-366, 1989.
53. Yergason RM: Supination sign, *J Bone Joint Surg* 13A:60, 1931.

SECTION C Anterior and Multidirectional Glenohumeral Instability

The phenomenon of gross instability of the glenohumeral joint has been well documented and described over the centuries. Recently the subtleties of instability have been appreciated and it has been realized that the symptoms of shoulder pain and dysfunction may be secondary to an unstable joint even in the absence of a frank dislocation.

Overhead athletic activities require complex adaptive mechanisms and a high level of neuromuscular coordination to stabilize the glenohumeral joint, while providing a platform to perform the athletic activities with the abducted arm. After a traumatic instability episode, many athletes require surgical intervention because of functional impairment. Many overhead athletes who are diagnosed with rotator cuff disease and/or chronic impingement have concomitant anterior instability of the glenohumeral joint. The athlete who is found to have instability and impingement typically has instability as the primary problem and underlying rotator cuff tendinitis or impingement as a secondary sequela.

If the primary dysfunction is recognized early, the majority of the injuries (perhaps up to 95%) can be treated conservatively with success.

HISTORICAL REVIEW

Instability of the glenohumeral joint is not a new phenomenon. It was well known to Hippocrates, who described the anatomy of the shoulder and treated problems of glenohumeral dislocations with a corrective surgical procedure.[1] Hippocrates described a technique using a red hot iron poker placed into the anterior inferior shoulder to produce a cicatrix to prevent recurrent dislocations. In 1861 Flower[7] described the humeral head defect that was reported 79 years later by Hill and Sachs.[14] Perthes[43] suggested that the separated labrum and capsule were responsible for the pathologic anatomy in unstable shoulders, and he demonstrated a technique using drill holes through the rim of the glenoid to reattach the separated labrum and capsule.

Bankart[3] reported on the surgical technique of reattaching the avulsed capsule and labrum to the glenoid, as well as stressed the importance of correcting this "essential lesion." Rowe and associates[46] reported on the long-term results of the Bankart procedure. The technique described by Rowe involved detachment of the coracoid process and the subscapularis muscle for improved exposure and reattachment of the separated anterior capsule to the glenoid rim with sutures placed through three holes along the anterior glenoid rim. Although there was only a 3.5% redislocation rate, only 33% of those involved in overhead athletics returned to their previous level of activity. The Bankart lesion has also been repaired with staples, as described by Sisk and Boyd.[50] In their review of the Du Toit staple capsulorrhaphy, only 58% of their patients returned to their previous athletic activities.

The use of a bone block for correction of glenohumeral instability was described by Eden[6] and Hybbinette.[18] They suggested that the use of a bone block was best performed in cases where there was a deficiency of glenoid bone secondary to recurrent dislocations. The bone graft would be placed into a periosteal pocket, located along the anterior glenoid rim. Helfet[13] described a technique of transplantation of the coracoid process and its attached conjoined tendon through an opening in the subscapularis to the anterior inferior aspect of the glenoid rim. The procedure was given Bristow's name and was later modified by May.[32]

The modified Bristow procedure stabilizes the shoulder by the dynamic sling effect of the conjoined tendon and substitution of the inferior subscapularis muscle for the inferior glenohumeral ligament.[14,27] Lombardo and associates[27] reported a 2% redislocation rate with an average loss of 11° of external rotation and an unsuspected inability to return to competitive throwing. They also showed that the success rate diminished in subluxating shoulders with the absence of a frank dislocation or with patients who had a hyperelastic or attenuated capsule and multidirectional laxity.

Osmond-Clarke[41] did not recognize the Bankart lesion as the sole cause of recurrent dislocation and thought that stretching of the anterior structures, especially the capsule and ligaments, also resulted in instability. The Putti-Platt surgical repair, as described by Osmond-Clarke, transects the conjoined tendon for exposure. The subscapularis muscle is detached 2.5 cm medial to its point of insertion and is retracted medially. The capsule is opened near the glenoid rim. The lateral subscapularis muscle and capsule are then sutured to the anterior glenoid with the shoulder in internal rotation. A loss of external rotation of 20° to 25° is one goal of the Putti-Platt procedure. The athlete's throwing ability, however, is impaired with this procedure.[21,49]

Neer and Foster[39] described a surgical procedure to correct multidirectional and inferior glenohumeral joint laxity. Their procedure demonstrated the importance of the capsular repair to correct the pathologic anatomy of a lax inferior caspular recess and stretched glenohumeral ligaments.

Basic science researchers have also looked at the problem of instability. Turkel and associates[52] demonstrated by anatomic dissection the importance of the glenohumeral ligaments. As the shoulder approaches 90° abduction, the inferior glenohumeral ligament provides the major static restraint against dislocation during external rotation. This explains the mechanism of anterior glenohumeral instability in a joint with ligamentous attenuation but an intact labrum. When a Bankart lesion is present, the ligamentous restraints fail because of a lack of continuity with the glenoid via the labrum.

Schwartz and associates[49] demonstrated the importance of the capsular structures and their role in glenohumeral stability. Selective arthroscopic transections of various components of the capsule were performed on cadaver shoulder models. They pointed out that instability was usually associated with both anterior and posterior capsular lesions. The anterior inferior glenohumeral ligament, along with the posterior inferior capsule, was also found to provide the primary restraint to anterior translation of the humeral head. The middle glenohumeral ligament was shown to provide a secondary restraint in anterior translation, and the posterior inferior capsule provided the primary restraint to posterior translation. They also demonstrated that the posterior superior capsule and the anterior superior glenohumeral ligament provided a secondary restraint to posterior translation of the humeral head.

Thus a common historical thread in both clinical and basic science is that instability (i.e., symptomatic capsular and ligamentous laxity) is at the core of most problems. Thus an ideal treatment would be to tighten these structures without significantly compromising the functional range of motion. Such a treatment would work for problems of dislocation and subtle instability. The anterior capsulolabral reconstruction (ACLR) used at the Kerlan-Jobe Orthopaedic Clinic was designed with this in mind. The goal of this procedure is to form a new capsulolabral complex by tightening the lax inferior glenohumeral ligament and capsule. This is done without detaching, shortening, or transferring any muscle. The procedure will be discussed in detail later; a summary is in order here. A split is made in the capsule, and the capsule is then pulled over itself in a vest-over-pants fashion and reattached to the anterior glenoid with sutures and bone anchors. The shoulder is mobilized immediately within a safe zone determined at surgery and is then splinted in abduction and external rotation between rehabilitation exercises. The procedure has been performed on many skilled overhead athletes and has consistently allowed them to return to their previous level of competition.[19,22]

Shoulder arthroscopy continues to prove itself a valuable tool for both diagnostic and therapeutic purposes. Probably the greatest contribution of shoulder arthroscopy has been its ability to better outline the articular anatomy and pathology. This is especially true with lesions that are often missed by other diagnostic techniques, such as capsular laxity and attenuation, and labral and chondral lesions.

Techniques for arthroscopic stabilization of the shoulder have continued to evolve since the original work performed by Johnson.[24] Arthroscopic staple-capsulorrhaphy, although initially popular, has not been satisfactory because of the high recurrence rates in glenohumeral instability and the potential for hardware complications.[31] This method appears to work best on unidirectional traumatic dislocation where the need for shifting the capsule and ligaments is not present.

In an attempt to avoid the complications caused by metal implants, Morgan[34] and Caspari[5] developed suture techniques designed to reduce the failure rate by getting better fixation of soft tissue to bone. Morgan's technique involved placing suture pins through the detached anterior capsule and labrum. The pins, with sutures, are passed posteriorly to the posterior glenoid neck, allowing the sutures to be tied posteriorly. Caspari, using a suture punch instrument, described placing multiple sutures in the anterior capsule and passing those sutures through a single transglenoid drill hole. The sutures are then tied over the posterior shoulder muscle fascia. Successful results (albeit with relatively short follow-up) have been reported in more than 90%, provided that the patient population was carefully selected to include only those patients with unidirectional traumatic anterior instability, with a distinct Bankart lesion and absence of significant capsular laxity.[35] Additional methods of fixation have also been advocated, including the use of biodegradable tacks[53] and metallic suture anchors.

CLASSIFICATION

Before classifying a patient with instability, it is important to remember that laxity does not mean instability. Many individuals have generalized ligamentous laxity with the ability to bring the thumb to the forearm and demonstrate increased translation of the glenohumeral joint. When evaluating the patient, the physician must be sure that the patient's normal laxity is not confused with pathologic instability. This is accomplished by performing a careful physical examination[12,15] and correlating the findings on examination to the patient's history. Patients who are extremely hypermobile with marked congenital glenohumeral laxity are usually asymptomatic but may experience shoulder subluxation with activities of daily living in the absence of traumatic or microrepetitive traumatic events. In this group there has been no stretching, tearing, or alteration of the patient's normal labral ligamentous anatomy. Symptoms attributable to a patient's congenitally lax capsule do occasionally require treatment. However, these patients usually respond to a nonoperative exercise program.

Instability of the glenohumeral joint can be classified by direction, cause, degree, and control (voluntary vs. involuntary) (Box 7-1).

BOX 7-1

CLASSIFICATION OF SHOULDER INSTABILITY

A. Direction
1. Anterior
2. Posterior
3. Inferior
4. Multidirectional

B. Cause
1. Traumatic
2. Atraumatic

C. Degree
1. Dislocation
2. Subluxation

D. Control
1. Involuntary
2. Voluntary
   a. Normal psychologically
   b. Abnormal psychologically

The most common classification of instability in the shoulder is an anterior dislocation produced by significant trauma. This usually results from the tremendous forces occurring when the arm is forced into maximum abduction and external rotation that then overcomes the capsular and labral restraints. Typically, anterior instability injuries result from traumatic episodes such as falling onto an outstretched arm (e.g., while skiing) or having an arm forced into further extension when it is in the air (e.g., when a basketball player goes in for a lay-up and the arm is blocked and pushed into further extension). After a traumatic anterior shoulder dislocation, patients frequently experience intermittent subluxation and/or dislocation associated with subsequent minor trauma.

Inferior instability normally accompanies either anterior or posterior instability. Significant inferior instability is usually a sign of multidirectional laxity and does not usually occur as an isolated event, except in patients who have undergone a previous surgical repair.

Multidirectional instability is typically seen in individuals with hyperelasticity, although it may also occur in patients who have had multiple traumatic instability episodes that stretch the capsular restraints.

Atraumatic instability occurs insidiously and is not attributable to one specific traumatic event. Typically, atraumatic instability results from chronic microrepetitive injuries, such as those seen in the throwing athlete. Atraumatic instability may also be associated with generalized soft-tissue laxity that allows abnormal excursion in multiple planes accentuated by subtle microrepetitive injuries. Atraumatic instability of the shoulder typically produces progressive subtle subluxation that may be unrecognized and usually occurs without a history of dislocation.

Most patients' instability is involuntary, and the patient has no control over the shoulder subluxation or dislocation. The instability occurs when the arm is placed in certain positions and subjected to excessive forces or trauma. Some patients, however, can voluntarily dislocate or sublux the shoulder joint. The ability may be preceded by a traumatic event, or it may occur in the shoulder with atraumatic multidirectional laxity. Most patients with voluntary control of their instability develop a habitual mechanism for subluxating the shoulder with muscular control (see Chapter 9). It is important to separate this group of patients from patients who sublux their shoulder joint for psychiatric reasons and secondary gain. Patients with a psychiatric component sublux the shoulder willfully and therefore compromise any surgical repair or rehabilitation program. These patients need psychiatric counseling to address the underlying problem and reasons for their secondary gain.

CLINICAL EVALUATION

Athletes with atraumatic subluxation of the glenohumeral joint are usually involved in overhead sports, which include baseball, volleyball, water polo, javelin, overhead racquet sports, and swimming.[42] They are usually young (i.e., between the ages of 16 and 35 years old), and primary pathologic changes under the coracoacromial arch are absent.

The history and physical examination are critical for establishing the diagnosis. When rotator cuff inflammation is present, the athlete shows signs of impingement. There is tenderness along the joint line posteriorly, positive impingement signs, and a positive impingement test result.[21] It is important to note that relief of pain during the impingement test (administration of 10 ml of local anesthetic into the subacromial bursa) confirms that there is inflammation within the subacromial space, but it does not indicate that the underlying causative factor is a primary impingement syndrome.

The rotator cuff[38,39] should always be evaluated for the possibility of a complete tear. Typical symptoms and signs are night pain, significant atrophy of the supraspinatus and infraspinatus, and weakness on resisted abduction and external rotation of the shoulder. If indicated clinically, an arthrogram or an MRI scan[28,40] may be performed to rule out a complete rotator cuff tear. A complete rotator cuff tear is rarely found in the young, overhead athlete. In particular, the MRI scan must be evaluated very carefully because of its sensitivity for showing pathologic changes within the rotator cuff tendon. The MRI signal visible on the scan from an intact rotator cuff with tendinitis, insubstance tears, or fibrosis can be misinterpreted as a complete tear of the rotator cuff.

The pain experienced by the athlete with glenohumeral subluxation usually occurs during the overhead phase of activity, specifically in throwing during the late cocking and acceleration phases. Often the pain is felt proximally along the posterior aspect of the glenohumeral joint and may be mistaken for infraspinatus tendinitis. The "dead-arm" symptoms of weakness, paresis, or paresthesias are usually absent. The shoulder should be evaluated for both an apprehension sign and palpable subluxation. Posterior or multidirectional instability should always be considered in the differential diagnosis.[39]

When anterior instability (subluxation) is present, the relocation test is painful on the posterior joint line until posterior pressure on the humeral head is given to relocate the head and relieve the rotator cuff impingement on the posterior rim, but does not produce a sense of panic or impending dislocation that is usually present in the patient with traumatic dislocation. It is important to always compare the involved with the uninvolved shoulder to differentiate normal laxity from pathologic instability. The relocation test has been very helpful in eliciting the presence of anterior instability and posterior joint line impingement of the rotator cuff. The posteriorly directed force on the proximal humerus relocates the humeral head within the glenoid fossa and reduces or eliminates the athlete's pain. On manual palpation of the shoulder, there may be demonstrable increased humeral head translation in both an anterior and anterior/inferior direction. On occasion, even in the presence of atraumatic subluxation, all or some of these findings may be absent.

What makes the diagnosis of atraumatic glenohumeral subluxation difficult is that the signs of subluxation may be extremely subtle. When the rotator cuff is inflamed, the impingement signs are very obvious and dramatic, and therefore the underlying diagnosis may often be obscured. Plain radiographs should always be evaluated for evidence of instability, such as a bony Bankart lesion, Hill-Sachs lesion, or pathologic subacromial findings. Results of diagnostic tests such as computed axial tomography, MRI scanning, and arthrography often are negative and do not usually help determine the diagnosis. The typical findings seen in the patient with traumatic instability such as a Bankart lesion or labral tear are usually absent in the throwing athlete with atraumatic instability. However, there may be evidence of a stretched anterior capsule. To establish and/or confirm the diagnosis in many cases, an examination under general anesthesia and arthroscopic evaluation may be necessary.

Thus, when evaluating the overhead athlete with shoulder pain, silent atraumatic glenohumeral instability must be ruled out. When instability is present, it should be addressed as a primary lesion; impingement symptoms caused by rotator cuff impingement within the subacromial space or along the posterior rim of the glenoid, and rotator cuff fatigue are treated as a secondary problem. The arthroscope plays an important role in evaluating both the glenohumeral joint and subacromial bursa when the diagnosis is unclear. Anteroinferior labral pathology, rotator cuff fraying, anteroinferior glenohumeral ligament laxity, and enlarged bare spots on the posterior humeral head are the most common pathologic findings. An acromioplasty[8] for chronic subacromial impingement should only be considered after eliminating the diagnosis of instability with secondary internal impingement and confirming the presence of pathologic conditions along the coracoacromial arch. Likewise, the problem could result from excessive thickening of the anterolateral band of the coracoacromial ligament.[4] Such a problem can be both diagnosed and treated arthroscopically.

TREATMENT OF GLENOHUMERAL INSTABILITY

Management of the unstable shoulder is shown in Box 7-2.

BOX 7-2

MANAGEMENT OF THE UNSTABLE SHOULDER

A. Examination
1. Document direction
2. Check for occult subluxation (especially easy to misdiagnose in the athlete)
3. Rule out brachial plexus injury

B. Radiologic Studies
1. Review plain films (including axillary or scapular lateral)
2. Obtain computed arthrography or MRI scan, if necessary, to complement roentgenographic findings

C. Diagnostic Arthroscopy
1. When diagnosis is subtle or unclear
2. Always before performing a reconstruction

D. Treatment
1. Conservative (four phases in progressive rehabilitation program: rest, strengthening, endurance, sport-specific activity)
2. Surgical reconstruction indications:
   a. For patients with recurrent dislocation/subluxation
   b. For patients with failed rehabilitation
   c. In the presence of a complete Bankart lesion
   d. In the presence of a complete rotator cuff tear

Dislocation

Conservative Treatment

Patients with a documented initial dislocation of the glenohumeral joint are usually treated by a closed reduction and immobilization. After reduction of the joint, the arm is immobilized in a sling or shoulder immobilizer for 3 weeks. Ice and appropriate analgesic agents are used to help reduce the initial pain and swelling. The patient should be assessed to determine whether there is any evidence of associated neurovascular or rotator cuff injury associated with the dislocation. Generally a dislocated shoulder should be reduced as soon as possible. Delay in treatment causes increased pain and makes reduction more difficult, secondary to increasing muscle spasm. Force must never be used to reduce the dislocation, since this may cause further problems such as an iatrogenic fracture. Whenever possible, a complete set of radiographs should be obtained before reduction to rule out any associated bony injuries. The extent of anesthesia required to accomplish a reduction depends to some extent on the amount of trauma that produces dislocation, the time since the dislocation, and the presence of an initial vs. a recurrent dislocation. First time dislocations usually cause more soft tissue trauma. A number of closed methods can be used to reduce the glenohumeral joint.[17,26,33,37,44] In each method the same principles are used, including adequate gentle muscle relaxation, avoidance of force, and progressive delivery of the shoulder into a distracted position to allow external rotation to occur. Then internal rotation to reduction is accomplished. After reducing the glenohumeral joint, new x-rays should be obtained to verify the reduction and to evaluate the shoulder for fractures. The patient's neurologic and functional status should be checked again.

The amount of time for postreduction immobilization of the glenohumeral joint has been controversial. McLaughlin[33] reported that prolonged immobilization did not change the incidence of recurrence. In most reported studies 3 weeks has been used for immobilization after an initial dislocation. Various studies have recommended a range of 2 to 5 weeks in young patients and shorter periods of immobilization for patients over the age of 30 because of the lesser predilection for recurrence and greater tendencies for shoulder stiffness in the older group.[44,54,57]

After 3 weeks, the sling is discarded and the patient begins a progressive range-of-motion and strengthening program. The program emphasizes strengthening of the rotator cuff and parascapular musculature. After range of motion and strength are regained, the patient begins specific activities to reproduce the stresses that occur in their activities of daily living, work activities, and athletic endeavors. A strengthening program for as long as 3 months may be required before an athlete with traumatic instability can perform at the preinjury level.

Surgical Treatment

There are a few absolute indications for early surgery in the treatment of anterior glenohumeral dislocation. An open surgical procedure is rarely required at the time of the initial treatment of a dislocation. Surgery as the initial treatment may be required when the joint is irreducible because of soft-tissue interposition such as a torn rotator cuff, capsule, or biceps tendon. Occasionally a fracture of the lesser tuberosity may block or prevent an acceptable anatomic reduction. If this occurs, an open reduction is generally required. Typically, dislocation associated with fractures around the glenohumeral joint can be reduced closed with subsequent fracture management as necessary.

There are indications for performing an early reconstruction of the glenohumeral joint after an initial dislocation and closed reduction. The relative indication for an early reconstructive procedure involves patients whose activities require an absolutely stable joint and patients who are expected to have recurrent instability of the glenohumeral joint, such as an overhead athlete. The patient's age at the time of the initial dislocation has a major effect on the incidence of redislocation. McLaughlin[33] observed that 95% of 181 primary traumatic dislocations in teenagers recurred. Patients who are younger than age 20 experience recurrent instability between 80% and 92% of the time according to Rowe[45] and McLaughlin.[33] However, the incidence of recurrent instability for patients who are older than 40 years of age drops sharply to between 10% and 15%.[31] Matsen[30] noted that injuries sustained by young patients with traumatic dislocations are unlikely to yield a stable shoulder. This is secondary to inappropriate healing of the avulsed glenohumeral ligaments from the anterior glenoid rim. With this in mind, early surgery should be considered for patients who require absolute stability of the glenohumeral joint for their occupations, such as people involved in vigorous, overhead labor activity or young, competitive, overhead athletes.

Baker's[2] study evaluated arthroscopic findings after acute dislocation of the shoulder. The largest group in this study was shown to be grossly unstable under anesthesia with the complete disruption and separation of the glenohumeral ligament and labrum (Bankart lesion). In Baker's report,[2] 11 of 12 unoperated patients were reevaluated after an average of 3 years. Of those 11, 7 patients went on to have recurrent dislocation or subluxation of the shoulder. Of 16 patients who underwent a surgical repair, 13 were reevaluated and one had a subsequent subluxation or dislocation. These results were similar to those of Wheeler[55] in an evaluation of West Point cadets who had a 22% redislocation rate in those treated with arthroscopic surgery in comparison to a 92% redislocation rate in those treated nonoperatively.

Young, competitive athletes who require the use of their shoulder for overhead activities and athletes involved in contact sports should be considered for early surgery. These athletes should have a closed reduction and be treated conservatively to allow swelling and capsular irritation to subside before surgery. If a diagnostic arthroscopy reveals a complete Bankart lesion, a reconstruction is recommended. Athletes should be allowed to complete a current season, provided they respond to a conservative program and do not have further clinical episodes of instability. At the end of the season, patients with any residual instability findings should undergo diagnostic arthroscopy, and those who are found to have a residual unhealed complete displacement of their capsulolabral complex (Bankart lesion) need to have the Bankart lesions repaired. An open reconstruction should be performed, since the proven success rate is higher and more predictable than the success rate for patients who have been treated with arthroscopic repair. In the future, as arthroscopic fixation techniques improve, allowing for a more stable repair and early motion, arthroscopy may become the standard form of treatment after an acute initial anterior shoulder dislocation. At this time, however, arthroscopic stabilization is not the procedure of choice.

Patients who have a history of recurrent traumatic instability of the shoulder and who did not have early surgery often progress to the point that a dislocation or subluxation results from trivial trauma or by merely placing the arm in a position that places stress on the anterior capsule. The problem does not respond to an exercise program; surgical reconstruction is required to stabilize the joint and prevent progressive arthrosis secondary to repeated traumatic instability. Before proceeding with the surgical reconstruction, the patient must complete a thorough evaluation to ascertain the direction of instability, whether a multidirectional component also exists, and whether there is possibly a psychiatric component.

Protective devices have not proved helpful upon resumption of athletics in the overhead population because these devices are too restrictive to allow adequate athletic function. Restrictive protective devices provide a limited role for patients involved in activities where overhead reaching is required. These recommendations are logical in young, vigorous, competitive athletes because the recommendations allow these athletes to return to their sport and help prevent them from missing an additional season. This is a limited group, however, and in the general, nonathletic population the patient is more likely to be treated conservatively until they have demonstrated evidence of either a recurrent subluxation or a dislocation.

Subluxation

Conservative Treatment

In athletes who have recurrent subluxation[9] the initial treatment is a systematic conservative program after a comprehensive evaluation. This approach allows most athletes to avoid reconstructive surgery.[23] These athletes should be placed on a rehabilitation program that is divided into the following four phases: rest from their sport, strengthening program, endurance program, and sport-specific program. During the initial treatment, the athlete must not participate in the offending activity to allow an inflamed and stretched capsule to calm down and to reduce the inflammation of the rotator cuff muscles. A comprehensive discussion of the conservative treatment can be found in Chapter 7F. The majority of athletes (as many as 95%) can return to their prior level of competition with a conservative program and without surgery. This depends on an early diagnosis before progressive anatomic changes occur to the glenohumeral ligaments. When this treatment fails, surgery is necessary.

Historical Review of Surgical Treatment

For athletes who do not respond to a well-managed and supervised rehabilitation program, surgical reconstruction may be required. The indications for surgical reconstruction in the athlete with atraumatic instability include failure of a rehabilitation program and the desire to return to overhead athletics, but an inability to do so without surgery. Rare cases of atraumatic instability with a complete Bankart lesion and/or complete tear of the rotator cuff should also be considered for surgical reconstruction, even before attempting a rehabilitation program. If a complete rotator cuff tear is found in the process of evaluating the patient or at the time of the patient's diagnostic arthroscopy, it must be addressed at surgery.

Historical Procedures

Many procedures have been developed to correct glenohumeral instability. The total overall success of surgical stabilization in preventing further occurrences of instability has been high (greater than 90% for anterior instability and 60% to 80% for posterior instability). The lower rate for posterior instability repair reflects the fact that the capsular tissue available for repair is relatively thin and often attenuated.

The overall success with surgical stabilization, including allowing athletes to play again at a competitive level, has been less satisfactory.

Bristow Procedure

For many years the Bristow procedure was considered the procedure of choice. As previously noted, Lombardo[27] demonstrated excellent results for traumatic anterior dislocations but greater unpredictability for those with recurrent subluxation and loss of the functional ability to return to competitive throwing sports. The Bristow procedure has also been criticized because of the potential complications from screw migration and breakage, nonunion of the transferred coracoid, and the distortion of the normal anatomy that makes a revision procedure technically more difficult with increased risk to the underlying neurovascular structures. In addition, the Bristow procedure does not allow for treatment of capsular laxity, which is often found to be a component of those who have a subluxing joint from overhead activity.

Bankart Procedure

The Bankart procedure[3,46] has been recommended by many surgeons for the treatment of instability in the athlete with the goal of obtaining an anatomic repair. In the Bankart procedure, shoulder stability is restored by securing the avulsed anterior capsule back to the anterior rim of the glenoid fossa using sutures through drill holes. The Bankart procedure may be combined with a capsular shift (Figs. 7-31 and 7-32) in patients who have both anterior and inferior instability or multidirectional instability with anterior predominance. The classic Bankart procedure requires detachment of the subscapularis muscle (Fig. 7-33) for exposure and reattachment of the subscapularis muscle at the completion of the procedure. This carries the potential for shortening of the subscapularis and an ultimate loss of external rotation,

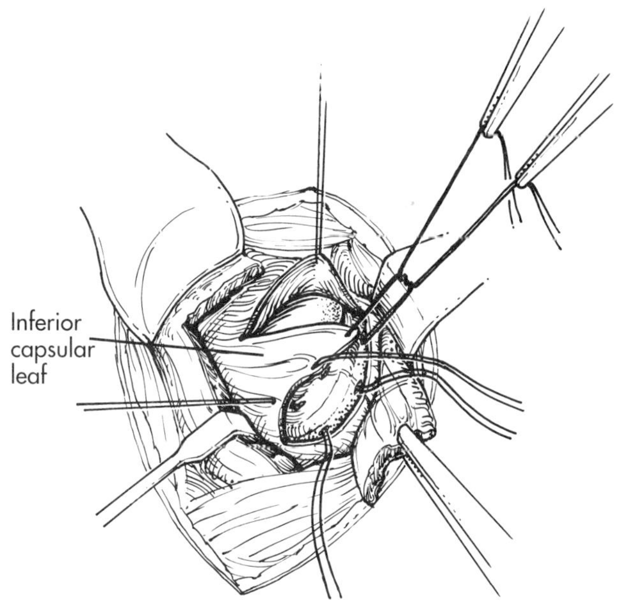

FIGURE 7-31 Bankart repair of the anterior capsule with a capsular shift.

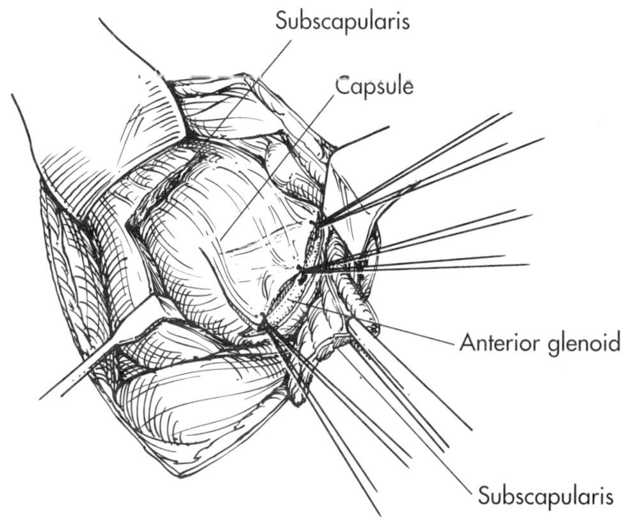

FIGURE 7-32 Completed Bankart repair with a capsular shift.

which may compromise the athlete's ability to return to overhead sports. In addition, to protect the repair of the subscapularis at the completion of the procedure, the range of motion must be limited, including the passive external rotation and active internal rotation of the shoulder, for 4 to 6 weeks. Failure of the subscapularis repair, although rare, is a devastating complication that not only diminishes shoulder function but often causes an excellent reconstruction to fail because of lack of the dynamic stabilization provided by the subscapularis.

The Bankart procedure is designed to restore the

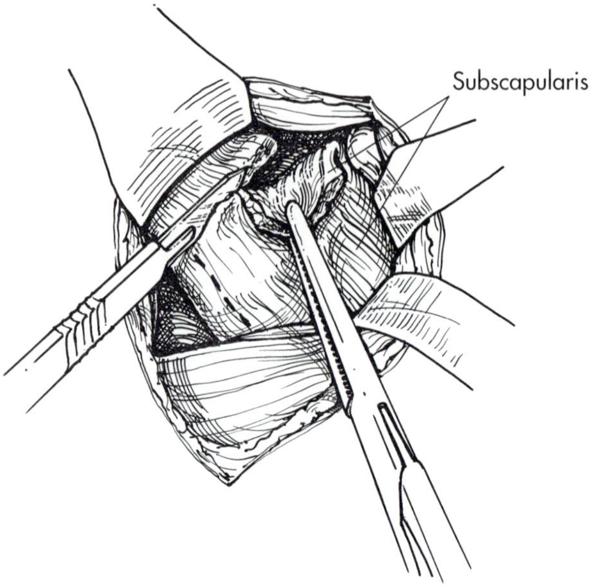

FIGURE 7-33 Detachment of the subscapularis tendon and muscle.

pathologic anatomy to a near-normal anatomic location and works well with the nonthrowing population. Unfortunately, this procedure does not restore the normal capsular labral complex to the glenoid rim, rather the joint is entered through a vertical incision 0.5 cm lateral to the glenoid rim. After preparation of the glenoid neck and placement of drill holes, the lateral capsule is repaired to the prepared glenoid rim. This accomplishes a repair of the capsule to the glenoid rim but ultimately shortens the capsule by 1 cm and, in addition, does not restore the labrum and its immediate adjacent capsule to the glenoid rim. A stable joint is created, but losing 1 cm of the capsule creates a loss of external rotation, which may be further compromised by shortening of the subscapularis tendon after its repair.

SURGICAL TREATMENT: THE ANTERIOR CAPSULOLABRAL RECONSTRUCTION

The anterior capsule labral reconstruction (ACLR) forms a new capsulolabral complex by imbricating the capsule and the inferior glenohumeral ligament through sutures and bone anchors placed into the anterior glenoid rim.[19-21] This is performed without detaching, shortening, or transferring any muscle. The shoulder is mobilized immediately within a "safe" zone determined during surgery and is splinted in abduction and external rotation. Rehabilitation begins the day after surgery. This hastens the return to functional motion and shortens the rehabilitation time.

Two reviews of the anterior capsular reconstruction[20,21] have demonstrated the improved success rate in allowing overhead athletes to return to their previous level of competition.

Indications

Sometimes an examination under general anesthesia and an arthroscopic evaluation are necessary to confirm the diagnosis of instability (see Chapter 7B), especially when secondary rotator cuff tendinitis is present.[10,11] What makes the diagnosis difficult is the subtleness of the signs of subluxation. With secondary rotator cuff tendinitis and fraying, the signs of impingement are more obvious and dramatic, often obscuring the diagnosis of instability. Overhead athletes who show signs of instability and impingement have instability as their primary problem and underlying rotator cuff tendinitis as a secondary problem. Those who have been treated for an impingement syndrome, without the instability having been addressed, continue to have symptoms. As a result, the instablity must be addressed first. This usually eliminates the impingement symptoms without further treatment. Such an evaluation is usually followed immediately by the definitive surgery for instability in those cases that fail a conservative trial of rehabilitation. If there is significant inferior instability, closure of the rotator interval is very helpful and may be combined with the ACLR. Two sutures are usually enough to close the interval.

Procedure

Positioning

The patient is placed in the supine position at the edge of the operating table with two folded towels beneath the scapula for stabilization. The arm is centered on and supported by an arm board. The involved extremity is draped free to allow for control of shoulder motion and arm position during the procedure. Fig. 7-34 shows the instruments that are required for the procedure to be performed.

Approach

An axillary incision is made beginning 2 to 3 cm distal and lateral to the coracoid process and extending distally into the anterior axillary crease in the skin line. The skin is undermined to provide access to the deltopectoral groove. This allows visualization of the deltoid muscle, the pectoralis muscle, and the deltopectoral groove (Fig. 7-35). Occasionally, it is difficult to determine the location of the deltopectoral groove. Dissection toward the coracoid process in a superomedial direction under the medial skin flap allows better delineation of this interval. Located within the interval is the cephalic vein, which is reflected laterally to avoid the many tributaries that drain the deltoid muscle. The deltopectoral interval is then developed with blunt and sharp dissection by undermining and retracting the deltoid muscle and cephalic vein laterally and the pectoralis muscle medially. Modified Goelet retractors are used to expose the clavipectoral fascia, conjoined tendon, and coracoid process.

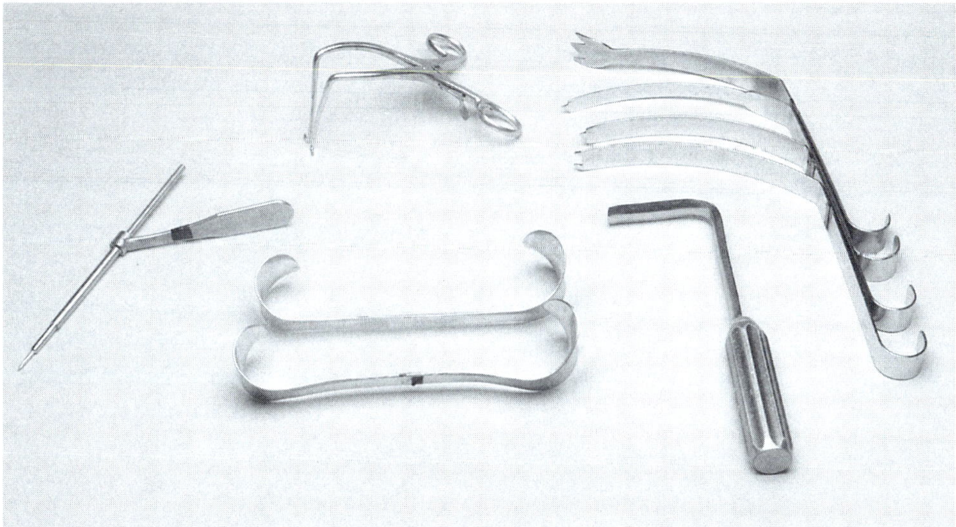

FIGURE 7-34 Surgical instruments for the anterior capsulolabral reconstruction.

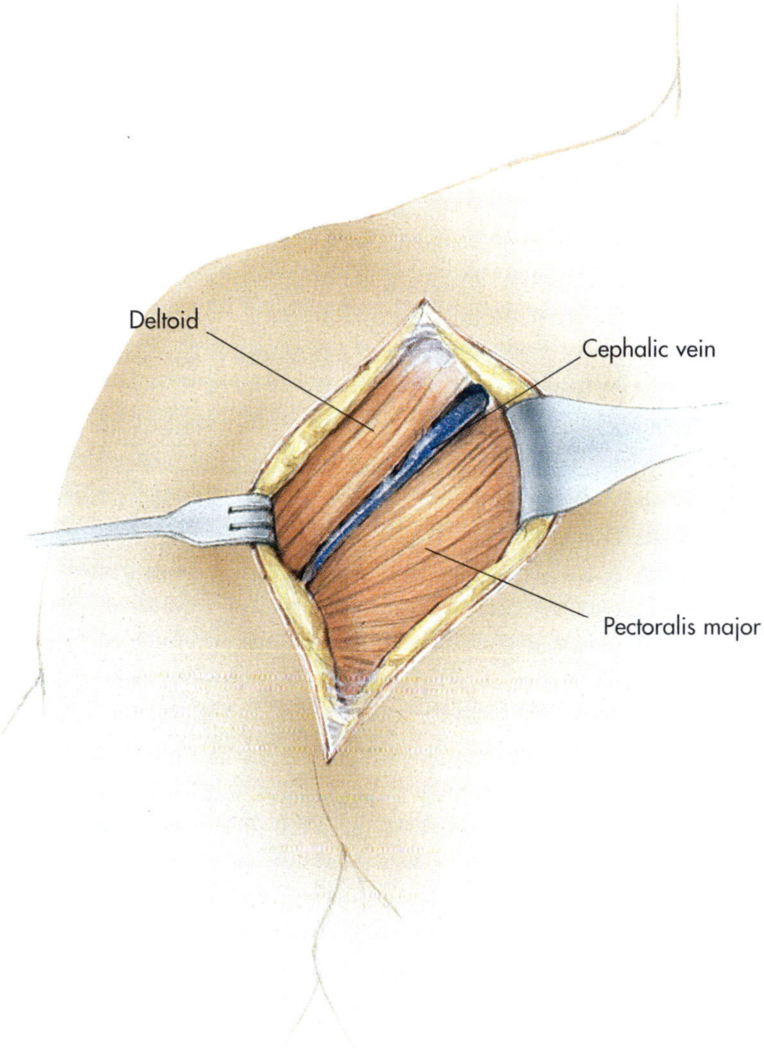

FIGURE 7-35 Deltopectoral interval exposure.

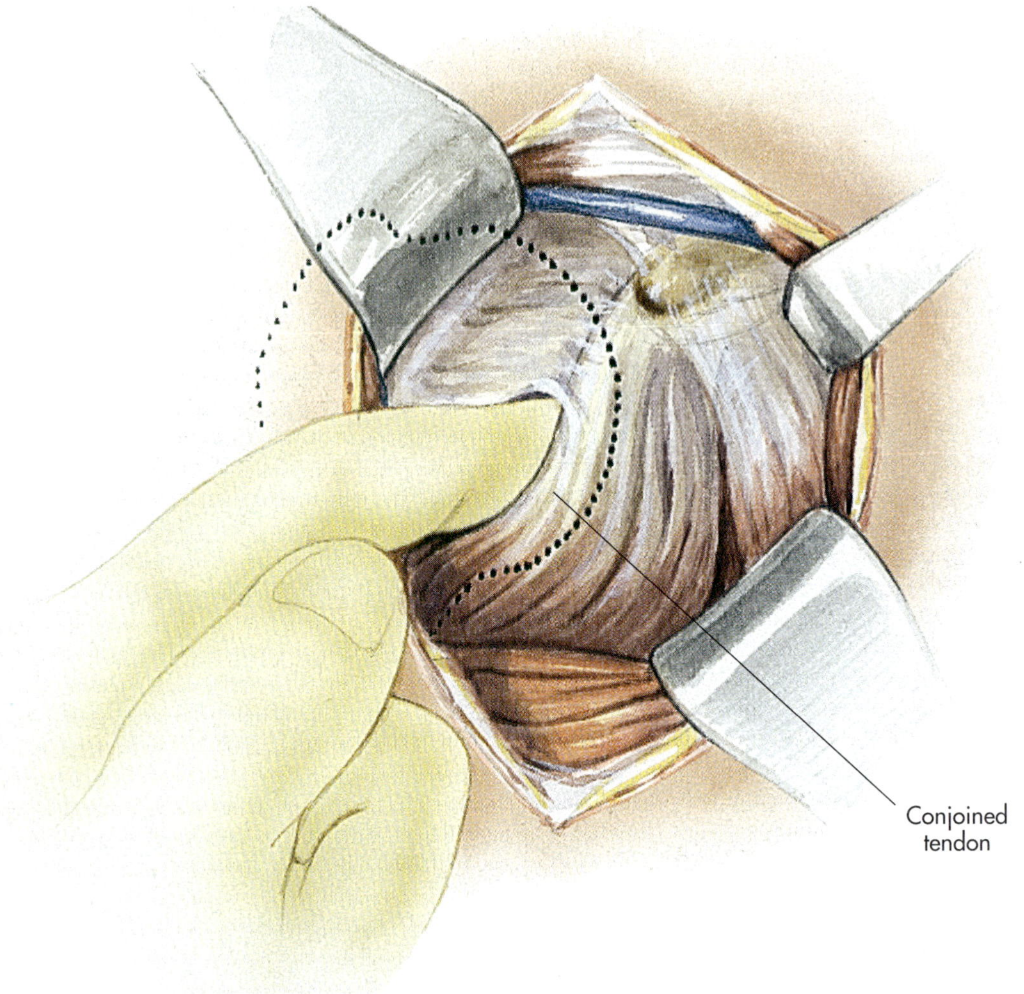

FIGURE 7-36 Retraction of the conjoined tendon.

Medial Retraction of the Conjoined Tendon

The clavipectoral fascia is incised along the lateral margin of the conjoined tendon, beginning at the level of the inferior margin of the humeral head and extending proximally to the coracoid process (Fig 7-36). Careful attention is needed to ensure that the dissection begins lateral to the fleshy portion of the coracobrachialis muscle, rather than medially at the lateral border of the tendinous short head of the biceps muscle. The conjoined tendon must be retracted as a single unit to allow visualization of the subscapularis muscle. Blunt dissection is used to undermine and free the conjoined tendon, which is retracted medially with a long, narrow right-angle retractor.

Division and Dissection of the Subscapularis Muscle

The subscapularis muscle and tendon are brought into view by externally rotating the arm. Careful palpation delineates the bicipital groove, the lesser tuberosity, and the superior and inferior borders of the subscapularis muscle. The subscapularis tendon and muscle are then split longitudinally (Fig. 7-37, *A*) along the course of their fibers using a needle-point bovie, and the capsule and tendon are separated (Fig. 7-37, *B*). The tendon split is made between the lower third and upper two thirds of the subscapularis tendon but not so deep as to penetrate the capsule. The interval between the subscapularis and capsule is easily identified if the dissection under the subscapularis is begun medially within the muscular portion. When the interval has been identified, the capsular exposure is extended laterally with sharp and blunt dissection, and then medially with blunt dissection. A modified Gelpi retractor is used to retract the split subscapularis tendon laterally, and a Goelet retractor is then placed between the two prongs of the Gelpi retractor to retract the deltoid laterally. A three-pronged pitchfork retractor is placed on the anterior glenoid neck to retract and separate the subscapularis muscle medially. Care

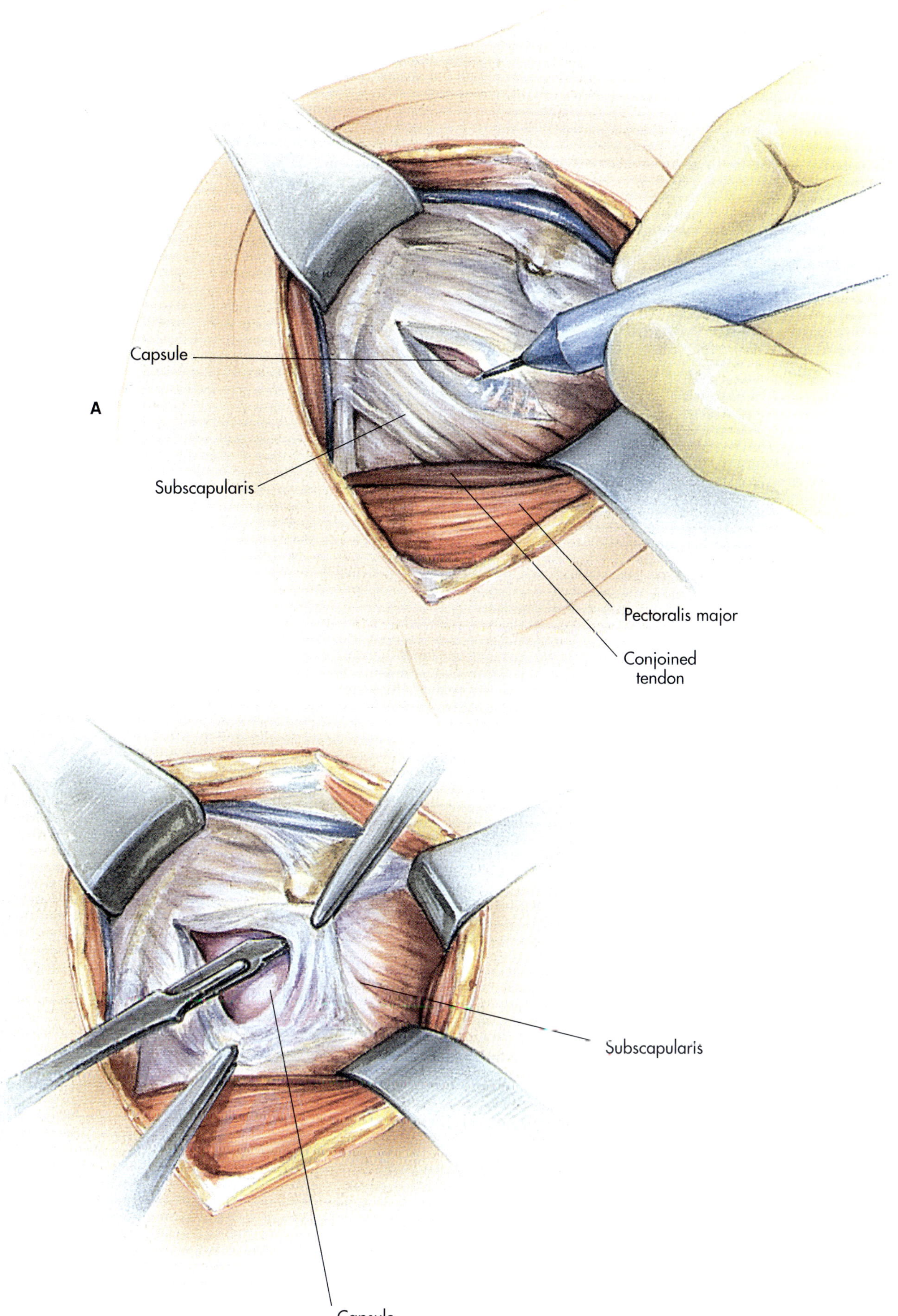

FIGURE 7-37 **A,** Division of the subscapularis tendon and muscle, **B,** Separation of capsule and tendon.

must be taken when placing the pitchfork retractor; it must be placed, under direct vision, lateral to the conjoined tendon and between the inferior and superior subscapularis muscle bellies to avoid injury to neurovascular structures. After the pitchfork retractor is seated on the scapular neck, the long, narrow Richardson retractor can be removed along with the medial Goelet retractor.

Division of the Anterior Capsule

The capsule is held with a long tissue forceps to avoid scoring the humeral head. Using a long-handled #15 blade, the surgeon incises the capsule (Fig. 7-38) longitudinally and parallel to the division of the subscapularis tendon, beginning laterally and extending medially down to but not through the anterior labrum. Tag sutures are placed at the capsule margin just lateral to the labrum.

Before the capsule is divided, the capsule and the glenoid rim are palpated. When there is a large redundant capsule, it is easy to misdirect the capsular incision as one proceeds from the lateral to medial aspect. If the capsular incision is not placed appropriately, it tends to drift either too far inferiorly or superiorly rather than being completed along the midanterior glenoid rim at about the 4 o'clock position. It is important not to violate the anterior labrum during the capsulotomy. Exposure may be facilitated by inserting a single-prong narrow humeral head retractor between the humeral head and the posterior rim of the glenoid. This allows the humeral head to be displaced laterally, yielding increased exposure of the glenoid, the anterior capsule, and the anterior labrum. The synovial layer is cut, and the fibrous layer is subperiosteally elevated (Fig. 7-39). The capsulotomy may be completed down to the level of the glenoid labrum, and at this time the joint may be inspected along with palpation of the glenoid articular surface, glenoid labrum, and capsule. At this point the small retractor can be replaced by the larger two-prong humeral head retractor. With both the subscapularis pitchfork and the humeral head retractor in place, the retraction can be balanced between the two instruments to increase the exposure and facilitate the decision-making process before proceeding with the reconstruction.

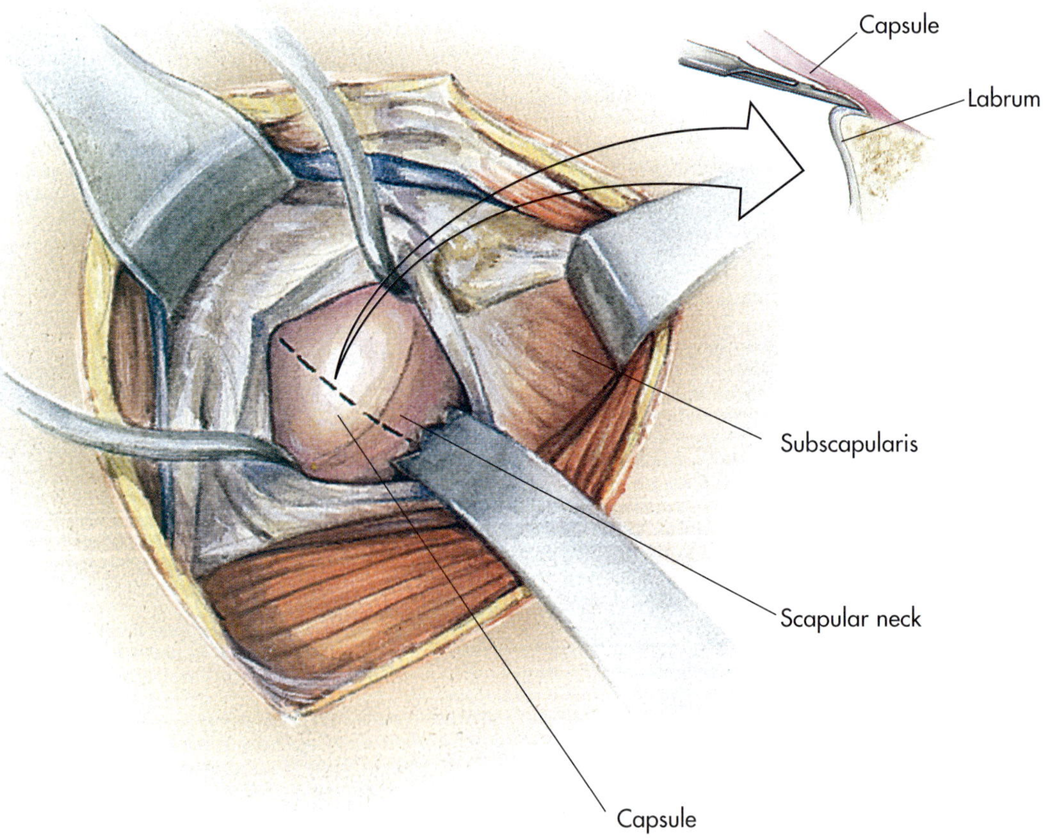

FIGURE 7-38 Anterior capsule incision.

Decision Making: Addressing the Capsular and Labral Pathology

At this point the surgeon is required to make a decision based on the patient's history, findings on physical examination, and operative findings. The surgeon must decide the degree of capsular redundancy present and the need for capsular shift. In addition, the surgeon must determine the presence or absence of a Bankart lesion.

It is common for the athlete who has had isolated traumatic events in the absence of chronic microrepetitive trauma to have an isolated, complete Bankart lesion without significant capsular laxity. In this case the Bankart lesion itself may be repaired without performing a capsular shift. The Bankart lesion may subsequently be repaired through the exposure gained by the longitudinal capsulotomy. This allows the Bankart lesion to be repaired anatomically, preserving the underlying labrum if it is not damaged, and without shortening the capsule to effect a repair to bone. When a complete Bankart lesion is observed at the patient's diagnostic arthroscopy, repairing the lesion must become a part of the surgical plan. If the labrum is severely damaged and altered anatomically, it may be removed. In chronic cases the labrum may be absent and the avulsed capsule is repaired directly. Even in the presence of an excellent capsular shift performed laterally at the humeral head, one of the most common causes of reconstructive failures has been well documented to be the presence of an unrepaired Bankart lesion.[30,36,47,48]

At the time of the patient's diagnostic arthroscopy, the integrity of the glenohumeral ligaments is evaluated. The importance of evaluating the ligaments in the patient with atraumatic instability has been emphasized, but the physician should also realize that the patient with traumatic instability and the presence of the Bankart lesion may have pathologic laxity and attenuation of the glenohumeral ligaments and capsule as well. In the presence of significant capsular laxity, repairing the Bankart lesion alone will not yield a stable joint, and problems of subluxation will continue.

When the longitudinal capsulotomy has been completed and the joint has been exposed, the glenoid labrum and capsule should be reevaluated to confirm the impressions gained at the examination under general anesthesia and the arthroscopic evaluation. The glenoid labrum should be carefully palpated with a small probe to determine the presence or absence of a Bankart lesion that may not have been appreciated at the time of arthroscopy. The capsule must be palpated for its integrity, volume, and ability to tighten and buttress the anterior inferior joint margin during external rotation of the arm. At this time the surgeon decides the amount of the capsular shift. The operation may be tailored to the patient's degree of laxity.

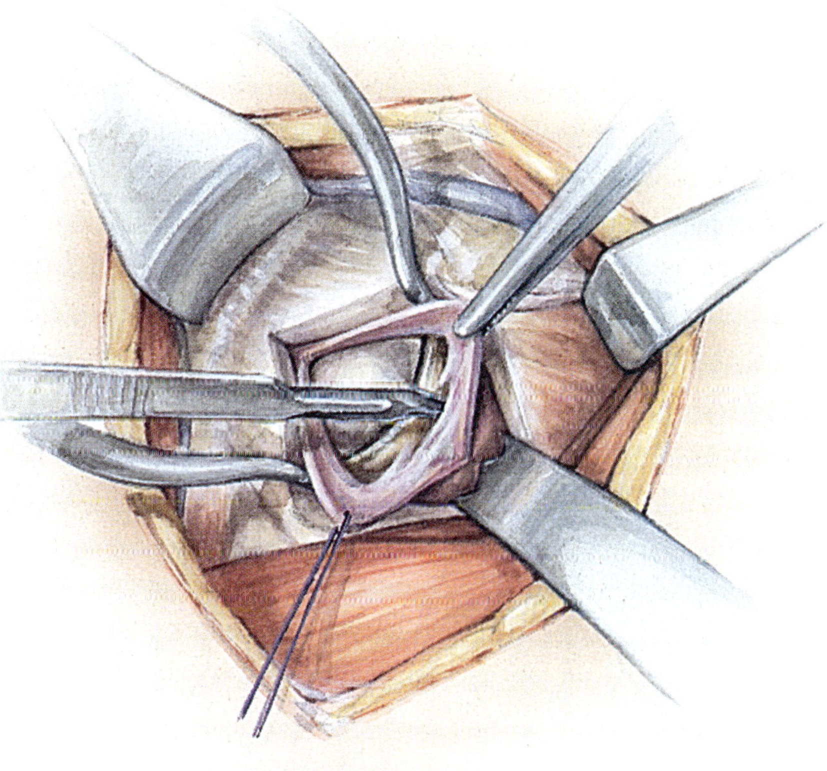

FIGURE 7-39 Exposure of the glenohumeral joint.

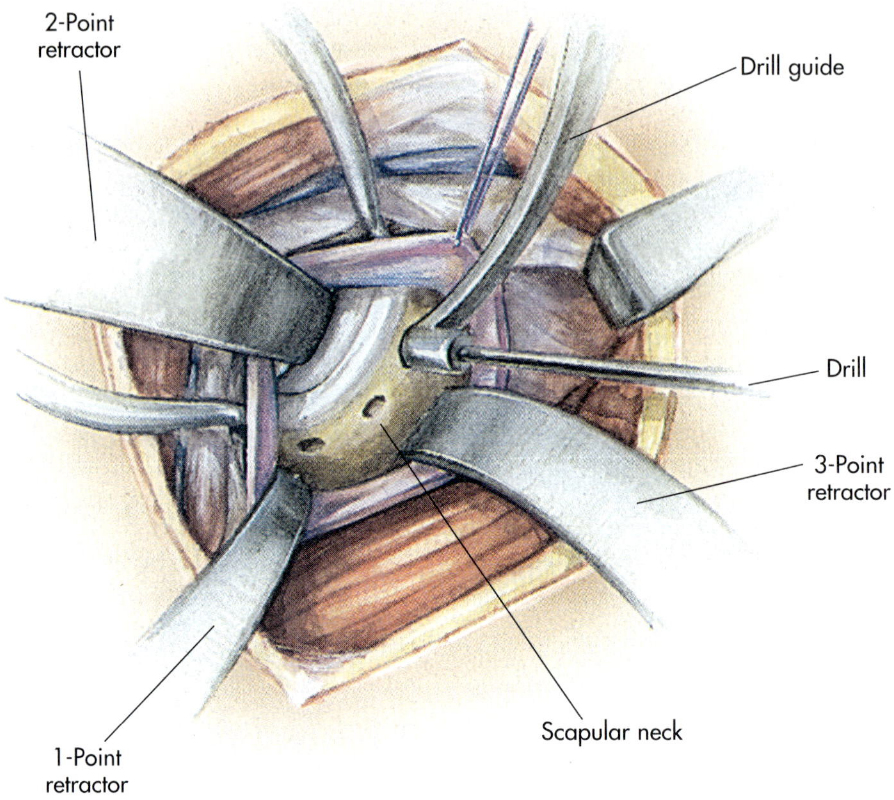

FIGURE 7-40 Drilling of the suture anchor holes.

Treatment of a Bankart Lesion

If a Bankart lesion (detachment of the anterior labrum and capsule) is present, the undersurface of the labrum should be roughened to promote healing of the labrum. The soft tissue and periosteum underneath and medial to the avulsed labrum and capsule is stripped to expose the bony anterior scapular neck. A curette and power burr may be used to abrade the anterior scapular neck and glenoid rim to provide a healing surface for fixation of the Bankart lesion.

The Bankart lesion is repaired by suture fixation to the prepared anterior scapular neck. This may be performed with the use of a curved spike-awl, as described by Rowe,[46] or by using a right-angle drill.[20] The holes along the anterior glenoid rim are usually placed at 3, 4, and 5 o'clock positions for the right shoulder (Fig. 7-40) and 9, 8, and 7 o'clock positions for the left shoulder. The preferred technique at this time for suture placement employs bony anchors* (Fig. 7-41). The bone anchor allows for accurate placement of the sutures along the anterior scapular neck even in the presence of a significant glenoid deficiency. An additional significant advantage of the bone anchor is the fact that the articular cartilage, along with anterior glenoid, does not have to be violated, as required with the use of standard Bankart instruments. The only disadvantage to using the bone anchor is the need for placement of a small metallic fixation device within the cancellous bone of the glenoid neck.

The #2 nonabsorbable suture should be used to reattach the avulsed labrum and capsule anatomically to the prepared scapular neck. By reattaching the labrum and medial capsule anatomically to the scapular neck, capsular shortening is avoided, and the potential for lost range of motion is minimized. The humeral head retractor is then removed, and the lateral portion of the capsule can be closed anatomically or with minimal overlap.

Treatment of Capsular Laxity

After the joint has been exposed and the initial longitudinal capsulotomy performed, the capsule is inspected and palpated. At this point the capsule is confirmed as being lax or incompetent, thereby determining the decision to perform the capsular shift. In patients with microrepetitive atraumatic instability, the findings of capsu-

*Mitek Surgical Anchor Products, Norwood, MA.

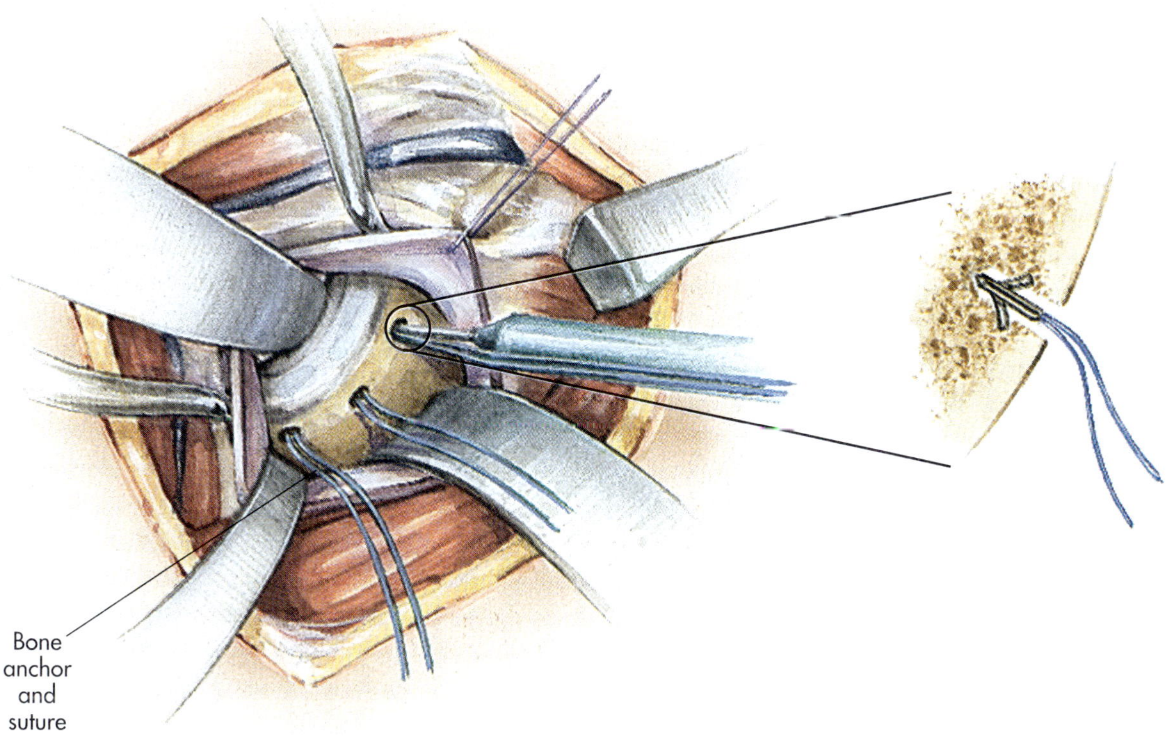

FIGURE 7-41 Placement of the suture anchor.

lar laxity are typical in the absence of a Bankart lesion. The capsule must then be overlapped to obliterate the redundancy and allow the return of external rotation that is required for athletic function at the same time. This is accomplished by incising the capsule down onto the labrum and medial glenoid neck for subperiosteal elevation. This obviates a need for capsular shortening during its repair. Tag sutures have been placed at the margin of the capsulotomy just lateral to the labrum for easy identification.

At this time, exposure is facilitated by inserting a single-prong, narrow humeral head retractor. The humeral head retractor should be placed so the small, single prong is behind the inferior glenoid rim. Inferiorly, the axillary nerve is protected by using this retractor.

The inferior leaf of the capsular tissue contains most of the inferior glenohumeral ligament. This portion of the capsule is used to reconstruct the inferior ligament by advancing the tissue along the anterior glenoid rim and shifting it proximally. This technique also reinforces and adds to the anterior buttress and density of the labrum. The superior leaf of the capsule will later be brought distally over the inferior leaf and labrum, and then it will rest along the anterior scapular neck. The capsular repair is maintained by #2 nonabsorbable sutures from the anterior glenoid bone anchors (e.g., Mitek bone anchor).

Before the sutures are placed in the capsule, the capsule is advanced along the anterior glenoid rim and labrum in a superior direction again, avoiding any medial shortening of the capsule. The location of the capsule as it corresponds to the three previously placed sutures is noted to mark the location for a proper placement of the sutures in the inferior capsular leaf (Fig. 7-42). Beginning with the inferior suture, the sutures are brought through the medial edge of the capsule in the previously marked position with careful attention to protect the axillary nerve inferiorly with the use of the small single-point retractor. The sutures are always brought through capsular tissues under direct visualization. After the sutures have been placed, the repair should be tested by pulling tightly on the suture and noting the position of the capsule. The inferior capsular leaf should be noted to have been drawn superiorly, along the anterior rim of the glenoid, without moving the capsule medially along the scapular neck. The sutures are then tied, but not cut, because they will be used to anchor the superior capsular flap.

The superior capsular leaf is pulled over the inferior capsule repair (Fig. 7-43). As in the preparation of the inferior capsule, the location of the superior capsule and its relative position to the sutures are noted, and careful attention is paid to avoid moving the capsule medially as the sutures are brought through its substance. The

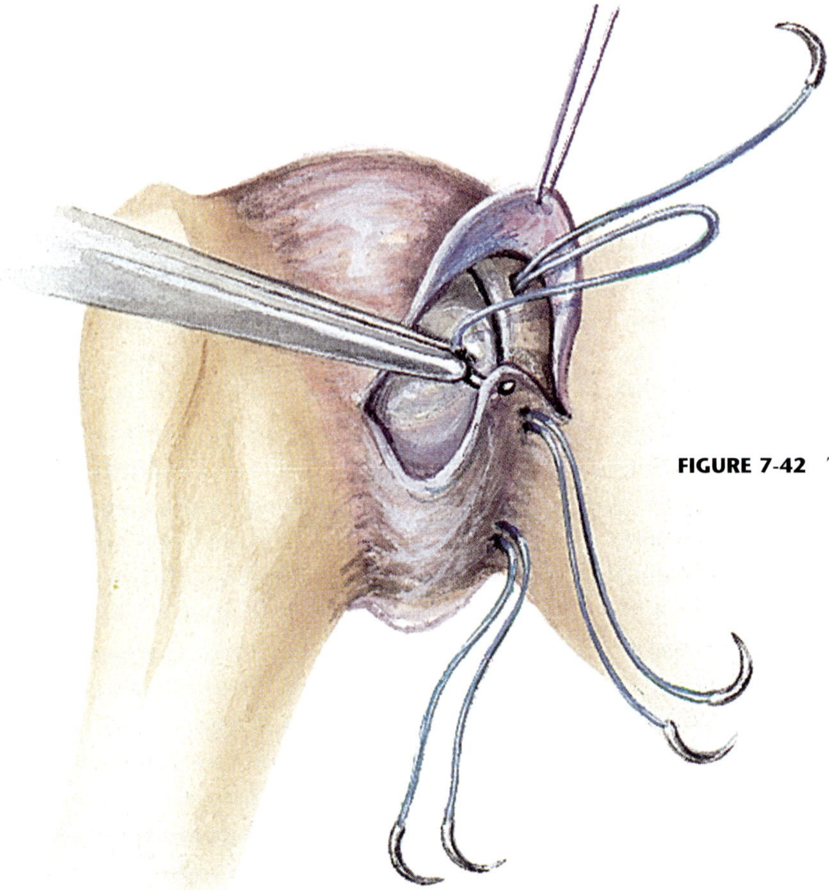

FIGURE 7-42 The inferior leaf is secured superiorly.

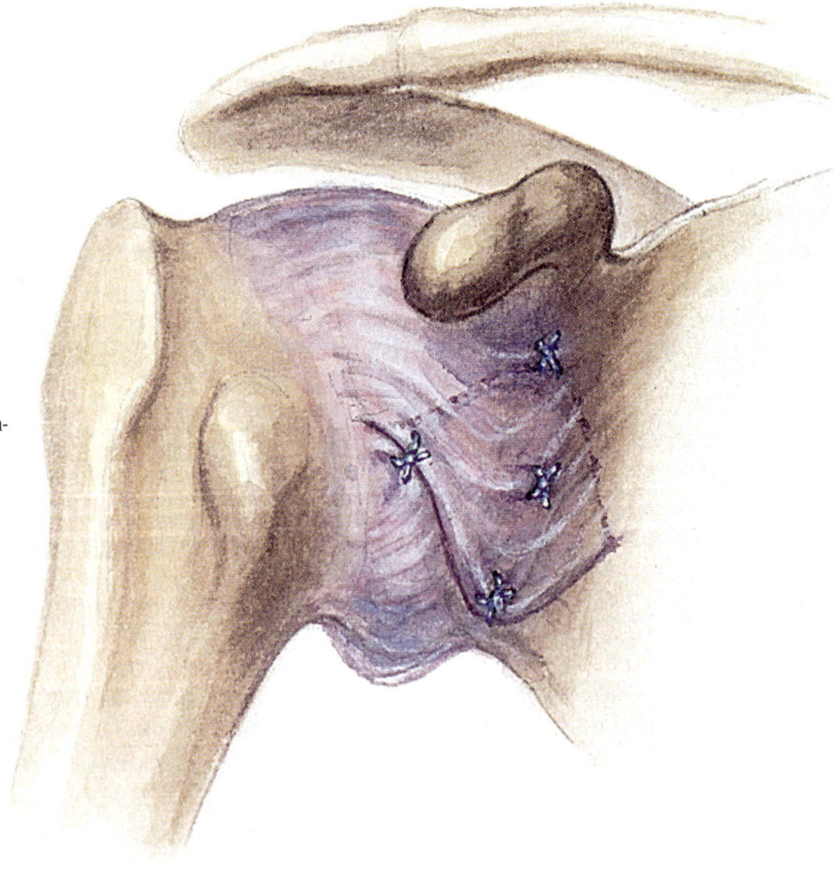

FIGURE 7-43 The superior leaf is secured inferiorly.

humeral head retractor is then removed and the shoulder is brought through a range of motion to ensure that the repair of the superior capsule has not compromised the postoperative safe zone for range of motion. The sutures are tied and cut. The lateral expansion of the capsule is then repaired by bringing the superior capsule loosely over the inferior capsule with a vest-over-pants technique using nonabsorbable suture.

Treatment of a Combined Bankart Lesion and Capsular Laxity

Because of the multitude of instability episodes, there may be distortion of the anatomy, including absence of the anterior glenoid labrum and/or a defect in the anterior glenoid rim. In the presence of a Bankart lesion (capsular avulsion from the anterior glenoid rim) or in the absence of the glenoid labrum, the repair is performed by securing the capsule to a prepared anterior scapular neck. Typically the capsule has become redundant, which necessitates not only a reattachment of the capsule to the scapular neck, but also a capsular shift. When performing a capsular shift in the absence of a labrum, the surgeon must ensure that the capsular shift reduces the anteroinferior capsular recess without excessively moving the capsule medially and losing postoperative range of motion.

Safe Zone Range of Motion Test

On completion of the capsular closure, the arm is taken through a range of motion to determine the point where tension is placed on the repair. The patient may move within this safe zone after surgery without jeopardizing the reconstruction. This allows the athlete to begin an early range-of-motion program and avoid the complications of adhesions, capsular contraction, and atrophy, but at the same time protect the repair. This safe zone usually allows abduction above 90° in the scapular plane and external rotation beyond 45° before tension is placed along the repair. If at the completion of the procedure, an adequate safe zone is not allowed, the repair should be taken down and the sutures replaced. Usually when an adequate safe zone is not possible, it is because the sutures have been placed too lateral within the capsular flaps ultimately moving those capsular repairs medially or because the overflap is too tight.

Closure and Reapproximation of Subscapularis Muscle

After completion of the capsular repair and observation of the safe zone, the Gelpi and pitchfork retractors are removed and replaced by a Goelet retractor laterally and a long Richardson retractor medially. The subscapularis is then reapproximated with several interrupted #0 absorbable sutures (Fig. 7-44). All retractors are then removed after a thorough irrigation of the operative field. The deltoid and pectoralis muscles fall into place and typically do not require suture reapproximation. The skin is closed in a subcuticular manner, sterile adhesive strips (Steri-Strips) are applied, and then a sterile dressing is applied.

The arm may then be placed in an adjustable orthotic device that splints the arm in abduction and external rotation, but the arm is removed for postoperative range of motion and bathing. The purpose of the splint is to prevent contraction of the capsule and loss of range of motion. In patients who have generalized ligament laxity, a shoulder abduction pillow at 45° is used because range of motion has been easy to gain. Patients with global multidirectional instability and generalized soft-tissue laxity do not require an abduction splint because their tissues stretch easily and they are able to regain postoperative range of motion.

SURGICAL TREATMENT: ARTHROSCOPY

The techniques for arthroscopic stabilization[29,31,53,56] continue to improve as does the success, provided that the patient population is carefully selected. Many authors have recommended against the use of arthroscopic stabilization in the athlete involved in collision sports because of an increased recurrence rate.[25,42] Most published reports concerning arthroscopic stabilization have recommended that the procedure not be performed in patients with capsular laxity in the absence of a Bankart lesion. The results to date for arthroscopic reconstruction in the face of atraumatic instability have been poor, and arthroscopic reconstruction is not recommended in the overhead athlete with atraumatic instability.[25,31,34]

Two recent arthroscopic surgical techniques[53,56] have enjoyed an early success rate but lack long-term follow-up and have only been applied to a carefully selected patient population with a clean Bankart lesion in the absence of significant capsular laxity. The suture anchor technique[56] uses arthroscopically placed sutures to transfix a Bankart lesion and an arthroscopically placed Mitek bone anchor. Early results of this procedure in 20 patients demonstrated no complications and no recurrences of instability. The arthroscopic Bankart repair using a cannulated absorbable fixation device[53] uses an absorbable tack of polyglyconate, which is absorbed over 6 weeks. The overall recurrence rate of instability using this procedure in 26 patients has been 8%. Both of these procedures require postoperative immobilization for 3 to 4 weeks.

Unfortunately, the success rate of arthroscopic reconstruction to date has not matched the success rate for open procedures, especially in the athletic population. The duration of postoperative immobilization is greater in the arthroscopic technique than in the open technique. Undoubtedly, as arthroscopic techniques continue to develop with improved fixation in conjunction with

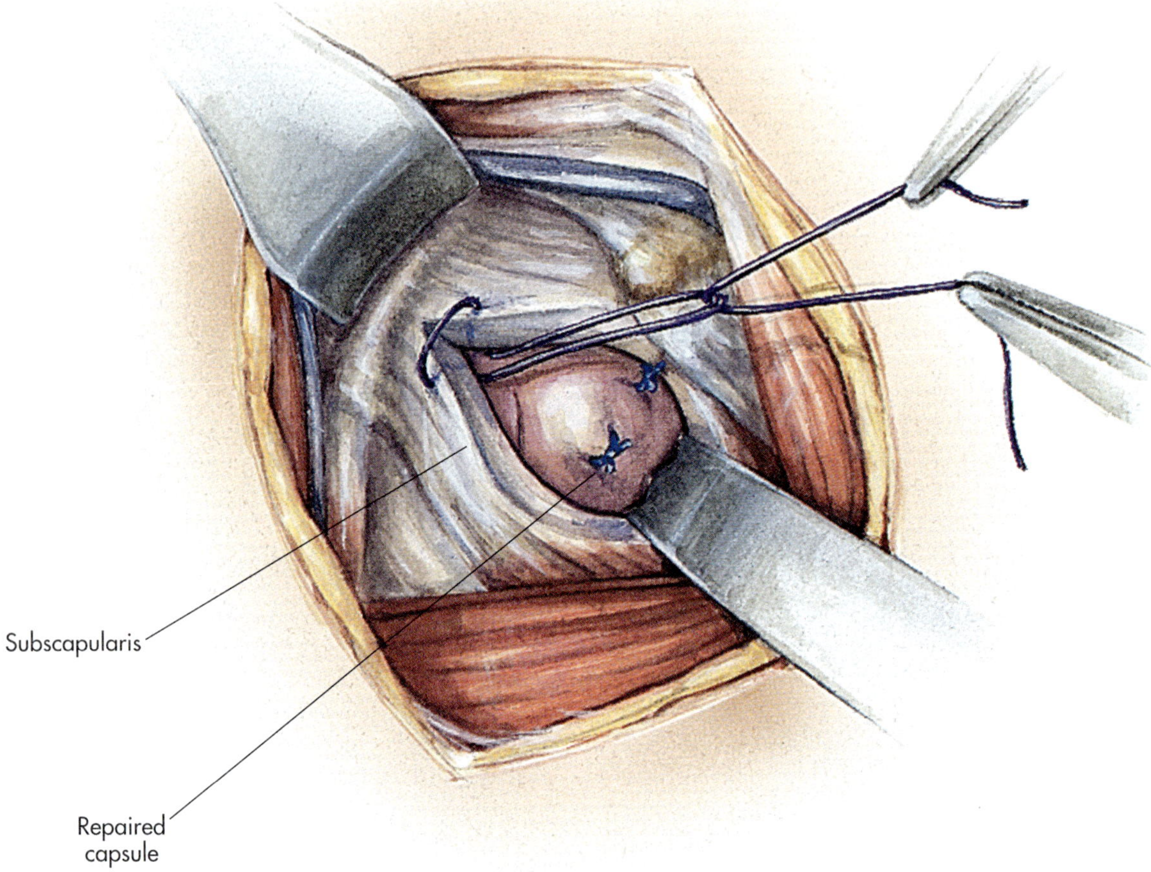

FIGURE 7-44 Closure of the subscapularis.

earlier range of motion, the role and indications for arthroscopic stabilization will continue to expand.

Labral lesions may certainly occur in the absence of obvious glenohumeral instability. Tears of the superior labrum may result from a superiorly directed force such as a fall on the outstretched arm. Snyder[51] has described an injury involving the superior aspect of the glenoid labrum beginning posteriorly and extending anteriorly (SLAP lesion). This area of the labrum was noted to be functionally important because it serves as an anchor for the insertion of the long head of the biceps tendon. SLAP lesions are not common, but when present they may be confused with anterior instability of the glenohumeral joint because of the presence of pain associated with overhead activities and the fact that often they may only be diagnosed at the time of arthroscopy. They frequently occur in conjunction with anterior instability and internal impingement.

The pain caused by a labral lesion is usually anterior, and there is often a "click" associated with range of motion. SLAP lesions are often seen in pitchers and overhand athletes; internal impingement of the rotator cuff against the superior rim in overhead activities appears to be a common cause of this condition.

The SLAP lesion has been divided into the following four types: type 1 lesions involve fraying of the superior labrum with an intact peripheral labral edge and biceps tendon anchor, type 2 lesions involve fraying of the labrum, as well as detachment of the superior labrum and biceps tendon from the underlying glenoid, type 3 lesions demonstrate a bucket-handle tear of the superior labrum with an intact peripheral attachment and biceps tendon anchor, and type 4 lesions involve a bucket-handle tear of the superior labrum that extends into the biceps tendon and anchor.[51] The SLAP lesions involving an intact biceps tendon and labral attachment to the glenoid (types 1 and 3) may be treated with simple arthroscopic débridement of the torn labrum. When the biceps tendon and labral attachment to the glenoid have been disrupted (types 2 and 4), the treatment of choice is reattaching the biceps tendon and labral complex to the superior glenoid surface. The open technique to repair a type 2 or 4 SLAP lesion requires an osteotomy of the acromion and an approach in the interval between the supraspinatus and subscapularis. The displaced SLAP lesion can be treated with decortication of the superior glenoid rim and transfixation of the biceps tendon and labral complex with a cannulated absorbable fixation device[53] (Surtac) or fixation with sutures transfixed to a Mitek bony anchor.[56]

SUMMARY

The shoulder joint is vulnerable to traumatic and atraumatic instability because of the lack of bony constraints, and the joint's stability depends on the capsuloligamentous complex. Obtaining an accurate history and physical examination is critical in establishing the diagnosis of instability, as well as the direction and nature of pathologic laxity. Arthroscopic evaluation is sometimes necessary to confirm the diagnosis, especially when occult subluxation is present. Treatment is predicated on an accurate diagnosis and begins with a well-supervised rehabilitation program. Surgery is reserved for patients who fail conservative therapy, except in unique circumstances where failure is predictable without surgery. Surgical reconstruction is very effective in controlling instability, and recent techniques have allowed athletes involved in overhead sports to return to their former competitive level. Arthroscopy has played an important role in the evaluation of the glenohumeral joint and the treatment of mechanical lesions, such as a superior labral tear. An open anterior capsulolabral reconstruction is currently the preferred technique for athletes with symptomatic anterior and multidirectional instability of the glenohumeral joint.

References

1. Adams FL: *The genuine work of hippocrates,* vols 1 and 2, New York, 1986, William Wood.
2. Baker CL, Uribe JW, Whitman C: Arthroscopic evaluation of acute initial anterior shoulder dislocation, *Am J Sports Med* 18: 25, 1990.
3. Bankart ASB: The pathology and treatment of the recurrent dislocation of the shoulder joint, *Br Surg* 26:23, 1939.
4. Bigliani LU et al: Arthroscopic coracoarcromial ligament resection for impingement in the overhead athlete, presented at American Shoulder and Elbow Surgeons Closed Meeting, Manchester, Vt, 1994 (abstract)
5. Caspari RB: Arthroscopic stabilization for shoulder instability: operative techniques in shoulder surgery, Gaithersburg, Md, 1991, Aspen, pp. 57.
6. Eden R: Zur operation der habituellen schulterluxation unter mitteilung eines neuen verfahrens beim abriss am inneren pfannenrande, *Dtsch Zeitschr Chir* 144:269, 1918.
7. Flower WH: On pathologic changes produced in the shoulder joint by traumatic dislocation, *Trans Path Soc London* 12:179, 1961.
8. Fly WR et al: Arthroscopic subacromial decompression in athletes less than 40 years old, American Shoulder and Elbow Surgeons Sixth Open Meeting, New Orleans, La, February, 1990 (abstract).
9. Garth WP, Allman FL, Armstrong WS: Occult anterior subluxation of the shoulder in noncontact sports, *Am J Sports Med* 15: 579, 1987.
10. Glousman RE: Instability versus impingement syndrome in the throwing athlete, *Orthop Clin North Am* 24, 1993.
11. Glousman RE et al: Dynamic electromyographic analysis of the throwing shoulder with glenohumeral instability, *J Bone Joint Surg* 70(A):220, 1988.
12. Hawkins RJ, Hobeika P: Physical examination of the shoulder, *Orthopaedics* 6:12, 1983.
13. Helfet AJ: Coracoid transplantation for recurring dislocation of the shoulder, *J Bone Joint Surg* 40B:198, 1958.
14. Hill HA, Sachs MD: The grooved defect of the humeral head. A frequently unrecognized complication of dislocations of the shoulder joint, *Radiology* 35:690, 1940.
15. Hoppenfeld S: *Physical examination of the spine and extremities,* New York, 1976, Appleton-Century-Crofts.
16. Hovelius L, Gavle JT, Fredin LH: Recurrent anterior dislocation of the shoulder: results after the Bankart and Putti-Platt operations, *J Bone Joint Surg* 61A:566, 1979.
17. Hussein MD: Kocher's method is 3,000 years old, *J Bone Joint Surg* 50B:669, 1968.
18. Hybbinnette S: De la transplantation d'un fragment osseux pour remedier aux luxations recidivantes de l'epaule. Constatations et resultats operatoires, *Acta Chir Scand* 71:411, 1932.
19. Jobe FW et al: Anterior capsulolabral reconstruction of the shoulder in athletes in overhand sports, *Am J Sports Med* 19:428, 1991.
20. Jobe FW, Glousman RE: Anterior capsulolabral reconstruction, *Tech Orthop* 3:29, 1989.
21. Jobe FW, Glousman RE: Anterior capsulolabral reconstruction. In Paulos LE, Tibone JE, editors: *Operative technique in shoulder surgery,* Gaithersburg, Md, 1992, Aspen Publishing.
22. Jobe FW, Glousman RE: *Anterior instability in the throwing athlete,* instructional course lecture, American Orthopaedic Society For Sports Medicine, Palm Desert, Calif, June, 1988.
23. Jobe FW, Moynes DR: Delineation of diagnostic criteria and a rehabilitation program for rotator cuff injuries, *Am J Sports Med* 10:336, 1982.
24. Johnson LL: *Shoulder arthroscopy: arthroscopic surgery: principles in practice,* St Louis, 1986, Mosby.
25. Johnson LL: Symposium on open versus arthroscopic techniques for shoulder instability, presented at the American Shoulder and Elbow Surgeons, Fourth Open Meeting, Atlanta, February, 1988.
26. Kiviluoto O et al: Immobilization after primary dislocation of the shoulder, *Acta Orthop Scand* 51:915, 1980.
27. Lombardo SJ et al: The modified Bristow procedure for recurrent dislocation of the shoulder, *J Bone Joint Surg* 58A:256, 1976.
28. Macha TJ et al: MRI and ultrasound of suspected rotator cuff tears: clinical correlation with arthroscopy and arthrography, *Orthop Trans* 13(1):153, Spring, 1989.
29. Maki NJ: Arthroscopic stabilization: suture technique, *Oper Tech Orthop* 1:180, April 1991.
30. Matsen FA, Thomas SC, Rockwood CA: Anterior glenohumeral instability. In Rockwood CA, Matsen FA, editors: *The shoulder,* Philadelphia, 1990, WB Saunders.
31. Matthews LS et al: Arthroscopic staple capsulorrhaphy for recurrent anterior shoulder instability, *Arthroscopy* 4:106, 1988.
32. May VR Jr: A modified Bristow operation for anterior recurrent dislocation of the shoulder, *J Bone Joint Surg* 52A:1010, 1970.
33. McLaughlin HL, MacLellan DI: Recurrent anterior dislocation of the shoulder. II. A comparative study, *J Trauma* 7:191, 1967.
34. Morgan CD: Arthroscopic transglenoid Bankart suture repair, *Oper Tech Orthop* 1:171, April 1991
35. Morgan CD, Bodenstab AB: Arthroscopic Bankart suture repair: technique and early results, *Arthroscopy* 3:111, 1982.
36. Morrey BF, Jones JM: Recurrent anterior dislocation of the shoulder: long-term follow-up of the Putti-Platt and Bankart procedures, *J Bone Joint Surg* 58A:252, 1976.
37. Nash J: The status of Kocher's method of reducing recent anterior dislocation of the shoulder, *J Bone Joint Surg* 16:535, 1934.
38. Neer CS II: Anterior acromioplasty for the chronic impingement syndrome in the shoulder: a preliminary report, *J Bone Joint Surg* 54(A):41, 1972.

39. Neer CS II, Foster CR: Inferior capsular shift for involuntary inferior and multidirectional instability of the shoulder: a preliminary report, *J Bone Joint Surg* 62A:897, 1980.
40. Nelson MA et al: Evaluation of the painful shoulder: a prospective comparison of magnetic resonance imaging, computerized tomographic arthrography, metra sonography, and operative findings, *J Bone Joint Surg* 73A:707, 1990.
41. Osmond-Clarke H: Habitual dislocation of the shoulder: the Putti-Platt operation, *J Bone Joint Surg* 30B:19, 1948.
42. Perry J, Glousman RE: Biomechanics of throwing. In Nicholas JA, Hershman EB, editors: *The upper extremity in sports medicine,* St Louis, 1990, Mosby.
43. Perthes G: Uber operationen der habituellen schulterluxation, *DTZ Chir* 85:199, 1906.
44. Rockwood CA: Part 2: dislocations about the shoulder fractures, ed 2, vol 1, Philadephia, 1984, JB Lippincott.
45. Rowe CR: Prognosis in dislocations of the shoulder, *J Bone Joint Surg* 38A:957, 1956.
46. Rowe CR, Patel D, Southmyd WW: The Bankart procedure, *J Bone Joint Surg* 60A:1, 1978.
47. Rowe CR, Zarins B, Ciullo JV: Recurrent anterior dislocation of the shoulder after surgical repair: apparent causes of failure and treatment, *J Bone Joint Surg* 66A:159, 1984.
48. Rowe CR, Zarins B: Recurrent transient subluxation of the shoulder, *J Bone Joint Surg* 63A:863, 1981.
49. Schwartz RR et al: *Capsular restraints to anterior-posterior motion in the shoulder,* American Shoulder and Elbow Surgeons Fourth Open Meeting, Atlanta, 1988.
50. Sisk TD, Boyd HB: Management of recurrent anterior dislocation of the shoulder: Du Toit type of staple capsulorrhaphy, *Clin Orthop* 103:150, 1974.
51. Snyder SJ et al: SLAP lesions of the shoulder, *Arthroscopy* 6:274, 1990.
52. Turkel SJ et al: Stabilizing mechanisms preventing anterior dislocation of the glenohumeral joint, *J Bone Joint Surg* 63A:1208, 1981.
53. Warner JP, Warren RG: Arthroscopic Bankart repair using a cannulated, absorbable fixation device, *Oper Tech Orthop* 1:192, April, 1991.
54. Warren RF: Subluxation of the shoulder in athletes, *Clin Sports Med* 2:339, 1983.
55. Wheeler JH et al: Arthroscopic versus nonoperative treatment of acute shoulder dislocation in young athletes, *Arthroscopy* 5:213, 1989.
56. Wolf EM, Wilk RM, Richmond JC: Arthroscopic Bankart repair using suture anchors, *Oper Tech Orthop* 1:184, 1991.
57. Yoneda B, Welsh RP, MacIntosh DL: Conservative treatment of shoulder dislocation in young males (proceedings), *J Bone Joint Surg* 64B:254, 1982.

SECTION D Subacromial Impingement: Clinical Assessment and Treatment

Subacromial impingement refers to encroachment of the rotator cuff by surrounding bony and soft-tissue structures, leading to mechanical wear and symptoms of shoulder pain. Traditionally such impingement has been described, classified, and treated in an older, relatively nonathletic population in which it is the most common cause of chronic shoulder disability.[34] However, impingement symptoms (caused by undersurface cuff-labral impingement at the posterior, superior labral rim) recently has been found in younger patients as well and is considered among the most common causes of shoulder pain in the population under the age of 35. It is particularly common among individuals involved in repetitive overhead activities such as baseball, swimming, racquet sports, and volleyball.

Although Neer's theory of impingement has been effective in the older population (in whom it was originally described), it has proven less helpful in understanding or successfully treating younger (less than 35 years) athletes with impingement. Differences in patient age and activity, as well as in physical examination and arthroscopic findings, have led to a better understanding of the impingement process. In the previous sections of this chapter, distinctions were drawn between the younger and older athlete with shoulder pain. Although age alone is not an indicator of the etiology of shoulder pain, when impingement is being considered as a primary or secondary phenomenon, age is a useful starting point.

In this chapter the focus is on patients with primary impingement, excluding from consideration the younger athlete with underlying instability. The clinical presentation and evaluation of impingement have been previously covered. The purpose of this chapter is to review the etiology and diagnosis of impingement, with emphasis on the nonoperative and operative treatment of subacromial impingement in the usually older athlete with isolated impingement and no evidence of underlying instability.

ETIOLOGY

Impingement Theory

Since 1972, Neer's theory of impingement has greatly advanced our understanding, diagnosis, and treatment of patients with shoulder pain, particularly in the older population in whom rotator cuff pathology is so prevalent. Neer synthesized what for many years has served effectively as a unifying theory of rotator cuff pathology,[36] in which mechanical wear of the cuff by constricting surrounding structures leads to impingement.

Arising from the scapula, the subscapularis, supraspinatus, infraspinatus, and teres minor coalesce as a tendinous "cuff" that inserts on the lesser and greater tuberosities of the proximal humerus (Figs. 7-45 and 7-46). Coordinated muscle tension within this cuff exerts a compressive force on the humeral head, centering it within the glenoid fossa and thereby providing a fulcrum for deltoid function throughout the available range of shoulder movement. The subacromial bursa provides a frictionless interface between (1) the rotator cuff and long head of the biceps below, and (2) the coracoacromial arch, consisting of the acromion, acromioclavicular (AC) joint, and the undersurface of the coracoclavicular (CA) ligament, above. Normal overhead movement results in the rotator cuff's bursal surface (including the biceps tendon located within the rotator interval) gliding smoothly against the bursa's lining along the fibrous acromial undersurface, CA ligament, and AC joint.

Any process that either (1) interferes with cuff mechanics (resulting in failure to maintain humeral head/glenoid relationship) or (2) compromises the normal "outlet" of the coracoacromial arch through which the otherwise normal cuff passes can lead to encroachment or impingement of the rotator cuff. Compressive "wear" damage of the cuff's superior (bursal side) surface

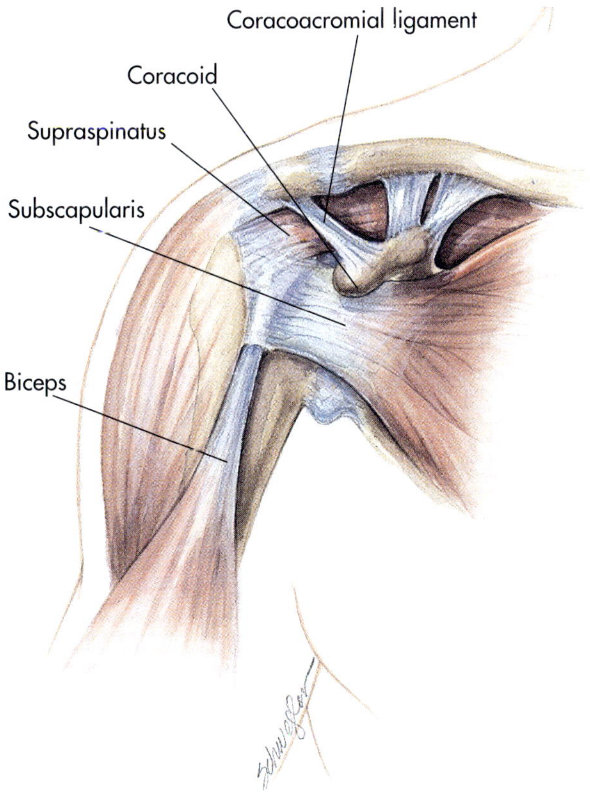

FIGURE 7-45 The subscapularis tendon anteriorly arises from the subscapular fossa and inserts onto the lesser tuberosity of the proximal humerus. The coracoacromial ligament arises from the coracoid and attaches to the anterior inferior acromion.

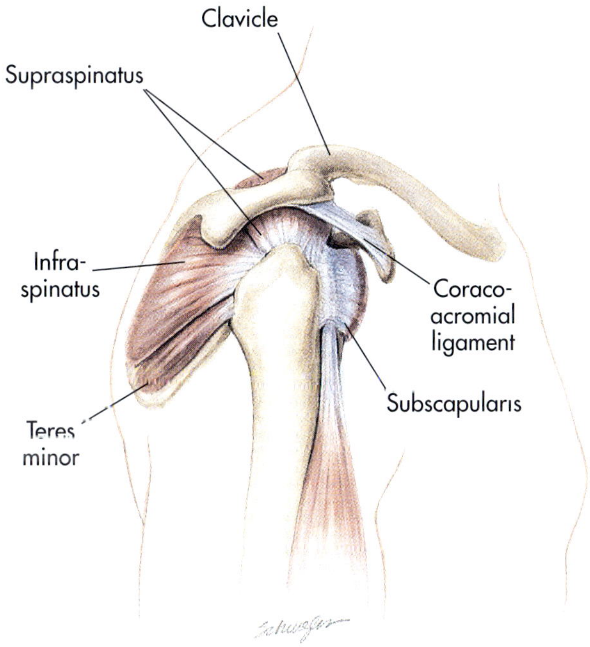

FIGURE 7-46 From the lateral view, the remainder of the cuff can be seen, including the supraspinatus superiorly and the infraspinatus and teres minor posteriorly. These three muscles attach through their tendinous insertion onto the greater tuberosity. The CA ligament and anterior acromion form the coracoacromial arch.

against the outlet structures may, over time, result in progressive injury.

Neer divided the causes of impingement into either "outlet" or "nonoutlet."[35] Narrowing of the supraspinatus "outlet" (the space beneath the anterior acromion, coracoacromial ligament, and AC joint) is the most frequent cause of impingement[34] (Fig. 7-47). Specific outlet causes reported by other investigators include abnormal acromial tilt, slope, or morphology.[36,55] Bigliani and Morrison described three types of acromia: type I is flat; type II is curved; and type III is "hooked"[4,29] (Fig. 7-48). The reported association of a type III acromion with rotator cuff tear has been reported by many investigators, although some have suggested that such acromial morphology is a consequence of traction stress on the CA ligament and not causally related to impingement.[35,36] Understanding the contribution of acromial morphology to cuff pathology is further complicated by the variability in acromial classification simply resulting from differences in radiographic technique. Outlet impingement also may occur secondary to structural abnormalities at the acromioclavicular (AC) joint (i.e., joint hypertrophy from posttraumatic or age-related arthritis).

In nonoutlet impingement, the cuff functions in abnormal proximity to the outlet, resulting in friction and mechanical cuff wear. Although encountered less frequently than outlet impingement, nonoutlet impingement may be due to a variety of etiologies. Neurologic injury to the scapular rotators results in failure of the humeral head to clear the obstructing nonmobile acromion as the arm is brought into abduction. Acute trau-

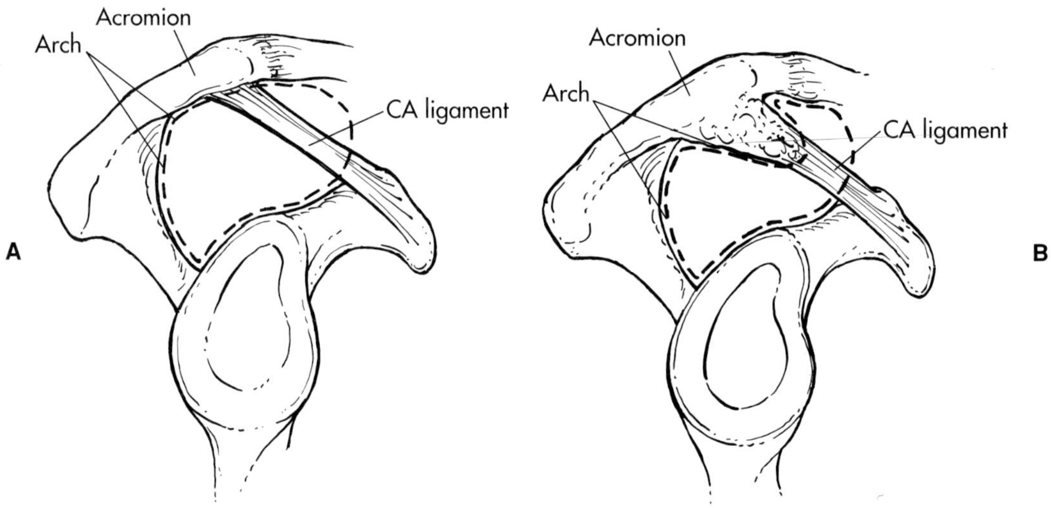

FIGURE 7-47 **A,** The normal coracoacromial arch outlet is composed of the acromion, the AC joint, and the CA ligament. Notable is the space available for cuff mobility. **B,** The constriction of the arch, known as *outlet type impingement* of the arch, is caused by osteophyte impingement into the arch at the CA ligament attachment.

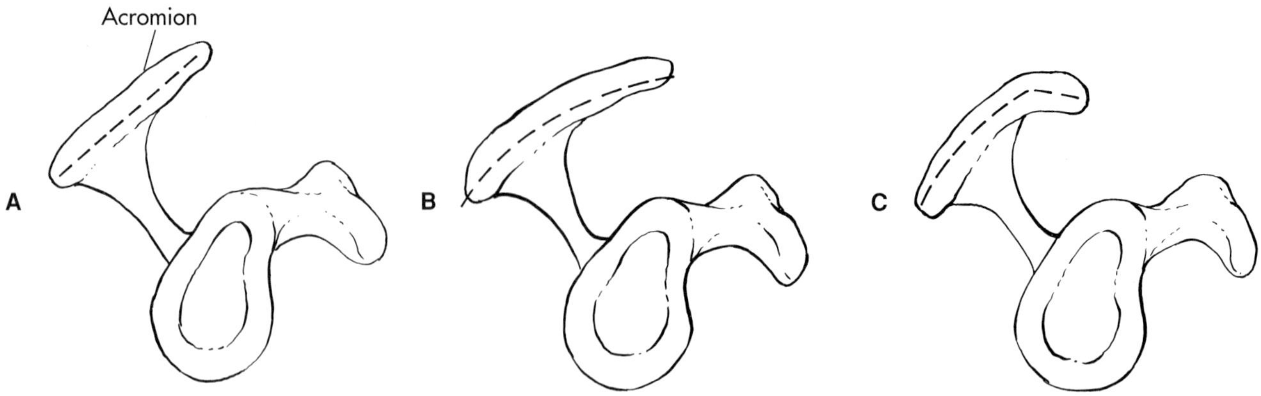

FIGURE 7-48 Acromia have been classified according to their shape on a Y-shaped lateral outlet view and are, **A,** flat, **B,** curved, and, **C,** hooked.

matic injury to the rotator cuff resulting in contusion or strain can lead to relative dysfunction and loss of the normal force couple. Other nonoutlet causes include prominence of the greater tuberosity (malunion or nonunion), loss of humeral head depressors (cuff tear or biceps rupture), loss of glenohumeral fulcrum (such as occurs in patients with ligamentous laxity or instability), loss of the normal suspensory mechanism of the shoulder (old AC separation), defects of the acromion (unfused acromial epiphysis—os acromiale),[33,37] thickened bursa or cuff (calcium deposit or bursitis), and loss of the lower extremities (paraplegia, amputation, arthritis) resulting in transfer of the weight-bearing function to the upper extremity.

Clinical and lab investigators have identified other mechanisms by which "impingement" may occur. Unlike Neer, who considered that 95% of cuff tears were due to subacromial impingement, some investigators believe that cuff wear reflects intrinsic pathology with age-related thinning, degeneration, and weakening.* According to Uhthoff et al, for example, rotator cuff tears are unlikely to be due to primary impingement but rather a consequence of an "intrinsic degenerative tendinopathy."[25,38] Pathology within the tendon itself (including tendinopathy and partial or small complete tears) permits proximal migration of the humeral head into the arch, leading to secondary impingement. This may then create a vicious circle, ultimately leading to significant full-thickness cuff tears.

Researchers have described a "critical zone" of vascular insufficiency within the supraspinatus tendon just proximal to its insertion on the greater tuberosity, which theoretically contributes to attrition, tendon degeneration, and cuff rupture.[24,44] There is evidence that contradicts this theory of relative vascular insufficiency.[13,31,48,49] Most investigators believe that a combination of vascular, degenerative, traumatic, and mechanical processes leads to rotator cuff pathology.

Other Theories of Impingement

Neither Neer's theory of impingement nor our observations of occult instability by themselves comprehensively explain all forms of "impingement." Impingement symptoms encompass several different conditions that may independently, and in some cases interdependently, result in pathology of the rotator cuff.

Impingement syndrome therefore is multifactorial in origin, with many underlying contributing etiologies ultimately manifesting themselves in a clinically similar manner. The contributing factors include mechanical wear (subacromial impingement, glenoid impingement) with or without overt underlying instability. Most of these mechanisms initially may be reversible. With continued activity, however, progressive fiber failure, abnormal mechanics, cuff dysfunction, and structural changes within the glenohumeral joint perpetuate the process, leaving residual pathologic damage.

Classification

Regardless of the specific etiology, impingement has been classified into three theoretically distinct but practically overlapping stages.[21] Stage I reflects reversible cuff edema, and hemorrhage is usually seen in younger patients. In stage II, fibrosis and tendinitis have become, to some degree, irreversible. In stage III, a tear (either partial or complete) has developed in the cuff, with some degree of irreversibility.

CLINICAL EVALUATION

Thorough evaluation of the athlete with subacromial impingement relies on a comprehensive history, physical examination, and pertinent radiographic imaging studies. Because impingement pain so often overlaps with instability and rotator cuff tear, evaluation and diagnosis of these disorders are reviewed in a previous chapter. In this section the most relevant findings in those patients with classic subacromial impingement are only briefly identified.

History

Overhead activity with related shoulder pain that is often poorly localized and resolves with rest is the hallmark complaint of the individual with impingement.

Physical Examination

Observation of the patient during overhead elevation may demonstrate scapulohumeral dysrhythm or a painful arc of motion, with discomfort in the overhead position usually from between 70° to 120°. Focal tenderness may be present over the anterior or lateral subacromial space, anteriorly over the biceps, or posteriorly over the cuff but is nonspecific. Range of motion is not significantly restricted in subacromial impingement, although some mild limitation is not uncommon.

The most commonly used physical examination techniques for eliciting subacromial impingement are those described by Neer[36] or Hawkins.[16] In Neer's impingement sign, the affected arm is elevated in the sagittal plane against the scapula, which is immobilized by the examiner's other hand (Fig. 7-49). Theoretically, the cuff is compressed against the unyielding subacromial arch. This sign, however, is generally nonspecific; it may, in fact, reflect internal impingement of the rotator cuff as it is compressed against the superior rim of the glenoid. In the maneuver described by Hawkins, the shoulder is flexed forward 90° while adducting and forcibly internally rotating the upper arm against the fixed scapula. This test is thought to be more specific in eliciting subacromial impingement, because the cuff is compressed beneath the subacromial arch.

*References 6, 8, 21, 25, 38, 51.

The integrity of the cuff musculature in subacromial impingement is difficult to determine by physical examination alone. Pain with supraspinatus and/or external rotation strength testing is not specific for cuff pathology, although painless normal strength probably precludes tendon involvement. Supraspinatus testing is performed by resisting the patient's shoulder elevation in the scapular plane, with the thumb pointing downward.

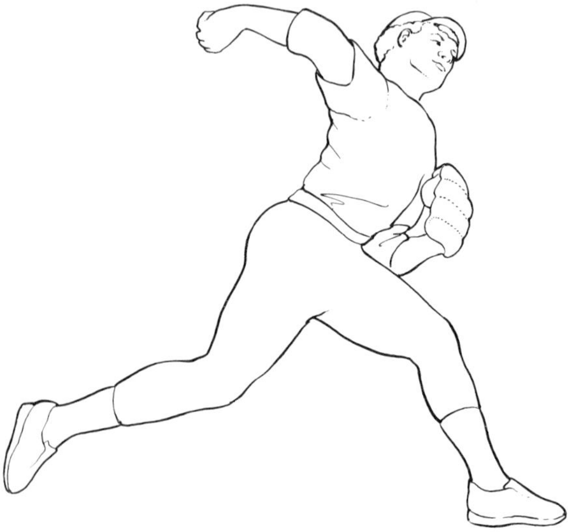

FIGURE 7-49 The Neer impingement sign is elicited by raising the patient's arm in forward flexion while holding the scapula fixed, thereby impinging the cuff and reproducing symptoms of pain when positive.

Radiographic Examination

Typical radiographic findings in subacromial impingement include acromial sclerosis, spurring of the distal clavicle or AC joint, and a "pseudocyst" within the greater tuberosity adjacent to the cuff insertion (Fig. 7-50). Narrowing of the acromiohumeral interval often is a late finding associated with large or massive rotator cuff tears.

Impingement Injection Test

This test originally was described as a valuable method for separating impingement lesions from other causes of shoulder pain.[34] In this test, symptomatic relief after the injection of 10 ml of 1% lidocaine into the subacromial bursa indicates the likelihood that pathology within this space is responsible for the symptoms. If after injection of the lidocaine, "the painful arc is considerably reduced or abolished, it establishes the anatomical site of the lesion but does not give an indication of the precise pathology or extent of the lesion."[21] We have not found this test helpful in distinguishing those with subacromial impingement from those with symptoms of impingement caused by underlying instability. Subacromial injection of lidocaine often will provide temporary relief even

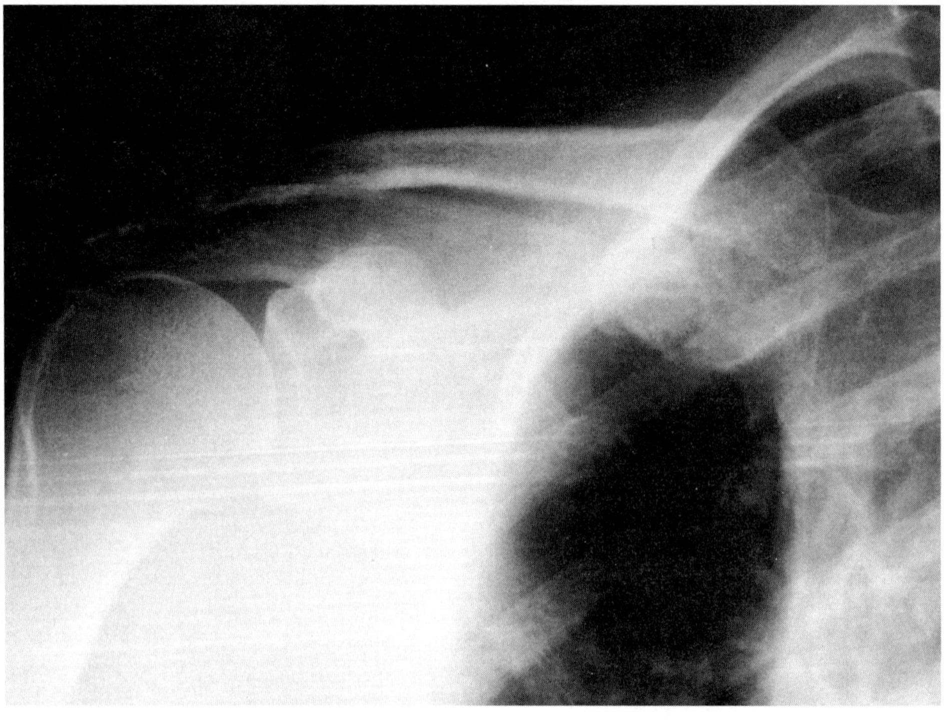

FIGURE 7-50 An AP shoulder x-ray with typical findings of impingement. Notable are the subacromial and greater tuberosity sclerosis and the proximal humeral lucency, the so-called pseudocyst of the greater tuberosity. The acromiohumeral interval is preserved.

in athletes in whom subsequent arthroscopy reveals underlying instability and a normal subacromial bursa. It may be that lidocaine in the bursa nonspecifically anesthetizes most or all of the cuff's pain fibers.

Arthrography, MRI, and Ultrasound

Sophisticated imaging techniques are neither necessary nor cost effective early in the evaluation of subacromial impingement. However, persistent symptoms may mandate use of one or more of these tests. Their indications, interpretations, and limitations are more fully discussed in previous chapters.

MANAGEMENT

Foremost in the management of the patient with impingement is the elimination of shoulder pain. In the treatment of athletes, however, successful management means more than simply pain relief, because the ability to return to the preinjury activity level determines the success of treatment. The single best chance for returning patients to preinjury levels of activity is to accurately identify the cause of the impingement symptoms. Beyond that, explaining the cause and treatment strategy to the athletes in a way they can understand and follow is critical to successful treatment. This often requires the involvement of the trainer and skilled physical therapist. Nonoperative rehabilitation programs designed to decrease inflammation and restore motion and muscle strength generally have met with a high level of success. Therefore a structured, supervised rehabilitation program is essential for at least 3 months before considering surgical intervention.

Nonsurgical Treatment

Principles of Nonoperative Treatment

Prevention of this syndrome is the most effective form of treatment and is based on a carefully designed training program emphasizing proper mechanics and warm-up, flexibility, strength, and conditioning. Preventive sport-specific rehabilitation protocols have been the focus of several reports.[17,32] For example, swimmers should do an easy warm-up for 20 to 30 minutes before sprinting and should change strokes frequently. Baseball players should toss lightly before throwing hard and should be placed on a program for rotator cuff and scapular rotator strengthening.

If impingement already is present, the specific program for the treatment of impingement depends on the stage. Although initial treatment for all stages is similar, the duration of the symptoms dictates further diagnostic or therapeutic initiatives. For patients in whom impingement or shoulder pain is secondary to suspected instability, the reader is referred to the chapters on instability (anterior, multidirectional, and posterior), in which the specific protocols used in this athletic population are outlined. For the less common, usually older patient in whom primary impingement (without cuff tear, i.e., stages I and II) has occurred without instability, the principles of nonoperative intervention follow with specific rehabilitation protocol in later chapters.

The principles of rotator cuff impingement treatment are (1) eliminate inflammation, (2) restore range of motion, (3) improve strength of cuff and scapular rotators, (4) optimize scapulohumeral rhythm and coordination, (5) implement conditioning, (6) reinitiate similar biomechanical motion/activity, attending to and correcting activity mechanics as necessary, and (7) gradually return the athlete to activity.

Elimination of Inflammation

Rest is a relative term. Considering the loads imparted to the athlete's shoulder during many activities,[40,41] particularly during overhead-throwing sports, simply avoiding the athletic activity itself constitutes some degree of "rest." Whether it involves throwing, serving, or performing the butterfly stroke, the athlete must stop the offending activity to allow the inflammation to subside.

During this initial rest period, antiinflammatory modalities are useful. Prescription of a nonsteroidal antiinflammatory agent for the first 3 to 4 weeks of rehabilitation is thought to further decrease inflammation and potentiate the benefits of therapy. Local modalities, including ice, heat, and alternating (contrast) therapy, may decrease the discomfort associated with the offending activity and are useful throughout the rehabilitation program. Cold therapy has been shown to be useful in the treatment of inflammatory conditions.[28] Heat seems effective when used in preparation for activity.

Restoration of Range of Motion/Stretching

Because of capsular tightness associated with impingement, some patients will require a stretching program to restore their motion to normal. This is particularly true in the older athlete with primary impingement, in whom posterior capsular tightness actually can exacerbate impingement during forward elevation. However, caution must be used in the younger athlete in whom underlying instability is so frequently the cause of shoulder pain; in these patients, shoulder positions that place the joint at risk for instability (such as the position of abduction and external rotation) should be avoided. If there is any possibility of anterior instability, exercises in which anterior structures may be stretched should be eliminated from the program. Specific techniques in stretching will be discussed in a later chapter.

Role of Technique/Activity/Mechanics Alterations

Specific recommendations regarding any individual's sport technique are beyond the scope of this text. With a "team" approach, incorporating the professional expertise of athletic trainers, coaches, and other professionals, however, return to athletics is achieved and further problems are avoided. Modification of the throwing motion, tennis stroke, racquet tension, amount of body roll, or breathing pattern in swimming may reduce the risk of recurrence of the impingement phenomenon.

Role of Steroid Injections

Because of concern about possible tendon damage resulting from corticosteroid injection,[20] such injections are used infrequently. If corticosteroid injection is used, the number of injections for any condition is limited to three. In such a case, the athlete is discouraged from aggressively participating in sports for 7 days thereafter (10 to 14 days according to Leach[22]). Rehabilitation exercises should continue during this period.

Duration of Physical Therapy

The duration of therapy depends on several factors, including symptom onset and severity; presence of stiffness, weakness, or dysfunctional rhythm; stage of impingement; presence and degree of underlying instability/laxity; endurance; previous treatment; and patient goals. Therapy is initiated under the supervision of a physical therapist or the athlete's trainer. Exercise frequency and intensity are individually determined. Therapy may last only 3 to 4 weeks for the minimally symptomatic athlete who simply "overdid it." However, prolonged treatment for several weeks to a few months may be needed for the chronically symptomatic athlete with recurrent impingement. The decision to intervene surgically depends on a combination of factors, including the patient's underlying diagnosis, treatment, stage of involvement, response to treatment, and goals for return to activity. As a general principle, we do not consider surgery on any patient who has not undergone at least 3 months of supervised rehabilitation. Exercises in a supervised setting may continue for more than 6 months, particularly under the watchful eye of the trainer. Techniques in warm-up, stretching, and strengthening should continue throughout the athlete's career.

Results of Nonoperative Treatment

The majority of patients with impingement will respond to a nonoperative rehabilitation program.* However, most of these reports involve the care of nonathletes. There are few studies that have objectively reviewed impingement in an athletic population to determine whether, in fact, they were capable of returning to their previous level of performance. This is critical because in this group of high-demand athletes, failure to maintain the same speed, force, or accuracy of throwing, or any seemingly insignificant loss of strength, flexibility, or coordination can mean the difference between excellence in performance and failure to continue at their position.

Return to Activity

In some patients, symptoms persist despite treatment and interfere with their ability to return to their previous activity or at their desired level of performance. In the athlete unable to return to activity despite appropriate supervised rehabilitation, returning to a different position or changing to another sport entirely may be an acceptable alternative to surgical intervention.

*References 8, 10, 19, 22, 34, 35, 39, 53.

Preferred Surgical Treatment

Surgical treatment is indicated for those patients in whom nonoperative management has been ineffective at eliminating symptoms and/or allowing them to return to their activity. Surgery is designed to address the underlying problem. In the athletic population, particularly overhead-throwing athletes, this most commonly involves the treatment of the underlying occult instability; in older athletes, this means the treatment of primary impingement. Be sure you are dealing with subacromial impingement before carrying out a subacromial decompression.

A subacromial decompression, including an acromioplasty and coracoacromial (CA) ligament resection, is indicated in patients with persistent subacromial impingement unresponsive to adequate conservative treatment for at least 3 months' duration. Acromioplasty is rarely performed under the age of 40.

Surgical Procedures and Results

Both open and arthroscopic operative methods have been described to treat impingement. These include subacromial bursectomy, coracoacromial ligament resection, anterior acromioplasty, AC joint inferior osteophyte resection, distal clavicle resection, and combinations of these procedures.

Subacromial Bursectomy

Isolated subacromial bursectomy has not been shown effective in the treatment of this condition. We have no experience with this procedure and suspect it has a limited place in the treatment of "true" impingement pain, if any.

Coracoacromial Ligament Excision

There are reports of success with isolated CA ligament excision, most commonly in younger athletes involved in such activities as swimming, tennis, and throwing.[9,16,22] However, the effectiveness of this procedure in the athlete has been questionable,[18] and this procedure currently has no role in the authors' treatment protocol because it does not address the pathology in either the young or the old athlete.

Arthroscopic Findings

For the patient with primary impingement, glenohumeral arthroscopy usually demonstrates normal shoulder joint structures, although there may be minimal fibrillation of the cuff's undersurface. The striking arthroscopic finding, however, is found in the subacromial space, where inflammation, fibrosis, and scarring are evident.

Subacromial Decompression

The principles of surgical decompression of the coracoacromial arch include (1) preservation of the deltoid origin, (2) excision of the subacromial bursa, (3) acromioplasty of the anteroinferior acromion, (4) resection of the coracoacromial ligament, (5) resection of any spurs on the undersurface of the distal clavicle, (6) decompression with excision of the acromioclavicular joint as needed in cases of AC joint arthritis, and (7) inspection and further treatment as necessary of any rotator cuff pathology. Whether such goals are achieved arthroscopically or by more conventional open techniques depends on the surgeon, the patient, and the degree of pathology present. Both arthroscopic and open techniques and their results will be described.

Subacromial Arthroscopy

After examining the glenohumeral joint, the examiner arthroscopically inspects the subacromial space. One may reposition the arm for subacromial inspection and decompression by adjusting the traction into a position of approximately 20° abduction in the coronal plane of the body. Current techniques of arthroscopic subacromial decompression are essentially unchanged from the description provided by Ellman.[12] The arthroscope sheath and its obturator are withdrawn from the glenohumeral joint and cuff muscles and are redirected through the same posterior portal into the subacromial space. Gently moving the obturator and sheath back and forth reveals the degree of fibrosis within the space, and when the fibrosis is significant, can open up fibrotic areas, allow increased visualization, and facilitate an otherwise difficult bursoscopy.

A second portal is established anterolaterally approximately 3 cm lateral to the anterolateral acromion, along a line connecting the anterior acromion and AC joint. After Marcaine infiltration and incision with a #11 blade, the surgeon introduces a disposable 7-mm plastic cannula with blunt obturator, and using the principle of triangulation, sweeps the subacromial space. Before instilling irrigation fluid into the space through the scope sheath, visualize the colored cannula. Inflow is begun, and in cases of minimal fibrosis, the subacromial space is inspected. Inspection begins with the bursa, which, when disease-free, is a delicate, thin, areolar, transparent membrane extending from the acromial undersurface tissue to the bursal side of the cuff. The musculotendinous junction of the cuff often is visible, as is the tendinous insertion of the cuff laterally. The undersurface of the acromion, AC joint capsule, and coracoacromial ligament are visualized. A probe introduced through the anterolateral portal allows palpation of acromial or AC joint spurs or bursal-side cuff damage. If the subacromial space has a pristine appearance without evidence of fibrosis or cuff wear, no further surgery is performed because this suggests that subacromial impingement is not the cause of the symptoms. In our opinion, there is no role for an isolated coracoacromial ligament resection. Arthroscopic instruments are removed, and the portals are closed routinely.

In the presence of pathology, however, a motorized 5.5-mm shaver is introduced through the anterolateral portal, and a bursectomy is performed under direct visualization. Inflow commences through the arthroscopic sheath. Because such inflow often is inadequate to keep pace with the shaver's suction, a third portal for additional irrigation inflow also may be established. The surgeon makes a stab incision approximately 3 cm posterolateral from the posterolateral tip of the acromion after infiltrating the skin with 0.25% Marcaine and epinephrine. The arthroscope is removed and reintroduced through this new posterolateral portal, with the accessory inflow portal placed posteriorly. After confirming visualization of the accessory portal, the surgeon commences inflow through this portal (Fig. 7-51). Alternatively, an arthroscopic pump may be useful to facilitate inflow, using an arthroscope sheath with both inflow and pressure monitor connected, and outflow connected to the lateral instrumentation portal. However, when using the pump, the surgeon must watch for soft-tissue swelling. The absence of a true compartment of the shoulder can allow ongoing fluid extravasation throughout the soft tissue with no anatomic restricting barrier, leading to significant swelling of the shoulder and torso. Additionally, the intermittent "surge" of inflow produced by the pump may make targeting of bleeding points by the electrocautery device or laser difficult and frustrating. For these reasons, we have continued to use overhead gravity irrigation for arthroscopic decompressions.

Whether normal saline or lactated Ringer's solution is used for irrigation fluid, 1 ampule of epinephrine (1:1000) is added to each 3-L bag to minimize bleeding in the subacromial space. Because such bleeding can prevent visualization and make this procedure arthroscopically impossible, we coordinate with the anesthetist to maintain the patient's systolic pressure at approximately 100 mm Hg when possible, which has been shown

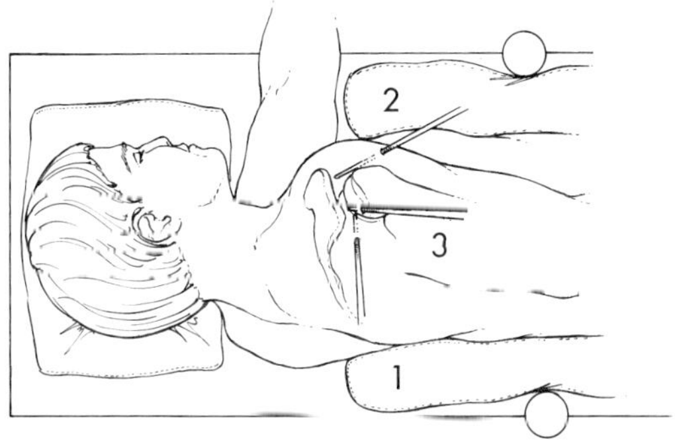

FIGURE 7-51 In the usual operative setup, the patient is placed in the lateral decubitus position for shoulder arthroscopy. Portal *1* is the usual posterior shoulder scope portal. Portal *2* is the "working" anterolateral portal for the decompression. Portal *3* is sometimes used as a third portal for placement of the scope, thereby relegating portal *1* to providing an accessory inflow function.

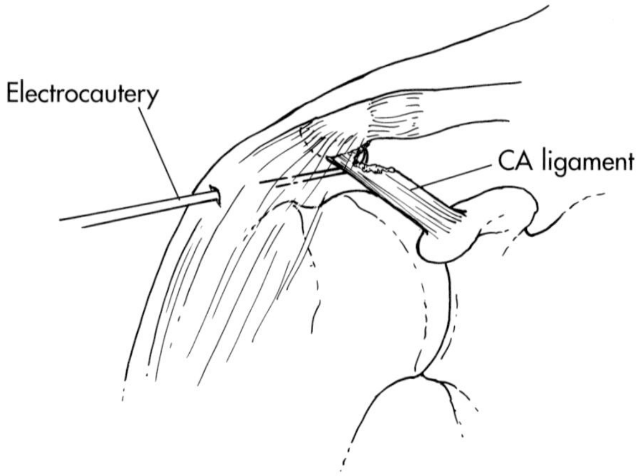

FIGURE 7-52 Through the anterolateral portal, the electrocautery facilitates arthroscopic CA ligament resection.

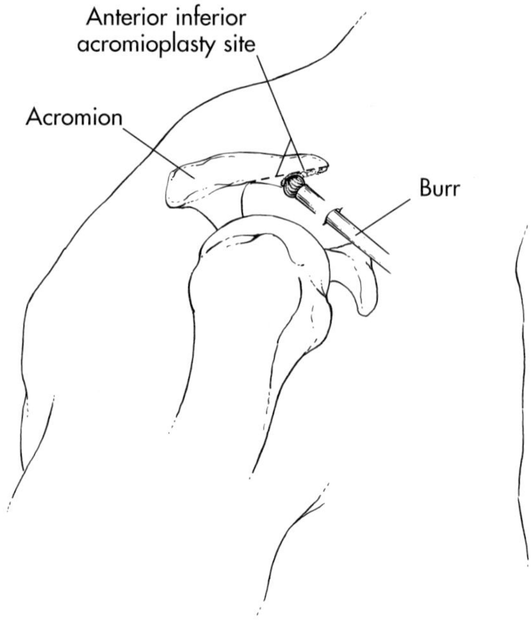

FIGURE 7-53 A motorized arthroscopic burr removes the anteroinferior undersurface of the acromion.

effective at optimizing visualization.[30] Insulated cautery devices designed for use in this procedure facilitate hemostasis and thus optimal visualization.

Soft tissue from the acromial undersurface is debrided with curettes and the shaver through the anterolateral portal. Spinal needles introduced at the AC joint and the lateral acromion mark the limits of attachment of the coracoacromial ligament. Electrocautery with an insulated curved tip detaches the CA ligament under direct vision (Fig. 7-52). Care is taken to progressively cut through this ligament layer by layer to ensure hemostasis of the acromial branch of the thoracoacromial artery.[11] When this vessel is injured, the bleeding will challenge the most gifted arthroscopist.

The ligament is released in its entirety, and the spinal needles are removed. Baskets may be used to morselize the remaining ligament, which is then completely excised, followed by use of the motorized shaver. Next, the acromioplasty is performed by introducing a 6-mm oval burr through the anterolateral portal (Fig. 7-53). The burr is seated to a depth that depends on the thickness of the patient's acromion and degree of pathology. Such a decision should be based on the preoperative radiographs. Approximately 5 to 8 mm of bone is removed from the anteroinferior acromion. The acromioplasty is carried out systematically, beginning in the front anterolaterally, tapering posteriorly, and progressively moving medially until the acromioplasty is complete. Care is taken to ensure that the acromion undersurface is smooth with no remnant osteophytes or irregularities.

Débridement of the AC joint capsule depends on the presence of AC joint involvement or osteophytes along the distal clavicle. If the AC joint is involved, the inferior capsular soft tissues are debrided first, followed by burring of the inferior distal clavicle, AC joint, and acromion as necessary. The shaver may be introduced through the anterior portal established at the level of the AC joint to facilitate AC joint débridement. If a distal clavicle excision is needed, it is carried out either arthroscopically or by an open approach.

On completion of the acromioplasty, the subacromial space is inspected for any remaining impingement or bleeding. The rotator cuff is inspected both immediately under the acromion at its musculotendinous junction, and laterally at its tendinous insertion. A probe helps determine the degree of cuff involvement, especially when the cuff is partially torn. What type of treatment, if any, should be performed on the partially torn or fibrillated cuff remains unclear at this time. Some authors recommend débridement of partial-thickness tears down to bleeding muscle-tendon tissue.[2] The authors débride any partial tear to determine its extent and significance but remain unconvinced that such débridement serves any therapeutic purpose.

The arm may be disengaged from its suspension and moved to observe the site of cuff insertion and the relationship of this site to the acromial undersurface. Any remaining impingement should be definitively addressed at this time.

Instruments are removed, and the portals are closed with #3 nylon simple interrupted sutures followed by disconnection of the suspension apparatus and application of a sterile compressive dressing and a sling.

The available outcome studies have focused predominantly on nonathletes and, with few exceptions, have ignored the ability to return to preinjury level of activity. In the few reports that address an athlete's outcome after arthroscopic subacromial decompression, results are less favorable.[1,7,26,46]

In the largest reported series of athletes undergoing this procedure to date, Lowe and Tibone[26] reported on the outcome of a group of 79 patients, 71 of whom (90%) were actively involved in sports. Although 71% of all patients were rated satisfactory, only 54% of those under age 35 achieved this rating. Younger patients had a significantly worse result than those in the older group. Of the entire group, 68% returned to the same level of activity, 23% continued to play their sport but at a lower level, and 9% were unable to return. In closer analysis by sport, only two of five (40%) baseball pitchers, four of seven (57%) swimmers, and two of five (40%) volleyball players had a satisfactory result. Conversely, those involved in nonpitching baseball positions or racquet sports had a higher likelihood of return. Unrecognized subtle glenohumeral instability was the most common reason for failure in this series, with nearly half of the patients with unsatisfactory results having detectable instability at follow-up.

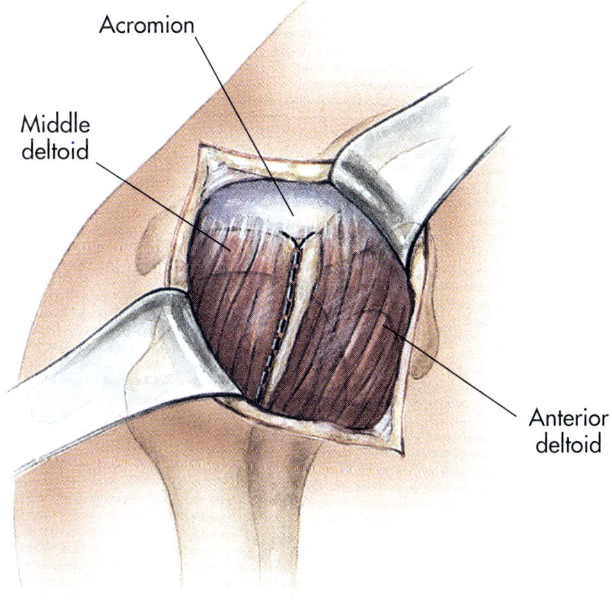

FIGURE 7-54 After an anterior "strap" incision is made between the AC joint and lateral acromion, the deltoid is split for 3 cm along the line of its fibers between the anterior and middle deltoid heads.

Open Subacromial Decompression Technique and Results

The surgical procedure is essentially the same as originally described by Neer in 1972,[36] with only a few minor modifications. Advantages of an open acromioplasty include a more thorough and reliable subacromial decompression with some surgeons, as well as direct tactile evaluation of the cuff. If torn, "the cuff can be better repaired through an open approach."[34]

Open acromioplasty may be performed in either the "beach chair" or lateral decubitus position, depending on the surgeon's preference. Because the authors usually perform an arthroscopic examination first, the procedure is preferably performed in the lateral decubitus position, using the Vacu-Pak (Olympic Medical, Seattle, WA) to maintain position. After carefully padding the downside extremity and placing an axillary roll (described in the preceding section on arthroscopic acromioplasty), the authors detach the affected extremity from the suspension overhead traction device and place a sterile stockinette over the hand and forearm such that the extremity is draped freely. If necessary, the shoulder and axilla are reprepared and draped, and 0.25% Marcaine with epinephrine is used to infiltrate the intended incision. An anterior saber ("strap") incision is made from the superior acromion midway between the AC joint and the lateral acromion and carried distally 5 cm from the anterior acromial edge (Fig. 7-54). Sharp dissection is performed subcutaneously, raising medial and lateral flaps and achieving hemostasis with electrocautery. The interval between the anterior and middle deltoid is developed but is split no more than 5 cm distal to the anterior acromion (to avoid damage to the axillary nerve). Electrocautery is used to subperiosteally elevate the deltoid-fascial attachment proximally along the anterior acromion, a "deltoid-on" approach, preserving continuity of the deltoid muscle fascia and trapezioacromial fascia. Occasionally, limited exposure mandates a "T" extension of the incision of the deltoid's anterior attachment, medially toward the AC joint and laterally to the anterolateral acromion. When detached in this manner, a sleeve of trapeziodeltoid fascia is left intact to facilitate secure deltoid reattachment.

A bursectomy is performed to facilitate exposure of the cuff, CA ligament, and undersurface of the distal clavicle and acromion. The surgeon then performs an acromioplasty using either a sagittal saw or an osteotome and resects the anteroinferior aspect of the acromion (Fig. 7-55). The surgeon then excises the osteotomized anterior acromial fragment along with its attached coracoacromial ligament, resecting the ligament from its coracoid attachment (Fig. 7-56). Care is taken to ensure that all bone anterior to the distal clavicle and AC joint is removed, along with any protruding osteophytes beneath the acromion and/or AC joint. The surgeon resects the AC joint at this time if clinically indicated, removing a sufficient amount to decompress the joint but preserving the coracoclavicular ligaments (usually 1 to 2 cm of distal clavicle). The surgeon confirms the absence of projecting osteophytes by finger palpation; a file may be helpful to smooth the acromial and distal clavicular undersurfaces and eliminate any potential for future cuff abrasion.

Having decompressed the arch, the surgeon now inspects the rotator cuff, which can be examined visually in its entirety by gentle manipulation of the arm. For

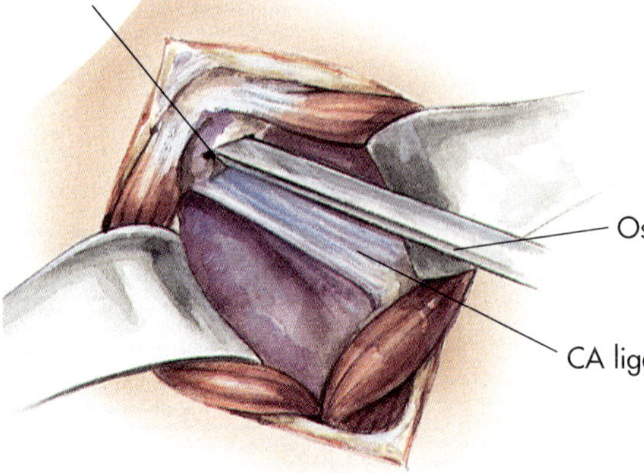

FIGURE 7-55 Through the deltoid split, the anteroinferior acromion is exposed and resected, here with an osteotome.

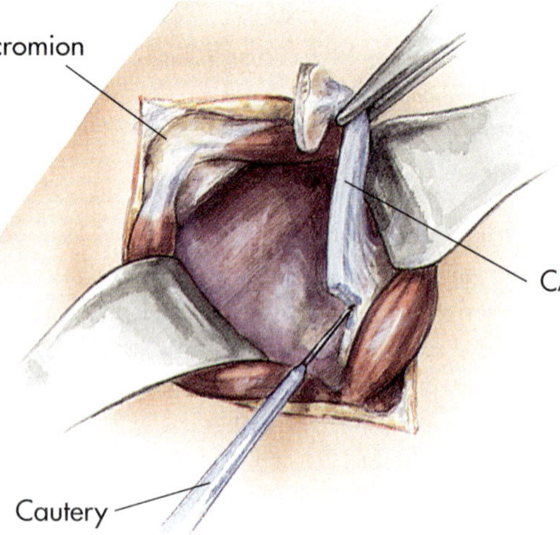

FIGURE 7-56 The CA ligament is resected, incised from its coracoid attachment, and removed with the excised acromion.

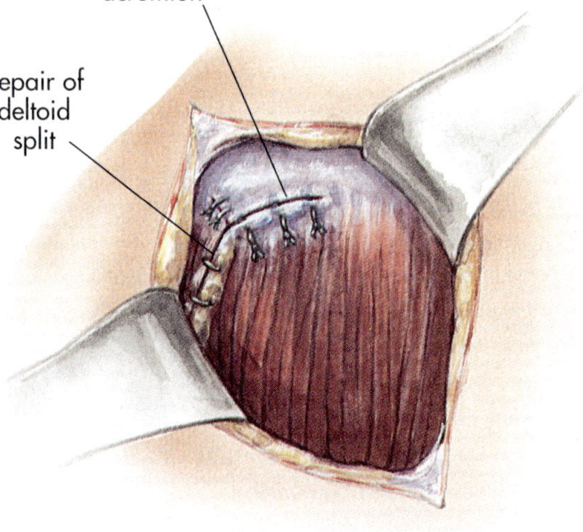

FIGURE 7-57 The deltoid is repaired with figure-of-eight sutures. If it is detached, it is reattached through drill holes to the anterior acromion.

definitive treatment of any identified partial- or full-thickness cuff tears, the reader is referred to the chapter on rotator cuff tears.

The wound is irrigated thoroughly, and attention is directed to deltoid repair (Fig. 7-57). If detached, the deltoid is repaired with #1 nonabsorbable suture on a cutting needle through drill holes in the anterior acromion. Vertical mattress sutures facilitate restoration of the normal deltoid attachment orientation and minimize impingement by pulling the deltoid onto the anterior, rather than the inferior, lip of the acromion. Several interrupted simple nonabsorbable sutures reapproximate the deltoid split. A sterile dressing is applied after wound closure, and an axillary pad is placed for comfort and hygiene. Finally, an arm sling is used for support and comfort.

Differences in patient selection (athletes, laborers, workers' compensation patients), mechanism of injury (acute, repetitive overuse), severity of symptoms (duration, nocturnal awakening, interference with activities), stage of disease, presence or absence of cuff tear (partial or full thickness), duration and type of nonoperative treatment, operative treatment itself (open, detachment, splitting deltoid [deltoid-on], resection of distal clavicle, débridement of cuff, deltoid repair quality, rehabilitation protocol), patient demands (activities of daily living versus professional major league pitcher), and rating system make outcome reports difficult to interpret.[23]

As in arthroscopic decompression studies, most outcome reports after open acromioplasty involve nonathletic populations. Nevertheless, anterior acromioplasty for impingement syndromes (stages I and II unresponsive to nonoperative care) in a nonathletic population generally has enjoyed a high rate of success.*

Of those studies in which athletes' outcomes were examined, results were less encouraging.[15,47,50] Of 41 recreational athletes undergoing open acromioplasty, only 27 (66%) were able to return to sports without any limitation by 3 years after surgery.[47]

Tibone et al published the only outcome study of a young (under 40 years old) group of athletes undergoing open acromioplasty for impingement.[50] This study included only patients with impingement unresponsive to conservative treatment for a minimum of 4 months and without evidence of cuff tear. Although 89% of the athletes were considered improved compared with their

*References 3, 5, 11, 14, 16, 34-36, 42, 43, 45, 47, 54.

preoperative status, the majority (76%) still had difficulties with throwing or overhead activity (pain, loss of velocity). The overall results were 43% good, 34% fair, and 23% poor. In the subset of patients involved in pitching and throwing, the results were even less satisfactory, with only four (22%) good, eight (44%) fair, and six (34%) poor results. Of the six swimmers' shoulders, four were fair and two were poor results. The only group that had uniformly good results was the tennis players, all four of whom had good results. Because none of these cases were preceded by arthroscopic examination, the incidence of underlying instability is not known, but in this throwing population, underlying instability undoubtedly would explain the poor results in treatment. In conclusion, Tibone et al noted that "surgical decompression of the coracoacromial arch is satisfactory for pain relief but commonly does not allow an athlete to return to his former competitive status."[50]

Open Versus Arthroscopic Acromioplasty

Currently only two reported studies have compared outcomes of open with arthroscopic acromioplasty,[27,52] with both studies finding superior results in arthroscopic acromioplasty. However, neither study was randomized or prospective, and the number of athletes and the rate of their return to activity were not given. The procedure with which the surgeon feels more comfortable will likely be the most effective.

Postoperative Rehabilitation

The specific postoperative rehabilitation to be prescribed depends on several considerations, including the type of surgery (arthroscopic or open), the nature of the deltoid repair (if detached), the extent of preoperative disability (stiffness, weakness), and the individual patient's goals. Given this caveat against routine "cookbook" prescription orders, there are several principles of postoperative therapy. These are summarized as (1) minimizing inflammation, including that induced by the "trauma" of surgery; (2) restoring or maintaining active and assistive range of motion of the operative extremity's hand, wrist, and elbow immediately after surgery; (3) restoring or maintaining shoulder range of motion as quickly as possible beginning with Codman's passive-assistive pendulum exercises on the first postoperative day and advancing accordingly; (4) progressing to strengthening exercises; (5) restoring scapulohumeral rhythm; and finally (6) returning to activities in planes above the horizontal in the "impingement arc."

The specific rehabilitation protocol employed after subacromial decompression is discussed in detail elsewhere. The following discussion highlights the differences in protocol in arthroscopic techniques versus open techniques. These differences in protocol are the result of technical considerations clinicians need to evaluate.

Arthroscopic Protocol

The primary advantage of the arthroscopic technique is preservation of the deltoid muscle origins, which allows early rehabilitation and earlier return to activities and, for the athlete, competition. Deltoid preservation allows almost immediate unrestricted activities, limited only by patient symptoms. Therefore the authors encourage active use of the arm as soon as the patient is comfortable. Patients squeeze a ball or putty to maintain hand and wrist strength. They are instructed in active elbow exercises. Although slings are applied in the recovery room, patients are encouraged to discard them as soon as they are comfortable, usually within the first postoperative week. In addition to a narcotic analgesic for pain, a steroidal antiinflammatory medication is very helpful if patients tolerate it and have no gastrointestinal contraindications. Patients begin a postoperative rehabilitation program the first day after surgery, emphasizing restoration of range of motion through active and assistive exercises in addition to isometric strengthening of the deltoid and rotator cuff. Patients begin progressive strengthening of the rotator cuff and scapular rotators using either surgical tubing or light weights during the second postoperative week and increase as tolerated. Patients generally begin progressive resistive exercises and incorporate isokinetic and eccentric strengthening exercises the fourth postoperative week. A return to activities of daily living is encouraged as tolerated. Return to sport-specific retraining begins with restoration of normal active motion, including scapulohumeral rhythm, strength of the deltoid, and rotator cuff and scapular stabilizers that are comparable to the opposite normal side (90%). In addition, there must be no pain in the overhead position (or the usual position for performing sport activity). Athletes generally do not return to repetitive overhead activities before the sixth postoperative week.

Open Protocol

The open acromioplasty postoperative protocol is in theory identical to the arthroscopic protocol, but because of the limited deltoid detachment, some precautions are required in activities that could compromise the repair. Specifically, care is taken to avoid deltoid compromise during active forward flexion or elevation. Thus the patient is not permitted to actively forward flex, abduct, elevate, or strengthen the anterior and middle deltoid for 6 weeks after surgery. Such precautions limit the possible rehabilitation and may indicate the most significant advantage of the arthroscopic technique. With a "deltoid-on" approach, the decreased likelihood of detachment may facilitate a more aggressive rehabilitation program.

SUMMARY

Since the term was originally coined by Neer, *impingement* has proven a useful concept in the treatment of patients with anterior shoulder pain. Despite overall good results in the nonoperative management of older patients with impingement, however, younger athletes treated through either nonoperative or operative techniques have not enjoyed comparable satisfactory results.

Impingement in athletes appears to occur in two distinct clinical populations. In the older athlete, impingement appears to be subacromial, as described by Neer, occurring as a result of mechanical cuff compression under the coracoacromial arch with repetitive overhead activity. In the younger athlete, impingement most commonly is due to underlying glenohumeral instability, with progressive functional fatigue or structural attenuation of the static capsular restraints and secondary impingement on the posterior rim of the glenoid. Evaluation and treatment of impingement depend on the careful selection of patients to obtain maximal benefit from the treatment prescribed.

References

1. Altchek DW et al: Arthroscopic acromioplasty, *J Bone Joint Surg* 72A:1198-1207, 1990.
2. Andrews JR, Broussard TS, Carson WG: Arthroscopy of the shoulder in the management of partial tears of the rotator cuff: a preliminary report, *Arthroscopy* 1:117, 1985.
3. Bigliani LU et al: Anterior acromioplasty for subacromial impingement in patients under forty years of age, *Clin Orthop* 246:112-116, 1989.
4. Bigliani LU, Morrison DS, April EW: The morphology of the acromion and its relationship to rotator cuff tears, *Orthop Trans* 10:228, 1986.
5. Bjorkenheim JM, Paavolainen PA, Juhani ASP: Subacromial impingement decompressed with anterior acromioplasty, *Clin Orthop* 252:150-155, 1990.
6. Brewer DBN: Aging of the rotator cuff, *Am J Sports Med* 7:102-110, 1979.
7. Burns TP, Turba JE: Arthroscopic treatment of shoulder impingement in athletes, *Am J Sports Med* 20(1)13-16, 1992.
8. DePalma AF: Biologic aging of the shoulder. In Pederson D, editor: *Surgery of the shoulder,* ed 3, Philadelphia, 1983, JB Lippincott.
9. DePalma AF: Injuries of the shoulder in sports. In: *Surgery of the shoulder,* ed 3, Philadelphia, 1983, JB Lippincott.
10. Ellman H: Diagnosis and treatment of incomplete rotator cuff tears, *Clin Orthop* 254:64-74, 1990.
11. Ellman H: Shoulder arthroscopy: current indications and techniques, *Orthopaedics* 11:45, 1988.
12. Ellman H: *Arthroscopic subacromial decompression: a preliminary report,* presented at the First Open Meeting of the American Shoulder and Elbow Surgeons, Las Vegas, Nev, Jan 23, 1985.
13. Gerber C, Schneeberger AG, Vinh TS: The arterial vascularization of the humeral head: an anatomical study, *J Bone Joint Surg* 72A: 1486-1494, 1990.
14. Hawkins RJ et al: Acromioplasty for impingement with an intact rotator cuff, *J Bone Joint Surg* 70B:795-797, 1988.
15. Hawkins RJ, Brock RM: Anterior acromioplasty: early results for impingement with intact rotator cuffs, *Orthop Trans* 3:274, 1979.
16. Hawkins RJ, Kennedy JC: Impingement syndrome in athletes, *Am J Sports Med* 8:151-158, 1980.
17. Janda DH, Loubert P: A preventative program focusing on the glenohumeral joint in basic science and clinical application, *Athlete's Shoulder Clin Sports Med* 10(4):955-971, 1971.
18. Jobe FW, Ling B: The shoulder in sports. In Post M, editor: *The shoulder: surgical and nonsurgical management,* ed 2, Philadelphia, 1988, Lea & Febiger.
19. Jobe FW, Moynes DR: Delineation of diagnostic criteria and a rehabilitation program for rotator cuff injuries, *Am J Sports Med* 10(6):336-339, 1982.
20. Kennedy JC, Willis RB: The effects of local steroid injections on tendons: a biomechanical and microscopic correlative study, *Am J Sports Med* 4:11-21, 1976.
21. Kessel L: *Clinical disorders of the shoulder,* Edinburgh, 1982, Churchill Livingstone.
22. Leach RE: The impingement syndrome. In Zarins B, Andrews JR, Carson WG, editors: *Injuries to the throwing arm,* Philadelphia, 1985, WB Saunders.
23. Lirette R, Morin F, Kinnard P: The difficulties in assessment of results in anterior acromioplasty, *Clin Orthop* 278:14-16, 1992.
24. Loehr JF, Uhthoff HK: The microvascular pattern of supraspinatus tendon, *Clin Orthop* 254:35-38, 1990.
25. Loehr JF, Uhthoff HK: The pathogenesis of degenerative rotator cuff tears, *Orthop Trans* 11(2):237, 1987 (presented to the American Shoulder and Elbow Surgeons, Jan, 1987).
26. Lowe WR, Tibone JE: Arthroscopic acromioplasty: long-term results, submitted to *J Shoulder Elbow Surg,* 1992.
27. Lucie S, Hardy P, Hopkins RD: A comparison of arthroscopic anterior acromioplasty vs open anterior acromioplasty for the treatment of subacromial impingement syndrome, *Orthop Trans* 15(1):61, 1991 (presented to the Eastern Orthopedic Association Oct, 1991).
28. McMaster WC, Liddle S, Waugh TR: Laboratory evaluation of various cold therapy modalities, *Am J Sports Med* 6:291-294, 1978.
29. Morrison DS, Bigliani LU: The clinical significance of variations in acromial morphology, *Orthop Trans* 11:234, 1987 (presented to the American Shoulder and Elbow Surgeons, Jan, 1987).
30. Morrison DS, Schaefer RK: Relationship between subacromial space pressure, blood pressure and visual clarity during arthroscopic subacromial decompression, *Orthop Trans* 14(3):564, 1990 (presented to the American Academy of Orthopaedic Surgeons, Feb, 1990).
31. Moseley HF, Goldie I: The arterial pattern of the rotator cuff, *J Bone Joint Surg* 45B:780, 1963.
32. Moynes DR: Prevention of injury to the shoulder through exercises and therapy, Symposium on Injuries to the Shoulder in the Athlete, *Clin Sports Med* 2(2):413-422, 1963.
33. Mudge MK, Wood VE, Frykman GK: Rotator cuff tears associated with os acromiale, *J Bone Joint Surg* 66A:427-429, 1984.
34. Neer CS II: *Shoulder reconstruction,* 1990, Philadelphia, WB Saunders.
35. Neer CS II: Impingement lesions, *Clin Orthop* 173:170, 1983.
36. Neer CS II: Anterior acromioplasty for the chronic impingement syndrome in the shoulder: a preliminary report, *J Bone Joint Surg* 54A:41-50, 1972.
37. Neer CS II et al: The relationship between the unfused acromial epiphysis and subacromial impingement lesions, *Orthop Trans* 7:138, 1983.
38. Ogata S, Uhthoff HK: Acromial enthesopathy and rotator cuff tear: a radiologic and histologic post mortem investigation of the coracoacromial arch, *Clin Orthop* 254:39-48, 1990.
39. Paulos LE, Franklin JL: Arthroscopic shoulder decompression development and application: a five year experience, *Am J Sports Med* 18:235-244, 1990.
40. Perry J: Anatomy and biomechanics of the shoulder in throwing, swimming, gymnastics, and tennis, Symposium on Injuries to the Shoulder in the Athlete, *Clin Sports Med* 2:247-270, 1983.
41. Poppen NK, Walker PS: Normal and abnormal motion of the shoulder, *J Bone Joint Surg* 58A:195, 1976.

42. Post M, Cohen J: Impingement syndrome: a review of late stage II and early stage III lesions, *Clin Orthop* 207:126-132, 1986.
43. Raggio CL, Warren RF, Sculco T: Surgical treatment of impingement syndrome: four year follow-up, *Orthop Trans* 9:58, 1985.
44. Rathbun JB, MacNab I: The microvascular pattern of the rotator cuff, *J Bone Joint Surg* 52B:540, 1970.
45. Rockwood CA, Lyons FR: Surgical treatment of the shoulder impingement syndrome: a modification of the Neer anterior acromioplasty in 71 shoulders, *Orthop Trans* 14(2):251, 1990 (presented to the American Shoulder and Elbow Society, Feb, 1990).
46. Speer KP, Lohnes J, Garrett WE: Arthroscopic subacromial decompression: results in advanced stage II impingement syndrome, *Orthop Trans* 14(2):246, 1990 (presented to the American Orthopaedic Society for Sports Medicine, June, 1989).
47. Stuart MJ, Azevedo AJ, Cofield RH: Anterior acromioplasty for treatment of the shoulder impingement syndrome, *Clin Orthop* 260: 195-200, 1990.
48. Swiontkowski MF: Intraoperative assessment of rotator cuff vascularity using laser Doppler flowmetry. In Post M, Morrey BF, Hawkins RJ, editors: *Surgery of the shoulder,* St Louis, 1990, Mosby-Year Book.
49. Tada H et al: Microvascular study of a human rotator cuff of the shoulder: the shoulder joint, *Jpn Shoulder Sox* 10:1-4, 1986.
50. Tibone JE et al: Shoulder impingement syndrome in athletes treated by an anterior acromioplasty, *Clin Orthop* 188:134-140, 1985.
51. Uhthoff HK, Sarkar K: Classification and definition of tendinopathies, basic science and clinical application in the athlete's shoulder, *Clin Sports Med* 10(4):707-720, 1991.
52. Van Holsbeeck E, De Rijcke J, Declercq G: Subacromial impingement—open vs arthroscopic decompression, *Orthop Trans* 14(3): 659, 1990 (presented to the American Orthopaedic Association, June, 1990).
53. Watson KC, Corbitt DK: Conservative treatment of subacromial impingement, *Orthop Trans* 11(1):173, 1987 (presented to the Clinical Orthopaedic Society, Oct, 1987).
54. Watson M: Rotator cuff function in the impingement syndrome, *J Bone Joint Surg* [Br] 71B:361-366, 1989.
55. Zuckerman JD et al. The influence of coracoacromial arch anatomy on rotator cuff tears, *J Shoulder Elbow Surg* 1:4-14, 1992.

SECTION E Rotator Cuff Tear: Clinical Assessment and Treatment

INTRODUCTION AND PHILOSOPHY

Well beyond the age of 40, athletes are actively participating in competitive and recreational sports. The repetitive overhead use of the arm required in many of these sports, such as baseball, softball, tennis, and swimming, depends on the integrity and function of a normal rotator cuff. Although asymptomatic rotator cuff tears have been noted in individuals past the age of 40,[80,81] it is unlikely that those individuals were athletes engaged in sport activities. If the rotator cuff of an athlete is torn, shoulder function will inevitably be impaired.

In the younger athletic population, particularly throwing athletes, our understanding of the incidence and etiology of rotator cuff tears continues to evolve.

The nonsurgical "repair" of a partial rotator cuff tear by proper rehabilitation is certainly preferred over surgical intervention whenever possible. Although some physicians have recommended nonsurgical care for the management of complete cuff tears, this chapter will emphasize the need to restore normal rotator cuff function to provide athletes with the ability to return to their sport, which usually will mandate early surgical repair when a full-thickness rotator cuff tear is identified. When surgery is necessary, the mechanism by which the tear has occurred should be determined, and the normal anatomy should be restored as closely as possible. Finally, a well-supervised postoperative rehabilitation program is critical to the patient's successful recovery.

DYNAMIC FUNCTION OF THE ROTATOR CUFF

The musculotendinous rotator cuff plays two important dynamic roles in shoulder function: (1) stabilization of the humeral head within the glenoid fossa and (2) rotation of the humerus. Looked at simply, the stabilization and positioning of the humeral head in the glenoid are accomplished by the action of several major balanced muscle force couples.* Balance of these force couples achieves an equilibrium that maintains the fulcrum of the humeral head centered within the glenoid (Fig. 7-58). Although many other factors are involved, this equilibrium will be lost when the rotator cuff is damaged or torn.

Providing or resisting internal and external rotation of the humerus throughout the full range of shoulder motion is the second function of the rotator cuff. Internal rotation of the humerus on the glenoid by the subscapularis muscle is assisted by the pectoralis major, teres major, and latissimus dorsi muscles. On the other hand, 80% of humeral external rotation strength is attributed to the infraspinatus muscle.[75,82,94] Active external rotation is mandatory for functional overhead use of the arm, and it is essential in almost all sports.[26,75] Although a symptomatic athlete may be able temporarily to continue participation in sports with a torn supraspinatus tendon, extension of the tear into the infraspinatus tendon will dramatically impair shoulder function and compromise an athlete's athletic performance.

*References 5, 15, 26, 46, 49, 75.

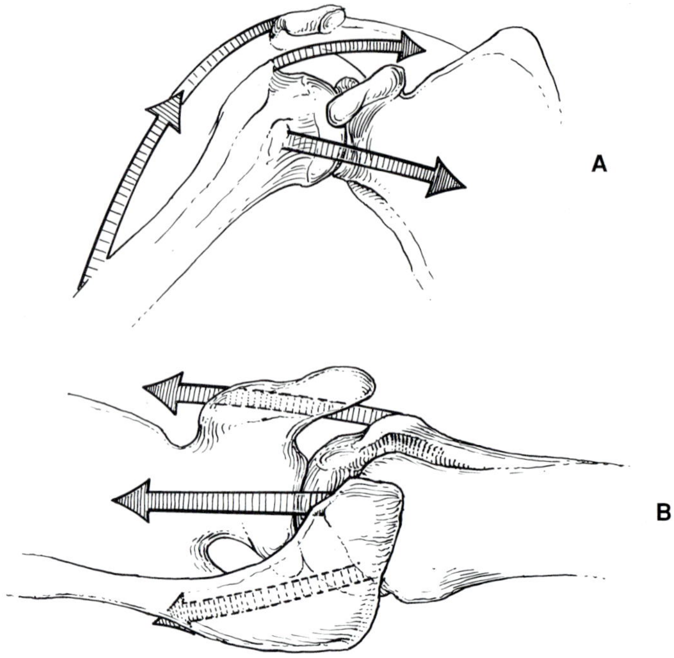

FIGURE 7-58 Diagrams of the balanced muscular force couples created by the rotator cuff that center the fulcrum of the glenohumeral joint on the glenoid. **A,** The vector forces in the coronal plane. **B,** The vector forces in the transverse plane.

CLASSIFICATION

Many classifications for rotator cuff tears have been reported. Tears often are divided by the duration of symptoms into acute tears, chronic tears, and chronic tears with an acute extension. The American Shoulder and Elbow Surgeons classification describes the extent of the tear by the size of the defect: small tears, less than 1 cm; medium tears, 1 to 3 cm; large tears, 3 to 5 cm; and massive tears, greater than 5 cm. Cuff tears often are further described based on the thickness of the tear (full or partial thickness) and the shape of the tear (transverse, linear, L-shaped, triangular, or crescent)[27,30] (Fig. 7-59). Massive tears usually are described by the size of the defect and the number of tendons involved[9] (Fig. 7-60).

Partial-thickness rotator cuff tears are classified anatomically as articular surface, intratendinous, and bursal surface. Rotator cuff tears found during arthroscopy have been classified based on the depth of the tear as A (articular surface partial tear), B (bursal surface partial tear), or C (complete-thickness tear) and further described by the size of the tear (grade 0 to 4).[92]

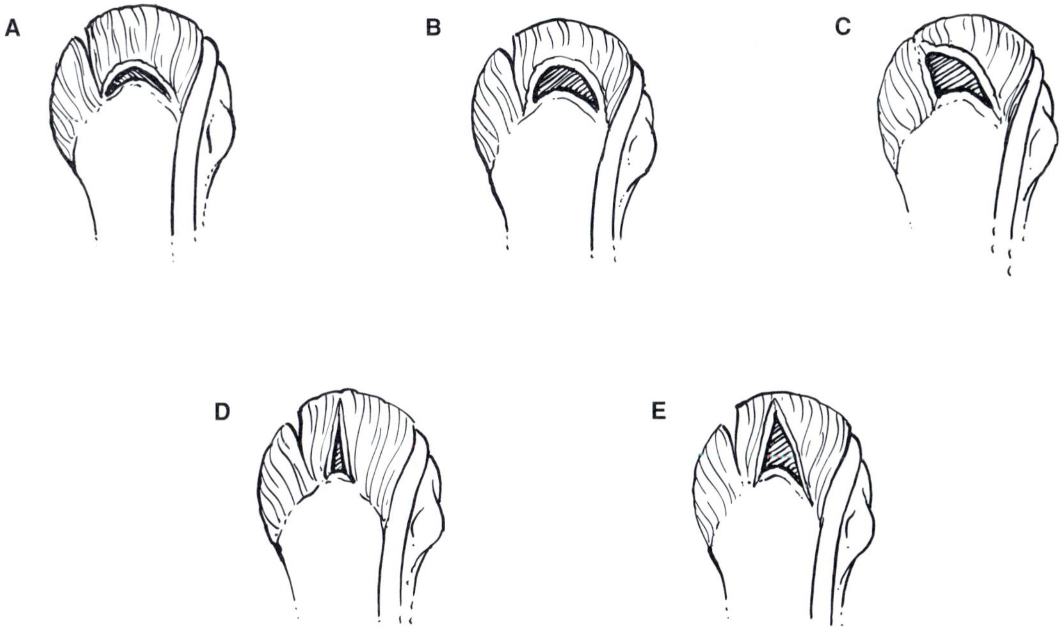

FIGURE 7-59 Diagram of the pattern variation of rotator cuff tears. **A,** Transverse-shaped tear, **B,** crescent-shaped tear, **C,** L-shaped tear, **D,** linear-shaped tear in line with the tendon fibers, and **E,** triangular-shaped tear.

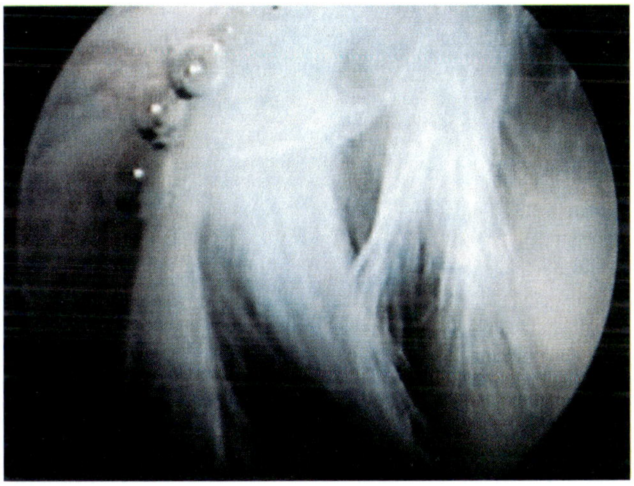

FIGURE 7-60 An articular surface partial-thickness rotator cuff tear involving the superior margin of the infraspinatus tendon

The authors document the tendons involved, the depth of the tear, the extent of the tear, the quality of the remaining tendon tissue, the condition of the long head of the biceps, and the ability to advance the tendons to their original insertion sites. Further, the authors classify the mechanism of injury to the cuff as follows: tears secondary to primary outlet impingement, tears associated with occult instability, tears after direct trauma, tears after acute dislocations, and tears caused by degenerative change.

INCIDENCE

The incidence of complete rotator cuff tears found in cadaveric studies has been reported as high as 20% to 26%.[5,101] This has led some authors to conclude that asymptomatic, unrecognized cuff tears are prevalent in the active general population, and therefore many patients with documented tears should be able to recover without surgical repair.

In contrast, clinical studies have shown that complete tears rarely occur in individuals less than 40 years of age.[9,10,30,45] The incidence of tears found in cadaveric studies increases significantly with age, and, accordingly, the higher the average age of the cadaveric specimens, the higher the expected incidence of complete tears.[30,36,45,75] The average age of most cadaveric specimens is much higher than the average age of the active general population.[75,80] Finally, several large cadaveric studies have reported the incidence of complete tears at only 7%.[36,37,75] Complete, full-thickness cuff tears in active individuals, particularly those involved in sports that demand normal shoulder function, probably will almost always become symptomatic.

In a series of 249 cadaveric shoulder dissections, partial-thickness cuff tears have been identified in 33 (13%) with intratendinous lesions found more frequently than bursal-side or articular-side lesions.[37] Others have reported a similar incidence of partial-thickness rotator cuff tears[74,75] and have demonstrated that the frequency of partial tears increases with age.[97]

Recently, arthroscopy,[1,2,38,92] and magnetic resonance imaging[14] have brought attention to partial tears occurring in young overhead athletes. The occurrence of partial-thickness cuff tears in young athletes is now well accepted.

MECHANISM OF INJURY

Age and Cuff Tear Pathogenesis

The pathomechanics of shoulder problems in young athletes (less than 35 years of age) differs from that of older athletes (more than 35 years of age). Therefore two separate subgroups should be considered when evaluating an athlete for a possible rotator cuff injury.[52,53,55-59] In the younger age group, impingement and partial or complete rotator cuff tears usually occur as a result of occult anterior shoulder instability and secondary impingement of the articular side of the cuff along the posterosuperior rim of the glenoid.[50,55,56] Primary "supraspinatus outlet" impingement and degenerative disease are still thought to be responsible for many rotator cuff problems in the older age group.[10,55,69,72,75]

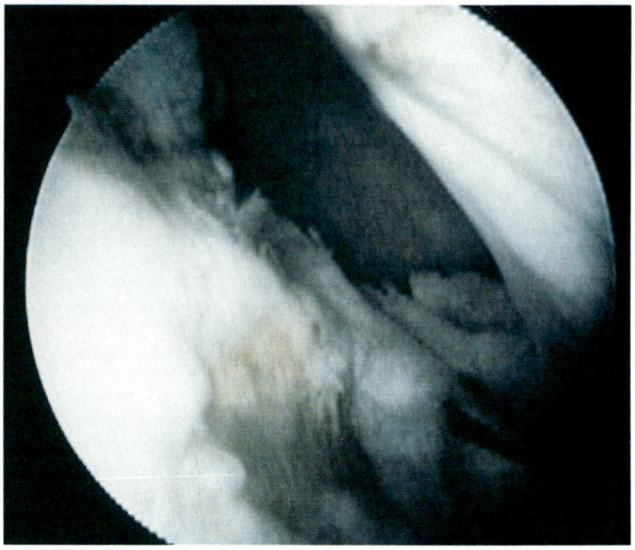

FIGURE 7-61 This 2-cm full-thickness rotator cuff tear in the nondominant arm of a 27-year-old professional baseball shortstop occurred when he fell on the point of his shoulder while diving for a ground ball.

Under 35 Years

Full-thickness rotator cuff tears rarely occur in patients less than 40 years of age[9,10,30,45,72]; however, arthroscopy and magnetic resonance imaging have demonstrated that partial-thickness tears are relatively common in the young throwing athlete with shoulder pain.[1,2,14,38,92] The mechanism by which partial-thickness rotator cuff tears occur in the younger population is probably multifactorial and is still not completely understood. However, current understanding does imply that any process that weakens the stabilizing capsular ligaments or significantly alters the force couple produced by the normal rotator cuff muscles will result in abnormal anterior humeral head translation on the glenoid. This may then lead to injury in the cuff by impingement of the articular surface of the cuff along the posterior superior glenoid rim[50,55] when the arm is angulated posteriorly (see Fig. 7-60).

Because of the repetitious, high-velocity, chronic, mechanical stress placed on the shoulder, the overhead athlete is at considerable risk for rotator cuff injuries.[56] Although several explanations for this increased risk have been reported, the most likely is the occurrence of a cascade of events caused by the stress applied to the anterior shoulder during overhead activities. Repetitive microtrauma occurring within the stabilizing anterior capsular ligaments may result in microscopic tears and eventually, attenuation of the ligaments and capsule. This leads to occult anterior subluxation (instability) of the humeral head on the glenoid during the late cocking and acceleration phases of throwing.[55,56] In this setting, impingement is thought to occur along the upper one third of the posterior glenoid.[50] This concept has been referred to as the internal impingement and is discussed in detail in preceding chapters.

Outlet impingement was formerly considered the primary cause of impingement and rotator cuff tears in the young throwing athlete.[69,72] It is now recognized that this mechanism occurs much less frequently than previously thought if at all. Tibone et al. reported the results of open acromioplasty and rotator cuff repair in 45 athletes who were less than 40 years of age. Only 56% were able to return to their previous level of sport participation without pain.[95] Unrecognized instability in this young athletic population probably accounted for such poor results.

Rarely, direct major trauma, such as a hard fall on the outstretched arm or onto the point of the shoulder, may compress the cuff tendons against the acromion forcefully enough to cause an acute tear of the cuff tendons (Fig. 7-61). Less severe trauma produces acute traumatic subacromial bursitis and may eventually lead to thickening of the bursa, persistent outlet impingement, and eventually a small tear in the rotator cuff.[69,75,94] Major trauma more commonly causes tuberosity fractures, glenohumeral joint dislocations, and acromioclavicular joint separations.

Over 35 Years

Even though occult instability must still be considered, in an athlete over 35 years of age, a rotator cuff tear will more likely be due to chronic outlet impingement. This condition is characterized by a narrowed supraspinatus outlet and impingement of the bursal surface of the cuff tendons along the anterior edge of the acromion.[21,72,75,87]

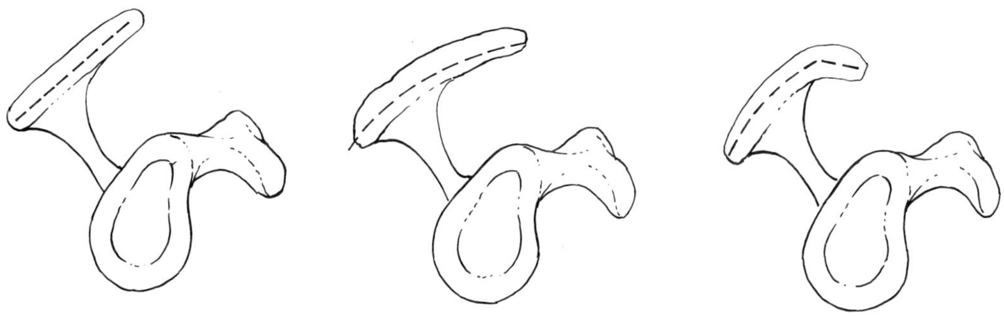

FIGURE 7-62 Variations of acromial morphology. Type I is flat, type II is curved, and type III is hooked.

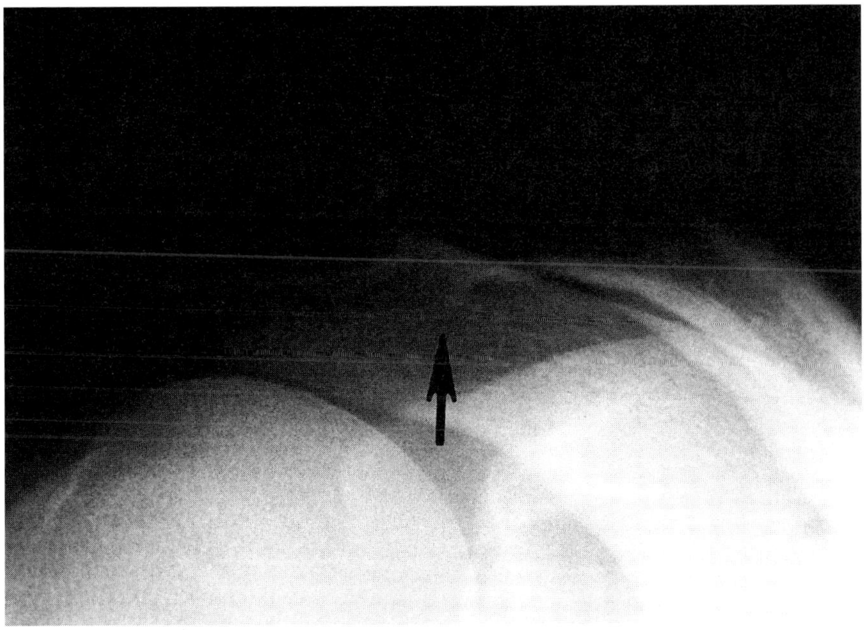

FIGURE 7-63 Radiograph of a distally pointing acromioclavicular joint osteophyte.

Outlet factors, which cause narrowing of the supraspinatus outlet beneath the coracoacromial arch, and nonoutlet factors, which influence the impingement process by methods other than narrowing of the outlet, have been classified and are discussed in preceding chapters.[71,75]

Attrition,[63] ischemia,[17,18,20,67,05] trauma,[19,69,75,94] occupation,[19,20,68] and sport[7,10,78,95,96] also have been shown to contribute to outlet impingement and rotator cuff tears.

The variable anatomic shape and tilt of the acromion have been well described by several authors[3,11,104] and are separated into three types: type I is flat, type II is curved, and type III is hooked[11] (Fig. 7-62). Rotator cuff tears were most commonly identified with the type III acromion and a low-angle acromial tilt.[11,104] An association between distally pointing acromioclavicular osteophytes and complete tears of the supraspinatus tendon also has been demonstrated[80] (Fig. 7-63).

Rotator cuff tears begin with failure of the tendon fibers near the articular surface of the cuff adjacent to the tendon insertion on the tuberosity.[20,37,47,63,75] As fibers fail, greater stress is borne by adjacent fibers. This leads to further fiber failure as the cycle persists. Loss of fiber attachment decreases muscle strength and allows proximal head migration. Impingement wear disrupts more fibers. The relatively poor vascular supply is further diminished, weakening the remaining fibers and leading to additional fiber failure.[63] These attritional and ischemic changes eventually may lead to small complete tears. Most large tears will subsequently develop from an acute extension within this compromised tissue.[9,30,45,63,75] Ultimately, even minor trauma is capable of creating a massive tear.

The Biceps Tendon

The long head of the biceps tendon originates on the supraglenoid tubercle and passes beneath the rotator interval and the transverse humeral ligament into the bicipital groove. Because the biceps tendon and the up-

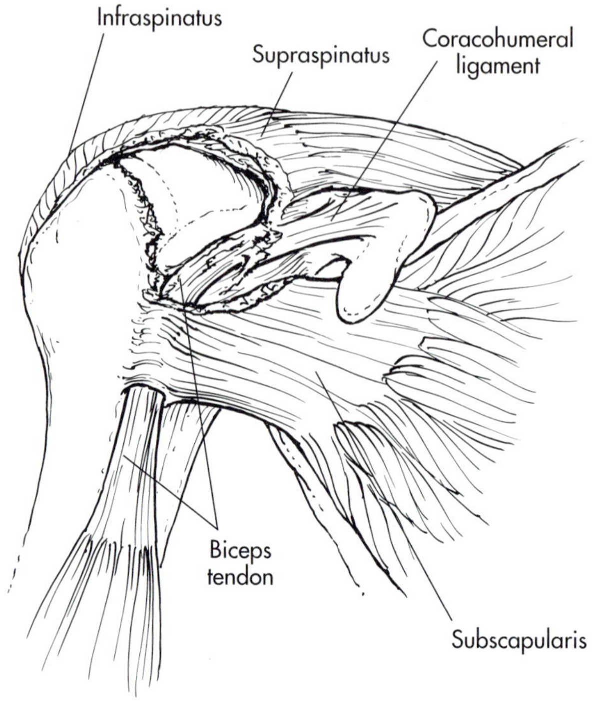

FIGURE 7-64 A massive rotator cuff tear involving the subscapularis, supraspinatus, and infraspinatus muscle tendons. There is retraction of the supraspinatus tendon, subluxation of the biceps tendon, and contraction of the coracohumeral ligament.

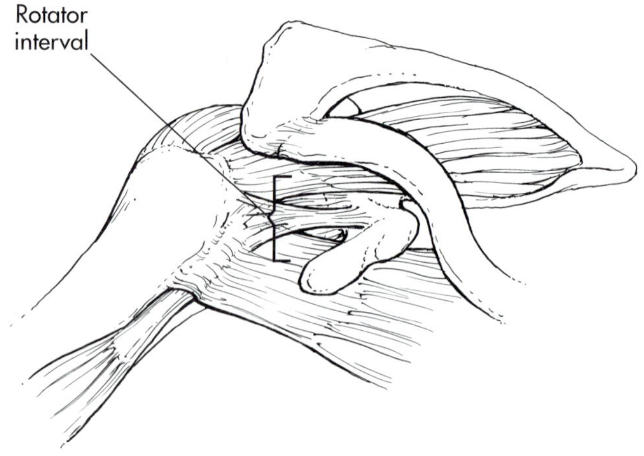

FIGURE 7-65 The rotator interval between the subscapularis tendon and supraspinatus tendon contains the coracohumeral ligament and the superior joint capsule.

per portion of the bicipital groove pass under the coracoacromial arch within the "impingement zone" during forward flexion of the humerus, flattening, fraying, or rupture of the tendon may occur secondary to the same chronic impingement process that results in rotator cuff tears.[73,75] Hypertrophy of the tendon often is noted in the presence of cuff tears and probably occurs to compensate for the loss of the depressor function of the cuff tendons.[20] When the biceps tendon ruptures, it may retract distally, completely, partially, or not at all. Biceps tendon subluxation and dislocation are extremely rare but may be seen in older patients with large cuff tears that include the upper subscapularis tendon and the transverse humeral ligament[75] (Fig. 7-64).

The Rotator Interval

No tendinous fibers are present within the "rotator interval" located between the subscapularis and the supraspinatus tendons. However, the coracohumeral ligament, the joint capsule, and portions of the superior glenohumeral ligament, which all provide support for the rotator interval, are susceptible to injury[17,18,75,79] (Fig. 7-65). Tears occurring within this interval usually are associated with anterior instability.[75] A "ballooning-out enlargement" of the rotator interval has been seen in javelin throwers with multidirectional glenohumeral instability. In the older athlete after an acute glenohumeral dislocation, rotator interval injuries have been observed as longitudinal tears in the interval occasionally associated with small tears in the upper subscapularis tendon.[75]

Two types of injuries involving the rotator interval have been described.[79] Type 1 results in contraction of the interval and loss of shoulder motion after a superficial injury and subsequent inflammation. Type 2 results in glenohumeral instability caused by complete separation of the deeper layers of the interval. Although our understanding of problems of the rotator interval has improved, there is still much to be explained.

CLINICAL PRESENTATION

History

The evaluation of the athlete with a possible rotator cuff injury must begin with a precise and detailed history. Age profoundly influences the etiology of cuff tears in athletes and should be noted early. The examiner also must consider any previous history of "bursitis," "tendinitis," stiffness, trauma, dislocation, the duration of recent symptoms, the type and duration of any previous treatment (including the number of prior steroid injections), the demands of the patient's occupation or sport on the involved shoulder, and the impairment caused by the presenting symptoms (e.g., change in the athlete's recent performance).

The most common presenting complaints from athletes with rotator cuff injuries are pain at rest, painful motion, crepitation, weakness, and decreased performance.[7,56,69] Pain with activity is noted with either cuff tendinitis or cuff tears, but pain at night is considered a hallmark of a complete tear. Traditionally, the pain is vaguely located in the anterior shoulder and may radiate to the lateral arm. Frequently, the athlete can precisely recount the activity that causes pain. Throwing and overhead athletes with occult instability and secondary rotator cuff injuries typically experience pain in the posterior aspect of the glenohumeral joint during the late cocking and acceleration phases of motion.[56] Forceful abduction and overhead reaching will be painful in athletes with traumatic tears resulting from collision sports.

The athlete may describe crepitation deep in the anterior shoulder when the arm is elevated and the supraspinatus tendon passes under the anterior edge of the acromion. A painful catch or "jog" may lead the examiner to suspect a tear in the supraspinatus tendon; however, this sign is not reliable and may be caused by thickened subacromial bursa.

Weakness may or may not be present, depending on the location and extent of the tear. When the infraspinatus tendon becomes torn, the athlete will report a dramatic loss of shoulder function both at the side and overhead (e.g., a tennis player may be unable to hit a backhand stroke, reach for a forehand stroke, or serve overhead because of the loss of external rotation strength). Classically, active range of motion is impaired while passive motion is preserved when a complete cuff tear is present. However, stiffness is common in the presence of a partial-thickness tear, particularly when the bursal side is involved.[35,75]

Acute full-thickness tears in the young athlete are small and usually follow major trauma, such as a fall on the shoulder or a direct blow in collision sports.[7,75] Clinical examination may be unreliable. Loss of strength and function may be immediate and dramatic, or performance may be minimally affected initially. As secondary impingement and bursitis develop from local inflammation and the loss of adequate humeral head depression, performance becomes impaired.

Special Imaging Studies

This chapter emphasizes early surgical repair of full-thickness rotator cuff tears in athletes. This mandates early conclusive evaluation of the cuff when proper rehabilitation evaluation fails to produce significant improvement of symptoms in 6 weeks. Although the presence of a complete tear may be suspected after a thorough examination, a special imaging study, such as arthrography, ultrasonography, magnetic resonance imaging, and arthroscopy, often is required to confirm the diagnosis.

Shoulder arthrography is still considered the gold standard and may be performed with single and double contrast or combined with plain or computed tomography (Fig. 7-66). With single- and double-contrast arthrography, sensitivity is reported between 87% and 100%.[45,63,66,83] Cuff tear size may be closely estimated, providing useful data for preoperative planning.[25,41,43]

Ultrasonography is of little value in documenting partial-thickness cuff tears[12,23,66]; however, it may become a useful noninvasive screening tool for evaluating athletes suspected of having a full-thickness tear.[12,65] Unfortunately, the recent results in the community setting have not duplicated the results from major centers.[23,66]

Magnetic resonance imaging is very sensitive and specific for both partial- and full-thickness cuff tears,[33,47,103] and has the ability to document musculotendinous retraction, muscular atrophy, acromial morphology, acromial and clavicular osteophytes, and acromioclavicular capsular hypertrophy[47,89] (Fig. 7-67). The

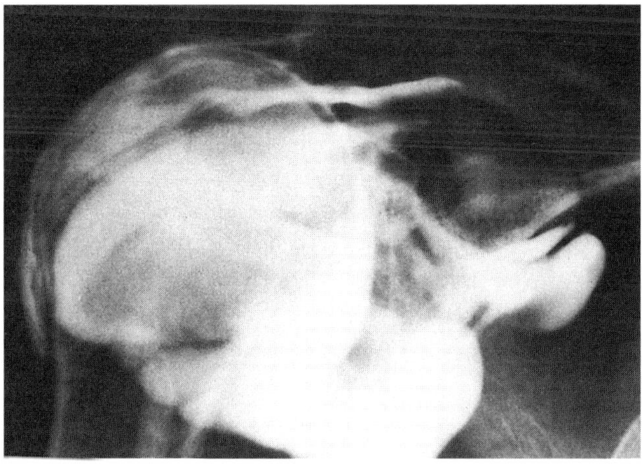

FIGURE 7-66 Single-contrast arthrographic radiography demonstrating a massive full-thickness rotator cuff tear.

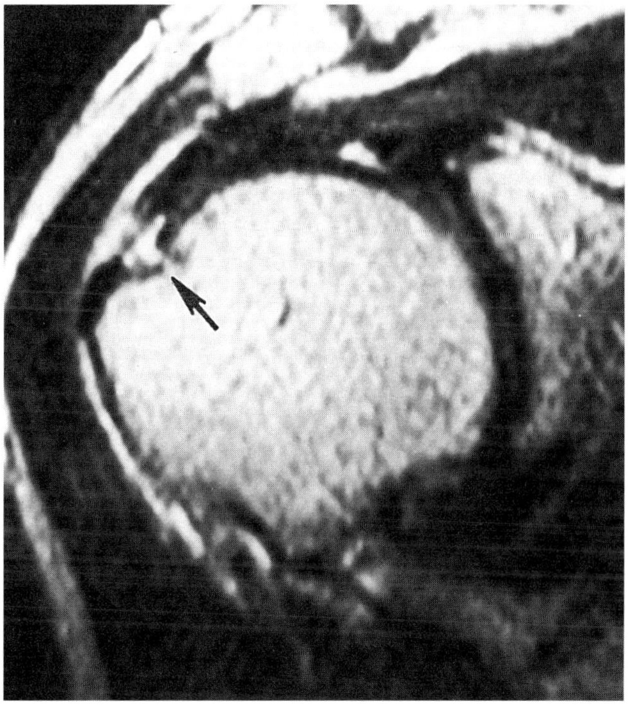

FIGURE 7-67 Magnetic resonance imaging study demonstrating a full-thickness rotator cuff tear in the supraspinatus tendon.

use of magnetic resonance imaging to evaluate cuff pathology is increasing; however, the experience of the radiologist, the availability of dedicated surface coils, and the comfort of the patient affect the reliability and availability of this tool.

Diagnostic shoulder arthroscopy reliably documents the presence and size of both partial- and full-thickness rotator cuff tears.[2,38,92] Associated pathology, such as biceps tendon tears, SLAP lesions, degenerative glenohumeral arthritis, labral tears, and glenohumeral instability, also may be identified.

The authors use arthroscopy where there is any question about the diagnosis or the possibility of a second diagnosis, particularly in a young athlete. Arthroscopy is performed just before the open repair.

DIFFERENTIAL DIAGNOSIS

Clearly, the most critical information to obtain in the evaluation of an athlete with rotator cuff pathology is an accurate and *complete* diagnosis. Even when a torn cuff is conclusively documented, other conditions may coexist and, if unrecognized, may compromise the resultant treatment.

The most common conditions to consider in the younger athlete include anterior glenohumeral instability, acromioclavicular joint arthritis, vascular obstruction, suprascapular neuropathy, and brachial plexopathy. The older athlete also may be affected by these conditions as well as cervical radiculopathy, adhesive capsulitis, and glenohumeral joint arthritis.

TREATMENT RATIONALE

Introduction

The primary goals in caring for an athlete with an injured rotator cuff are an accurate diagnosis, rapid relief of pain, restoration of shoulder strength and function, prevention of injury recurrence or progression, and a timely return to sport or occupation.

The patient's age, the duration of symptoms, the described or apparent mechanism of injury, and the possible presence of occult instability, muscle weakness, or neurovascular compromise must be determined. The athlete's sports and competitive level, the mechanics involved in those sports, and the demands on the athlete to return rapidly to play also must be considered because these also may affect management.

The Young Athlete

Occult anterior shoulder instability is responsible for the vast majority of rotator cuff injuries in young overhead athletes, and full-thickness cuff tears are rare.[61] The more commonly seen partial-thickness tears infrequently require repair because of their good potential to heal after proper shoulder rehabilitation and/or an operative stabilization procedure.* Furthermore, aggressive débridement of partial-thickness tears found during diagnostic arthroscopy is discouraged because of the potential of further thinning of the cuff tendons.[51] Full-thickness tears identified in association with anterior instability should be repaired early, along with capsulolabral reconstruction.

In those few young athletes with partial- or full-thickness cuff tears that are thought to have occurred as a result of chronic outlet impingement or direct trauma, a careful examination under anesthesia and diagnostic arthroscopy often are necessary to document the absence of subtle anterior instability. All full-thickness tears should be surgically repaired, with the mechanism of injury determining the need for an acromioplasty.

Partial-thickness tears caused by outlet impingement or trauma in young patients may be treated successfully with a nonoperative rehabilitation program.[72] Nevertheless, conservative care for longer than 6 months is of little benefit and may simply waste precious time from the athlete's career. When proper rehabilitation is ineffective or sport participation is impaired, surgical intervention is indicated.

The Older Athlete

Now more than ever, patients past the age of 35 are participating at professional, elite, and recreational levels in a wide variety of sports. Although their expectations may be different from those of younger athletes, the goal of treatment is still to return these athletes to their previous level of function. Rarely is nonoperative management of a documented full-thickness rotator cuff tear an acceptable option when the patient desires to remain active and participate in overhead sports. Very little data are available in the literature concerning the postoperative performance of older athletes[1,2,10,95]; however, because of the high demands on the shoulder, return to sports such as baseball, softball, or swimming is likely to be more difficult than return to tennis, racquetball, golf, or bicycling after rotator cuff repair.[10]

Because the etiology of rotator cuff pathology in many of these older athletes is chronic outlet impingement, surgical management will routinely require decompression of the coracoacromial arch via acromioplasty and removal of any thickened subacromial bursa.[48] Arthroscopic subacromial decompression followed by a limited anterior deltoid splitting approach for cuff repair is a viable surgical alternative when a small rotator cuff tear is diagnosed.[62] Larger tears are much more reliably repaired through a classic, open anterior superior approach as described by Neer and others.†

Associated conditions such as an unstable os acromiale, acromioclavicular joint arthritis, and glenohumeral

*References 53, 56, 59, 60, 72, 75.

†References 42, 45, 72, 83, 87, 96.

instability should be recognized before surgery because these problems can and should be treated at the time of rotator cuff repair.

How to reliably recognize and manage tears occurring in the rotator interval is still unclear. A history of a recent anterior shoulder dislocation in the older athlete should raise the index of suspicion for an injury in this interval, particularly when the athlete has symptoms of recurrent instability.[75,79] Unfortunately, capsulolabral ligament and rotator cuff tendon injury resulting from the dislocation may cause similar anterior instability symptoms. Because tears within the rotator interval may potentially heal without repair, conservative care, including 6 weeks of relative rest followed by aggressive rehabilitation, is recommended.[75] Infrequently in the older athlete, the rotator interval defect or the anterior capsular ligaments will require repair to restore joint stability and normal shoulder function.[79]

Early Surgical Repair

The need for surgical repair of all documented tears in the rotator cuff is still controversial. Pain relief after the nonoperative treatment of full-thickness cuff tears has varied from 33% to 90% of patients in various reports,* and Hawkins has noted that "most patients" diagnosed with a rotator cuff tear are "not treated surgically."[45] Based on these and similar reports in the literature, some authors have argued for the conservative care of complete rotator cuff tears. However, these arguments ignore the importance of an intact, balanced, functioning rotator cuff to the active individual who requires vigorous use of the arm away from the body and overhead.[8,56,58,75]

Furthermore, continued activity risks the progression of small tears to large or massive tears,[9,30,45,63,75] and, indeed, larger cuff tears become more difficult to repair.[9,30] Ellman reported that the more prolonged the duration of preoperative pain, the larger the size of the cuff tear.[30] Bassett and Cofield reported that patients with acute tears that were repaired less than 3 weeks after injury had better strength and active range of motion than patients in whom the tears were repaired 6 to 12 weeks after injury. They concluded that acute tears should be repaired within 3 weeks of injury for best results, particularly "in patients who place high demands on their shoulders."[6] Many authors have reported better results after the repair of small tears than after the repair of large tears,† and early surgical repair frequently is recommended in active patients with a documented complete tear of the rotator cuff.‡

Matsen et al postoperatively evaluated 105 repairs of the rotator cuff with ultrasonography to determine the integrity of the repair. Of the tears that involved only the supraspinatus tendon, 20% had a recurrent defect, whereas 50% of the tears involving more than the supraspinatus tendon alone had recurred. Active range of motion, strength, and functional use of the arm away from the body and overhead correlated with the integrity of the tendon repair.[42]

Based on this data, the "wait-and-see" conservative approach to the management of complete rotator cuff tears cannot be justified in an individual who desires to remain active and involved in sports. The critical role of the rotator cuff in active shoulder motion mandates that normal or near-normal cuff anatomy and function be restored whenever possible. A trial of conservative care for 6 weeks is appropriate when a chronic tear is suspected, but if significant improvement does not occur, special studies should be obtained to evaluate the tear. Acute symptoms of pain and weakness, implying an extension of an existing tear, must be evaluated immediately to document the status of the rotator cuff. A full-thickness tendon defect repaired within 3 weeks of injury often provides the best results.[21,45,69,77]

*References 13, 44, 45, 64, 88, 93, 102.
†References 4, 22, 30, 39, 40, 83, 99.
‡References 6, 21, 45, 69, 77, 83.

INDICATIONS FOR SURGERY

Surgery is indicated for any active or previously active patient with a documented symptomatic full-thickness rotator cuff tear who has acceptable anesthetic risks, who is able to participate in an appropriate postoperative rehabilitation program, and who desires to return to his or her prior activity level. Indications for surgically repairing a partial-thickness cuff tear largely depend on the mechanism of injury, the presence of associated conditions, the response to conservative care, and the functional demand of the patient's activities. In general, a partial-thickness tear in a young athlete can be left alone if the anterior instability or other pathology is corrected so that the cuff is no longer at risk of further damage. These factors are discussed in preceding chapters.

SURGICAL MANAGEMENT

Principles for Surgical Repair of the Rotator Cuff

Limit the Release of the Anterior and Middle Deltoid Origin

The anterior and middle deltoid muscles become increasingly effective as humeral elevators when humeral abduction increases. In addition, there are no muscles that may adequately substitute for the deltoid if function is impaired.[75,82] Because extensive release of the deltoid origin may result in permanent deltoid weakness, the extent of anterior and middle deltoid origin release must be limited in patients who desire to return to overhead activities.[7,21,51,75]

Removing the deltoid origin by subperiosteal dissection from the superior, anterior, and inferior acromial edge more reliably preserves adequate tissue for subsequent repair (Fig. 7-68). Nonabsorbable braided sutures passed through both the outer and deep deltoid fascia and then through bone tunnels in the acromion lessen the risk for loss of deltoid reattachment during the postoperative period (Fig. 7-69).

Protect the Axillary Nerve

A 5-cm "safe zone" from the edge of the acromion usually is described for dissection in the deltoid muscle. However, the axillary nerve may lie as close as 3 cm from the acromial edge.[16,90] Shoulder abduction further decreases the distance between the nerve and the acromion. A more acceptable absolute "safe zone" is probably less than 3 cm, and care should be taken if dissection is performed with the arm abducted.[16,90] A suture placed in the apex of the deltoid muscle dissection limits unrecognized distal extension during retraction.

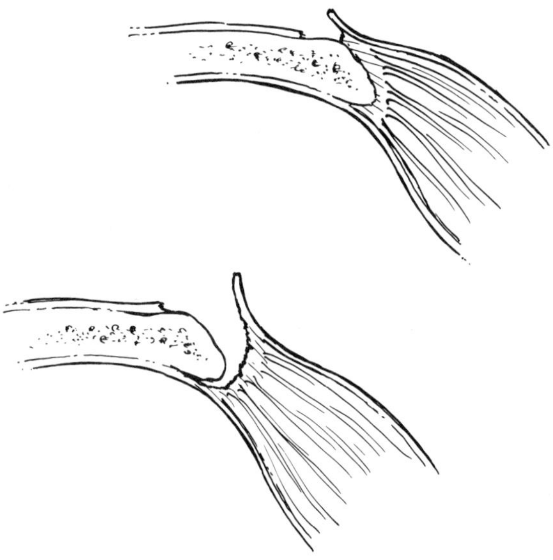

FIGURE 7-68 Subperiosteal dissection of the deltoid muscle origin from the anterior acromion.

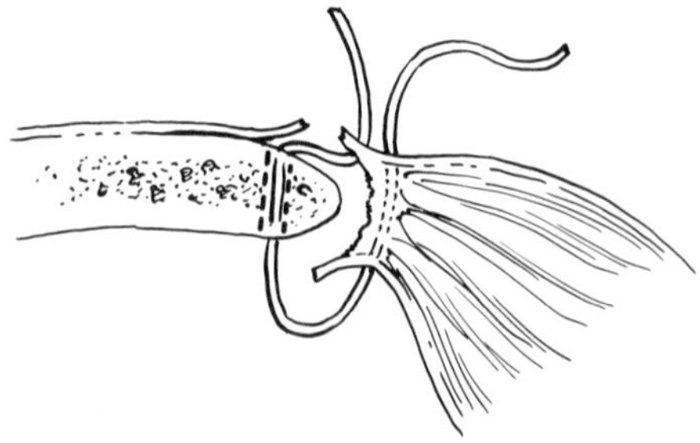

FIGURE 7-69 Reattachment of the deltoid muscle origin onto the acromion with suture passing through the outer and deep fascia of the deltoid and through a bony tunnel in the acromion.

Protect the Suprascapular Nerve

Superiorly, the suprascapular nerve is relatively fixed to the floor of the supraspinatus fossa, averaging 3 cm from the superior glenoid rim, and may be tethered by the spinoglenoid ligament.[98] Posteriorly, the average distance from the glenoid rim is 2 cm.[91,98]

Dissection medially under the supraspinatus and infraspinatus muscles to mobilize a torn, retracted tendon may injure the suprascapular nerve. Based on cadaveric studies, a standard anterosuperior approach will safely allow only 1 cm of tendon mobilization for either the supraspinatus or the infraspinatus tendons.[98] Either tendon may be mobilized up to 3 cm through the advancement technique of Debeyre, but safe advancement is limited by tension in the motor branches of the suprascapular nerve.[98]

Perform an Adequate Acromioplasty When Indicated

Radical acromionectomy is never indicated because of loss of deltoid function and poor results after this procedure.[70] However, anterior acromioplasty, as described by Neer[72] and modified by Rockwood,[86] is conventionally required during rotator cuff tendon repair surgery in patients with outlet impingement.[72,75] Failure to adequately enlarge the area beneath the coracoacromial arch will allow continued outlet impingement after tendon repair and ultimately diminish the results of surgery. In young overhead athletes with occult anterior subluxation and secondary rotator cuff tendon pathology, restoring glenohumeral joint stability prevents further impingement, making an acromioplasty unnecessary and contraindicated.[54,56,59] Infrequently, the mechanism of tendon injury in the young athlete is from either acute trauma or outlet impingement. Therefore in those cases only a limited acromioplasty may be required at the time of tendon repair.

Important surgical findings that indicate the necessity of an acromioplasty in young athletes include: bursal surface partial-thickness rotator cuff tears, coracoacromial ligament fraying, hypertrophic subacromial bursa, radiographic evidence of low-angle acromial tilt, type II or type III acromial morphology, and os acromiale.[11,75]

Preserve Large Os Acromiale Fragments When Possible

The acromion forms by the fusion of four separate epiphyses, and the epiphyses may fail to close at any of these four levels: preacromion, mesoacromion, meta-acromion, and basiacromion.[75] Motion eventually may occur at the unfused level, and the presence of an unstable os acromiale has been recognized as a potential cause of supraspinatus outlet impingement.

Resection of a small preacromial fragment probably results in minimal loss of deltoid function. However, resection of larger fragments is functionally equivalent to performing a radical acromionectomy and is discouraged because of the potentially severe impairment of deltoid function.[70,94] Although fusion is frequently difficult to obtain, open reduction, internal fixation, and bone grafting are recommended when possible.[75,84]

Resect the Distal Clavicle for Arthritis or Exposure

Routine distal clavicle resection during rotator cuff repair surgery is discouraged. However, untreated symptomatic acromioclavicular joint arthritis associated with rotator cuff pathology will diminish the result of tendon repair. The condition of the acromioclavicular joint and the need for resection should be determined preoperatively through a carefully performed physical exam, and when indicated, a lidocaine injection test, plain radiographs, and a pinhole columnated bone scan.

Distal clavicle resection also is indicated infrequently when greater exposure of the supraspinatus tendon is required to allow tendon mobilization and repair.

Inspect and Preserve the Biceps Tendon

Tendinitis and deformity of the biceps tendon result from outlet impingement beneath the coracoacromial arch and often are noted in association with supraspinatus tendon tears. The function of the biceps tendon as an active depressor of the humeral head warrants specific emphasis on preserving the tendon whenever possible despite apparent pathology.

Flattening, hypertrophy, erythema, fraying, and incomplete rupture of the biceps tendon are easily noted by inspecting the tendon through the defect in the cuff tendons at the time of rotator cuff tendon repair. The rotator interval may be divided, allowing access to the tendon when the cuff tear is small and visualization of the biceps tendon is inadequate for proper assessment.

Acromioplasty effectively relieves biceps tendon impingement. When applicable, débridement of the tendon to allow movement within the biceps tendon groove is preferred to tenodesis. However, tenodesis may be required when extensive damage to the tendon has occurred or the function of the tendon as a humeral head depressor is lost. Unfortunately, this may preclude the athlete from returning to overhead activities such as pitching.

Release Coracohumeral Ligament for Tendon Mobilization and External Rotation

The coracohumeral ligament is a broad, thick, fibrous structure that runs from the coracoid process to the humerus in the rotator interval and forms a portion of the roof of the biceps tendon[17,18] (see Fig. 7-65). The ligament normally tightens during external rotation and may become contracted in diseased states.[75,79] The coracohumeral ligament frequently must be released to restore external rotation and sometimes to mobilize the subscapularis and supraspinatus tendons during rotator cuff repair.

Carefully Handle and Repair the Rotator Cuff Tendons

Regardless of the extent of the tear, the torn edges of the rotator cuff should be gently handled to avoid further injury and loss of tissue strength. Multiple horizontal mattress sutures placed along the tendon edge with a tapered needle produce the least amount of damage when mobilizing the tendon for repair. Kocher or similar clamps should not be placed along the margins of the tendon edge.

Minimal débridement of the frayed edge of a torn tendon is advised. However, resection of the torn edge to the level of bleeding tissue results in the loss of repairable tendon tissue and may prevent repair of the tendon with the arm at the side. Whenever possible, the tendon edge should be brought back to its original anatomic insertion site and repaired under normal tension with the arm adducted at the side of the body. Repairs that require abduction of the arm away from the side to maintain the tendon edge in the bone trough are more likely to fail.

The extent of postoperative shoulder mobilization must be based on the quality of the tendon tissue and the integrity of the repair (Box 7-3).

Treatment Options

Arthroscopic Subacromial Decompression Without Tendon Repair

An older patient with outlet impingement and a full-thickness rotator cuff tear may be treated with arthroscopic acromioplasty and débridement of the tear. The technique is modified from the original descriptions by Ellman.[29,31] Standard diagnostic shoulder arthroscopy is performed with visualization of the articular and bursal

BOX 7-3

PRINCIPLES FOR SURGICAL REPAIR OF THE ROTATOR CUFF

- Limit the release of the anterior and middle deltoid origin.
- Protect the axillary nerve.
- Protect the suprascapular nerve.
- Perform an appropriate acromioplasty when indicated.
- Preserve large os acromiale fragments when possible.
- May resect the distal clavicle for arthritis or exposure.
- Inspect and preserve the biceps tendon.
- Release coracohumeral ligament for mobilization or rotation.
- Carefully handle and repair the rotator cuff tendons.

surfaces of the rotator cuff. The location, depth, and extent of the tear are determined. A limited débridement of the frayed tendon edge is performed with a motorized rotary shaver, and arthroscopic subacromial decompression then is performed as described in the preceding chapter. This procedure works especially well on an elderly person with low demands who prefers pain relief over functional use.

Arthroscopic Subacromial Decompression and Limited Open Tendon Repair

Partial-thickness or unretracted small cuff tendon tears may be considered for arthroscopic-assisted repair through a small lateral incision. After arthroscopic subacromial decompression, extremity traction is removed and the arm is placed into a sterile impervious stockinette and covered with an Ace wrap. A 5-cm saber incision is made beginning along the lateral edge of the acromion and extending 2 cm anterior to the acromion. The deltoid muscle is exposed and carefully split with blunt dissection in line with the muscle fibers. The axillary nerve is protected by placing a suture at the apex of the divided deltoid muscle 3 cm from the acromial edge. Retractors are placed, and the entire rotator cuff is inspected by rotation of the humeral head.

After limited débridement of the frayed margins of the tear, primary repair of the tendon may be performed tendon-to-tendon or tendon-to-bone, depending on the size and shape of the tear. Longitudinal tears are easily repaired side-to-side. Crescent-shaped, L-shaped, and triangular tears should be repaired into a shallow bone trough along the articular margin. Postoperative shoulder mobilization begins during the first 24 hours after surgery.

Conventional Open Anterior Acromioplasty and Tendon Repair

Positioning

A Vacu-Pak positioning bag, two table posts (or two kidney rests), an axillary roll, and two pillows are required for positioning. The Vacu-Pak bag is placed on the operating room table, and the patient is positioned onto the table in the supine position. After adequate general endotracheal anesthesia is achieved, a careful examination is performed under anesthesia.

The patient is then rolled into the lateral decubitus position and secured with the Vacu-Pak bag and either table posts or kidney rests. An axillary roll is placed beneath the chest wall at the level of the axilla, and distal pulses are checked. A pulse oximeter may be used to ensure adequate perfusion of the contralateral extremity. The patient's head is supported to prevent traction on the brachial plexus, and pads are placed both beneath and between the legs to avoid pressure on the peroneal nerves. The bed is then repositioned into a 20° reverse Trendelenburg position, allowing gravity to assist traction on the arm (Fig. 7-70). The patient is allowed to drift slightly posteriorly so that the operative shoulder is at the table's edge. The surgeon stands at the patient's neck and has no difficulty visualizing the wound. The assistant can position the arm with ease.

An impervious split drape is then placed about the shoulder. The entire arm and shoulder are prepared and draped in the usual sterile fashion. A cotton stockinette and an Ace wrap are used to cover the arm. The arm is left at the side, and an assistant provides rotation and traction of the arm during the procedure.

Incision

The bony landmarks over the shoulder are outlined with a marking pen. A 10-cm anterior superior saber incision is made beginning just anterior to the posterior acromial edge and approximately 5 mm medial to the lateral acromial edge. The incision is extended anteriorly along the lateral border of the acromion and ends approximately 4 cm anterior to the acromion and just lateral to the coracoid (Fig. 7-71). A more medial placement

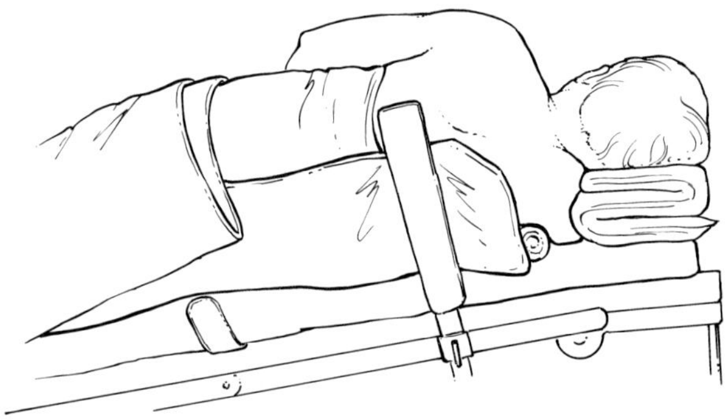

FIGURE 7-70 A patient in the lateral decubitus position on the operating room table in 15° of reverse Trendelenburg position. The patient is secured with a Vacu-Pak bean bag and table posts.

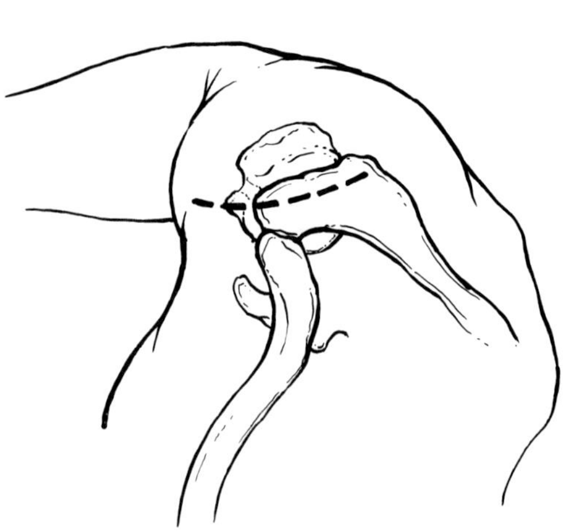

FIGURE 7-71 Placement of the anterior superior saber incision over the acromion and anterior shoulder.

of this incision may be used when distal clavicle resection is anticipated.

Approach

The deltoid fascia is identified, and full-thickness skin flaps are developed, taking care to leave the deltoid and trapezius fascia intact. Kocher clamps are placed in the dermis of the lateral flip and rotated laterally for self-retaining retraction. A retractor may be used for medial retraction, affording excellent exposure of the anterior lateral acromion and the anterior and middle deltoid muscle fibers.

The raphe between the anterior and middle deltoid muscles is identified; it usually is seen as a thickened fascia originating at the anterior lateral corner of the acromion (Fig. 7-72). A key elevator may be used to divide this raphe. However, use of a needle-point bovie electrocautery will maintain hemostasis. The outer fibers of the raphe are divided. To protect the underlying rotator cuff, a hemostat clamp is placed at the anterior lateral corner of the acromion and passed underneath the acromion. The clamp is then turned laterally underneath the remaining fibers of the deltoid raphe, and with the clamp open, the deeper deltoid fasica is divided; this reduces the risk of injury to the underlying bursa or rotator cuff tendons.

Careful dissection is carried through the raphe, and a suture is placed 3 cm from the edge of the acromion to prevent further dissection distally, thereby protecting the axillary nerve.

Deltoid Detachment

Careful subperiosteal detachment of the deltoid beginning 1 cm from the anterior edge of the acromion and 0.5 cm from the lateral edge of the acromion will maintain adequate tissue for appropriate deltoid repair at the completion of the cuff repair (see Fig. 7-68). Low-voltage needle-point electrocautery facilitates dissection and minimizes bleeding.

Digital dissection or use of a blunt elevator usually is required to free the adherent underlying bursa from the deep deltoid fascia. Additionally, frequent adhesions within the subacromial space must be released for better exposure of the bursa and rotator cuff. Narrow right-angle retractors are placed for retraction (Fig. 7-73). With traction on the arm distally, the subacromial space is well exposed.

Coracoacromial Ligament Resection

The interval between the deep fascia of the anterior deltoid muscle and the coracoacromial ligament is developed, permitting adequate exposure of the ligament for resection near the coracoid. The acromial branch of the thoracoacromial artery usually is encountered anteriorly over the coracoacromial ligament, and bleeding may be avoided by using electrocautery.

Acromioplasty

The acromioplasty is performed in two steps (Fig. 7-74). The first step requires the removal of the anterior edge of the acromion using a rongeur until the anterior acromion is flush with the anterior edge of the distal clavicle. This step removes the anterior projection of the acromion, allows estimation of the thickness of the acromion, and provides a flat surface for an osteotome or oscillating bone saw during the second step of the acromioplasty.

During the second step, a Darrach or other flat retractor is placed beneath the acromion and over the humeral head to protect the bursa and rotator cuff. Under direct vision, a thin ½-inch osteotome or a thin-blade oscillating bone saw is used to resect the anterior 2 cm of the undersurface of the acromion. Soft-tissue attachments are released, and the acromial fragment is removed. A high-speed burr or flat rasp may be used to further resect or

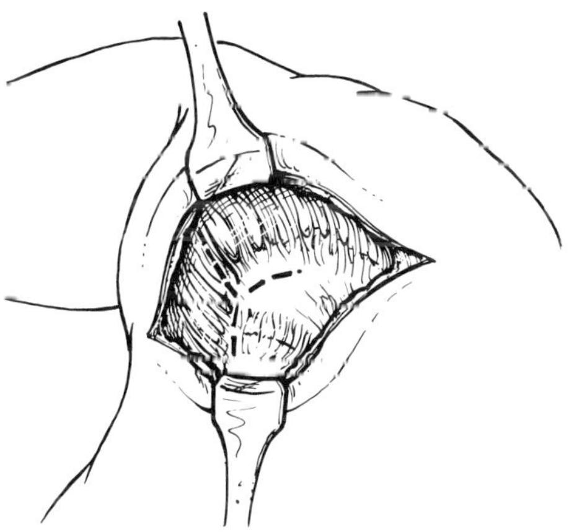

FIGURE 7-72 Exposure of the deltoid muscle and acromion. The deltoid muscle raphe is divided and the deltoid origin is dissected from the acromion along the dashed line.

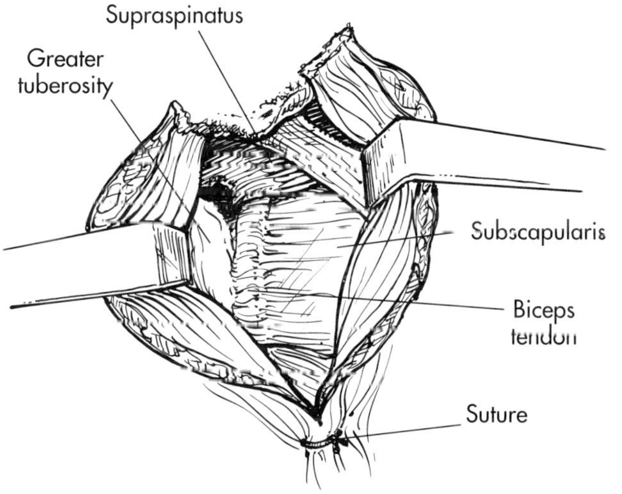

FIGURE 7-73 Exposure of the subacromial space. Suture ties at the distal apex of the split in the deltoid muscle raphe minimize risk to the axillary nerve during retraction.

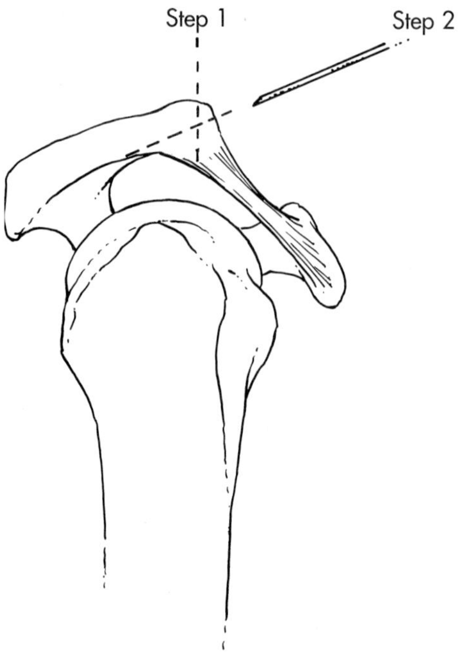

FIGURE 7-74 Two steps are required for partial anterior acromioplasty. Step 1 is resection of the anterior edge of the acromion. Step 2 is resection of the undersurface of the anterior lateral acromion with a thin osteotome.

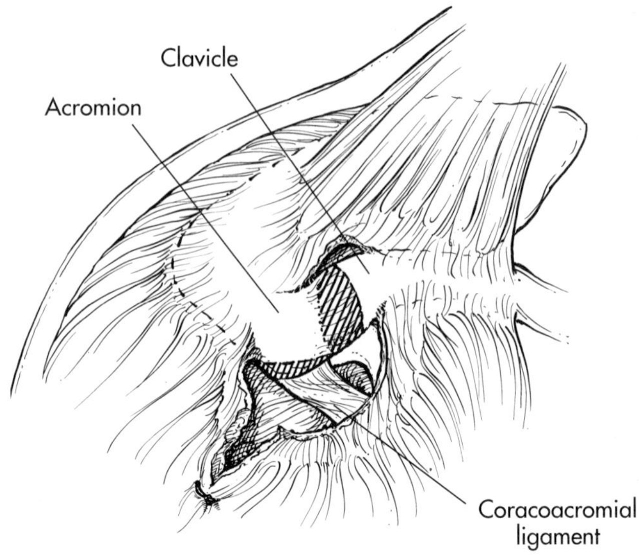

FIGURE 7-75 Resection of the distal clavicle and anterior edge of the acromion. Removal of the distal clavicle improves exposure to allow mobilization of the supraspinatus tendon.

contour the undersurface of the acromion. The surgeon must pay attention to the medial edge of the acromion and the undersurface of the acromioclavicular joint because prominent osteophytes may be present and require resection.

Subacromial Inspection

The size and condition of the subacromial and subdeltoid bursa are apparent with rotation of the humerus. The bursa should be divided and preserved for later repair when the bursa appears normal. More commonly, the bursa will be hypertrophic and require some resection.

After removal or reflection of the bursa, the rotator cuff tendons are brought into the wound for inspection by rotation of the humerus. The cuff tear is identified and classified according to the location, size, and shape. The quality of the remaining tendon and the condition of the biceps tendon also are noted.

Acromioclavicular Joint

If the patient has symptomatic acromioclavicular joint arthritis or greater exposure is required, the distal clavicle may be resected at this time (Fig. 7-75). Dissection over the deltoid and trapezius fascia is performed, and retractors are placed to expose the distal clavicle. Needle-point electrocautery is used to divide the deltotrapezius aponeurosis and clavicular periosteum over the distal clavicle extending across the acromioclavicular joint in line with the fibers of the acromioclavicular ligament. Care is taken not to "T" the incision over the acromioclavicular joint so that the acromioclavicular ligament remains intact.

The distal clavicle is exposed by reflecting the fascia and periosteum anteriorly and posteriorly. Elevators or flat retractors are placed beneath the clavicle to further subperiosteally expose the distal end of the bone. A microoscillating bone saw is used to resect the outer 1 cm of the distal clavicle, and bone wax is placed onto the cut end of the clavicle. Impingement of the distal clavicle against the acromion or scapular spine is prevented by dividing the clavicle from superior lateral to inferior medial in the coronal plane, and from anterior lateral to posterior medial in the transverse plane. The deltotrapezial fascia is repaired by use of a purse-string suture to pull surrounding soft tissue into the acromioclavicular defect.

Os Acromiale

Small, unstable, anterior os acromiale fragments should be resected. One should attempt to preserve larger, unstable os acromiale fragments at this point with internal fixation. The technique uses cannulated 4-mm cancellous screws, #5 nonabsorbable suture, and bone graft (Fig. 7-76). The anterior acromial os is reduced onto the posterior acromion. The first screw guide pin is placed from anterior to posterior along the lateral border of the acromion, with care to avoid penetration into the subacromial space. The second pin is placed along the medial border of the acromion in a similar fashion. The pins are replaced with two 4-mm cannulated partially threaded cancellous screws. After the defect is compressed, the screws are exchanged for fully threaded 4-mm screws to prevent motion about the narrow proximal screw shaft.

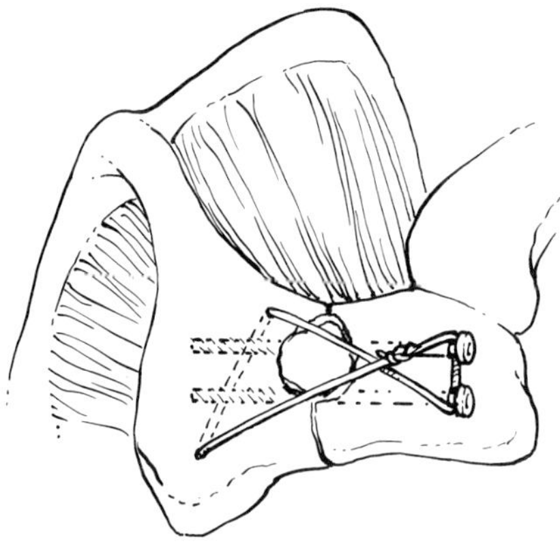

FIGURE 7-76 Open reduction, internal fixation, and bone grafting of a large unstable os acromiale fragment.

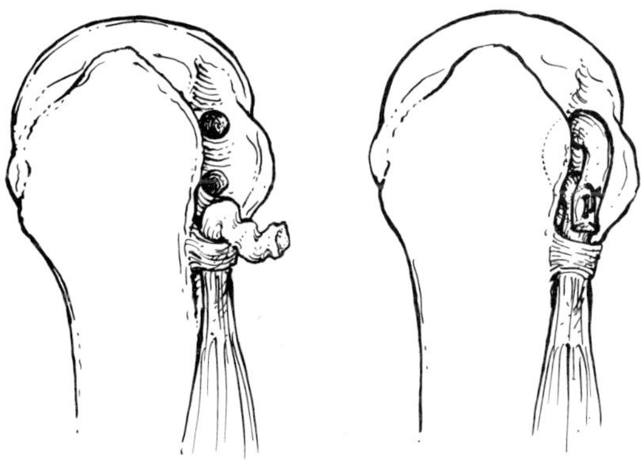

FIGURE 7-77 Biceps tendon tenodesis within the bicipital groove. (See the text for a more detailed description.)

Two drill holes are placed through the posterior acromion into the subacromial space, staying just lateral to the shaft of the medial screw and just medial to the shaft of the lateral screw. Two #5 nonabsorbable braided sutures are passed into the subacromial space through one of the holes and then brought back out through the other.

A trough created between the two screws in the failed union site of the acromion using a high-speed burr. Bone graft from the distal clavicle, the anterior acromial osteophyte, or the iliac crest may be used and is packed into the trough. The two #5 nonabsorbable sutures then are placed in a figure 8 underneath the screw heads and tied over the top of the acromion. Tension band fixation is achieved, and the suture maintains the graft in proper position.

Biceps Tendon Rupture

The biceps tendon is evaluated before rotator cuff tendon repair. Minor fraying of the biceps tendon may be débrided. Extensive hypertrophy of the tendon may require partial resection of the margin of the tendon to allow the tendon to move within the biceps groove. Severe deformity and near-total rupture of the tendon are managed by biceps tenodesis using bone tunnels within the biceps groove and suturing the tendon back onto itself (Fig. 7-77).

Partial-Thickness Tears

Partial-thickness rotator cuff tears involving the bursal surface of the tendon are easily recognized. Articular-surface partial-thickness tears can be identified by injecting the glenohumeral joint with a dilute solution of methylene blue and saline as described by Fukuda.[36] A bluish discoloration in the tendon is noted in the area where the rotator cuff is thinned by the partial-thickness tear. Intratendinous lesions are more difficult to identify and may require division of the tendon in line with its fibers to allow inspection when a tear is suspected but not easily recognized.

Excision of the frayed or degenerative edges of the partial-thickness tear followed by side-to-side repair of the tendon fibers usually is adequate to obtain repair.

Small and Medium Tears

Small and medium-size tears may occur in many shapes, including simple transverse, crescent, L-shaped, and triangular, and rarely require extensive mobilization for repair. Resection of the bursa and division of the adhesions between the tendon and overlying trapezius or deltoid musculature usually allows mobilization of the torn edges for repair. Tendon-to-tendon, tendon-to-bone, or combined inverted "Y" side-to-side and tendon-to-bone repair is performed, depending on the pattern of the tear (Fig. 7-78).

Transverse and crescent-shaped tears are repaired by creating a shallow trough with a rongeur or high-speed burr along the humeral head articular margin. Drill holes are placed in the trough and tuberosities to create bone tunnels for suture repair. Nonabsorbable, braided, #1 sutures then are placed horizontally through the tendon and brought out through the bone tunnels in the tuberosity. The rotator cuff tendon edge is pulled into the bone trough, and each suture is tied individually over a bony bridge lateral to the tuberosity (Fig. 7-79).

L-shaped tears generally require mobilization of the more retracted portion of the tendon down to a bony trough, followed by side-to-side repair of the split along the tendinous fibers.

Triangular tears are best repaired by converting the V-shape of the tear to a Y shape. This allows side-to-side repair of a significant portion of the tear, and the two arms of the "Y" then are brought down into a bony trough through mattress sutures (Fig. 7-80).

Large tears

Large tears commonly involve more than one rotator cuff tendon and usually are accompanied by greater tendon retraction. When the tear has been present for a long time, more aggressive mobilization techniques are required to advance the tendon and achieve an adequate repair.

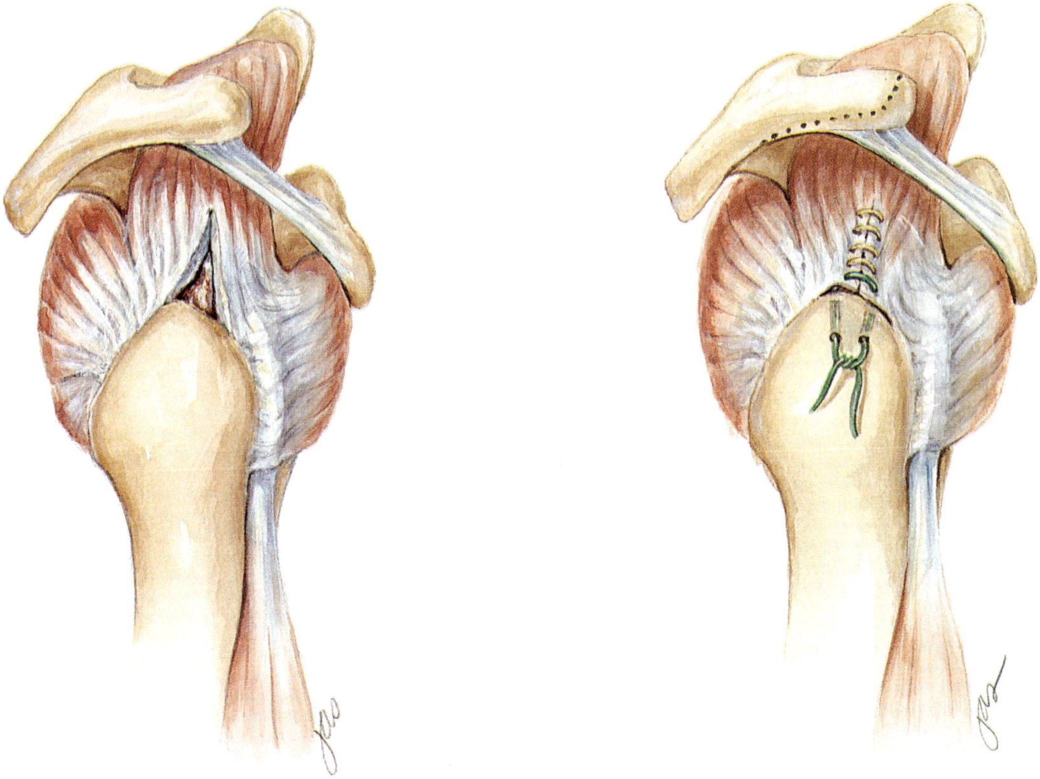

FIGURE 7-78 **A,** A small triangular-shaped rotator cuff tear. **B,** Tendon-side-to-tendon-side and tendon-edge-to-bone sutures are used for repair.

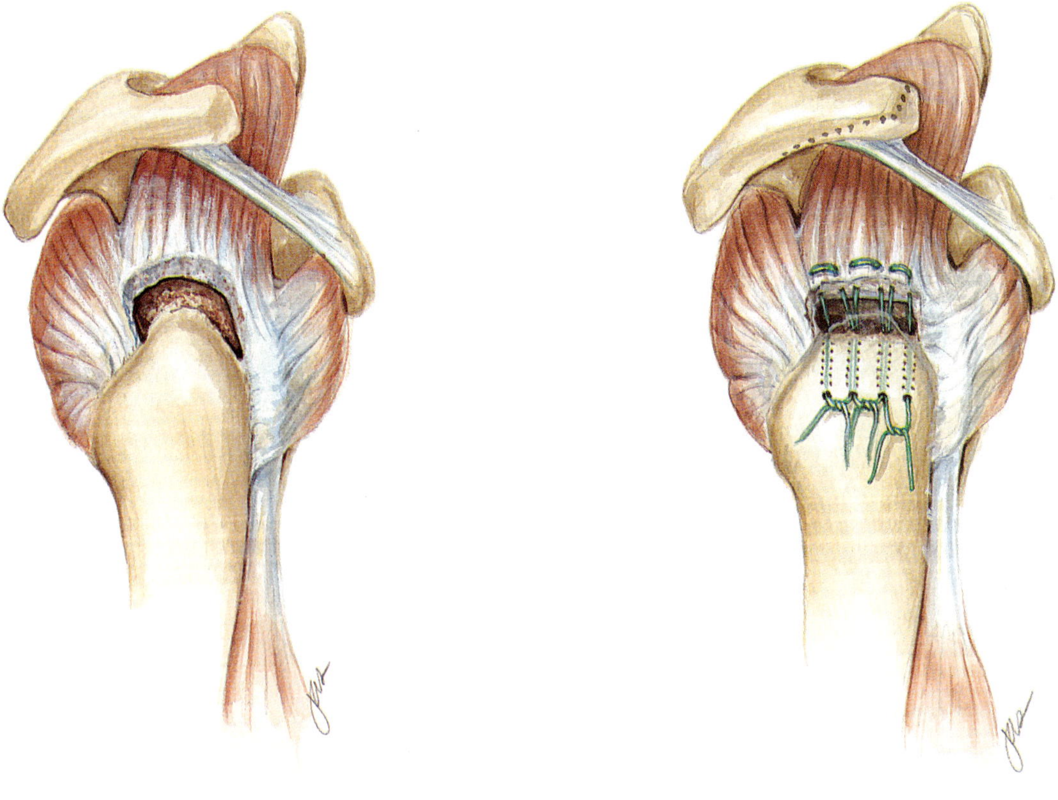

FIGURE 7-79 **A,** A medium-size, crescent-shaped rotator cuff tear involving the supraspinatus tendon. **B,** The free tendon edge is mobilized and reattached into a trough at the articular margin of the humeral head. Mattress sutures passed through bone tunnels are tied over bone bridges.

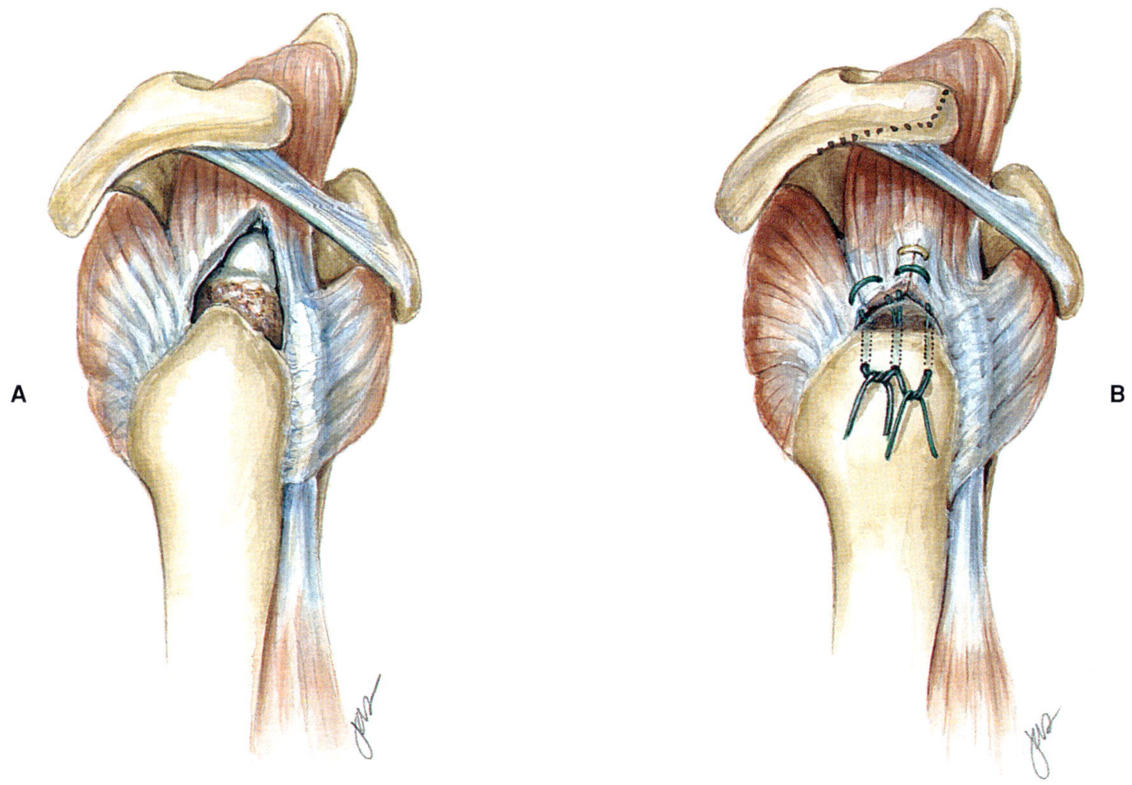

FIGURE 7-80 **A,** A medium-size triangular-shaped rotator cuff tear involving the supraspinatus tendon. **B,** The V shape of the triangular tear is converted into a Y shape with tendon-side-to-tendon-side sutures. The remaining free edge of the tear is reattached into a trough at the articular margin of the humeral head with sutures through bone tunnels.

Intramuscular adhesions between the rotator cuff muscles and overlying trapezius or deltoid muscles are released by use of a blunt elevator. Occasionally, the subscapularis will be involved and will require release of adhesions between the subscapularis muscle and the deltoid and pectoralis muscles. Constant traction on the tendon for up to 15 to 20 minutes, using multiple sutures along the tendon edges, may allow stress relaxation within the muscle fibers to lengthen the tissue for repair.

Exposure and release of the coracohumeral ligament from the coracoid greatly facilitates advancement of the subscapularis and supraspinatus tendons. Furthermore, adhesions between the posterior coracoid and the supraspinatus tendon are released.

Glenohumeral joint capsule contracture is best managed by release of the capsule from the superior glenoid margin (Fig. 7-81). Care is taken during mobilization of the muscle from the glenoid to avoid injury to the suprascapular nerve. Finally, a relaxing incision may be made in the medial tendinous fibers of the rotator cuff to increase lateral mobilization of the tendon edge.

Preferentially, the mobilized tendon edges then are placed into a bony trough along the margin of the articular suface of the humeral head-articular glenoid margin through methods similar to those described for small and medium tears (Fig. 7-82). The arm may be abducted away

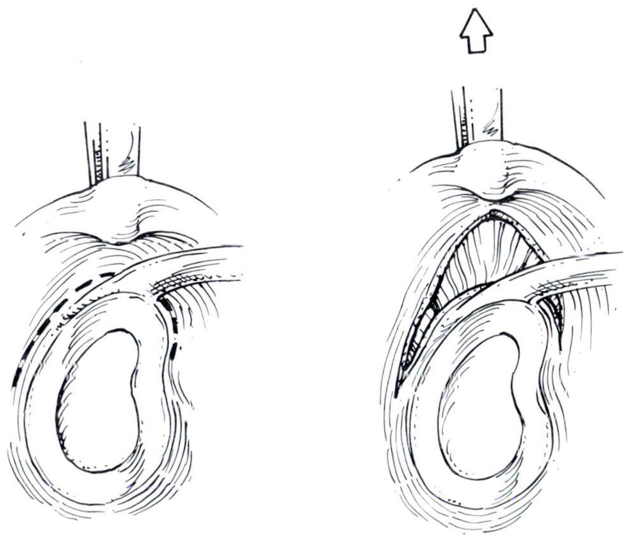

FIGURE 7-81 Release of the contracted glenohumeral joint capsule from the superior margin of the glenoid. (See the text for a more detailed discussion.)

from the side of the body when the sutures are tied, but normal tension within the muscle unit should be achieved, and the tendon edge should be able to reach the bone trough in the humeral head with the arm at the side. This may occasionally require reattaching of the ten-

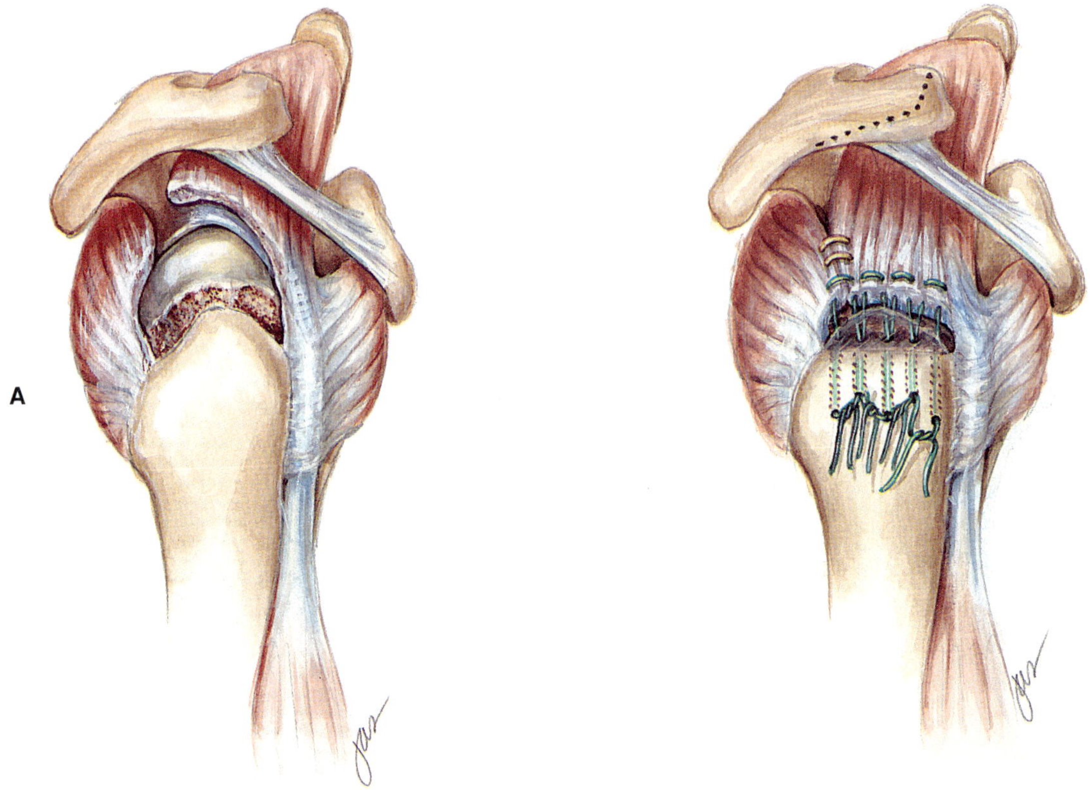

FIGURE 7-82 **A,** A large rotator cuff tear involving the supraspinatus and infraspinatus tendons. **B,** The retracted tendon edges are mobilized. (See the text for a more detailed discussion.) Tendon-side-to-tendon-side and tendon-edge-to-bone sutures are used for the repair.

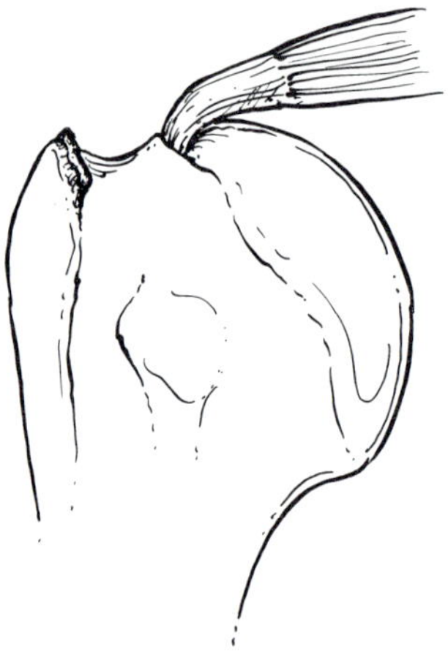

FIGURE 7-83 Repair of a medially retracted supraspinatus tendon that cannot be mobilized to the articular margin of the humeral head. The tendon is reattached to a bone trough created medially on the humeral head with mattress sutures passed through bone tunnels.

don edges into a bony trough created medial to the anatomic insertion site on the humeral head, recognizing that active abduction and forward flexion may be diminished after surgery (Fig. 7-83).

Massive Tears

Massive tears may involve three or four rotator cuff tendons and usually mandate greater exposure for mobilization and repair. Greater exposure may be obtained by three methods.

Resection of the distal clavicle will improve exposure superiorly and anteriorly, but requires extended release of the anterior deltoid muscle. Improved posterior exposure may be gained by the release of an additional 1 cm of the lateral deltoid muscle from the lateral border of the acromion. The surgeon must realize that these two methods may cause permanent postoperative deltoid muscle weakness resulting from extensive detachment of the deltoid origin, if the repair is not performed properly.

A posterior incision over the scapular spine with release of the posterior deltoid muscle origin may be used to increase posterior exposure and to gain access to the supraspinatus and infraspinatus tendons. Careful release of the infraspinatus and supraspinatus muscles from the body of the scapula will increase tendon mobilization up to 1 cm and avoid injury to the suprascapular nerve.[98] Postoperative deltoid muscle weakness is less apparent after release of the deltoid from the scapular spine.

The methods of tendon mobilization described previously for the repair of large rotator cuff tendon tears also apply to the repair of massive tears. Additional measures also may be considered. However, these measures require altering normal rotator cuff anatomy and should be avoided when possible.

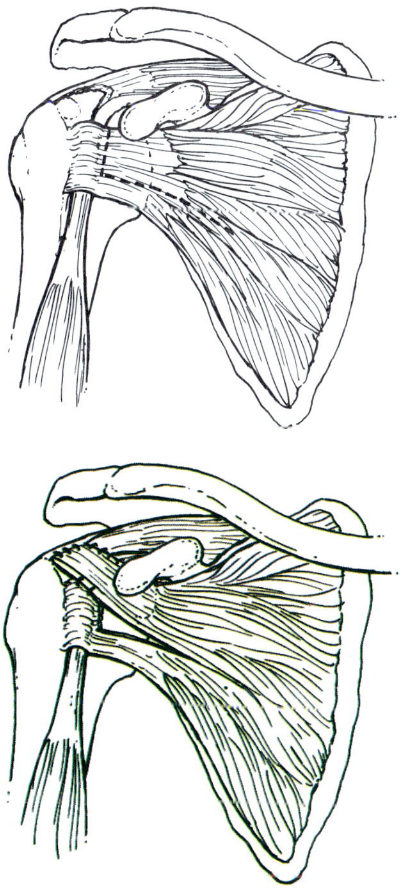

FIGURE 7-84 Superior advancement of the upper two thirds of the subscapularis muscle tendon to cover an area defect caused by severe retraction of the supraspinatus tendon.

The upper two thirds of the subscapularis tendon may be released sharply from the lesser tuberosity and advanced superiorly to fill an area defect created by retraction of the supraspinatus tendon (Fig. 7-84). Similarly, the upper one half of the infraspinatus teres minor conjoined tendon may be released and advanced superiorly onto the humeral head. The infraspinatus and the subscapularis muscles both are weakened after tendon transfer. Although other muscles are available to provide internal rotation strength, the infraspinatus provides most of the shoulder external rotation strength, and loss of external rotation power will limit the use of the arm away from the side.

Use of the biceps tendon in the repair of massive cuff tears has been advocated when biceps tenodesis already is considered because of severe deformity of the tendon. A functioning biceps tendon is not considered to be available for this purpose. Before the tendon is incorporated into the repair, the biceps tendon must be divided away from the glenoid. During shoulder external rotation, the biceps groove moves away from the glenoid and the biceps tendon must be able to slide within the groove. Tenodesis of the biceps tendon onto the humeral head, whether in the biceps groove or in a more lateral position, may result in postoperative external rotation loss.

A posterior incision over the scapular spine with complete release of the infraspinatus and supraspinatus muscle origins from the scapula is described by Debeyre.[24] Up to 3 cm of mobilization may be obtained; however, this method weakens both muscles and places the suprascapular nerve at risk for permanent injury.

Finally, there are many options for free grafts to repair massive tears, but the complication rate is quite high. Thus these grafts currently are not a desirable option.

RESULTS OF TREATMENT

Partial-Thickness Rotator Cuff Tears

Several authors have advocated arthroscopic subacromial decompression and limited débridement without cuff repair for the management of incomplete rotator cuff tears in stage II subacromial impingement.[31,38,92] The average patient age ranged from 40 to 49 years and represents a significantly younger population than reported in most series on the repair of complete tears.[9,10,30,45,72] Satisfactory results were reported in 85% of cases, but previous activity level or sport was not noted. Of athletes less than 40 years of age treated similarly by Fly et al,[34] 77% returned to their level of sport participation. Incomplete tears did not affect results; however, half the patients with labral tears or instability continued to have moderate to severe pain with sport participation.

Andrews reported the results of an even younger athletic population (average age, 22 years), of which 64% were pitchers. After arthroscopic cuff débridement and postoperative rehabilitation, 76% returned to the same level of sport activity. Superior labral injury was noted in all patients.[2] Articular-surface cuff tears and superior labral fraying suggest the occurrence of "inside impingement" caused by unrecognized subtle anterior instability.[6,51]

The repair of incomplete cuff tears, exploiting a limited anterior approach after arthroscopic partial acromioplasty, has been described.[28,76] However, 25% of patients in one study had unsatisfactory results and required additional surgery.[28] Open partial acromioplasty and repair of incomplete rotator cuff tears was recommended for older patients with incomplete-thickness tears that fail to respond to conservative care over 3 to 6 months. The studies did not mention activity level, but patient age averaged 45 years, and 92% obtained a satisfactory result.[36]

Full-Thickness Rotator Cuff Tears

Satisfactory results were obtained in 56% to 65% of older patients with full-thickness cuff tears treated with arthroscopic partial acromioplasty and limited débridement.[1,31,38] The rotator cuff tears were not repaired, and the results were inferior to those reported after conventional open acromioplasty and tendon repair.[9,22,30,45,68]

Repair of complete tears of the rotator cuff through a limited anterior approach after arthroscopic subacromial decompression has been described.[62] The average age was 57 years, and there were no data regarding sport participation. Overall, good to excellent results were achieved in 80% of cases, and 100% of small and medium tears obtained a satisfactory result.[62]

Significant pain relief has been reported in 84% to 96% of patients after conventional open partial acromioplasty and primary rotator cuff repair.[9,22,30,45,68] Complete pain relief has been obtained less frequently, and has been reported at 65% to 77%.[9,22,68,75] Unfortunately, little mention of the patient's preinjury or postoperative activity is presented.

Ellman et al[30] analyzed the prognostic significance of preoperative strength and active range of motion. An unsatisfactory result was nine times greater in patients with preoperative active abduction less than 100 degrees. Additionally, the risk of an unsatisfactory result was seven times greater in patients with a rating of grade 3 or less in external rotation strength.[30] Comparing preoperative external rotation strength with the arm at the side to the size of the tear found at surgery, Hawkins et al[45] demonstrated that patients with a large or massive tear were statistically weaker than patients with a small or moderate tear. Others have reported similar findings.[32] Although up to 50% of patients continue to have weakness after tendon repair,[45] the benefit of tendon repair has been displayed by significant gains in strength ratings measured in forward flexion, abduction, and external rotation after surgery.[30,75]

Complete rotator cuff tears in athletes only recently have gained attention as a separate group. Tibone et al[95] reported on 45 athletes less than 40 years old (average age 29) with partial or complete tears treated by open partial acromioplasty and tendon repair. Overall, 76% reported pain relief, 56% returned to sport, and 40% returned to throwing. Only 32% of the group of throwers participating at the college and professional levels were able to return to the same level of competition. Fourteen athletes had a complete tear 1 cm or greater, and of these, four of five throwers returned to throwing and 71% overall returned to their previous level of sport activity. This series was studied between 1976 and 1982, before the concept of an injury continuum progressing from instability to impingement to rotator cuff tear was appreciated.

Bigliani et al[10] reported on 23 tennis players, with an average age of 58 years, with complete rotator cuff tears managed with open partial acromioplasty and tendon repair. Nineteen patients (83%) returned to their previous level of participation, three returned to play at a lower level, and only one was unable to play tennis. The etiology of these tears was thought to be outlet impingement.

Massive Tears

Good results after acute repair of massive tears have been reported by several authors,[9,10,30,72,83] but longstanding massive tears with retraction, scarring, contracture, and cuff tear arthropathy frequently are irreparable and associated with a higher rate of failure.[9,45] Bigliani et al[9] reported on 61 patients with massive cuff tears treated with open partial acromioplasty, tendon mobilization, and cuff reattachment to bone. Overall, 85% had a satisfactory result and 52% were rated excellent. Repair within 6 months of reported trauma in patients less than 60 years of age is correlated with better results. Complete release of the coracohumeral ligament improved tendon mobilization.

Reasons for Failure

The most commonly reported causes of persistent pain and poor shoulder function after cuff tendon repair are inadequate acromioplasty, excessive acromioplasty, failed deltoid muscle reattachment, failed tendon repair, residual postoperative weakness, lost active or passive range of motion, and neurologic injury (axillary or suprascapular nerves). Moreover, unrecognized associated conditions also often diminish the quality of the result. These conditions include: subtle anterior shoulder instability, acromioclavicular joint arthritis, an unstable os acromiale, glenohumeral joint arthritis, significant coracoid impingement, and cervical radiculopathy.

COMPLICATIONS

Complications may result from either nonoperative or operative factors. The most common nonoperative complication is progression of the lesion.[63] When a patient desires conservative care for a complete cuff tear, the patient must be cautioned about the risk of enlargement of the tear and the possibility of a poor result from a later repair. Massive tears that have been present for a long time may develop cuff tear arthropathy. This extensive disease is rarely seen in active individuals.

The most frequently reported complications of rotator cuff repair surgery are failure of deltoid reattachment, failure of tendon repair, and axillary nerve injury. Limiting the initial extent of deltoid detachment, obtaining good suture purchase in both the inferior and superior deltoid fascia, and reattaching the deltoid onto the acromion through drill holes with nonabsorbable suture usually will prevent loss of deltoid attachment.

Failure of tendon repair has been reported in over 50% of tears involving more than one tendon.[63] When the tendon edge cannot be brought into a bony trough with the arm at the side, failure of the repair can be anticipated.

Axillary nerve injury can be avoided by limiting dissection away from the acromion to 3 cm.[16] A protective suture placed at the apex of the division in the deltoid will prevent unrecognized propagation of the muscle split during retraction. Less frequently, the suprascapular nerve may be injured by overzealous attempts to mobilize the supraspinatus and infraspinatus tendons, either off the neck of the glenoid or by advancing the tendons as described by Debeyre.[24]

Superior humeral head dislocation after débridement of a massive cuff tear has been reported,[100] and resection of the coracoacromial ligament probably increases the risk of this complication.

Postoperative wound infections, which usually are superficial and respond to local care and oral antibiotics, are a relatively rare problem after cuff repair surgery but have been reported as high as 6%.[9,30,32,40,83] Foreign body reaction to suture material in the subcutaneous tissues has been implicated as a source of infection and has led some authors to recommend closing only the skin after deltoid reattachment.

SUMMARY

Overhead use of the arm in sports requires intact rotator cuff tendons and balanced rotator cuff muscle forces. In the younger athlete, rotator cuff tendon injury commonly results from either occult anterior glenohumeral instability or direct local trauma. In the older athlete, primary supraspinatus outlet impingement is most often responsible.

Treatment mandates an accurate diagnosis followed by relief of pain, recovery of shoulder strength and function, prevention of recurrence, and return to sport. Normal rotator cuff anatomy and muscle strength must be restored for recovery of shoulder function.

In the younger athlete with a partial-thickness rotator cuff tear, nonoperative treatment often is effective; however, underlying conditions such as occult instability must be recognized and treated. In the older athlete, surgical care is much more often indicated, and full-thickness tears should be repaired when documented.

Careful attention to surgical principles will aid in preventing unsatisfactory results or complications. Finally, an individualized daily rehabilitation program in supervised and home settings cannot be neglected if the athlete desires to return to his previous level of sport participation.

References

1. Altchek DW et al: Arthroscopic acromioplasty, *J Bone Joint Surg* 72A(8):1198-1207, 1990.
2. Andrews JR, Broussard TS, Carson WG: Arthroscopy of the shoulder in the management of partial tears of the rotator cuff: a preliminary report, *Arthroscopy* 1(2):117-122, 1985.
3. Aoki M, Ishii S, Usui M: The slope of the acromion and rotator cuff impingement, *Orthop Trans* 10(2):228, 1986.
4. Bakalim G, Pasila M: Surgical treatment of the ruptured rotator cuff tendon, *Acta Orthop Scand* 46:751-757, 1975.
5. Bassett RW et al: Glenohumeral muscle force and mechanics in a position of shoulder instability, *J Biomech* 23:405, 1990.
6. Bassett RW, Cofield RH: Acute tears of the rotator cuff: the timing of surgical repair, *Clin Orthop* 175:18-24, 1983.
7. Bateman JE: Cuff tears in athletes, *Orthop Clin North Am* 4:721-745, 1973.
8. Bateman JE, Welsh RP: *Surgery of the shoulder,* Philadelphia, 1984, BC Decker.
9. Bigliani LU et al: Operative repair of massive rotator cuff tears: long-term results, *J Shoulder Elbow Surg* 1(3):120-130, 1992.
10. Bigliani LU et al: Repair of rotator cuff tears in tennis players, *Am J Sports Med* 20(2):112-117, 1992.
11. Bigliani LU, Morrison DS, April EW: The morphology of the acromion and its relationship to rotator cuff tears, *Orthop Trans* 10(2):228, 1986.
12. Brenneke SL, Morgan CJ: Evaluation of ultrasonography as a diagnostic technique in the assessment of rotator cuff tears, *Am J Sports Med* 20(3):287-289, 1992.
13. Brown JT: Early assessment of supraspinatus tears, procaine infiltration as a guide to treatment, *J Bone Joint Surg* 31B:423-425, 1949.
14. Burk DL et al: MR imaging of shoulder injuries in professional baseball players (1), *J Mag Res Imaging* 1(3):385-389, 1991.
15. Burkhart SS: Arthroscopic treatment of massive rotator cuff tears: clinical results and biomechanical rationale, *Clin Orthop* 267:45-56, 1991.
16. Burkhead WZ, Scheinberg RR, Box G: Surgical anatomy of the axillary nerve, *J Shoulder Elbow Surg* 1(1):31-36, 1992.
17. Clark JM, Harryman DT: Tendons, ligaments, and capsule of the rotator cuff, *J Bone Joint Surg* 74A(5):713-725, 1992.
18. Clark J, Sidles JA, and Matsen FA: The relationship of the glenohumeral joint capsule to the rotator cuff, *Clin Orthop* 254:29-34, 1990.
19. Codman EA: *The shoulder,* Malabar, Fla, 1984, RE Kreiger Publishing.
20. Codman EA: The classic: rupture of the supraspinatus tendon, *Clin Orthop* 254:3-26, 1990 (reprinted from *Boston Med Surg J* clxiv[2]:708-710, May 18, 1911).
21. Cofield RH: Current concepts review: rotator cuff disease of the shoulder, *J Bone Joint Surg* 67A(6):974-979, 1985.
22. Cofield RH, Hoffmeyer P, Lanzer WL: Surgical repair of chronic rotator cuff tears, *Orthop Trans* 14(2):251, 1990.
23. Conway JE, Watson KC: Ultrasonographic detection of incomplete rotator cuff tears, *Orthop Trans* 11(3):585, 1987.
24. Debeyre J, Patte D, Emelik E: Repair of ruptures of the rotator cuff with a note on advancement of the supraspinatus muscle, *J Bone Joint Surg* 47B:36-42, 1965.
25. DesMarchais JE, Vezina J: The accuracy of double-contrast arthrotomography in evaluating the size of rotator cuff tears, *Orthop Trans* 9(1):49, 1985.
26. DiGiovine NM et al: An electromyographic analysis of the upper extremity in pitching, *J Shoulder Elbow Surg* 1(1):15-25, 1992.
27. Ellman H: Surgical treatment of rotator cuff rupture. In Watson MS, editor: *Surgical disorders of the shoulder,* Edinburgh, 1991, Churchill Livingstone, pp 283-291.
28. Ellman H: Diagnosis and treatment of incomplete rotator cuff tears, *Clin Orthop* 254:64-74, 1990.
29. Ellman H: Arthroscopic subacromial decompression: a preliminary report, *Orthop Trans* 9(1):49, 1985.
30. Ellman H, Hanker G, Bayer M: Repair of the rotator cuff: end-result study of factors influencing reconstruction, *J Bone Joint Surg* 68A(8):1136-1144, 1986.
31. Ellman H, Kay SP: Arthroscopic subacromial decompression: 2 to 5 year result, *Orthop Trans* 13(2):239, 1989.
32. Essman JA, Bell RH, Askew M: Full-thickness rotator-cuff tear: an analysis of results, *Clin Orthop* 265:170-177, 1991.
33. Farley TE: Full-thickness tears of the rotator cuff of the shoulder: diagnosis with MR imaging, *Am J Radiol* 158:347-351, 1992.

34. Fly WR et al: Arthroscopic subacromial decompression in athletes less than 40 years old, *Orthop Trans* 14(2):250, 1990.
35. Fukuda H, Mikasa M, Yamanaka K: Incomplete thickness rotator cuff tears diagnosed by subacromial bursography, *Clin Orthop* 223:51-58, 1987.
36. Fukuda H, Craig EV, Yamanaka K: Surgical treatment of incomplete thickness tears of rotator cuff: long-term follow-up, *Orthop Trans* 11(2):237-238, 1987.
37. Fukuda H et al: The partial thickness tear of the rotator cuff, *Orthop Trans* 7(1):137, 1983.
38. Gartsman GM: Arthroscopic acromioplasty for lesions of the rotator cuff, *J Bone Joint Surg* 72A(2):169-180, 1990.
39. Godsil RD Jr, Linscheid RL: Intratendinous defects of the rotator cuff, *Clin Orthop* 69:181-188, 1970.
40. Gore DR et al: Shoulder-muscle strength and range of motion following surgical repair of full-thickness rotator-cuff tears, *J Bone Joint Surg* 68A(2):266-272, 1986.
41. Hamada K: Roentgenographic findings in massive rotator cuff tears: a long-term observation, *Clin Orthop* 254:92-97, 1990.
42. Harryman DT et al: Repairs of the rotator cuff: correlation of functional results with integrity of the cuff, *J Bone Joint Surg* 73A(7):982-989, 1991.
43. Hattrup SJ et al: Shoulder arthrography for determination of size of rotator cuff tear, *J Shoulder Elbow Surg* 1(2):98-105, 1992.
44. Hawkins RJ et al: Failed anterior acromioplasty, *Clin Orthop* 243:106-111, 1989.
45. Hawkins RJ, Misamore GW, Hobeika PE: Surgery for full-thickness rotator-cuff tears, *J Bone Joint Surg* 67A(9):1349-1355, 1985.
46. Hawkins RJ, Bokor DJ: Clinical evaluation of shoulder problems. In Rockwood CA, Matsen FA, editors: *The shoulder,* Philadelphia, 1990, WB Saunders, pp 149-177.
47. Iannotti JP et al: Magnetic resonance imaging of the shoulder, *J Bone Joint Surg* 73A(1):17-29, 1991.
48. Iannotti JP, editor: *Rotator cuff disorders,* Rosemont, Ill, 1991, American Academy of Orthopaedic Surgeons.
49. Inman VT, Saunders JB, Abbott LC: Observations on the function of the shoulder joint, *J Bone Joint Surg* 26A:1, 1944.
50. Jobe CM, Sidles J: *Evidence for a superior glenoid impingement upon the rotator cuff: anatomic, kinesiologic, MRI and arthroscopic findings,* Fifth International Conference on Surgery of the Shoulder, Paris, France, July 12, 1992.
51. Jobe FW: Personal communication, 1994.
52. Jobe FW, Bradley JP, Pink M: Impingement syndrome in overhand athletes: part I, Surg Rounds Orthop, *Sports Med Series* 19-24, 1990.
53. Jobe FW: Impingement problems in the athlete. In Barr JS, editor: *Instructional Course Lecture,* XXXVIII, Boston, 1989, AAOS, pp 205-209.
54. Jobe FW, Jobe CM: Painful athletic injuries of the shoulder, *Clin Orthop* 173:117-124, 1983.
55. Jobe FW, Kvitne RS: Shoulder pain in the overhand or throwing athlete: the relationship of anterior instability and rotator cuff impingement, *Orthop Rev* XVIII(9):963-975, 1989.
56. Jobe FW, Bradley JP: Rotator cuff injuries in baseball prevention and rehabilitation, *Sports Med* 6:378-387, 1988.
57. Jobe FW, Bradley JP, Pink M: Impingement syndrome in overhand athletes: part II, Surg Rounds Orthop, *Sports Med Series* 39-41, September, 1990.
58. Jobe FW, Bradley JP: Impingement syndrome in overhand athletes: part III, Surg Rounds Orthop, Sports Med Series, 24-26, October, 1990.
59. Jobe FW, Bradley JP: The diagnosis and nonoperative treatment of shoulder injuries in athletes, *Clin Sports Med* 8(3):419-437, 1989.
60. Jobe FW, Moynes DR: Delineation of diagnostic criteria and a rehabilitation program for rotator cuff injuries, *Am J Sports Med* 10(6):336-339, 1982.
61. Kvitne R, Jobe F: The diagnosis and treatment of anterior instability in the throwing athlete, *Clin Orthop* 291:107-123, 1993.
62. Levy HJ, Uribe JW, Delaney LG: Arthroscopic assisted rotator cuff repair: preliminary results, *Arthroscopy* 6(1):55-60, 1990.
63. Matsen FA, Arntz CT: Rotator cuff tendon failure. In Rockwood CA, Matsen FA, editors: *The shoulder,* Philadelphia, 1990, WB Saunders, pp 647-677.
64. McLaughlin HL: Rupture rotator cuff, *J Bone Joint Surg* 44A:979-983, 1962.
65. Middleton WD: Ultrasonographic evaluation of the rotator cuff and biceps tendon, *J Bone Joint Surg* 68A(3):440-450, 1986.
66. Misamore GW, Woodward C: Evaluation of degenerative lesions of the rotator cuff, *J Bone Joint Surg* 73A(5):704-706, 1991.
67. Moseley HF, Goldie I: The arterial pattern of the rotator cuff of the shoulder, *J Bone Joint Surg* 45B(4):780-789, 1963.
68. Neer CS, Flatow EL, Lech O: Tears of the rotator cuff: long term results of anterior acromioplasty and repair, *Orthop Trans* 12:735, 1988.
69. Neer CS, Welsh RP: The shoulder in sports, *Orthop Clin North Am* 8(3):583-591, 1977.
70. Neer CS, Marberry TA: On the disadvantages of radical acromionectomy, *J Bone Joint Surg* 63A(3):416-419, 1981.
71. Neer CS, Poppen NK: Supraspinatus outlet, *Orthop Trans* 11(2): 234, 1987.
72. Neer CS: Anterior acromioplasty for the chronic impingement syndrome in the shoulder, *J Bone Joint Surg* 54A(1):41-50, 1972.
73. Neer CS, Bigliani LU, Hawkins RJ: Rupture of the long head of the biceps related to subacromial impingement, *Orthop Trans* 1:111, 1977.
74. Neer CS: Impingement lesions, *Clin Orthop* 173:70-77, 1983.
75. Neer CS: *Shoulder reconstruction,* Philadelphia, 1990, WB Saunders, pp 26, 27, 74.
76. Neviaser TJ, Neviaser RJ: The diagnosis and treatment of incomplete rotator cuff tears, *Orthop Trans* 13(2):239, 1989.
77. Neviaser RJ: Ruptures of the rotator cuff, *Orthop Clin North Am* 18(3):387-394, 1987.
78. Noah J, Gidumal R: Rotator cuff injuries in the throwing athlete, *Orthop Rev* XVII(11):1091-1096, 1988.
79. Nobuhara K, Ikeda H: Rotator interval lesion, *Clin Orthop* 223:44-50, 1987.
80. Petersson CJ, Gentz CF: Ruptures of the supraspinatus tendon, *Clin Orthop* 174:143-148, 1983.
81. Pettersson G: Rupture of the tendon aponeurosis of the shoulder joint in anterior inferior dislocation, *Acta Chir Scand (Suppl)* 77:1-184, 1942.
82. Poppen NK, Walker PS: Forces at the glenohumeral joint in abduction, *Clin Orthop* 135:165-170, 1978.
83. Post M, Silver R, Singh M: Rotator cuff tear: diagnosis and treatment, *Clin Orthop* 173:78-91, 1983.
84. Post M: Complications of rotator cuff surgery, *Clin Orthop* 254:97-104, 1990.
85. Rathbun JB, Macnab I: The microvascular pattern of the rotator cuff, *J Bone Joint Surg* 52B(3):540-553, 1970.
86. Rockwood CA, Lyons FR: Surgical treatment of the shoulder impingement syndrome: a modification of the Neer anterior acromioplasty in 71 shoulders, *Orthop Trans* 14(2):251, 1990.
87. Rockwood CA, Lyons FR: Shoulder impingement syndrome: diagnosis, radiographic evaluation, and treatment with a modified Neer acromioplasty, *J Bone Joint Surg* 75A(3):409-424, 1993.
88. Samilson RL, Binder WF: Symptomatic full thickness tears of the rotator cuff: an analysis of 292 shoulders in 276 patients, *Orthop Clin North Am* 6(2):449-466, 1975.
89. Seeger LL: Magnetic resonance imaging of the shoulder, *Clin Orthop* 244:48-59, 1989.
90. Seltzer D et al: Anatomy of the axillary nerve: relationship to surgical approaches to the rotator cuff, unpublished data, 1992.

91. Shaffer B et al: Infraspinatus-splitting incision in posterior shoulder surgery: an anatomic and electromyographic study, *Am J Sports Med* 22(Jan/Feb):113-120, 1993.
92. Snyder SJ et al: Partial thickness rotator cuff tears: results of arthroscopic treatment, *Arthroscopy* 7(1):1-7, 1991.
93. Takagish N: Conservative treatment of the ruptures of the rotator cuff, *J Jpn Orthop Assoc* 52:781-787, 1978.
94. Thorling F, Hovelius L: Surgical treatment of rotator cuff impingement. In Watson MS, editor: *Surgical disorders of the shoulder*, New York, 1991, Churchill Livingstone, pp 271-282.
95. Tibone JE et al: Surgical treatment of tears of the rotator cuff in athletes, *J Bone Joint Surg* 68A(6):887-891, 1986.
96. Tibone JE et al: Shoulder impingement syndrome in athletes treated by an anterior acromioplasty, *Clin Orthop* 198:134-140, 1985.
97. Uhthoff HK, Loehr J, Sarkar K: The pathogenesis of rotator cuff tears. In: *Proceedings of the Third International Conference on Surgery of the Shoulder*, Fukuoka, Japan, October 27, 1986.
98. Warner JJP et al: Anatomy and relationships of the suprascapular nerve: anatomical constraints to mobilization of the supraspinatus and infraspinatus muscles in the management of massive rotator-cuff tears, *J Bone Joint Surg* 74A(1):36-45, 1992.
99. Watson M: Major ruptures of the rotator cuff: the results of surgical repair in 89 patients, *J Bone Joint Surg* 67B(4):618-624, 1985.
100. Wiley AM: Superior humeral dislocation: a complication following decompression and débridement for rotator cuff tears, *Clin Orthop* 263:135-141, 1991.
101. Wilson CL, Duff GL: Pathologic study of degeneration and rupture of the supraspinatus tendon, *Arch Surg* 47:121-135, 1943.
102. Wolfgang GL: Surgical repair of tears of the rotator cuff of the shoulder, factors influencing the result, *J Bone Joint Surg* 56A:14-26, 1974.
103. Zlatkin MB et al: Rotator cuff tears: diagnostic performance of MR imaging, *Radiology* 172(1):223-229, 1989.
104. Zuckerman JD et al: The influence of coracoacromial arch anatomy on rotator cuff tears, *J Shoulder Elbow Surg* 1(1):4-13, 1992.

SECTION F Conservative and Postoperative Management of Shoulder Problems

Treating a high-caliber athlete with an injured shoulder requires an understanding of normal motion at the scapulothoracic and glenohumeral joints. If movement, strength, coordination, and proper biomechanics are not restored to the physiologic preinjury level, sophisticated function will be impossible. This chapter will discuss the early diagnosis and treatment of shoulder injuries. This chapter will mention what the authors have done in the past and why some of these procedures have been changed; the chapter also will cover the optimal physical therapy treatment for patients with anterior instability and for those with primary, subacromial impingement. At the end of the chapter is an example of an evaluation form and some protocols to use for sport-specific exercise (baseball, tennis, golf) in the final stages of rehabilitation.

For athletes and indeed for most patients, early treatment is better treatment. In the past, the main treatment for many orthopedic injuries was rest, with the ultimate in "rest" being immobilization. Today, clinicians understand better the role played by flexible tissues and well-conditioned muscles in the final outcome of the treatment program. Adherence to the old rest routine leads to tenacious adhesions that are difficult to elongate and painful to move. Disuse contributes to muscular atrophy, reduced strength, diminished endurance, and decreased coordination. Any one or more of these problems mandates a longer recovery. Early attention to controlled and specific mobility leads to the formation of what we call "flexible scar tissue." Such tissue lends itself more readily to the extensibility athletes need if they wish to return to serious competition. Shoulder joints with full, unrestricted range of motion can be strengthened throughout their arc, rather than just within a restricted section of it.

In the past, impingement problems and unstable

shoulders were treated as two unrelated kinds of pathology. Rotator cuff disease, when recognized (and not misdiagnosed as bursitis, bicipital tendinitis, or shoulder osteoarthritis) was treated with exercise by the therapist and subacromial decompression by the orthopedist. These patients were classified by the presence and size of their tears. Some of these patients improved, some were unchanged, and some became worse. For a long time, examiners were unable to distinguish retrospectively which antecedent factors were responsible for each of these outcomes.

The diagnosis of shoulder instability was made much less often. The treatment goal, after the diagnosis was made, was simple: Stabilize the shoulder to keep it from coming out of the joint again. To that end, therapists most often saw patients postoperatively who had undergone a Bankart repair, modified Bristow repair, or other stabilizing procedure. These patients, in addition to their surgery, had undergone a period of immobilization that varied by procedure and by surgeon. The patients' shoulders were managed in a sling, with minimal motion allowed for several weeks to several months. Regaining function was an arduous and time-consuming task for patient and therapist. Full flexibility seldom was attained, despite the best efforts of both. Patients requiring a full or an extended range of motion found themselves unable to return to their preinjury level of performance because most operative procedures offered stability at the expense of mobility.

Thus there were two groups of patients with a number of unsatisfactory outcomes among them: patients with impingement whose pain did not decrease with the standard exercises and/or subacromial decompression and patients with unstable shoulders who never were able to regain enough motion postoperatively to function effectively in their desired sports.

INSTABILITY

Classification

Younger, athletic patients with shoulder pain and signs of impingement have a problem that falls somewhere along an instability continuum. These repeated physiologic demands test the limits of the patient's strength and endurance. When either is found wanting, brief episodes of anterior instability ensue. In addition, with repeated anterior translation of the humeral head, a tightened posterior capsule is often seen, which contributes its own impetus to the other anteriorly directed forces. The humeral head, now placed less than optimally, rides anteriorly and superiorly in the glenoid, thereby leading to both labral pathology and impingement posteriorly; continued impingement can result in a frank tear of the rotator cuff tissue.

For classification purposes in young overhead athletes without complete dislocation, this continuum is divided into four functional categories. Group 1 has pure impingement with no antecedent or underlying instability. Group 2 patients have instability with impingement as a secondary phenomenon. Group 3 demonstrates generalized ligamentous laxity and also has evidence of impingement secondary to this laxity. Group 4 patients have an incident, usually traumatic, in their history that has caused them an episode of instability. No impingement is present.

ANTERIOR INSTABILITY

Conservative Management

A conservative program for patients in groups 2, 3, and 4—all of whom have anteriorly unstable shoulders—focuses on restoring the strength of the scapular muscles, rotator cuff, and anterior wall muscles along with the normal scapulohumeral rhythm. This rhythm depends on synergistic timing, adequate strength, and sufficient endurance. The first part of the goal, the easy part, is to see whether the muscles responsible for providing stability during motion can be strengthened to provide some dynamic restraint to the anteriorly translating humeral head. The second and more important part of the program is to give these muscles enough endurance to perform that task of dynamic stabilization repeatedly with no degradation in the quality of the output.

All rehabilitation programs should have two goals: strengthening the dynamic stabilizers so that these muscles can exert the desired control and contract with the necessary synergistic action and restoring the flexibility of structures that may be restricting the joint excursion necessary for optimal performance. Overall strength and endurance must be adequate for vocational and avocational use. However, if the anterior joint capsule and ligaments are attenuated and the glenoid labrum is frayed or torn, exercises alone may not be able to restore the original integrity of either of these structures.

Flexibility

Tightness in either the posterior or inferior structures can contribute to instability and secondary impingement. A tight posterior capsule can push the humeral head forward and, in the face of inadequate anterior restraints, may lever the head far enough forward during motion to produce symptoms. Posterior capsular structures should be stretched or mobilized to facilitate posterior gliding of the humeral head so that it resumes its normal orientation to the glenoid fossa.

The most commonly used posterior cuff stretch is produced by pulling the arm across the chest, into extreme horizontal adduction (Fig. 7-85). Some patients, especially those who have some associated rotator cuff or bicipital irritation, find this stretch uncomfortable. One gentle, alternative method is shown in Fig. 1-1. Lying supine with the shoulder abducted to 90°, the arm is passively internally rotated, allowing the humeral head to stretch the posterior tissues.

Another effective posterior capsular stretch requires the patient to lie on the uninvolved side, with the shoulder horizontally abducted and the scapula adducted. The examiner fixes the axillary border of the scapula and horizontally adducts the humerus (Fig. 7-86), stretching both the posterior capsule and the posterior deltoid.

Strength

The rotator cuff, serratus anterior, deltoid, trapezius, rhomboids, pectoralis major, and latissimus dorsi are the primary muscles controlling the various aspects of shoulder function. Chapter 5 covers some of the research data detailing specifics of the function of these muscles during athletic activities.

The rotator cuff muscles depress the humeral head and compress it in its position on the glenoid. When this position is attained, the deltoid elevates the humerus. Obtaining and maintaining this optimal glenoid position are very important in the prevention of dysfunction. The supraspinatus works in synergy with the deltoid to produce elevation, the subscapularis controls adduction and internal rotation, and the cuff as a whole works to depress the humeral head and counteract the upward force of a strong deltoid. In Figs. 1-2, 1-3, 1-4, 1-6, 1-8, and 1-9 illustrate strengthening exercises for the supraspinatus, the subscapularis, and the infraspinatus/teres minor complex.

Another method of strengthening the supraspinatus has been described by Blackburn.[2] He suggests that the patient lie prone with the involved extremity hanging off the side of the table. The patient abducts the arm horizontally while in external rotation (Fig. 7-87). Blackburn believes that there is more supraspinatus activity during this maneuver than there is during the "empty beer can" supraspinatus exercise. A recent study by Ballatyne et al[1] does not support this conclusion. In addition, the humeral head is levered forward during this exercise, which is an undesirable position. Finally, this exercise also strengthens the posterior cuff and deltoid. The clinician must make certain that relative posterior structure tightness has been rectified before proceeding so that strengthening of these muscles does not perpetuate the capsular imbalance so often found in these patients' shoulders.

For these reasons, the scapular plane elevation ("scaption") exercise should still be used for the supraspinatus. When this exercise is performed properly, with careful attention to positioning and prevention of more than 90° of elevation, most patients can perform it without pain. In the early stages, just lifting the arm against gravity provides enough resistance. When 20 to 30 repetitions are

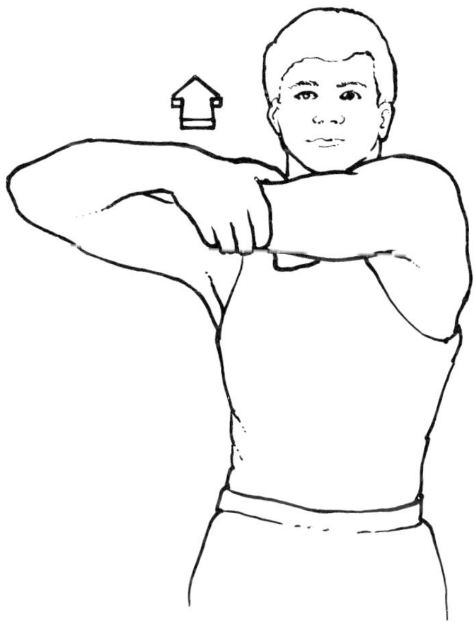

FIGURE 7-85 Posterior cuff stretch.

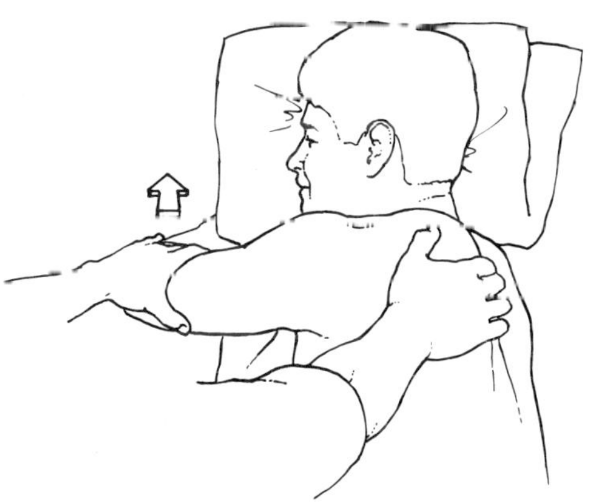

FIGURE 7-86 Side-lying posterior cuff stretch.

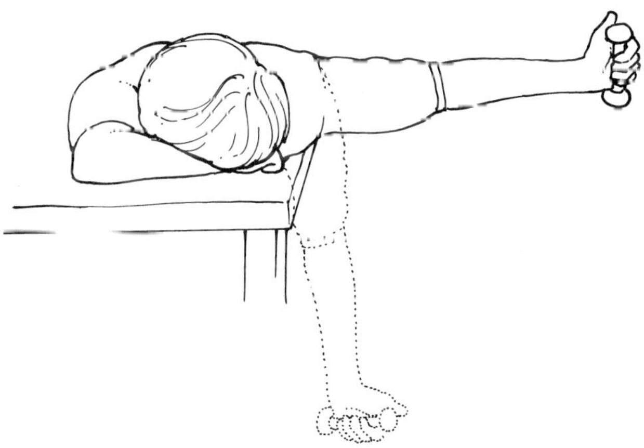

FIGURE 7-87 Prone supraspinatus strengthening exercise.

possible without pain, weights are added, ½ pound at a time. Although patients almost always have unilateral pathology, bilateral performance of this and the other elevation exercises (forward flexion and abduction) facilitates normal scapulohumeral rhythm.

Strengthening the subscapularis may pay another dividend. Anatomically, the subscapularis lies anterior to the glenohumeral joint and, when contracted, it acts as an anterior wall to restrict the amount of anterior translation possible by the humeral head. However, this restrictive function occurs only with the arm below 75° to 80° of abduction and external rotation. With increased abduction, the muscle's line of pull relative to the joint no longer produces an effective restraint.[14]

External rotation is controlled by the infraspinatus and teres minor. Such motion must be consistently performed and appropriately timed to allow the greater tuberosity to clear the coracoacromial arch without mechanical interference. There are several ways to strengthen the external rotators of the shoulder. The therapist must consider the stage of rehabilitation when choosing exercises. Some of the choices are side-lying with the arm at the side and hand weights for resistance; standing, with the arm at the side, using rubber tubing for resistance; prone, with the arm abducted 90° and using the weight of the arm moving into internal and external rotation for resistance; isokinetic exercise with the arm at the side in the loose-packed position; and isokinetic exercise with the arm abducted to 90°.

Exercising with the arm at the side has been criticized for contributing to decreased blood flow in the relatively avascular zone of the supraspinatus tendon as it inserts onto the humerus.[12] Many clinicians advocate that the humerus be placed in the loose-packed position for arm-at-the-side exercises; this is approximately 30° of forward flexion to the scapular plane, to faciliate blood flow through the supraspinatus at its musculotendinous junction. Other authors advocate exercising the internal and external rotators with the arm in 90° of abduction, allowing unrestricted or uncompressed blood flow. However, 90° of abduction is a vulnerable position for the glenohumeral joint; thus this position must be considered cautiously.

Another objection to the arm-at-the-side exercises is that this position is not a functional one and therefore does not prepare the patient to return to preinjury activities, especially if such an activity profile includes overhead sports or occupational activity wherein the arm is abducted with rotation. In addition, the teres minor is not optimally exercised in this position. Despite these concerns, isokinetic exercise for rotation in a position of abduction may not be the best choice. During isokinetic exercise in this posture, the elbow pad supporting the arm does not permit the rotator cuff musculature to perform its primary function, that is, depressing the humeral head in the glenoid fossa while rotating the humerus. Also, as patients progress and gradually resume their functional activities, the rotator cuff muscles become stronger in their functional range.

Exercise in the prone position certainly does not meet the functional requirement. The prone position may allow the patient to work against gravity more than in other positions, requiring more effort to rotate the humerus externally. It can, however, put additional strain across the anterior capsular structures, as previously mentioned. For that reason, caution should be exercised when this maneuver is used.

The arm-at-the-side posture offers several advantages. First and perhaps most important, it allows the patient to isolate specific muscles and strengthen them as needed before combining these rotators with other shoulder girdle groups to work for endurance and function. Second, with the arm in this position, it is easier to modify exercise motion minutely and prevent anterior translation of the humeral head. The patient will more likely be pain free in this position and be able to keep the humeral head centrally located in the fossa.

The serratus anterior, whose functions are outlined in the previous chapter, can be strengthened as depicted in Fig. 1-14 or, alternatively, with a military press, performed as described in Fig. 7-88.

The lower portion of the serratus anterior, responsible for upward rotation, helps to preserve contact between the glenoid fossa and the humerus during arm elevation. When this contact is maintained, the deltoid can act at a mechanical advantage. Conversely, inadequate strength in the lower serratus anterior makes it difficult to main-

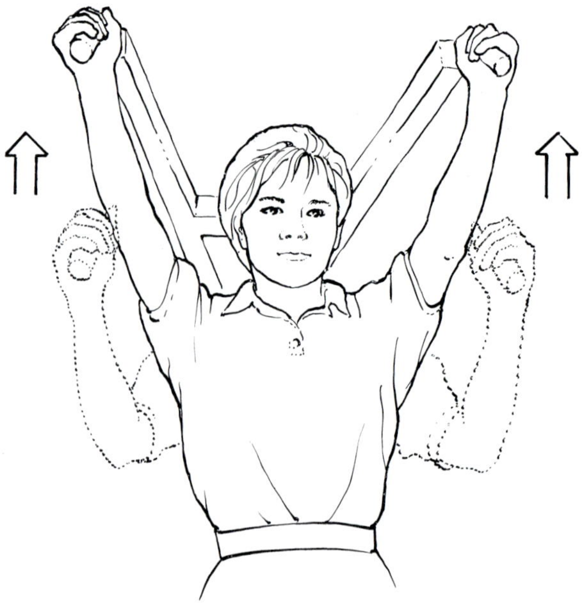

FIGURE 7-88 Military press.

tain the appropriate relationship between the humeral head and glenoid; the deltoid must function at a relative mechanical disadvantage. An efficient strengthening program consists of push-ups with maximal scapular protraction at the end of the motion (push-ups "plus") and military presses in 125° to 135° of forward flexion.

Exercises for the latissimus dorsi and the teres major must be included in this conservative rehabilitation program for patients in groups 2, 3, and 4. These muscles (part of the "power group") are especially active during the late cocking and acceleration phases of throwing, contracting eccentrically to decelerate the humerus while functioning as humeral head depressors to center the head in the glenoid fossa.[5] As motion proceeds into acceleration, the latissimus dorsi and the teres major contract concentrically to rotate the humerus internally. Subjective complaints of posterior glenohumeral joint pain may result from overuse and weakness of these muscles in the face of continued demand. Tenderness may be present and palpable at the proximal half of the axillary scapular border.

Exercises to strengthen the latissimus dorsi and teres major muscles can be performed either prone or in the standing position and are illustrated in Chapter 1. The patient starts with free weights and progresses gradually to heavier weights before going on to weight-training equipment. As mentioned during the discussion on rotator-cuff strengthening, exercise of these muscles can exacerbate or perpetuate anterior instability if it is performed too soon or too vigorously or without careful monitoring of the end position. During horizontal abduction, the patient must try not to lift the arm behind the plane of the trunk (Fig. 7-89). In the early stages, the patient should lift only to the scapular plane (i.e., about 30° in front of the coronal plane).

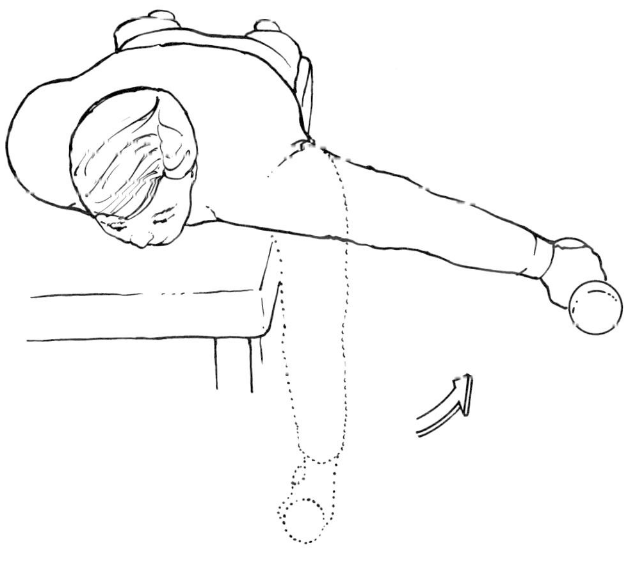

FIGURE 7-89 Prone horizontal abduction.

Endurance

Even though the patient may have the flexibility to permit full external rotation and the strength to maintain the humeral head within the glenoid fossa, problems may occur if endurance is insufficient for the specific task at hand. Fatigue—and its companion ineffectiveness—are most likely to occur in the anatomically smaller muscles first, specifically, those of the rotator cuff. The larger deltoid will continue to function, pulling the humeral head even more superiorly onto the posterior superior labrum, because the counterbalancing humeral head depressors are no longer effective.

A pitcher, the most demanding user of the shoulder, throws many times over many years. During the late cocking phase, the arm is abducted and externally rotated, forcing the humeral head to translate anteriorly and thereby loading the static stabilizers. Active, strong dynamic stabilizers may be able to compensate for this degree of anterior shift. With continued demand (i.e., continued throwing), muscles not trained to adequate levels of endurance will fatigue and no longer provide the dynamic compensation for the anterior shift. The humeral head, no longer located centrally, rotates on a new axis. The new axis is less efficient and demands higher output from the dynamic stabilizers, leading to even more fatigue and a progressive downward spiral of inefficiency and ineffectiveness.

Early in the rehabilitation period, endurance may be improved effectively with either an upper body ergometer or an isokinetic machine. The latter should include work for the internal and external rotators, horizontal abductors and adductors, flexors and extensors, and abductors and adductors. The shoulder should be positioned to avoid any anterior excursion of the humeral head. High speeds (e.g., 200° per second and higher) should be used to approximate those speeds necessary for functional output.

Later in the rehabilitation program, performing functional activities appropriate for a given patient is the most efficient way to improve endurance. When strength and motion permit, the therapist should begin throwing activities with a baseball player; ground strokes with a racquet sport player; chip, putt, and short shots with a golfer; and so on.

Postoperative Management

Sometimes, despite the most vigorously executed and biomechanically appropriate conservative care, repair of the underlying structure is required. The exact timing of the rehabilitation sequence depends on the specifics of the operative findings (e.g., the degree of laxity, presence or absence of coexisting impingement). Because no muscles have been cut, active range of motion within a safe zone can begin the first day after surgery. It is critical to attain full range of motion within 2 months. If full range of motion is not attained within 2 months, it

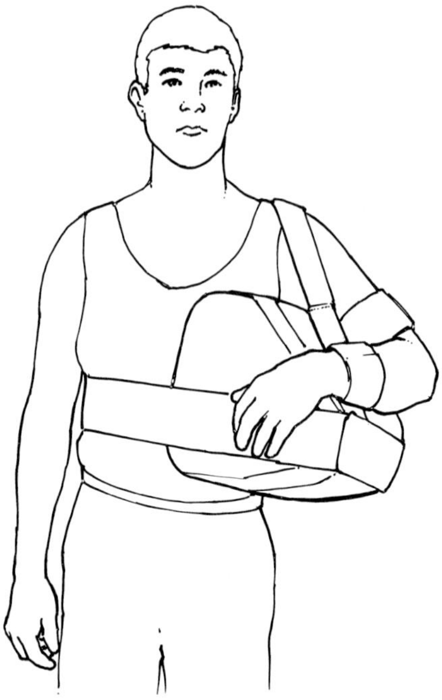

FIGURE 7-90 Pillow abduction splint.

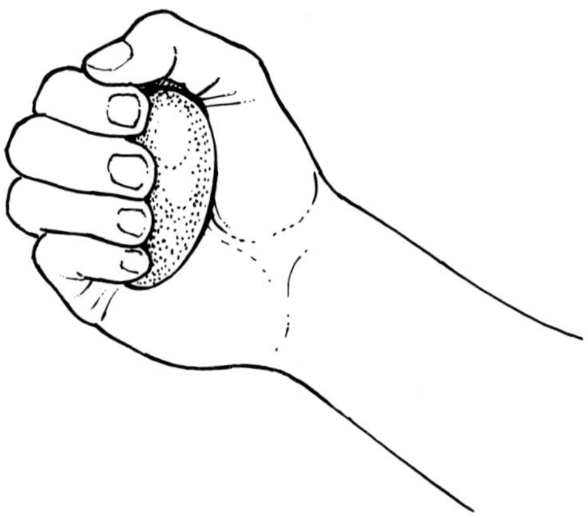

FIGURE 7-91 Hand-strengthening exercise.

becomes extremely difficult ever to reach that level. In setting this goal, the therapist should consider what is "full" motion for a patient. For example, if the patient is a throwing athlete, more external rotation will be needed on the throwing side than on the nonthrowing side.[3]

After an anterior capsulolabral reconstruction, the patient may be in a pillow abduction splint or an "airplane"-type splint for 1 or 2 weeks during the first phase of rehabilitation (Fig. 7-90). Other patients for whom excessive connective tissue laxity is a concern wear a sling after surgery.[6]

During this immediate postoperative period, the patient removes the sling or splint for active and active assisted elevation exercises. On the first day, the patient lifts the arm up and out of the splint. Active elbow flexion and extension and wrist motion begin on the first postoperative day. Patients should begin squeezing a ball or an egg-shaped plastic exerciser immediately (Fig. 7-91).

As soon as the splint or sling is discarded, wand exercises are added for elevation and multiple-angle isometric exercises for internal rotation, external rotation, abduction, flexion, and extension (Fig. 7-92).

Isotonic resisted exercises begin by week 3. The first group of exercises includes active resisted internal (Fig. 7-93, *A*) and external (Fig. 7-93, *B*) rotation with the arm at the side using elastic resistance bands or tubing. Active shoulder extension may be performed either prone (Fig. 7-94) or standing while bending forward at the waist. The patient extends the arm, with the elbow straight, to the plane of the trunk. The patient should not go beyond this plane. When horizontal adduction is added 1 or 2 weeks later, the patient starts in the supine position with the humerus supported so that the exercise begins in the scapular plane and the ending position does not extend beyond this plane (Fig. 7-95).

The second phase of the rehabilitation program emphasizes progressive strengthening, beginning with the shoulder rotators. The patient moves from elastic band resistance of increasing difficulty to side-lying external rotation (Fig. 7-96) with free weights. The therapist must take care to position the arm during internal rotation with a bolster under the lateral chest wall. The patient should perform supraspinatus exercise in a pain-free range only.

The clinician should continue strengthening the anterior deltoid; work above 110° should be included. Active abduction is limited to 90° because deltoid activity peaks at that angle during abduction.[8]

Active horizontal abduction (with the same position options as extension, i.e., prone or leaning forward from the waist) is limited to the plane of the trunk. Scapular adduction and trunk rotation can mimic some degree of horizontal abduction, making it appear that more of horizontal abduction is accomplished than is really the case.

By the third postoperative month, eccentric rotator cuff exercises, vigorous elbow and wrist strengthening, and military presses with the arms in front of the chest (see Fig. 7-88) all are part of the program. For the serratus anterior, the patient should begin with wall push-ups, move on to modified hands-and-knees push-ups, and then progress to regular military push-ups (Fig. 7-97). All styles should emphasize scapular protraction at the end of each repetition.

Isokinetic training is begun when the patient is able to lift 5 to 10 pounds in external rotation and 15 to 20 pounds in internal rotation with no pain and no swelling. Endurance training with an upper-body ergometer begins with an easy 5-minute program: 1 minute forward, 1 minute rest, 1 minute backward, 1 minute rest, and 1 minute forward. The exercise increases in 1-minute increments. The ergometer can be used earlier for upper-extremity mobility work, setting it for extremely low resistance.

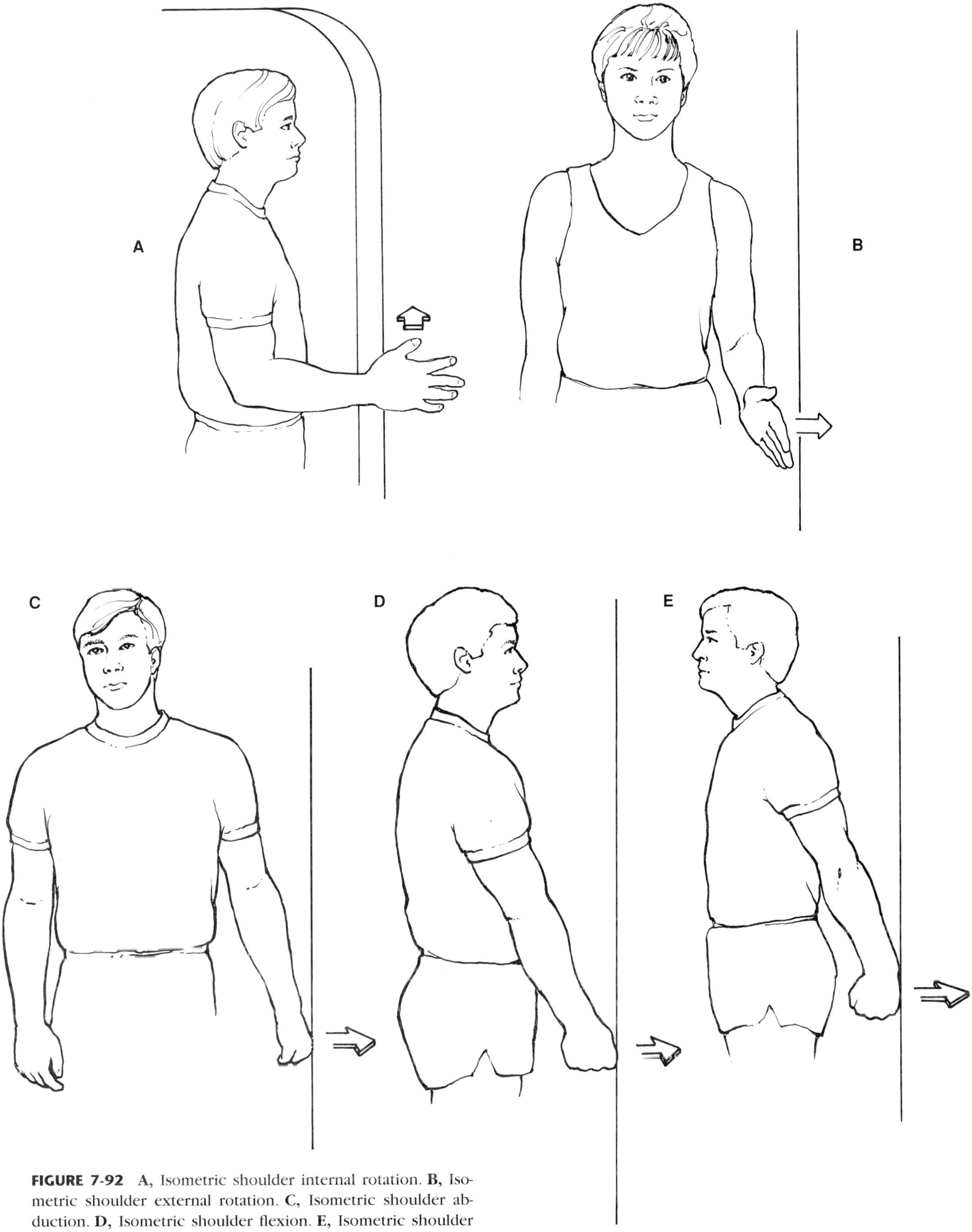

FIGURE 7-92 **A,** Isometric shoulder internal rotation. **B,** Isometric shoulder external rotation. **C,** Isometric shoulder abduction. **D,** Isometric shoulder flexion. **E,** Isometric shoulder extension.

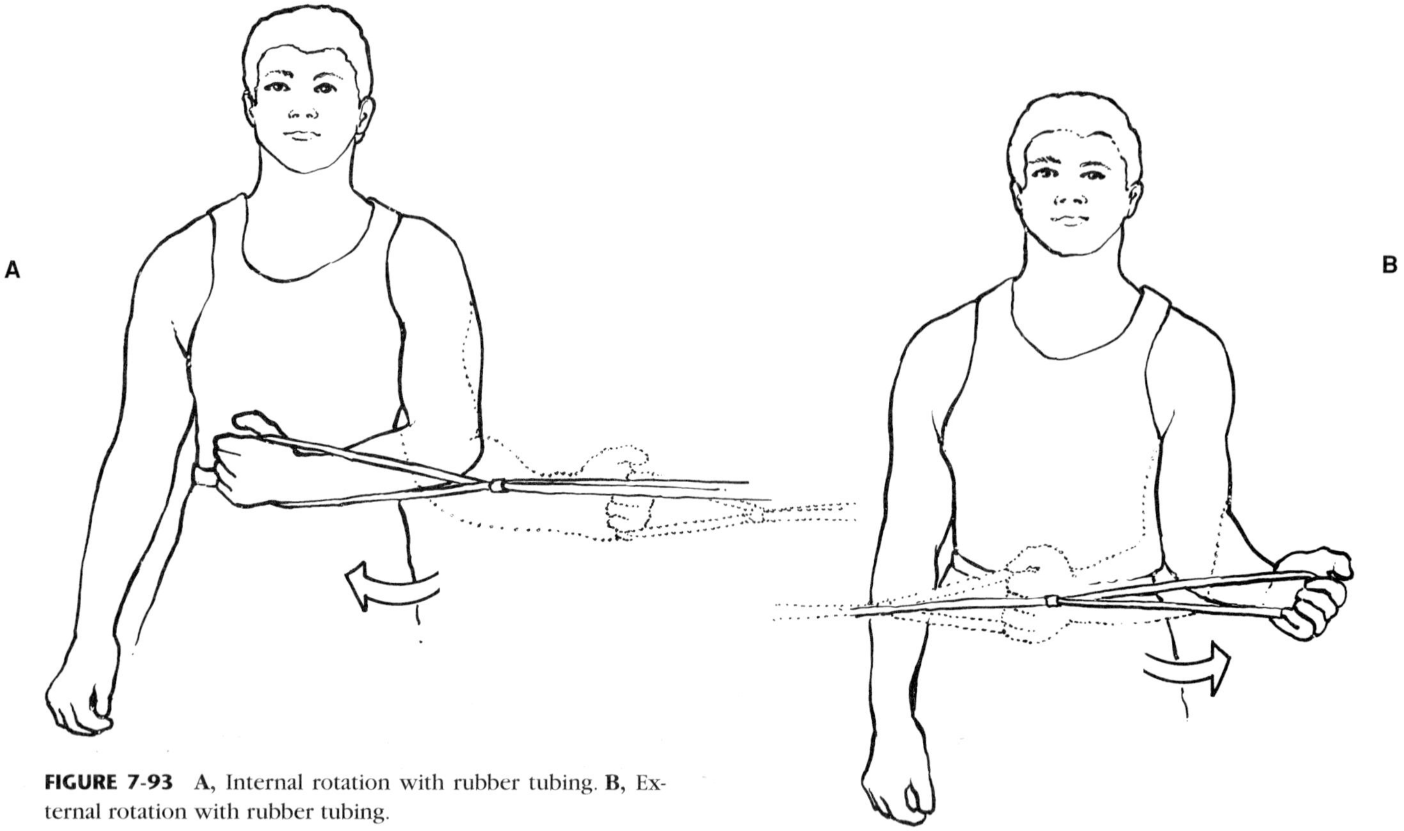

FIGURE 7-93 **A,** Internal rotation with rubber tubing. **B,** External rotation with rubber tubing.

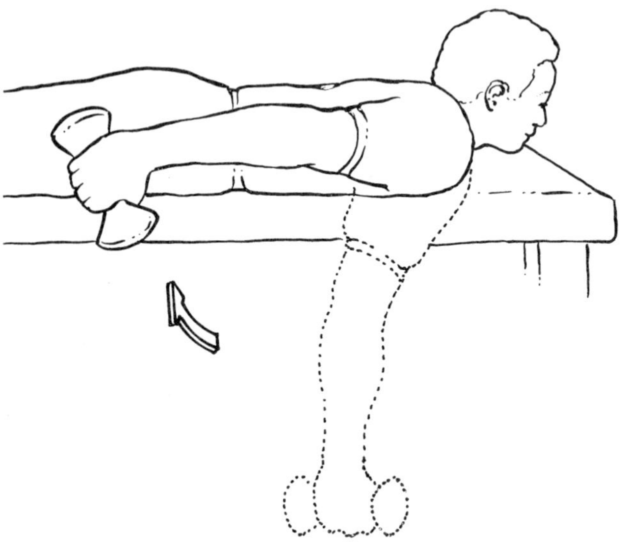

FIGURE 7-94 Prone shoulder extension.

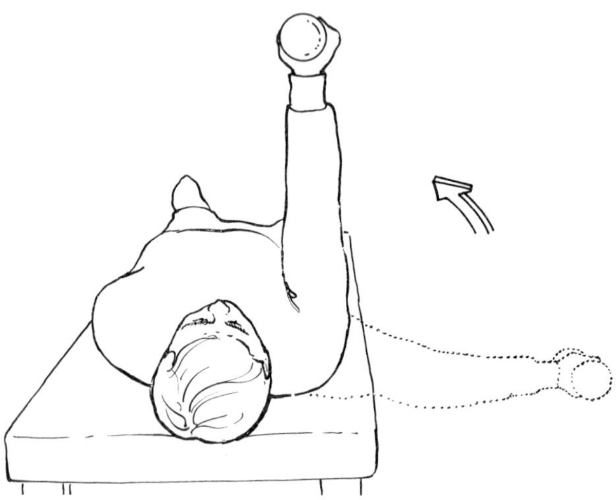

FIGURE 7-95 Horizontal adduction.

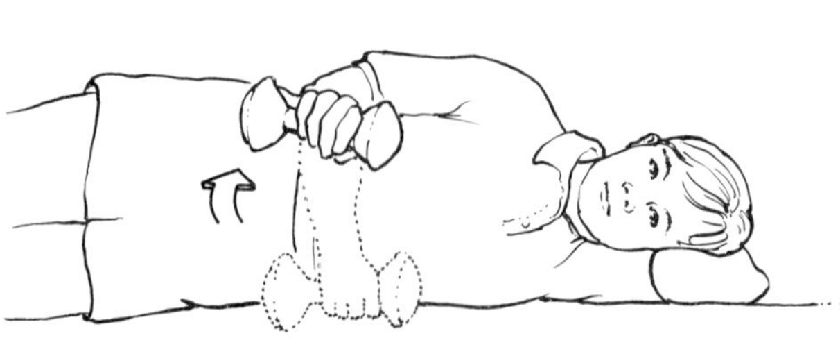

FIGURE 7-96 Side-lying external rotation.

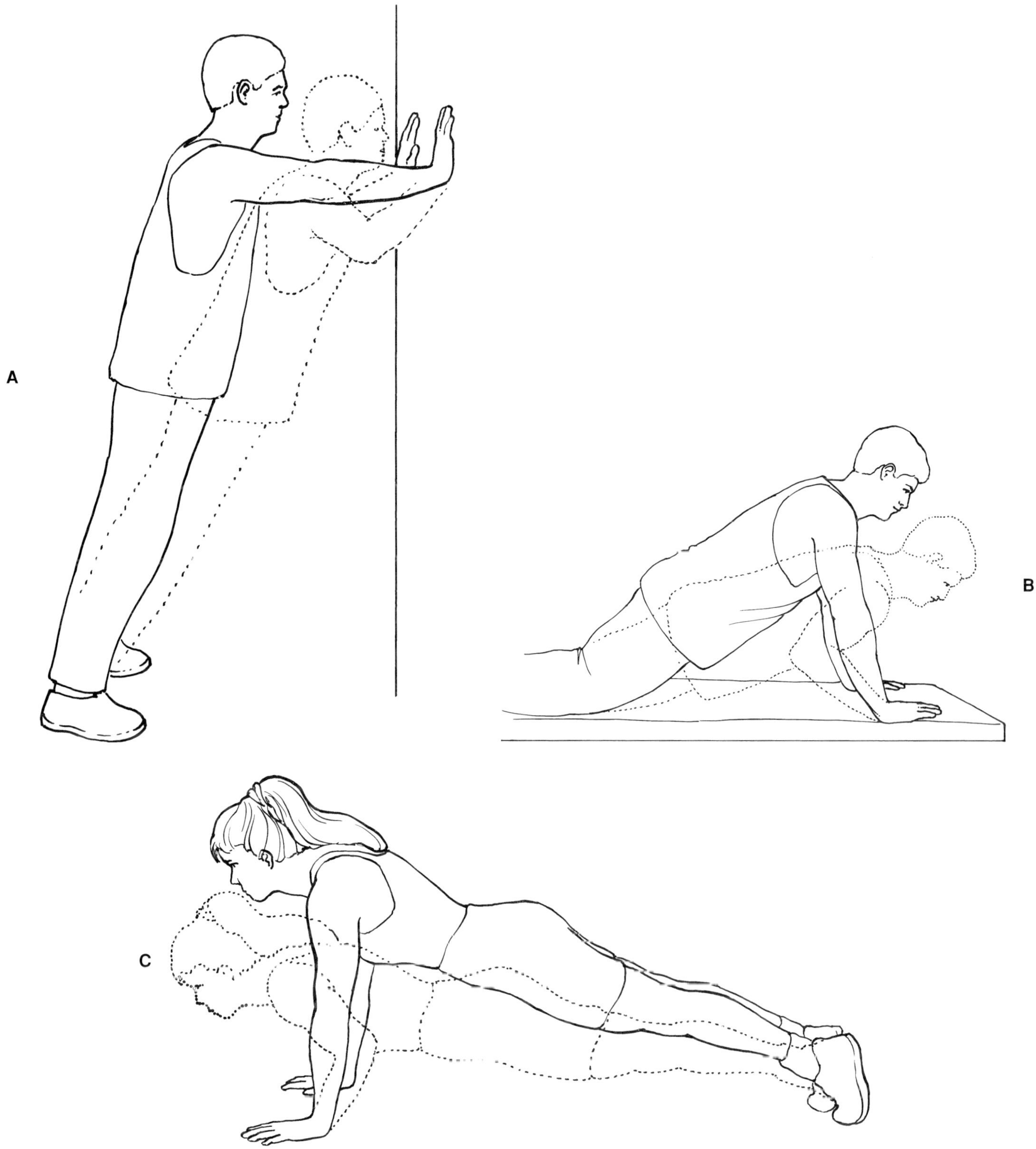

FIGURE 7-97 **A,** Wall push-ups. **B,** Modified hands-and-knees push-ups. **C,** Military push-ups.

At about 4 months after surgery (and if isokinetic testing has verified that the involved shoulder has at least 70% of the strength of the uninvolved shoulder), the third phase—sport-specific rehabilitation—begins. Throwing athletes, tennis players, and golfers begin an appropriate program. (See the rehabilitation protocols for throwers, tennis players, and golfers. These protocols are located at the end of this chapter.) The patient may proceed from one step to the next step of a sport-specific program as long as there is no pain. The number of throws, speed, distance, or number of days spent practicing should decrease depending on the patient's progress or complaints. For throwers, the speed should be three fourths of the maximum speed until about 7 months after surgery; full speed is not a reasonable goal until almost a year after surgery. This allows adequate time for the reconstructed tissues to heal and adapt to the stresses placed on them during throwing.

PRIMARY AND SECONDARY IMPINGEMENT

Impingement syndrome is a common shoulder disorder often associated with periods of repetitive overhead activities. In people over 35 years of age, this syndrome may occur when the rotator cuff and subacromial bursa become trapped against the coracoacromial arch.[6,7,11] Supraspinatus point tenderness, biceps tendon inflammation, and painful overhead motions are the most commonly presented symptoms. Conservative management may include antiinflammatory medication, corticosteroid injection into the subacromial space, and/or exercise for rotator cuff strengthening and scapulohumeral rhythm.[4,6] If this condition persists, rotator cuff tears may result.

However, the symptoms of an impingement syndrome, although part of the younger patient's presenting complaints, often are the secondary effects of an underlying anterior instability. Many patients may be unaware of their instability and offer no subjective complaints of subluxation.

In a throwing athlete, the impingement is most often internal (i.e., inside the glenohumeral joint), and occurs as the supraspinatus rubs against the posteriosuperior rim of the glenoid when the arm is posteriorly angulated (extreme horizontal abduction) and externally rotated. A SLAP lesion may be present if the same condition occurs more superiorly. Early diagnosis and early conservative intervention (stop throwing and initiate rotator cuff strengthening exercises) can alleviate the impingement in 95% of the patients.

Conservative Management

To reduce inflammation, the patient must modify or refrain from activities that aggravate the condition.[10,13] The therapist will apply pain-relief modalities to reduce pain and swelling as needed and perform or direct range-of-motion exercises. Pay special attention to the posterior capsule to allow the humeral head to sit back in the fossa instead of sliding anteriorly and superiorly.[14]

Active strengthening exercises for internal and external rotation are performed with the arm at the side and the elbow fixed to 90° using surgical tubing or other elastic bands for resistance. If necessary, the external rotation exercise can be modified by limiting the degree of rotation; this will prevent excessive translation of the humeral head in the fossa and reduce discomfort. If pain continues, isometric exercise can begin, keeping the arm in the same position (i.e., near the side with the elbow flexed to 90°). If this still causes discomfort, the shoulder position can be adjusted to allow a bit of abduction and flexion—the loose packed position.

As pain decreases and strength increases, free weights are the next step. Internal rotation is best performed lying on the involved side with a bolster under the lateral chest wall to decrease the joint compression on the involved shoulder (Fig. 7-98). Again, the therapist should limit excursion into external rotation on the eccentric portion of the exercise to minimize stress on the anterior capsule. External rotation is performed while lying on the uninvolved side (see Fig. 7-96). The same caution applies about avoiding excessive anterior translation of the humeral head by limiting the degree of external rotation performed. If pain is still a problem, a pillow or towel roll can be placed under the patient's involved shoulder to obtain a position of some abduction and flexion. If 90° elevation is available in the scapular plane, supraspinatus exercise can be added. These exercises are alternated with active shoulder flexion throughout the pain-free range of motion and with shoulder abduction performed in the scapular plane. At some point in the rehabilitation program, attention must be paid to developing strength and, more important, endurance in the anterior and middle deltoid in the overhead (above 90°) position (Fig. 7-99). These exercises must be performed without irritating the cuff structures or the long head of the biceps.

Shoulder extension can be performed as illustrated earlier in the section on instability (i.e., either standing

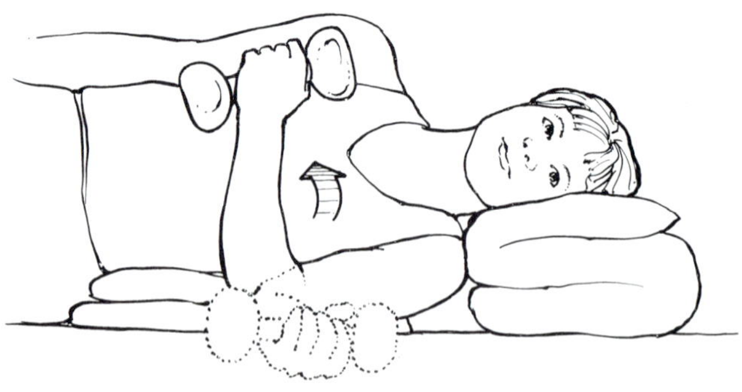

FIGURE 7-98 Side-lying internal rotation.

or prone). The shoulder extensors also function as depressors of the humeral head and thus resist the upward migration of the humeral head, decreasing the likelihood of further impingement.[9]

Shoulder shrugs can be a problem for the patient with primary impingement. When the glenohumeral space is decreased, it is necessary to apply gentle, controlled traction to the humerus to keep it from riding up in the glenoid fossa during the exercise. When excessive laxity is present and is multidirectional, this corrective traction is contraindicated.

Finally, even in the early stages of rehabilitation, shoulder endurance exercises should be included. As soon as adequate pain-free range of motion is present, arm ergometer work can be added. The patient begins with short-duration, low-intensity work and frequent rest periods, increasing duration and intensity as recovery and tolerance permit.

Later in the conservative program, the patient continues to work on posterior cuff and capsule stretching as indicated. When pain is gone, the patient begins isokinetic workouts for both strength and endurance. The patient should use speeds greater than 200° per second for shoulder internal and external rotation. The best and safest position is standing with the dynamometer head tilted and the shoulder in the scapular plane, arm at the side.

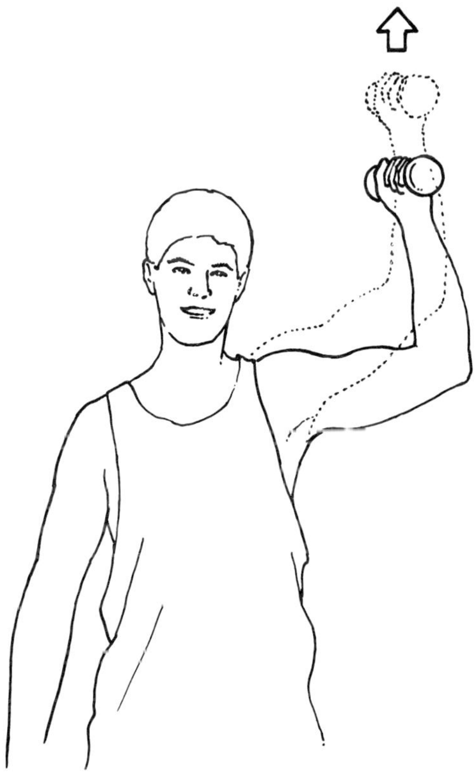

FIGURE 7-99 Anterior and middle deltoid strengthening exercise.

The free-weight portion of the exercise program emphasizes eccentric contraction of the rotator cuff and the posterior shoulder girdle musculature. Active horizontal adduction exercise is added, with the starting position in the scapular plane. Both military presses and push-ups (see Figs. 7-88 and 7-97) are added now. Wall push-ups may be the first phase, concentrating on protraction of the scapula. The patient should pay special attention to getting full extension of the elbows and the extra "push" into full scapular protraction at the end of the exercise and should not lower the trunk below elbow level. For patients, skill development or retrieval feels like the most important part of the program. At this time, the patient begins at a low-intensity level in the specific sport or activity (e.g., volleyball, basketball, work hardening) and progresses logically and carefully. Progress involves intensity, distance, and endurance in an interrelated fashion. It would be unwise to increase all of these variables in a single session.

Throwers initiate their programs with emphasis on technique and endurance. The actual number of throws and the time spent throwing should be small initially and increased only as tolerated. If pain occurs or recurs with any progression, the patient should retreat to the previous level until equilibrium is restored. (See the throwing protocols located at the end of this chapter for more details.)

Conditioning for the rest of the body is appropriate, remembering to include exercises for the forearm, wrist, and fingers. Although not part of the pathologic process, these structures usually have become weakened because the entire extremity has been used less during the injury and recovery periods. Lunges (Fig. 7-100), squats, trunk strengthening and flexibility, and general cardiovascular conditioning should be added now. Isokinetic testing of the shoulder internal and external rotators may be indicated at this point as a marker in the rehabilitation process.

The last stage of the program is continuation of the total body conditioning program and progressively more intense sport-specific workouts. The patient emphasizes the eccentric phase of the rotator cuff strengthening and progressively more difficult isotonic exercises and increases the amount of time spent on the arm ergometer. Skill refinement continues, along with extended workout times. A second isokinetic test for internal and external rotation, as well as one for flexion and extension, may be warranted.

Postoperative Management

When conservative care is insufficient, a surgical repair may be indicated. Such procedures will address the underlying pathology of inadequate glenohumeral joint space, excessive joint laxity, or frank muscle tears. The timing of the rehabilitation program, but not its principles, depends on the specifics of the surgery.

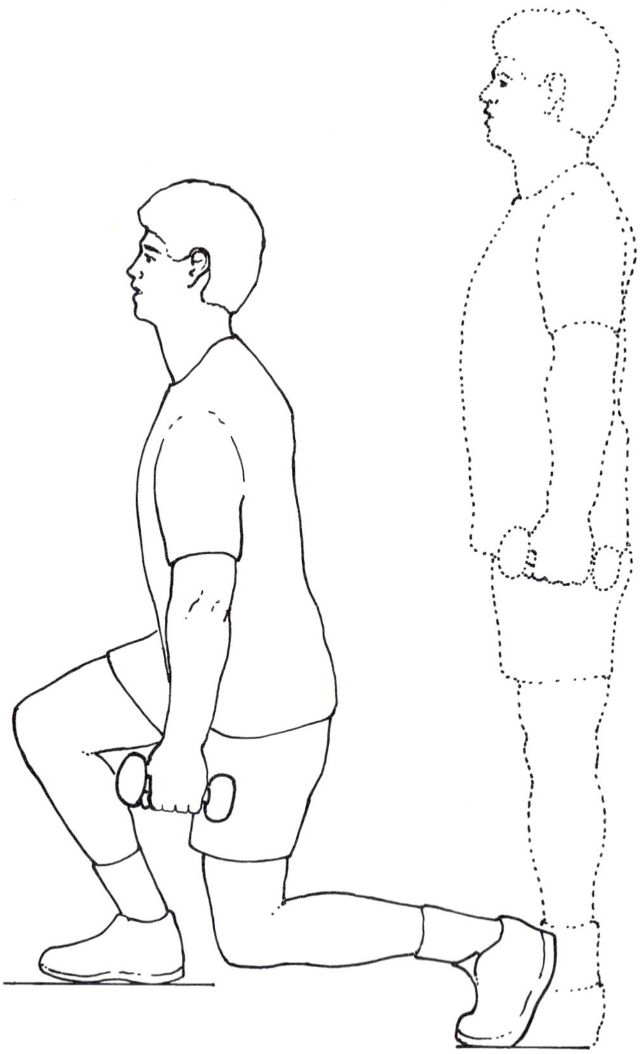

FIGURE 7-100 Lunges.

If the patient has had an open rotator cuff repair, passive shoulder flexion or abduction is allowed for the first month. Immobilization is applied for comfort, using a sling, except for gentle passive range of motion in flexion, abduction, and external rotation. With the arm at the side and the elbows extended, active shoulder internal and external rotation is permitted. Modalities and mobilizations may be used for pain control, if necessary. Active exercises include shoulder shrugs, pendulum exercises, and putty squeezes to strengthen the hand, wrist, and forearm.

If the patient has had an anterior capsulolabral reconstruction in addition to a rotator cuff repair, the protocol for the period after the first month of immobilization is followed.

SUMMARY

Guiding design and execution of rehabilitation protocols is an attempt to link the underlying functional biomechanics of the shoulder with the contents of an exercise program. A complete and thorough evaluation is critical in planning a successful rehabilitation program. Emphasis is placed on strengthening the rotator cuff muscles, restoring normal scapulohumeral rhythm, and avoiding undue stress in the direction of instability. Successful return to full function and previous athletic level depends on maintaining the integrity of the static stabilizers, increasing the strength and endurance of the dynamic stabilizers, restoring flexibility to the appropriate structures, and improving mechanics during activity.

REHABILITATION THROWING PROGRAM FOR PITCHERS*

Step 1: Toss the ball (no wind-up) against a wall on alternate days. Start with 25 to 30 throws, build up to 70 throws, and gradually increase the throwing distance.

Number of Throws	Distance (ft)
20	20 (warm-up phase)
25-40	30-40
10	20 (cool-down phase)

Step 2: Toss the ball (playing catch with easy wind-up) on alternate days.

Number of Throws	Distance (ft)
10	20 (warm-up)
10	30-40
30-40	50
10	20-30 (cool-down)

Step 3: Continue increasing the throwing distance while still tossing the ball with an easy wind-up.

Number of Throws	Distance (ft)
10	20 (warm-up)
10	30-40
30-40	50-60
10	30 (cool-down)

Step 4: Increase throwing distance to a maximum of 60 feet. Continue tossing the ball with an occasional throw at no more than half speed.

Number of Throws	Distance (ft)
10	30 (warm-up)
10	40-45
30-40	60-70
10	30 (cool-down)

Step 5: During this step, gradually increase the distance to 150 feet maximum.

Phase 5-1:	Number of Throws	Distance (ft)
	10	40 (warm-up)
	10	50-60
	15-20	70-80
	10	50-60
	10	40 (cool-down)

Phase 5-2:	Number of Throws	Distance (ft)
	10	40 (warm-up)
	10	50-60
	20-30	80-90
	20	50-60
	10	40 (cool-down)

Phase 5-3:	Number of Throws	Distance (ft)
	10	40 (warm-up)
	10	60
	15-20	100-110
	20	60
	10	40 (cool-down)

Phase 5-4:	Number of Throws	Distance (ft)
	10	40 (warm-up)
	10	60
	15-20	120-150
	20	60
	10	40 (cool-down)

*Patients start at the step that is appropriate for them. Postsurgical patients begin at step 1. Patients progress depending on the maintenance of their pain-free status and their strength and endurance.

Continued.

REHABILITATION THROWING PROGRAM FOR PITCHERS—cont'd

Step 6: Progress to throwing off the mound at one-half to three-fourths speed. Try to use proper body mechanics, especially when throwing off the mound:

- Stay on top of the ball
- Keep the elbow up
- Throw over the top
- Follow through with the arm and trunk
- Use the legs to push

Phase 6-1:	Number of Throws	Distance (ft)
	10	60 (warm-up)
	10	120-150 (lobbing)
	30	45 (off the mound)
	10	60 (off the mound)
	10	40 (cool-down)

Phase 6-2:	Number of Throws	Distance (ft)
	10	50 (warm-up)
	10	120-150 (lobbing)
	20	45 (off the mound)
	20	60 (off the mound)
	10	40 (cool-down)

Phase 6-3:	Number of Throws	Distance (ft)
	10	50 (warm-up)
	10	60
	10	120-150 (lobbing)
	10	45 (off the mound)
	30	60 (off the mound)
	10	40 (cool-down)

Phase 6-4:	Number of Throws	Distance (ft)
	10	50 (warm-up)
	10	120-150 (lobbing)
	10	45 (off the mound)
	40-50	60 (off the mound)
	10	40 (cool-down)

At this time, if the pitcher has successfully completed phase 6-4 without pain or discomfort and is throwing approximately three-fourths speed, the pitching coach and trainer may allow the pitcher to proceed to step 7: "up/down bullpens." Up/down bullpens is used to simulate a game. The pitcher rests between a series of pitches to reproduce the rest period between innings.

Step 7: Up/down bullpens: (one-half to three-fourths speed)

Day 1:	Number of Throws	Distance (ft)
	10 warm-up throws	120-150 (lobbing)
	10 warm-up throws	60 (off the mound)
	40 pitches	60 (off the mound)
	Rest 10 minutes	
	20 pitches	60 (off the mound)

Day 2: Off

Day 3:	Number of Throws	Distance (ft)
	10 warm-up throws	120-150 (lobbing)
	10 warm-up throws	60 (off the mound)
	30 pitches	60 (off the mound)
	Rest 10 minutes	
	10 warm-up throws	60 (off the mound)
	20 pitches	60 (off the mound)
	Rest 10 minutes	
	10 warm-up throws	60 (off the mound)
	20 pitches	60 (off the mound)

Day 4: Off

Day 5:	Number of Throws	Distance (ft)
	10 warm-up throws	120-150 (lobbing)
	10 warm-up throws	60 (off the mound)
	30 pitches	60 (off the mound)
	Rest 8 minutes	
	20 pitches	60 (off the mound)
	Rest 8 minutes	
	20 pitches	60 (off the mound)
	Rest 8 minutes	
	20 pitches	60 (off the mound)

At this point the pitcher is ready to begin a normal routine, from throwing batting practice to pitching in the bullpen. This program can and should be adjusted as needed by the trainer or physical therapist. Each step may take more or less than listed, and the program should be monitored by the trainer, physical therapist, and physician. The pitcher should remember that it is necessary to work hard but not overdo it.

REHABILITATION PROGRAM FOR CATCHERS, INFIELDERS, AND OUTFIELDERS

Note: Perform each step three times.
All throws should have an arc or "hump."
The maximum distance thrown by infielders and catchers is 120 feet.
The maximum distance thrown by outfielders is 200 feet.

Step 1: Toss the ball with no wind-up. Stand with your feet shoulder-width apart and face the player to whom you are throwing. Concentrate on rotating and staying on top of the ball.

Number of Throws	Distance (ft)
5	20 (warm-up)
10	30
5	20 (cool-down)

Step 2: Stand sideways to the person to whom you are throwing. Feet are shoulder-width apart. Close up and pivot onto your back foot as you throw.

Number of Throws	Distance (ft)
5	30 (warm-up)
5	40
10	50
5	30 (cool-down)

Step 3: Repeat the position in step 2. Step toward the target with your front leg and follow through with your back leg.

Number of Throws	Distance (ft)
5	50 (warm-up)
5	60
10	70
5	50 (cool-down)

Step 4: Assume the pitcher's stance. Lift and stride with your lead leg. Follow through with your back leg.

Number of Throws	Distance (ft)
5	60 (warm-up)
5	70
10	80
5	60 (cool-down)

Step 5: *Outfielders:* Lead with your glove-side foot forward. Take one step, crow hop, and throw the ball.
Infielders: Lead with your glove-side foot forward. Take a shuffle step and throw the ball. Throw the last five throws in a straight line.

Number of Throws	Distance (ft)
5	70 (warm-up)
5	90
10	100
5	80 (cool-down)

Step 6: Use the throwing technique used in step 5. Assume your playing position. Infielders and catchers do not throw farther than 120 feet. Outfielders do not throw farther than 150 feet (mid-outfield).

Number of Throws	Infielders' and Catchers' Distance (ft)	Outfielders' Distance (ft)
5	80 (warm-up)	80 (warm-up)
5	80-90	90-100
5	90-100	110-125
5	110-120	130-150
5	80 (cool-down)	80 (cool-down)

Step 7: Infielders, catchers, and outfielders all may assume their playing positions.

Number of Throws	Infielders' and Catchers' Distance (ft)	Outfielders' Distance (ft)
5	80 (warm-up)	80-90 (warm-up)
5	80-90	110-130
5	90-100	150-175
5	110-120	180-200
5	80 (cool-down)	90 (cool-down)

Step 8: Repeat step 7. Use a fungo bat to hit to the infielders and outfielders while in their normal playing positions.

REHABILITATION PROGRAM FOR TENNIS PLAYERS

The following tennis protocol is designed to be performed every other day. Each session should begin with the warm-up exercises as outlined below. Continue with your strengthening, flexibility, and conditioning exercises on the days you are not following the tennis protocol.

Warm-Up

Lower extremity:

- Jog four laps around the tennis court.
- Stretches:
  - Gastrocnemius
  - Achilles tendon
  - Hamstring
  - Quadriceps

Upper extremity

- Shoulder stretches:
  - Posterior cuff
  - Inferior capsule
  - Rhomboid
- Forearm/wrist stretches:
  - Wrist flexors
  - Wrist extensors

Trunk

- Side bends
- Extension
- Rotation

Forehand ground strokes:

Hit toward the fence on the opposite side of the court. Do not worry about getting the ball in the court.

During all of the strokes listed above, remember these key steps:

- Bend your knees.
- Turn your body.
- Step toward the ball.
- Hit the ball when it is out in front of you.

Avoid hitting with an open stance because this places undue stress on your shoulder. This is especially more stressful during the forehand stroke if you have had anterior instability or impingement problems. This is also true during the backhand if you have had problems of posterior instability.

On the very first day of these sport-specific drills, start with bouncing the ball and hitting it. Try to bounce the ball yourself and hit it at waist level. This will allow for consistency in the following:

- How the ball comes to you.
- Approximating your timing between hits.
- Hitting toward a target to ensure follow-through and full extension.
- Employing the proper mechanics, thereby placing less stress on the anterior shoulder.

Week 1

Day 1: 25 forehand strokes
25 forehand strokes

Day 2: If there are no problems after the first-day workout, increase the number of forehand and backhand strokes.
50 forehand strokes
50 backhand strokes

Day 3: 50 forehand strokes (waist level)
50 backhand strokes (waist level)
25 high forehand strokes
25 high backhand strokes

Week 2

Progress to having the ball tossed to you in a timely manner, giving you enough time to recover from your deliberate follow-through (i.e., wait until the ball bounces on the other side of the court before tossing another ball). Always aim the ball at a target or at a spot on the court.

If you are working on basic ground strokes, have someone bounce the ball to you consistently at waist height.

If you are working on high forehands, have the ball bounced to you at shoulder height or higher.

Day 1: 25 high forehand strokes
50 waist-height forehand strokes
50 waist-height backhand strokes
25 high backhand strokes

Day 2: 25 high forehand strokes
50 waist-height forehand strokes
50 waist-height backhand strokes
25 high backhand strokes

Day 3: Alternate hitting the ball cross court and down the line, using the waist-high and high forehand and backhand strokes.
25 high forehand strokes
50 waist-height forehand strokes
50 waist-height backhand strokes
25 high backhand strokes

Week 3

Continue the three-times-per-week schedule. Add regular and high forehand and backhand volleys. At this point, you may begin having someone hit tennis balls to you from a basket of balls. This will allow you to get the feel of the ball as it comes off another tennis racket. Your partner should wait until the ball that you hit has bounced on the other side of the court before hitting another ball to you. This will give you time to emphasize your follow-through and not hurry to return for the next shot. As always, emphasis is placed on proper body mechanics.

Day 1: 25 high forehand strokes
50 waist-height forehand strokes
50 waist-height backhand strokes
25 high backhand strokes
25 low backhand and forehand volleys
25 high backhand and forehand volleys

Day 2: Same as day 1, week 3.

REHABILITATION PROGRAM FOR TENNIS PLAYERS—cont'd

Day 3: Same as day 2, week 3, with emphasis on direction (i.e., down the line and cross court). Remember, good body mechanics is still a must:
- Keep knees bent.
- Hit the ball on the rise.
- Hit the ball in front of you.
- Turn your body.
- Do not hit the ball with an open stance.
- Stay on the balls of your feet.

Week 4

Day 1: Continue having your partner hit tennis balls to you from out of a basket. Alternate hitting forehand and backhand strokes with lateral movement along the baseline. Again, emphasis is on good mechanics as described previously.

Alternate hitting the ball down the line and cross court. This drill should be done with a full basket of tennis balls (100 to 150 tennis balls).

Follow this drill with high and low volleys using half a basket of tennis balls (50 to 75 balls). This drill also is performed with lateral movement and returning to the middle of the court after the ball is hit.

Your partner should continue allowing enough time for you to return to the middle of the court before hitting the next ball. This is to avoid your rushing the stroke and using faulty mechanics.

Day 2: Same drill as day 1, week 4.

Day 3: Same drills as day 2, week 4.

Week 5

Day 1: Find a partner able to hit consistent ground strokes (able to hit the ball to the same area consistently, e.g., to your forehand with the ball bouncing about waist height).

Begin hitting ground strokes with this partner alternating hitting the ball to your backhand and to your forehand. Rally for about 15 minutes, then add volleys with your partner hitting to you from the baseline. Alternate between backhand and forehand volleys and high and low volleys. Continue volleying another 15 minutes. You will have rallied for a total of 30 to 40 minutes.

At the end of the session, practice a few serves while standing along the baseline. First, warm up by shadowing for 1 to 3 minutes. Hold the tennis racquet loosely and swing across your body in a figure 8. Do not swing the racquet hard. When you are ready to practice your serves using a ball, be sure to keep your toss out in front of you, get your racquet up and behind you, bend your knees, and hit up on the ball. Forget about how much power you are generating, and forget about hitting the ball between the service lines. Try hitting the ball as if you are hitting it toward the back fence.

Hit approximately 10 serves from each side of the court. Remember, this is the first time you are serving, so do not try to hit at 100% of your effort.

Day 2: Same as day 1, week 5, but now increase the number of times you practice your serve. After working on your ground strokes and volleys, return to the baseline and work on your second serve: Hit up on the ball, bend your knees, follow through, and keep the toss in front of you. This time hit 20 balls from each side of the court (i.e., 20 into the deuce court and 20 into the ad court).

Day 3: Same as day 2, week 5, with ground strokes, volleys, and serves. Do not add to the serves. Concentrate on the following:
- Bending your knees.
- Preparing the racket.
- Using footwork.
- Hitting the ball out in front of you.
- Keeping your eyes on the ball.
- Following through.
- Getting in position for the next shot.
- Keeping the toss in front of you during the serve.

The workout should be the same as day 2, but if you emphasize the proper mechanics listed previously, you should feel as though you had a harder workout than in day 2.

Week 6

Day 1: After the usual warm-up program, start with specific ground-stroke drills, with you hitting the ball down the line and your partner on the other side hitting the ball cross court. This will force you to move quickly on the court. Emphasize good mechanics as mentioned previously.

Perform this drill for 10 to 15 minutes before reversing the direction of your strokes. Now have your partner hit down the line while you hit cross court.

Proceed to the next drill with your partner hitting the ball to you. Return balls using a forehand, then a backhand, then a put-away volley. Repeat this sequence for 10 to 15 minutes. End this session by serving 50 balls to the ad court and 50 balls to the deuce court.

Continued.

REHABILITATION PROGRAM FOR TENNIS PLAYERS—cont'd

Day 2: Day 2 should be the same as day 1, week 6, plus returning serves from each side of the court (deuce and ad court). End with practicing serves, 50 to each court.

Day 3: Perform the following sequence: warm-up; cross-court and down-the-line drills; backhand, forehand, and volley drills; return of serves; and practice serves.

Week 7

Day 1: Perform the warm-up program. Perform drills as before and practice return of serves. Before practicing serving, work on hitting 10 to 15 overhead shots. Continue emphasizing good mechanics. Add the approach shot to your drills.

Day 2: Same as day 1, week 7, except double the number of overhead shots (25 to 30 overheads).

Day 3: Perform warm-up exercises and cross-court drills. Add the overhead shot to the backhand, forehand, and volley drill, making it the backhand, forehand, volley, and overhead drill.

If you are a serious tennis player, you will want to work on other strokes or other parts of your game. Feel free to gradually add them to your practice and workout sessions. Just as in other strokes, the proper mechanics should be applied to drop volley, slice, heavy topspin, drop shots, and lobs, offensive and defensive.

Week 8

Day 1: Warm-up and play a simulated one-set match. Be sure to take rest periods after every third game. Remember, you will have to concentrate harder on using good mechanics.

Day 2: Perform another simulated game but with a two-set match.

Day 3: Perform another simulated game, this time a best-of-three-set match.

If all goes well, you may make plans to return to your regular workout and game schedule. You also may practice or play on consecutive days if your condition allows it.

REHABILITATION PROGRAM FOR GOLFERS

This sport-specific protocol is designed to be performed every other day. Each session should begin with the warm-up exercises outlined here. Continue the strengthening, flexibility, and conditioning exercises on the days you are not playing or practicing golf. Advance one stage every 2 to 4 weeks, depending on the severity of the shoulder problem, as each stage becomes pain free in execution.

Warm-Up

Lower extremities: Jog or walk briskly around the practice green area three or four times; stretch the hamstrings, quadriceps, and Achilles tendon.

Upper extremities: Stretch the shoulder (posterior cuff, inferior cuff, rhomboid) and wrist flexors and extensors.

Trunk: Do sidebends, extension, and rotation stretching exercises.

Stage 1	Putt	50	3 times/week
	Medium long	0	0 times/week
	Long	0	0 times/week
Stage 2	Putt	50	3 times/week
	Medium long	20	2 times/week
	Long	0	0 times/week
Stage 3	Putt	50	3 times/week
	Medium long	40	3 times/week
	Long	0	0 times/week

Not more than ⅓ best distance

Stage 4	Putt	50	3 times/week
	Medium long	50	3 times/week
	Long	10	2 times/week

Up to ½ best distance

Stage 5	Putt	50	3 times/week
	Medium long	50	3 times/week
	Long	10	3 times/week
Stage 6	Putt	50	3 times/week
	Medium long	50	3 times/week
	Long	20	3 times/week

Play a round of gold in lieu of one practice session per week.

REHASAMPLE EVALUATION FORM
SHOULDER SUBJECTIVE EVALUATION FORM

Name: ____________________ Date: ____/____/____
Diagnosis: ____________________ Date of birth: ____/____/____
Referring physician: ____________________ Date of injury: ____/____/____
Occupation: ____________________ Date of surgery: ____/____/____

A. General Information

1. Hand dominance: (circle one) Right Left
2. Currently working? (circle one) Yes No
   If no, date last worked: ____/____/____
3. Job requirements: (circle all activities that apply)
   Driving
   Overhead work
   Carrying objects
   Lifting objects
   Repetitive movements
   Pulling objects
   Pushing objects
   Other: ____________________

B. Sports and Recreation

1. Sport(s) participate in: (circle all activities that apply)
   Basketball Hockey Soccer
   Volleyball Tennis Racquetball
   Baseball Golf Softball
   Football Track Swimming
   Other: ____________________
2. Level of competition: (circle)
   Professional
   College
   Recreational
   Amateur
   High school
   None of the above
3. Number of times per week participated: ____________________
4. Date last participated: ____________________

C. Major Complaint

1. Date problem began: ____/____/____
2. How did the problem develop? ____________________
   ____
   ____
3. Have you ever had this or a related problem before? (circle one) Yes No
   If yes, then
   a. Date of the previous problem: ____/____/____
   b. What type of problem was it? ____________________
   ____
4. Have you ever had surgery for this or a related problem before? (circle one) Yes No
   If yes, then
   a. Date of previous surgery: ____/____/____
   b. Type of surgery: ____________________
   ____
5. Have you ever had treatment for this or a related problem before? Yes No
   If yes, then
   a. Dates of treatment: __________ To __________
   b. Type of treatment: ____________________
   ____
   c. Results of the treatment: ____________________
   ____

D. Pain

1. Do you experience pain? (circle one) Yes No
   If yes, then

Continued.

SAMPLE EVALUATION FORM
SHOULDER SUBJECTIVE EVALUATION FORM—cont'd

2. What is your current pain level? (circle one number)
   0 = No pain 10 = Pain that would require hospitalization
   1 2 3 4 5 6 7 8 9 10
3. How often do you experience pain? (circle one)
   Constant (24 hr/day) Intermittent (some periods of relief)
4. What does your pain feel like? (circle)
   Sharp Burning Throbbing
   Dull Ache Other: ________________
5. Within the last month, has your pain: (circle one)
   Increased Decreased Remained unchanged
6. Indicate on the diagram below where your pain is located:

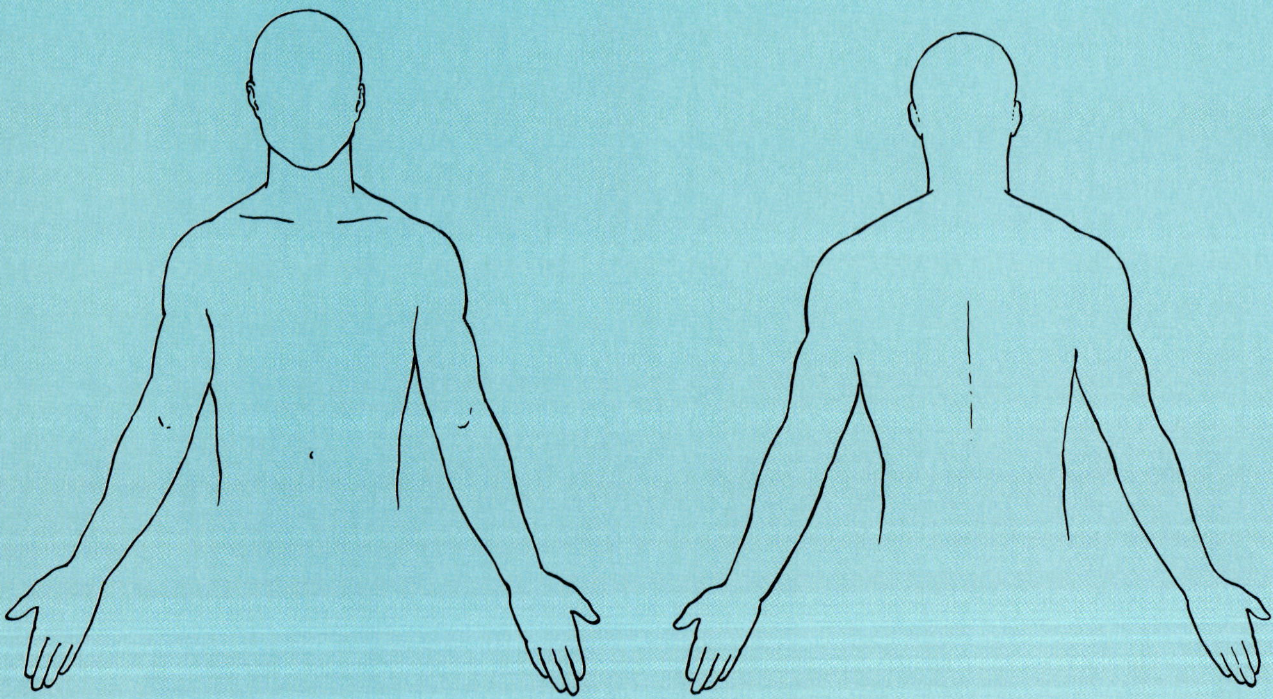

SAMPLE EVALUATION FORM
SHOULDER SUBJECTIVE EVALUATION FORM—cont'd

E. Tingling

1. Do you experience any tingling? (circle) Yes No
   If yes, then
   a. What is your current level of tingling? (circle one)
      None Mild Moderate Severe
   b. How often do you experience tingling? (circle one)
      Constant (24 hr/day) Intermittent (some relief)
   c. In the last month, has your tingling: (circle one)
      Increased Decreased Remained unchanged
   d. Indicate on the diagram below where your tingling is located:

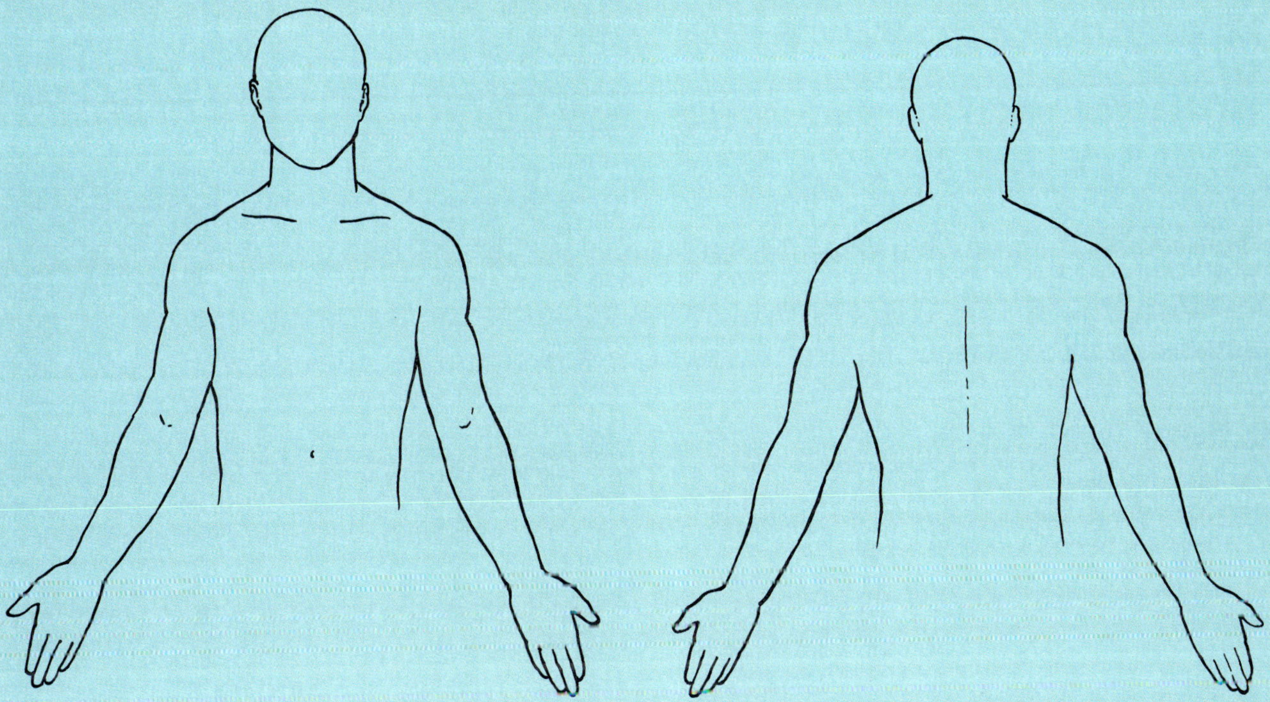

Continued.

SAMPLE EVALUATION FORM
SHOULDER SUBJECTIVE EVALUATION FORM—cont'd

F. Numbness

1. Do you experience any numbness? (circle one) Yes No
   a. How often do you experience numbness? (circle one)
      Constant (24 hr/day) Intermittent (some relief)
   b. In the last month, has your numbness: (circle one)
      Increased Decreased Remained unchanged
   c. Indicate on the diagram below where your numbness is located:

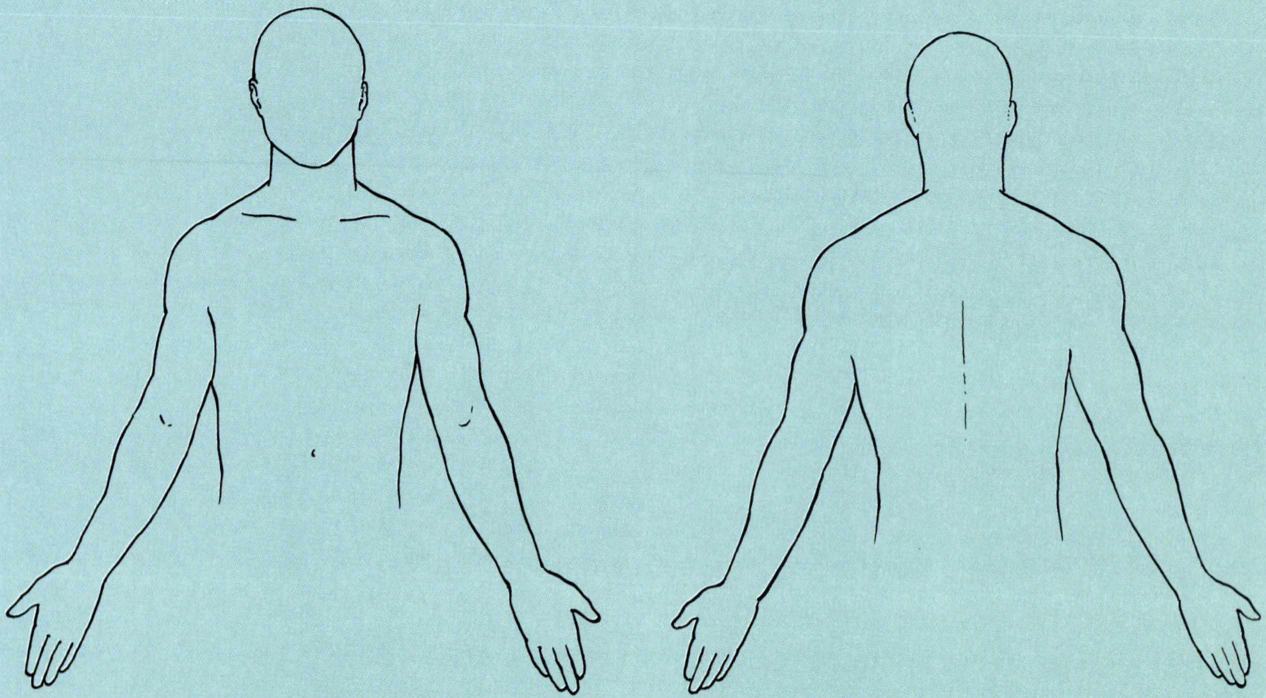

G. Aggravating Factors

Which of the following activities make any of your symptoms worse? (circle all that apply)

Dressing and Daily Activities:

Putting on: Tucking in shirt Washing your:
Pants Hooking bra Back
T-shirt Eating with utensils Underarm
Coat Accepting change Face
Coughing Opening a jar Right shoulder
Sneezing Brushing your teeth/hair Left shoulder
Taking a deep breath Managing toilet activities Dishes
Turning a door knob Pouring from a pitcher Car
Turning a key Drinking from a cup Cooking/stirring

Cleaning Activities:

Ironing Sweeping Vacuuming
Wringing out clothes

[redacted]

SAMPLE EVALUATION FORM
SHOULDER SUBJECTIVE EVALUATION FORM—cont'd

Positional Activities:

Hanging from a bar Pushing objects Pulling objects
Reaching: Carrying objects: Lifting objects:
Across your face Above your head Above your head
Up to a high shelf Below your shoulders Below your shoulders
Into your back seat Quick movements Sitting
Into your back pocket Grasping objects Standing
Lying on your: Bending your: Neck movements:
Back Wrist Looking up
Stomach Elbow Looking down
Right side Straightening your: Right side bend
Left side Wrist Left side bend
With hands behind head Elbow Right rotation
Behind your back In hands and knees position Left rotation

Functional Activities:

Writing Typing Driving

Sports and Recreational Activities:

Tennis: Golf: Basketball:
Serve Driving Shooting
Forehand Putting Dribbling
Backhand Chipping Passing
Baseball: Volleyball: Swimming:
Batting Serving Front crawl
Overhand throwing Setting Breast stroke
Underhand throwing Spiking Back stroke
Catching Passing Diving
Bowling Bicycling Push-ups
Dips Chin-ups Pull-ups
Working out with weights

H. Factors That Relieve Symptoms

Which activities, positions, modalities (e.g., ice) help relieve your symptoms?

____
____
____

I. Miscellaneous

1. Do you wake up at night because of pain? (circle one)
   Yes No If yes, then answer 2 and 3.
2. What type of mattress do you sleep on? (circle one)
   Firm Medium Soft Waterbed
3. How many pillows do you use? ____________
   a. Where are they placed? ______________________
4. When are your symptoms worse? (circle)
   When you wake up in the morning At night
   As the day progresses No difference
5. Do you suffer from neck pain? (circle one) Yes No

Continued.

SAMPLE EVALUATION FORM
SHOULDER SUBJECTIVE EVALUATION FORM—cont'd

6. Do you wear a sling or other type of support? (circle one)
   Yes No If yes, then
   a. What type is it? ______
   b. How often do you wear it? ______
   c. Does using it give you any relief? (circle one)
      Yes No
7. Do you have a feeling of weakness? (circle one)
   Yes No If yes, then
   a. Where? (circle)
      Arms Legs Neck
      Hands Feet Back

J. Other Medical History

1. Do you have any of the following conditions? (circle all that apply)
   Diabetes High blood pressure Heart disease
   Epilepsy Arthritis Respiratory disease
   Fainting spells Hypoglycemia
   Other: ______ Other: ______
   Other: ______ Other: ______
2. What medications are you currently taking?
   ______ ______
   ______ ______
   ______ ______
3. Have you had any of the following tests? (circle all that apply)
   X-rays MRI CT scan
   Arthrogram Myelogram Nerve conduction tests
   Bone scan EMG studies

SAMPLE EVALUATION FORM
SHOULDER OBJECTIVE EVALUATION FORM

Name: ______________________________ Date: ____/____/____
Diagnosis: ______________________________ Date of birth: ____/____/____
Referring physician: ______________________________ Date of injury: ____/____/____
Social Security no.: ________/______/________ Date of surgery: ____/____/____

I. Objective findings

A. Observations: Denote all that apply: R = right, L = left, B = bilateral, and 0 = absent.

Step deformity	________	Asymmetrical scapula	________	Edema	________
Depressed shoulder	________	Muscular atrophy	________	Skin changes	________
Forward shoulder	________	Sprengel's deformity	________	Scars	________
Bruising	________	Supportive equipment	________	Incision	________

Comments: ____
____

B. Scapulohumeral rhythm: Note whether the timing is early, late, or normal.

	Early	**Late**	**Normal**
0°-30°	________	________	________
30°-90°	________	________	________
90°-180°	________	________	________

Comments: ____
____

C. Scapular mobility: Denote: "+" for increased mobility, "−" for decreased mobility, and "N" for normal movement.

	Right	**Left**	**Comments:**
Elevation	________	________	____________________
Depression	________	________	____________________
Protraction	________	________	____________________
Retraction	________	________	____________________
Upward rotation	________	________	____________________
Downward rotation	________	________	____________________

D. Glenohumeral range of motion: Note pain location/intensity on 0-10 pain scale.

	AROM			**PROM**		
	Right	**Left**	**Comments:**	**Right**	**Left**	**Comments:**
Flexion	_____	_____	__________	_____	_____	__________
Extension	_____	_____	__________	_____	_____	__________
Abduction	_____	_____	__________	_____	_____	__________
Internal rotation	_____	_____	__________	_____	_____	__________
External rotation	_____	_____	__________	_____	_____	__________
Internal rotation (90° abduction)	_____	_____	__________	_____	_____	__________
External rotation (90° abduction)	_____	_____	__________	_____	_____	__________
Horizontal abduction	_____	_____	__________	_____	_____	__________
Horizontal adduction	_____	_____	__________	_____	_____	__________

Continued.

SAMPLE EVALUATION FORM
SHOULDER OBJECTIVE EVALUATION FORM—cont'd

E. Strength: Give numeric grade and note location/intensity of pain on 0-10 scale.

	Right	Left	Comments:
Flexion			
Extension			
Abduction			
Abduction with internal rotation			
Internal rotation			
External rotation			
Horizontal abduction			
Horizontal adduction			
Protraction			
Retraction			
Grip			

F. Reflexes: Denote "+" for increased, "–" for decreased, and "N" for normal.

	Right	Left	Comments:
Pectoralis major (C6-C7)			
Biceps (C5-C6)			
Brachioradialis (C6)			
Triceps (C7)			

G. Special tests and signs: Denote: "+" for positive and "–" for negative.

	Right	Left		Right	Left
Yergason's test			Anterior apprehension test		
Speed's test			Posterior apprehension test		
Drop arm test			Allen maneuver		
Ludington's test			Adson maneuver		
Neer impingement test			Halstead maneuver		
Forced flexion test			Costoclavicular syndrome		
Jobe's test			Apley's scratch (external rotation)		
Sulcus sign			Apley's scratch (internal rotation)		
			Hawkins test		

Comments: ______________________________

H. Accessory motion: Denote "+" for increased laxity, "–" for decreased laxity, and "N" for normal. Also note location/intensity of pain on 0-10 scale.

Glenohumeral:	Right	Left	Comments:
Long axis traction			
Lateral distraction			
Caudal glides			
Anterior glides			
Posterior glides			
Acromioclavicular joint:			
Sternoclavicular joint:			

SAMPLE EVALUATION FORM
SHOULDER OBJECTIVE EVALUATION FORM—cont'd

I. Sensation: Note any significant findings on the diagram below.

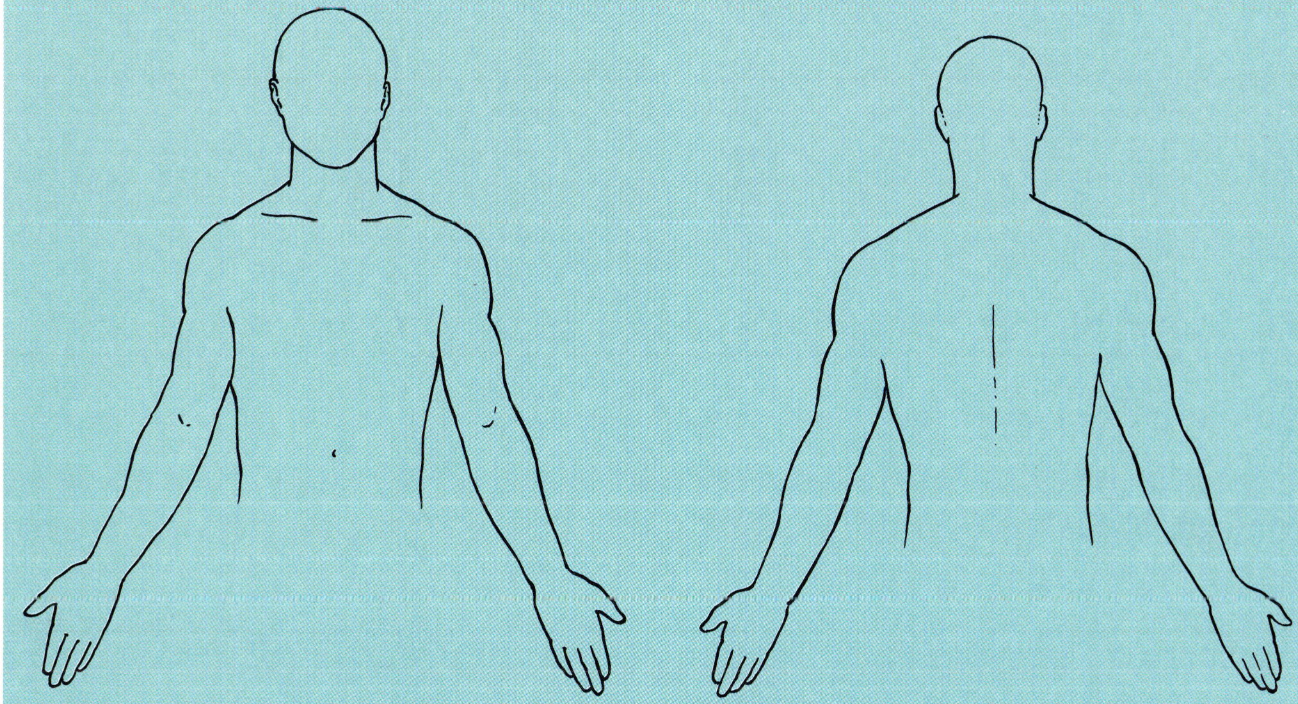

J. Palpation: Rate intensity of pain on 0-10 scale. Note significant findings below.

Muscular:	**Right**	**Left**
Upper trapezius	_____	_____
Supraspinatus	_____	_____
Infraspinatus	_____	_____
Rhomboids	_____	_____
Pectoralis major	_____	_____
Pectoralis minor	_____	_____
Biceps	_____	_____
Triceps	_____	_____
Latissimus dorsi		
Subscapularis	_____	_____
Teres major	_____	_____

Tendinous:	**Right**	**Left**
Supraspinatus	_____	_____
Biceps: long head (origin)	_____	_____
Biceps: short head (origin)	_____	_____
Triceps	_____	_____
Posterior cuff insertion	_____	_____
Pectoralis major	_____	_____
Subscapularis	_____	_____
Latissimus dorsi	_____	_____

Bony:	**Right**	**Left**
Clavicle	_____	_____
Sternoclavicular joint	_____	_____
Acromioclavicular joint	_____	_____
Coracoid process	_____	_____
Sternum	_____	_____

Ligamentous:	**Right**	**Left**
Transverse humeral	_____	_____

Other:		
Subdeltoid bursa	_____	_____
Subacromial bursa	_____	_____

Comments: ____

____

____

Continued.

SAMPLE EVALUATION FORM
SHOULDER OBJECTIVE EVALUATION FORM—cont'd

II. *Other joints: Denote "+" for increased symptoms, "−" for decreased symptoms, or 0 for no effect on symptoms.*

Cervical spine:	**Right**	**Left**
Flexion	_____	_____
Extension	_____	_____
Right lateral flexion	_____	_____
Left lateral flexion	_____	_____
Right rotation	_____	_____
Left rotation	_____	_____
Compression	_____	_____
Distraction	_____	_____

Further cervical spine evaluation needed?
Yes No

Elbow:	**Right**	**Left**
Flexion	_____	_____
Extension	_____	_____
Pronation	_____	_____
Supination	_____	_____

Wrist:	**Right**	**Left**
Radial deviation	_____	_____
Ulnar deviation	_____	_____

Further elbow evaluation needed?
Yes No

References

1. Ballantyne BT et al: Electromyographic activity of selected shoulder muscles in commonly used therapeutic exercises, *Phys Ther* 73: 668, 1993.
2. Blackburn TA et al: EMG analysis of posterior rotator cuff exercises, *Athl Train* 25:40, 1990.
3. Brown LP et al: Upper extremity range of motion and isokinetic strength of the internal and external shoulder rotators in major league baseball players, *Am J Sports Med* 16:577, 1988.
4. DePalma AF: *Surgery of the shoulder,* ed 3, Philadelphia, 1983, JB Lippincott.
5. Glousman R et al: Dynamic electromyographic analysis of the throwing shoulder with glenohumeral instability, *J Bone Joint Surg* 70A:220, 1988.
6. Kerr R: Shoulder impingement syndrome, *Orthopedics* 10:637, 1987.
7. Kessel L, Watson M: The painful arc syndrome, *J Bone Joint Surg* 59B:166, 1977.
8. Kronberg M, Nemeth G, Brostrom L: Muscle activity and coordination in the normal shoulder, *Clin Orthop* 257:76, 1990.
9. Moynes DR: Electromyography motion analysis of the upper extremity in sports, *Phys Ther* 66:1905, 1985.
10. Mulligan E: Conservative management of shoulder impingement syndrome, *Athl Train* 23:348-353, 1988.
11. Neer CS: Anterior acromioplasty for the chronic impingement syndrome in the shoulder: a preliminary report, *J Bone Joint Surg* 54A:41, 1972.
12. Rathbun JB, MacNab I: The microvascular pattern of the rotator cuff, *J Bone Joint Surg* 52B:540, 1970.
13. Thein LA: Impingement syndrome and its conservative management, *J Orthop Sports Phys Ther* 11:183, 1989.
14. Turkel SJ et al: Stabilizing mechanisms preventing anterior dislocation of the glenohumeral joint, *J Bone Joint Surg* 63A:1208, 1981.

CHAPTER 8

Posterior Glenohumeral Instability

JAMES E. TIBONE
CLIVE E. BREWSTER

Posterior glenohumeral joint instability is seen in the young athletic population, but it is not as common as anterior instability. True dislocations are rare, as most athletes present with chronic posterior subluxation rather than recurrent posterior dislocations. The diagnosis can be difficult, because the signs and symptoms often are subtle. Therefore the treating physician must be aware of this entity, especially in young athletes.

MECHANISM AND INCIDENCE OF INJURY IN SPECIFIC SPORTS

Posterior subluxation can occur among two different athletic populations. The first is the throwing or overhead athlete.

The mechanism of injury in this population is usually repetitive microtrauma resulting from overuse. The throwing athlete may stretch the posterior capsule during the follow-through phase of pitching or throwing.[23]

Posterior glenohumeral joint instability also can be seen among contact-sport athletes. In contact sports, such as football, trauma usually initiates the instability, with either a fall on the outstretched hand or a force to the anterior shoulder that pushes the humeral head posteriorly. Among football players, posterior subluxation usually occurs in an offensive lineman when performing blocking maneuvers with the arms in a forward flexed position. The upper extremities get "jammed," and the humeral head gets pushed posteriorly, causing posterior subluxation. This can occur after one specific incident that stretches the capsule and damages the posterior labrum, or can occur over time with repetitive blocking maneuvers.

The true incidence of this entity never has been documented in the literature. Rowe reported an incidence rate of 2% for posterior instability compared with 98% for anterior instability. However, his series did not study athletes, and the patients had dislocations rather than subluxations. The true incidence of subluxation therefore remains unknown.

CLINICAL PRESENTATION

These athletes usually present with pain rather than instability. The pain may be anterior, posterior, or both. Pain in the region of the biceps tendon may be an indicator of subtle posterior instability, just as infraspinatus and teres minor pain may be a symptom of anterior instability. The most common complaint is pain with the arm held in the forward-flexed, internally rotated position. A throwing athlete may complain of increased fatigue or lack of endurance in his affected arm. A swimmer may be unable to accumulate the usual training mileage. Pain associated with falling on the shoulder or pain with blocking is a common complaint of football players with posterior instability. Objectively, these athletes usually present with subtle signs. There may be diffuse tenderness about the shoulder joint or only localized tenderness over the biceps tendon. The shoulder range of motion usually is within normal limits. Impingement signs are mild if present and generally are not as common as with anterior instability. Less than one half of these athletes are able to voluntarily demonstrate their posterior instability. This instability is demonstrated by subluxing the joint with the arm flexed forward and internally rotated and then reducing the joint by bringing the arm into extension and external rotation. This may be confusing, because the subluxation episode usually is painless, but the reduction is painful and occurs with a "clunk." The inexperienced examiner may think that the patient is demonstrating an anterior subluxation. However, voluntary anterior subluxation is extremely rare in the athletic population. On examination, these patients exhibit more anterior posterior translation than in the contralateral "normal" shoulder. This increased translation makes the subluxation easier to demonstrate with the patient supine, because this partially stabilizes the scapula. The humeral head then can be pushed anteriorly and posteriorly. One hand grasps the humeral head while the other is placed around the acromion and the coracoid. Another method is to load the joint axially and attempt to displace it posteriorly.

CLASSIFICATION

Chronic posterior glenohumeral subluxation can be classified according to traumatic and atraumatic etiologies (Box 8-1). Traumatic subluxation can be further subdivided into macrotrauma (single traumatic event) or microtrauma (recurrent minor injuries). In addition, posterior subluxation can be classified as either involuntary or voluntary subluxation. Voluntary subluxation can be further subdivided as psychologically abnormal, consisting of individuals who sublux their shoulder for secondary gain, and the positional subluxation, which is common in the athlete, who can demonstrate the instability in certain positions, usually forward flexion and internal rotation. This classification does not include the athlete with multidirectional instability, in which posterior subluxation is just one component of the instability.

BOX 8-1
CLASSIFICATION OF POSTERIOR GLENOHUMERAL SUBLUXATION*

Etiology

Macrotrauma (traumatic): single traumatic event
Microtrauma (repetitive): recurrent minor injuries
Atraumatic: spontaneous onset

Volition

Involuntary

Athlete cannot demonstrate instability
Instability is demonstrable only by examiner

Voluntary

Psychological
- Using selective muscular control
- Usually with arm at the side
- Usually with ligamentous laxity

Positional
- Usually in forward flexion and internal rotation
- Usually in athletes

*These two basic classification systems (one by etiology and one by volition) are not mutually exclusive. Functionally, these systems are intertwined. Any of the etiologies can be involuntary or voluntary.

SPECIAL ASSESSMENT

All athletes should be evaluated with standard radiographic views, including anterior/posterior and axillary views. Although plain radiographs usually are normal, stress radiographs in the axillary projection sometimes can demonstrate posterior subluxation. However, these films must be compared with the normal contralateral shoulder. CT arthrograms and MRI scans, unfortunately, have not been very helpful in this athletic population. The primary pathology is capsular and ligamentous stretching, because bony deficiencies are uncommon. An examination under anesthesia and arthroscopes may be necessary to establish the diagnosis. Under anesthesia, the involved shoulder usually exhibits increased anteroposterior translation compared with the normal shoulder. Arthroscopic findings are largely unremarkable, because the only findings may include capsular stretching or minor posterior labral damage. Rotator cuff tears associated with posterior instability are extremely rare, although undersurface rotator cuff fraying may be encountered. Of interest, posterior Bankart lesions occur in less than 5% of all cases. The true value of arthroscopy lies in the assessment of the anterior glenohumeral ligaments and the anterior glenoid labrum to determine the major direction of instability.

NONSURGICAL TREATMENT

Conservative treatment of posterior shoulder subluxation in athletes consists of an extensive physical therapy exercise program. This program emphasizes strengthening of the external rotators, namely the infraspinatus, teres minor, and posterior deltoid.

The physical therapy rehabilitation for posterior shoulder instability varies in duration depending on factors such as the following:

- Degree of shoulder instability/laxity
- Acute versus chronic condition
- Length of time immobilized
- Strength/range of motion status
- Performance/activity demands

The rehabilitation program is outlined in three phases. Phases can overlap (phase I-II, phase II-III) depending on the progress of each individual.[8,10,19,24,25]

Phase I (1 to 2 months): The emphasis during this phase is on reducing pain, restoring range of motion, and initiating strengthening exercises. Caution must be applied to avoid placing undue stress on the posterior joint capsule until the dynamic joint instability is restored.

- Apply modalities as needed (e.g., heat, ice, electrotherapy)
- Perform range-of-motion (ROM) exercises (passive, active-assistive) for flexion, abduction, horizontal abduction, and external rotation (as needed).
- Shoulder stretch: apply anterior cuff/capsule stretch (as needed).
- Add joint mobilization (e.g., emphasis on glenohumeral joint anterior glides) as needed.
- Active external rotation may be performed from 0° rotation to full external rotation. Arm is positioned at side with elbow flexed at 90°. Resistance is achieved with the use of tubing.

  Modifications: Limit the degrees of internal rotation to protect the posterior joint capsule. The shoulder position may be adjusted to allow a pain-free muscle contraction to occur.

  Progression: As strength improves, progress to using free weights while side-lying with arm at side. ROM is from 0 degrees to full external rotation.
- Add active internal rotation performed from full external rotation to 0° rotation using tubing. Limiting the degrees of internal rotation is necessary to avoid excessive stress to the posterior joint capsule.

  Progression: Using free weights, the patient performs this while side-lying with the involved side resting on the plinth. Elevate or support the lateral chest wall (e.g., with pillow, bolster) to minimize the joint compression on the involved shoulder.

  Modifications: If there is pain with active movements, strength can be maintained by performing an isometric contraction. The shoulder position may be adjusted by placing it more in the scapular plane to allow a pain-free muscle contraction to occur.
- Add supraspinatus exercise if adequate range of motion is available (0° to 90°). The shoulder is positioned in the scapular plane approximately 20° to 30° forward of the coronal plane.
- Add active shoulder flexion exercise through available pain-free range of motion.
- Add active shoulder abduction exercise to 90°.
- Add shoulder shrug exercise; avoid traction in the glenohumeral joint between repetitions by not allowing the arms to drop completely. This will avoid an excessive inferior glide of the humeral head.
- Add active horizontal abduction exercise (posterior deltoid) in a prone-lying position. Avoid excessive stress to the posterior capsule by limiting movement from 45° of horizontal adduction to full horizontal abduction.
- Add forearm strengthening exercises (elbow, wrist).

Phase II (2 to 3 months): This intermediate phase focuses on progressive strengthening exercises as pain subsides and full normal range of motion is restored. Modalities and stretching are continued only as needed. Isokinetic strengthening and endurance training may begin during this phase.

- Continue anterior cuff/capsule stretch, mobilization, and range-of-motion exercises (as necessary).
- Continue shoulder strengthening (emphasis on rotator cuff and posterior deltoid) with tubing and/or free weights. Emphasis should be placed on the eccentric contractions of the rotator cuff.
- Add push-ups. Movement should be pain-free with emphasis on protecting the posterior joint capsule. Shoulders are positioned in 80° to 90° of abduction. *Caution is applied during the ascent phase of the push-up to avoid excessive stress to the posterior capsule* by not raising the body beyond the scapular plane. Begin with wall push-ups.

  Progression: As strength improves, progress to floor push-ups: first on hands and knees then to hands and feet (military style).
- Add isokinetic strengthening and endurance exercises (at high speeds; ≥200°/sec) for shoulder internal and external rotation with the arm positioned at the side and the shoulder in the scapular plane.
- Horizontal abduction may be performed through an increased range (starting at 90° of horizontal adduction as tolerated).
- Add arm ergometer for endurance exercise.

- Add total body conditioning with emphasis on strength and endurance. Include flexibility exercises as needed.

Phase III (3 to 4 months): The emphasis during this advanced stage is on returning the individual to the prior level of activity (e.g., work, recreational activity, sports). Exercises and drills are initiated to simulate the tasks and abilities needed to achieve full recovery.

- Continue anterior capsule stretching (as needed).
- Continue to emphasize the eccentric phase in strengthening the rotator cuff.
- Add military press. Press the weight directly over or behind the head.
- Add isokinetic test. Perform isokinetic strength and endurance test in shoulder internal/external rotation (arm at side). To perform this test, strength requirements of the rotator cuff are 5 to 10 lb for external rotation and 15 to 20 lb for internal rotation. The shoulder should be pain free and have no significant amount of swelling. Test results for internal/external rotation and horizontal abduction should demonstrate at least 90% strength and endurance (as compared with the uninvolved side) before the patient proceeds to exercises specific to the activity setting.

  Warner et al. found a significant difference in the internal-rotation-to-external-rotation ratio in a study including asymptomatic throwers and non–upper-extremity athletes. He compared nondominant to dominant shoulder strength and found a 30% greater internal rotator strength in the dominant shoulder.
- Add isokinetic strengthening for horizontal abduction/adduction, flexion/extension, and abduction/adduction as needed.
- Continue arm ergometer training.
- Continue total body conditioning program with emphasis on the shoulder (rotator cuff, posterior deltoid).
- Skill mastery. Begin practicing skills specific to the activity (e.g., work, recreational activity, sport). *For example, throwing athletes (e.g., pitchers) may proceed to a throwing program.*

Biofeedback may have a place in the treatment of voluntary posterior instability. Beall et al.[1] stimulated the posterior deltoid muscle with surface electrodes in an effort to control posterior instability. Biofeedback may allow patients to recognize an abnormally relaxed posterior deltoid muscle to reeducate the muscles to contract in a protective manner. Studies in our biomechanics laboratory showed that during voluntary posterior subluxation, the rotator cuff is relatively silent.[12] The deltoid muscle is responsible for both the subluxation and the reduction maneuvers as the anterior deltoid allowed for subluxation of the shoulder and the posterior provided the reduction.

The exercise program is continued for at least 6 months in an attempt to strengthen the shoulder musculature and decrease the athlete's functional disability. In the authors' experience, approximately 70% of athletes will improve with this conservative program. Commonly, however, the instability is not eliminated, but the functional disability during athletics is improved. This usually allows athletes to return to their sports as they adapt to their instability and require no further treatment.

SURGICAL TREATMENT

The management of athletes who fail conservative care is both complex and exceedingly difficult. Surgical procedures that are designed to enable them to perform at a highly competitive level unfortunately have a low success rate. Indications for surgery include pain and instability that interfere with activities of daily living. Athletes contemplating surgery to regain the ability to compete at a high level must be informed that surgery, unfortunately, is not highly successful. The diagnosis of an isolated posterior instability must be confirmed before surgery. Any increased inferior humeral translation compared with the normal shoulder may be an indication that multidirectional instability also is present; in this case other treatment would be more appropriate.

Historical View

Historically, surgical treatment for posterior instability has included subscapularis transfers, biceps tendon transfer with staple capsulorrhaphy, reverse Bankart repair, reverse Putti-Platt repair, infraspinatus advancement, posterior/inferior capsular shift, glenoid osteotomy, humeral osteotomy, posterior bone block, posterior staple capsulorrhaphy, and combinations of the above.

In 1944, Rowe and Yee[16] described a posterior approach to the shoulder to allow for a reverse Bankart procedure in which the torn labrum was sutured to bone. In the two cases described, both regained "normal function." Fried,[5] in 1949, reported on five patients treated with an extracapsular bone block, all with good results. Subsequently, Jones[11] presented a case report where a posterior bone block procedure allowed a soldier to return to full activity after having suffered symptomatic subluxations. Mowery[15] presented five patients with recurrent posterior dislocations treated with an extracapsular bone block from the iliac crest. Screw fixation to the glenoid was used. Four patients rated an excellent result; one patient, however, sustained a subsequent anterior dislocation.

In 1952, McLaughlin[14] reported good results in six patients with posterior instability stabilized with transfer of the subscapularis into a reverse Hill-Sachs defect in the anterior aspect of the humeral head. McLaughlin[13] then followed up on these original patients in 1962, noting that a sharp distinction should be made between fixed and recurrent posterior dislocations or subluxations of the shoulder. He stated that fixed posterior dislocations with substantial anterior humeral head defects do well with a subscapularis transfer. For recurrent subluxations, however, posterior capsular plication and bone block was the preferred procedure.

A reverse Putti-Platt procedure with reconstruction of the posterior capsule and infraspinatus advancement has been used with varying results. In 1952, Severin[18] presented two cases in which the infraspinatus tendon was divided and advanced laterally after a capsular plication. In 1950, DePalma[4] reported that advancement of the teres minor and infraspinatus laterally in three patients demonstrated satisfactory results. Using a modification of this technique, Hawkins presented good results with no recurrences in 15 patients. Bell,[2] in 1991, also noted good results with this procedure.

Tibone[21] reported on posterior staple capsulorrhaphy without detachment or advancement of the infraspinatus or teres minor in athletes. In the initial series of 10 athletes, none returned to their former level of throwing, and 3 athletes (30%) had recurrence of their posterior instability. Tibone concluded that this procedure should be supplemented in "ligamentously lax" individuals. In 1990, additional follow-up of 20 athletes further emphasized that the failure rate was unacceptably high.[22] Nine patients had satisfactory results, 6 patients had recurrence of their posterior instability, and 3 patients still had moderate or severe pain. Only 1 patient was able to return to former competitive level. Researchers concluded that posterior staple capsulorrhaphy is not an acceptable treatment for posterior subluxation of the shoulder because of an unfortunately high rate of failure and complications.

Recently, rotational osteotomy of the humerus for posterior instability has been presented. Surin[20] reported on 10 patients (12 shoulders) who presented with recurrent painful posterior instability treated by external rotation osteotomy of the humerus. Only 3 patients (4 shoulders) participated in overhead sports. Subjectively, 10 of the 12 shoulders rated good to excellent. Objectively, 2 shoulders were rated excellent, 8 as good, and 2 as fair. There was recurrent instability in 1 patient with multidirectional instability.

Scott,[17] in 1967, used a posterior glenoid osteotomy for posterior instability. Three patients who presented with recurrent posterior subluxations were treated with a glenoplasty in which the glenoid retroversion was corrected by redirecting it anteriorly. Scott believed that the glenoplasty provided a stable buttress without disruption of the basic shoulder mechanism while a concomitant capsulorrhaphy or bone block procedure could be performed to augment the glenoplasty. Two patients did well and resumed their military activities, but one immediate dislocation that required reduction was noted. The remaining patient still had recurrent subluxation episodes and pain. Many surgeons have since used this technique with varying results. In 1984, Hawkins presented surgical results using a glenoplasty (17 shoulders), reverse Putti-Platt plication (6 shoulders), or biceps transfer (3 shoulders). The results of these surgical reconstructions were generally poor, with a 50% recurrence rate (13 of 26 shoulders). There were 5 complications out of the 26 that had undergone surgery. Of the 26 shoulders, 16 had no improvement in their athletic impairment. The glenoplasties were augmented with a capsular plication and infraspinatus overlap procedures. Seven of 17 patients had recurrences of instability, and 5 complications, including one case of avascular necrosis of the osteotomized glenoid, were reported.

Recently, a posteroinferior capsular shift has been reported that has demonstrated improved success rates for posterior instability. Goss[7] and Bigliani[3] have described their use of a posteroinferior capsular shift for posterior instability. In 1989, Fronek and Warren[6] presented the use of a posterior capsulorrhaphy augmented with an extraarticular bone block in 5 of 11 surgically treated patients. Their indications for a posterior bone block included a severely deficient posterior glenoid, or an attenuated posterior capsule or infraspinatus tendon. The one patient who did develop recurrent instability 4 years after posterior capsulorrhaphy did not have a concomitant bone block. Overall, a success rate of 91% was noted. However, of the operative group of patients who returned to sports, 70% participated at a lower level of competition or changed their position.

Because this appears to be a capsular problem, it should be treated with a capsular operation. Posterior capsulorrhaphy with suture fixation is the current treatment of choice. This treatment was performed with staples in the past. However, staples have caused metal complications about the shoulder and are no longer recommended.

Operative Technique

The patient is placed in the lateral decubitus position with the involved shoulder accessible (Fig. 8-1). The patient is held in this position with a Vacu-Pak* and kidney rests. The inferior leg is padded to prevent pressure on the peroneal nerve. Arthroscopy is performed before the posterior reconstruction to assess the articular cartilage and to rule out an associated anterior labral tear, because this would be a contraindication for a posterior procedure. The arthroscopy is performed through a conventional posterior portal.

After the arthroscopy is completed, the patient is released from traction and the arm is rested at the side

*Olympic Vacu-Pak, Seattle, WA.

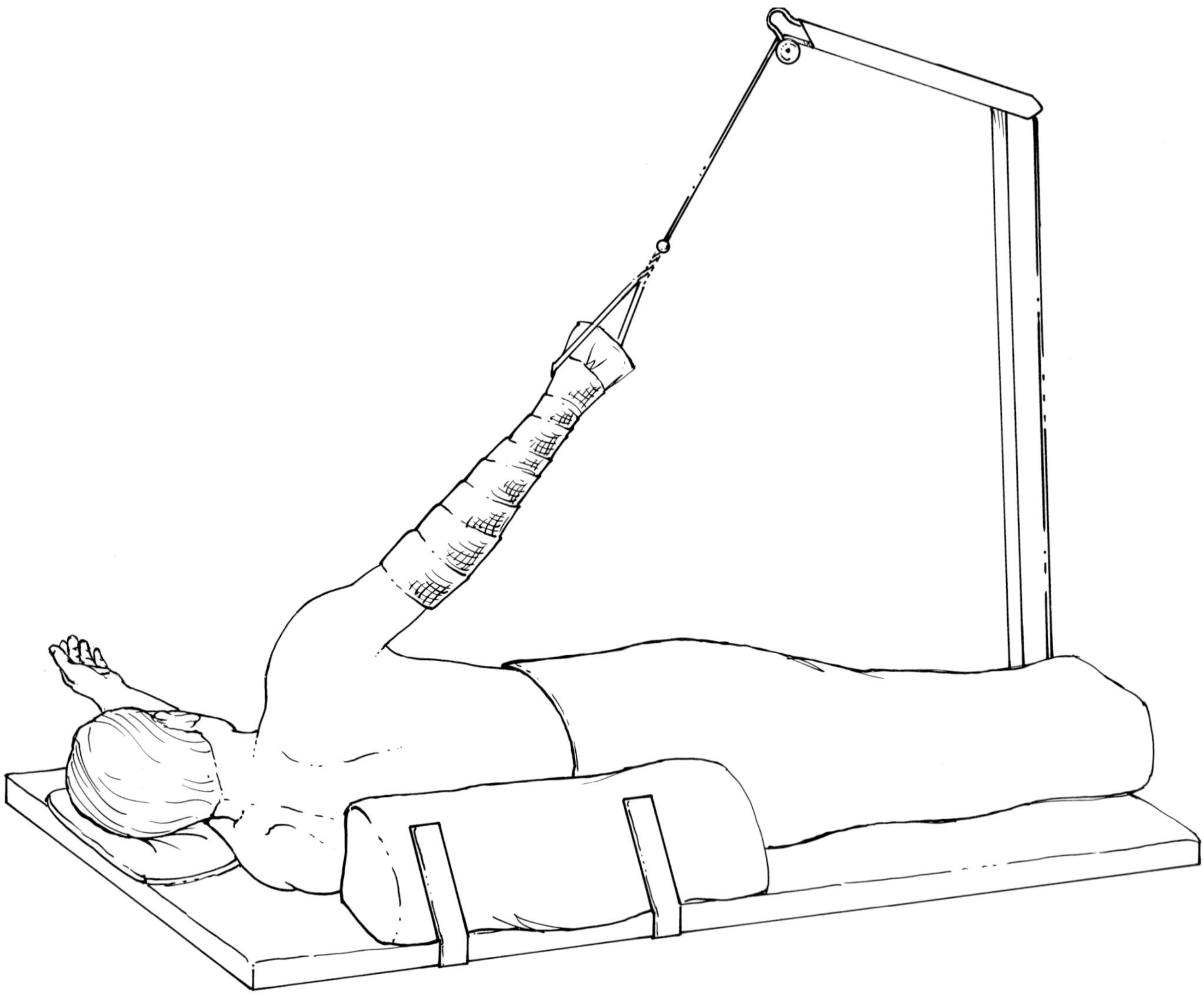

FIGURE 8-1 Patient in lateral decubitus position with traction set up for arthroscopy of the shoulder.

with the patient retained in the same lateral decubitus position. Repreparing and redraping usually is not necessary.

The landmarks for the skin incision include the posterior aspect of the acromioclavicular joint, an area just medial to the posterior lateral corner of the acromion, and the posterior axillary fold. A 10-cm saber-cut incision is made beginning at the posterior aspect of the acromioclavicular joint, proceeding approximately 2 cm medial to the posterolateral corner of the acromion, and continuing inferiorly toward the posterior axillary fold (Fig. 8-2). The skin flaps are raised, exposing the underlying deltoid muscle. The deltoid muscle is split distally (approximately 6 cm) in line with its fibers from the spine 2 to 3 cm medial to the posterolateral corner of the acromion (Fig. 8-3). The deltoid need not be detached from the spine of the scapula or the acromion. The deltoid is retracted with Goelet retractors or a self-retaining Balfur retractor. This exposes the underlying teres minor and infraspinatus muscles. A heavy fascia layer covers these muscles, and one must divide this layer to better visualize the muscles. The interval between the teres minor and the infraspinatus is poorly defined. The interval between the two heads of the infraspinatus may be a better landmark. The infraspinatus is a bipennate muscle with a fat stripe between the two heads. This interval is an excellent area for exposure of the underlying capsule (Fig. 8-4). The infraspinatus is divided between its two heads from its lateral tendinous insertion to just medial to the glenoid. Care is taken not to divide the muscle more than 1.5 cm medial to the glenoid to avoid damage to branches of the suprascapular nerve, which also innervate the infraspinatus muscle. The infraspinatus is then dissected from the underlying capsule using sharp dissection laterally and a periosteal elevator medially. The infraspinatus must be completely separated from the

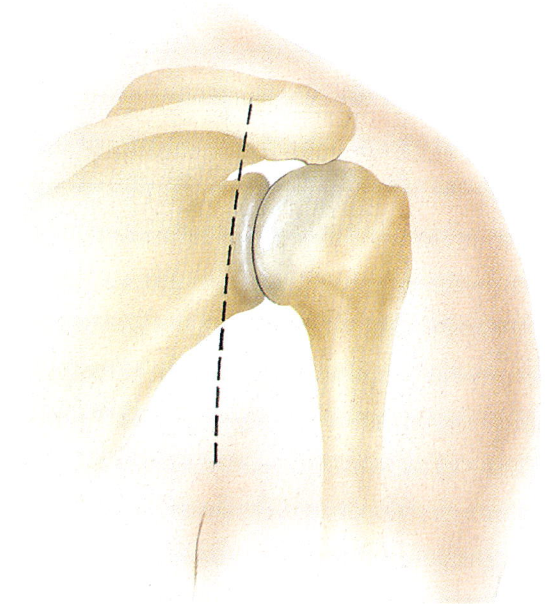

FIGURE 8-2 Skin incision outline from the posterior aspect of the AC joint toward the posterior axillary fold.

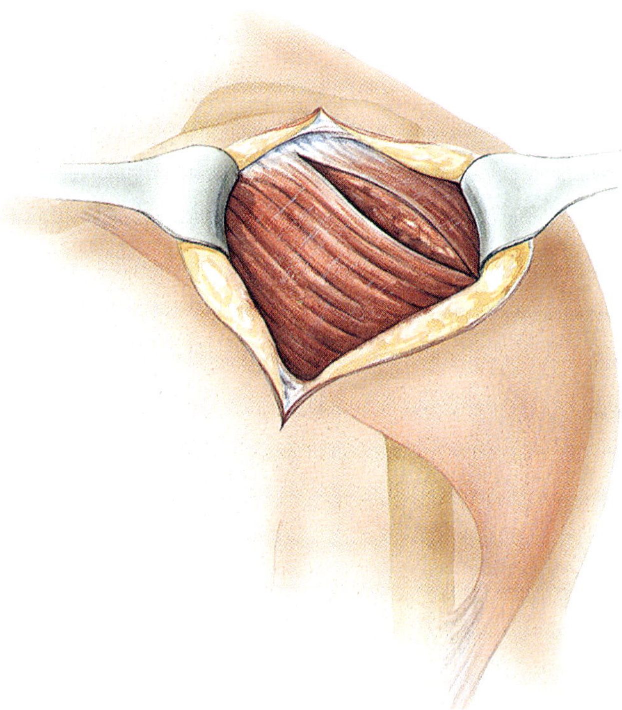

FIGURE 8-3 The deltoid is exposed and split in line with its fibers from the spine of the scapula distally 6 cm.

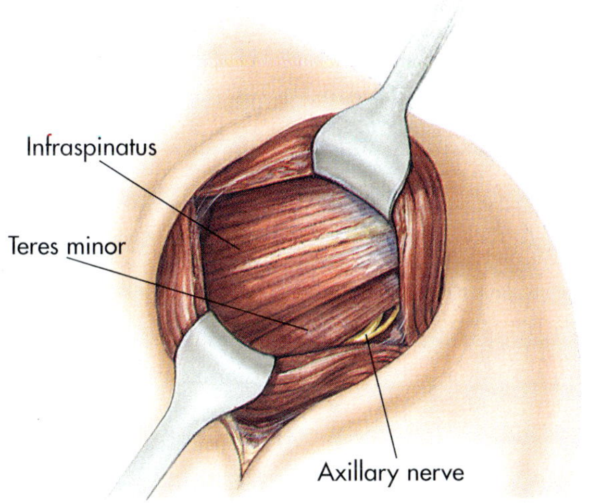

FIGURE 8-4 The deltoid is retracted, exposing underlying infraspinatus and teres minor muscles. The fat stripe separating the two heads of the infraspinatus is a useful surgical landmark.

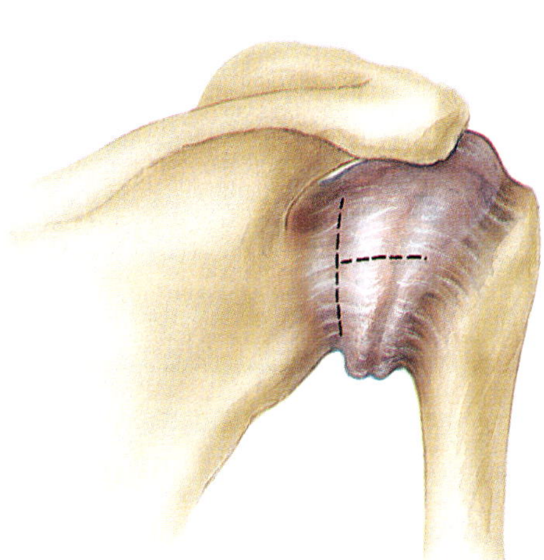

FIGURE 8-5 The "T" incision in the capsule is outlined.

capsule to allow the capsule to be sufficiently mobilized. A Gelpi retractor is placed laterally between the two heads of the infraspinatus, and a pitchfork retractor is inserted onto the glenoid neck to aid in the exposure of the underlying capsule (Fig. 8-5). The capsule is divided from lateral to medial in its midportion to the edge of the posterior glenoid labrum. In the majority of cases (approximately 95%), the labrum is intact and can be used to hold sutures when advancing the capsule. Next, the capsule is cut medially along the edge of the glenoid labrum, creating superior and inferior flaps (Fig. 8-6). These flaps then are tagged with sutures for further mobilization and for retraction. Three or four #1 Ethibond sutures are used for the repair, and these are passed sequentially through the glenoid labrum from an inferior to a superior direction. The inferior capsular flap is placed superiorly and medially, and the Ethibond sutures are placed through the capsule, beginning inferiorly (medially) and proceeding superiorly. The sutures then are tied with the arm in neutral rotation (Fig. 8-7). The supe-

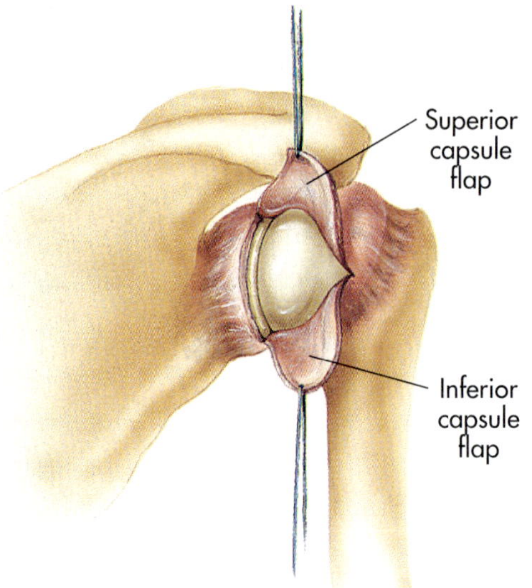

FIGURE 8-6 The superior/inferior capsule flaps are demonstrated after the "T" incision is made in the capsule along the glenoid margin.

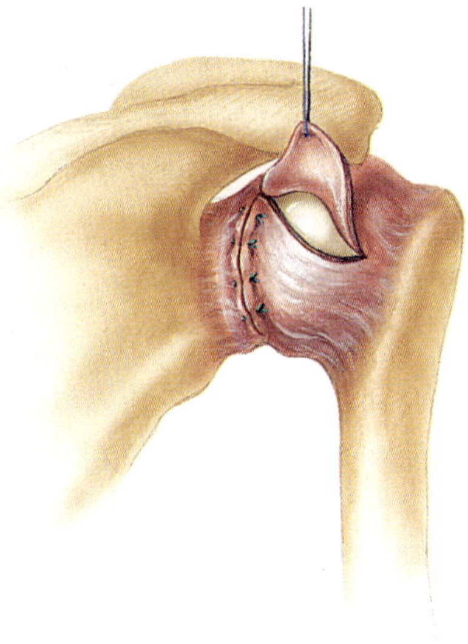

FIGURE 8-7 The inferior capsular flap is advanced superiorly and sutured to the glenoid rim.

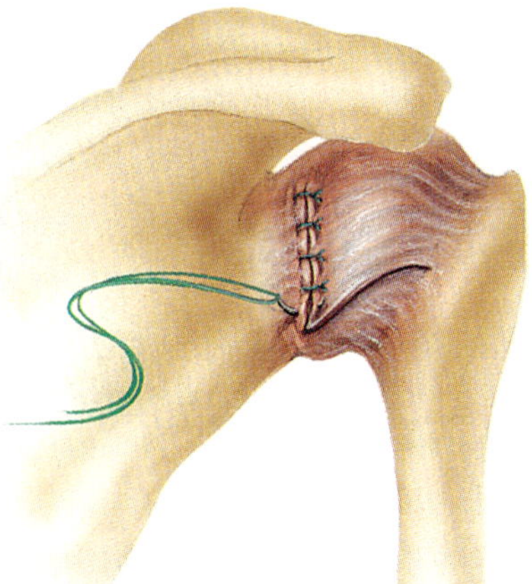

FIGURE 8-8 The superior capsular flap is advanced inferiorly and sutured over the inferior capsular flap.

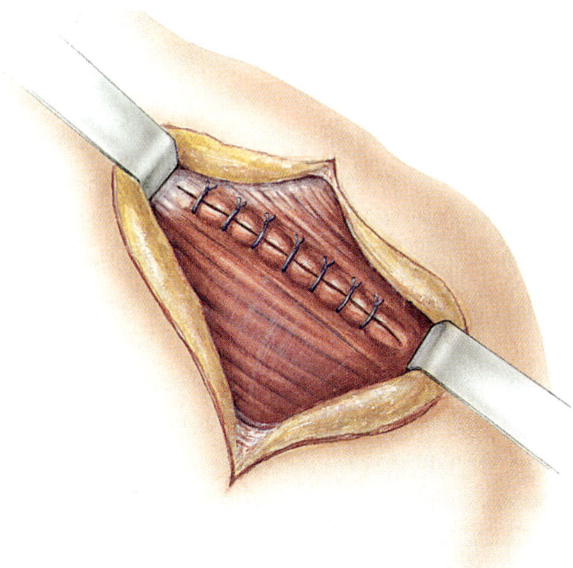

FIGURE 8-9 The split in the deltoid is repaired.

rior flap is advanced distally and slightly medial over the inferior flap. The same Ethibond sutures that were previously tied then are placed through the superior flap (Fig. 8-8). This creates a double layer of capsule at the rim of the glenoid. The lateral split in the capsule then is repaired in a pants-over-vest fashion with #1 absorbable suture. (In those instances where the labrum is damaged and there is a reverse Bankart lesion, the procedure is performed in a similar fashion except that the labrum is resected and the Ethibond sutures are fixed to the glenoid rim through drill holes, as in a conventional Bankart repair, or with Mitek suture anchors). The split in the infraspinatus is closed with #1 absorbable suture. The split in the deltoid is closed with a running absorbable suture through the superficial fascia (Fig. 8-9). The subcutaneous tissue and skin are closed routinely. A subcuticular skin closure leaves a cosmetically acceptable scar. A sterile dressing is applied, and the patient is placed in an abduction pillow. The elbow is kept posterior to the coronal plane of the body, and care is taken to avoid humeral rotation and horizontal adduction (cross-body adduction) for approximately 3 weeks to decrease stress on the repair. With the elbow in this position, the pillow keeps the shoulder in neutral rotation.

Postoperative Management

As the nonsurgical treatment, the physical therapy rehabilitation program after posterior shoulder subluxation/dislocation surgical repair will vary in length depending on factors such as the following:

- Degree of shoulder instability/laxity
- Acute versus chronic condition
- Length of time immobilized
- Strength/range of motion status
- Performance/activity demands

The rehabilitation program is presented in four phases. Overlapping of phases is permitted (e.g., phase II-III, phase III-IV), depending on the progress of the patient.[10,19,25]

Phase I: This initial phase is divided into time-dependent sections to account for the different phases in the healing process. Caution is used to avoid stressing the posterior joint capsule. During the first 2 weeks after surgery, an immobilizer is used. Emphasis is placed on reducing pain, decreasing swelling, and providing gentle passive range of motion. During the second part of this initial phase, the patient is no longer required to use the immobilizer. Active-assistive range of motion exercises are performed, and strengthening exercises are initiated.

Initial 2 weeks after surgery:

- The patient is immobilized during the initial 2 weeks after surgery.
- The immobilizer may be removed for gentle passive range-of-motion exercises for shoulder flexion, abduction, horizontal abduction, and external rotation. Perform two times per day with emphasis on protecting the posterior joint capsule. *Passive internal rotation is not allowed at this time to protect the posterior capsule.*
- Provide pain-relief modalities as needed.
- Provide mobilization of the glenohumeral joint for pain relief.
- Avoid active shoulder elevation or internal rotation in the first month. Elevation is prohibited to allow the deltoid, which was incised, to heal, and internal rotation is avoided to minimize the stresses placed on the posterior capsule (Shields).[19]

Phase I (2 to 6 weeks after surgery):

- If the physician gives permission, the patient is no longer required to wear the immobilizer.
- Continue use of modalities as needed (heat, ice, electrotherapy).
- Continue gentle passive range-of-motion exercises. Add range-of-motion exercises for shoulder internal rotation as needed.
- Add active-resistive range-of-motion exercises (e.g., wand exercises).
- Continue gentle joint mobilization for pain relief and range of motion as needed.
- Add shoulder shrug exercise. Avoid traction of the glenohumeral joint by not allowing the arms to drop completely. This will avoid excessive inferior glide of the humeral head.
- Add isometric internal and external rotation with arm at side and elbow flexed at 90° according to the patient's tolerance. Isometric shoulder flexion and extension may be added as needed.

  Modifications: To allow a pain-free muscle contraction, place the shoulder more into the scapular plane (approximately 20° to 30° anterior to the coronal plane).
- As strength improves, active external rotation, with the arm positioned at the side, may be added. Use tubing for resistance. If there is pain with active movements, continue with isometric strengthening.
- Add active horizontal abduction while lying prone. Restrict movement to 45° of horizontal adduction to full horizontal abduction to avoid excessive stress to the posterior capsule.

Phase II (1½ to 3 months): Stretching exercises to attain full range of motion are continued as needed. Strengthening exercises and the restoration of normal glenohumeral and scapulothoracic biomechanics are targeted, provided that full range of motion has been achieved. Protect the posterior capsule as needed until dynamic stability is reestablished.

- Continue passive and active-assistive range-of-motion exercises. Wall climbs may be added for shoulder flexion and abduction. The patient should have full range of motion by the end of this phase.
- Continue mobilization as needed.
- As strength improves, progress to free weights for external rotation in the side-lying position with arm at side.

  Modifications: Limit the degrees of internal rotation to protect the posterior capsule.
- Add supraspinatus exercise if movement is pain free and adequate range of motion is available (0° to 90°). The shoulder is positioned in the scapular plane approximately 20° to 30° forward of the coronal plane.
- Add active internal rotation using tubing. Movement is performed while standing with the arm at the side and elbow flexed at 90 degrees.

  Progression: Using free weights, perform internal rotation in the side lying position with the arm at the side and elbow bent to 90°.

  Modifications: Limit the amount of internal rotation to avoid excessive stress to the posterior joint capsule. To avoid excessive compressive forces on the glenohumeral joint, elevate the lateral chest wall using a bolster or pillow.
- Add active shoulder flexion through available range of motion.
- Add active shoulder abduction to 90°.
- Add push-ups. Movement should be pain free with

emphasis on protecting the posterior joint capsule. Shoulders are positioned in 80° to 90° of abduction. *Caution is applied during the ascent phase of the push-up to avoid excessive stress to the posterior capsule.* Do not raise the body beyond the scapular plane. Begin with wall push-ups. As strength improves, progress to floor push-ups (modified, hands and knees; or military, hands and feet) as tolerated by the patient.
- Horizontal abduction may be performed through an increased range (with starting position of 90° of horizontal adduction as tolerated).
- Add arm ergometer as tolerated during the latter portions of this phase.

Phase III (3 to 4 months): This phase focuses on progressive strengthening exercises. Isokinetic strengthening and endurance training may begin during this stage.
- Continue to progress weights as tolerated (e.g., rotator cuff, horizontal abduction/adduction, flexion, abduction). Emphasis may be placed on the eccentric phase of contraction in strengthening the rotator cuff.
- Add active horizontal adduction for endurance exercise.
- Continue arm ergometer for endurance exercise.
- Add isokinetic strengthening and endurance exercises (high speeds, ≥200°/sec) for shoulder internal/external strength (arm at side). Prerequisite strength requirements of the rotator cuff are 5 to 10 lb for external rotation and 15 to 20 lb for internal rotation. The shoulder should be pain free and have no significant amount of swelling.
- Add military press. Press the weight directly over or behind the head.
- Add total body conditioning with emphasis on strength and endurance.

Phase IV (4 to 5 months): The emphasis during this advanced stage is on returning individuals to their prior level of activity (e.g., work, recreational activity, sports). Exercises and drills are initiated to simulate the tasks and abilities needed to achieve full recovery.
- Add the isokinetic test. Perform the isokinetic strength and endurance test for the following suggested movement patterns: internal/external rotation (arm at side), horizontal abduction/adduction, and abduction/adduction.
- Continue to progress isotonic and isokinetic exercises.
- Continue strengthening the rotator cuff, emphasizing the eccentric phase.
- Isokinetic exercises for shoulder flexion/extension and abduction/adduction may be added.
- Continue arm ergometer.
- Continue total-body conditioning with emphasis on the shoulder (rotator cuff, posterior deltoid).
- Add skill mastery. Begin practicing skills specific to the activity (e.g., work, recreational activity, sports). See the guidelines in the progressive shoulder throwing program presented in Chapter 7, Section F.

Results

Of 40 athletes who underwent posterior capsulorrhaphy and who were reviewed at the Kerlan-Jobe Orthopaedic Clinic, only 50% had a good or excellent result and could return to their same level of competition. Of the 40, 16 patients (40%) were considered failures. Of the 16 failures, 11 had a recurrence of instability (8 posterior and 3 anterior). Five patients failed secondary to recalcitrant pain. Of the 11 patients who had recurrent instability, 9 were "ligamentous lax" individuals, while only 2 of the 29 athletes with "normal collagen" had recurrence of their instability after surgery. Researchers concluded that if ligamentous laxity was encountered in an athlete, a posterior capsulorrhaphy may not be sufficient. In this situation, the capsulorrhaphy must be augmented with a capsular shift or possibly a bone block; however, the best procedure for this ligamentously lax population is currently unknown.

SUMMARY

The initial treatment of posterior subluxation of the shoulder in athletes requires a detailed history and physical examination. Multidirectional instability must be eliminated. After an isolated posterior subluxation is diagnosed, the ideal treatment is a supervised exercise program. This is successful in the majority of cases.[9] If the athlete fails conservative care, the options for treatment are limited. Pain with activities of daily living usually can be corrected with a surgical procedure. However, surgery on a high-level athlete cannot guarantee return to the prior level of activity. When surgery is indicated, a soft-tissue procedure, such as a posterior capsulorrhaphy with suture fixation, is recommended to eliminate the laxity in the posterior capsule. Athletes with multidirectional instability and ligamentous laxity are associated with an unacceptable rate of surgical failure. The proper operation in these individuals is unknown. Rehabilitation after surgery is important and requires a slow, well-structured program that usually lasts 1 year.

References

1. Beall MS Jr, Diefenbach G, Allen A: Electromyographic biofeedback in the treatment of voluntary posterior instability of the shoulder, *Am J Sports Med* 15(2):175-178, 1987.
2. Bell RH, Noble JS: An appreciation of posterior instability of the shoulder, *Clin Sports Med* 10(4):887-899, 1991.
3. Bigliani LU, Endrizzi DR, McIlveon SJ: Operative management of posterior shoulder instability, Presented at American Shoulder and Elbow Surgeons Fifth Open Meeting, Las Vegas, *Orthop Trans* 13:232, 1989.
4. DePalma AF: *Surgery of the shoulder,* Philadelphia, 1950, JB Lippincott.
5. Fried A: Habitual posterior dislocation of the shoulder joint: a case report on 5 operated cases, *Acta Orthop Scand* 18:329, 1949.
6. Fronek J, Warren RF, Bowen M: Posterior subluxation of the glenohumeral joint, *J Bone Joint Surg* 71A:205-216, 1989.
7. Goss TP, Costello G: Recurrent symptomatic posterior glenohumeral subluxation, *Orthop Rev* 17:1024-1028, 1988.
8. Hart DL, Carmichael SW: Biomechanics of the shoulder, *J Orthop Sports* 6(4):229-234, 1985.
9. Hurley JA et al: Posterior shoulder instability: surgical vs nonsurgical results, *Orthop Trans* 11(3):458, 1987.
10. Jobe FW, Moynes DR, Brewster CE: Rehabilitation of shoulder joint instabilities, *Orthop Clin* 18(3):473-482, 1987.
11. Jones V: Recurrent posterior dislocation of the shoulder: report of a case treated by posterior bone block, *J Bone Joint Surg* 40B:203-207, 1958.
12. McFarland EG et al: Electromyographic analysis of recurrent posterior instability of the shoulder, Presented at the Fifth Annual Open Meeting of the American Shoulder and Elbow Surgeons, Las Vegas, *Orthop Trans* 13(2):230, 1989.
13. McLaughlin HL: Follow up notes on articles previously published in the journal, posterior dislocation of the shoulder, *J Bone Joint Surg* 44A:1477, 1962.
14. McLaughlin HL: Posterior dislocation of the shoulder, *J Bone Joint Surg* 34A:584-590, 1952.
15. Mowery CA et al: Recurrent posterior dislocation of the shoulder: treatment using a bone block, *J Bone Joint Surg* 67A:777-781, 1985.
16. Rowe CR, Yee LB: A posterior approach to the shoulder, *J Bone Joint Surg* 26:580-584, 1944.
17. Scott DJ Jr: Treatment of recurrent posterior dislocations of the shoulder by glenoplasty, *J Bone Joint Surg* 49A:471-476, 1967.
18. Severin E: Anterior and posterior recurrent dislocation of the shoulder: the Putti-Platt operation, *Acta Orthop Scand* 23:14, 1985.
19. Shields CL: *Manual of sports surgery,* New York, 1987, Springer-Verlag, pp 32-37.
20. Surin V et al: Rotational osteotomy of the humerus for posterior instability of the shoulder, *J Bone Joint Surg* 72A:181-186, 1990.
21. Tibone JE et al: Staple capsulorrhaphy for recurrent posterior shoulder dislocations, *Am J Sports Med* 9(3):135-139, 1981.
22. Tibone JE, Ting A: Capsulorrhaphy with a staple for recurrent posterior subluxation of the shoulder, *J Bone Joint Surg* 12A:999-1002, 1990.
23. Tullos HS, King JW: The throwing mechanism in sports, *Orthop Clin North Am* 4:709-720, 1973.
24. Turkel SJ et al: Stabilizing mechanisms preventing anterior dislocation of the glenohumeral joint, *J Bone Joint Surg* 63A:1208-1217, 1981.
25. Warner JP et al: Patterns of flexibility, laxity and strength in normal shoulders and shoulders with instability and impingement, *Am J Sports Med* 18(4):366-375, 1990.

Bibliography

Ahlgreen SA, Heplung T, Nistor L: Idiopathic posterior instability of the shoulder joint: results of operation with posterior bone graft, *Acta Orthop Scand* 49:600-603, 1978.

Boyd HB, Sisk TD: Recurrent posterior dislocation of the shoulder, *J Bone Joint Surg* 54A:779-786, 1972.

Bradley JP, Perry J, Jobe FW: The biomechanics of the throwing shoulder, *Perspect Orthop Surg* 1(2):49-59, 1990.

Bradley JP, Tibone JE: Electromyographic analysis of the muscle action about the shoulder, *Clin Sports Med* 10(4):789-805, 1991.

Brewer BJ, Wubben RC, Carrera FG: Excessive retroversion of the glenoid cavity, *J Bone Joint Surg* 68A:724-731, 1986.

Chaudhuri GK, Sengupta A, Saha AK: Rotation osteotomy of the shaft of the humerus for recurrent dislocation of the shoulder: anterior and posterior, *Acta Orthop Scand* 45:193-198, 1974.

DePalma AF: *Surgery of the shoulder,* ed 2, Philadelphia, 1973, JB Lippincott.

Dugas RW, Scerpella TA, Clancy WG: Surgical treatment of symptomatic posterior shoulder instability, Presented at The American Orthopaedic Sports Medicine Fifteenth Annual Meeting, Traverse City, Michigan, *Orthop Trans* 14(2):245, 1990.

English E, Macnab I: Recurrent posterior dislocation of the shoulder, *Can J Surg* 17(3):147-151, 1974.

Gerber C, Ganz R: Clinical assessment of instability of the shoulder with special reference to anterior and posterior drawer tests, *J Bone Joint Surg* 66B:551-556, 1984.

Gerber C, Ganz R, Vinh TS: Glenoplasty for recurrent posterior shoulder instability: an anatomic reappraisal, *Clin Orthop* 216:70-79, 1987.

Greenhill BJ: Persistent posterior shoulder dislocation: its diagnosis and its treatment by posterior Putti-Platt repair, *J Bone Joint Surg* 54B:763, 1972.

Hawkins RJ: Unrecognized dislocations of the shoulder. In Stauffer ES editor: *Instructional Course Lecture, The American Academy of Orthopaedic Surgeons,* vol 34, St Louis, 1984, CV Mosby, p 258.

Hawkins RJ, Koppers G, Johnston G: Recurrent posterior instability (subluxation) of the shoulder, *J Bone Joint Surg* 66A:169-174, 1984.

Hawkins RJ, McCormack RG: Posterior shoulder instability, *Orthopaedics* 11:101-107, 1988.

Hernandez A, Drez D: Operative treatment of posterior shoulder dislocations by posterior glenoplasty, capsulorrhaphy, and infraspinatus advancement, *Am J Sports Med* 14:187-191, 1980.

Hindenach JCR: Recurrent posterior dislocation of the shoulder, *J Bone Joint Surg* 29A:582-586, 1947.

Jobe FW et al: An EMG analysis of the shoulder in pitching: a second report, *Am J Sports Med* 12(3):218-220, 1984.

Kretzler HH Jr: Scapular osteotomy for posterior shoulder dislocations. In Proceedings of the Western Orthopaedic Association, *J Bone Joint Surg* 56A:197, 1974.

Matsen FA III: Glenohumeral instability. In Evarts CM: *Surgery of the musculoskeletal system,* vol 2, New York, 1983, Churchill Livingstone, pp 49-75.

Neer CS II, Foster CR: Inferior capsular shift for involuntary inferior and multidirectional instability of the shoulder, *J Bone Joint Surg* 62A:897-908, 1980.

Norris TR: Diagnostic techniques for shoulder instability. In: American Academy of Orthopaedic Surgeons Instructional Course Lecture, 34:239-257, 1985.

Norwood LA, Terry GC: Shoulder posterior subluxation, *Am J Sports Med* 12(1):25-30, 1984.

Rockwood CA Jr: Subluxation and dislocation about the shoulder. In Rockwood Jr CA, Green DP, editors: *Fractures in adults,* vol 1, Philadelphia, 1984, JB Lippincott, pp 722-780.

Rowe CR: Prognosis in dislocations of the shoulder, *J Bone Joint Surg* 38A:957-977, 1956.

Rowe CR, Pierce DS, Clark JG: Voluntary dislocation of the shoulder. A preliminary report on a clinical, electromyographic, and psychiatric study of twenty six patients, *J Bone Joint Surg* 55A:445-460, 1973.

Shaffer BS et al: *Infraspinatus splitting incision in posterior shoulder surgery. An anatomic and electromyographic study,* presented at the American Academy of Orthopaedic Surgeons 59th Annual Meeting, Washington, DC, 1992.

Tibone JE: Posterior capsulorrhaphy for posterior shoulder subluxation. In Paulos LE, Tibone JE, editors: *Operative techniques in shoulder surgery,* Gaithersburgh, Md, 1991, Aspen, pp 143-147.

Vegter J, Marti RK: Treatment of posterior dislocation of the shoulder by osteotomy of the neck of the scapula, *J Bone Joint Surg* 63B: 288, 1981.

Warren RF: Subluxation of the shoulder in athletes, *Clin Sports Med* 2(2):339-354, 1983.

Zuckerman JD, Matsen FA III: Complications about the glenohumeral joint related to the use of screws and staples, *J Bone Joint Surg* 66A:175-180, 1984.

CHAPTER 9

Voluntary Glenohumeral Instability

EDWARD G. MCFARLAND

Voluntary shoulder instability is the least-common type of shoulder instability encountered in patients, including athletes. Because of continued confusion and controversy over what constitutes voluntary instability, the exact incidence, presentation, symptoms, evaluation, and treatment remain vague. This chapter will clarify these issues, particularly as they may relate to athletes.

MECHANISM AND INCIDENCE

The patient with voluntary shoulder instability usually is experiencing a subluxation of the shoulder and not a true dislocation of the entire humeral head. This subluxation, which can occur in an anterior, posterior, inferior, or combination of directions, can be produced willfully and intentionally by the patient. Patients who voluntarily *dislocate* their shoulders are rare, but they do exist (Fig. 9-1). In this group there is usually a history of severe trauma, seizure disorder, neuromuscular disease (e.g., syringomyelia), or other medical conditions. Hereafter in this chapter, voluntary instability will refer to the patients who *subluxate* their shoulders.

The incidence of voluntary shoulder instability is unknown for a variety of reasons. No study has specifically addressed the incidence of this disorder. Many of these patients are asymptomatic and probably do not seek medical evaluation. During their careers, most physicians will rarely see patients with this disorder. Studies of this condition usually report on only a few patients or tend to include groups of patients with a variety of instability patterns. In most series of patients with voluntary subluxation, the majority of patients are merely subluxating their shoulders posteriorly. According to Rowe, only 16 cases of voluntary instability were reported before 1962.[24] The largest series of patients with posterior subluxation, consisting of 41 shoulders in 35 patients, was reported by Hawkins in 1984.[13] In his study, 80% of patients could demonstrate the instability. Voluntary shoulder instability among athletes is less common and composes only a small subgroup in most reported series (Table 9-1). Rowe

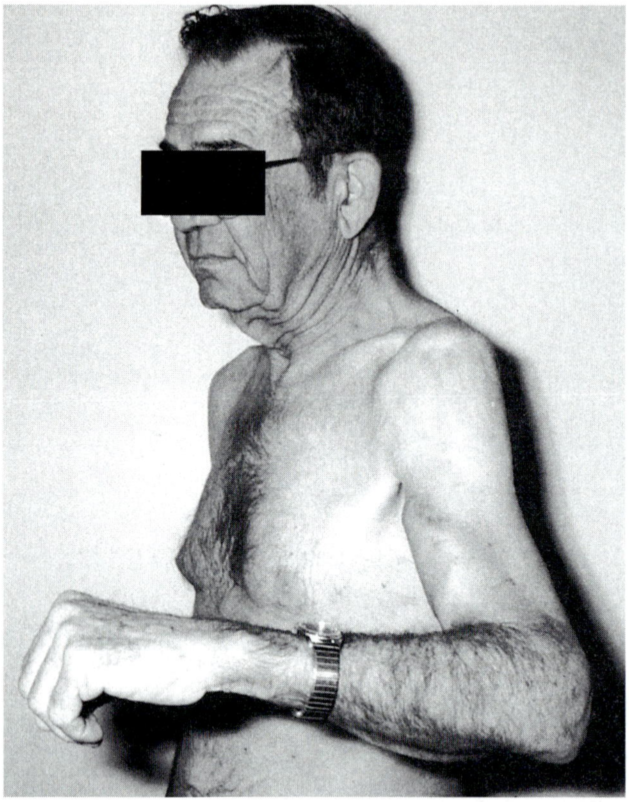

FIGURE 9-1 A 60-year-old man, who could voluntarily dislocate his shoulder anteriorly, with a seizure disorder and multiple anterior and posterior dislocations. He reduced the shoulder with traction to the arm.

reported that several of his 26 patients with voluntary subluxations noted onset of their subluxation with sports, such as throwing or swimming.[24] In his series of 35 patients with posterior subluxations, Hawkins reported that only 9 could participate in sports with no limitations, but almost all of the patients were unaffected in activities of daily living.[13] Fronek et al reported that 17 of their 24 patients with posterior shoulder instability developed instability with sports, but only 12 of their patients were considered to have voluntary instability. In addition, 6 patients' instability occurred after severe trauma, usually a blow to the arm in an adducted and forward-flexed position. Typical cases would be a lineman whose shoulder is pushed posteriorly while blocking or a player who falls directly on an adducted arm. Repetitive microtrauma with sports was implicated in 8 of their patients.[7]

The microtraumas of swimming, throwing, and racquet sports have been proposed as the cause of posterior subluxation in athletes.[4,7,13,16,29] Swimmers were most symptomatic with the pull-through phases of the freestyle or butterfly strokes. Racquet-sport athletes were most symptomatic in the follow-through of a serve or backhand shot, and weight lifters were most symptomatic with bench-press or push-up maneuvers. Throwers noticed the instability in the follow-through phase of pitching.[7] In their 50 patients with instability, Hurley et al reported instability in 25 patients caused by repetitive trauma such as blocking in football, and in 19 patients caused by overhead sports such as baseball, tennis, or swimming. All of their patients sought treatment because of the involuntary component of their instability.[16] Re-

TABLE 9-1
Summary of Pertinent Literature on Voluntary Instability

Series and Year	Total # Patients	# Voluntary Instabiltiy	History of Trauma (All Patients)	Involuntary Compartment	Muscular Intent	Age
Rowe et al, 1973	26	26 patients	11	N/A	26 patients	All <26 yr
Hawkins et al, 1984	35*	40 shoulders	11	35 shoulders	10 shoulders	16 yr (average)
Norwood, Terry, 1984	21	N/A	14	Not stated	2 patients	23.1 yr (average)
Fronek et al, 1989	24	12 patients	24†	24 patients	8 shoulders	20 yr (average)
Tibone, Ting, 1990	20	5 patients	6	N/A	N/A	All <30 yr
Hurley et al, 1992	47‡	37 patients (80%)		47 patients	All could demonstrate	No surgery: 16.3 yr average Surgery: 18.3 yr average

N/A, Not applicable.
*50 shoulders.
† 14 with major trauma.
‡ 50 shoulders.

current posterior subluxation caused by the microtrauma of drawing a bow, "archer's shoulder," also has been reported.[8]

The exact mechanism leading to the subluxations has yet to be elucidated. In 1984, Sjovall found that the posterior capsule had to be lax to allow posterior subluxation. In cadavers, he found that releasing the posterior capsule allowed the head to lever out posteriorly as the lesser tuberosity pushed the humerus out of the glenoid.[27] Many authors have noted at surgery that most of these patients have posterior capsular laxity, whereas posterior Bankart lesions are uncommon.* Mollerud and Fried have postulated that when the arm is raised, the posterior rotator cuff muscles are lax and cannot resist the force of the antagonists.[6,21] Samilson and Miller studied with cineradiography two patients with voluntary posterior shoulder subluxations. They found that the patients first set the scapula in an abnormally "winged" or horizontal position. As the arm was flexed and internally rotated, the greater tuberosity cleared the acromion, and the shoulder subluxed posteriorly.[25]

Electromyographic (EMG) studies of voluntary shoulder instability have provided insight into the mechanism of instability. Rowe et al using high-speed cameras and electromyography, evaluated 11 patients who could subluxate their shoulders anteriorly, posteriorly, or inferiorly. They found that the patients used different muscles depending on the direction of instability. Although they could make no definite statements, they found that, in general, voluntary posterior subluxations had high activity in the anterior deltoid and supraspinatus. They concluded that abnormal muscle coordination was necessary to produce the subluxations. Stabilization of the scapula on the thorax allowed one side of the force couple to relax while the opposing muscles contracted, thus causing the subluxation.[24]

Other studies have used surface EMGs to evaluate small numbers of patients with voluntary posterior subluxations.[1,18,19,23] Beall et al studied three patients but did not systematically evaluate the mechanism of subluxation.[1] Pande and Hawkins studied four patients with surface EMGs and with an electrogoniometer attached to the distal humerus. Two patients subluxated their shoulders with their arms in abduction and external rotation, positions that are more typical of anterior instability. In these two patients, the muscles active at the time of subluxation were the infraspinatus and the posterior deltoid. In their other two patients, a more classic position of abduction and internal rotation was used by each patient to subluxate his shoulder posteriorly. In these patients, the anterior deltoid was active during subluxation, but the pectoralis major and rotator cuff muscles were not active. They concluded that the subjects had learned how to contract their muscles selectively to produce subluxation.[23]

In the Biomechanics Laboratory of Centinela Hospital, Inglewood, California, muscle activity was studied in eight patients with posterior voluntary shoulder instability; the study used indwelling fine-wire electrodes and cinematography at 50 frames per second.[19] The patients were asked to subluxate and reduce their shoulders. The muscle activity for eight muscles was determined as a percentage of the normalization base (% MMT). The patients were photographed in three planes, and the film was synchronized with the EMGs.

The patients used a variety of maneuvers to posteriorly subluxate and reduce their shoulders. A majority used a motion described by many previous authors (Fig. 9-2) that involves abduction, forward flexion, and internal rotation.[1,6,7,14,25] This was called the *arm up* position. This position also is typical of what some authors call *positional* subluxation.[12] As the arm was raised, the shoulder subluxated with ease and the prominence of the humeral head could be seen posteriorly. The shoulder began to subluxate at an average of 94° of abduction (range, 0° to 115°), 84° of flexion (range, 47° to 125°), and 55° of horizontal flexion (range, 27° to 95°). When the subluxation was complete, the arm generally moved into more adduction and internal rotation. Reduction was achieved by abducting and horizontally extending the arm. This usually produced a visible reduction as the humeral head was levered back into the glenoid.

Like previous studies, this study found highly variable muscle activity among patients. In most patients, the anterior deltoid fired consistently as the arm was raised into the position in which the shoulder subluxated. Patients used the posterior deltoid to reduce the shoulder as they extended their arms (Fig. 9-3). The pectoralis major muscle fired when the arm was adducted and had no relationship to the subluxation. The supraspinatus activity occurred when the arm was raised. The subscapularis and infraspinatus muscles had no consistent firing patterns among the patients and did not appear to play an active role in producing the subluxation or the reduction.

Two patients also could subluxate their shoulders posteriorly with their arms at their sides (Fig. 9-4). This involved forward flexion of 40° to 60° and internal rotation of the shoulder. There was no consistent muscle-firing pattern between these two patients. Two additional patients could subluxate their shoulders anteriorly (Fig. 9-5). In both these patients, the pectoralis major and latissimus dorsi muscles contracted as the shoulder subluxated. The firing pattern among the other muscles was inconsistent.

Patients with voluntary shoulder instability appear to have learned how to subluxate their shoulders with selective muscle activity. These patients show high variability in the position and technique used to subluxate

*References 2, 6, 15, 21, 25, 29.

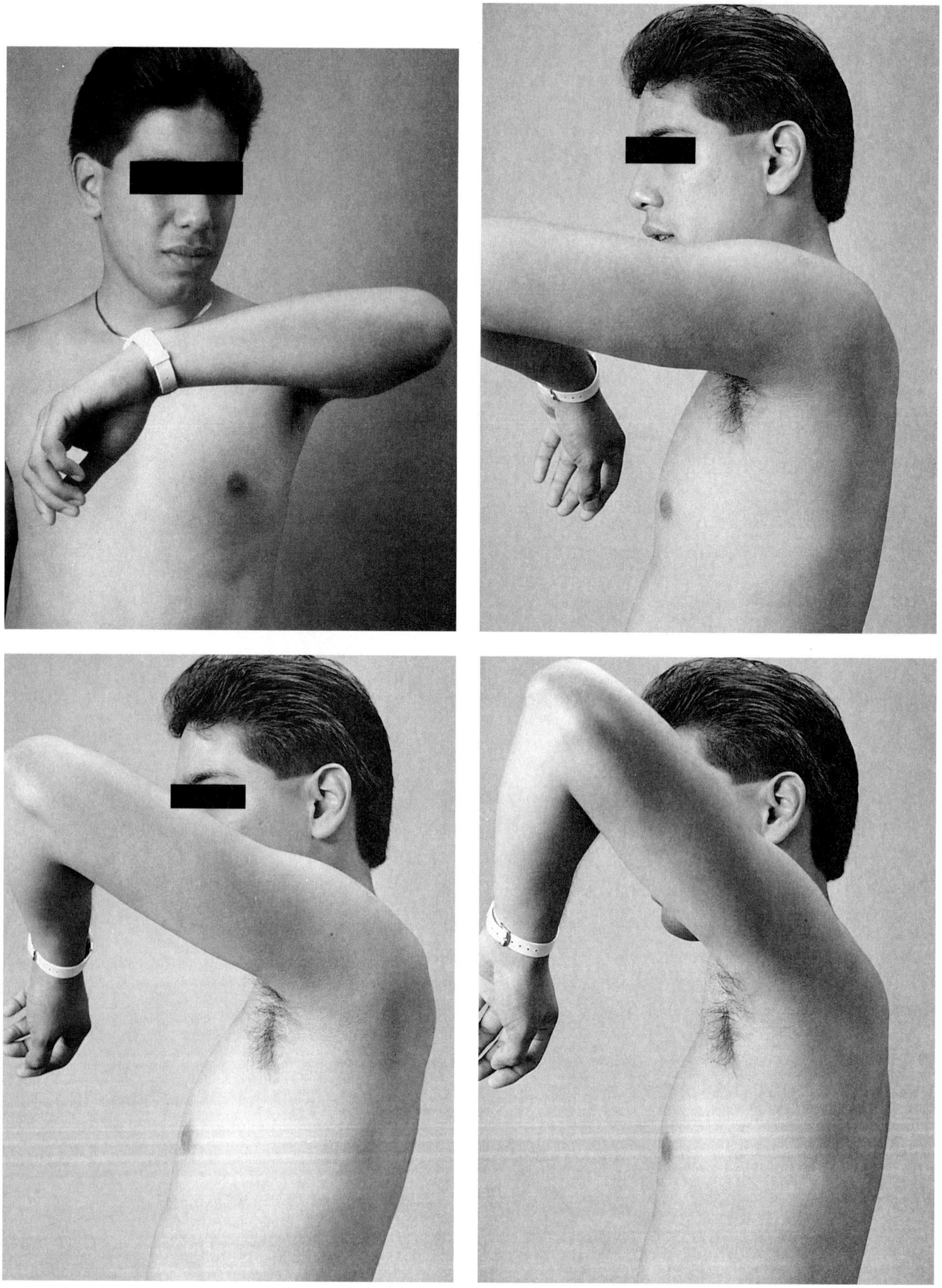

A B C D

FIGURE 9-2 Classic position and maneuver for *arm up* or *positional* voluntary shoulder instability. **A,** Frontal view of arm position when subluxation is completed. **B,** The arm often is rested in horizontal adduction and internal rotation. **C,** The patient produces reduction extending the shoulder with some abduction. This patient used more abduction and internal rotation than most patients. **D,** When the reduction is complete, the humeral head prominence posteriorly has disappeared.

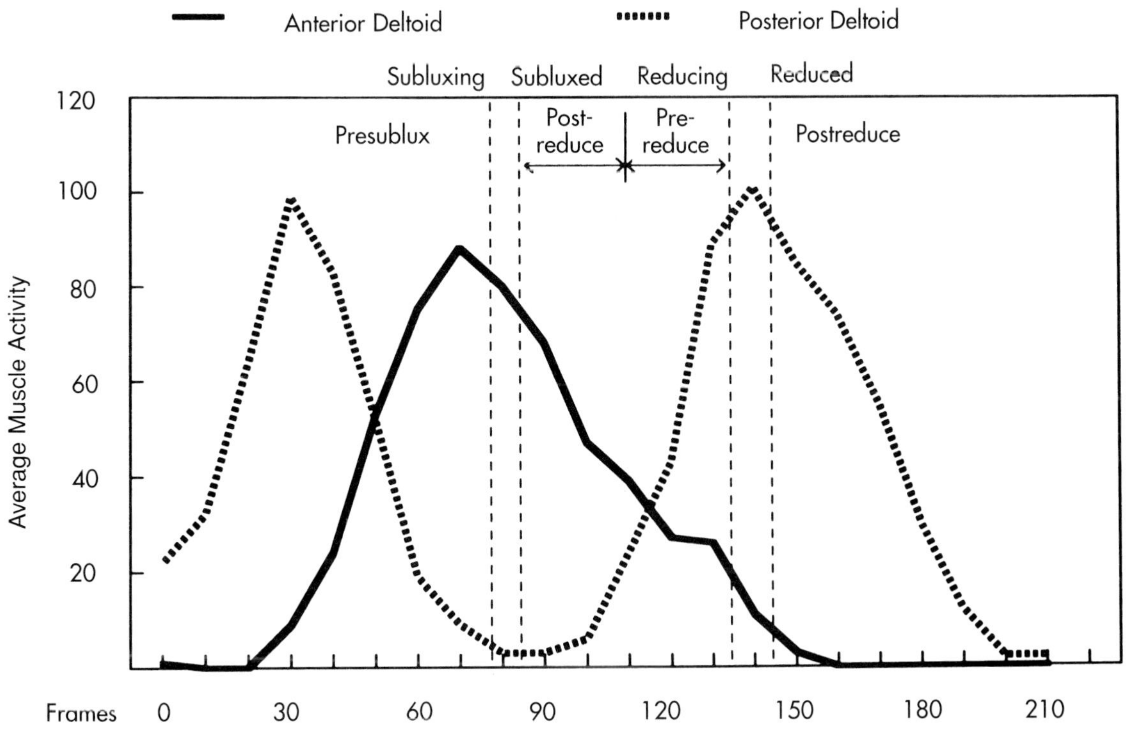

FIGURE 9-3 Muscle activity in the anterior and posterior deltoid when posteriorly subluxating the arm. *SB*, Beginning of subluxation, *SD*, completely subluxated; *RG*, beginning of reduction; *RD*, end of reduction.

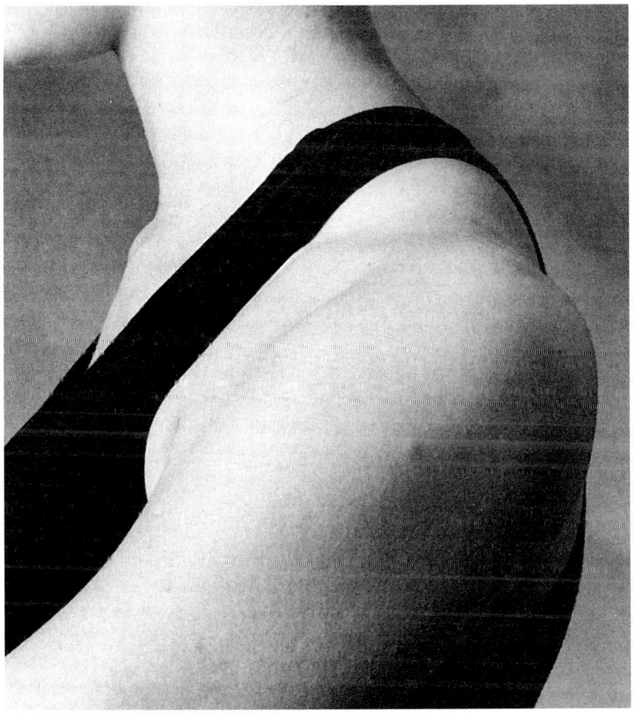

FIGURE 9-4 *Arm down* position for voluntary posterior subluxation.

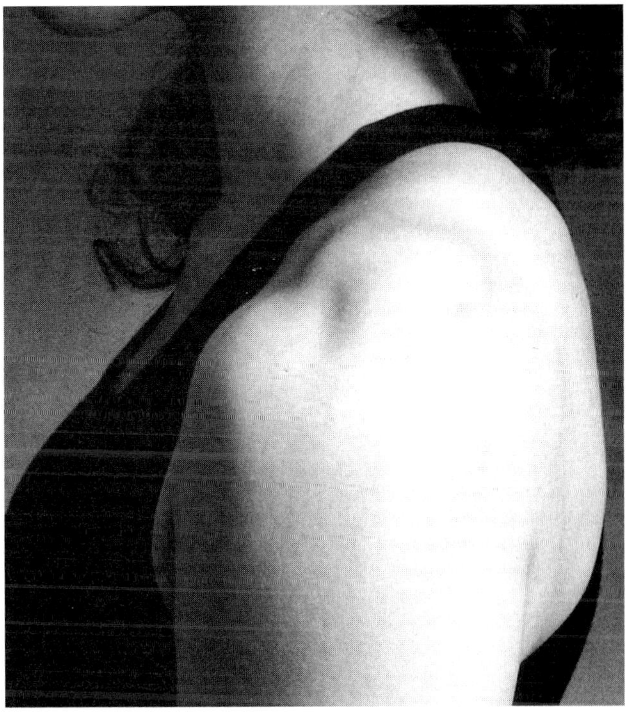

FIGURE 9-5 Anterior or anteroinferior voluntary subluxation.

TABLE 9-2
Spectrum of Posterior Instability

	Pure Voluntary	Voluntary-Involuntary	Pure Involuntary
Demonstrable	Yes	Yes	No
Symptomatic	Usually not	Yes	Yes
History of trauma	Usually not	Usually	Usually
Direction	Any	Usually posterior	Usually posterior
Psychiatric history	More common	Less common	Less common
Willful component	Yes	No	No
Other names	Muscular, habitual	Positional, unintentional	Occult subluxation

their shoulders. The study could not determine whether the muscles are actively pulling or pushing the humeral head or merely placing it in a position to subluxate. However, the rotator cuff muscles did not seem to consistently serve a particular function to push or pull the humeral head out of the glenoid. The findings of this study agree with those of other studies that a combination of posterior ligamentous laxity and selective muscle contraction contributes to the ability of the patient to demonstrate the instability. This study neither refutes nor supports studies that have suggested that the instability can be controlled through biofeedback and physical therapy.[1,18]

CLINICAL PRESENTATION

There are basically three groups of patients with voluntary instability (Table 9-2). Patients with pure voluntary instability usually are younger, and they have no history of trauma. These individuals discover that they can subluxate their shoulders at will. These patients may be able to subluxate their shoulders anteriorly, posteriorly, or in a combination of directions. The instability is almost uniformly asymptomatic and rarely causes symptoms. Many of these patients seek physicians primarily to learn what their shoulders are doing. Some of these patients may demonstrate the instability to their friends or to gain attention. The psychiatric evaluation of this group of patients is important, because some may have a history of psychiatric illness or derive important secondary gains from their shoulder problem.[24] These patients generally have good muscular control over their shoulders and the subluxations.

The second group of patients with voluntary instability is those who have an involuntary component (i.e., subluxation occurs when the patient does not want it to occur). Although the patient may be able to demonstrate the position in which the shoulder subluxates, most of the time the subluxation is not performed intentionally. A patient in this group typically has a history of some trauma that leads to the instability. The trauma usually is relatively minor, but the instability also can be due to major trauma or repetitive microtrauma. The patient experiences subluxations of the shoulder when the arm is raised in either sports or activities of daily living. Subluxation and reduction often are symptomatic, and usually the involuntary nature of the subluxation is what causes the patient to seek treatment. These patients usually do not have a history of psychiatric illness or any apparent secondary gain from their instability.

The last group of patients consists of those with purely involuntary posterior subluxations, who cannot demonstrate voluntarily their instability. This group usually is the most difficult to diagnose because they often present with only pain or a click in certain positions. Pain may be felt posteriorly, anteriorly, or diffusely.[7] In these patients, the posterior subluxation under examination reproduces their symptoms. This group will not be discussed further in this chapter because these patients are discussed elsewhere (see Chapter 8).

CLASSIFICATION

Voluntary shoulder instability has been difficult to classify because many patients overlap in terms of their histories, presentations, and results of treatment. The wide clinical spectrum has made it difficult to create a workable classification system. This difficulty continues to this day, complicating the assessment and treatment of these patients.

The confusion began when Sjovall and Mollerud suggested that Blumenthal's classification of patellar instability be applied to the shoulder.[21,27] Acute dislocations were separated into the following groups:

1. Fresh luxations—acute dislocations caused by trauma
2. Recurrent luxations—dislocations that occurred spontaneously at short or long intervals as sequelae of the "primary luxation"
3. Permanent luxations
   a. Habitual—when the joint luxates with every motion

b. Constant—when the joint is never in a normal relationship

In this classification scheme, a constant luxation is essentially a locked, missed dislocation. Traumatic anterior dislocations were typically "recurrent luxations."

Patients with recurrent shoulder instability with a history of minimal or no trauma were difficult to place within this system. Sjorall reported the case of a 22-year-old man who had posterior dislocations of his shoulder but no history of trauma, calling this condition "habitual-voluntary."[27] Hildenach noted that the recurrent and permanent-habitual types overlapped. He aptly concluded that "the classification of the disability is confused."[15]

Rowe distinguished between involuntary, recurrent dislocations, which were usually traumatic, and voluntary recurrent dislocations, which usually occurred spontaneously or with minimal trauma. He divided the voluntary group into the psychologically normal and the psychologically abnormal. For psychologically normal patients who remained symptomatic despite prolonged physical therapy, he recommended surgical stabilization. Surgery was not successful in symptomatic patients who were psychologically abnormal.[24]

Hawkins recommended that chronic instability be divided into several subgroups. He distinguished between voluntary and involuntary recurrent subluxations. Voluntary subluxators either (1) were habitual (psychologically abnormal) or (2) could contract their muscles intentionally to subluxate their shoulders (psychologically normal). Thus he cautions that "the voluntary (intentional) subluxor should not be confused with the habitual subluxor."[13] Patients who could demonstrate subluxation by placing the arm in a certain position were considered "positional" and thus were involuntary. In this classification system, the main basis for distinction between muscular and positional types of instability is the conscious, directed effort the patient makes to subluxate and reduce the shoulder.[12,13]

Warren et al recommended dividing voluntary posterior shoulder instability into groups on the basis of the frequency, etiology, direction, and degree of the instability. In their study of 24 patients, all had posterior subluxation of the arm when it was raised. However, only eight patients were considered "voluntary," whom Warren et al divided in two groups. In the "positional" type, the humeral head subluxated posteriorly when the arm was flexed and adducted by the patient. The second "muscular" type produced a posterior subluxation with the arm at the side by selectively firing certain muscles.[7]

Rockwood divided shoulder instability (subluxation) into four groups based on a history of a traumatic event.[4] All four groups can be further subdivided by the direction of the instability, such as anterior, posterior, or multidirectional. In this schema, the instability is involuntary if it occurs unintentionally. Voluntary and involuntary instability also may coexist.

These conflicting classification systems reflect the protean nature of this group of patients. Important characteristics by which to distinguish among these groups include history of trauma (major, minor, or none), psychiatric status, presence or absence of symptoms, unidirectionality or multidirectionality of subluxation, and the degree of intention in subluxating. This author favors a classification system based on a patient profile of symptoms and intent (see Table 9-2) that reflects the spectrum of presentations of these patients. In this schema, any patient who can demonstrate instability is by definition a voluntary subluxator to some degree. It is possible that the term *demonstrable* should be substituted for the term *voluntary*. The terms *habitual, positional,* and *muscular* are not helpful distinctions among patients. The major bases for distinguishing among patients are the presence or absence of symptoms and the presence or absence of unwanted, unintentional subluxations. However, these distinctions may converge when the pathology and the surgical results are considered. Hopefully, a classification system will be developed in the future that is based on more objective, measurable laxities and more definitive anatomic lesions.

ASSESSMENT

All of these factors should be assessed with a careful history and physical examination. Frequent assessments of the patient are important for noting the accuracy and repeatability of the history and examination, and also for gauging the patient's motivation and character.

A patient who can subluxate the shoulder at will should be asked about the circumstances of the first subluxation. The severity of the initial trauma is an important factor. When a patient can demonstrate the instability, there is usually little question about its direction. However, the patient should be questioned carefully about other positions that cause symptoms or sensations of shifting, especially with sports. Symptoms of pain or grinding may indicate repetitive trauma or subluxations. The effects of instability on sports and activities of daily living are important. A history of seizures or a previous history of psychiatric problems, substance abuse, or neuromuscular disorder should be noted.

The physical examination must be complete to rule out other etiologies of the subluxation. Observation of atrophy, range of motion, and position of the arm and body at the time of subluxation and reduction is important. The patient should be asked to demonstrate the instability. Care should be taken not to mistake subacromial or scapulothoracic crepitus or catching for voluntary instability. An assessment of the degree of discomfort experienced by the patient can be obtained while observing the subluxation and reduction.

A neurologic examination of the upper extremity is recommended, including reflexes when indicated. Impingement testing is usually negative unless the patient has an inflamed shoulder. Instability testing, either sitting or supine, is recommended. The testing should include the sulcus sign, clunk test, apprehension test, and anterior and posterior drawer tests (see Chapter 7B).

Posterior shoulder laxity is best examined supine, and both shoulders should be examined.[9] The laxity should be graded, for which this author favors a modified Hawkins classification.[11] Type I laxity is normal, and although the humeral head can be brought up to the rim, it cannot be subluxated over the rim. Type II laxity describes a shoulder in which the head can be subluxated over the rim and reduced. Posterior laxity, including subluxation, may be more common as a normal variant than previously appreciated. In a study of 388 shoulders of asymptomatic adolescent male and female athletes (average age of 16 years), 55% of the shoulders were type II and 45% were type I.[20] Asymmetric posterior laxities were demonstrated by 10%, with half of those showing more laxity in the dominant shoulder. Emery and Mullasji studied 75 schoolchildren and found that 55% of the shoulders had a positive posterior drawer test.[5] Consequently, the presence of posterior subluxation on examination does not suffice as the only criterion for posterior instability. Normal posterior laxity should not be misinterpreted as instability.[10,20] Other factors, such as symptoms and functional disability, must be considered when evaluating these patients.

Posterior apprehension is uniformly negative in most patients. Based on our EMG and cinematography study, there are two reasons for this. First, most patients seem to have a fairly specific arm position that produces subluxation. This position is difficult for the examiner to reproduce, even where the patient can demonstrate the subluxation. Second, posterior apprehension tests are described with the arm horizontally adducted and internally rotated.[12,14,26,27] Based on the authors' study, this is not the position in which the subluxation occurs, but it is the position most patients use to rest the arm after the subluxation is complete.[19] Finally, muscle relaxation should be complete to reproduce the subluxation, and many of these patients will not relax when their subluxations are painful.

In patients with previous surgery, careful notation should be made of any limitation of range of motion, especially if there has been excessive loss of external rotation that might be contributing to the posterior subluxations.[12] Patients also should be evaluated for signs of generalized ligamentous laxity, although neither Rowe nor Warren could find any correlation between ligamentous laxity and voluntary shoulder instability.[13,24]

Radiographic assessment of the shoulders in patients with voluntary shoulder instability should include standard anteroposterior radiographs in internal and external rotation and an axillary view. In most cases, these radiographs will be normal.[4,12,13,24] Occasionally, there may be some blunting of the glenoid rim caused by repetitive subluxations, but this blunting is not as common in these patients as in those with traumatic instability.[22] Some patients may demonstrate calcifications along the posterior glenoid in the axillary or Stryker notch views.[7]

Stress radiographs to demonstrate the subluxation(s) usually are not necessary unless the diagnosis is in question. If they are needed, then axillary radiographs will best demonstrate the subluxation.[17] Likewise, fluoroscopic evaluation is not commonly needed but can be used if the diagnosis remains elusive.[13]

CT scanning and CT arthrography may be indicated in some patients. Several authors have suggested that excessive glenoid retroversion may be a factor in posterior subluxations.[13,16,17] Recently Hurley et al reported that CT scans revealed that their patients with posterior instability had significantly more glenoid retroversion than did 10 control patients. However, there was no difference in glenoid retroversion between those treated operatively and those treated nonoperatively, nor was there any difference between the glenoid versions of the symptomatic (subluxing) shoulder and the asymptomatic shoulder.[17] These findings suggest that more factors are involved than glenoid version alone. However, CT scanning can be useful in evaluating patients with previous surgery, those with glenoid abnormalities on plain radiographs, and those rare patients in whom glenoid osteotomy is being considered.

Magnetic resonance imaging (MRI) is less useful in patients with voluntary instability. Posterior Bankart lesions are uncommon in this group of patients.* Although some patients may have fraying of the posterior labrum, this fraying generally is not to a degree that can be demonstrated using current MRI technology. Patients with bony glenoid abnormalities are better examined with CT scanning. Cine-MRI may have a place in evaluating difficult cases when the technology becomes both more available and less costly.

NONSURGICAL TREATMENT

Treatment for pure voluntary instability often involves simply reassuring the patient that there is nothing seriously wrong with the shoulder. If possible, these patients should avoid activities that make the instability worse, or they should attempt to make adjustments in their sports techniques. Younger patients who frequently perform their shoulder subluxations should be cautioned to cease the maneuver to prevent inflammation or chronic symptoms. Patients suspected of psychiatric illness or other psychologic problems should be encouraged to seek appropriate counseling.

Physical therapy programs may help many of these patients symptomatically, although the programs may not

*References 2, 6, 7, 13, 15, 29.

prevent the subluxations.[4,7,16] A physical therapy program designed to strengthen the rotator cuff and scapular stabilizers is recommended. Some patients feel stable as long as they comply with the rehabilitation program.[7] Burkhead and Rockwood recommend a three-phase therapy program using progressive resistance exercises.[4] With this program, their type III-B patients (voluntary instability with no psychologic problems) obtained good to excellent results in 14 out of 16 cases. In their group IV patients, 87% had good to excellent results. In both of these groups, only half of those with either voluntary or involuntary anterior subluxation (four of eight patients) had good to excellent results.[4] Any coexisting tendinitis or impingement also may be treated with cryotherapy and antiinflammatory medication.

Patients with an involuntary component to their voluntary instability also may respond favorably to a physical therapy program. A majority of Rowe's patients responded to a therapy program.[24] Hawkins reviewed 24 patients treated with therapy alone, and most patients became asymptomatic in activities of daily living. Four of the patients had to modify their sports activities.[13] Fronek et al found that 63% of their patients had less pain or instability after a therapy program. However, only 37% were able to return to sports, even at reduced levels of competition.[7] Hurley et al reported similar results in their 25 patients with involuntary posterior shoulder instability treated with a rehabilitation program. Although 96% of these patients had recurrence of their instability, 68% felt subjectively improved. Overall, there was slight improvement in the ability of these patients to participate in sports, with 20% performing all sports, 24% performing at a decreased level, and 52% limited to no overhead sports.[16]

Several authors have recommended biofeedback to prevent or control voluntary shoulder instability.[1,18] Beall et al reported that three patients were helped with biofeedback and muscle reeducation.[1] With surface EMG monitoring, the patients were taught how to perform an isolated contraction of the posterior deltoid. They were then taught to raise the arm to a position of instability and resist the subluxation using the posterior deltoid. The biofeedback program was 4 weeks long and superimposed on an isometric strengthening program. This author's experience is that biofeedback does not add significantly to an exercise program alone.

OPERATIVE TREATMENT

Operative treatment is rarely needed for the patient with pure voluntary instability because a majority of these patients respond to nonoperative treatment. Patients with recognized psychiatric or psychologic conditions should not be offered an operation.[4,24] Unfortunately, the underlying emotional problem sometimes is not exposed or is not diagnosed until well after the operation. Patients with multiple operations who consistently fail their operative procedures should be evaluated carefully and approached with caution.[4,12,24,27,29]

Patients who develop symptomatic voluntary-involuntary instability may be considered as surgical candidates after failing 4 to 6 months of a supervised rehabilitation program.[4] Surgical options include a posterior capsulorraphy (or Bankart), a posterior bone block, posterior infraspinatus tenodesis (or Putti-Platt), posterior glenoid osteotomy, or a combination of these.* This author favors a posterior capsular shift, as described in Chapter 8, as the initial procedure in most patients. Postoperatively, a splint brace is used to prevent internal rotation and cross horizontal adduction for 3 to 4 weeks. A structured rehabilitation program as described in Chapter 8 is then followed. Patients are advised that surgery may provide stability but may not return them to the same level of competitive sports.[7,13,16,29]

Patients who fail surgical treatment must be evaluated carefully, and the diagnosis must be reconsidered. Other instability patterns may be present or may have resulted from the index operation. Secondary gain or psychologic factors also must be considered. Studies to evaluate nerve dysfunction or abnormal glenoid version may be indicated. Patients who have failed one operation have a lesser chance of returning to competitive sports. Consequently, a supervised rehabilitation program should be the initial treatment in these patients. In those who have failed previous surgery, further surgical intervention should be directed to the appropriate pathology only after a careful evaluation and thorough counseling of the patient.

SUMMARY

Voluntary shoulder instability is a protean disorder that presents a significant challenge to the orthopedic surgeon. The treating physician should strive to understand as completely as possible the severity of the patient's symptoms and goals. Nonoperative treatment is recommended for a majority of these patients. Surgical treatment may be successful in some but does not currently offer an athlete complete return to sports.

References

1. Beall MS Jr, Diefenbach G, Allen A: Electromyographic biofeedback in the treatment of voluntary posterior instability of the shoulder, *J Sports Med* 15:175, 1987.
2. Boyd HB, Sisk TD. Recurrent posterior dislocation of the shoulder, *J Bone Joint Surg* 54A:779, 1972.
3. Brewer BJ, Webber RC, Carrera FG. Excessive retroversion of the glenoid cavity, *J Bone Joint Surg* 68A:724, 1986.
4. Burkhead WZ, Rockwood CA: Treatment of instability of the shoulder with an exercise program, *J Bone Joint Surg* 74A:890-896, 1992.

*References 3, 7, 13, 14, 16, 22, 26, 28, 29.

5. Emery RJH, Mulloji AB: Glenohumeral joint instability in normal adolescents, *J Bone Joint Surg* 73B:406-408, 1991.
6. Fried A: Habitual posterior dislocation of the shoulder joint: a case report on five operated cases, *Acta Orthop Scand* 18:329, 1949.
7. Fronek J, Warren RF, Bowen M: Posterior subluxation of the glenohumeral joint, *J Bone Joint Surg* 71A:204, 1989.
8. Fukada J, Warren RF, Bowen M: Posterior subluxation of the glenohumeral joint, *J Bone Joint Surg* 71A:204, 1989.
9. Gerber C, Ganz R: Clinical assessment of instability of the shoulder with special reference to anterior and posterior drawer tests, *J Bone Joint Surg* 71A;205, 1989.
10. Harryman DT et al: Laxity of the normal glenohumeral joint: a quantitative in vivo assessment, *J Shoulder Elbow Surg* 1:66-76, 1992.
11. Hawkins RJ, Bellow RM: *Posterior instability of the shoulder,* Instructional Course Lecture 30:211, Chicago, 1989, American Academy of Orthopaedic Surgeons.
12. Hawkins RJ, Bokos DJ: Clinical evaluation of shoulder problems. In Rockwood CA, Matsen FA, editors: *The shoulder,* Philadelphia, 1990, WB Saunders.
13. Hawkins RJ, Koppers G, Johnston G: Recurrent posterior instability (subluxation) of the shoulder, *J Bone Joint Surg* 66A:169, 1984.
14. Hernandez A, Drez D: Operative treatment of posterior shoulder dislocations by posterior glenoplasty, capsulorrhaphy, and infraspinatus advancement, *Am J Sports Med* 14:187, 1980.
15. Hindenach JCR: Recurrent posterior dislocation of the shoulder, *J Bone Joint Surg* 29A:582, 1947.
16. Hurley JA et al: Posterior shoulder instability, *Am J Sports Med* 20:396-400, 1992.
17. Jones V: Recurent posterior dislocation of the shoulder: report of a case treated by posterior bone block, *J Bone Joint Surg* 40B:203, 1958.
18. Leffert RD et al: Treatment of voluntary dislocation of the shoulder by therapeutic exercise based on video-electromyographic analysis, *Orthop Trans* 7:141, 1983.
19. McFarland EG et al: Electromyographic analysis of recurrent posterior instability of the shoulder. In Post M, Morrey BF, Hawkins RJ editors: *Surgery of the shoulder,* Chicago, 1990, Mosby.
20. McFarland EG, Campbell G, and McDowell J: Posterior shoulder laxity in asymptomatic adolescent athletes, American Orthopaedic Society for Sports Medicine Meeting, Palm Desert, Calif, July, 1994.
21. Mollerud A: A case of bilateral habitual luxation in the posterior part of the shoulder joint, *Acta Chir Scand* 94:181-186, 1946.
22. Norwood LA, Terry GC: Shoulder posterior subluxation, *Am J Sports Med* 12:25, 1984.
23. Pande P, Hawkins R, Peat M: Electromyography in voluntary posterior instability of the shoulder, *Am J Sports Med* 17:644, 1989.
24. Rowe CR, Pierce DS, Clark JG: Voluntary dislocation of the shoulder: a preliminary report on a clinical, electromyographic, and psychiatric study of twenty-six patients, *J Bone Joint Surg* 55A:445, 1973.
25. Samilson RL, Miller E: Posterior dislocations of the shoulder, *Clin Orthop* 32:69-86, 1964.
26. Scott DJ Jr: Treatment of recurrent posterior dislocations of the shoulder by glenoplasty, *J Bone Joint Surg* 49A:471, 1967.
27. Sjovall H: A case of spontaneous backward subluxation of the shoulder joint, operated ad modum Clairmont-Ehrlich, *Nordisk Med* 21:474-476, 1944.
28. Tibone JE: Posterior capsulorrhaphy for posterior shoulder subluxation. In Paulos LE, Tibone JE, editors: *Operative techniques in shoulder surgery,* Gaithersberg, Md, 1991, Aspen Publishing, pp 143-147.
29. Tibone JE, Ting A: Capsulorrhaphy with a staple for recurrent posterior subluxation of the shoulder, *J Bone Joint Surg* 12A:999, 1990.

CHAPTER 10

Bony Injuries of the Scapula and Clavicle

ROBERT W. CHANDLER
JOHN T. KAO

The shoulder girdle, consisting of the scapula and clavicle, is a unique structure that aids in maximizing motion at the shoulder while also offering a solid foundation for the upper extremity (Fig. 10-1). Motion at the sternoclavicular joint, acromioclavicular joint, and scapulothoracic interface combined with glenohumeral motion makes the shoulder the most mobile joint in the body. The broad scapula, resting congruently on the rib cage, is well supported with musculature that helps it to establish a stable base for the upper extremity.

Injury to the shoulder girdle usually is caused by high-energy trauma. Scapular or clavicular fracture, acromioclavicular or sternoclavicular dislocation, or scapulothoracic dissociation may result from such a trauma. Treatment of shoulder girdle injuries should be directed toward the maintenance of scapular function by providing a stable, but mobile, foundation. In addition, because the rotator cuff muscles take their origin from the scapula, treatment of these injuries must preserve rotator cuff function.

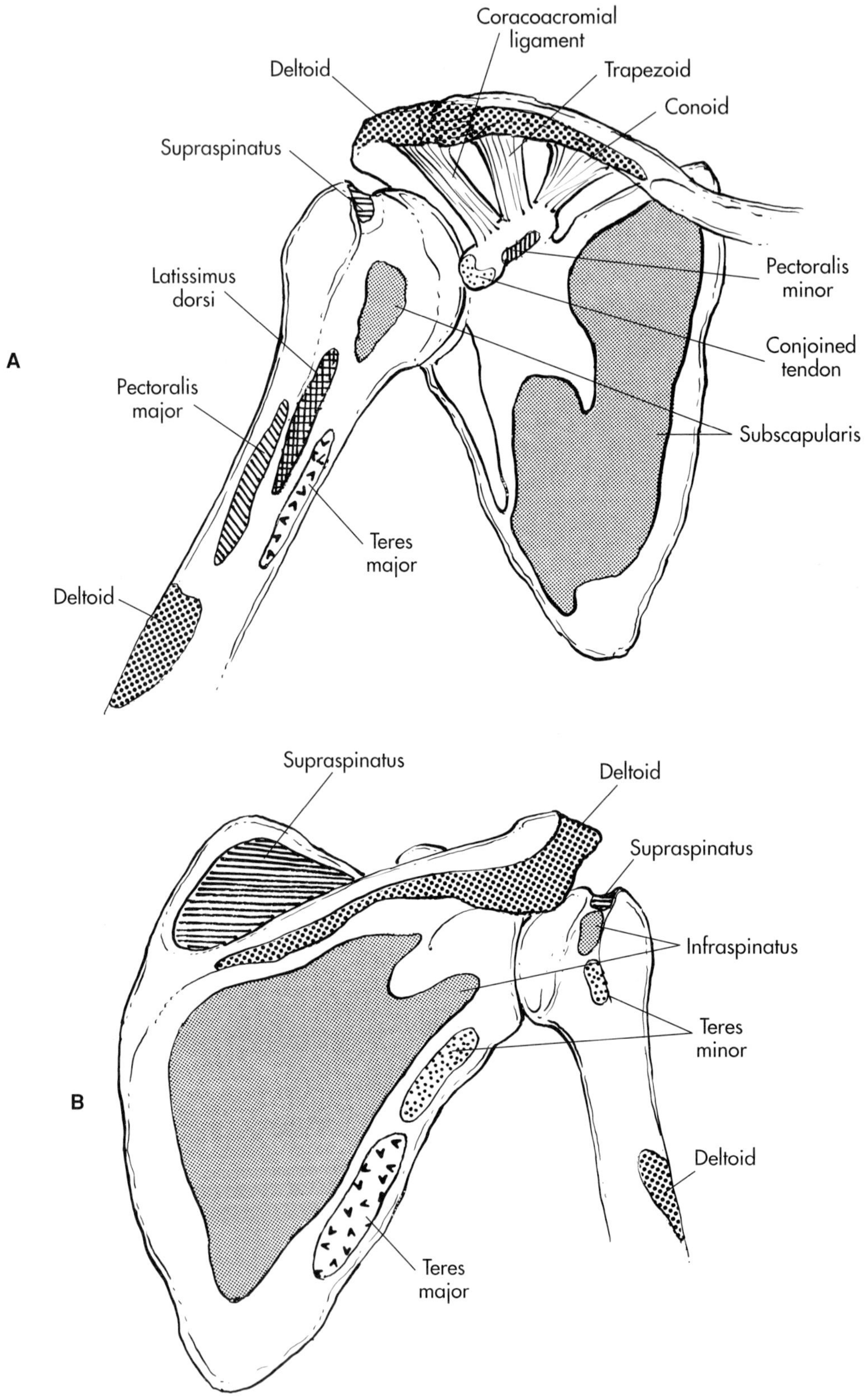

FIGURE 10-1 Shoulder girdle anatomy with ligamentous and muscular attachments. **A,** Anterior view. **B,** Posterior view.

SCAPULAR FRACTURES

Scapular fractures are rare injuries that usually are caused by motor vehicle accidents or falls. They account for 3% to 5% of shoulder girdle injuries and 0.4% to 1% of all fractures.[27,59,67] The scapula appears to resist fracture because of its mobility, the support of the rib cage, and the protection of the surrounding muscular envelope. The average age of the patient with a scapular fracture is 35 to 40 years.[4] Often, the fracture is initially missed or picked up only after routine chest x-rays are obtained. Studies have reported a 90% or greater incidence of a more serious associated injury, which may account for the missed diagnosis.*

One of the earliest descriptions of these fractures was given by Desault,[17] was translated into English by Charles Caldwell, and was published in the United States in 1805. Desault described fractures of the acromial process and the scapular body, along with reduction maneuvers and techniques of immobilization. The Desault device held the arm against the chest and applied an upwardly directed compression force to hold the humeral head against the acromion to resist gravity. Later, Gross[25] and Findlay[20] described successful nonoperative treatment of some of these fractures near the turn of the last century.

Subsequent studies have further documented successful conservative treatment of scapular fractures, but recently surgical reconstruction has been recommended for some fractures to ensure the best possible functional result.†

Mechanism

Scapular body fractures often are caused by direct trauma, such as falls and gunshot wounds, and indirect trauma, such as falls on an outstretched arm and shoulder dislocations. Displacement usually is minimal because of the stabilization provided by investing musculature.

Because of the intimate relationship of the scapula with the rib cage, scapular fractures often are associated with rib fractures, with an incidence reported to be as high as 54%.[72] Cardiopulmonary injury, neurovascular injury, or other fractures also have been reported in the literature.[4,26,32,44] A mortality rate of 14% has been reported in cases involving scapular fractures resulting from blunt trauma.[72]

Muscular and ligamentous attachments of the coracoid process consist of the pectoralis minor, the coracobrachialis, the short head of the biceps brachii, and the coracoclavicular and coracoacromial ligaments. Similarly, the soft-tissue attachments of the acromial process are three heads of the deltoid muscle, the coracoacromial ligament, and the acromioclavicular ligaments. As described by Desault and others, apophyseal fractures of the scapula, acromion, and coracoid process are caused by direct impact or by avulsion through ligamentous or muscular traction.[17,29,37,51,69]

Fractures involving the glenoid articular surface usually are caused by violent force imparted to the articular surface directly through the humeral head or from a shoulder dislocation. Falls on or blows to the lateral aspect of the shoulder, a blow to the anterior or posterior shoulder causing dislocation, and an abduction–external rotation shoulder injury causing dislocation all may produce glenoid fracture.

This force can result in medialization and angulation of the glenohumeral joint, stepoff of the articular surface, or avulsion of the glenoid rim. Displacement may be limited by supporting structures, but joint instability or significant articular stepoff may occur.

Physical Examination

Scapular fractures often are missed at initial presentation because the close proximity of the rib cage minimizes any gross deformity. A careful physical examination, however, will reveal swelling, local tenderness, contusion, and pain with crepitus during shoulder range of motion. The patient usually holds the arm adducted and resists active motion, especially abduction. The shoulder may appear flattened, and pain with deep inspiration may be noted.

Nevaiser has described a "pseudorupture of the rotator cuff muscles" secondary to a scapular fracture.[56] Muscle dysfunction comes from spasm and hemorrhage underneath and within the muscle and resolves after several weeks. If symptoms persist, further investigation is warranted to identify a rotator cuff tear.

Associated injuries such as rib fractures (27% to 54%), concussions (20% to 24%), clavicular fractures (23% to 39%), pulmonary contusion (11% to 54%), pneumothorax (11% to 38%), brachial plexus injury (5% to 13%), and a myriad of other soft-tissue and bony injuries often dominate the clinical picture and outrank the scapular injury on the priority list.* Recognition and treatment of these associated injuries are critical.

Radiographs

Scapular views include the following:

1. An anteroposterior view with the arm in neutral to visualize the scapular neck and body.
2. An anteroposterior view with the arm in 90° of abduction to visualize the lateral border of the scapula.[52]
3. A true scapular anteroposterior view (Grashey projection[24]) with the cone directed medial to lateral 40° to visualize intraarticular extensions of the fracture.

*References 4, 26, 32, 44, 72, 74.
†References 1, 13, 21, 26, 27, 74.

*References 4, 22, 32, 43, 44, 71, 76.

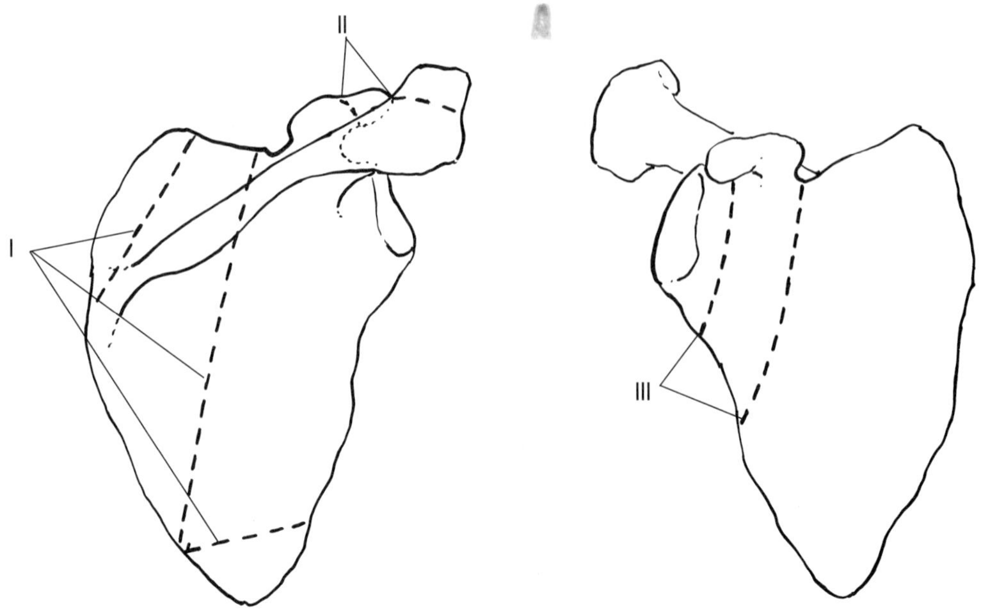

FIGURE 10-2 DeCoulx classification for scapular fractures. *I,* Body fractures; *II,* apophyseal fractures; *III,* superolateral angle fractures.

4. A scapular lateral view to identify body fractures with displacement, coracoid fractures, or acromial fractures.

Additional views may be necessary to identify relevant fracture elements:

1. An axillary view to better visualize intraarticular stepoff, coracoid fractures, or acromial fractures.
2. A West Point view to help identify a bony Bankart lesion in those patients with anteroinferior shoulder instability.[24]

The West Point view is obtained with the patient prone and the arm hanging off the table. The cone is directed at a 25° angle into the axilla and a 25° angle in a posterior-to-anterior direction.

If surgical reconstruction is being contemplated and the fracture pattern appears complex, tomograms or a CT scan is of value in planning surgery. Tomograms may be difficult to interpret because of the angle and anatomy of the scapula. Computerized axial tomograms are relatively simple and have the added advantage of allowing for reconstructed images that may be used for generation of three-dimensional views of the fracture.

Classification

Anatomic classification systems described by DeCoulx, Hardegger, Ada, and Ideberg are in current use.[1,15,27,31,75] DeCoulx has classified scapular fractures into: (1) fractures of the body, (2) fractures of the apophysis, and (3) fractures through the superolateral angle (Fig. 10-2). This classification scheme offers relative simplicity, but the type III group is too broad, encompassing a large variety of fracture patterns that cannot all be treated in a similar fashion.

Hardegger et al further break down scapular fractures into eight types denoted by letters. These are (A) body, (B) glenoid rim, (C) glenoid fossa, (D) anatomic neck, (E) surgical neck, (F) acromion, (G) spine, and (H) coracoid process fractures (Fig. 10-3). This system is more detailed and gives an excellent morphologic description as well as adequate grouping of patterns to help assign treatment.

Similar to Hardegger, Ada and Miller have described (IA) acromion, (IB) base of the acromion and spine, (IC) coracoid, (IIA) neck lateral to the acromial base, (IIB) neck extending into the acromial base, (IIC) transverse neck, (III) intraarticular glenoid, and (IV) body fractures (Fig. 10-4).

Ideberg further classified intraarticular glenoid fractures into five types. Type I fractures are anterior-margin avulsions usually caused by shoulder dislocations (Fig. 10-5). Type II fractures are transverse fractures through the fossa with a displaced inferior triangular component (Fig. 10-6). Type III fractures are oblique fractures exiting in the mid-superior region and usually associated with acromioclavicular injury (Fig. 10-7). Type IV fractures are horizontal fractures through the entire scapular body, and type V fractures are a combination of a type II and type IV fracture (Figs. 10-8 and 10-9).

Treatment Options

Most scapular fractures are properly treated without surgery. Wilber and Evans reported on 40 scapular frac-

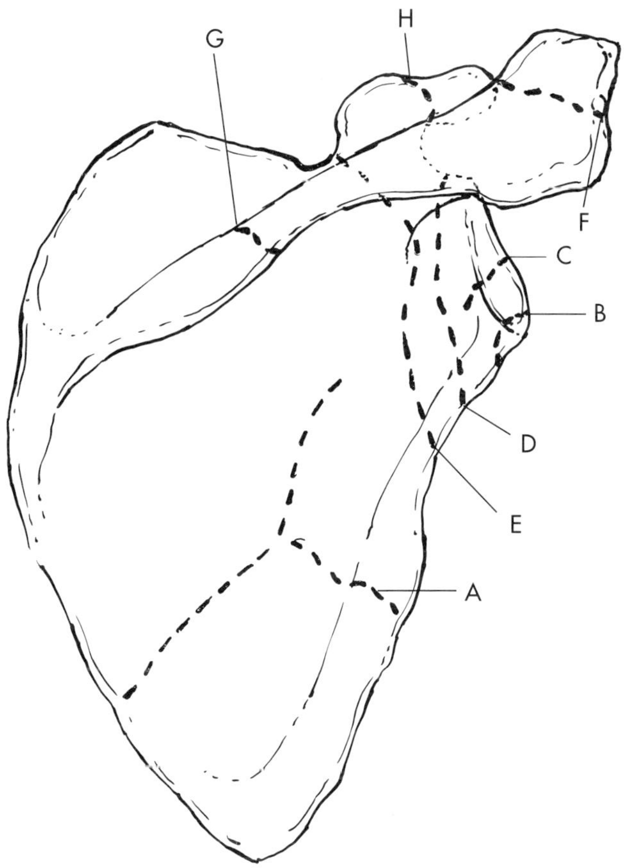

FIGURE 10-3 Hardegger classification for scapular fractures. *A,* Body; *B,* glenoid rim; *C,* glenoid fossa; *D,* anatomic neck; *E,* surgical neck; *F,* acromion; *G,* spine; *H,* coracoid process.

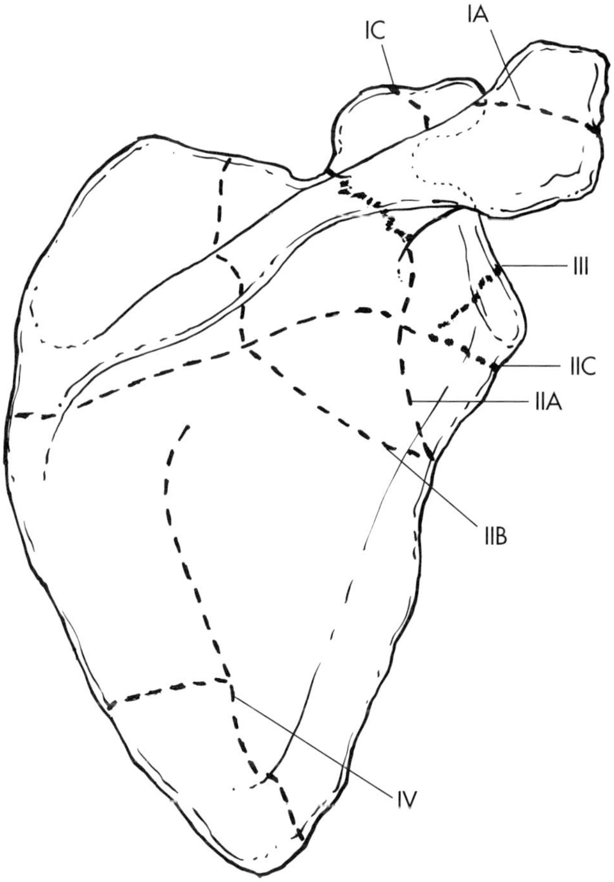

FIGURE 10-4 Ada and Miller classification for scapular fractures. *IA,* Acromion; *IB,* acromion and spine base; *IC,* coracoid; *IIA,* neck lateral to acromial base; *IIB,* neck extending into acromial base; *IIC,* transverse neck; *III,* intraarticular glenoid; *IV,* body fracture.

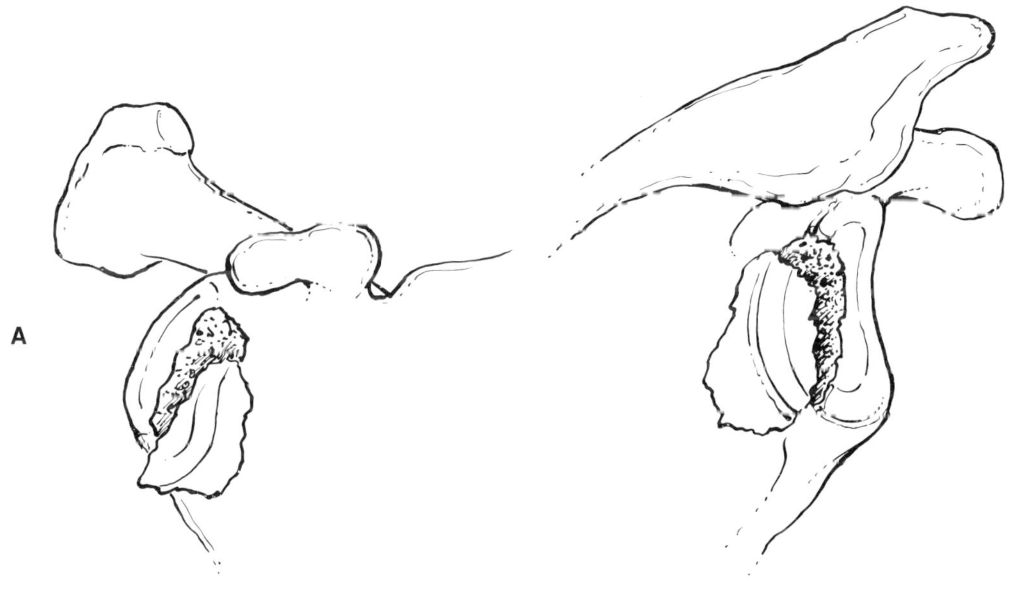

FIGURE 10-5 Ideberg classification type I. **A,** Anterior margin avulsion. **B,** Posterior margin avulsion.

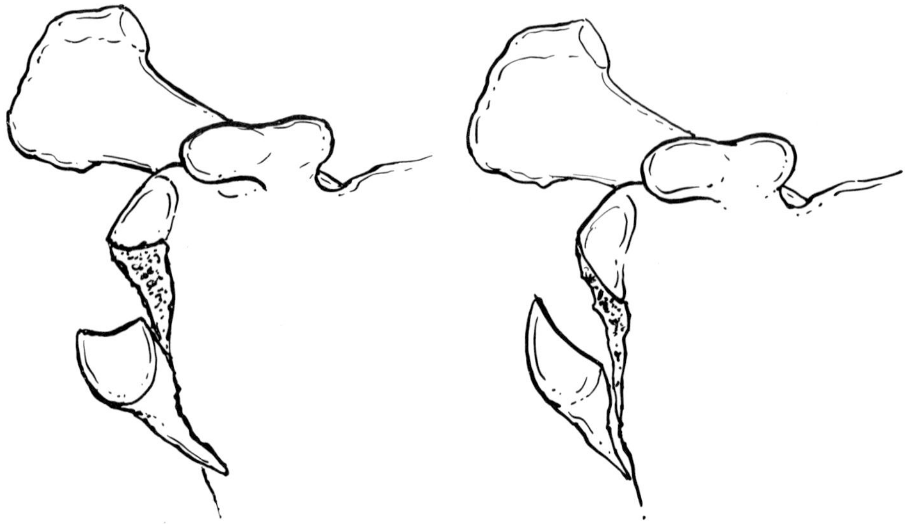

FIGURE 10-6 Ideberg classification type II. **A,** Transverse fracture through the glenoid fossa. **B,** Oblique fracture through the glenoid fossa.

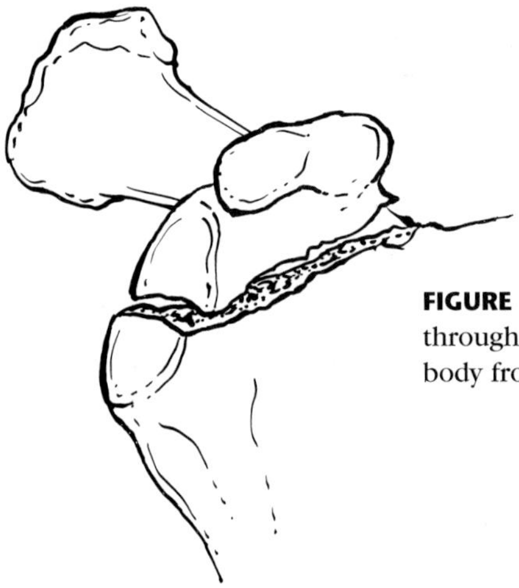

FIGURE 10-7 Ideberg classification type III. Oblique fracture through the superior region with separation of the scapular body from the apophyses and superior glenoid.

tures treated conservatively with mostly good results.[73] In their study, fractures involving a glenoid fossa split-socket, a glenoid fracture dislocation, or a coracoid fracture associated with acromioclavicular separation required surgical reconstruction.

Hardegger[27] reported on 37 fractures treated with open reconstruction, with 79% good or excellent results. Indications for surgery were glenoid fracture-dislocations, unstable fractures of the scapular neck, and significantly displaced apophyseal fractures.

Ada and Miller[1] reported good preliminary results with the open treatment of displaced shoulder neck fractures angulated more than 40° or displaced medially more than 1 cm. Fig. 10-10 illustrates internal fixation of a complex displaced glenoid neck fracture with an associated dislocation of the glenohumeral joint.

Treatment of intraarticular glenoid fractures should be directed toward maintenance of a congruent articular surface.[6,64] Ideberg type I fractures have satisfactory outcome when treated nonoperatively if minimal displacement is present. Open reduction and internal fixation is advised if more than one quarter of the surface area is involved and instability is present.[5,36,63]

Type II to V fractures have a poor prognosis if treated without anatomic realignment and rapid rehabilitation. Early mobilization may improve functional results while anatomic reconstruction of the joint delays arthritis. Figs. 10-12 through 10-18 suggest internal fixation strategies for each of the Ideberg fracture types. Figs. 10-11 through 10-17 give strategies for internal fixation of the Ideberg group of injuries, with one illustrative case.

Minimally displaced acromial fractures are treated with a sling for 3 weeks or more, depending on the pain at the fracture site. Occasionally, a displaced fracture may require open reduction and internal fixation to relieve neurovascular compromise, prevent impingement, or repair a nonunion.[45,47]

Fixation, which must adequately control the large tension forces present, usually can be achieved with the use of plate osteosynthesis along the scapular spine or the

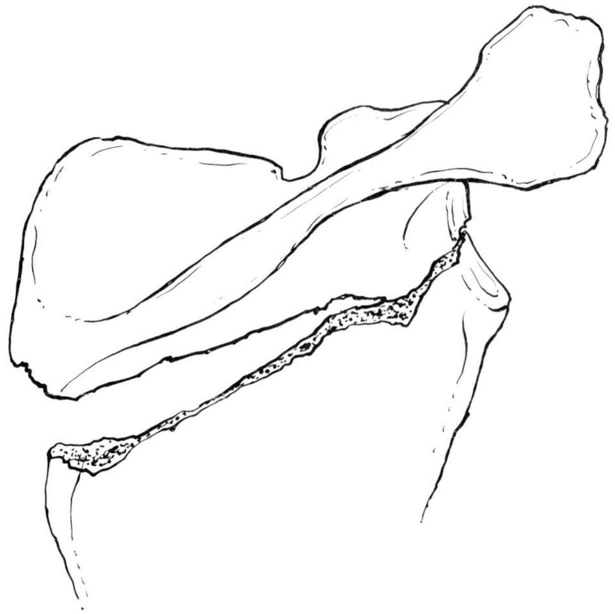

FIGURE 10-8 Ideberg classification type IV. Horizontal fractures through body.

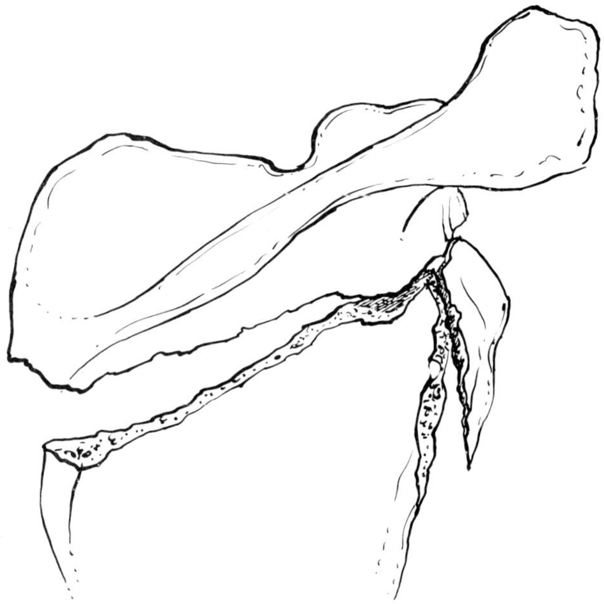

FIGURE 10-9 Ideberg classification type V. Combination of type II and IV fractures.

use of a tension band system. If the fracture represents a very small portion of the acromion, excision and reattachment of the deltoid to the remaining acromion is indicated. Care must be taken not to excise a significant portion of the acromion because instability and shoulder weakness may result from deltoid dysfunction. Poor, slow, or painful recovery may indicate a rotator cuff tear requiring decompression or suture.

Coracoid fractures do not require surgery often. Asymptomatic fibrous nonunion may result after coracoid fracture and may be left alone. The exception is a widely displaced coracoid fracture associated with acromioclavicular injury. Several reports document the need for acromioclavicular stabilization and immobilization to ensure a good functional result.[10,23,38,50,75]

Coracoid-process stress fracture secondary to repetitive microtrauma has been described in athletes. Benton and Nelson[8] have presented an 18-year-old male tennis player who experienced pain with his overhead serve. After failure of conservative treatment, the patient underwent excision of the coracoid fragment with reattachment of the conjoined tendon. Boyer[12] has described a competitive trapshooter who responded to rest and later returned to his sport.

Conservative Treatment

Nonoperative treatment options include a sling, a sling and swathe, and a spica cast. Local treatment with ice and compression along with relative immobilization is the goal. Most scapular body fractures and minimally displaced apophyseal or glenoid fractures do well treated with a sling or sling and swathe. Wilber and Evans,[74] however, reported poor results with significant loss of glenohumeral motion in fractures involving the acromion, coracoid, and glenoid neck. They recommended spica casting with the shoulder in 60° of abduction for 6 weeks allowing for active abduction at 3 weeks. Regardless of the form of immobilization that is chosen, immobilization is maintained for only 3 to 6 weeks. Isometric exercises are begun as early as can be tolerated by the patient.

Operative Treatment

Indications for surgery are the following:

1. Glenoid fracture associated with shoulder instability (Ideberg I, Hardegger B)
2. Glenoid fossa fractures displaced more than 2 mm (Ideberg types II to V, Hardegger C, Ada and Miller III)
3. Unstable fractures of the scapular neck (DeCoulx III, Hardegger types D to E, Ada and Miller types IIA and IIB)
4. Widely displaced apophyseal fractures associated with acromioclavicular separation (DeCoulx II, Hardegger H, Ada and Miller IC)

Surgical reconstruction may include plate osteosynthesis, interfragmentary screw fixation, or a combination of these techniques. Most often, a pelvic reconstruction plate is used for scapular body and neck fractures to allow for easier plate contouring to the scapular surface.

The scapula may be approached anteriorly through a deltopectoral approach to fix anterior glenoid avulsion fractures, coracoid fractures, and some glenoid fossa fractures. More often, the scapula must be approached from the posterior aspect to allow for extensile exposure of the scapular body and glenoid neck. Lastly, acromial frac-

Text continues on p. 302

A B C D

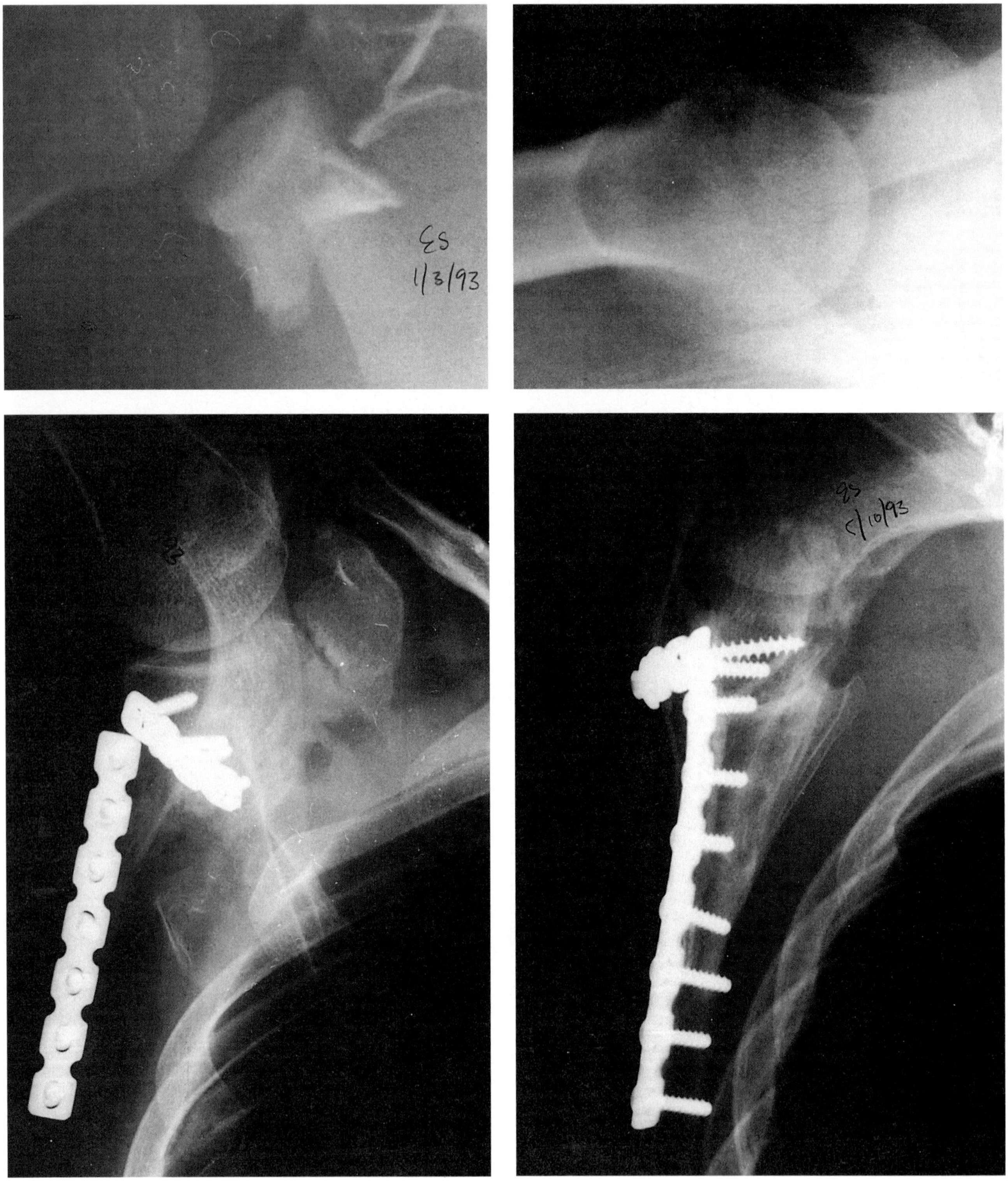

FIGURE 10-10 **A,** AP view of a displaced glenoid fracture in a 21-year-old male downhill skier who hit a tree and suffered an unstable fracture of the glenoid neck with dislocation of the glenohumeral joint. **B,** Axillary view showing no glenoid joint surface in approximation with the humeral head. **C** and **D,** Postoperative views showing reconstruction of the joint and stabilization of the scapular fracture fragments with 3.5-mm reconstruction plates.

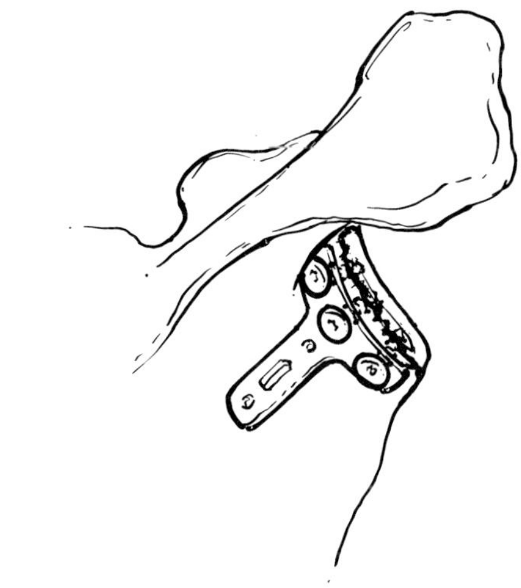

FIGURE 10-11 Open reduction and internal fixation of an Ideberg I fracture. Reconstruction of a large anterior joint fragment with a 3.5-mm "T" plate and lag screws. Lag screws alone are sufficient for most anterior fracture dislocations.

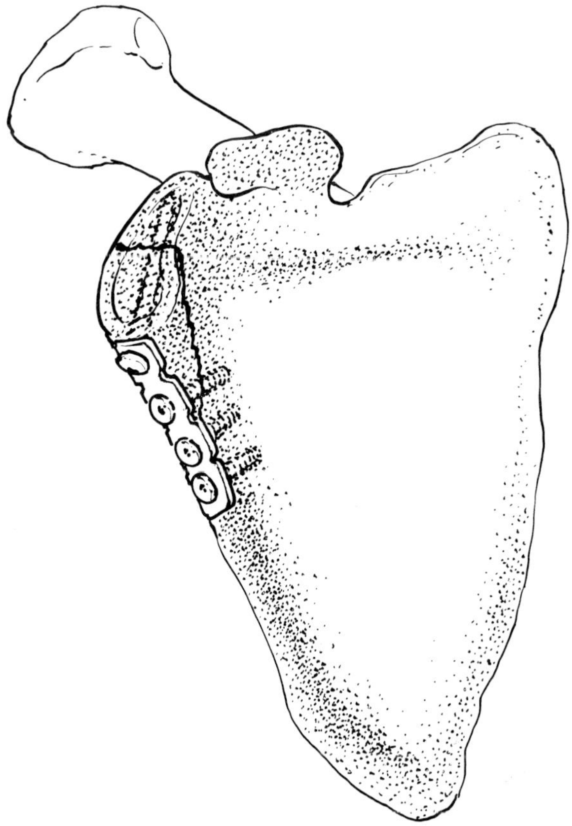

FIGURE 10-12 Open reduction and internal fixation of an Ideberg II fracture. Fixation with a four-hole 3.5-mm reconstruction plate and two 3.5-mm cortical lag screws through the plate.

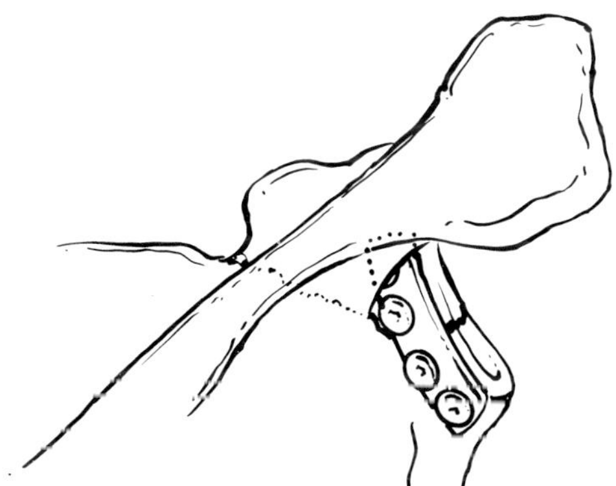

FIGURE 10-13 Open reduction and internal fixation of an Ideberg IIIa fracture. Fixation through a posterior approach using a 3.5-mm reconstruction plate.

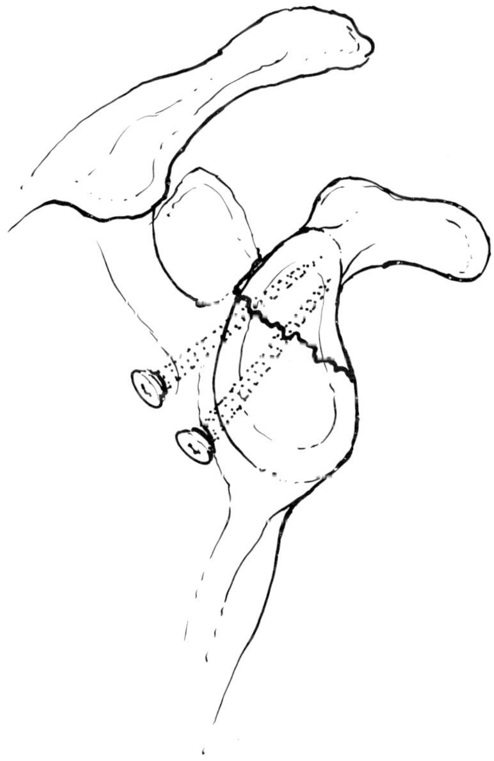

FIGURE 10-14 Open reduction and internal fixation of an Ideberg IIIb fracture. Fixation with two cortical lag screws.

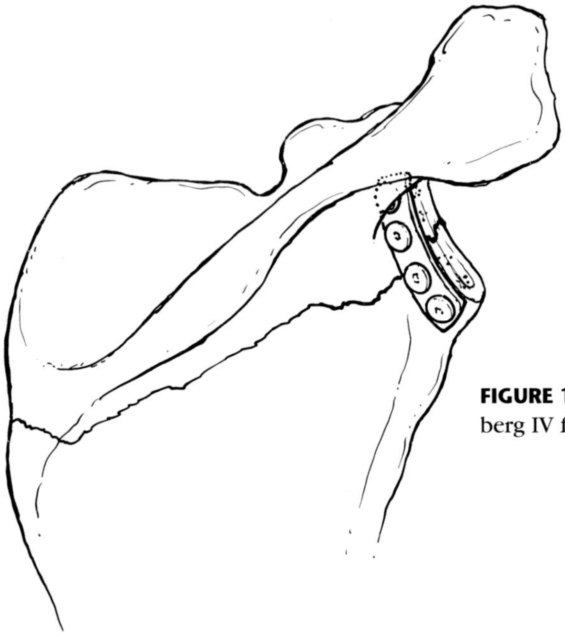

FIGURE 10-15 Open reduction and internal fixation of an Ideberg IV fracture. Fixation with a 3.5-mm reconstruction plate.

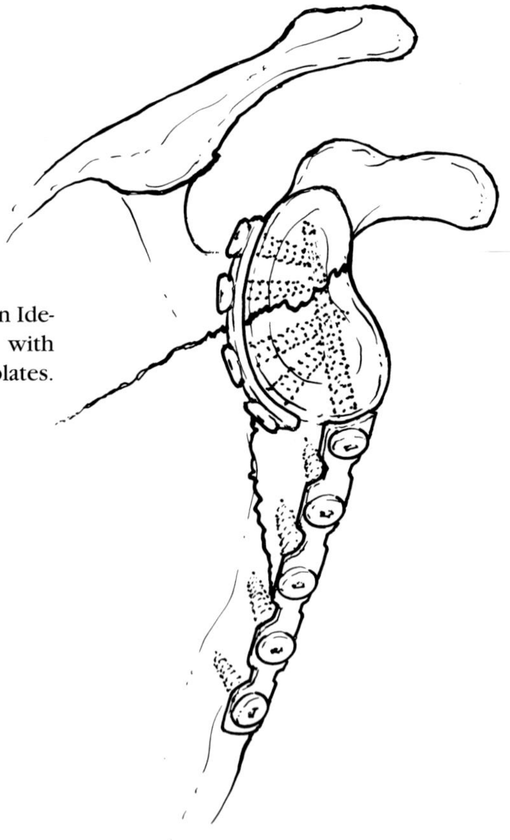

FIGURE 10-16 Open reduction and internal fixation of an Ideberg V fracture. Multiple unstable segments are linked with 3.5-mm reconstruction plates and lag screws through the plates.

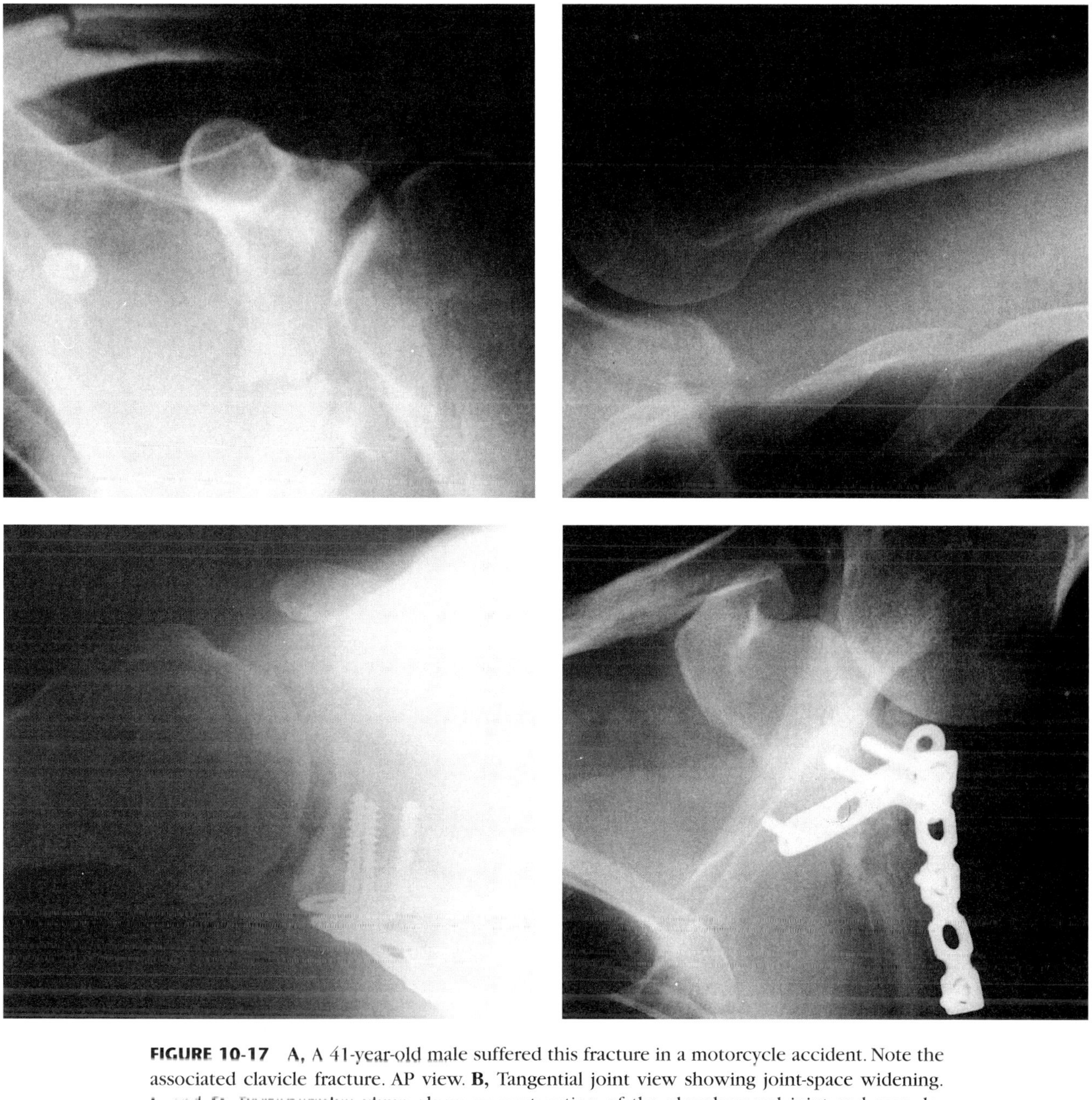

FIGURE 10-17 **A,** A 41-year-old male suffered this fracture in a motorcycle accident. Note the associated clavicle fracture. AP view. **B,** Tangential joint view showing joint-space widening. **C** and **D,** Postoperative views show reconstruction of the glenohumeral joint and scapular body components.

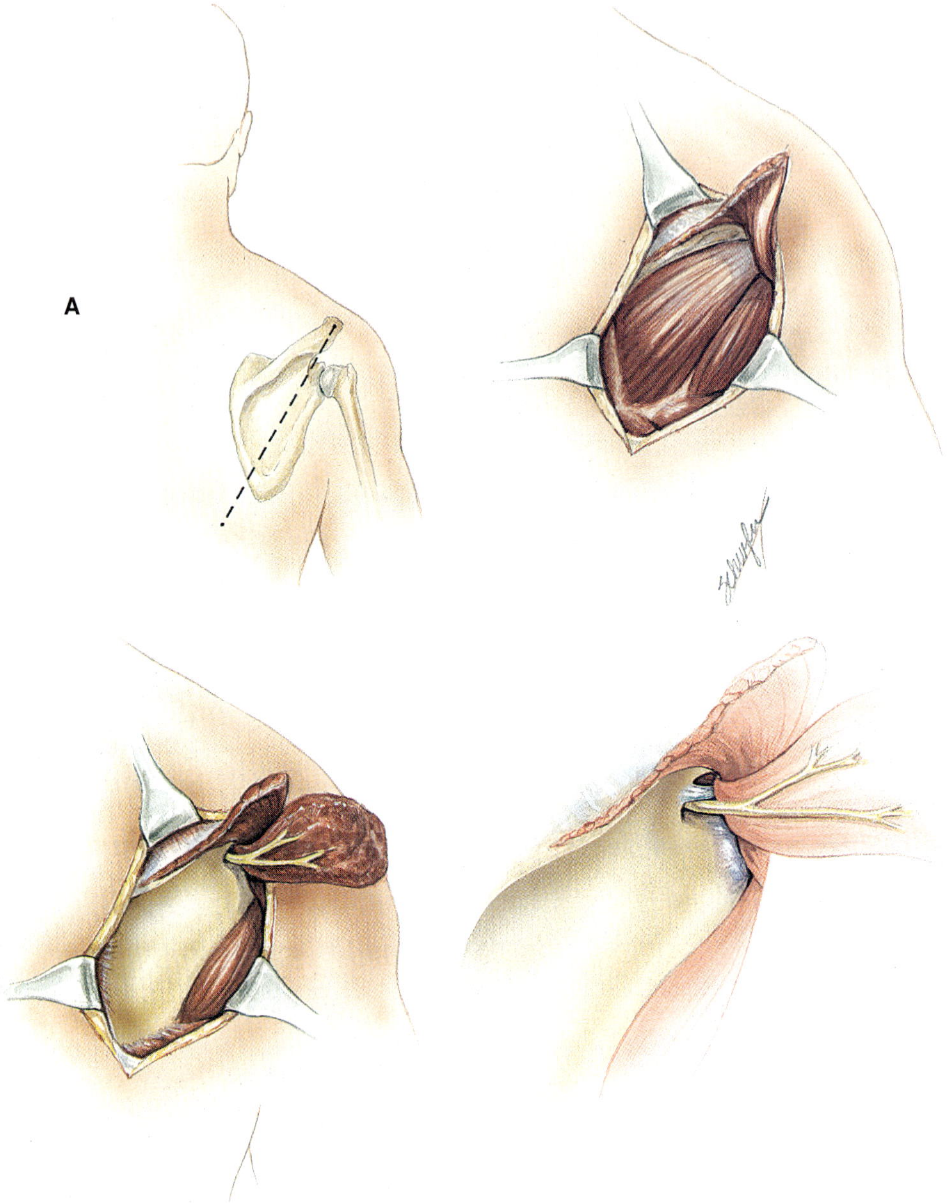

FIGURE 10-18 **A,** Posterior aspect of the shoulder illustrates the line of the skin incision. **B,** The deltoid has been partially reflected, exposing the infraspinatus and teres minor. **C,** The infraspinatus has been reflected with its neurovascular pedicle intact, exposing the infraspinous portion of the scapular body and posterior glenoid. **D,** Close-up view of the suprascapular notch showing exit of the suprascapular nerve from the notch into the infraspinatus muscle. The teres minor is innervated by a branch of the axillary nerve.

tures can be approached through a saber-type approach centered directly over the acromion.

Deltopectoral Approach

The deltopectoral approach allows excellent visualization of the shoulder's anterior portion. It is used for anterior shoulder reconstruction, coracoid-process fracture repair, relocation of anterior shoulder dislocations, and anterior glenoid-rim avulsion fracture repair.

The approach uses a saber-type incision parallel with Langer's lines. The interval between the deltoid innervated by the axillary nerve and the pectoralis major innervated by the medial and lateral pectoral nerves is identified by locating the cephalic vein, which lies within this interval. The vein is retracted laterally with the deltoid, and the pectoralis major is retracted medially to expose the underlying clavipectoral fascia. The fascia is then incised along the lateral border of the underlying conjoined tendon. The conjoined tendon is retracted medially to expose the subscapularis.

Care must be taken not to excessively retract the tendon to avoid injuring the musculocutaneous nerve. The subscapularis is then split horizontally through electrocautery along its fibers at the junction of the upper two thirds and lower third of the muscle. This plane lies between the innervation of the upper and lower subscapular nerves. The flaps are developed to allow visualization of the underlying anterior capsule. The capsule is then incised horizontally to allow exposure of the glenoid articular surface. Further exposure may be obtained by making a T-type capsulotomy medially or stripping the capsule off the anterior glenoid neck. After open reduction and internal fixation, care must be taken to securely reattach the anterior capsule down to bone, to minimize the possibility of anterior instability after the procedure.

Posterior Approach

Major articular disruptions (Ideberg types II to V) and scapular neck fractures should be repaired through a posterior approach. The posterior approach requires that the patient be positioned prone with the affected arm draped free.[49] The skin incision may be either a saber-type incision within Langer's lines or an incision along the lower border of the scapular spine (see Fig. 10-18). The deltoid is then subperiosteally dissected away from the spine, and the infraspinatus is dissected off the lower border of the spine. Care must be taken not to inadvertently wander lateral to the base of the spine to avoid injury to the suprascapular nerve. The medial border of the infraspinatus is then incised and dissected subperiosteally from medial to lateral until the lateral border of the scapular body is visualized.

This approach allows for excellent visualization of the entire posterior scapular body and scapular neck by rotating the infraspinatus on a superior and laterally based neurovascular pedicle. Fixation usually is best obtained along the undersurface of the spine, the glenoid neck, and the lateral border of the scapular body. A small posterior capsulotomy also may be made, if necessary, to visualize intraarticular pathology. Closure requires repair of the infraspinatus and deltoid back down to bone with sutures placed through the scapula spine. A drain often is necessary, given the extensive exposure of bone.

Complications

The most commonly seen complications after scapular fracture include loss of motion, shoulder pain, subscapular crepitus, malunion, and, rarely, nonunion.

Loss of Motion

Loss of shoulder motion is probably the most common complication after scapular fracture. McGinnis and Denton[46] reported on 40 scapular fractures treated nonoperatively and noted loss of motion in five patients out of 26 patients (19%) with adequate follow-up. Of these five, three had less than 90 degrees of abduction. Their fracture patterns included an isolated coracoid-process fracture combined with numerous associated injuries and a delay in range-of-motion therapy, an intraarticular glenoid and spine fracture, and a severely comminuted body fracture. This suggests the importance of early range-of-motion exercises but demonstrates that no single pattern was responsible for loss of motion.

Ada and Miller[1] reported on 116 scapular fractures treated conservatively, with the majority being scapular body fractures. Their study included follow-up on 24 patients with displaced scapular neck, comminuted spine, and intraarticular fractures. They noted that 3 of the 16 patients (19%) with scapular neck fractures, 5 of 11 scapular spine fracture patients (45%), and all 6 intraarticular fractures had loss of shoulder motion. Hardegger[27] reported on 37 patients with scapular fractures treated operatively and noted that 12 of 33 patients (36%) with adequate follow-up had some loss of motion. The fracture types of these patients included apophyseal fractures, glenoid intraarticular and rim fractures, and scapular neck fractures. Loss of motion appears to be a common complication after scapular fracture, with loss of abduction being the most common complaint. More often than not, the loss is minimal (less than 30°), however, and the patient remains functional.

Shoulder Pain

Ada and Miller[1] reported that 21 of 24 patients (88%) with scapular spine or neck fractures experienced some degree of pain. This pain was thought to be caused by rotator cuff dysfunction either from a loss of the normal biomechanical advantage of the cuff caused by medialization or rotation of the glenoid articular surface, or from direct soft-tissue trauma itself. Intraarticular fractures also were painful because of articular-surface injury or a displaced articular surface.

Hardegger[27] reported that 8 of 33 patients (24%) undergoing surgical intervention had resultant pain that usually was associated with activity. This study demonstrates that even patients undergoing open reduction and internal fixation with good anatomic reconstruction still may have postoperative pain.

Malunion

Significant malunion of scapular fractures often is without consequence. However, Nordqvist and Petersson[61] reported 8 of 20 patients (40%) with scapular body and neck malunions with resultant pain. Ada and Miller[1] reported that 2 of 52 patients (4%) with scapular body fractures experienced grating with scapulothoracic motion without significant pain. Numerous complaints of pain were noted, however, in patients with displaced scapular-neck fractures. Malunion at the glenoid articular surface often resulted in glenohumeral osteoarthritis and pain.

Nonunion

Nonunion is a rare complication of scapular fractures. Presumably, the large muscle envelope encircling the scapula provides an excellent blood supply. Ada and Miller[1] reported only 1 of 116 fractures (0.9%) going on to nonunion. This patient was treated successfully with surgical repair. Only a few isolated cases of scapular nonunion are found in the literature.[13,27] These patients reportedly do well and go on to union with surgical reconstruction and bone grafting.

CLAVICULAR FRACTURES

Clavicular fractures, unlike scapular fractures, are very common fractures and compose 1 in 20 of all fractures occurring anywhere in the body and two thirds of all fractures involving the shoulder.[14,16] Fractures of the clavicle can be divided into three groups: (1) fractures of the medial third of the clavicle, (2) fractures of the middle third of the clavicle, and (3) fractures of the lateral third of the clavicle. Fractures of the medial third of the clavicle are rare injuries, while fractures of the lateral third account for only approximately 15% of all clavicular fractures. The large majority of clavicular fractures are within the middle third, or diaphyseal portion, of the clavicle.

The S-shaped clavicle functions to improve upper-extremity power, stability, and range of motion. It also affords a stable base for attachment of the trapezius, deltoid, sternocleidomastoid, pectoralis major, and subclavius. Lastly, it also offers some bony protection to the vital neurovascular structures of the upper extremity.

Clavicular fractures also are the most common fractures in childhood.[14] The fracture may present as a limp arm at childbirth or a painful deformity as a teenager. Conservative care usually is the treatment of choice and should be aimed at reducing discomfort while using local modalities and reducing the deformity with a cast or brace. One must remember that acromioclavicular or sternoclavicular separations are rare in children and that physeal injuries are generally the rule. With the healing and remodeling potential of children, clavicular fractures universally do well, and surgery is indicated for only open fractures and rare situations with neurovascular compromise.

Mechanism

The mechanism of injury is either an indirect or a direct load on the clavicle.[71] The indirect load is the most common mechanism, and this results from a fall on an outstretched arm. This mechanism accounts for approximately 80% of all clavicle fractures, and almost all of these fractures occur within the middle third of the clavicle. The direct-load mechanism involves a blow to the clavicle itself, usually from a fall. Fractures caused by this mechanism account for the remaining 20% of clavicular fractures and the majority of clavicular fractures of the medial and lateral third.

Because of the anatomy surrounding the clavicle and its subcutaneous location, several injuries have been associated with these fractures. These injuries include open fracture, pneumothorax, axillary artery injury, brachial plexus injury, and soft-tissue interposition preventing adequate reduction.* These injuries are directly related to the energy of injury, which determines the degrees of displacement, comminution, and injury to surrounding vital structures.

Physical Examination

Clavicular fractures usually are much easier to diagnose than scapular fractures. The fracture usually is apparent with deformity, swelling, ecchymosis, and local tenderness. Because of the upward pull of the sternocleidomastoid muscle and the trapezius, the medial fragment usually displaces cephalad while the weight of the upper extremity displaces the lateral fragment caudad. The patient usually holds the arm against his or her body for support and to prevent excess motion. Shoulder motion often is limited by pain, and a painful shoulder-adduction maneuver may be an indication of intraarticular involvement of the acromioclavicular joint.

All open wounds near the fracture must be assumed to be caused by an open fracture because of the subcutaneous location of the clavicle. These injuries require urgent irrigation and débridement, followed by internal fixation if appropriate. A careful examination of the chest and affected upper extremity is necessary to rule out associated injury. Neurovascular injury as well as pneumothorax may occur, although these complications are rare. Soft-tissue interposition may maintain wide displacement, necessitating operation. These problems warrant more aggressive fracture management with strong consideration of immediate open exploration with reduction and internal fixation.

Radiography

Fracture location and cephalad or caudal displacement can be determined with an anteroposterior view of the clavicle. A better anteroposterior view of lateral-third fractures may be obtained with a Zanca view with the cone angled 15° cephalad.[24]

Anterior or posterior displacement in middle-third and medial-third fractures can be determined based on a serendipity view with the cone angled 45° cephalad and the cassette approximately 60 inches above the clavicle.[24] Anterior or posterior displacement of lateral-third clavicular fractures can be determined with an axillary view of the shoulder. Intraarticular involvement of either

*References 33, 42, 48, 57, 68, 73.

the acromioclavicular or sternoclavicular joints may be further evaluated with a CT scan.

Classification

Clavicular fractures are classified by region. Type I fractures involve the medial third of the clavicle, type II fractures involve the middle third, and type III fractures involve the lateral third of the clavicle.[14] Type III, or lateral-third, fractures are subdivided into four subtypes.[2,28,53] Subtype I is a minimally displaced fracture with intact coracoclavicular ligaments. Subtype IIa is a displaced fracture with intact ligaments. Subtype IIb is a displaced fracture with a torn conoid ligament and an intact trapezoid ligament attached to the distal fragment. Subtype III is an intraarticular fracture.

Treatment

Great debate about the ideal method of treating clavicular fractures characterizes work published on the subject. By 1929, more than 200 methods of treatment had been described.[39]

Most methods fall within two general groups. One group emphasizes closed reduction with casting or bandaging to maintain the fracture reduction. The other group emphasizes local care for control of pain followed by early range of motion while accepting the deformity resulting from fracture displacement.

Some displaced fractures are reducible with a hematoma block and manipulation. Unfortunately, this position is difficult to maintain, and the reduction inevitably is lost. Plaster casts such as the Billington Yoke[9] or a variety of shoulder spica casts or bandaging techniques have been described, but none are successful at maintaining the reduction.[3,35,52,63,66] Therefore it is imperative to emphasize to the patient, regardless of the treatment technique used, that deformity is expected but that a full return of shoulder function also is expected.

Fractures of the medial third of the clavicle usually are only minimally displaced. These minimally displaced fractures do well with local ice and support of the arm in a sling.[70] Early range of motion usually is well tolerated, and union is almost universally noted at 6 to 8 weeks. Open treatment is required only in patients with neurovascular injury, skin compromise, or open fractures. Open treatment should be directed at costoclavicular stabilization. Usually no hardware is required, and suture fixation is adequate.

Fractures of the middle third of the clavicle are almost universally treated without surgery. A figure-of-eight harness and/or a shoulder sling will restore some length to the shortened clavicle. Local treatment with ice also is beneficial. A great deal of explanation often is required to allay the apprehensions of patients after they have seen their radiographs or noted displaced bone ends. Rarely, a small spike of bone must be excised if compounding is threatened. Patients are informed that malunion is the standard outcome after such fractures, and nonunion, although rare, may occur and require surgical repair.

Indications for open treatment include soft-tissue interposition, neurovascular injury, open fracture, and possibly cosmesis in certain isolated situations.[77,78] Forequarter instability with associated scapular and clavicular fractures also is a good indication for clavicular osteosynthesis. In these cases, the clavicle, rendered stable with plate osteosynthesis, may help to support an unstable extremity.

Nevaiser[58] has described fixation with a Knowles pin. In this procedure, a 5 cm incision is made along the upper border of the clavicle. The fracture is reduced with minimal soft-tissue stripping. A Knowles pin then is introduced through the posterolateral corner of the lateral clavicle approximately 4 cm from the acromioclavicular joint. The pin is directed down the canal, into the medial fragment, and out the anteromedial surface. This technique allows for maintenance of fracture fixation and compression at the fracture site. Other intramedullary techniques have been applied successfully.[14]

Fatalities have been described after a smooth, straight pin has migrated into the mediastinum and thorax.[40,60]

Given the broad range of clavicle fracture configurations and the complex shape of the clavicle, plate-and-screw osteosynthesis often will control instability better than intramedullary devices. Fracture reduction and fixation is technically easier through an incision parallel to the long axis of the clavicle, but a saber incision also may be used. Small fragment (3.5-mm) LC-DC plates fit the clavicle well anteriorly, and in some regions may be contoured to fit on the cranial surface. Transverse and oblique fractures are ideal for axial and interfragmentary compression techniques. Comminuted fractures require bridge plating, possibly supplemented with autogenous bone graft.

Complications

Long-term complications of clavicular fractures include malunion, late neurovascular compromise, posttraumatic arthritis, and nonunion. Treatment of these complications depends on the severity of the symptoms.

Malunion

Malunion is the expected outcome after treatment of clavicular fractures. The malunion usually has no undesirable effect on shoulder function, and cosmesis may be the only resulting problem. If deformity is a major problem, the patient must be willing to accept a possibly unsightly scar and the risks of surgery for removal of the bump. If surgery is elected, usually only excision of the prominent bone is necessary to remedy the situation. Rarely will open reduction be necessary to correct the problem.

Late Neurovascular Compromise

Late neurovascular compromise has been reported in the literature.[7,78] The callus from the healed fracture, a malunion, or a nonunion may cause compression on the brachial plexus, the subclavian artery, or the subclavian vein. Patients may present with neuritic or neuropathic problems in the affected extremity. Diagnosis can be confirmed with angiography, electromyography, nerve conduction studies, and magnetic resonance imaging (MRI). We have used MRI to identify brachial plexus compression in one patient.

Treatment consists of removal of the compressive structure by callus excision and corrective osteotomy, or realignment and internal fixation of nonunion. Great care must be used when undertaking these cases, and the services of a thoracic surgeon may be beneficial.

Posttraumatic Arthritis

Posttraumatic arthritis may occur in either the sternoclavicular joint or the acromioclavicular joint. This is usually the result of intraarticular fracture. Treatment should be directed at pain relief and initially should consist of nonsteroidal antiinflammatory medications, rest, and steroid injections. If these conservative measures fail, the medial or lateral clavicle may be resected. When performing these procedures, the surgeon must leave the costoclavicular ligaments medially or the coracoclavicular ligaments laterally to avoid destabilizing the joint.

Nonunion

Clavicular nonunion is reported in only 1% to 4% of all clavicular fractures.[11,19,34,41,54] If these nonunion cases remain asymptomatic and the patient is pain free with normal shoulder function, the patient may be left alone. Otherwise, open reduction and fixation with plate and screws is the procedure of choice. An interposition bone graft may be necessary to restore proper length and soft-tissue tension. With proper technique, these fractures usually will go on to union without significant problems.

SCAPULOTHORACIC INJURY

Injuries to the scapulothoracic junction are uncommon injuries that rarely have been reported in the literature.[18,30,55] Two types have been described: scapulothoracic dislocation with locking of the inferior angle of the scapula between two adjacent ribs, and a scapulothoracic dissociation with traumatic lateral translation of the entire shoulder girdle.

Scapulothoracic dislocation with locking of the inferior angle of the scapula between adjacent ribs has been reported by Nettrour[55] and Hollinshead.[30] This injury is thought to be caused by direct blunt trauma, usually to the posterior aspect of the shoulder. Motor and sensory neurologic involvement has been described with this injury. If the dislocation is treated acutely, closed reduction usually is possible if adequate muscle relaxation is used and full return of neurologic function has been reported. Nettrour[55] reported the need for open reduction in an 11-year-old boy with a 6-week delay in diagnosis. Any offending structure, such as an osteochondroma as reported by Hollinshead,[30] must be removed to prevent future locking or snapping.

Scapulothoracic dissociation has been reported with translation of the entire shoulder girdle laterally by Oreck[62] and Ebraheim.[18] The injury, usually a result of violent blunt trauma and traction on the shoulder girdle, can be diagnosed with a true anterior-posterior radiograph of the chest. The distance from the spine to the medial border of the scapula will be significantly increased with a dissociation.

Motor vehicle and motorcycle accidents are responsible for most of these injuries, usually with the patient ejected from the vehicle while attempting to hold onto the steering wheel or handlebar. The injury is a closed amputation of the upper extremity with bony, neurovascular, and muscular involvement. The acromioclavicular joint, sternoclavicular joint, or clavicle is affected with dislocation or fracture. The subclavian vein usually is torn, and avulsion or a traumatic aneurysm may be noted in the subclavian or axillary artery. The brachial plexus also is partially or completely avulsed. Rupture of the deltoid, pectoralis major, rhomboids, levator scapulae, trapezius, and latissimus dorsi also is noted.

These injuries require immediate attention for preservation of life and limb, and the usual principles for management of the multitrauma patient must be followed. Ebraheim[18] reported a mortality rate of 20%, with two patients dying from exsanguination and one from a cardiac arrest 10 days after the injury.

After resuscitation and hemodynamic stabilization, an arteriogram should be performed to determine the extent of vascular involvement. Any vascular injury can then be surgically repaired with exploration of the brachial plexus and fracture fixation.

Patients with complete disruption of the brachial plexus have a very poor prognosis and should be offered a primary above-the-elbow amputation. These patients will end up with flail arms, and the best results are in patients undergoing above-the-elbow amputations, early fitting with a prosthesis, and aggressive physical and occupational therapy.

Shoulder arthrodesis was reported to be beneficial by some authors[18] but was thought to be questionable by Rorabeck.[65] Patients noted to have only a partial brachial plexus injury have a much better prognosis, and delayed muscle transfers may be performed to improve functional results.

SUMMARY

Bony injuries to the shoulder girdle often are high-energy injuries that may affect both the mobility and stability of the upper extremity. Injury may occur to the scapula, clavicle, or any of the associated articulations. The bony lesion is not always obvious, especially when the scapula is involved because of severe associated injuries.

Diagnosis requires a detailed history and physical examination along with appropriate radiographic studies. Classification of the fracture pattern may help to determine whether surgical intervention is required. When surgery is necessary, standard principles of fixation must be obeyed and attention should be placed on obtaining stability to allow early motion and on reducing any articular displacement to minimize the possibility of future arthritis.

With both conservative and surgical treatment, complications such as loss of motion, malunion, pain, and crepitus may occur, and the orthopedist must inform the patient of these possibilities and be prepared to treat them.

References

1. Ada JR, Miller ME: Scapular fractures analysis of 113 cases, *Clin Orthop* 269:174-180, 1991.
2. Allman FL: Fractures and ligamentous injuries of the clavicle and its articulation, *J Bone Joint Surg* 49A:774-784, 1967.
3. Andersen K, Jensen PO, Lauritzen J: Treatment of clavicular fractures: figure-of-eight bandage versus a simple sling, *Acta Orthop Scand* 58:71-74, 1987.
4. Armstrong CP, VanderSpuy J: The fractured scapula: importance and management based on a series of 62 patients, *Injury* 15:324-329, 1984.
5. Aston JW, Gregory CF: Dislocation of the shoulder with significant fractures of the glenoid, *J Bone Joint Surg* 55:1531-1533, 1973.
6. Aulicino PL, Reinert C, Kornberg M: Displaced intra-articular glenoid fractures treated by open reduction and internal fixation, *J Trauma* 26:1137-1141, 1986.
7. Barger WL, Marcus RE, Ittleman FP: Late thoracic outlet syndrome secondary to pseudoarthrosis of the clavicle, *J Trauma* 24:857-859, 1984.
8. Benton J, Nelson C: Avulsion of the coracoid process in an athlete, *J Bone Joint Surg* 53A:356-358, 1971.
9. Billington RW: A new (plaster yoke) dressing for fracture of the clavicle, *South Med J* 24:667, 1931.
10. Binazzi R, Assiso J, Vaccari V: Avulsion fractures of the scapula: report of eight cases, *J Trauma* 33:785-789, 1992.
11. Boehme D, Curtis RJ, Dehaan JT: Non-union of fractures of the midshaft of the clavicle. Treatment with a modified Hagie intramedullary pin and autogenous bone-grafting, *J Bone Joint Surg* 73A:1219-1226, 1991.
12. Boyer DW: Trapshooter's shoulder: stress fracture of the coracoid process, *J Bone Joint Surg* 57A:862, 1975.
13. Butters KP: The scapula. In Rockwood CA, Matsen FA: *The shoulder,* ed 1, Philadelphia, 1990, WB Saunders.
14. Craig EV: Fractures of the clavicle. In Rockwood CA, Matsen FA: *The shoulder,* ed 1, Philadelphia, 1990, WB Saunders.
15. DeCoulx MP, Minet P: Omoplate, *Lille Chir* 11:215-217, 1956.
16. Dameron TB, Rockwood CA: Fractures of the shaft of the clavicle. In Rockwood CA, Wilkins KE, King RE: *Fractures in children,* Philadelphia, 1984, JB Lippincott.
17. Desault PJ: *A treatise on fractures, luxations, and other affections of the bones,* Philadelphia, 1805, Fry & Kammerer.
18. Ebraheim NA, An HS, Jackson WT: Scapulothoracic dissociation, *J Bone Joint Surg* 70A:428-432, 1988.
19. Eskola A, Vainionpaa S, Myllynen P: Surgery for ununited clavical fractures, *Acta Orthop Scand* 57:366-367, 1986.
20. Findlay RT: Fractures of the scapula, *Ann Surg* 93:1001-1008, 1931.
21. Fischer WR: Fractures of the scapula requiring open reduction, *J Bone Joint Surg* 21:459-461, 1939.
22. Fischer RP, Flynn TC, Miller PW: Scapular fractures and associated major ipsilateral upper-torso injuries, *Curr Concepts Trauma Care* 1:14-16, 1985.
23. Fromison AI: Fractures of the coracoid process of the scapula, *J Bone Joint Surg* 60A:710-711, 1978.
24. Greenspan A: *Orthopedic radiology,* ed 1, Philadelphia, 1988, JB Lippincott.
25. Stimson: *LA. treatise on fractures,* Philadelphia, 1883, Henry C Lea's Co.
26. Guttentag IJ, Rechtine GR: Fractures of the scapula, a review of the literature, *Orthop Rev* 17:147-158, 1988.
27. Hardegger FK, Simpson LA, Weber BG: The operative treatment of scapular fractures, *J Bone Joint Surg* 66B:725-731, 1984.
28. Heppenstall RB: Fractures and dislocations of the distal clavicle, *Orthop Clin North Am* 6:477-486, 1975.
29. Heyse-Moore GH, Stoker DJ: Avulsion fractures of the scapula, *Skeletal Radiol* 9:27-32, 1982.
30. Hollinshead R, James KW: Scapulothoracic dislocation (locked scapula), *J Bone Joint Surg* 61A:1102-1103, 1979.
31. Ideberg R: Fractures of the scapula involving the glenoid fossa. In Bateman JE, Welsh RP: *Surgery of the shoulder,* Philadelphia, 1984, BC Decker.
32. Imatani RJ: Fractures of the scapula: a review of 53 fractures, *J Trauma* 15:473-478, 1975.
33. Jablon M, Sutker A, Post M: Irreducible fracture of the middle third of the clavicle, *J Bone Joint Surg* 61A:296-298, 1979.
34. Jupiter JB, Leffert RD: Non-union of the clavicle: associated complications and surgical management, *J Bone Joint Surg* 69A:753-760, 1987.
35. Kinni MG: A simple method of ambulatory treatment of fractures of the clavicle, *J Bone Joint Surg* 23:795-798, 1941.
36. Kummel BM: Fractures of the glenoid causing chronic dislocation of the shoulder, *Clin Orthop* 69:189-191, 1970.
37. Laing NA, Dee R: Fracture symposium, *Orthop Rev* 13:717-720, 1984.
38. Lasda NA, Murray DG: Fracture separation of the coracoid process associated with acromioclavicular dislocation: conservative treatment: a case report and review of the literature, *Clin Orthop* 134:222-224, 1978.
39. Lester CW: The treatment of fractures of the clavicle, *Ann Surg* 89:600-606, 1929.
40. Lyons FA, Rockwood CA: Migration of pins used in operations on the shoulder, *J Bone Joint Surg* 72A:1262-1267, 1990.
41. Manske DJ, Szabo R: The operative treatment of mid-shaft clavicular non-unions, *J Bone Joint Surg* 67A:1367-1371, 1985.
42. Matz SO, Welliver PS, Welliver DI: Brachial plexus neuropraxia complicating a comminuted clavicle fracture in a college football player, *Am J Sports Med* 17:581 583, 1989.
43. McLennen JG, Ungersma J: Pneumothorax complicating fractures of the scapula, *J Bone Joint Surg* 64A:598-599, 1982.
44. McGahan JP, Rab GT, Dublin A: Fractures of the scapula, *J Trauma* 20:880-883, 1980.
45. McGahan JP, Rab GT: Fracture of the acromion associated with an axillary nerve deficit: a case report and review of the literature, *Clin Orthop* 147:216-218, 1980.
46. McGinnis M, Denton JR: Fractures of the scapula: a retrospective study of 40 fractured scapulae, *J Trauma* 29:1488-1493, 1989.
47. Mick CA, Weiland AJ: Pseudoarthrosis of a fracture of the acromion, *J Trauma* 23:248-249, 1983.
48. Miller DS, Boswick JA: Lesions of the brachial plexus associated with fractures of the clavicle, *Clin Orthop* 64:145-149, 1969.
49. Miller ME, Ada JR: Injuries of the shoulder girdle. In Browner BD, Jupiter JB, Levine AM, editors: *Skeletal trauma,* Philadelphia, 1992, WB Saunders.

50. Montgomery SP: Avulsion fractures of the coracoid epiphysis with acromioclavicular separation, *J Bone Joint Surg* 59A:963-965, 1977.
51. Neer CS II: Fractures about the shoulder. In Rockwood CA, Green DP, editors: *Fractures,* Philadelphia, 1984, JB Lippincott.
52. Neer CS II: Fractures of the clavicle. In Rockwood CA, Green DP, editors: *Fractures in adults,* Philadelphia, 1984, JB Lippincott.
53. Neer CS II: Fractures of the distal third of the clavicle, *Clin Orthop* 58:43-50, 1968.
54. Neer CS II: Non-union of the clavicle, *JAMA* 172:1006-1011, 1960.
55. Nettrour LF, Krufky EL, Mueller RE: Locked scapula: intrathoracic dislocation of the inferior angle: a case report, *J Bone Joint Surg* 54A:413-416, 1972.
56. Neviaser JD: Injuries in and about the shoulder joint. *Instr Course Lect* 13:187-216, 1956.
57. Neviaser JS: Injuries to the clavicle and acromioclavicular joint, *Orthop Clin North Am* 18:433-438, 1987.
58. Neviaser RJ, Neviaser JS, Neviaser TJ: A simple technique for internal fixation of the clavicle, *Clin Orthop* 109:103-107, 1975.
59. Newell ED: Review of over 2,000 fractures in the past seven years, *South Med J* 20:644-648, 1927.
60. Nordback I, Markkula H: Migration of Kirschner pin from clavicle into ascending aorta, *Acta Chir Scand* 151:177-179, 1985.
61. Nordqvist A, Petersson C, Redlund-Johnell I: The natural course of lateral clavicle fracture 15 (11-21) year follow-up of 110 cases, *Acta Orthop Scand* 64:87-91, 1993.
62. Oreck SL, Burgess A, Levine A: Traumatic lateral displacement of the scapula: a radiographic sign of neurovascular disruption, *J Bone Joint Surg* 66A:758-763, 1984.
63. Packer BD: Conservative treatment of fracture of the clavicle, *J Bone Joint Surg* 26:770-774, 1944.
64. Rockwood CA: Management of fractures of the scapula, *J Bone Joint Surg* 10:219, 1986.
65. Rorabeck CH: The management of the flail upper extremity in brachial plexus injuries, *J Trauma* 20:491-493, 1980.
66. Rowe CR: An atlas of anatomy and treatment of midclavicular fractures, *Clin Orthop* 58:29-42, 1968.
67. Rowe CR: Fractures of the scapula, *Surg Clin North Am* 43:1565-1571, 1963.
68. Schwarz N, Hocker K: Osteosynthesis of irreducible fractures of the clavicle with 2.7 mm ASIF plates, *J Trauma* 33:179-183, 1992.
69. Smith DM: Coracoid fracture associated with acromioclavicular dislocation: a case report, *Clin Orthop* 108:165-167, 1975.
70. Stanley D, Norris SH: Recovery following fractures of the clavicle treated conservatively, *Injury* 19:162-164, 1988.
71. Stanley D, Trowbridge EA, Norris SH: The mechanism of clavicular fracture, *J Bone Joint Surg* 70B:461-464, 1988.
72. Thompson DA, Flynn TC, Miller PW: The significance of scapular fractures, *J Trauma* 25:974-977, 1985.
73. Tse DH, Slabaugh PB, Carlson PA: Injury to the axillary artery by a closed fracture of the clavicle, *J Bone Joint Surg* 62A:1372-1374, 1980.
74. Wilber MC, Evans EB: Fractures of the scapula, *J Bone Joint Surg* 59A:358-362, 1977.
75. Wolf AW: Unusual fractures of the coracoid process, *J Bone Joint Surg* 58A:423-424, 1976.
76. Zdravkovic D, Damholt VV: Comminuted and severely displaced fractures of the scapula, *Acta Orthop Scand* 45:60-65, 1974.
77. Zeni E, Krieg J, Rosen M: Open reduction and internal fixation of clavicular fractures, *J Bone Joint Surg* 63A:147-151, 1981.
78. Zuckerman JD: *Fractures, nonunions, and dislocations of the clavicle,* Instructional Course Lecture, AAOS annual meeting, San Francisco, 1993.

CHAPTER 11

Fractures of the Proximal Humerus

SCOTT E. POWELL
ROBERT W. CHANDLER

In the young athletic patient, proximal humerus fractures represent severe trauma that can be debilitating, particularly if coupled with neurovascular injury or complicated by nonunion or avascular necrosis. The shoulder is the most mobile joint in the body[1] (Fig. 11-1), and stiffness and limitation of shoulder motion often develop despite adequate treatment of these problem fractures. The development of subacromial impingement or secondary fracture displacement further worsens the prognosis.

Some fractures and fracture-dislocations may require prosthetic replacement, and unfortunately the expectations and functional requirements of the young athlete often are incompatible with the limitations imposed by a hemiarthroplasty or total shoulder replacement. Even nondisplaced fractures, which make up the vast majority of proximal humerus fractures, may result in considerable loss of function. To understand these injuries and deal with them effectively, relevant anatomy and mechanics will be reviewed, followed by fracture classifications and treatment recommendations.

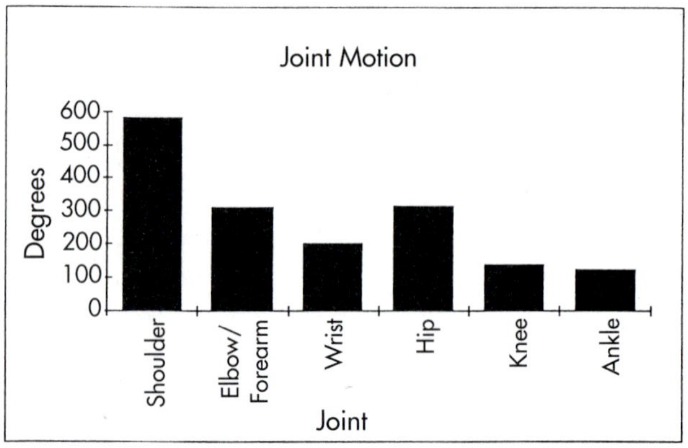

	Shoulder	Elbow / Forearm	Wrist	Hip	Knee	Ankle
Flexion	180	150	80	120	135	20
Extension	60	0	70	30	0	50
Abduction	180	0	20	45	0	15
Adduction	0	0	30	30	0	35
Internal Rotation	70	80		45	0	0
External Rotation	90	80		45	0	0
Total Arc =	580	310	200	315	135	120

FIGURE 11-1 Joint motion. The shoulder has almost twice the mobility of the next most mobile articulation.

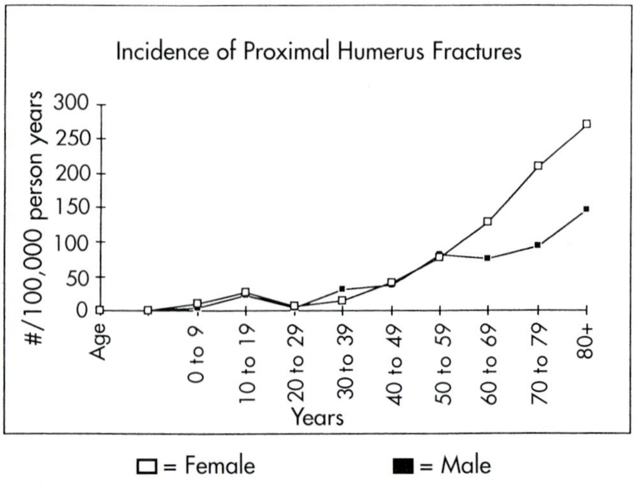

FIGURE 11-2 Incidence of proximal humerus fractures by sex and age.

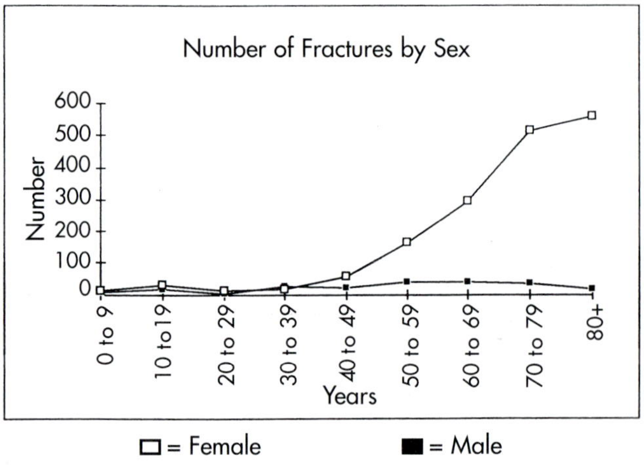

FIGURE 11-3 Number of proximal humerus fractures by sex and age.

EPIDEMIOLOGY

Incidence

Fractures of the proximal humerus comprise approximately 5% of adult fractures. Data collected over a 5-year period in Denmark established an incidence of 73 per 100,000 population, with 21% of those having a fracture requiring surgery.[15]

Age and Gender Distribution

In Neer's original series of 300 patients, the average age of patients was 55.6 years.[22] Lind found that three fourths of his patients were over 60 years old[16] (Fig. 11-2). In reviewing 41 patients with proximal humerus fractures treated operatively at the Kerlan-Jobe Orthopaedic Clinic, over half (51%) of patients were under age 50, and 10 of 41 (24%) were under age 40.

An epidemiologic study from the Mayo Clinic identified a predominance of proximal humerus fractures in women at a ratio of 1.5:1.[30] Lind noted a female:male ratio of 3:1, with an even higher ratio in the age group over 70[16] (Fig. 11-3).

Associated Medical Conditions

Factors that appear to be independently associated with an increased risk of fracture include a recent decline in overall health status, infrequent walking, insulin-dependent diabetes mellitus, and indicators of neuromuscular weakness, including an inability to stand with the feet in a tandem position for more than a few seconds.[11] Recent studies have suggested an increasing incidence of these fractures in the elderly, requiring increased hospitalization and allotment of resources.[16]

MECHANISM OF INJURY

Minor falls produce greater than 80% of proximal humerus fractures in patients over the age of 40 years.[30] Overall, only 29% of proximal humerus fractures were the result of severe trauma, compared with 63% of diaphyseal and 69% of distal humerus fractures. Of the group who sustained fractures as the result of severe trauma, 31% were the result of motor vehicle accidents and 26% the result of a fall. In another study, 20% of patients under the age of 40 years sustained their injury during athletic activity, primarily basketball.[27] In our review of 41 proximal humerus fractures, skiing accounted for 15% of proximal humerus fractures. Another 15% were the result of automobile, motorcycle, or off-road vehicle accidents. Three patients (7%) sustained fractures while riding or training horses, and one fracture occurred while bodysurfing. In this group, only 39% occurred with minor falls; the remainder occurred during athletic activity or heavy labor.

RADIOGRAPHIC EVALUATION

Accurate determination of the location and orientation of proximal humeral fracture fragments is essential in determining proper treatment. Evaluation of shoulder fractures with plain x-rays can be difficult in the injured patient when pain and discomfort preclude correct positioning for accurate studies. Neer proposed two standard radiographic projections for injured patients, one view parallel and a second view perpendicular to the scapular plane.[22] A clear anterior posterior radiograph combine with an axillary view is usually adequate, but additional views may be necessary. An apical oblique view may permit more accurate diagnosis of fractures and dislocations.[29]

Computed tomography has been used to evaluate linear displacement and rotation and has provided clinically useful information, altering treatment regimens[3] (Fig. 11-4). Volumetric three-dimensional imaging has been helpful in evaluating complex fractures about the shoulder girdle by eliminating overlapping structures and allowing focus on the region of interest.[14] MRI can help identify soft-tissue injury, such as rotator cuff tear, in the presence of bony injury (Fig. 11-5). Recently, ultrasound has been used effectively to detect occult irregularity of the humeral cortex of the greater tuberosity, suggesting fractures in patients who had sustained recent trauma. A fracture had been missed on plain radiograph in 10 of 24 patients.[26]

Comparison of a similar radiographic view of the uninjured side sometimes can help assess displacement or angulation in cases where these parameters are equivocal on plain films. A reverse overlay of either transthoracic or anteroposterior views from the unaffected side can provide information on displacement and angulation as well as definition of comminuted fragments. A reasonable effort should be expended to procure adequate information with conventional studies. However, there should be no reluctance to obtain tomograms, CT, or MRI to better determine the details of the fracture.

As a three-dimensional object, the humeral head has three axes—coronal, axial, and sagittal planes (Fig. 11-6). Displacement can occur in a single plane, as in a surgical neck fracture (Fig. 11-7). A fracture of the greater tuberosity can displace in the axial, as well as the coronal plane (Fig. 11-8). A fracture-dislocation occurs with displacement in the axial, sagittal, and coronal planes (Fig. 11-9).

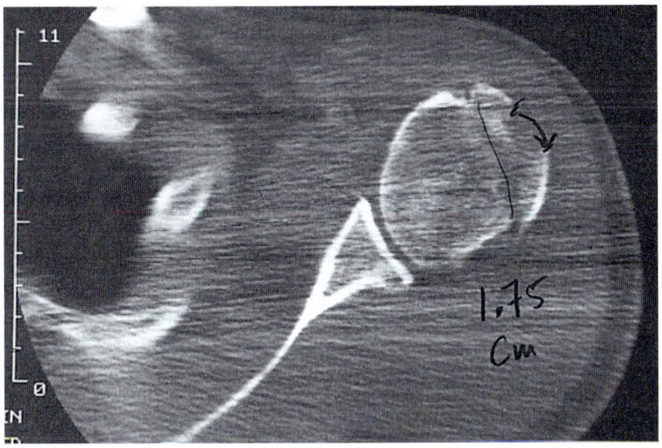

FIGURE 11-4 Axial computer tomographic view showing measurable displacement of the greater tuberosity of 1.75 cm, improving the precision of preoperative assessment.

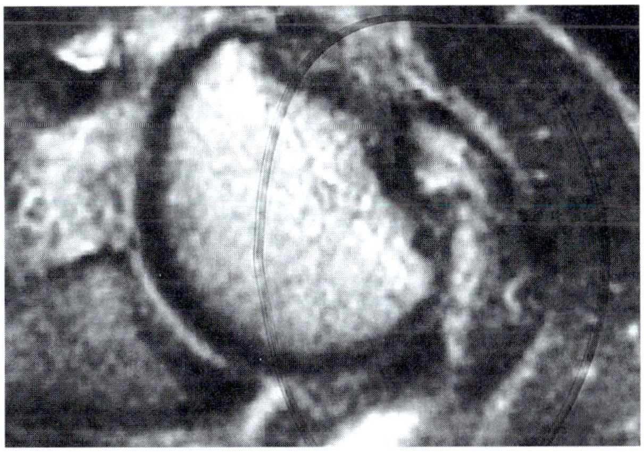

FIGURE 11-5 Magnetic resonance imaging shows detail similar to the CAT scan but yields additional information about the rotator cuff.

CLASSIFICATION

Codman

The classification of proximal humerus fractures has undergone several refinements since Codman introduced his concept based on the anatomic configuration of the proximal humeral epiphyses. In his system, fractures of the proximal humerus are composed of one, two, three, or four major segments: the shaft, the greater tuberosity, the lesser tuberosity, and the humeral head[5] (Fig. 11-10).

Neer

In 1970, Neer studied 300 displaced proximal humeral fractures and fracture-dislocations over a 14-year pe-

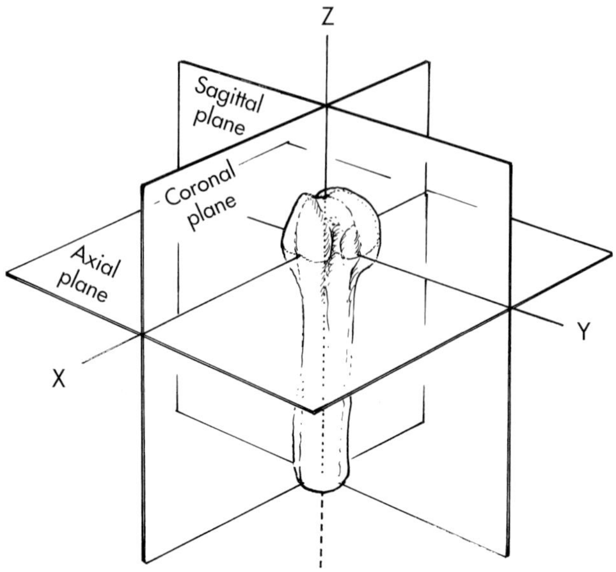

FIGURE 11-6 Planes of the shoulder. The proximal humerus is three-dimensional, and displacement and angulation must be evaluated in the axial, coronal, and sagittal planes.

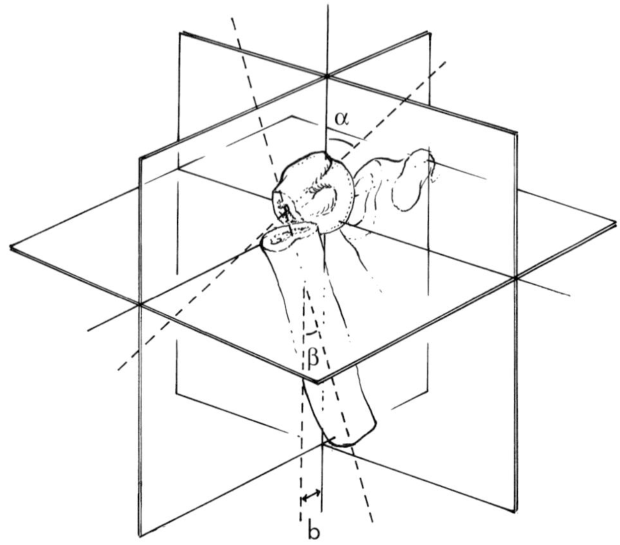

FIGURE 11-7 Two-part fracture deformity. Deformity in the two-part fracture of the proximal humerus is multiplanar. Varus deformity in the coronal plane is identified as angle α. In the sagittal plane, there is an apex-anterior angulation identified as angle β. Additional displacements may be measured. These displacements and angulations are maintained by wedging of the fragments into soft tissues. In this specific fracture configuration, the proximal shaft is driven into the pectoralis tendon, and at times the biceps tendon is incarcerated in the fracture.

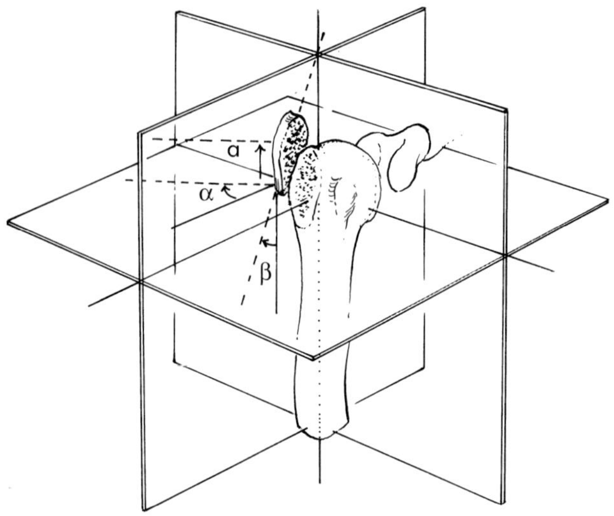

FIGURE 11-8 Two-part greater-tuberosity avulsion fracture. The greater tuberosity displaces cephalad distance *a*. There is rotation in the coronal plane given by angle α and rotation in the axial plane given by angle β.

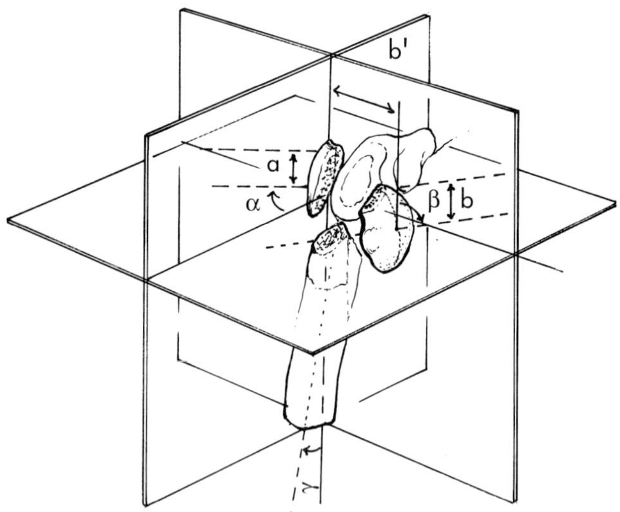

FIGURE 11-9 Three-part anterior fracture-dislocation. The head is displaced anteriorly distance *b*. The greater tuberosity is displaced cephalad distance *a* and is rotated in the coronal plane to angle α. The shaft is angulated angle γ.

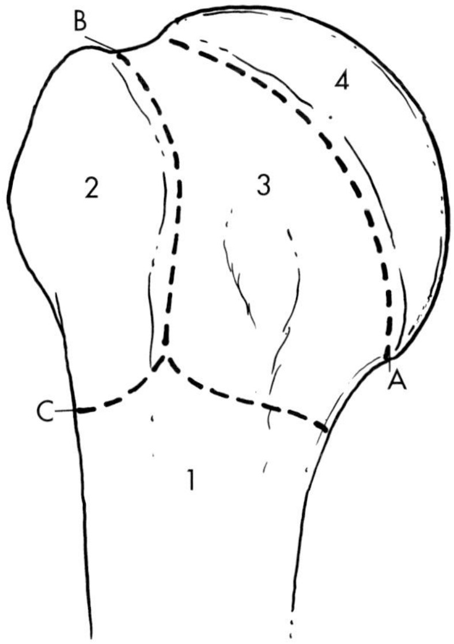

FIGURE 11-10 Codman classification: (*1*) shaft, (*2*) greater tuberosity, (*3*) lesser tuberosity, and (*4*) head.

riod.[22,23] By comparing roentgenograms and operative findings, Neer defined distinct categories. The four-segment classification is based on the presence or absence of displacement of one or more of the four major segments (Fig. 11-11). Six groups were defined.

Group I includes all fractures, regardless of location or number of fracture lines, that have displacement of less than 1 cm and angulation of less than 45°. This group of fractures represents the majority of all proximal humerus fractures,[18] ranging from 61%[9] to 85%.[22] Neer's rationale for including minimally displaced and angulated fractures in group I was as follows:

> Since all minimally displaced fractures pose analogous problems in treatment and prognosis, it seems logical that they be grouped together, regardless of the number of fracture lines. . . . The fractures are usually held together by soft tissue or are impacted, permitting early functional exercises, however, a brief period of immobilization may be required before the head and shaft rotate.[22]

Group II fractures consist of articular-segment displacement or anatomic neck fractures. These are rare lesions that can lead to malunion or avascular necrosis.

Group III is composed of surgical neck fractures with shaft displacement of more than 1 cm and angulation of greater than 45°. Three subtypes include: angulated, separated or unimpacted, and comminuted surgical neck fractures.

Group IV fractures constitute greater tuberosity fractures with displacement of more than 1 cm from the lesser tuberosity. This fracture pattern is pathognomonic of a rotator cuff tear.

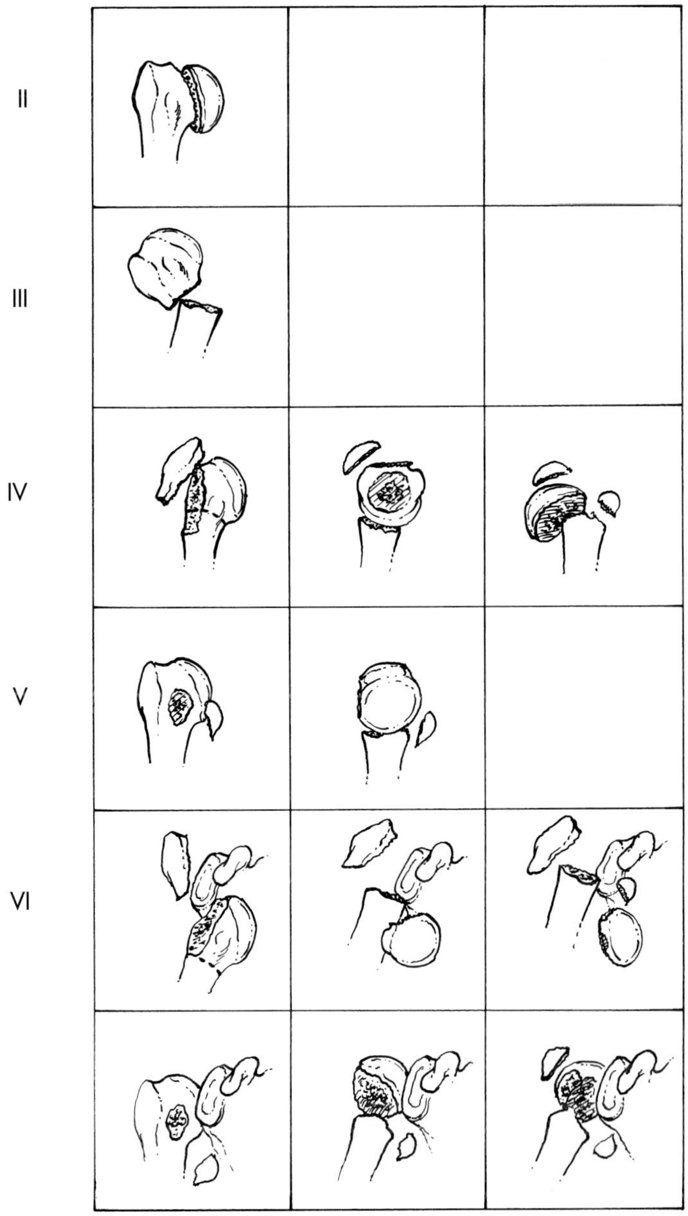

FIGURE 11-11 Neer classification. "One-part" fractures with angulation of less than 45° and displacement of less than 1 cm make up Group I.

Group V is composed of displaced lesser tuberosity fractures that occur as isolated avulsion fractures, such as after a seizure or electroconvulsive therapy or in association with a nondisplaced surgical neck fracture.

Group VI consists of fracture dislocations, either anterior or posterior, including impression fractures.

Dislocation implies extensive ligamentous damage and increased risk of pericapsular bone formation. Two-part or three-part fracture dislocations usually retain an adequate blood supply because of the attachment of one or the other of the tuberosities. In anterior three-part fracture dislocations, the lesser tuberosity remains attached, and in posterior dislocations, the greater tuberosity remains intact.

Impression fractures of the humeral head occurring in anterior or posterior dislocations are measured by the percentage of involvement of the articular surface. With a small Hill-Sachs lesion, early closed reduction is effective. With involvement of more than 20% of the humeral head, the head tends to redislocate and therefore often requires open treatment. Impression fractures involving more than 50% of the humeral head usually render the joint grossly unstable. A central impaction on the head produces a head-splitting fracture that may be extensively comminuted, requiring prosthetic replacement.

Arbeitsgemeinschaft für Osteosynthesefragen

In 1987 the Arbeitsgemeinschaft für Osteosynthesefragen/ Association for the Study of Internal Fixation (AO/ASIF) group developed a comprehensive classification scheme for all fractures, including the proximal humerus (Fig. 11-12). The guiding principle of the AO group is that "a classification is useful only if it considers the severity of the bone lesion and serves as a basis for treatment and for evaluation of results."[21] Proximal humerus fractures are divided into groups in order of increasing severity. The potential for avascular necrosis of the head also is considered. Group A fractures are extraarticular fractures with a single fracture line. Group B are extraarticular fractures but have two fracture lines. Group C includes all intraarticular fractures.

The A1 subgroup fractures consist of greater tuberosity fractures; these fractures also may involve a small portion of the articular cartilage but do not impair glenohumeral articulation.

The A2 fracture is an impacted metaphyseal fracture of the surgical neck, and an A3 fracture is a displaced surgical neck fracture.

Type B fractures have both metaphyseal and tuberosity fractures. Type B1 fractures consist of an impacted metaphyseal fracture with a displaced greater or lesser tuberosity. The prognosis can be affected by angulation of the metaphyseal fractures.

Type B2 fractures have an unimpacted metaphyseal segment and therefore are unstable to rotation. If the greater tuberosity is fractured, rotatory instability may be

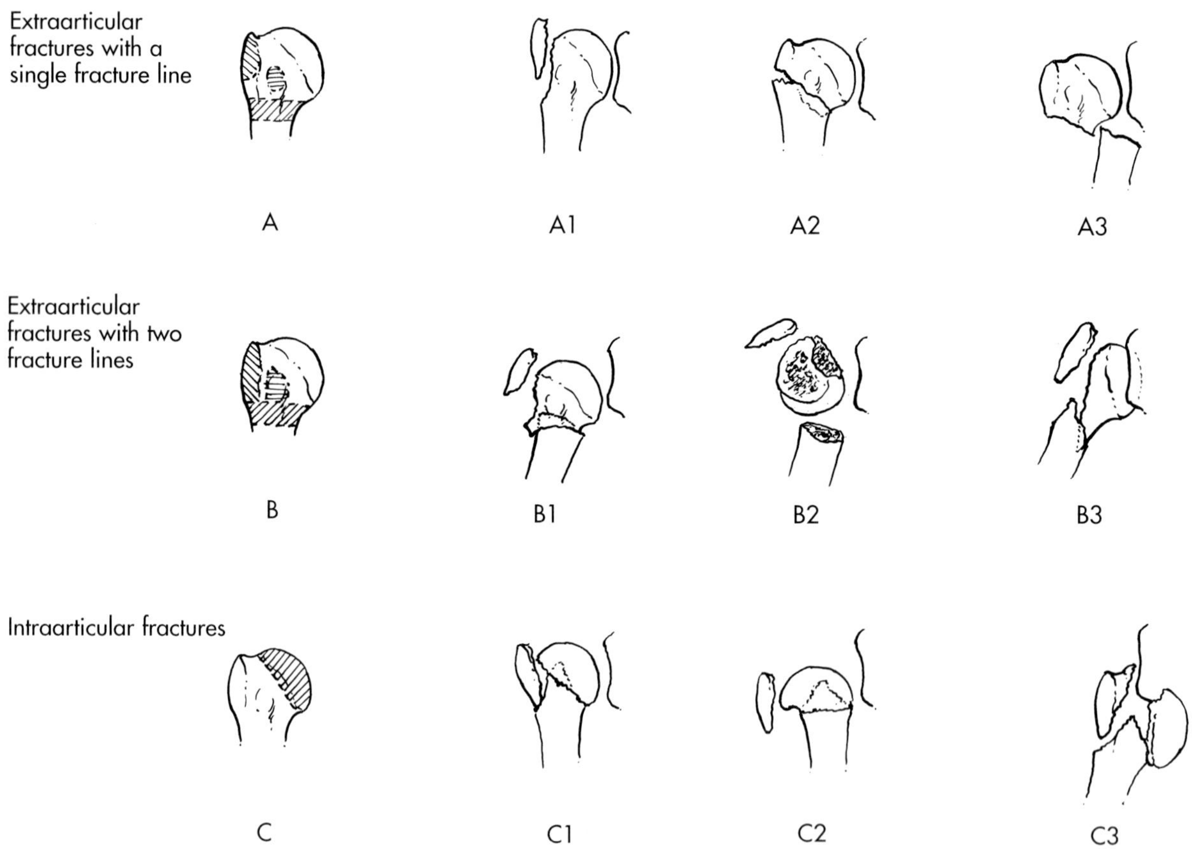

FIGURE 11-12 AO classification. Fractures are divided into the following three groups: extraarticular with a single fracture line, extraarticular with two fracture lines, and intraarticular fractures.

due to the unopposed pull of the subscapularis on the lesser tuberosity. If the lesser tuberosity is fractured, the unopposed pull on the greater tuberosity by the supraspinatus, infraspinatus, and teres minor gives rise to rotational instability. Finally, comminution of the metaphyseal segment can cause rotatory instability. This rotatory component of the fracture complicates reduction and compromises stability.

Type B3 fractures are extraarticular fractures of two fragments complicated by a dislocation of the humeral head. The first subgroup designates a fracture with a single fracture line that passes through both the greater tuberosity and the metaphysis and in which the head is dislocated. In a second group, the greater tuberosity is displaced, the surgical neck is fractured, and there is an associated glenohumeral dislocation. The third group consists of lesser tuberosity fractures with posterior dislocation of the humeral head.

Type C fractures include articular fractures that involve the anatomic neck of the humerus. Group C1 fractures are subdivided into impacted valgus, impacted varus, or isolated fractures of the anatomic neck. A second group of fractures is characterized by marked displacement of the head and impaction in valgus or varus (C2). Group C3 includes articular fractures associated with dislocation of the humeral head, whether anatomic neck, surgical neck and tuberosities, or marked comminution of the neck and head.

Reliability

The Neer classification has been studied to determine reliability of application. Wide interobserver variability has been found using conventional radiographs. Kristiansen et al found little agreement among four observers using anteroposterior and lateral radiographs.[12b] The experience level of the observer correlated positively with reliable use of the classification. Sidor et al found agreement on final classification in less than one third of cases in a study of five observers viewing the standard trauma series of radiographs.[33]

Intraobserver reliability in separate viewings 6 months apart ranged from 83% for a shoulder specialist to 50% for a skeletal radiologist in confirming their original classification selection. The addition of the scapular lateral and axillary radiographs had limited effect on improving interobserver and intraobserver reliability in evaluating the fracture pattern.[34]

EVALUATION SCALES

Neer developed a rating system for outcome of fractures based on a 100-point scale. Of these, 35 points represented pain, 30 points represented function, 25 points represented range of motion, and 10 points represented anatomic result. The most significant outcome parameter was pain. Excellent results were in the range of 89 to 100 points, satisfactory was over 80 points, unsatisfactory was from 70 to 79, and a failure was under 70 points.[22]

The Society of American Shoulder and Elbow Surgeons (ASES) has developed an evaluation scale in an attempt to compare treatment outcomes. A patient self-evaluation of function includes assessment of pain, type of medication and frequency, and presence or absence of a sensation of instability. Assessment of activities of daily living includes the following:

1. Put on a coat
2. Sleep on the affected side
3. Wash back/fasten bra
4. Manage toileting
5. Comb hair
6. Reach a high shelf
7. Lift 10 lb above shoulder
8. Throw a ball overhand
9. Perform usual work
10. Perform usual sport

Physician assessment includes evaluation of range of motion, tenderness, impingement signs, crepitus, atrophy, or deformity. Strength of forward elevation, abduction, external rotation, and internal rotation is recorded on a scale of 0 to 5, from no muscular activity to normal. Instability is graded on a scale of 0 to 3, from none to severe, for evaluation of anterior, posterior, or inferior translation. Apprehension, relocation test, and voluntary instability are also assessed. Presence or absence of neurologic deficit is noted.

TREATMENT AND RESULTS

Nondisplaced Fractures

Truly nondisplaced fractures of the proximal humerus should be treated with a rapid mobilization program. In our opinion, the hanging cast has no place in the management of humerus fractures of any type and is particularly inappropriate for the proximal humerus. For the first 2 to 3 weeks, patient comfort has the highest priority and is best achieved with a shoulder immobilizer and analgesics. Patients often learn they sleep best in a reclining chair or when propped up with pillows. Rehabilitation efforts are directed initially toward finger, wrist, and elbow function, with limited attention to the region of the fracture. Shoulder isometrics may be started along with passive forward flexion and abduction. Passive rotational activities and active motion are avoided.

As the fracture stabilizes, physical examination at 2 to 3 weeks after injury may demonstrate synchronous motion between the proximal and distal fragments, indicating sufficient healing to proceed to the next stage of treatment. The shoulder immobilizer is now discarded in favor of a sling, and gentle active-assisted range of motion in forward flexion and abduction is added.

Early radiographic and clinical evidence of union is typically present within 6 weeks after injury. Active mo-

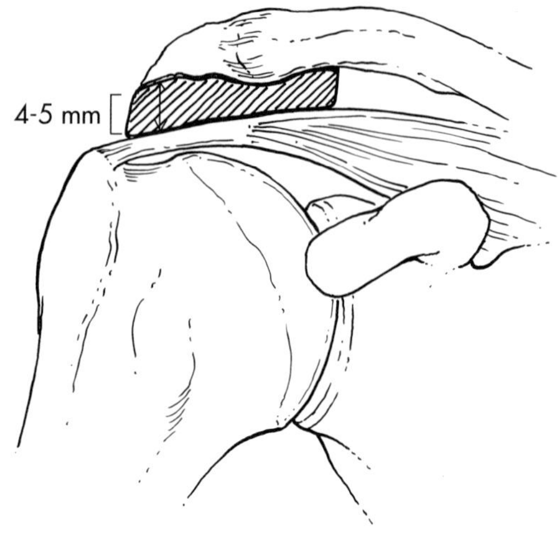

FIGURE 11-13 The acromial space has limited volume. Even minimal displacement of tuberosity fragments into the subacromial area results in obstructed motion.

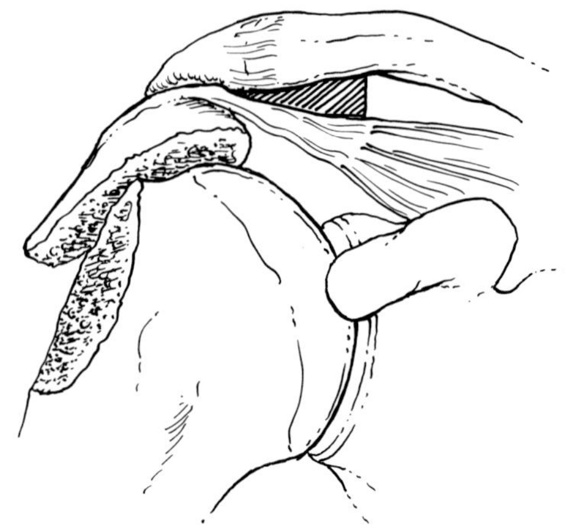

FIGURE 11-14 Displacement of a large greater-tuberosity fragment cephalad, producing subacromial obstruction and results in compensatory displacement of the humeral head.

tion is now encouraged in all planes, and gentle stretching is added. After complete radiographic union is present, more vigorous stretching is permitted, and a strengthening program is begun.

Since Neer's original classification scheme, most orthopedic literature on the subject has explored operative indications and results of three-part and four-part fractures. Little has been written about the so-called "one-part" proximal humerus fracture with displacement of less than 1 cm and angulation of less than 45°. A recent study has demonstrated a wide range of functional outcomes for this fracture pattern. Powell et al studied 102 proximal humerus fractures treated with early range of motion after a short period of immobilization.[27] Of these, 65% reported some limitation of function an average of 2 years after a standardized rehabilitation protocol. Despite an adequate recovery in range of motion (87% of forward elevation, 79% of external rotation, and 89% of internal rotation) compared with the opposite side, 67% of patients reported residual pain in the shoulder. In addition, 29% of patients continued to take pain medication 2 years after the initial fracture. Activities of daily living were significantly compromised. Nearly 40% of patients were unable to sleep on the affected side, 46% were unable to carry a 10 lb bag at their side, and more than half (51%) experienced difficulty in using their hand overhead.

The authors subdivided the fractures according to single or multiple fracture lines and according to displacement and angulation on x-ray. The results suggested that nondisplaced surgical neck fractures achieved almost 100% of motion. Fractures that approached angulation of 45° achieved 78% of motion. Nondisplaced greater tuberosity fractures recovered 91% of motion, and fractures displaced nearly 1 cm recovered 76% of motion. The rate of recovery of motion for fractures of combined surgical neck and greater tuberosity that satisfied Neer's criteria was only 62%. Functionally, these patients were able to perform only light housework and could use their hand overhead only with assistance. Increasing displacement and angulation resulted in decreased range of motion and decreased functional ability.

These results suggest the vast majority of proximal humerus fractures regarded as "one-part" fractures represent a spectrum of injury with a wide variation in outcomes.

Gray Zone Fractures

Somewhere between nondisplaced fractures and fractures with displacements of 1 cm or more lies a large group of injuries in which treatment selection can be very difficult.

Recent knowledge from traumatic and degenerative impingement syndrome and routine arthroscopic subacromial decompression suggests that a dimension of 4 to 5 mm is critical in the subacromial space (Fig. 11-13). Displacement of the greater tuberosity into the subacromial space (Fig. 11-14) can give rise to impingement and limit motion, primarily abduction. Loss of 30° of abduction may go unnoticed by most patients, but few will tolerate the loss of 45°. Angulation is usually varus and may be subtracted from abduction range to assess the need for correction.

In the young or more athletically inclined patients, the criteria for treatment of minimally displaced fractures should be narrowed. The following guidelines are pro-

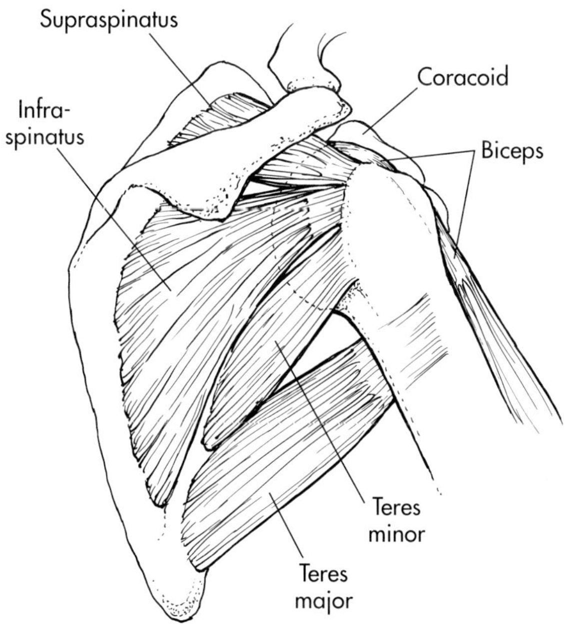

FIGURE 11-15 The posterior aspect of the shoulder. The low insertion of the teres minor on the surgical neck can displace fragments even when the tuberosity is anatomically reduced.

posed for the surgical treatment of these fractures in this population:

Angulation greater than 30°

Displacement greater than 5 mm

If a closed reduction cannot be achieved or cannot be maintained, open reduction and internal fixation is recommended. As more experience is gained with these injuries, new criteria may emerge.

Displaced Fractures

Operative Approaches

Most bony injuries of the proximal humerus may be adequately approached through three incisions. An extensile deltopectoral incision is used when fracture assembly is anticipated with a plate or a locking nail, or tension band is anticipated. A saber incision combined with a deltoid-splitting approach is used for simple avulsion fractures requiring access to the rotator cuff. If necessary, the saber incision may be extended into the deltopectoral interval. Finally, an anterior deltoid split approach is useful for septic cases and occasional two part fractures.

The Posterior Metaphysis

The long head of the biceps is an important landmark in approaching displaced fractures and is helpful in keying together the tuberosities at the front of the shoulder. The posterior aspect of the proximal humerus in displaced fractures is particularly problematic. Difficulty often is encountered in determining the origin of displaced posterior fragments, making reduction difficult. A clear knowledge of the posterior rotator cuff is helpful in approaching these problems surgically (Fig. 11-15). A recent study has demonstrated that the teres minor has muscular insertions on the surgical neck of the humerus 2 cm distal to the tendinous attachment on the tuberosity and may explain the displacement of posterior fragments even when the tuberosities themselves appear to be reconstituted.[3a]

Fixation Techniques

Proximal humerus fractures are a diverse group of injuries requiring a variety of internal fixation techniques. Active or athletic patients should receive anatomic restoration of displaced fractures. Unfortunately, no single method of fixation has proven to be reliable for the range of injuries encountered. A combination of tension wiring, lag screw and/or plate osteosynthesis, locking nail, and percutaneous 2.5-mm partially threaded pins may be necessary to treat these fractures (Table 11-1).

Reports in the literature seldom differentiate cases according to bone quality vs. fixation technique. Unfortunately, in large series, the number of fractures in patients under the age of 50 years is relatively small. As shown in Table 11-2, results of operative treatment are superior to nonoperative treatment for displaced fractures. Rigid fixation is more successful in younger patients with good bone stock.[20,31]

Lag Screw

Lag screws (Figs. 11-16 through 11-18) have limited application with proximal humerus fractures because success depends on the availability of solid bone. Occasionally screws may be used to internally fix a tuberosity avulsion fracture, but frequently the tendon is attached to a comminuted or soft tuberosity (Fig. 11-19). Tension-relieving fixation, such as heavy suture or wire, often is more appropriate and suitable than interfragmentary compression.

Tension Band

Tension-band techniques (Fig. 11-20) using heavy suture or wire are a fixation method applicable to avulsion-type injuries as well as some three-part fractures. Brunner and Weber have described a wire tension-band method for more complicated fractures.[2] If the head is impacted into the shaft and the greater tuberosity is avulsed, the tuberosity may be fixed to the shaft while at the same time stabilizing the head to the shaft.

If the head is unstable relative to the shaft, another technique, such as the technique described by Hawkins, should be selected.[8] The authors generally recommend

TABLE 11-1

Relative Merits of Internal Fixation Techniques

Technique	Advantages	Disadvantages
Lag screws	Excellent interfragmentary compression May be applied through small incision May be used for percutaneous fixation of anatomic neck fractures Rehabilitation in the first 2 weeks	Requires hard bone Poor control of tension force Requires large solid fragments For two-part fractures primarily unless combined with other fixation Large incision may be necessary.
Tension band	Excellent control of tension Captures the bone tendon junction Can be used with comminution Can be used for two-part and three-part fractures Rehabilitation in the first 2 weeks	
Plates	Can be used to assemble large well-fitting pieces Can be used for two-, three-, and four-part fractures Rehabilitation in the first 2 weeks	Requires hard bone Poor control of tension force Requires large solid fragments Technically demanding Large incision Bulky Poor control of torsional forces
Rush rod	Percutaneous technique for two-part fractures	Poor fixation at both ends Subacromial impingement Rehabilitation must be delayed until fracture stabilizes.
Enders plus wire	Applicable to two-, three-, and four-part fractures Not as bulky as plate	Intermediate stability Subacromial impingement Rehabilitation must be delayed until fracture stabilizes
Mouradian nail	Applicable to two-, three-, and four-part fractures Not as bulky as plate Applicable to comminuted fractures Good torsional control Rehabilitation in the first 2 weeks Good control of tension forces	Technically demanding Limited product development Impingement
Multiple pins (2.5 mm with end thread)	Applicable to two- and three-part fractures Percutaneous technique	Poor fixation in soft bone Rehabilitation hampered by pins Pin migration Technically demanding

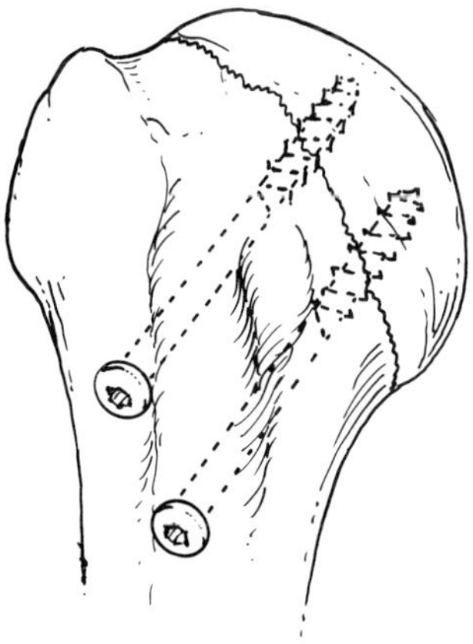

FIGURE 11-16 Lag screw technique. Two 6.5-mm cancellous screws can be used to fix a humeral head fracture.

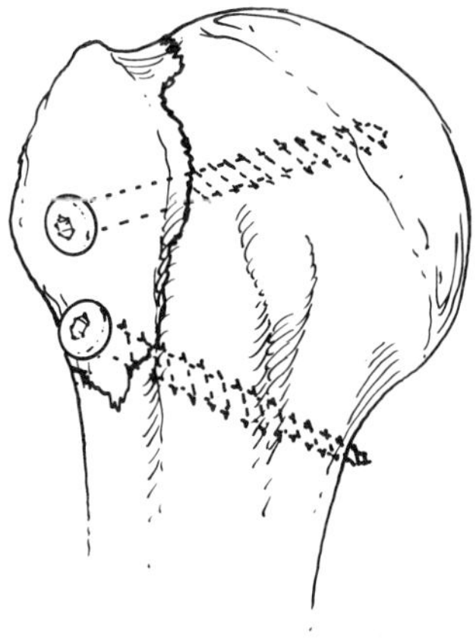

FIGURE 11-17 Two-screw fixation. Lag screws used to fix greater-tuberosity fractures should be divergent to prevent pullout and to control rotation.

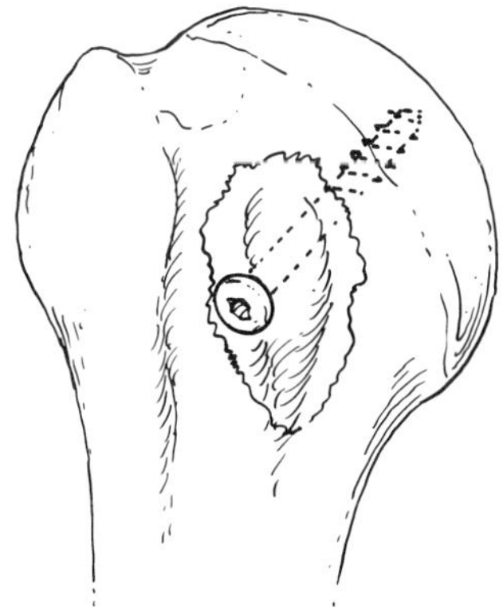

FIGURE 11-18 Single-screw fixation. Small fragments of bone may require that only one lag screw be used, as in this fixation of a lesser-tuberosity fracture.

A

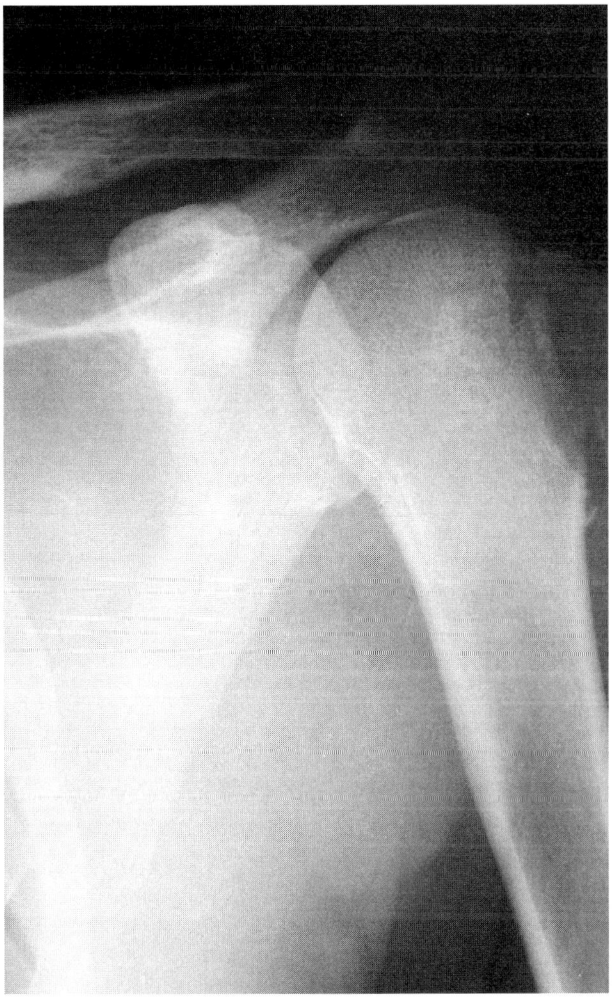

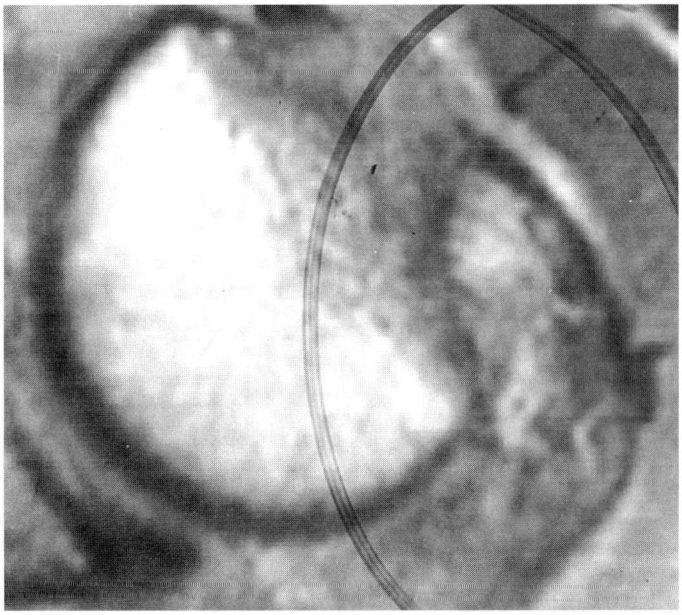

B

FIGURE 11-19 **A**, Marked displacement of a large greater tuberosity fragment in a young man with good bone quality fixed with two 6.5-mm cancellous lag screws. **B,** An MRI shows the extent of displacement. *Continued.*

C
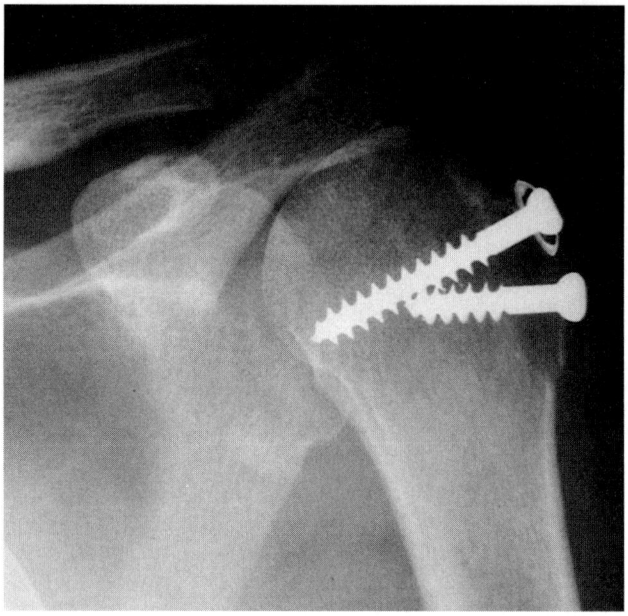
D
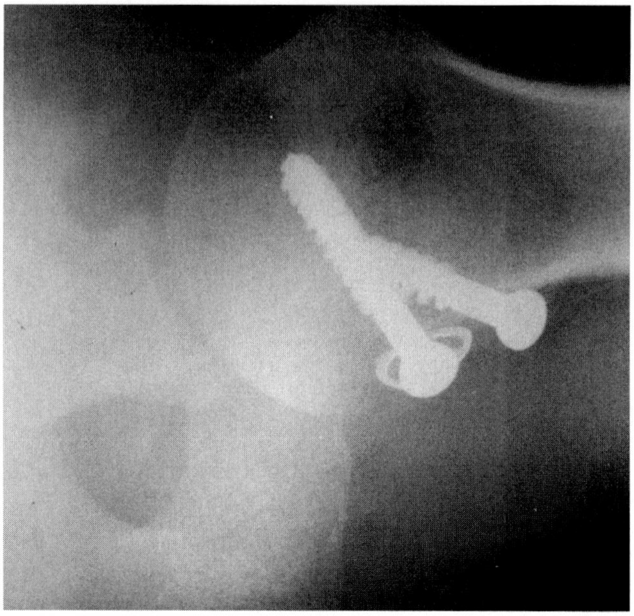

FIGURE 11-19—cont'd C, Postoperative AP x-ray. D, Postoperative axillary x-ray.

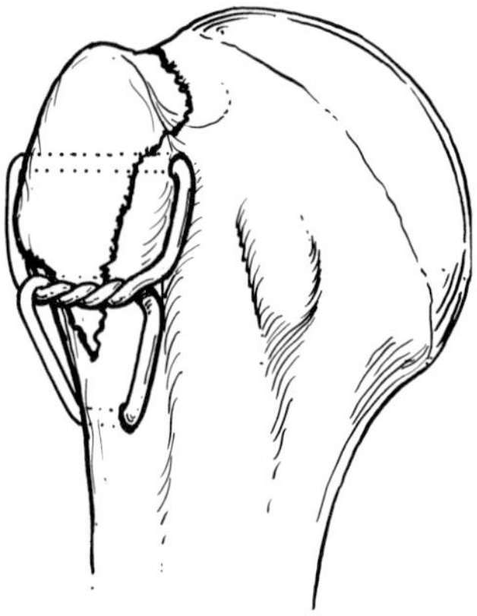

FIGURE 11-20 Tension band technique. This technique can be applied to tuberosity fractures and three-part fractures involving the shaft and the tuberosity.

that wire be avoided because of the possibility of irritation of the subdeltoid bursa, crepitation, and/or breakage (Fig. 11-21).

Displaced tuberosity fractures with rotator cuff injuries may be repaired with heavy suture such as #5 Ticron or #1 Ethibond, depending on the size of the fragment. Two-part fractures involving the greater or lesser tuberosity lend themselves to this fixation technique. Flatow reported 50% excellent and 50% good results in 12 patients with displaced two-part fractures treated with the suture technique.[6] Hawkins et al reported on 15 three-part fractures in patients ranging in age from 58 to 74 years who were treated with tension-band suture or wire.[8] Two patients had avascular necrosis, and one had impingement from wire fixation. There were no nonunions, infections, or secondary displacements. The study showed that these patients achieved an average forward flexion arc of 120° (range, 60° to 170°), an external rotation arc of 29° (range, 15° to 60°), and an abduction arc of 81° (range, 30° to 110°) after the treatment with tension-band suture or wire.

Plate

Plating (Figs. 11-22 and 11-23) has limited application to proximal humerus fractures for the majority of patients. Plates are bulky and technically difficult to apply. The

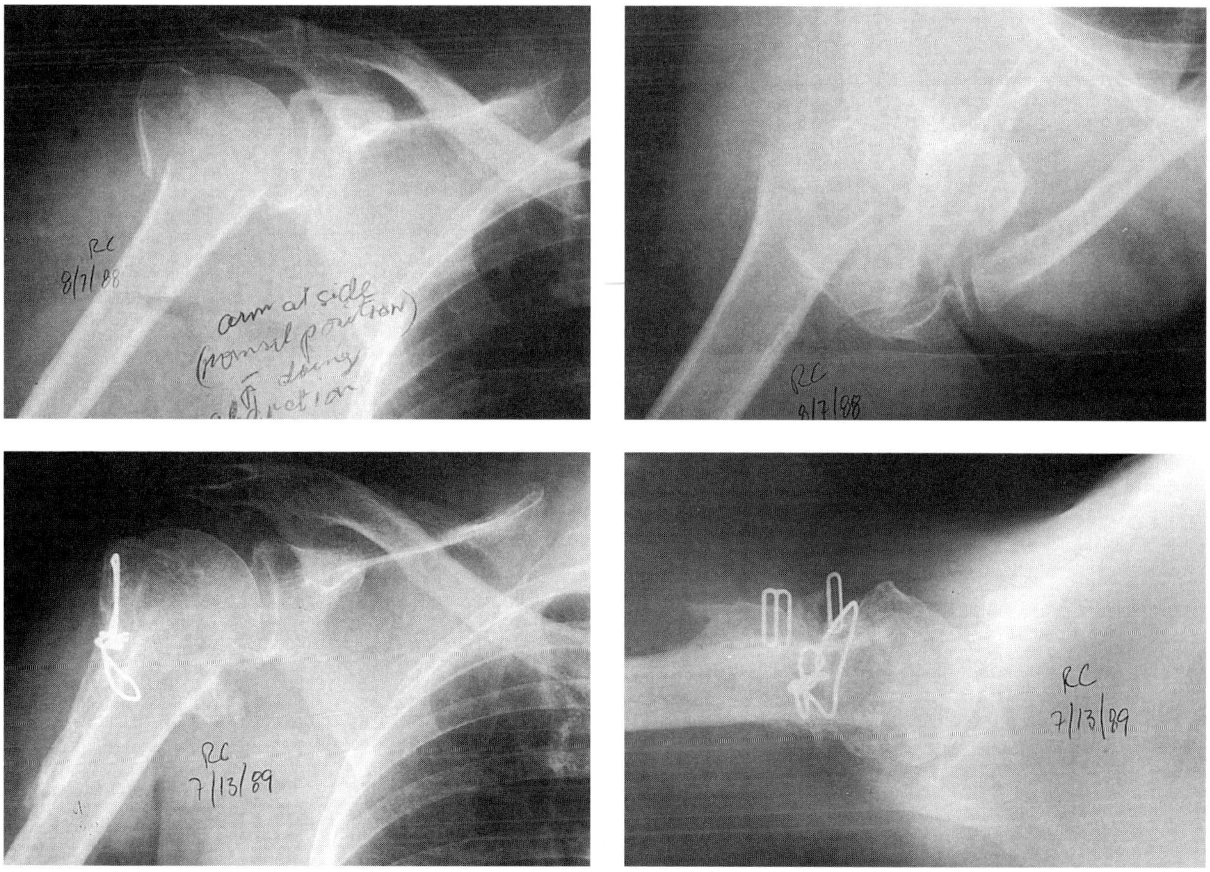

FIGURE 11-21 The wire tension band technique of Weber has been used in a fracture consisting of a valgus impacted head/neck component with associated tuberosity displacement. The tension band restores the approximate alignment of the tuberosities, avoiding the problem of subacromial impingement. The head should not be disengaged from the shaft during surgery on such fractures.

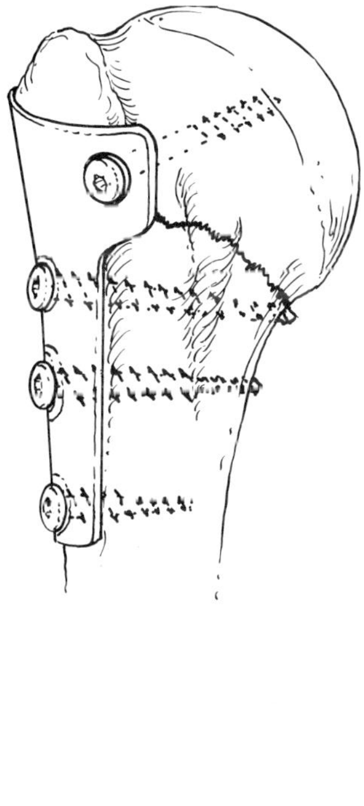

FIGURE 11-22 Buttress plate fixation. The plate functions as a neutralization plate device. Care must be taken not to injure the biceps tendon.

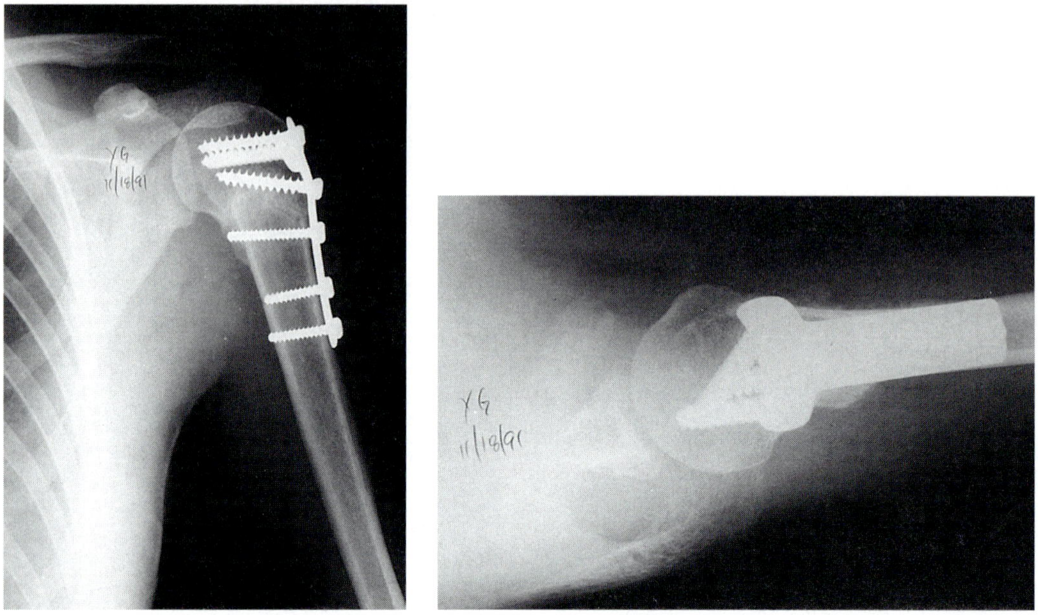

FIGURE 11-23 An ASIF buttress plate was used as a tension band device for a malpositioned pseudarthrosis. The patient, a veterinarian in her twenties, experienced pain and limitation of forward flexion and abduction. Treatment included derotating the head relative to the shaft and correcting varus. A tensioned T-plate and then an interfragmentary lag screw through the plate were applied.

TABLE 11-2
Results of Diverse Treatments for Displaced Proximal Humerus Fractures Using the Neer Criteria

Author	Year	Technique	Excellent (>89)	Satisfactory (80)	Unsatisfactory (70)	Poor (<70)
Mills[16a]	1985	Closed			47%	
Rasmussen[27a]	1992	Closed	2	10	7	23
Young[36a]	1985	Closed				
Kristiansen[13a]	1988	Closed reduction	1	3	2	4
Kristiansen[13]	1987	External fixation	3	6	2	0
Kristiansen[13a]	1988	External fixation	5	3	2	1
Mouradian[20]	1986	Nail				
Kocialkowski[12]	1990	K Wires	7	1	2	11
Paavolainen[25]	1983	Plate		23		8
Savoie[31]	1989	Plate				
Kristiansen[12a]	1986	Plate		9 of 20		11 of 20
Flatow[6]	1991	Suture	6	6	0	0
Hawkins[8]	1986	Suture				

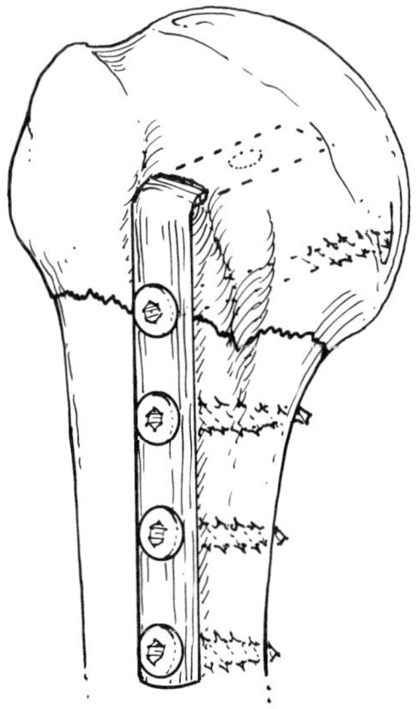

FIGURE 11-24 Blade plate fixation. Excellent bone quality is a prerequisite when attempting fixation with a blade plate.

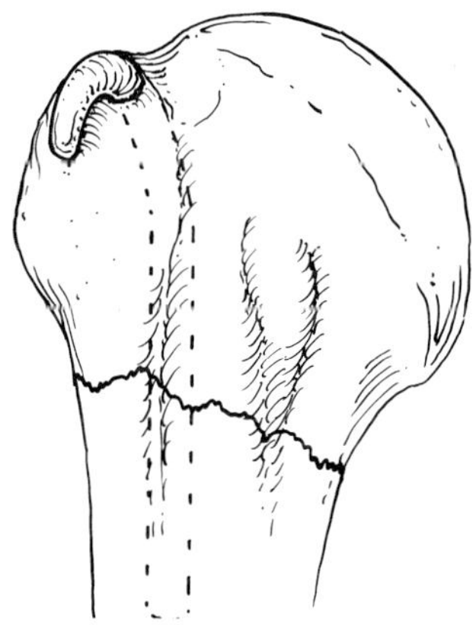

FIGURE 11-25 Rush rod technique. This technique has limited use because of its failure to control rotational instability and the potential complication of subacromial impingement.

mechanical forces operating on the proximal humerus with plates are primarily tension and torsion rather than compression, leading to loss of fixation in patients with soft bone.

Paavolainen et al reported 23 of 31 patients (74%) with good to excellent results by the Neer criteria using buttress plates and lag screws.[25] Savoie et al also successfully used similar techniques in a group of 9 patients with three-part fractures.[31] All 9 patients were followed for 2 years or more and had a satisfactory or better rating using the same Neer criteria. Patients averaged 110° of abduction (range, 100° to 170°), 130° of flexion (range, 100° to 170°), and 35° of external rotation (range, 10° to 60°). Combining both of these series, 9 of 40 patients subsequently had impingement (23%), 3 of 40 had avascular neurosis (8%), 1 of 40 had a deep infection (3%), and 2 of 40 patients had a superficial infection (5%). There were no nonunions (Table 11-2).

Special plates with a blade component have been designed for use in the proximal humerus (Fig. 11-24). Currently, they are not in widespread use but may have limited indications.[32]

Intramedullary Nail

The proximal humerus has a capacious intramedullary canal, making purchase with a conventional intramedullary device, tenuous. Humerus intramedullary nail devices such as Rush and Ender rods provide limited stability and generally should be avoided (Figs. 11-25 and 11-26). Enhanced fixation is possible by adding cerclage wire through the "eye" of an Ender rod. Intramedullary devices that penetrate the rotator cuff at the greater

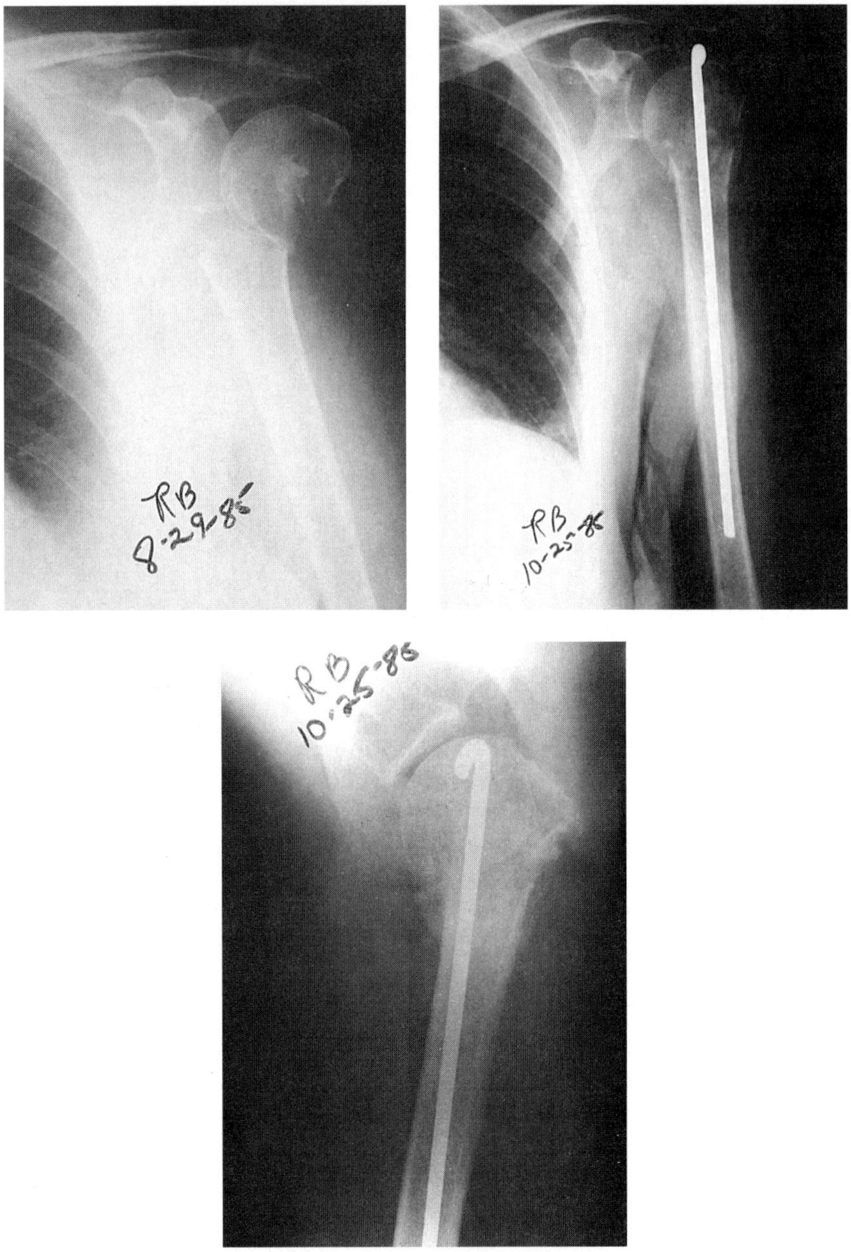

FIGURE 11-26 Although not a favored or reliable technique, a Rush rod was used to maintain position of this easily reduced, two-part neck shaft translocation fracture.

tuberosity may create mechanical subacromial impingement. Pain may result even if the device is countersunk beneath the level of the greater tuberosity.

Intramedullary devices with proximal locking mechanisms improve the quality of purchase proximally and are useful in some situations. The Mouradian nail has several advantages over other locking nails. The entry portal is located below the top of the greater tuberosity and may be countersunk within the substance of the tuberosity, decreasing impingement problems. Proximal fixation is provided by two large cancellous screws that seat within the proximal nail, adding torsional stiffness to the construct. Finally, the device may be used in some unstable three- and four-part fractures. In such cases, the head is linked to the shaft with the nail, and the tuberosities are repaired in a fashion similar to the technique employed in hemiarthroplasty (Figs. 11-27 through 11-29).

Mouradian reported on his nail for 6 two-part, 10 three-part, and 7 four-part acute fractures.[20] Results were presented as average Neer score by fracture grouping, with 6 patients with two-part fractures having 86.50, 7 with three-part fractures having 80.00, and 10 with

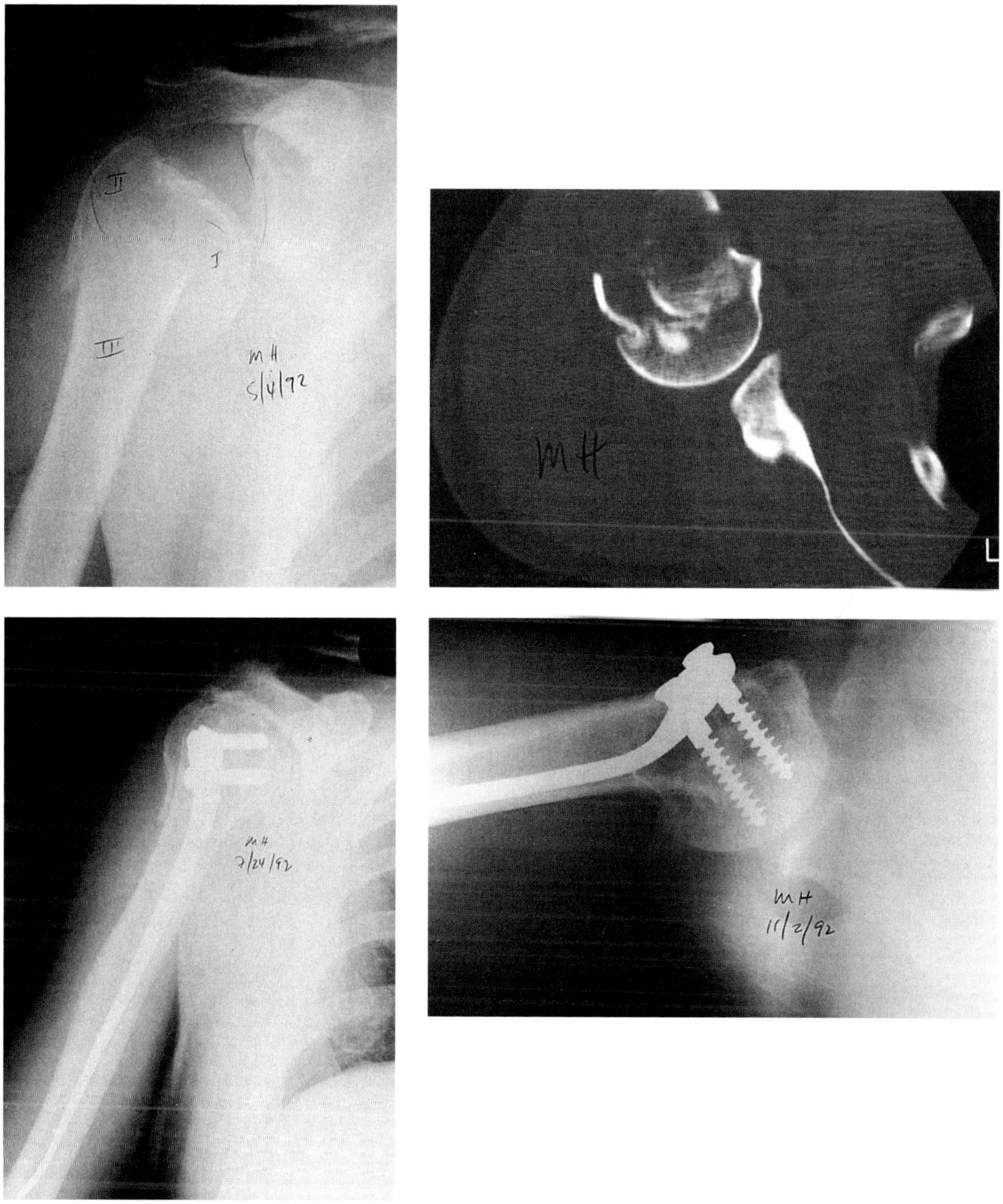

FIGURE 11-27 A 40-year-old cyclist suffered this three-part fracture with subluxation of the head. A Mouradian nail was used to reestablish continuity between the head and the shaft, and the greater tuberosity was sutured to the lesser tuberosity with heavy suture. A range-of-motion program was instituted within days of surgery, allowing recovery of a functional arc of motion.

three-part and four-part fracture dislocation having 80.80. All patients healed without infection, but there were 4 patients with radiographic evidence of avascular necrosis, 5 with impingement, and 2 with secondary displacement (see Table 11-2).

Multiple Pins

Retrograde fixation by means of percutaneous Kirschner wires or Steinmann pins has the advantage of less soft-tissue disruption than the aforementioned techniques. Jaberg et al have modified the technique by using three to five 2.5-mm pins that are threaded at their tips[10] (Fig. 11-30). Displaced fragments are manipulated percutaneously under fluoroscopic control to achieve a "closed reduction," then are transfixed with the manipulating pin. Considerable skill is required.

Two-, three-, and some four-part fractures have been treated successfully like this. Most of the fractures reported by Jaberg were two-part fractures in which reduction could not be maintained. Of 48 patients, 4 required reoperation because of loss of fixation, 2 developed global avascular necrosis, and 8 developed

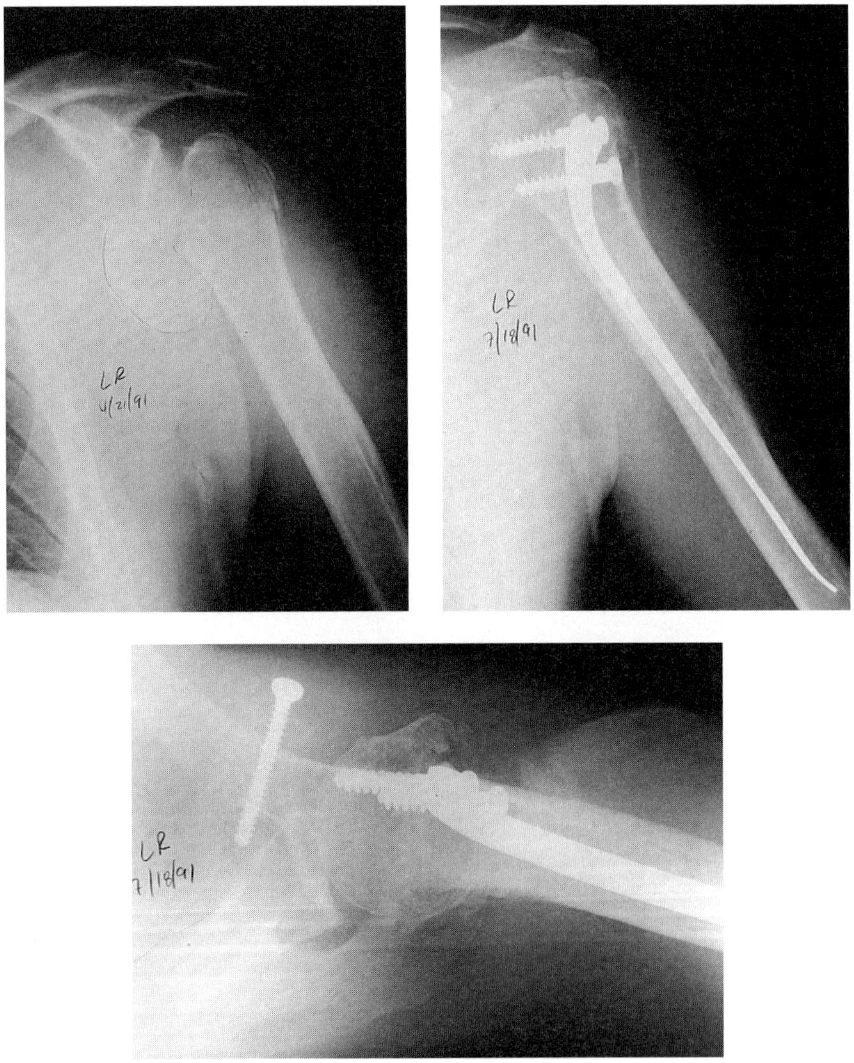

FIGURE 11-28 A three-part fracture-dislocation resulted from a fall off a ladder in a man in his late forties. His head was tightly wedged into the anterior glenoid, requiring removal of the coracoid process to free the trapped head without traumatically prying out the head. The coracoid later pulled free with no ill effect. The nail is placed within the substance of the tuberosity, reducing impingement.

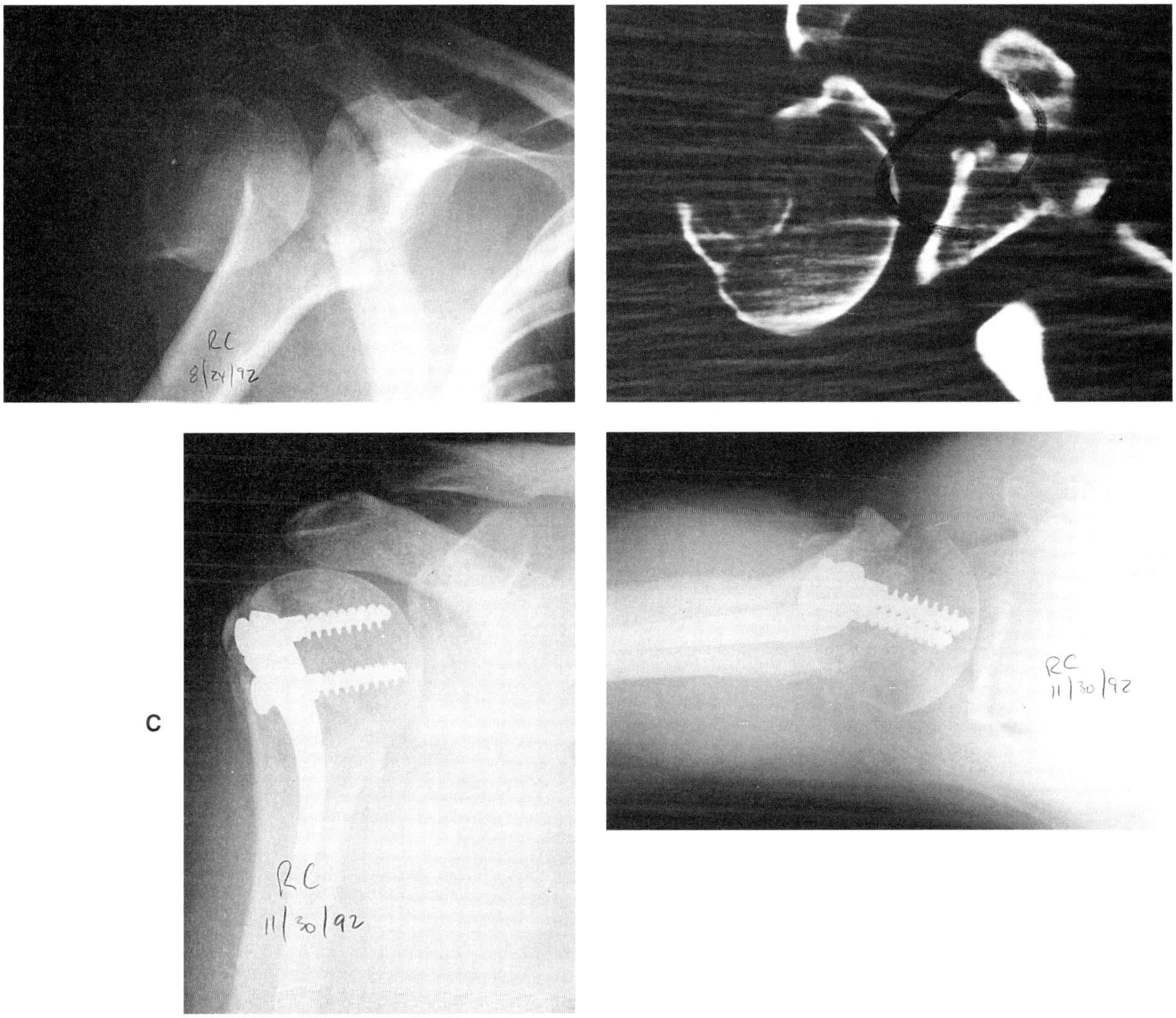

FIGURE 11-29 **A**, A man in his twenties rolled his three-wheeler, sustaining a three-part fracture-dislocation of the proximal humerus. **B**, The CAT scan shows posterior subluxation of the humeral head and an associated glenoid fracture. **C** and **D**, Open reduction was performed through an extended deltopectoral approach. The head had no intact greater or lesser tuberosity attachments but had an intact posterior cuff component.

focal avascular necrosis. According to a point-scale of Saillant, 70% of patients had good to excellent results; no data are offered on the outcome in terms of range of motion.

Kocialkowski used a retrograde smooth Steinmann pin in 18 patients with two-part fractures, 2 with three-part fractures, and 2 with four-part fractures.[12] His patients had 5 infections (23%), 9 secondary displacements (41%), 1 nonunion, and two cases of avascular necrosis. These combined problems led to unsatisfactory results using the Neer criteria in 13 (59%) patients (Table 11-3).

COMPLICATIONS

The complications of proximal humerus fractures include nerve damage, arterial injury, avascular necrosis, infection, loss of motion, heterotopic ossification, malunion, and nonunion (see Table 11-3).

Neurovascular

The neurovascular bundle is at risk during anterior fracture-dislocations and displaced surgical neck injuries when the humeral shaft is pulled anteromedially by the pectoralis major (Fig. 11-31,*A*). Axillary artery injury sec-

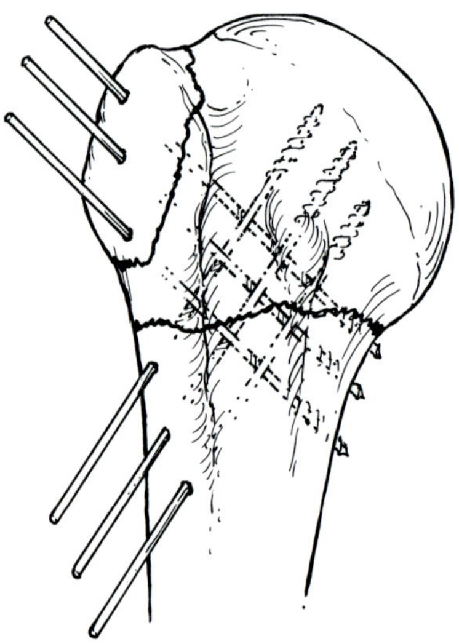

FIGURE 11-30 Multiple threaded pins. Percutaneous manipulation of fragments under fluoroscopy can reduce displaced two-part fractures; infection and secondary displacement remain significant complications.

TABLE 11-3
Complications After Treatment of Displaced Proximal Humerus Fractures

Author	Year	#	Two-part	Three-part	Four-part
Mills[16a]	1985	33	19		
Rasmussen[27a]	1992	42	16	17	9
Young[36a]	1985	64	32	3	
Kristiansen[12c]	1987	11			
Kristiansen[13]	1987	12	2	8	2
Kristiansen[12a]	1988	10			
Mouradian[20]	1986	22	6	10	7
Kocialkowski[12]	1990	22	18	2	2
Paavolainen[25]	1983	31	20	16	5
Savoie[31]	1989	9		9	
Kristiansen[12a]	1986	32	6		
Flatow[6]	1991	12	12	0	0
Hawkins[8]	1986	15		15	
TOTAL		315	131	80	25
			56%	34%	11%

AVN, avascular necrosis; *NDR,* no data recorded.

ondary to displaced proximal humerus fractures is rare but has been reported[37] (Fig. 11-31, *B* and *C*). The authors have seen 2 combined axillary artery and nerve injuries in a series of 41 displaced proximal humerus fractures for an incidence of 5%. The axillary artery was successfully repaired in both cases and had no effect on outcome.

The incidence of nerve injuries was 3 of 41 fractures, or 7%. In 1 of the 3 cases, there was complete return. One patient had permanent severe brachial plexus dysfunction, and the third was left with permanent deltoid atrophy resulting from axillary nerve damage.

In a study of four-part proximal humerus fractures, Stableforth noted that vascular injuries accompanied 4.9% of 81 patients, and brachial plexus injuries occurred in 6.1%.[35] Signs of nerve damage were delayed for 24 hours in 2 of the patients. Recovery was complete for 2 patients, but 3 patients had an incomplete recovery with no functional improvement more than 2 years after injury.

Urgent operative correction is mandatory on a neurologic as well as vascular basis (Fig. 11-32). Good anastomotic circulation is present in the upper extremity, so limb viability usually is maintained. Nerves may be stretched tightly over bone fragments, adding a time-related ischemic component to the initial kinetic insult. Observation should be the second treatment, after fracture stabilization. Electromyography is reserved for lesions that show no improvement 3 weeks after injury, because fibrillation potentials (the most sensitive indicator of motor axon loss) do not appear until then.

Heterotopic Ossification

Heterotopic ossification is an infrequent complication of proximal humerus fractures. Neer described the callus that forms around the extruded head of a fracture-dislocation as "pericapsular" bone.[23] This complication is rare except after a fracture-dislocation where there is ligamentous injury outside the joint. The bone disappears over time and rarely requires treatment other than observation. As in other sites of the body, resection of heterotopic bone is ill-advised before bone maturity as documented on bone scintigraphy.

Avascular Necrosis

Avascular necrosis of the humeral head is occasionally a debilitating complication of proximal humerus fractures. In extensively comminuted three-part fractures, four-part fractures, and fracture-dislocations, soft-tissue attachments to the head are traumatized, compromising blood supply to the head (Fig. 11-33). Avascular necrosis has been reported in 13% to 40% of three- and four-part fractures.[7,25] Frequently, the head revascularizes and does not require additional surgery. However, total collapse with severe arthrosis does occur and requires salvage with arthrodesis (Fig. 11-34) or arthroplasty.

Frozen Shoulder

In the younger patient, fractures of the proximal humerus can result in loss of motion with concomitant pain and limitation of function. Physical therapy is essential in regaining motion after injury but does not guarantee full recovery.[27] Manipulation under anesthesia is

Method	Infection	Secondary Displacement	AVN	Pseudarthrosis	Impingements
Closed					
Closed	0	0	5	5	
Closed Reduction	0	0	2	4	
External fixation	2	2	0	0	
External fixation	1	1	1	1	
Nail	0	2	4	0	5
PK wires	5	9	2	1	
Plate	3	2	0	0	6
Plate	0	0	3	0	
Plate	4	2	4	0	5
Suture	0	0	0	0	0
Suture	0	0	2	0	1
	6%	7%	4%		

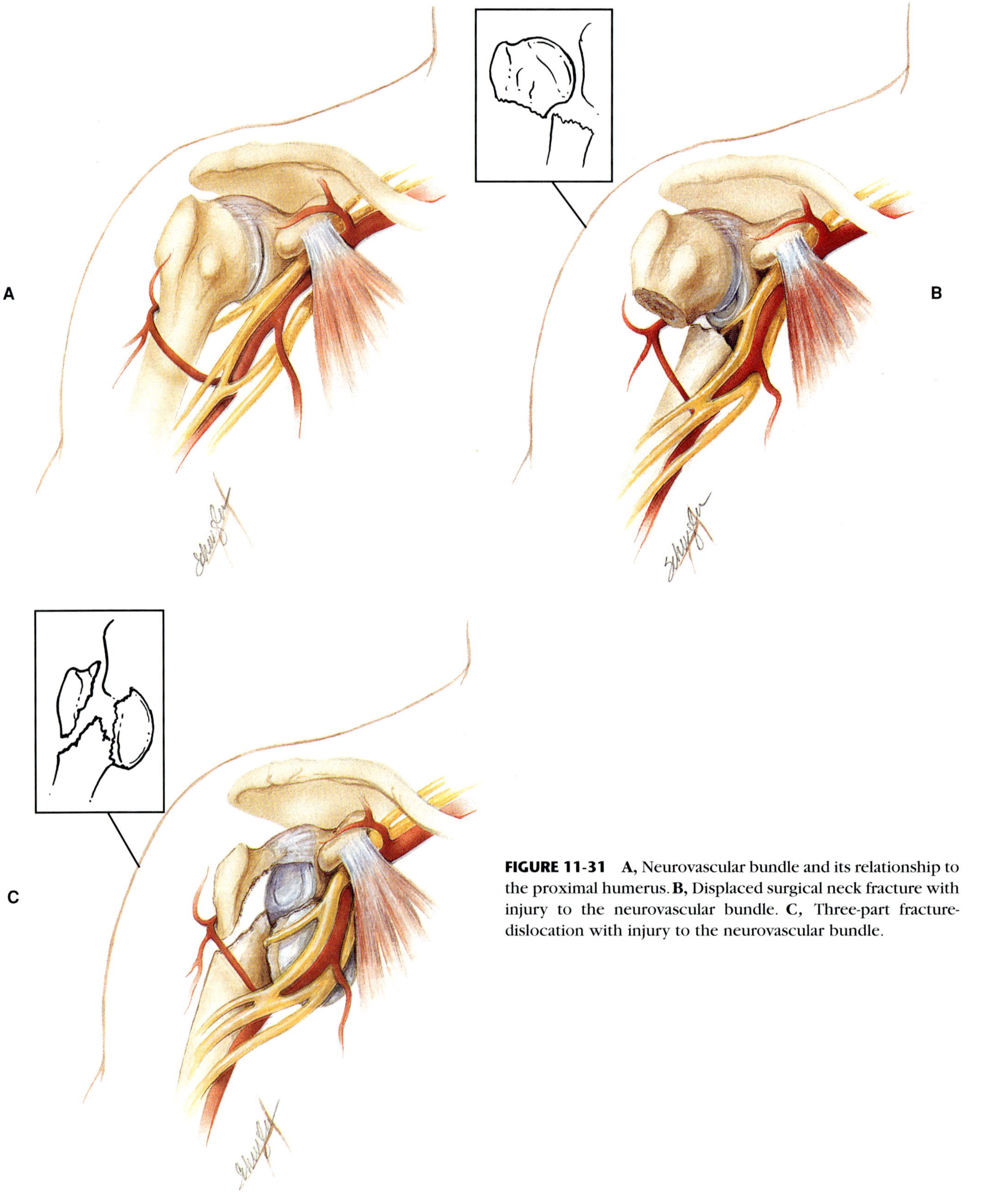

FIGURE 11-31 **A,** Neurovascular bundle and its relationship to the proximal humerus. **B,** Displaced surgical neck fracture with injury to the neurovascular bundle. **C,** Three-part fracture-dislocation with injury to the neurovascular bundle.

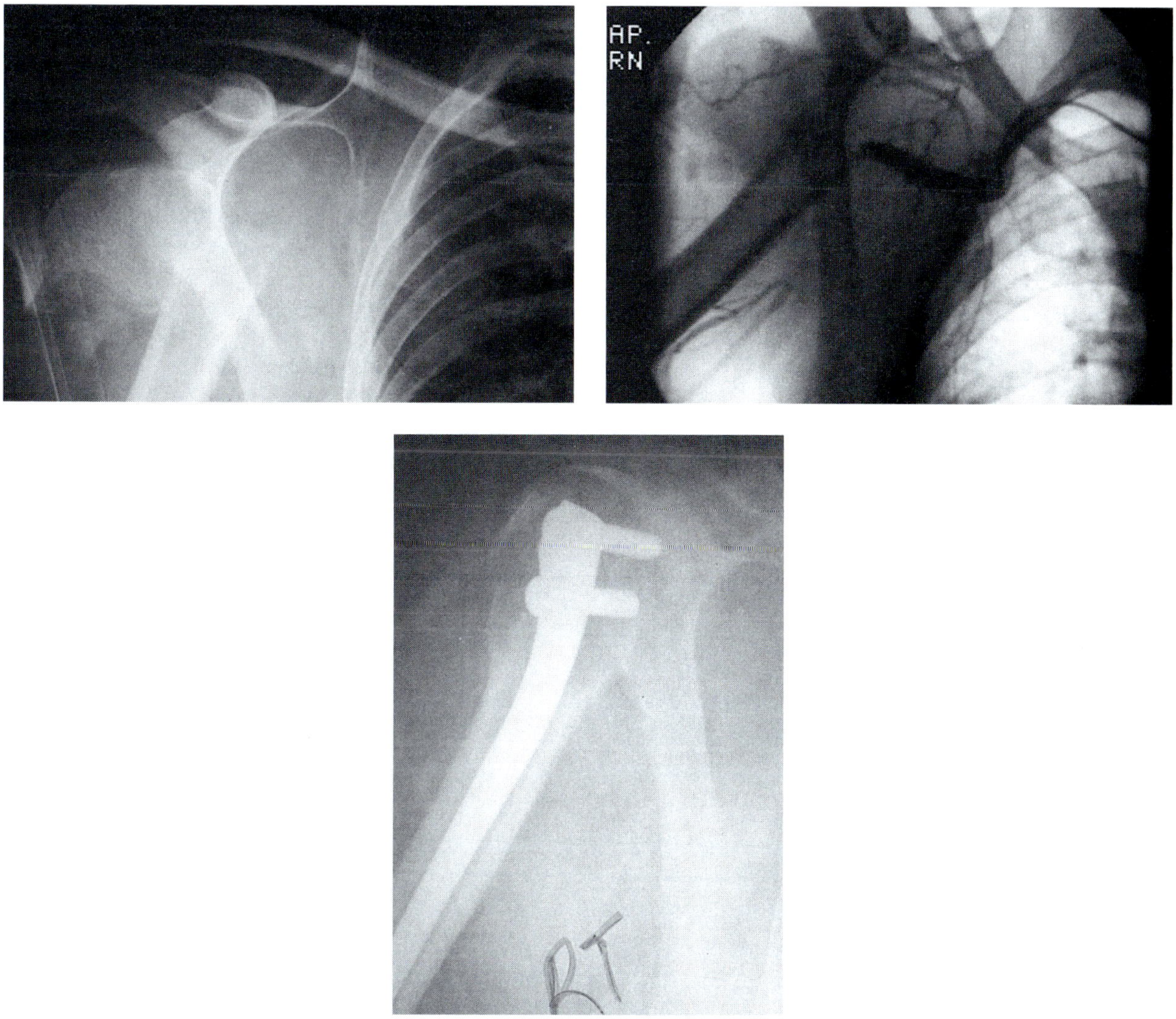

FIGURE 11-32 This four-part fracture-dislocation occurred when a thoroughbred race horse fell on the patient. The humeral shaft was violently thrust into the anteromedial soft tissues and penetrated the arterial adventitia, kinking the vessel but not causing a rupture or intimal lesion. In treatment, the bone was disengaged from the vessel and the vessel explored, but no lesion was identified. Normal flow ensued with no vascular sequelae. The humeral head has undergone union, with radiographic evidence of avascular necrosis without collapse. The patient's neurovascular deficit is profound and so dominates the clinical picture. The avascular process is relatively silent to date, 9 months after injury

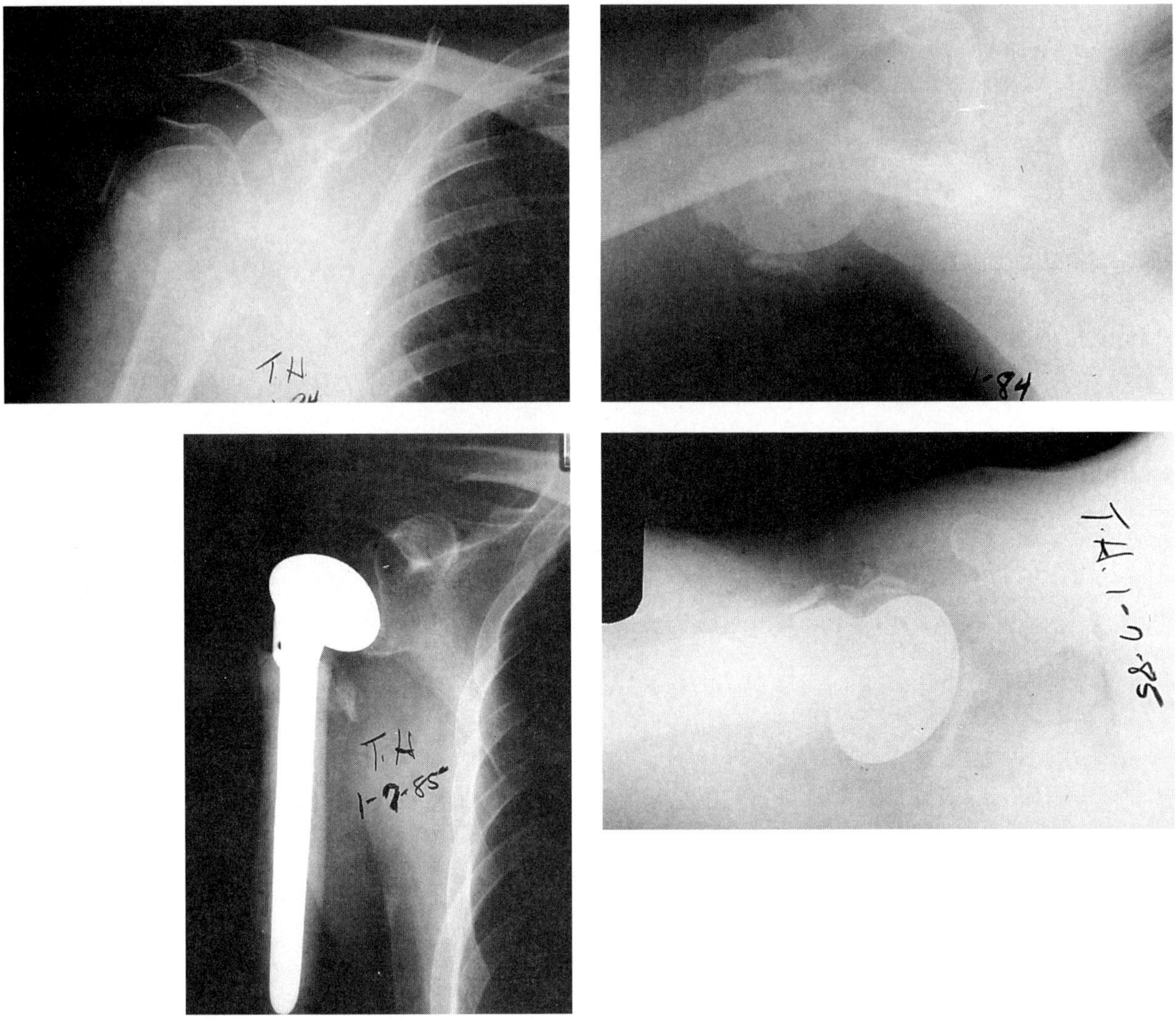

FIGURE 11-33 The humeral head is totally separated from its blood supply by this four-part fracture-dislocation. Because of the lack of blood supply, hemiarthroplasty was the selected technique. The patient is pain free at 8-year follow-up. Funtionally, he can play golf.

recommended if physical therapy fails to provide adequate ROM and is best performed after fracture union sometime between 3 and 6 months after injury.[24] Early passive and active range of motion must be achieved to prevent recurrence of fibrosis.

Malunion

Malunion of proximal humerus fractures, particularly the tuberosities, can lead to significant dysfunction. Displacement of the greater tuberosity can cause subacromial or glenoid impingement. Morris et al have presented successful outcomes after corrective osteotomy of symptomatic malunited tuberosity fractures by using screw fixation.[19] Correction of angular malunion also should be considered if functional limitation can be clearly attributed to malunion and not fibrosis. Malunion of comminuted three- or four-part fractures often requires revision to hemiarthroplasty (Fig. 11-35). Most authors recommend hemiarthroplasty as the initial treatment of comminuted three- or four-part fractures and fracture-dislocations.[4,17,23,28,36]

Nonunion

Pseudarthrosis occurs both after initial closed treatment and with initial surgery. Weber reported 7 proximal humeral pseudarthroses out of a total of 45 humeral pseudarthroses. Of the 7, 6 healed with plate osteosynthesis, and 1 failed to unite after arthrodesis of the shoulder combined with plate osteosynthesis of the pseudarthrosis.

As with acute fractures, no single operative plan applies uniformly to pseudarthroses of the proximal humerus. Hemiarthroplasty may be necessary if the head fragment is avascular or is insufficient for fixation. In a younger patient, destruction of the joint or severe deformity of the tuberosities may require arthrodesis. Simpler

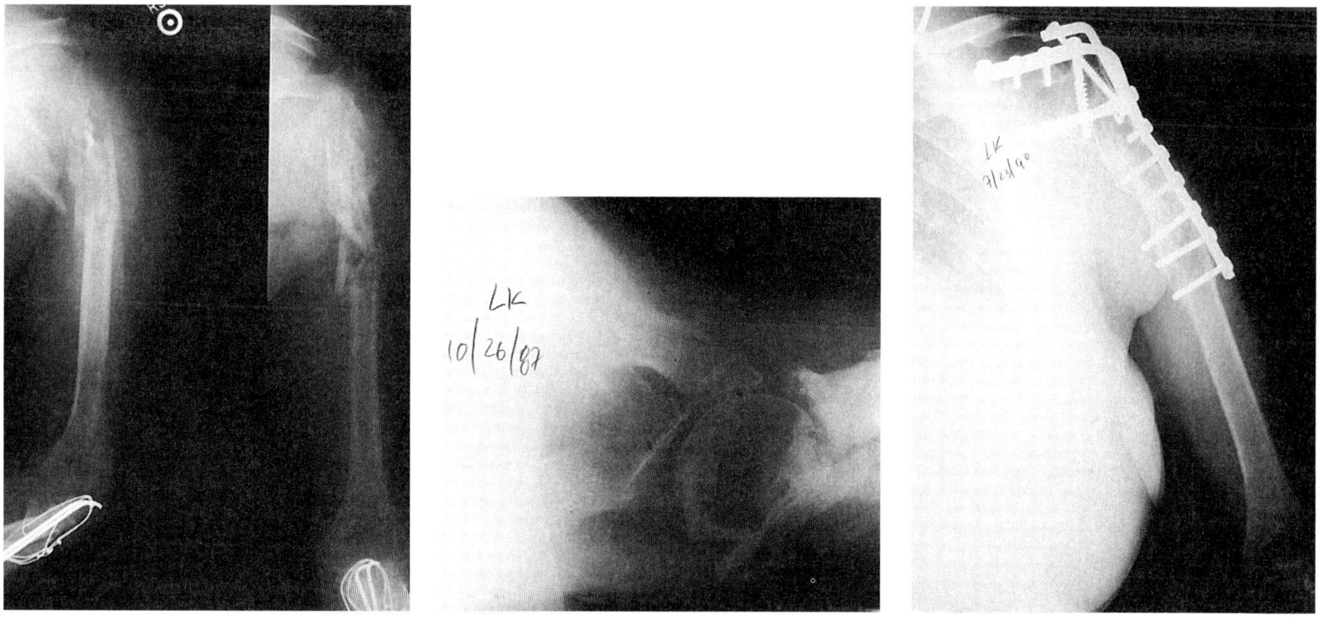

FIGURE 11-34 This former roller derby star was involved in vehicular trauma that produced a four-part proximal fracture with associated comminution of the shaft. A painful pseudarthrosis resulted. At surgery, the head was found to be deformed, with extremely poor-quality articular cartilage and bone. The joint was fused, and the pseudarthrosis was stabilized with a plate. The patient has restricted motion but is able to run her own catering business.

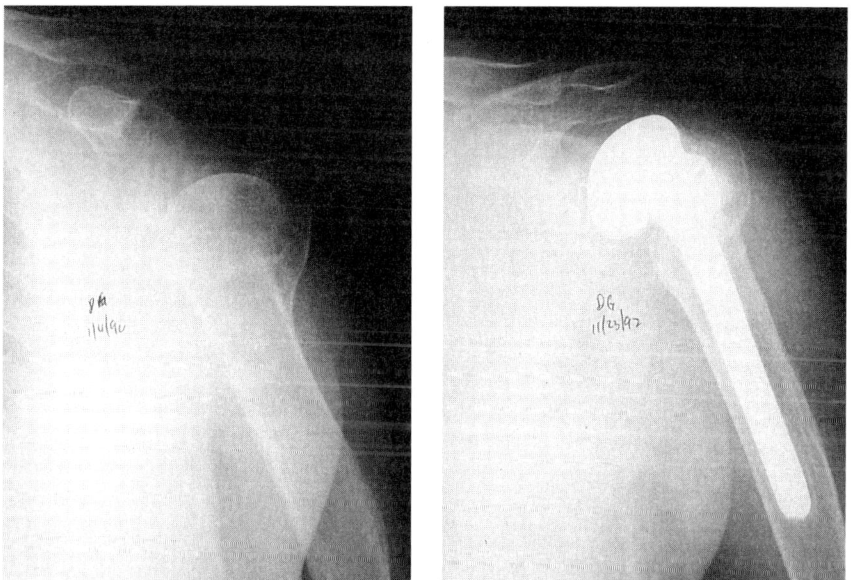

FIGURE 11-35 An impacted four-part fracture left the patient with painful limited motion. Arthroplasty substantially reduced the level of pain while increasing function.

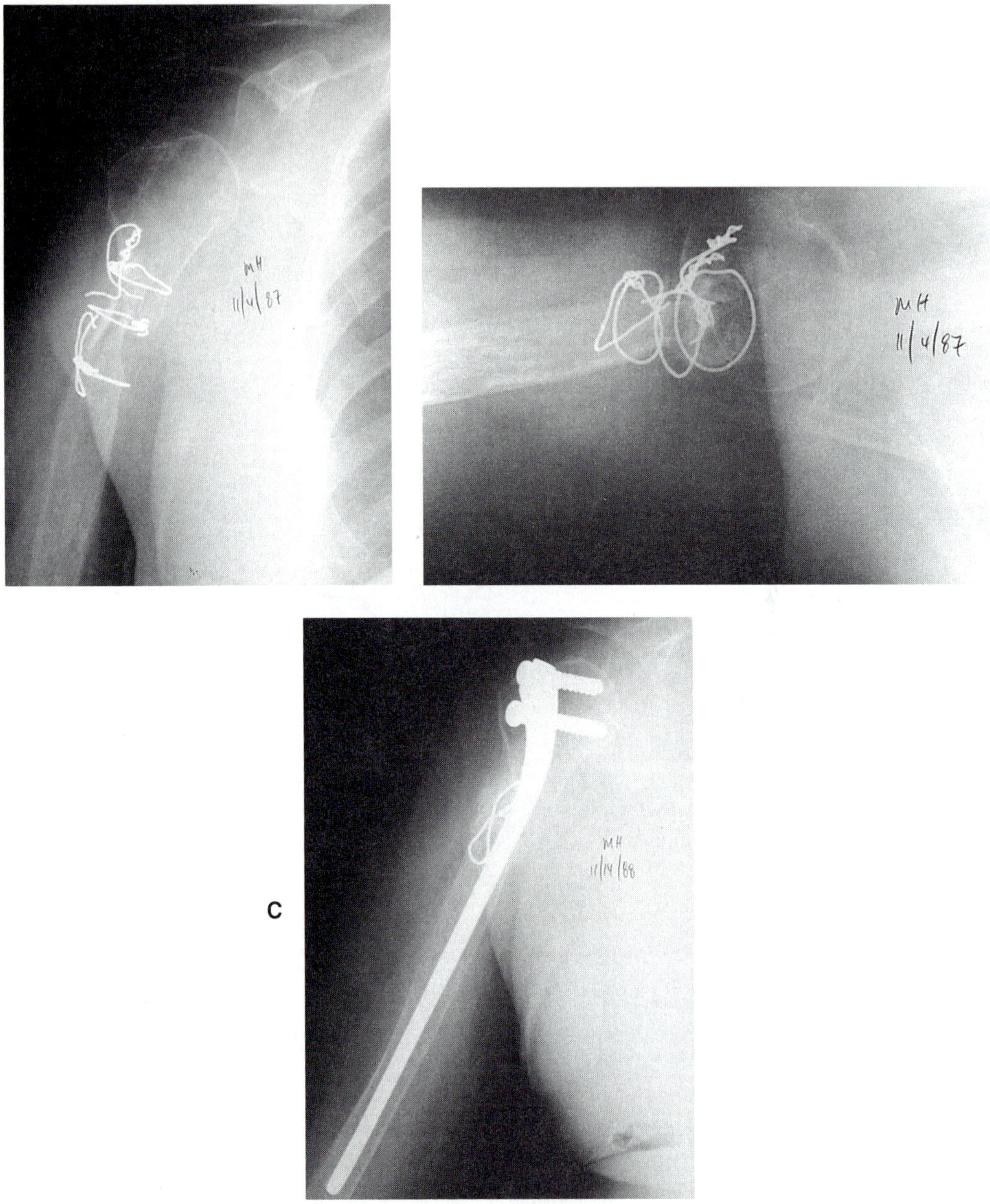

A

B

C

FIGURE 11-36 **A** and **B,** Preoperative AP and axillary views of a defect type nonunion reconstructed wtih a Mouradian nail. **C,** One graft and tension band wire.

infratuberous or surgical neck pseudarthroses can be repaired with plates or nails (Figs. 11-36 and 11-37).

Complications after treatment of displaced proximal humerus fractures are listed in Table 11-3.

SUMMARY

Proximal humerus fractures account for 4% to 5% of all fractures and are most common in elderly females. These fractures do occur in the young, athletically active population and in this population represent a higher level of trauma than in the elderly patient. Proximal humerus fractures represent a spectrum of injury from a benign fracture that heals with complete painless range of motion and full functional recovery to an extensively comminuted fracture requiring prosthetic replacement for pain-free but limited function.

An aggressive approach to diagnosis, treatment, and rehabilitation is essential to prevent the debilitating sequelae of these fractures. Complications such as stiffness, impingement, and limitation of motion are not uncommon with or without surgery. More serious complications, although rare, do occur and can be disastrous if neurovascular structures are compromised.

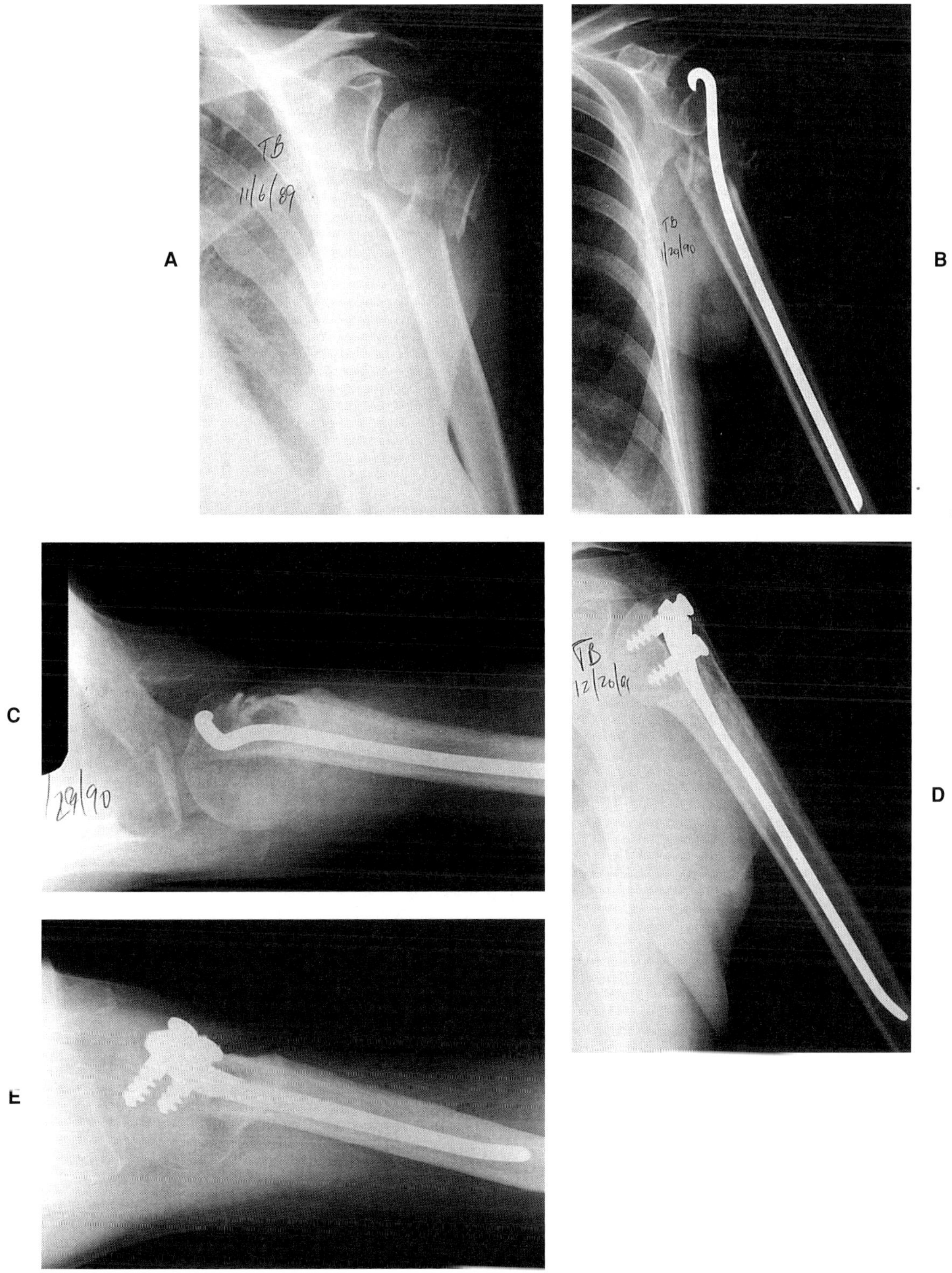

FIGURE 11-37 **A,** Displaced proximal humeral fracture with associated axillary artery injury. **B** and **C,** Initial treatment with Rush rod leading to nonunion. **D** and **E,** Salvage with Mouradian nail and bone graft. An intramedullary nail is also useful in the treatment of nonunion unamenable to plate and screw fixation because of poor bone quality.

Fixation techniques are varied and must be tailored to the fracture type and the surgeon's skills. New fixation methods, such as improved locking nails, may provide more consistent results. Further study will help identify better diagnostic, surgical, and rehabilitation techniques to improve functional outcome.

References

1. American Academy of Orthopaedic Surgeons: *Joint motion: method of measuring and recording,* Chicago, 1965, American Academy of Orthopaedic Surgeons.
2. Brunner CF, Weber BG: *Special techniques in internal fixation,* New York, 1982, Springer-Verlag.
3. Castagno AA et al: Complex fractures of the proximal humerus: role of CT in treatment, *Radiology* 165:759, 1987.

3a. Clark JM, Harryman DT: Tendons, ligaments and capsule of the rotator cuff, *J Bone Joint Surg* 74A:713, 1992.

4. Cofield RH: Comminuted fractures of the proximal humerus, *Clin Orthop* 230:49-57, 1988.
5. Codman EA: *The shoulder: rupture of the supraspinatus tendon and other lesions in or about the subacromial bursa,* Merbourn, Fla, 1984, Robert Krieger Publishers.
6. Flatow EL et al: Open reduction and internal fixation of two-part displaced fractures of the greater tuberosity of the proximal part of the humerus, *J Bone Joint Surg* 73A:1213-1217, 1991.
7. Frich LH, Sojberg JO, Sneppen O: Shoulder arthroplasty in complex acute and chronic proximal humeral fractures, *Orthopedics* 14(9): 949-954, 1991.
8. Hawkins RJ, Bell RH, Gurr K: The three-part fracture of the proximal part of the humerus, *J Bone Joint Surg* 68A:1410-1414, 1986.
9. Horak J, Nilsson B: Epidemiology of fractures of the upper end of the humerus, *Clin Orthop* 112:250-253, 1975.
10. Jaberg H, Warner JJP, Jakob RP: Percutaneous stabilization of unstable fractures of the humerus, *J Bone Joint Surg* 74A:509-515, 1992.
11. Kelsey JL et al: Risk factors for fractures of the distal forearm and proximal humerus, *Am J Epidemiol* 135(5):477-489, 1992.
12. Kocialkowski A, Wallace WA: Closed percutaneous K-wire stabilization for displaced fractures of the surgical neck of the humerus, *Injury* 21:209-212, 1990.

12a. Kristiansen B, Christiansen SW: Plate fixation of proximal humeral fractures, *Acta Orthop Scand* 57:320-323, 1986.

12b. Kristiansen B et al: The Neer classification of fractures of the proximal humerus, *Skeletal Radiology* 17: 420, 1988.

12c. Kristinasen B et al: External fixation of displaced fractures of the proximal humerus, *J Bone Joint Surg* 69:643, 1987.

13. Kristiansen B, Christiansen SW: Proximal humeral fractures: late results in relation to classification and treatment, *Acta Orthop Scand* 58:124-127, 1987.

13a. Kristiansen B, Kofoed H: Transcutaneous reduction and external fixation of displaced fractures of the proximal humerus: a controlled clinical trial, *J Bone Joint Surg (B)* 70(5):821-824, 1988.

14. Kuhlman JE et al: Complex shoulder trauma: three dimensional CT imaging, *Orthopedics* 11(11):1561, 1988.
15. Leyshon RL: Closed treatment of fractures of the proximal humerus, *Acta Orthop Scand* 55:48, 1984.
16. Lind T, Kroner K, Jensen J: The epidemiology of fractures of the proximal humerus, *Arch Orthop Trauma Surg* 108:285, 1989.

16a. Mills HJ, Horne G: Fractures of the proximal humerus in adults, *J Trauma* 25:801, 1985.

17. Moeckel BH et al: Modular hemiarthroplasty for fractures of the proximal part of the humerus, *J Bone Joint Surg* 74A(6):884, 1992.
18. Moriber LA, Patterson RL Jr: Fractures of the proximal end of the humerus, *J Bone Joint Surg* 49A:1018, 1967.
19. Morris ME et al: Humeral tuberosity fractures: evaluation by CT scan and management of malunion, unpublished.
20. Mouradian WH: Displaced proximal humerus fractures: seven years experience with a modified Zickel supracondylar device, *Clin Orthop* 212:209, 1986.
21. Mueller ME et al: *The comprehensive classification of fractures of long bones,* Berlin, 1990, Springer-Verlag.
22. Neer CS: Displaced proximal humeral fractures: part I, classification and evaluation, *J Bone Joint Surg* 52A:1077, 1970.
23. Neer CS: Displaced proximal humeral fractures: part II, treatment of three-part and four-part displacement, *J Bone Joint Surg* 52A:1090, 1970.
24. Ogilvie-Harris DJ: *Arthroscopic treatment of the frozen shoulder,* presented at the annual meeting of the Arthroscopy Association of North America, Monterey, Calif, 1992.
25. Paavolainen P et al: Operative treatment of severe proximal humeral fractures, *Acta Orthop Scand* 54:374, 1983.
26. Patten RM: Non-displaced fractures of the greater tuberosity of the humerus: sonographic detection, *Radiology* 182:201, 1992.
27. Powell SE et al: *One-part proximal humerus fractures: a prospective study of functional outcome,* presented at the annual meeting of the American Academy of Orthopaedic Surgeons, Washington, DC, 1992.

27a. Raumassen et al: Displaced proximal humerus fractures: results of conservative treatment, *Injury* 23:41, 1992.

28. Reckling FW: Posterior fracture-dislocation of the shoulder treated by a Neer hemiarthroplasty with a posterior surgical approach, *Clin Orthop* 207:133, 1986.
29. Richardson JB et al: Radiographs in shoulder trauma, *J Bone Joint Surg* 70B:457, 1988.
30. Rose SH et al: Epidemiologic features of humeral fractures, *Clin Orthop* 168:24, 1982.
31. Savoie FH, Geissler WB, VanderGriend RA: Open reduction and internal fixation of three-part fractures of the proximal humerus, *Orthopedics* 12:65, 1989.
32. Sehr JR, Szabo RM: Semitubular blade plate for fixation in the proximal humerus, *J Orthop Trauma* 2:327, 1992.
33. Sidor ML et al: Neer classification of proximal humerus fractures: assessment of inter- and intra-observer reliability, *J Bone Joint Surg* 75A:1745, 1993.
34. Sidor ML et al: The relative contribution of scapular lateral and axillary radiographs to Neer classification of proximal humerus fractures, *J Shoulder Elbow Surg* 3(1):24, 1994.
35. Stableforth PG: Four-part fractures of the neck of the humerus, *J Bone Joint Surg* 66B:104, 1984.
36. Tanner MW, Cofield RH: Prosthetic arthroplasty for fractures and fracture dislocations of the proximal humerus, *Clin Orthop* 179: 116, 1983.

36a. Young TB, Wallace WA: Conservative treatment of fractures and fracture-dislocation of the upper end of the humerus, *J Bone Joint Surg* 67B:373, 1985.

37. Zuckerman JD et al: Axillary artery injury as complication of proximal humerus fractures, *Clin Orthop* 189:234, 1984.

CHAPTER 12

Disorders of the Scapula and Clavice

RALPH A. GAMBARDELLA

NICK M. DIGIOVINE

Injuries to the acromioclavicular joint are common in all athletes. The prevalence is higher in those participating in contact sports such as football, hockey, rugby, and soccer. However, acromioclavicular injuries also occur frequently in such "noncontact" sports as cycling, baseball, and weight lifting.

In contrast, sternoclavicular and scapulothoracic injuries are rare in the athletic population. When they occur, however, these injuries may result in significant disability for the athlete.

This chapter reviews the disorders of these joints and articulations and focuses special attention on the clinical presentation and treatment of these disorders among athletes.

ANATOMY

The shoulder complex is made up of three "true" joints and two articulations: the glenohumeral joint, the acromioclavicular joint, the sternoclavicular joint, the scapulothoracic articulation, and the subacromial articulation (Fig. 12-1). Disorders of the glenohumeral joint and subacromial articulation will be discussed elsewhere. This chapter deals with the disorders of the clavicle, acromioclavicular joint, sternoclavicular joint, and scapulothoracic articulation.

Support for the upper extremity begins proximally at the sternoclavicular joint. The sternoclavicular joint is a diarthrodial joint. Less than 50% of the medial clavicle articulates with the clavicular notch of the sternum. This makes the sternoclavicular joint one of the more unstable in the body. Stability of the joint depends on the surrounding ligaments. These consist of the costoclavicular, interclavicular, and sternoclavicular ligaments, as well as the intraarticular disc ligament, which divides the joint into two separate compartments (Fig. 12-2, *B*). The sternoclavicular ligament is the first or primary stabilizer against upper displacement of the medial clavicle.[9]

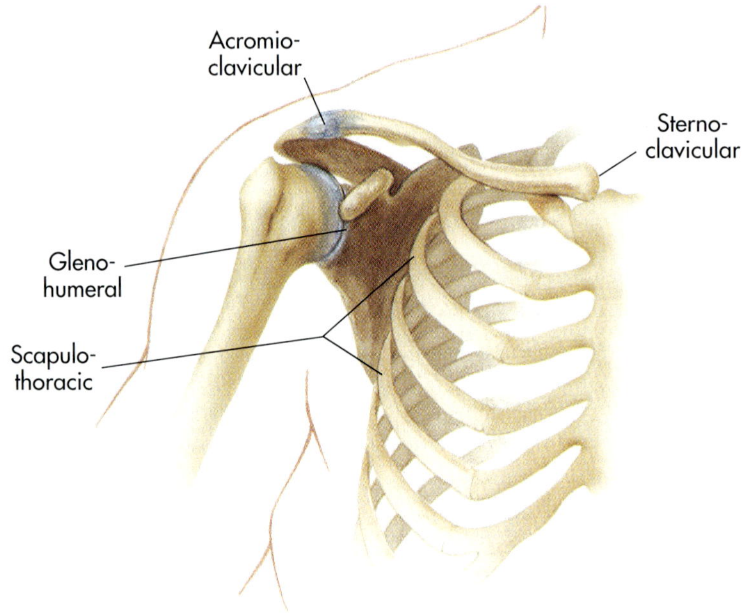

FIGURE 12-1 Shoulder joint complex: glenohumeral, acromioclavicular, sternoclavicular, scapulothoracic.

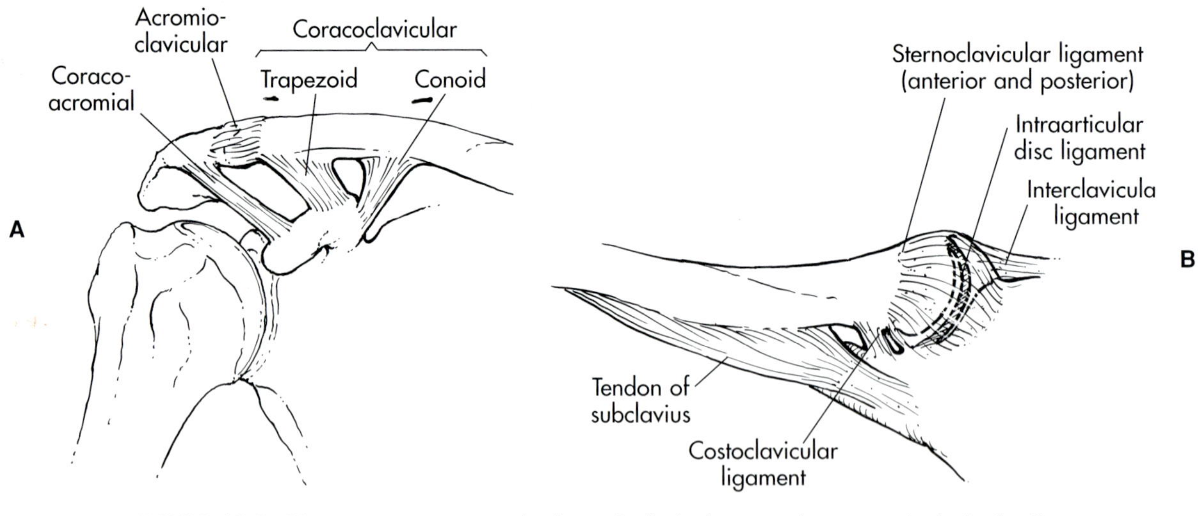

FIGURE 12-2 Ligamentous anatomy. **A,** Acromioclavicular complex: acromioclavicular ligament, coracoacromial ligament, coracoclavicular ligament. **B,** Sternoclavicular complex: sternoclavicular ligament, costoclavicular ligament, interclavicular ligament, intraarticular disc ligament.

Moving distally, the next most important structure is the coracoclavicular ligament. This ligament consists of two parts: the conoid and the trapezoid ligaments (Fig. 12-2, *A*). These ligaments stretch from the base of the coracoid process to the distal end of the clavicle. The conoid ligament is located more proximally and is thought to be the primary restraint to superior translation of the clavicle at the acromioclavicular joint. The trapezoid ligament is the primary restraint to acromioclavicular joint compression.[30]

The acromioclavicular ligament is the primary restraint to horizontal displacement.[30,67,82] The acromioclavicular ligament complex has four parts, including anterior, posterior, superior, and inferior ligaments.

As the shoulder moves, the scapula and clavicle rotate together. This is known as "synchronous scapuloclavicular rotation."[20,42] With forward flexion of the arm, the clavicle rotates upward 35°[39] (Fig. 12-3). Very little motion takes place at the acromioclavicular joint. By observing Kirschner wires drilled into the acromion and distal clavicle during range of motion, Rockwood[70] detected only 5° to 8° of motion at the acromioclavicular joint. This paucity of motion at the acromioclavicular joint also is supported by motion studies of shoulders with coracoclavicular arthrodesis[42] and acromioclavicular joint arthrodesis.[17]

The sternoclavicular joint permits motion in three planes (see Fig. 12-3). The clavicle is capable of 35° of upward elevation with full forward flexion. Abduction and extension result in 35° of anteroposterior displacement. Full forward elevation also results in 45° of rotation of the clavicle along its axis.[39] These motions are very common in the throwing athlete, and the sternoclavicular joint appears to withstand the repetitive stresses of overhead activities extremely well. This is probably due to the strength of the ligamentous structures that prevent displacement of the joint.

PROXIMAL AND DISTAL FRACTURES OF THE CLAVICLE

Mechanism of Injury

Fractures of the proximal and distal thirds of the clavicle are most common in contact sports, including football, rugby, soccer, ice and field hockey, and lacrosse. Fractures of the proximal clavicle usually occur with direct violence applied from the lateral aspect of the shoulder.[3] Fractures of the distal end of the clavicle, which are similar to acromioclavicular joint dislocations, commonly result from a fall on the point of the shoulder, driving the scapula and upper extremity in a caudad direction.[3]

Clinical Presentation

Patients with a clavicle fracture usually give a history of either direct or indirect trauma to the shoulder or upper extremity. A mechanism involving lateral compression or forced depression applied at the point of the shoulder is most common. Patients are seen with the involved extremities adducted by their sides, often supported by the other arm. Deformity, swelling, and ecchymosis are seen at the fracture site. Palpation reveals tenderness directly over the fracture site. Active and passive range of shoulder motion is accompanied by pain and crepitance. The physical examination also should focus on the possibility of associated injuries, including skeletal, lung, vascular, and brachial plexus injuries.[23]

Classification

Allman has classified clavicle fractures into three groups based on their location in the proximal, middle, or distal one thirds.[3] Craig has presented a useful classification system of clavicle fractures that further subdivides proximal and distal clavicle fractures into five different subtypes each.[23] This classification differs from the six-stage classification of acromioclavicular injuries to be discussed later.[24,29,35,56-58,62,68]

- Fracture of the middle third (80%)
- Fracture of the distal third (15%)
  - Type I—minimal displacement (interligamentous)
  - Type II—displaced secondary to a fracture medial to the coracoclavicular ligaments
    - Conoid and trapezoid attached
    - Conoid torn, trapezoid attached
  - Type III—fractures of the articular surface
  - Type IV—ligaments intact to the periosteum (children), with displacement of the proximal fragment
  - Type V—comminuted, with ligaments attached neither proximally nor distally, but to an inferior, comminuted fragment
- Fracture of the proximal third (5%)
  - Type I—minimal displacement
  - Type II—displaced (ligaments ruptured)
  - Type III—intraarticular
  - Type IV—epiphyseal separation (children and young adults)
  - Type V—comminuted

Treatment

Treatment of group II distal clavicle fractures is based on the degree of displacement and stability of the fracture fragments. Type I, type III, and type IV distal clavicle fractures usually can be treated nonoperatively with a sling and swathe.[34,68,69] In type II and type V distal clavicle fractures, the coracoclavicular ligaments have been detached from the proximal fragment, and there can be varying degrees of displacement and instability of the fracture fragments. With minimal displacement, these fractures can heal with nonoperative treatment[68,69] (Fig. 12-4). With significant displacement or instability, the risk of nonunion increases and primary open reduction and internal fixation is recommended.[29,57] Methods of internal fixation vary, but Craig[23] has described a method including in-

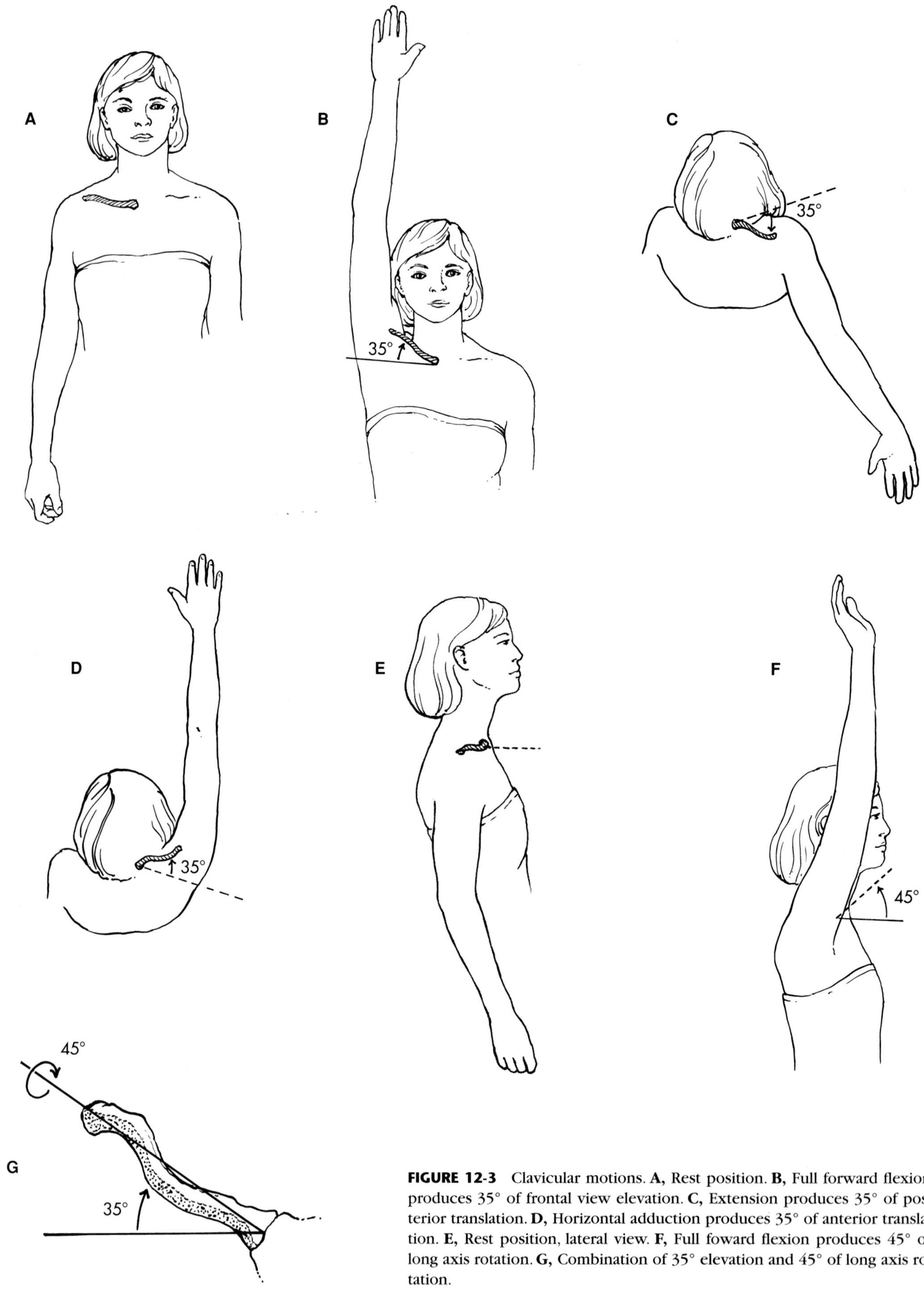

FIGURE 12-3 Clavicular motions. **A,** Rest position. **B,** Full forward flexion produces 35° of frontal view elevation. **C,** Extension produces 35° of posterior translation. **D,** Horizontal adduction produces 35° of anterior translation. **E,** Rest position, lateral view. **F,** Full foward flexion produces 45° of long axis rotation. **G,** Combination of 35° elevation and 45° of long axis rotation.

A

B

C

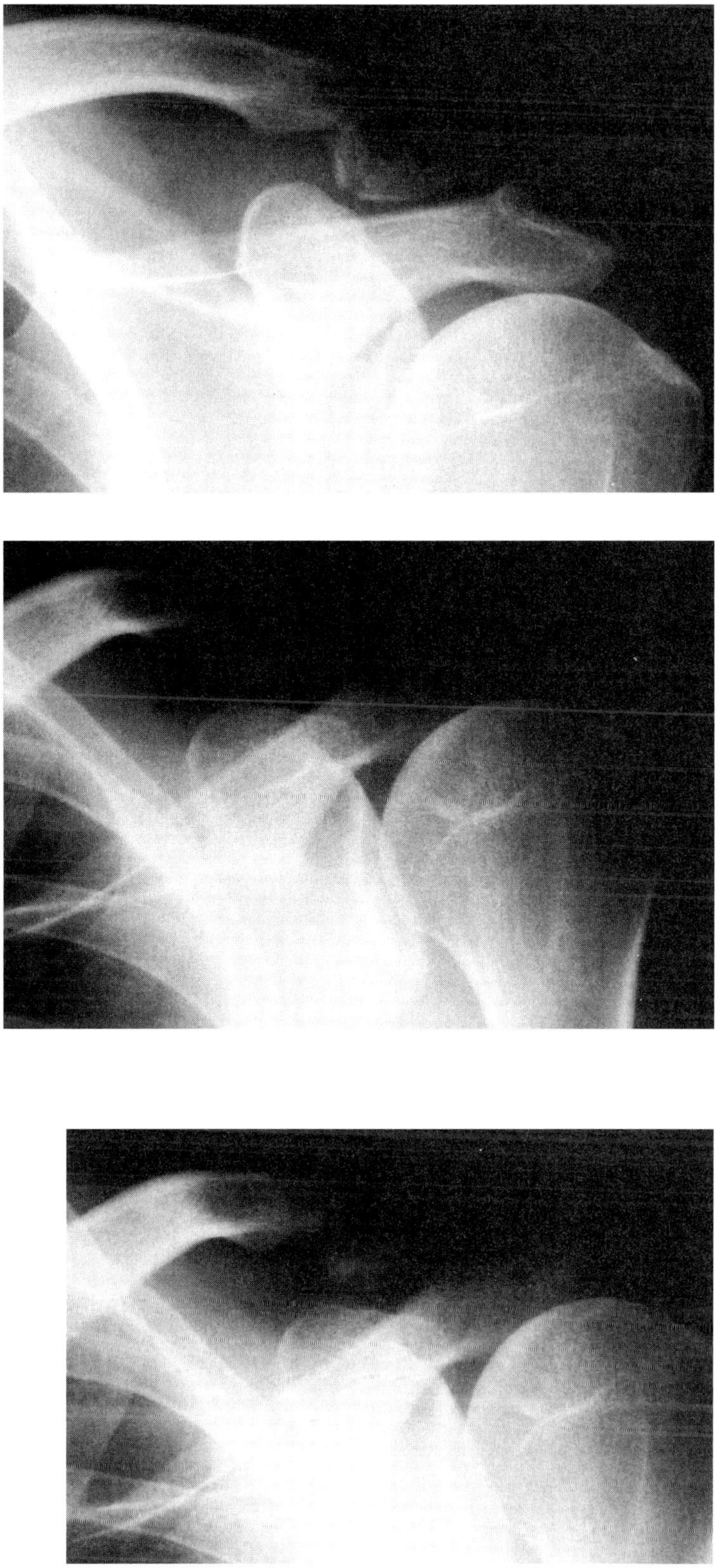

FIGURE 12-4 Type V distal clavicle fracture. **A,** Radiograph of a type V distal clavicle fracture in an elite triathlete. Patient refused operative treatment, discontinued his sling and began training at 1 week, and competed at 3 weeks after injury. **B,** Radiograph at $2\frac{1}{2}$ months after injury showing radiographic union. **C,** Radiograph at $1\frac{1}{2}$ years. Patient had no complaints, and his athletic performance had not suffered because of his injury.

tramedullary fixation with a Knowles pin augmented by Mersilene tape securing the proximal fragment to the coracoid process. This operative procedure is similar to the author's technique for the treatment of acromioclavicular ligament injuries (modified Weaver-Dunn procedure) and will be discussed later.

Group III fractures, or fractures of the proximal third of the clavicle, are rare and should be treated nonoperatively unless there is severe neurovascular compromise.

DISORDERS OF THE ACROMIOCLAVICULAR JOINT

Mechanism of Injury

Injury to the acromioclavicular joint occurs when one of four mechanisms occurs. The first and most common is a fall onto the point of the shoulder. This force drives the acromion downward and causes either a fracture of the clavicle's shaft, a fracture of the clavicle's distal one third, or a disruption of the acromioclavicular joint. This joint disruption results in a type I, II, III, or V injury (Fig. 12-5). A second mechanism is an indirect force applied to the acromioclavicular joint by a fall onto the outstretched upper extremity. A third mechanism of injury involves a force applied to the posterior aspect of the acromion or a posteriorly directed force applied to the distal clavicle. This can result in a type IV injury of the acromioclavicular joint. A fourth mechanism involves a severe abduction force applied to the upper extremity, resulting in a type VI acromioclavicular joint injury (see Fig. 12-5).

Clinical Presentation

The patient typically is seen with the injured extremity adducted at the side and often supported by the other hand. Depending on the degree of injury, there may be depression of the upper extremity with prominence of the distal end of the clavicle. Palpation may reveal tenderness at the acromioclavicular joint, in the coracoclavicular interspace, and along the distal one fourth of the clavicle near the attachment sites of the trapezius and deltoid muscles. Palpation also may reveal instability of the distal end of the clavicle. Pain with range of motion

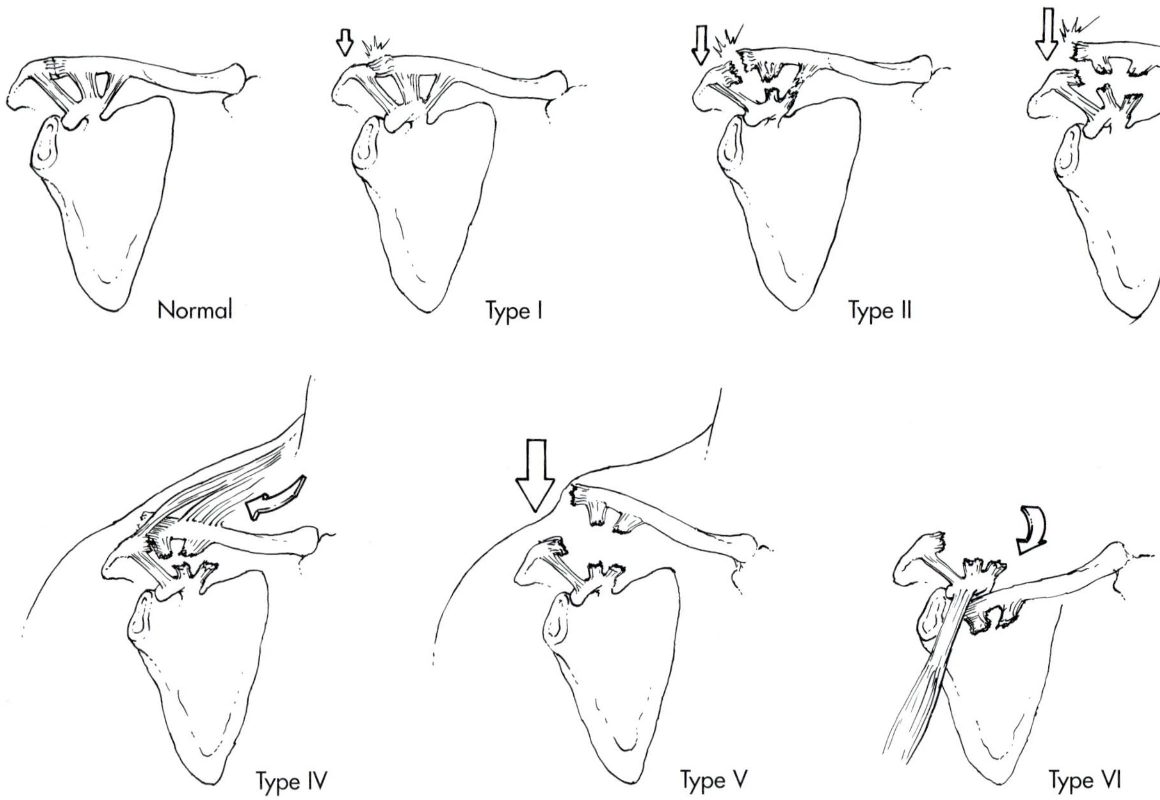

FIGURE 12-5 Classification of AC joint dislocations. Type I: A sprain of AC ligament. Type II: Tear of AC ligament and partial injury to coracoclavicular ligaments. Type III: Tear of AC ligament and tear of coracoclavicular ligaments. Type IV: Same as type III but with distal clavicle displaced posteriorly through trapezius. Type V: Same as type III but with disruption of deltoid and trapezius muscle attachments. Type VI: Same as type III but with distal clavicle wedged inferiorly below coracoid.

usually is noted and depends on the severity of the injury. A neurovascular examination always should be performed, but these injuries are uncommon except in type VI injuries, which involve a significant degree of trauma.

Classification

Classification of acromioclavicular (AC) joint injuries depends on the degree of soft-tissue injury and the degree of displacement between the distal clavicle and the scapula. The soft tissues involved usually include the acromioclavicular ligament, the coracoclavicular ligament, and the deltoid and trapezius muscle attachments to the distal one fourth of the clavicle.

Classification systems have evolved over time to include six major types of injuries[3,66,80] (see Fig. 12-5). Type I injuries involve a sprain of the acromioclavicular ligament. The acromioclavicular joint, the coracoclavicular ligaments, and the deltoid and trapezius muscles remain intact.

With a type II injury, the acromioclavicular ligaments are torn, the acromioclavicular joint is disrupted, and the coracoclavicular ligaments are sprained, but the deltoid and trapezius muscles remain intact.

With a type III injury, the acromioclavicular ligaments are torn, the acromioclavicular joint is disrupted, the coracoclavicular ligaments are torn, and the deltoid and trapezius muscles are detached from the distal end of the clavicle. The coracoclavicular interspace is no more than two times that of the normal opposite shoulder (Fig. 12-6).

In type IV injuries, the acromioclavicular ligaments are torn and the acromioclavicular joint is disrupted, with the distal clavicle displaced posteriorly into the trapezius muscle. The coracoclavicular ligaments also are torn, and the deltoid and trapezius muscles are disrupted.

A type V injury is essentially a type III injury with more than a 100% displacement of the coracoclavicular interspace when compared with a normal shoulder.

A type VI injury involves disruption of all soft-tissue elements previously mentioned, but displacement of the distal clavicle occurs below the coracoid.[47,63,74]

Another injury that can occur in conjunction with injuries to the acromioclavicular joint is a fracture of the base of the coracoid process. In this injury, the acromioclavicular ligaments are torn and the acromioclavicular joint is disrupted. The distal clavicle is superiorly displaced from the acromion, but the coracoclavicular interspace is normal.[18,86]

Radiographic Analysis

Evaluation of acromioclavicular joint injuries must include standard AP and axillary films. Anteroposterior films taken at 10° to 15° of cephalic tilt[89] will provide better delineation of the acromioclavicular joint. The most reproducible measurement of disruption of the acromioclavicular joint is the distance between the coracoid process and the upper aspect of the clavicle.[83] This distance should be measured in the injured shoulder and compared with the opposite normal shoulder. The coracoclavicular distance also can be measured as stress is applied to the upper extremities. In this method, 10 to 15 lb of weight should be suspended from the wrists, and the coracoclavicular distance should be measured and compared between the injured and uninjured shoulders. A difference of 40% to 50% is considered a complete disruption of the coracoclavicular ligaments.[8] Axillary films also are obtained to evaluate for the possibility

A

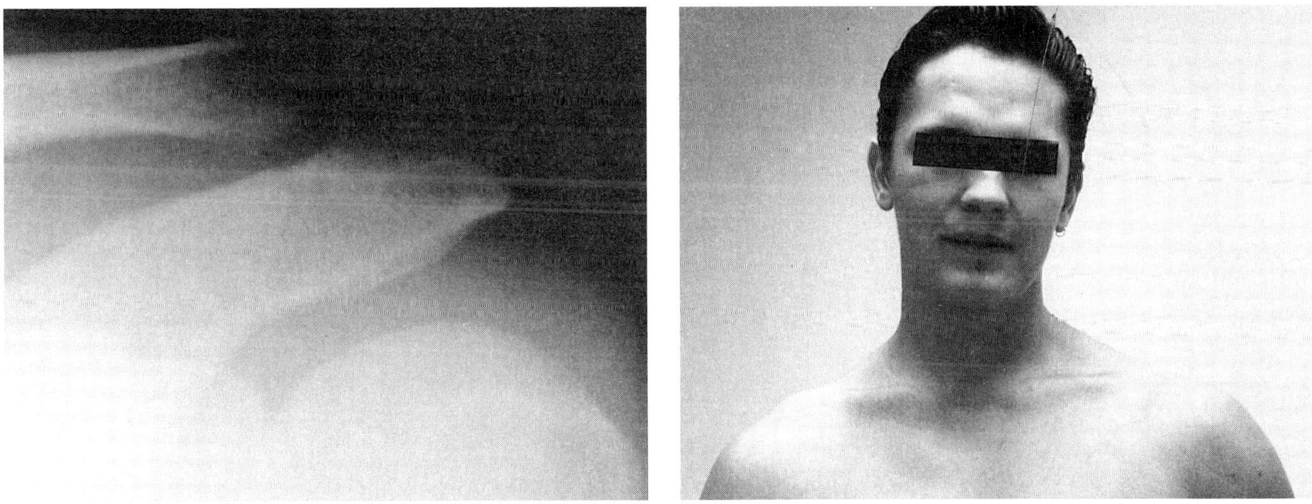

B

FIGURE 12-6 Type III AC dislocation. **A,** Radiograph. **B,** Clinical presentation.

of a type IVA to IVC joint injury, which is not appreciated on AP projections.

Treatment

Treatment of type I injuries consists of conservative measures including a sling for comfort, rest, ice, early overhead exercises, and a rapid return to sport at 2 to 14 days, as symptoms subside. Although most patients suffering a type I acromioclavicular injury have an excellent prognosis, some patients may experience persistent symptoms in the acromioclavicular joint. If symptoms persist, treatment can include rest, NSAIDs, steroid injections, or distal clavicle excision.[10,22]

Type II injuries are treated similarly to type I. A sling for comfort, rest, ice, and early overhead range of motion exercises are used. Previous authors have recommended the use of a "sling harness" device in an attempt to immobilize the acromioclavicular joint.[3] This type of treatment can be successful if the relocation force provided by the sling harness is uninterrupted. Patient compliance with these devices, however, makes this treatment option difficult. Return to sports usually occurs between 3 and 6 weeks and depends on the patient's symptoms and the physician's concern for reinjury. Most patients with type II injuries have an excellent prognosis.[11,61] As with type I injuries, some patients have persistent pain and stiffness.[10,22] These persistent symptoms also can be successfully treated with excision of the distal clavicle.[21,54]

Treatment of acute type III injuries remains controversial. Treatment options include (1) use of a sling for comfort, (2) sling-and-harness device designed to maintain a closed reduction of the acromioclavicular joint, and (3) immediate operative treatment. Sling-and-harness devices are difficult to use successfully because of lack of patient compliance. Nonsurgical treatment can be successful in type III injuries.* Immediate surgical treatment of acute type III injuries also is supported in the literature.[41,77,81] The operative procedures used include one or more of the following basic operations[70]:

1. Acromioclavicular joint fixation/repair/reconstruction
2. Coracoclavicular fixation/repair/reconstruction
3. Distal clavicle excision
4. Dynamic muscle transfers

The decision between immediate nonsurgical and surgical treatment remains controversial and is sometimes difficult. Guidelines are not rigid and are influenced by patient wishes and the inclinations of the surgeon.

Type IV, V, and VI injuries usually are treated with surgical intervention.[32,67,73] This includes operative reduction followed by surgical repair similar to the types of repairs that have been outlined with the treatment of acute type III injuries. Most repairs involve restoration of the coracoclavicular restraints and are modifications of the procedure described by Weaver and Dunn in 1972.[84]

*References 6, 11, 25, 33, 38, 43, 44, 78, 87.

Treatment of Choice

Our experience over the past several years has consistently shown that most, if not all, acute type III injuries can be treated nonoperatively, including professional and collegiate athletes who have injured their dominant arm. A sling is used initially for comfort in the early postinjury period, and immediate active range of motion as tolerated is allowed. A supervised physical therapy program is then begun within 3 weeks after injury to restore full range of motion and to strengthen shoulder girdle musculature. With this type of treatment, more than 90% of patients have been able to return successfully to their previous level of activity and sport without complications occurring.[11]

In patients who elect surgical repair for cosmetic purposes, our choice of treatment has been a modification of the procedure described by Weaver and Dunn (Fig. 12-7). This is also the procedure of choice for type V injuries.

Surgical Technique for Modified Weaver-Dunn Procedure

The patient is placed on the operating room table in a supine position or in a beach chair position with two folded towels under the scapula to help stabilize the shoulder girdle. The entire upper extremity should be prepared and draped free to allow full range of motion and control of the glenohumeral joint. A saber-type skin incision is made beginning at the level of the distal clavicle and extending approximately 8 cm toward the coracoid (see Fig. 12-7, *A*). This incision should be made parallel to Langer's lines to ensure the most optimal cosmetic appearance after surgery. The subcutaneous tissue is undermined to allow good visualization in all directions, and Goelet retractors are placed medially and laterally. The confluence of the deltoid and trapezius fascial layers over the superior aspect of the clavicle is then identified and split sharply through needle-tip cautery to produce one subperiosteal layer (see Fig. 12-7, *B*). This ensures one good thick layer to which the deltoid and trapezius muscles are reapproximated at the completion of the procedure. This dissection must be carried to at least the level of the acromion to allow adequate exposure of the fibrocartilaginous disc as well as the coracoacromial ligament. A longitudinal split is then made that parallels the deltoid fibers to the level of the coracoid and thereby exposes the underlying coracoacromial ligament and tip of the coracoid. The coracoclavicular ligaments usually can be visualized at this time; however, the ligaments often have been torn in their midsubstance and made unavailable for the repair.

A distal clavicle resection is then performed using the oscillating saw and removing approximately 1 cm of bone, taking care to rasp and bevel the remaining free edge of the distal clavicle (see Fig. 12-7, *C*). The fibrocartilaginous disc, which is often torn, is also excised at this time. The surgeon should check for the adequacy of the

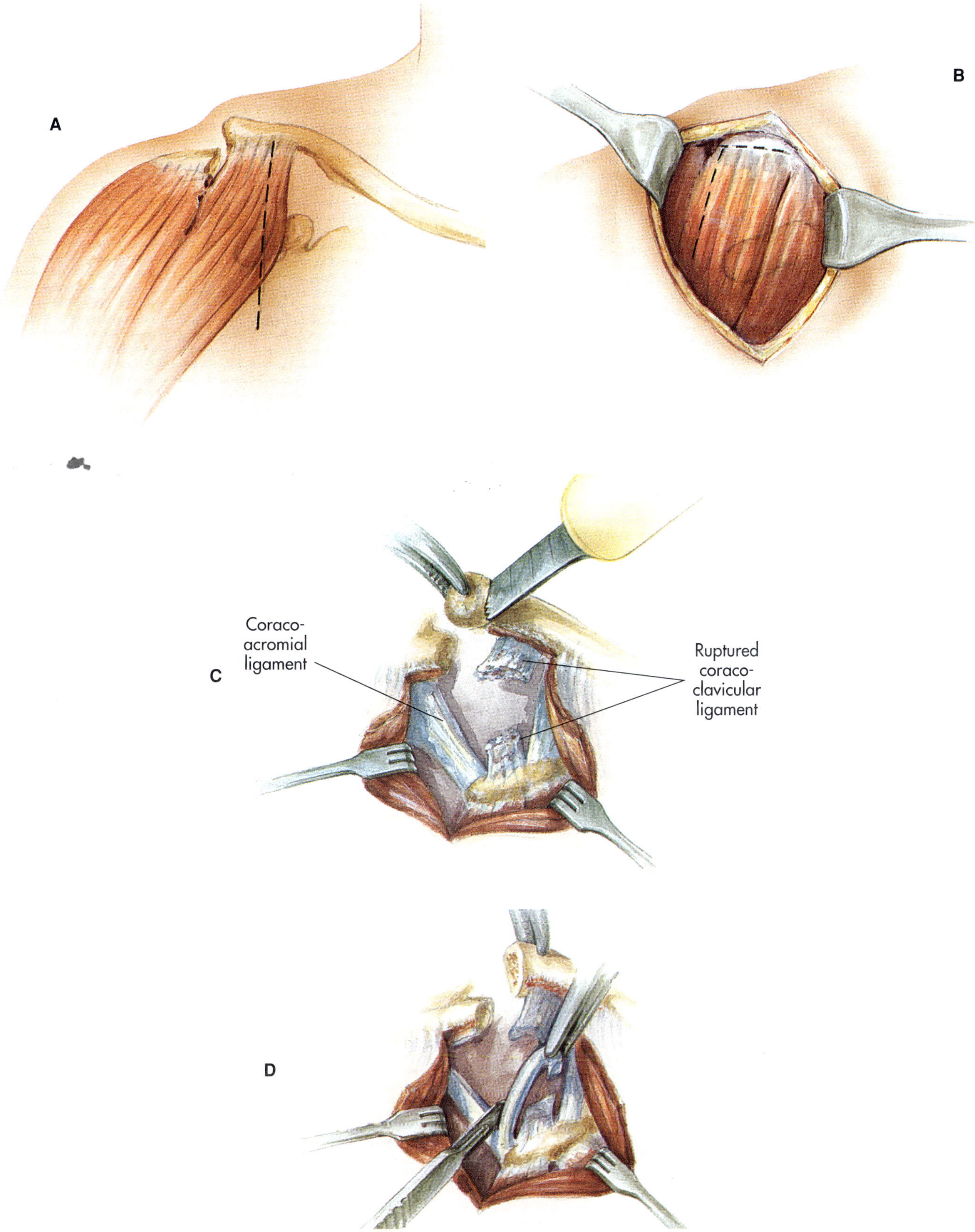

FIGURE 12-7 Modified Weaver-Dunn reconstruction. **A,** Skin incision following Langer's lines. **B,** Deltoid split. **C,** Distal clavicle resection. **D,** Portion of coracoacromial ligament released from acromion. *Continued.*

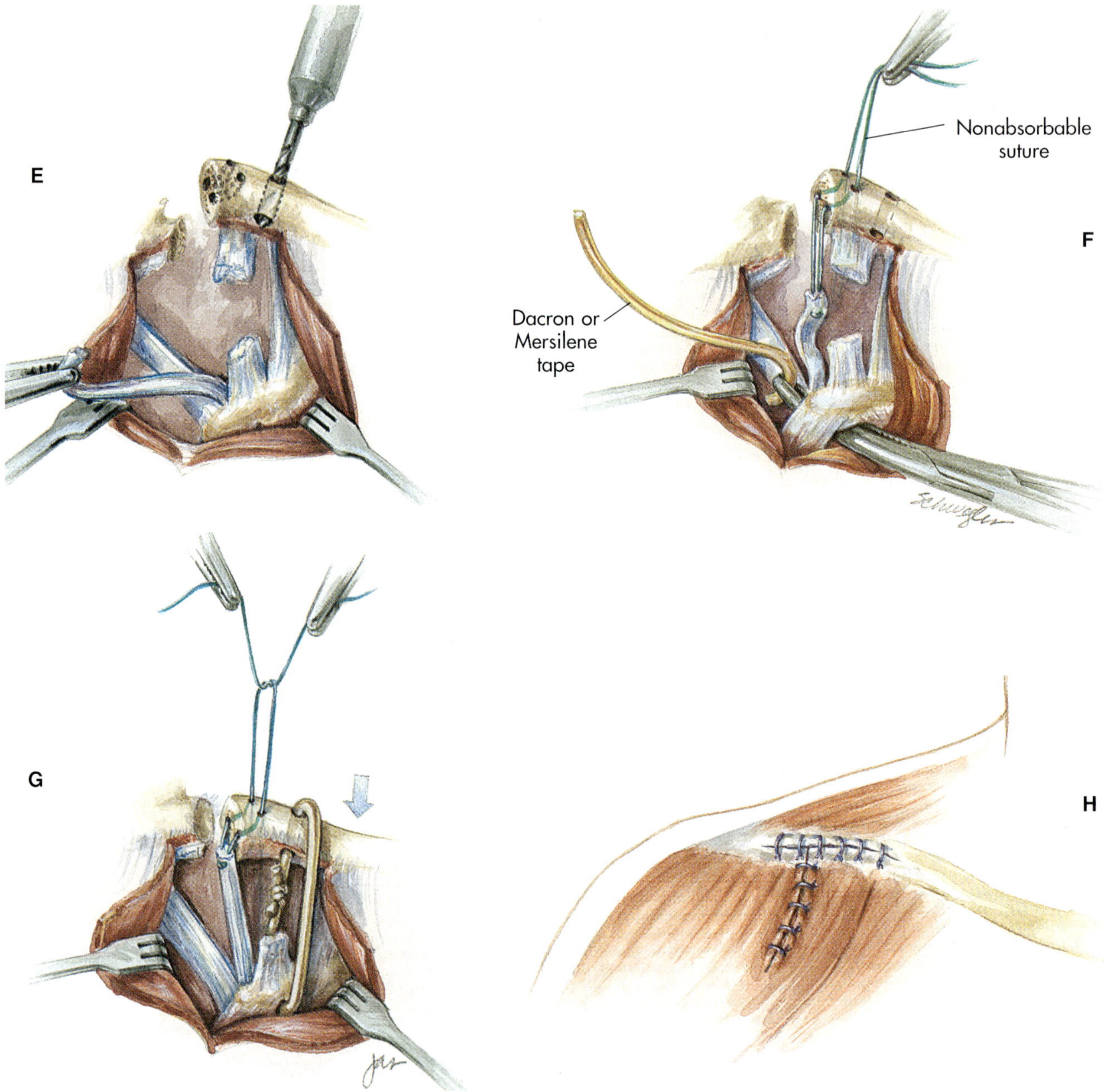

FIGURE 12-7—cont'd **E,** Drill holes placed in clavicle. **F,** Dacron tape passed around coracoid. **G,** Dacron tape tied and reinforced with coracoacromial ligament. **H,** Deltoid and trapezius closure.

decompression by manually reducing the clavicle and then clinically taking the upper extremity through a range of motion, including forward flexion across the chest to ensure that the acromion does not impinge on the free edge of the distal clavicle.

The acromial attachment of the coracoacromial ligament is then detached sharply (see Fig. 12-7, *D*). Number 1 Ethibond suture then is passed through the free edge of the coracoacromial ligament with a modified Kessler stitch. Two small drill holes are passed through the distal clavicle from superior to inferior and the #1 Ethibond suture then is passed from inferior to superior through these holes. The clavicle then is again reduced into position, and a third drill hole is made in the distal clavicle directly over the base of the coracoid, with the hole made in the anterior one third of the clavicle as visualized in the axial plane (see Fig. 12-7, *E*). A 1 mm Dacron tape or Mersilene tape then is passed in a circular fashion circumferentially around the base of the coracoid and through the hole placed in the clavicle. A right-angle clamp facilitates the passage of this material along the base of the coracoid beneath the short head of the biceps (see Fig. 12-7, *F*). Care must be taken while passing material along the base of the coracoid to avoid any intervening soft tissues.

The clavicle is then reduced into position, and the Dacron or Mersilene tape is tied (see Fig. 12-7, *G*). The reconstruction is then completed as the coracoacromial ligament is secured into position within the distal clavicle by tying the #1 Ethibond suture. The coracoclavicular interval is thereby restored using both the coracoacromial ligament and the augmentation with the synthetic material. The deltoid-trapezius interval then is reapproximated with heavy absorbable suture, which is similarly used to approximate the split in the anterior deltoid (see Fig. 12-7, *H*). Before closure, the wound should be irrigated to remove debris, and meticulous hemostasis should be achieved with the use of electrocautery. The subcutaneous tissues are closed with absorbable undyed suture, and the skin is closed with a running subcuticular Prolene suture.

Postoperative Rehabilitation

The involved extremity is placed in a sling with the sutures removed 7 to 10 days after surgery. Sling immobilization is continued for 4 to 6 weeks. During this period, daily mobilization of the wrist and elbow and finger gripping exercises are recommended.

After the 4 to 6 weeks of immobilization, an aggressive range-of-motion program is instituted with the help of supervised physical therapy on a three-times-a-week basis. Shoulder girdle strengthening activities commence after the first month of therapy. Most patients will require approximately 4 to 6 months of recovery from surgery before they can comfortably return to full activities without restriction.

Complications

Late complications of acromioclavicular injuries include osteolysis of the distal clavicle, acromioclavicular arthritis, and coracoclavicular ossification.

Osteolysis

Osteolysis of the distal clavicle can occur after traumatic injuries[40,45,55] and as a result of overuse without a history of acute trauma.[15,16,76] Most patients present with subjective complaints of pain with overhead use of the involved extremity and tenderness over the acromioclavicular joint. Early radiographic changes in the distal clavicle include osteoporosis, cyst formation, and loss of the subchondral cortical line.[16] Later radiographic changes include complete osteolysis and tapering of the distal clavicle[45] (Fig. 12-8). Additional radiographic studies, including bone scintigraphy[16] and MRI,[28] may help make the diagnosis.

Initial treatment should include rest from the aggravating activities and nonsteroidal antiinflammatories, and may include cortisone injection into the acromioclavicular joint. The judicious use of these types of medications can be very helpful in providing both short-term and long-term relief for problems involving the acromioclavicular joint. Care should be taken to perform these injections early, and frequent injections are not recommended. In general, the authors try to limit injections to a maximum of three. Should conservative measures fail to sufficiently resolve the patient's symptoms, excision of the distal clavicle may be indicated.

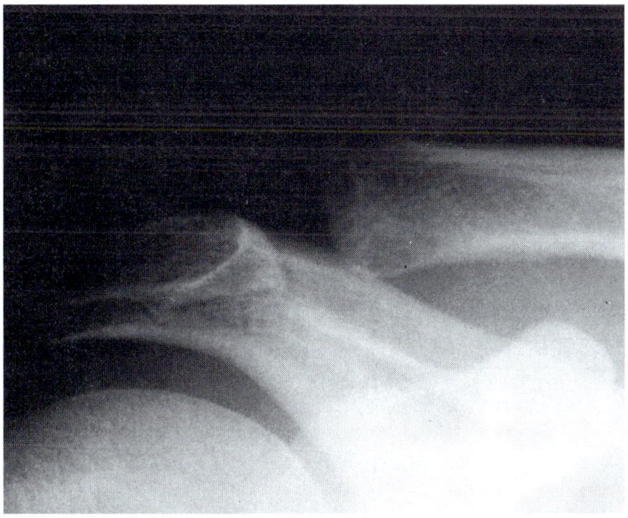

FIGURE 12-8 Osteolysis of distal clavicle.

Arthritis

Acromioclavicular arthritis has both a traumatic[54] and nontraumatic[64] origin (Fig. 12-9). Symptoms include aching pain aggravated by activities that require adduction or internal rotation and difficulty in using the extremity for overhead and repetitive activities. Initial treatments should include rest, nonsteroidal antiinflammatories, and steroid injections into the acromioclavicular joint. If symptoms persist, excision of the distal end of the clavicle yields excellent results.[21,54] Arthroscopic resection of the distal clavicle is comparable to open resection[31] (Fig. 12-10).

Ossification or calcification in the coracoclavicular interval[62] results from mild, moderate, and severe injuries.[4,52] Coracoclavicular ossification does not negatively influence the outcome of acromioclavicular injuries[2,85] and should be treated conservatively.

DISORDERS OF THE STERNOCLAVICULAR JOINT

Overview

Disorders of the sternoclavicular (SC) joint are relatively rare. In Cave's review of shoulder girdle injuries,[19] the incidence of sternoclavicular dislocations was 2.5%. However, Rockwood[70] reported that SC dislocation was not as

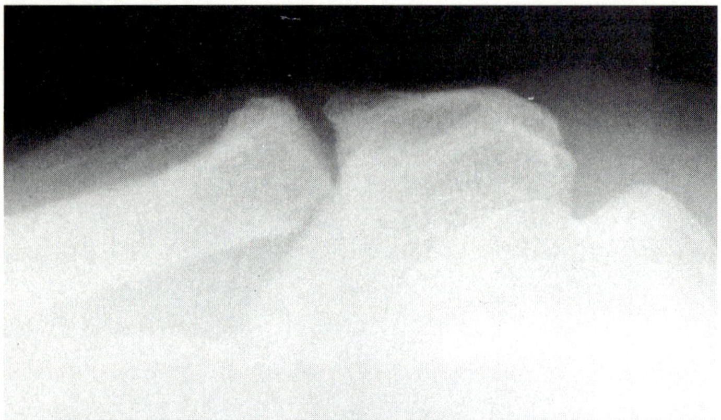

FIGURE 12-9 Acromioclavicular joint arthritis.

A B C D

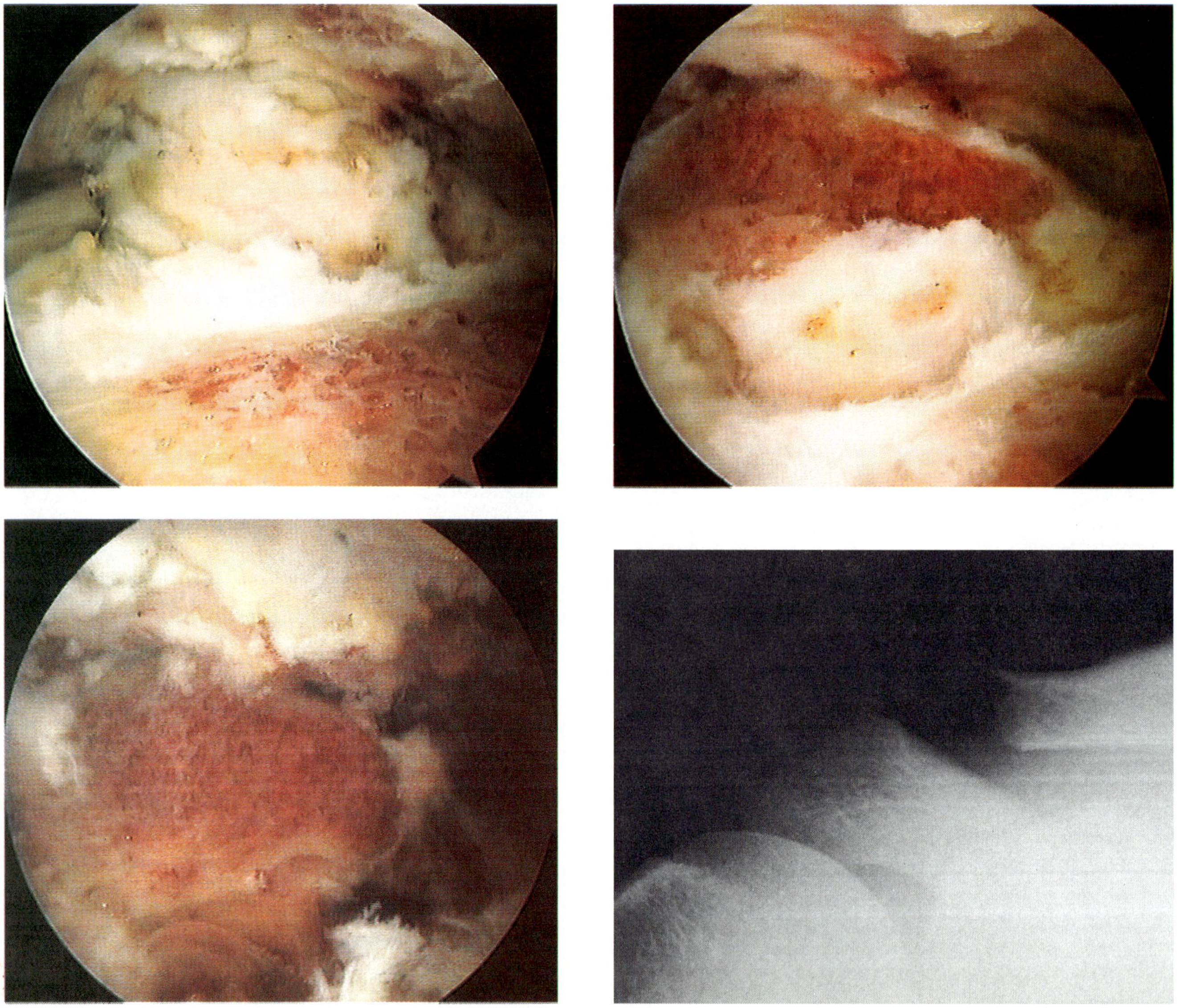

FIGURE 12-10 Arthroscopic resection of the distal clavicle. **A,** Distal clavicle unresected. **B,** Partially resected. **C,** Totally resected. **D,** Postoperative radiograph.

rare as posterior glenohumeral dislocation, which accounted for only 2% of all shoulder dislocations.

Anterior sternoclavicular dislocations are more common than posterior dislocations. Nettles and Linshcid's[59] study revealed a ratio of 20:1. However, Rockwood's series[70] showed a ratio of 3:1. Most published reports have focused on the rare and potentially life-threatening posterior dislocation, which can cause venous congestion with difficulty breathing or swallowing along with decreased peripheral circulation. The first report of a traumatic posterior dislocation was by Rodrigues in 1843.[72] Anterior dislocations, although more common, rarely have been reviewed in the literature.

Mechanism of Injury

In addition to motor vehicle accidents, the most common source of injury to the sternoclavicular joint is participation in sports.[60] The sternoclavicular joint may be traumatized by direct or indirect forces, resulting in sprains, dislocations, physeal injuries, or arthritis. Direct injuries usually are the result of a blow to the anteromedial aspect of the clavicle and will produce a posterior dislocation. However, an indirect mechanism occurs when a force is applied to either the anterolateral or posterolateral shoulder region. This indirect mechanism is the most common mechanism in producing both anterior and posterior injuries to the sternoclavicular joint. A force directed posterolaterally with the arm extended produces an anterior dislocation (Fig. 12-11, *A*). A force directed anterolaterally with the arm adducted and internally rotated results in posterior dislocation (Fig. 12-11, *B*). Football players may be most at risk for this type of injury, but falling on the abducted and slightly extended extremity in any sport may drive the shoulder medially, injuring the sternoclavicular joint.

Problems in the sternoclavicular joint also may occur without trauma and may be of spontaneous origin or secondary to congenital abnormalities. In the overhead athlete, these present as anterior subluxations or dislocations, which are usually asymptomatic. When the arm is abducted and externally rotated, the joint is subluxated anteriorly and/or superiorly; when the arm is brought back down to the side, the joint spontaneously reduces.

Clinical Presentation

The patient with a sternoclavicular joint disorder will complain of pain over the joint associated with movement of the ipsilateral upper extremity. In nontraumatic circumstances, the presenting complaint may be of a bulge or bump that occurs with overhead movement of the arm.

In acute traumatic sternoclavicular dislocations, the pain can be severe. The patient will tend to hold the affected arm across his body. Discomfort intensifies with supine positioning. In the more rare but dangerous posterior dislocation, there may be venous congestion in the neck or arm. The patient may experience difficulty with breathing or swallowing, and peripheral circulation may be impaired (Fig. 12-12).

Physical inspection and palpation of the SC joint usually can distinguish between anterior and posterior problems. With the more common anterior injury, the medial aspect of the clavicle is more visibly prominent and lies anterior to the sternum. However, Rockwood[70] has reported that clinical signs may be confusing, and x-ray evaluation is mandatory.

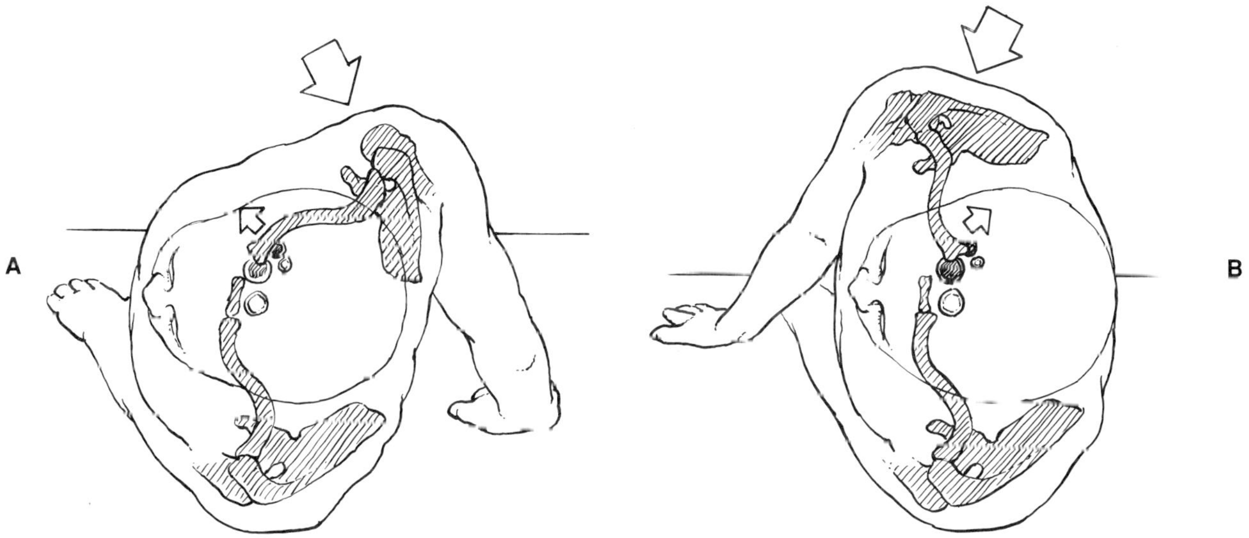

FIGURE 12-11 Sternoclavicular joint mechanism of injury. The athlete has fallen down and is lying on the ground and either, **A**, a posterior lateral compression force is applied to the extended arm, producing an anterior dislocation, or, **B**, an anterior lateral compression force is applied to the adducted arm, producing a posterior dislocation.

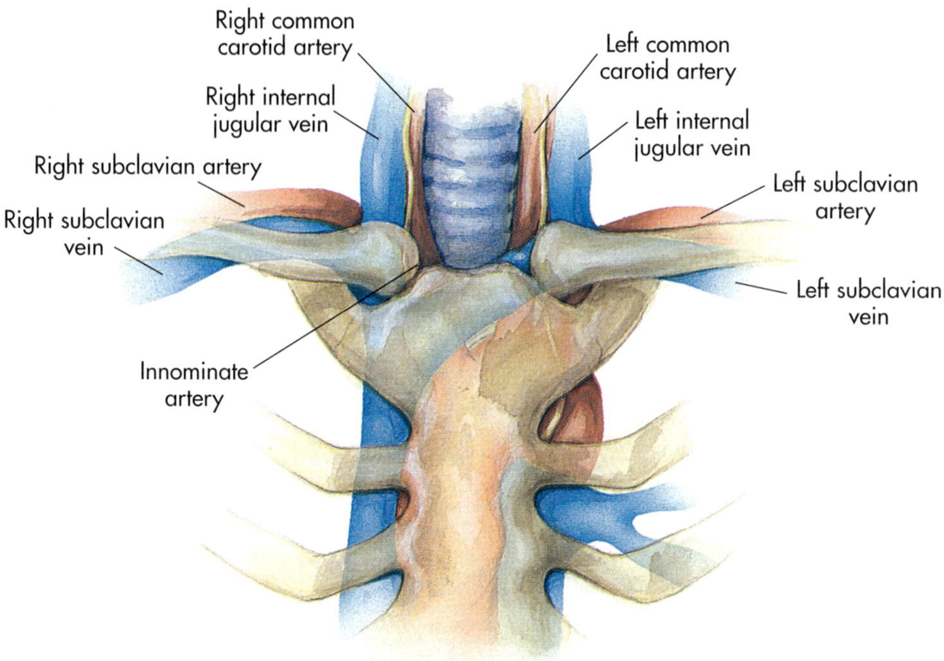

FIGURE 12-12 Sternoclavicular joint vascular anatomy. Association of sternoclavicular joint to the great vessels in the chest cavity is outlined: right and left subclavian vein, right and left subclavian artery, innominate artery, left common carotid artery, right and left internal jugular vein.

Radiographic Analysis

X-ray analysis is mandatory to confirm the direction of displacement in traumatic injuries of the sternoclavicular joint. Unfortunately, plain x-rays are difficult to interpret. The most effective technique is to use a view similar to an apical chest view, which is a 40-degree cephalic tilt view of both medial clavicles. Tomography is a more valuable tool in evaluating the direction of displacement and the presence of associated fractures but has been supplanted by CT and MRI.

Without a doubt, CT and MRI scanning techniques are currently the best and most accurate methods for evaluating the sternoclavicular joint. CT scanning displays the best bony detail, but MRI imaging may be even more helpful if posterior dislocation is suspected, because the underlying vessels and soft tissues can be better evaluated with MRI. In either situation, bilateral comparison films should be used to evaluate the positions of the normal and injured joint. In atraumatic conditions, it may be important to position the arm into abduction and external rotation to demonstrate the subluxation radiographically.

Treatment

Traumatic Disorders

Sprains

Sprains to the sternoclavicular joint can be easily managed with ice, analgesics, and a sling for initial pain relief. Early range of motion is encouraged, and recovery may be anticipated within 3 to 6 weeks, depending on the severity of the sprain. Patients with more severe sprains may be more comfortable with a figure-of-eight harness.

Anterior Dislocations

Traumatic anterior dislocations most often can be managed similarly to sprains. An attempt should be made at closed reduction, although in the vast majority of cases the reduction is unstable and redislocation may occur.

Closed reduction is accomplished with the patient supine and a few folded towels under the scapula. With a posteriorly applied force directed to the shoulder, the medial tip of the clavicle is manually pushed into position. If the dislocation spontaneously recurs, as is most often the case, the patient is treated in a sling or figure-of-eight harness, and early range of motion is instituted. The prognosis is good for a complete recovery and return to full activities.

Posterior Dislocations

Traumatic posterior dislocations should be treated as soon as possible with either closed or open reduction techniques. Closed reduction is performed with the patient supine and several folded towels between the shoulder blades (Fig. 12-13, *A*). A general anesthetic may be required. The involved extremity will need to be abducted and extended. Traction is applied to the abducted arm as the arm is slowly brought into more extension. It may be necessary to grasp the medial clavicle to obtain a reduction, and if the patient is properly anesthetized, a towel clip may be used effectively (Fig. 12-13, *B*). When

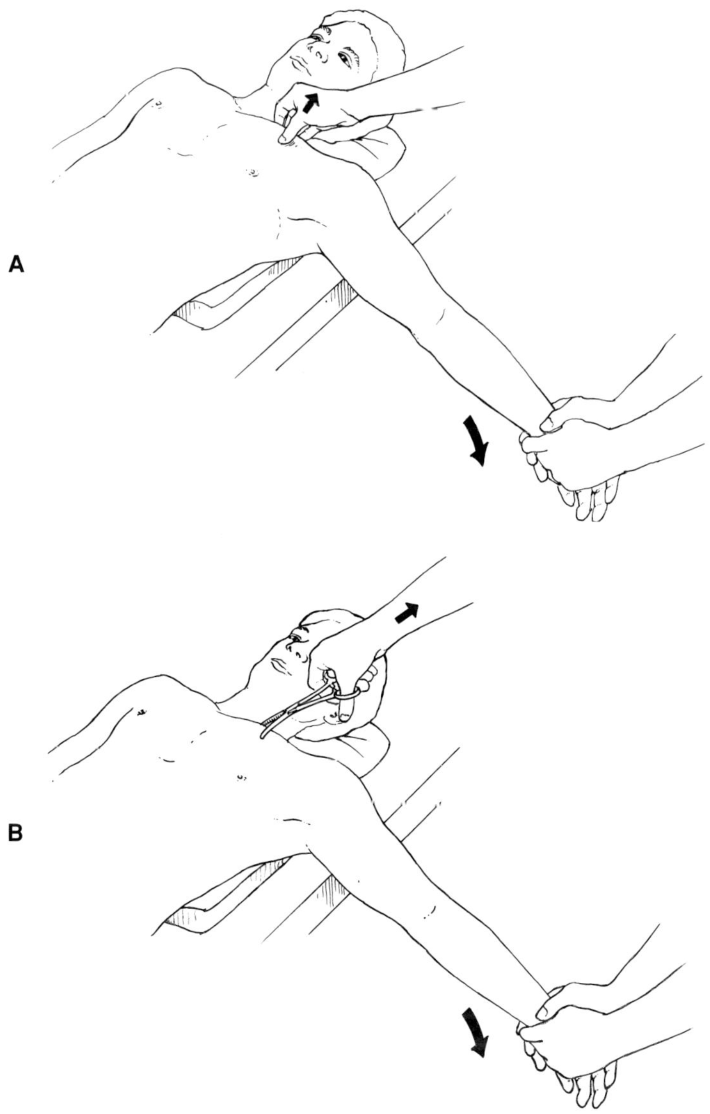

FIGURE 12-13 Technique of closed reduction of posterior dislocation sternoclavicular joint. The patient is supine with folded towels under scapula. The arm is abducted and extended with traction applied. **A,** The proximal end of the clavicle is grasped manually and elevated to dislodge it from the sternum. **B,** A sterile towel clip can be used to dislodged the proximal clavicle if necessary.

the joint is reduced, it is stable, and the patient is again treated in a figure-of-eight harness for comfort.

Open reduction should be performed if closed techniques are unsuccessful. This should be performed in conjunction with a thoracic surgeon because vital structures lie in close proximity. The key to a successful open reduction is maintaining the integrity of the anterior capsule. If the anterior capsular ligament is sacrificed, the joint probably will be unstable, necessitating medial clavicular resection and a costoclavicular ligament reconstruction (Fig. 12-14). Costoclavicular ligament reconstruction has best been accomplished with a 1-mm Dacron tape, according to Rockwood.[70]

K-wires, pins, or other metallic devices should *not* be used because there are many reports in the literature of migration of these devices. These complications are potentially catastrophic. Postoperative management after open reduction again includes a figure-of-eight harness, but motion is delayed for 4 to 6 weeks.

Physeal Injuries

Traumatic physeal injuries often are mistaken for dislocations of the sternoclavicular joint. The epiphysis on the medial end of the clavicle is the last epiphysis in the human body to close. It does not radiographically appear to ossify until approximately the eighteenth year of age and does not unite with the clavicle until age 25. The ma-

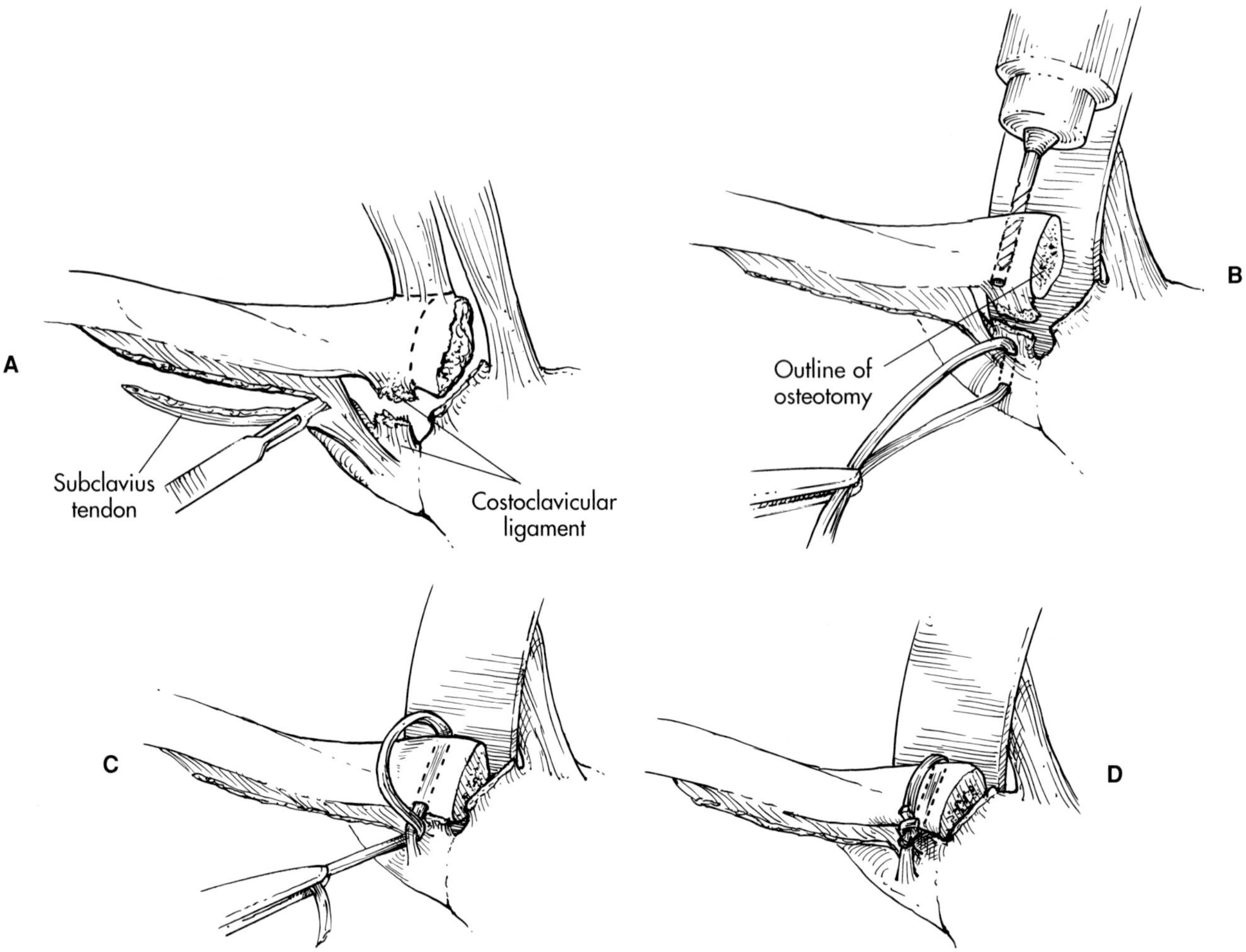

FIGURE 12-14 Sternoclavicular joint reconstruction. Surgical reconstruction consists of a proximal clavicle resection and reconstruction of the costoclavicular ligament with either, **A,** subclavius tendon or, **B,** 1-mm Dacron tape. **C** and **D,** The tendon or tape is looped through a drill hole placed in the proximal clavicle after resection.

jority of sternoclavicular injuries that occur in people under the age of 25 actually are physeal fractures. The majority of physeal injuries will heal with abundant callus, and no surgical intervention is needed. Again, as in the treatment of dislocations, anterior physeal injuries usually can be allowed to heal and remodel, but posterior physeal injuries should be reduced. This has been documented by several authors. Capsular ligaments are attached to the periosteum in both type I and type II physeal injuries, and it is from this intact periosteal layer that bone remodeling usually occurs. Therefore, despite displacement of the medial clavicle, the costoclavicular ligaments, capsular ligaments, and intraarticular disc ligament usually are not displaced and remain attached to the periosteal sleeve. The prognosis is good for complete healing and return to all functional activities.

Posttraumatic Arthritis

A small minority of patients develop posttraumatic arthritis as a result of anterior subluxation or dislocation of the SC joint. The vast majority of these patients can be managed with occasional use of analgesics, oral antiinflammatory medications, and/or occasional cortisone injection into the sternoclavicular joint.

In patients who fail this type of conservative management, operative resection of the medial clavicle has been described.[13,46,48,65] (Fig. 12-15). If this type of resection arthroplasty is performed, one must completely débride the intraarticular disc ligament. If the costocla-vicular ligament is damaged or attenuated, it is imperative to reconstruct this structure. The clavicle is best stabilized to the first rib with either Mersilene or Dacron tape. Detachment of the sternocleidomastoid clavicular head, as outlined in the technique of Burrows,[14] helps prevent further upward migration of the clavicle (see Fig. 12-14, *A*). Arthrodesis of the sternoclavicular joint for the treatment of posttraumatic arthritis should be avoided because this will result in significant restriction of shoulder motion.

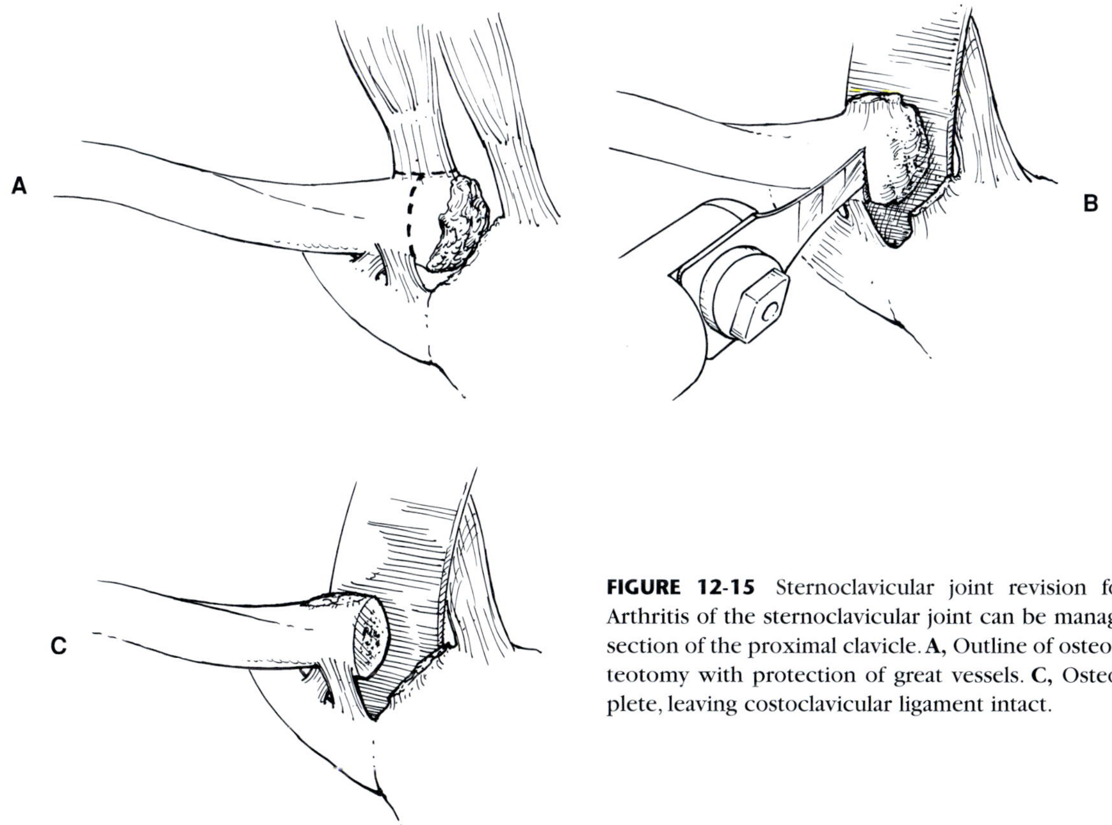

FIGURE 12-15 Sternoclavicular joint revision for arthritis. Arthritis of the sternoclavicular joint can be managed with resection of the proximal clavicle. **A,** Outline of osteotomy. **B,** Osteotomy with protection of great vessels. **C,** Osteotomy complete, leaving costoclavicular ligament intact.

Atraumatic Disorders

Atraumatic subluxation or dislocation of the sternoclavicular joint is best treated with patient education, and any type of operative management is best avoided. Episodic pain is best treated with the occasional use of oral antiinflammatory medications, and on occasion, patients may respond to isolated cortisone injection within the sternoclavicular joint. The majority of patients do not complain of pain but are concerned only with the clicking that is present. Patient education and understanding of this problem usually satisfy patients to the point that they can continue their athletic endeavors. The best review of operative and nonoperative management of this condition is by Rockwood and Odor.[71] At 8-year follow-up, 29 patients treated nonoperatively had no limitations of activity or lifestyle, as opposed to the eight patients who had been treated with surgery and had ongoing difficulty.

DISORDERS OF THE SCAPULOTHORACIC JOINT

Overview

Injury to the scapula is uncommon, accounting for less than 5% of all shoulder girdle injuries. High-energy trauma often is needed to produce injuries to the scapula and its articulation with the thorax. Therefore these injuries are extremely rare in sports. Injury can be produced by direct impact, usually leading to fracture of the scapula. However, scapulothoracic dissociation can occur as an indirect injury, usually through axial loading on the outstretched arm. Thompson[79] has devised a classification for scapular fractures, and Ideberg has proposed a separate classification for interarticular glenoid fractures.[36,37] Scapulothoracic dissociation has been described by Ebraheim,[27] but again, this is an exceedingly rare injury in which the scapula displaces laterally, usually with clavicle disruption and associated soft-tissue injury involving the neurovascular bundle.

Snapping Scapula Syndrome

Snapping scapula syndrome is perhaps the most common scapulothoracic disorder seen in the athletic population. Patients present with scapulothoracic pain and complaints of audible snapping that appears to arise from the scapulothoracic area. Milch[49,51] has written several articles on this disorder and notes that the intensity of the snapping does not correlate with the severity of symptoms nor with the presence of a definitive anatomic abnormality in the scapulothoracic area. Other presenting symptoms and signs may include a history of the scapula sliding in and out of place and clinical evidence of crepitance and winging of the scapula.

The most common anatomic abnormality producing

this syndrome is an osteochondroma of the scapula. This mass usually presents on the undersurface of the scapula projecting toward the thorax. Although these lesions may be seen radiographically with a scapulothoracic view, a CAT scan usually is required.

The most common soft-tissue abnormality that produces snapping scapula syndrome is abnormality of the subscapular bursae. The three bursae that commonly may be involved are one at the superior medial angle of the scapula, one at the inferior angle of the scapula, and a third between the serratus anterior and the lateral chest wall. How these bursae actually produce this syndrome is not well understood. One theory is that injury to the scapular area results in fibrosis or muscle atrophy of the shoulder girdle, which reduces the cushioning effect of the scapula on the thorax.

Treatment of choice involves conservative management, which may include postural exercises, pain-reducing modalities, and strengthening exercises emphasizing the scapular stabilizers. Corticosteroid injection into either trigger point areas or subscapular bursal regions has been extremely helpful. Patients with bony anatomic deformities, such as osteochondromas or rib exostoses, may require surgical treatment. However, surgical excision of the superomedial angle of the scapula has produced mixed results in the treatment of this syndrome when only soft-tissue etiologies have been suspected.[50] Recently, isolated cases of the treatment of these disorders with arthroscopic bursal excision have produced favorable outcomes.

References

1. Reference deleted in proofs.
2. Alldredge RH: Surgical treatment of acromioclavicular dislocations (abstract), *J Bone Joint Surg* 47A:1278, 1965.
3. Allman FL Jr: Fractures and ligamentous injuries of the clavicle and its articulation, *J Bone Joint Surg* 49A:774-784, 1967.
4. Arner O, Sandahl U, Ohrling H: Dislocation of the acromioclavicular joint: review of the literature and a report of 56 cases, *Acta Chir Scand* 113:140-152, 1957.
5. Reference deleted in proofs.
6. Bannister GC et al: The management of acute acromioclavicular dislocation: a randomized prospective controlled trial, *J Bone Joint Surg [Br]* 71(5):848-850, 1989.
7. Reference deleted in proofs.
8. Bearden JM, Hughston JC, Whatley GS: Acromioclavicular dislocation: method of treatment, *J Sports Med* 1(4):5-17, 1973.
9. Bearn JG: Direct observations on the function of the capsule of the sternoclavicular joint in clavicle support, *J Anat* 101:159-170, 1967.
10. Bergfeld JA, Andrish JT, Clancy WG: Evaluation of the acromioclavicular joint following first- and second-degree sprains, *Am J Sports Med* 6(4):153-159, 1978.
11. Bjerneld H, Hovelius L, Thorling J: Acromioclavicular separations treated conservatively: a 5-year follow-up study, *Acta Orthop Scand* 54:743-745, 1983.
12. Reference deleted in proofs.
13. Breitner S, Wirth CJ: Resection of the acromial and sternal ends of the clavicula, *Z Orthop* 125:363-368, 1987.
14. Burrows HJ: Tenodesis of subclavius in the treatment of recurrent dislocation of the sternoclavicular joint, *J Bone Joint Surg* 33B(2):240-243, 1951.
15. Cahill BR: Atraumatic osteolysis of the distal clavicle: a review, *Sports Med* 13(3):214-222, 1992.
16. Cahill BR: Osteolysis of the distal part of the clavicle in male athletes, *J Bone Joint Surg* 64A(7):1053-1058, 1982.
17. Caldwell GD: Treatment of complete permanent acromioclavicular dislocation by surgical arthrodesis, *J Bone Joint Surg* 25(2):368-374, 1943.
18. Carr AJ, Broughton NS: Acromioclavicular dislocation associated with fracture of the coracoid process, *J Trauma* 29(1):125-126, 1989.
19. Cave EF: *Fractures and other injuries,* Chicago, 1958, Year Book Medical Publishers.
20. Codman EA: Rupture of the supraspinatus tendon and other lesions in or about the subacromial bursa. In: *The shoulder,* Boston, 1934, Thomas Todd.
21. Cook FF, Tibone JE: The Mumford procedure in athletes: an objective analysis of function, *Am J Sports Med* 16(2):97-100, 1988.
22. Cox JS: The fate of the acromioclavicular joint in athletic injuries, *Am J Sports Med* 9(1):50-53, 1981.
23. Craig EV: Fractures of the clavicle. In: *The shoulder,* vol 1, Philadelphia, 1990, WB Saunders, pp 367-408.
24. Dameron TB Jr, Rockwood CA Jr: Fractures of the shaft of the clavicle. In Rockwood CA, Wilkins KE, King RE, editors: *Fractures in children,* Philadelphia, 1984, JB Lippincott, pp 608-624.
25. Dias JJ, Gregg PJ: Acromioclavicular joint injuries in sport: recommendations for treatment, *Sports Med* 11(2):125-132, 1991.
26. Reference deleted in proofs.
27. Ebraheim NA et al: Scapulothoracic dissociation, *J Bone Joint Surg* 70A:428-432, 1988.
28. Erickson SJ et al: Post-traumatic osteolysis of the clavicle: MR features, *J Comput Assis Tomogr* 14(5):835-837, 1990.
29. Eskola A et al: Outcome of operative treatment in fresh lateral clavicle fracture, *Ann Chir Gynaecol* 76(3):167-168, 1987.
30. Fukuda K et al: Biomechanical study of the ligamentous system of the acromioclavicular joint, *J Bone Joint Surg* 68A(3):434-439, 1986.
31. Gartsman GM et al: Arthroscopic acromioclavicular joint resection. An anatomical study, *Am J Sports Med* 19(1):2-5, 1991.
32. Gerber C, Rockwood CA Jr: Subcoracoid dislocation of the lateral end of the clavicle: a report of three cases, *J Bone Joint Surg* 69A(6):924-927, 1987.
33. Glick JM et al: Dislocated acromioclavicular joint: follow-up study of 35 unreduced acromioclavicular dislocations, *Am J Sports Med* 5(6):264-270, 1977.
34. Havranek P: Injuries of distal clavicular physis in children, *J Pediatr Orthop* 9(2):213-215, 1989.
35. Heppenstall RB: Fractures and dislocations of the distal clavicle, *Orthop Clin North Am* 6(2):477-486, 1975.
36. Ideberg R: Unusual glenoid fractures: a report on 92 cases, *Acta Orthop Scand* 58:191-192, 1987.
37. Ideberg R: Fractures of the scapula involving the glenoid fossa. In Bateman JE, Welsh RP, editors: *Surgery of the shoulder,* Philadelphia, 1984, BC Decker, pp 63-66.
38. Imatani RJ, Hanlon JJ, Cady GW: Acute complete acromioclavicular separation, *J Bone Joint Surg* 57A(3):328-332, 1975.
39. Inman VT, Saunders JG, Abbott LC: Observations on the function of the shoulder joint, *J Bone Joint Surg* 26:1-30, 1944.
40. Jacobs P: Post-traumatic osteolysis of the outer end of the clavicle, *J Bone Joint Surg* 46B:705-707, 1964.
41. Jalovaara P et al: Acute acromioclavicular dislocations treated by fixation of the joint and ligament repair or reconstruction, *Acta Orthop Belg* 57(3):296-305, 1991.
42. Kennedy JC, Cameron H: Complete dislocation of the acromioclavicular joint, *J Bone Joint Surg* 36B(2):202-208, 1954.

43. Larsen E, Bjerg-Nielsen A, Christensen P: Conservative or surgical treatment of acromioclavicular dislocation: a prospective, controlled, randomized study, *J Bone Joint Surg* 68A(4):552-555, 1986.
44. MacDonald PB et al: Comprehensive functional analysis of shoulders following complete acromioclavicular separation, *Am J Sports Med* 16(5):475-480, 1988.
45. Madsen B: Osteolysis of the acromial end of the clavicle following trauma, *Br J Radiol* 36(431):822, 1963.
46. McLaughlin H: *Trauma,* Philadelphia, 1959, WB Saunders.
47. McPhee IB: Inferior dislocation of the outer end of the clavicle, *J Trauma* 20(8):709-710, 1980.
48. Milch H: The rhomboid ligament in surgery of the sternoclavicular joint, *J Int Coll Surg* 17(1):41-51, 1952.
49. Milch H: Snapping scapula, *Clin Orthop* 20:139-150, 1961.
50. Milch H: Partial scapulectomy for snapping in the scapula, *J Bone Joint Surg* 32A:561-566, 1950.
51. Milch H, Burman MS: Snapping scapula and humerus varus, *Arch Surg* 26:570-588, 1933.
52. Millbourn E: On injuries to the acromioclavicular joint: treatment and results, *Acta Orthop Scand* 19:349-382, 1950.
53. Reference deleted in proofs.
54. Mumford EB: Acromioclavicular dislocation, *J Bone Joint Surg* 23:799-802, 1941.
55. Murphy OB et al: Post-traumatic osteolysis of the distal clavicle, *Clin Orthop* 109:108-114, 1975.
56. Neer CS II: Fractures of the clavicle. In Rockwood CA, Green DP, editors: *Fractures in adults,* Philadelphia, 1984, JB Lippincott, pp 707-713.
57. Neer CS II: Fractures of the distal third of the clavicle, *Clin Orthop* 58:43-50, 1968.
58. Neer CS II: Fracture of the distal clavicle with detachment of coracoclavicular ligaments in adults, *J Trauma* 3:99-110, 1963.
59. Nettles JL, Linscheid R: Sternoclavicular dislocations, *J Trauma* 8(2):158-164, 1968.
60. Omer GE: Osteotomy of the clavicle in surgical reduction of anterior sternoclavicular dislocation, *J Trauma* 7(4):584-590, 1967.
61. Park JP et al: Treatment of acromioclavicular separations: a retrospective study, *Am J Sports Med* 8(4):251-256, 1980.
62. Parkes JC, Deland JD: A three-part distal clavicle fracture, *J Trauma* 23(5):437-438, 1983.
63. Patterson WR: Inferior dislocation of the distal end of the clavicle, *J Bone Joint Surg* 49A:1184-1186, 1967.
64. Petersson CJ: Resection of the lateral end of the clavicle: a 3 to 30-year follow-up, *Acta Orthop Scand* 54:904-907, 1983.
65. Pridie K: Dislocation of acromioclavicular and sternoclavicular joints (proceedings), *J Bone Joint Surg* 41B(2):429, 1959.
66. Rockwood CA Jr: Acromioclavicular dislocation. In: *Fractures,* vol 1, ed 1, Philadelphia, 1975, JB Lippincott, pp 721-756.
67. Rockwood CA Jr: Injuries to the acromioclavicular joint. In: *Fractures in adults,* vol 1, ed 2, Philadelphia, 1984, JB Lippincott, pp 860-910.
68. Rockwood CA: Management of fracture of the clavicle and injuries of the SC joints, *Orthop Trans* 6:422, 1982.
69. Rockwood CA: Treatment of the outer clavicle in children and adults, *Orthop Trans* 6:472, 1982.
70. Rockwood CA, Matsen FA: *The shoulder,* vol 1, Philadelphia, 1990, WB Saunders.
71. Rockwood CA Jr, Odor JM: Spontaneous atraumatic anterior subluxations of the sternoclavicular joint in young adults: report of 37 cases, *Orthop Trans* 12(3):557, 1988.
72. Rodrigues H: Case of dislocation inwards of the internal extremity of the clavicle, *Lancet* 1:309-310, 1843.
73. Sondergard-Petersen P, Mikkelsen P: Posterior acromioclavicular dislocation, *J Bone Joint Surg* 64B(1):52-53, 1982.
74. Sage J: Recurrent inferior dislocation of the clavicle at the acromioclavicular joint, *Am J Sports Med* 10(3):145-146, 1982.
75. Reference deleted in proofs.
76. Scavenius M, Inversent BF: Nontraumatic clavicular osteolysis in weight lifters, *Am J Sports Med* 20(4):463-467, 1992.
77. Sunderaram N, Patel DV, Porter DS: Stabilization of acute acromioclavicular dislocation by a modified Bosworth technique: a long-term follow-up study, *Injury* 23(3):189-193, 1992.
78. Taft TN, Wilson FC, Oglesby JW: Dislocation of the acromioclavicular joint: an end-result study, *J Bone Joint Surg* 69A(7):1045-1051, 1987.
79. Thompson DA et al: The significance of scapular fractures, *J Trauma* 25:974-977, 1985.
80. Tossy JD, Mead NC, Sigmond HM: Acromioclavicular separations: useful and practical classification for treatment, *Clin Orthop* 28: 111-119, 1963.
81. Tsou PM: Percutaneous cannulated screw coracoclavicular fixation for acute acromioclavicular dislocations, *Clin Orthop* (243):112-121, 1989.
82. Urist MR: Complete dislocation of the acromioclavicular joint: the nature of the traumatic lesion and effective methods of treatment with an analysis of 41 cases, *J Bone Joint Surg* 28:813-837, 1946.
83. Vaatainen U, Pirinen A, Makela A: Radiological evaluation of the acromioclavicular joint, *Skeletal Radiol* 20(2):115-116, 1991.
84. Weaver JK, Dunn HK: Treatment of acromioclavicular injuries, especially complete acromioclavicular separation, *J Bone Joint Surg* 54A(6):1187-1197, 1972.
85. Weitzman G: Treatment of acute acromioclavicular joint dislocation by a modified Bosworth method: report on twenty-four cases, *J Bone Joint Surg* 49A(6):1167-1178, 1967.
86. Wilson KM, Colwill JC: Combined acromioclavicular dislocation with coracoclavicular ligament disruption and coracoid process fracture, *Am J Sports Med* 17(5):697-698, 1989.
87. Wojtys EM, Nelson G: Conservative treatment of grade III acromioclavicular dislocations, *Clin Orthop* (268):112-119, 1991.
88. Reference deleted in proofs.
89. Zanca P: Shoulder pain: involvement of the acromioclavicular joint: analysis of 1,000 cases, *AJR* 112(3):493-506, 1971.

CHAPTER 13

Muscle Ruptures of the Shoulder Girdle

JOHN D. KELLEY
NEAL S. ELATTRACHE

Musculotendinous injuries in the athlete are extremely common. Fortunately, most injuries only involve minor strains, but occasionally, actual ruptures or avulsions of muscle attachments do occur. Ruptures generally occur near the musculotendinous junction or at the tendon's insertion site either with or without an accompanying fragment of bone. According to McMaster,[57] ruptures through normal tendon do not occur. He found that approximately one half of a tendon's fibers had to be severed to permit rupture under severe strain. The implication is that for a tendon to rupture (i.e., the typical Achilles tendon rupture) a predisposing condition must be present that allows this to occur, according to authors who have evaluated muscle ruptures.[3,26,30,93] Whereas aging, rheumatoid changes, and decrease in tendon blood supply contribute to a large number of muscle and tendon ruptures in the population as a whole, these predisposing conditions occur less frequently in athletes. Etiologic factors, especially in overhead athletes, include excessive fatigue of muscle-tendon units through overuse and improper use. In this setting these muscle-tendon units may be less likely to resist sudden forces placed on them.

Taken as a whole, ruptures of muscles or tendons around the shoulder joint in athletes are uncommon. Far more common are the problems of tendinitis, bursitis, and instability. Muscle and tendon rupture occurring in the shoulder girdle are described in this chapter. Because rupture of certain muscles is rare, this discussion is not limited to the athletic population; rather it covers etiologic factors in general.

PECTORALIS MAJOR RUPTURES

Rupture of the pectoralis major muscle is uncommon. The first reported case was in 1822 by Patissier.[71] Since that time, 85 additional cases have been published.* McEntire[53] reported the largest review of pectoralis major ruptures in 1972, with 11 new cases added to 45 already in the literature. Only 22 of these 56 cases, including 8 of McEntire's 11, were treated operatively. The point was made that these may not all have been actual ruptures. Kretzler[39] reported 19 new cases in 1989, 16 of which were confirmed at surgery. The other, large series of new cases was published by Wolfe[97] in 1992 and included 14 cases, 7 of which were repaired. Most ruptures have occurred distally and involve the sternal head,† although complete ruptures of both heads‡ and muscle belly ruptures have also been reported.[37,53,55] Ruptures have most often been associated with a sudden overload to a contracting muscle, although "spontaneous" ruptures in elderly patients[65] and injury at childbirth[94] have been reported. Treatment has included nonoperative and operative means, each method having its proponents.

Anatomy

Gray's Anatomy[29] describes the pectoralis major muscle as being a "thick, triangular muscle arising from the anterior surface of the sternal half of the clavicle and the anterior surface of the sternum, as low down as the cartilage of the sixth or seventh ribs and from the aponeurosis of the oblique externum abdominis." It goes on to state that this muscle attaches by a double laminar tendon to the lateral lip of the intertubercular sulcus of the humerus. The anterior lamina is composed of the clavicular portion, while the posterior lamina is made up of the sternal and abdominal oblique portions. The sternal head

*References 6-8, 12, 13, 19, 21, 23, 33, 36-39, 41, 43, 46, 0, 55, 62, 69, 74-76, 80, 81, 86, 90, 92, 94, 97, 98.
†References 7, 13, 23, 39, 41, 49, 50, 53, 76, 82, 86, 97, 9
‡References 46, 48, 53, 69, 92, 97.

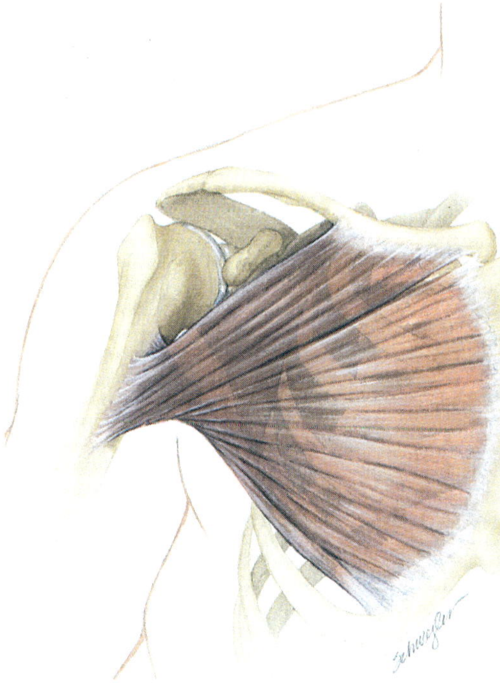

FIGURE 13-1 The sternocostal and abdominal portion of the muscle and tendon spiraling superiorly and posteriorly to insert posterior and deep to the more directly oriented clavicular head of the muscle.

fibers twist approximately 90° before inserting into the humerus via the posterior lamina. These fibers insert more proximally on the humerus than do those of the upper, clavicular head (Fig. 13-1). The lower border of the muscle forms the anterior axillary fold. To clarify the anatomy of the area of insertion, Kretzler[39] used cadaver dissections to show that the tendon was about 1 cm long on its anterior surface and 2.5 cm long on its posterior surface. In a more complete look at the muscle architecture, Wolfe[97] used cadavers to determine the fiber length at various points along the muscle both at rest and during a simulated bench-press maneuver. He showed a disproportionate stretching of the muscle's inferior fibers during extension of the humerus from 0° to 30° when compared with the superior fibers and with flexion of the humerus from 0° to 40°. The pectoralis major is innervated by the lateral and medial pectoral nerves.

Etiology

In the cases where a mechanism was given, the majority of ruptures have occurred secondary to a sudden force applied to the upper extremity, causing overload to a contracting pectoralis muscle. The single most common mechanism of this type has been the bench-press maneuver, representing 31 reported cases.* The majority of these cases occurred in body-builders and competitive

*References 7, 36, 39, 46, 49, 76, 92, 97, 98.

weight-lifters. Only five of these patients admitted to anabolic steroid use.[7,97] Attempting to stop a fall with the upper extremity has also been reported as a common cause of rupture. Ruptures have occurred in many sports other than weight-lifting such as wrestling, water skiing, football, rugby, boxing, sailboarding, skiing, basketball, and ice hockey. Most of the patients in these reports have a sudden force applied to the upper extremity in common. Direct blows account for a small percentage of injuries. In two elderly patients,[65] no known significant trauma occurred before the rupture.

All reports to date have involved males. In part this may be because women athletes and women in general have historically been involved with less violent activities. This may change now that more women are participating in sports like body-building and weight-lifting, in which rupture of the pectoralis appears more likely to occur. In the 67 cases where age was given the average age was 32.3 years, and approximately 80% of these causes occurred between the ages of 20 and 35.

Rupture most often involves the sternal portion of the muscle. This can be predicted, at least in the weight-lifting population, by Wolfe's[97] study showing excessive lengthening of the lower fibers during the humeral extension part of the bench press. Rupture by excessive tension usually occurs at the musculotendinous junction, within the tendon proper, or by avulsion from the humeral insertion. Complete rupture of both sternal and clavicular heads, although fewer in number, has been reported.* Muscle belly ruptures tend to result from a direct blow or crushing injury to the muscle.[37,53,55] Muscle belly rupture was a common finding in McEntire's review,[53] although it has been uncommon in other published reports.

*References 46, 48, 53, 69, 92, 97.

Documentation of the presence or absence of chronic symptoms in the area of the pectoralis major muscle before rupture is lacking in the literature. Marmor[50] suggests that attrition of the tendon does not normally occur, and rupture of the pectoralis major muscle may be presumed to be caused by trauma to a normal tendon.

Diagnosis

In the acute setting, patients have a history of a sudden force applied to the involved upper extremity or a direct blow to the upper arm or chest wall. The trauma is often associated with a tearing or burning sensation in the area of the pectoralis major tendon. Pain and swelling develop and limit active range of motion. Ecchymosis can be found in the area of rupture and can extend to the upper arm and anterior chest wall. In the unlikely event of rupture in the muscle belly or at the origin of the muscle medially, the ecchymosis may be concentrated more medially, away from the anterior axillary fold and upper arm. In the more common distal, sternal head rupture the sternal portion of the muscle retracts medially. As the acute swelling subsides, loss of the normal anterior axillary fold is seen. This defect is accentuated by active contraction of the muscle (Fig. 13-2).

After the acute period of pain and edema has passed, the major complaints of patients are weakness and the resultant cosmetic deformity. This is particularly true in patients involved in body-building or competitive weight-lifting. The greatest strength deficit is in humeral adduction in the scapular plane followed by humeral internal rotation. This was substantiated by Marmor[50] in a study of a patient with congenital unilateral absence of the sternal head of a pectoralis major muscle. Isokinetic testing of both upper extremities showed a loss in the involved arm of nearly 50% adduction strength in the scapular plane, as well as a "significant diminution of

A 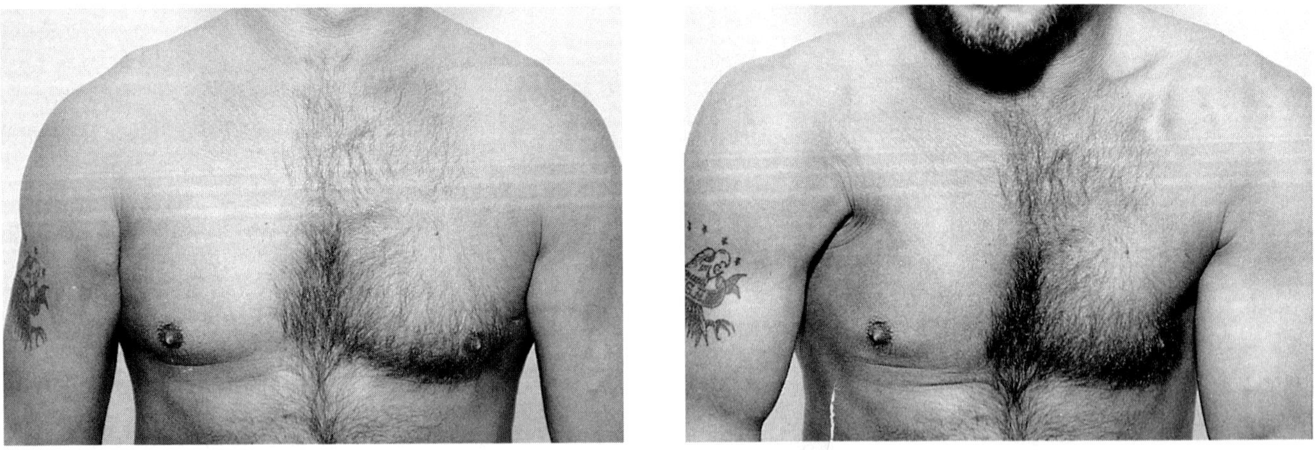 B

FIGURE 13-2 **A**, Normal chest contour with pectoralis major relaxed; **B**, Asymmetric chest contour resulting from medial retraction of the sternocostal head of the pectoralis major with active contraction of the muscle.

strength in internal rotation." Kretzler,[39] Roi,[80] Scott,[82] and Wolfe[97] used isokinetic testing to demonstrate weakness in adduction and internal rotation rupture. Many others have stated that weakness was evident on manual muscle testing after rupture.*

Chronic ruptures have a history of past injury, but without the acute findings of pain and swelling. Patients' complaints often center on weakness, cosmetic deformity, and in some cases difficulty with or inability to perform their occupation or sport. Generally these are patients with physically demanding jobs or sports requiring significant upper body strength. As expected, body-builders also complain of the loss of symmetry.

Associated findings include rupture of the anterior deltoid and tears of the rotator cuff reported by McEntire,[53] and myositis ossificans in a patient seen 4 months after rupture.[76] Kawashima[37] described a patient in whom a crush injury to the chest wall resulted in a pectoralis major rupture, brachial plexus injury, and ruptured latissimus dorsi muscle. Smith[86] reported a case of rhabdomyosarcoma at the site of a ruptured pectoralis major muscle 10 years after injury.

Radiographic examination is usually negative regarding the humerus. However, some authors have reported that loss of the normal axillary fold shadow on chest radiograph is a reliable sign of distal pectoralis major muscle rupture.[49,50,69] MRI has been used to assess rupture and soft-tissue injury to other musculotendinous units but has not to date been mentioned in the literature concerning pectoralis major muscle ruptures. In the future this might be a useful adjunct in cases where the diagnosis is unclear.

Treatment

Treatment of pectoralis major ruptures must be based on the specific diagnosis (i.e., partial ruptures, strains, and complete ruptures). Partial ruptures can be successfully treated by nonoperative methods.[80,90] Depending on the severity, treatment for partial ruptures consists of an initial period of immobilization for comfort followed by gradual mobilization as symptoms decrease. Strengthening can generally begin 4 to 6 weeks after injury.[80,90]

Complete ruptures can involve the muscle origin, muscle belly, musculotendinous junction, or insertion. The most common injury among athletes is a distal rupture of the sternal head. The type of individual who incurs this injury is often an athlete with high demands on upper-body strength. Most authors recommend surgical repair in patients who wish to continue in these activities at a high level or athletes requiring side-to-side symmetry of upper-body musculature.† Many of these authors extend their indications for surgery to include people whose occupation calls for repetitive activity requiring significant upper-body strength.

Acute surgical treatment consists of suture repair of the musculotendinous junction ruptures or repair of an avulsed distal tendon into the humeral insertion site via sutures through drill holes. Variations have included the use of a barbed staple by Egan,[23] pull-out wires by McEntire,[53] and suture of the tendon into a trough made at the humeral insertion site as described by Wolfe.[97] Postoperatively, immobilization is prescribed for 4 to 6 weeks followed by range-of-motion exercises. After 6 to 12 weeks, when most of the motion has been regained, strengthening exercises are begun.

Appropriate treatment of chronic ruptures is divided between authors favoring conservative means and those advocating late repair. Some authors have recommended nonoperative treatment secondary to expected difficulty with surgical dissection and repair. Roi[80] reported "... almost complete functional recovery. . ." in a weight-lifter with a chronic tear treated nonoperatively. Marmor[40] treated a wrestler conservatively who presented 3 years after injury and achieved good results. In the last 15 years several reports have been published suggesting that successful repair of chronic tears is possible.* Scott[82] noted that the operation was not "unduly difficult." Kretzler[39] reported successful repair in two cases 5 years after rupture. Postoperative treatment of chronic repairs has been similar to treatment for acute repairs.

Results of treatment are unfortunately in the form of case reports with objective data lacking in many cases. Park[69] in 1970 reviewed 30 cases of pectoralis major ruptures. He found that patients who were treated surgically had 80% excellent and 10% good results versus 17% excellent and 58% good results in patients with ruptures treated nonoperatively. They note that "complete recovery of strength and contour" is seldom obtained after conservative treatment. McEntire[53] reviewed 56 cases in the literature and found that surgical treatment yielded 70% excellent and 10% good results in comparison to 27% excellent and 47% good results in conservatively treated ruptures. Therefore he recommended conservative treatment for muscle belly ruptures and surgical management for distal ruptures. Jones[36] in 1988 looked at the results of treatment for 46 patients found that ruptures repaired within 7 days had 57% excellent and 30% good results, whereas those patients with delayed repair had no excellent and 60% good results. In addition, conservative treatment yielded no excellent and only 46% good results. Kretzler[39] in 1989 reported on 16 surgically repaired distal ruptures, 81% of which had full return of strength. Two patients repaired 5 years after injury had incomplete cosmetic correction. In a group of athletes with 14 ruptures, Wolfe[97] treated 7 surgically and 7 conservatively. He found noticeable deficits in peak torque

*References 7, 13, 36, 38, 74, 75, 81, 98.

†References 7, 8, 21, 22, 36, 39, 46, 48-50, 53, 69, 74, 75, 80, 90, 97, 98.

*References 7, 39, 46, 76, 81, 82, 97.

and work capacity in conservatively treated individuals as compared with those treated surgically.

Complications reported include a patient with limited abduction in Kretzler's series,[39] and a patient with postoperative fourth and fifth digit paresthesias noted by Wolfe.[97] The first reported case, in 1822, died secondary to an infected local hematoma followed by sepsis.[71]

Conclusions

Rupture of the pectoralis major muscle is uncommon. Among athletes, it most commonly occurs during the bench-press exercise. Most often the distal portion of the sternal head is injured. Muscle belly ruptures or partial disruption of the distal muscle heads may be treated conservatively with good results. Complete, distal ruptures of the sternal head, the clavicular head, or both can be repaired in the acute and in many cases the chronic setting with predictably good to excellent results in the majority of cases. Repair is recommended in competitive athletes and laborers requiring full strength for their activities. For activities of daily living and nonstrenuous upper extremity activity, conservative treatment results in satisfactory function in most instances.

TRICEPS RUPTURES

Triceps muscle or tendon ruptures are rare. Conwell[18] in 1937 and Waugh[89] in 1949 reported that the triceps was the least frequently ruptured muscle or tendon. Haldeman[30] in 1935 found only 2 of 61 upper-extremity muscle or tendon ruptures to involve the triceps. Anzel[3] in 1959 found 8 triceps ruptures in a review of 1014 cases of muscle and tendon ruptures, and 4 of these resulted from direct trauma. The first case report was by Partridge[70] in 1868. Since that time, there have been 49 cases reported in the English literature. Most ruptures occurred at the site of distal tendon insertion into the olecranon, although rupture at the musculotendinous junction,[5,26,83] rupture through the muscle belly,[40,60,72] and avulsion proximally[10,11] have been reported. Levy[44,45] pointed out the importance of associated injuries such as radial head fracture. Lee[42] described a case of distal radius fracture associated with triceps rupture. Farrar,[24] Lotem,[47] Preston,[73] and Searfoss[83] have linked chronic renal failure and associated secondary hyperparathyroidism with six cases of triceps rupture. Other medical problems associated with triceps rupture include anabolic steroid usage, by Bach,[5] and oral corticosteroid usage in a patient with rheumatoid arthritis, by one of the authors. Clayton[14] described a case of chronic olecranon bursitis in a patient with triceps rupture.

Anatomy

The triceps muscle lies in the posterior or extensor compartment of the arm. *Gray's Anatomy*[29] describes the triceps as being composed of three heads—the long head arising from the infraglenoid tubercle of the scapula, the lateral head arising from the posterior and lateral shaft of the humerus, and the medial head arising from the posterior and medial shaft of the humerus. The distal tendinous portion begins in the middle of the muscle and is initially composed of a smaller, superficial layer and a deeper, larger layer that combine above the elbow to insert together posteriorly onto the upper surface of the olecranon process of the ulna. Laterally, a band of fibers continues over the anconeus to blend with the antebrachial fascia. The long head also divides the quadrilateral space, containing the posterior humeral circumflex vessels and the axillary nerve from the triangular space, which contains the circumflex scapular vessels. Swelling associated with rupture of the long head proximally can simulate a quadrilateral space syndrome. The triceps is innervated by the radial nerve in the arm.

Etiology

The small number of published accounts of triceps rupture is probably partly because of its infrequent occurrence and the lack of clinical awareness of this injury. An indirect mechanism of injury, such as a fall onto the upper extremity, is the most common cause of triceps rupture.[44,45] This accounts for 29 of the 49 reported cases where the mechanism was known. In 8 of the 49 cases a direct blow to the triceps area was responsible for injury. Lotem[47] reported little or no trauma involved in two cases of rupture in patients with chronic renal failure and secondary hyperparathyroidism. Searfoss[83] described a patient with chronic renal failure who ruptured the triceps during a seizure. In 31 cases, males were involved; females were involved in 10 cases. This information was not given in 9 cases. The average age in those reported was 26 years old, ranging from 7 to 72 years old.[5]

Nine ruptures have occurred during athletic activities. Brumback,[11] Gilcreest,[26] and Bowerman[10] reported triceps injuries as a result of throwing. Kuniichi[40] described a triceps rupture occurring as the result of a volleyball serve. A weight-lifter ruptured his triceps during a "snatch" maneuver as reported by Bach.[5] Clayton[14] reported a triceps rupture resulting from a fall from a stationary bicycle. The remaining three cases involved direct blows to the triceps. One case resulted from a martial arts kick described by Kuniichi,[40] another involved a skiing accident in which a ski struck the arm during a fall reported by Farra,[24] a third involved a football player with a ruptured triceps that resulted from being kicked by another player as reported by Tarsney.[89]

Diagnosis

Patients with a ruptured triceps muscle complain of elbow pain after any one of the mechanisms mentioned earlier. Clinical suspicion should be increased in patients with chronic renal failure or those taking anabolic steroids or corticosteroids. Presentation is usually acute,

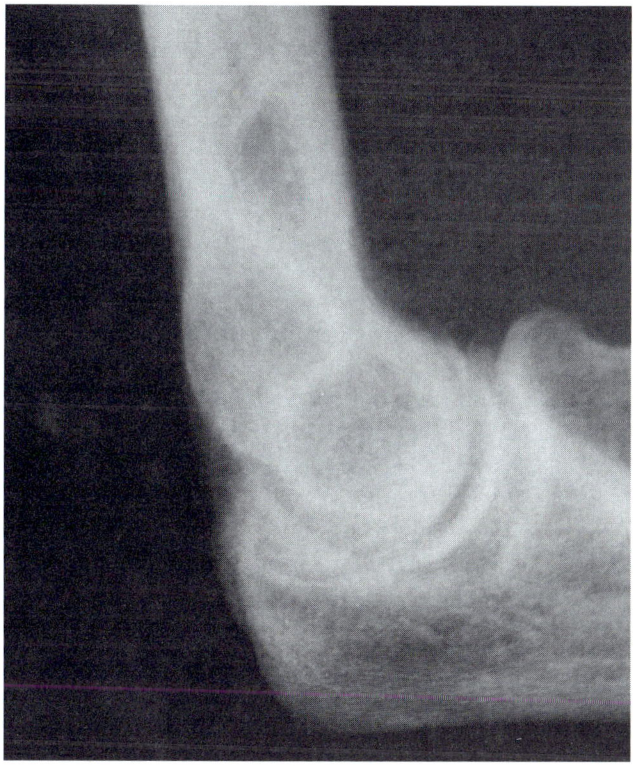

FIGURE 13-3 Lateral radiograph showing avulsion of a portion of the olecranon insertion of the triceps with retraction.

however, in some cases the diagnosis has been delayed for months.[1,68,84] Usually the pain is posterior, although when associated with radial head fracture the pain may also be lateral. Examination demonstrates swelling with or without ecchymosis, usually over the distal triceps area. In the rare cases of musculotendinous junction or muscle belly ruptures these findings are more proximal. In most cases a defect is palpable just proximal to the olecranon. This may be less obvious in acute cases associated with severe swelling. In these instances a repeat examination after the initial swelling has subsided may be useful. Active range of motion and strength testing usually demonstrate a significant extensor lag and weakness with complete ruptures. The clinical findings in partial ruptures are not as impressive.

Radiographic examination should include anteroposterior, lateral, and oblique views of the elbow The lateral film may show a "fleck of bone" proximal to the olecranon (Fig. 13-3). This may support the diagnosis of a complete distal tendon avulsion from its insertion.* Care should also be taken to exclude other fractures, especially a radial head fracture.[44,45,89] Although MRI is not mentioned in the current literature on triceps ruptures, it may be useful in questionable cases, since it has been helpful in diagnosing soft-tissue disruptions in other parts of the body.

*References 25, 42, 44, 47, 48, 68, 73, 89.

Treatment

Treatment of triceps ruptures, when discussed in the literature, has been mainly surgical. Three complete ruptures have been treated nonoperatively, including a midmuscle belly rupture of Kuniichi's,[40] a distal tendon avulsion in an adult treated by Farrar,[24] and a distal tendon avulsion in a 7-year-old reported by Levy.[44] Partial tears have been treated nonoperatively with immobilization by Levy[44,45] and Lotem.[47]

Operative treatment consists of suturing the avulsed distal tendon through drill holes into the olecranon. Absorbable,[5] nonabsorbable,[5] and wire sutures[1] have all been described for repair. Clayton[14] reported a "flap turn down" technique similar to that reported for repair of Achilles tendon ruptures. Postoperative immobilization consists of a cast or posterior splint with the elbow in 30° to 40° of flexion for an average of 3 to 4 weeks. Protected motion consisting of active flexion and passive extension is then begun. When the healing process is complete, more aggressive strengthening and range-of-motion exercises are used.

Results of treatment, whether for complete or incomplete ruptures, are described in the literature by such terms as "good or excellent," "normal motion and strength," "complete function," or "full recovery" with few exceptions. Unfortunately, reports including objective results such as isokinetic testing are limited.[5,84] The reported complications include loss of motion in extension of 5° to 20° in four patients.[1,5,45,89] Compartment syndrome was reported by Brumback[11] in a case of proximal avulsion. Olecranon bursitis was attributed to the use of wire suture in one patient.[68]

Conclusions

Triceps rupture or avulsion is an uncommon injury resulting from an indirect force to an actively extending elbow or from a direct blow. The majority of cases occur in non-sports-related activities and involve avulsion of the distal tendon from the olecranon. A palpable defect, extensor weakness, and extensor lag are commonly found during the examination. A "fleck of bone" on the lateral radiograph lends support to the clinical diagnosis. Treatment consists of surgical repair in complete rupture of avulsion and initial immobilization in partial rupture. Motion and strength are generally good to excellent after such treatment.

BICEPS RUPTURES

Long head tendon ruptures of the biceps are discussed in Chapter 7. Distal biceps tendon ruptures are covered in Chapter 22. This section discusses ruptures of the muscle belly.

Although rupture of the long head tendon of the biceps is not uncommon, especially for patients with rotator cuff disease, rupture of the muscle belly of the biceps is extremely unusual. One of the earliest documented cases of belly rupture was described by Mason[51] in 1924. Gilcreest[26] in 1925 and Conwell[18] in 1928 believed that muscle belly ruptures were frequently overlooked or misdiagnosed when compared with the more common long head tendon ruptures. In Gilcreest's[27] review of 106 cases of biceps tears or ruptures reported in 1934, complete belly ruptures accounted for 6 cases with 11 partial belly ruptures, for a total of 17 cases, or 16% of the total. This represents a much higher percentage compared with other authors' reports, which likely reflects both Gilcreest's high clinical suspicion and interest in this topic. Heckman[34] in 1978 presented his results in 48 muscle belly ruptures, all occurring in military parachutists.

Anatomy

The biceps brachii muscle[29] consists of two proximal heads of origin. The short head arises from the coracoid process along with the coracobrachialis. The long head takes origin from the supraglenoid tubercle at the apex of the glenoid cavity, continuous with the labrum. The long head tendon then exits the joint proper and passes between the humeral tuberosities and beneath the transverse humeral ligament. The muscle bellies from each head are joined approximately 7 cm proximal to the elbow joint. They terminate as a common distal tendon that inserts into the radial tuberosity. Both heads of the muscle receive innervation from the musculocutaneous nerve. The main functions of the biceps brachii are supination of the forearm and flexion of the elbow.

Etiology

Most reported muscle belly ruptures have resulted from direct trauma to the anterior aspect of the arm. Most of the cases were published by Heckman.[34] Each involved military parachutists and was caused by improper positioning of the static line across the upper arm at the beginning of the jump, causing a sudden, forceful compression on the muscle belly of the biceps. This injury is not common in recreational parachutists probably because the static line is less commonly used. Conwell[17] described a case caused by sudden forceful extension of a strongly flexed elbow.

Diagnosis

Diagnosis of biceps muscle belly rupture can be difficult because of its unusual occurrence and low clinical suspicion on the part of most clinicians. It can be difficult to distinguish long head tendon rupture from proximal muscle belly rupture, although belly ruptures are usually associated with more swelling because of significant hematoma formation.[26] A history of direct or indirect trauma should be given by the patient, as well as complaints of pain and swelling in the anterior arm. The pain is usually worse when attempting to move the elbow. Patients may complain of weakness with elbow flexion. Paresthesias in the distal distribution of the musculocutaneous nerve can be an additional feature. Heckman[34] reports that in chronic cases most patients complain of weakness and easy fatigability with repetitive elbow flexion. Physical examination demonstrates signs of contusion with noticeable local hematoma formation. Because of the noticeable swelling, a palpable defect within the muscle belly may be difficult to appreciate initially.[34] Acutely, patients may demonstrate flexion weakness, which might be ascribed to pain and swelling instead of acute rupture. In chronic cases a defect is usually both palpable and visible, especially with resisted flexion of the elbow. Weakness may also be elicited on examination. Heckman[34] points out that in a group of 28 patients with belly ruptures the examining physicians rated manual muscle testing as good or excellent in all 28. Ergometric testing in these same patients revealed flexion power to average only 53% of normal. Radiographic findings have been almost exclusively negative, with the exception of one case with an associated scapular neck fracture.[34] MRI may prove to be useful in differentiating a complete rupture from a less severe strain early, although no reports have yet been published.

Associated injuries include the above-mentioned scapular neck fracture and nine musculocutaneous nerve injuries reported by Heckman,[34] one of which showed persistent signs of denervation a year after injury. Interestingly, Heckman states that none of these patients complained of paresthesias or loss of sensation in the distal sensory distribution of the musculocutaneous nerve. Mellen[58] reported a case of muscle rupture in a paratrooper with an associated contusion and thrombosis of the brachial artery requiring saphenous vein grafting. This same patient had an ipsilateral partial triceps tear.

Treatment

Mason[48] in 1924 described open repair of a near-total belly rupture suffered from a direct blow to the arm. Postoperatively, the arm was immobilized in full flexion and supination for 3 weeks. Active range of motion and passive range of motion began at 3 weeks. Mason reported that the patient was discharged at 6 weeks "... the arm being satisfactory in every respect." Rocyn-Jones[79] in 1925 stated that "the only satisfactory treatment is to operate and suture the torn muscle." He described one case treated conservatively with poor results. Gilcreest[26] in 1925 recommended that surgery be performed without delay if an acute complete rupture was diagnosed. He began motion 3 weeks postoperatively also. In a more complete report on belly ruptures, Gilcreest[27] in 1934 recommended splinting in a fully flexed position for 2 to 3 weeks in partial belly ruptures and early repair of complete ruptures. Conwell[17,18] in 1928 and 1937 recommended immediate exposure of the ruptured muscle and suturing of the muscle and fascia. He described one complete rupture treated by repair, which had an excellent result and uneventful recovery. Heckman and Levine[34] in 1979 reported on the treatment of 48 cases of muscle belly rupture, all caused by static line injury in paratroopers. A group of 28 patients, who were treated conservatively with an average follow-up of 19 months, provided a relative natural history of this injury. They were treated with a sling for approximately 1 week, and then they gradually returned to activity. At final follow-up, 25 of 28 patients complained of weakness and early fatigue with elbow flexion. Twelve patients complained of pain, and 17 were bothered by the cosmetic deformity at the site of rupture. Flexion power of the involved side was only 53% of normal as measured by an ergometer. A group of six patients had late operations consisting of suture repair. Five of these six had follow-up, and three increased their flexion power from an average 42% preoperatively to an average 57% postoperatively. The second part of the study was a prospective, randomized look at 20 ruptures, also in paratroopers. Ten patients underwent operative repair within 72 hours; the other 10 underwent early aspiration of a hematoma from the rupture site. Each group was splinted in acute flexion, the operative group for 4 weeks and the nonoperative group for 6 weeks. The operative group was then splinted at 90° flexion for 2 additional weeks. Each group was allowed active range of motion beginning at 6 weeks, then gradually increasing activity at 8 weeks. Average follow-up for the group was 7.1 months for the conservatively treated group and 8.8 months for the operative group. All 10 in the conservative group were available for final follow-up, as well as 9 of 10 operative patients. All patients in each group had normal range of motion and were without neurologic complications. Two patients in the conservative group complained of mild or moderate weakness; three patients in the operative group complained of slight weakness. The person in the conservative group who complained of moderate weakness also complained of pain and cosmetic deformity. In the operative group, one patient complained of pain, and no one complained of cosmetic deformity. Strength measurements using ergometers showed 77% of normal strength in the conservative group versus 76.5% of normal strength in the operative group. Complications occurring in the operative group consisted of one deep wound infection requiring drainage and one postoperative hematoma that resolved by the 6-week follow-up examination.

Conclusions

Muscle belly rupture of the biceps brachii is an uncommon injury. Most reports in the literature are the result of direct injury to the arm, although indirect injury has also been described. With the Heckman and Levine[34] series as a guide, treatment in the acute setting should consist of aspiration of hematoma with a large-bore needle and splinting in acute flexion for 6 weeks. This is followed by gradual recovery of motion and strength and, finally, a return to normal activities. Partial ruptures may be treated similarly but with earlier return of motion and activity.[27,51] Consideration of operative treatment in cases that are nonacute should be based on the degree of functional limitations, since the results are not as good as with those treated acutely.[34]

SUBSCAPULARIS RUPTURES

Isolated rupture of the subscapularis muscle is uncommon. Smith[87] first reported such an injury in 1835 as a finding at cadaver dissection. Gilcreest[28] in 1939 credits Speed and Bull and Gilbert with reports of three cases of isolated subscapularis rupture, one of which was confirmed at surgery. Gilcreest[28] added a case that he treated surgically. McGuinness[54] also published a case report in 1939. Since that time there have been several additional accounts of subscapularis rupture with and without small avulsions of bone from the lesser tuberosity.*

Anatomy

The subscapularis muscle is described by *Gray's Anatomy*[30] as a large, triangular muscle that fills the subscapular fossa, which arises from its medial two thirds. The fibers converge into a tendon laterally, attaching to the lesser tuberosity of the humerus. The muscle is attached also to the anterior capsule of the glenohumeral joint laterally. DePalma[23] in a study looking at 122 cadavers found that the lateral 2 cm of the anterior capsule was inseparable from the overlying subscapularis tendon. The action of the subscapularis is to internally rotate the humerus. The subscapularis also plays a role in humeral adduction. The nerve supply to the muscle is the upper and lower subscapular nerves.

Etiology

Most reports of subscapularis rupture or avulsion have been associated with anterior shoulder dislocations.† Others have involved falls with a sudden load placed onto the contracting upper extremity, without dislocation.‡ Biondi[9] described a case of isolated subscapularis rupture in an arm wrestler. McGuinness[54] reported a case of lateral avulsion that occurred during convulsant therapy. White published the only report of avulsion in a child,[95] an abduction injury suffered while climbing a wall.

The subscapularis is an important structure in preventing anterior glenohumeral dislocation and has been

*References 2, 4, 9, 16, 31, 52, 56, 64-66, 77, 85, 95.
†References 22, 31, 38, 64-66, 85, 88.
‡References 2, 16, 28, 52, 77, 95.

found ruptured or lax in cases of recurrent or even initial anterior dislocations.* The humeral avulsion of glenohumeral ligaments (HAGL) lesion was first described by Nicola[65] in 1942 and involved the avulsion of the capsule laterally instead of medially or at the glenoid labrum. Since the lateralmost part of the subscapularis tendon is relatively inseparable from the underlying capsule,[22] in many instances the subscapularis is torn along with the lateral capsule. The HAGL lesion has been found in up to 19% of some series of anterior dislocations.†

Diagnosis

The most common cause of subscapularis rupture seems to be trauma associated with anterior glenohumeral dislocation. The injury occurs after a sudden abduction, external rotation force to the upper extremity, and documented anterior dislocation. Those without actual dislocation present after sudden eccentric loading to the upper extremity, usually in abduction, and many times associated with a fall. Most patients complain of anterior shoulder pain and an inability to abduct the arm secondary to pain. Internal rotation strength is significantly weaker than the uninjured side. Pain in the shoulder increases with passive external rotation and passive abduction.

Standard radiographs may show an avulsed fragment of the lesser tuberosity. In patients with a dislocation additional history findings, such as Hill-Sachs deformity, may be found. Other useful imaging modalities are CT arthrogram and MRI, either of which can confirm clinical suspicion of this injury and delineate any associated injuries when present.[9,16,64,85]

Associated injuries include a case of axillary nerve palsy reported by Andreasen[2] and two cases of medial, intraarticular dislocation of the long head of the biceps tendon described by Collier.[18] Chapter 7 provides a more detailed discussion of cases of nonisolated subscapularis ruptures, such as cases associated with rotator cuff tears.

Treatment

Most reports of isolated subscapularis rupture or avulsion have been individual cases that have been surgically treated.‡ Andreasen[2] described a 56-year-old woman who refused operation for an avulsion. She was treated in a splint with 45° of abduction, midinternal rotation, and 25° of forward flexion. After 2 months, she returned to work as a nurse with internal rotation weakness and "slight disability." At the 14-month follow-up, the small avulsed piece of bone from the lesser tuberosity had resorbed.

The reports of operative treatment* have involved suture repair of the tendon to the site of origin. In cases of tendon rupture, suture repair to the remaining stump has been used. When an avulsion includes a small piece of lesser tuberosity, the piece of bone can be placed into a trough cut into the humerus. Postoperatively, most authors immobilize the shoulder in internal rotation for a period of 2 to 3 weeks, and then protect the shoulder from motion. Strengthening exercises begin at 6 weeks.

When subscapularis rupture is associated with recurrent anterior shoulder dislocation, labral or capsular damage is repaired along with reattachment of the subscapularis to the lesser tuberosity.[22,63,88] Further discussion about operative techniques and postoperative rehabilitation after labral and capsular procedures can be found in later chapters.

Results of repair involving isolated subscapularis rupture or avulsion have lacked objective data. McGuinness[54] gave no results in his patient. Gilcreest[26] reported a satisfactory result and return to regular work in a 30-year-old laborer. Hauser[31] described the results of a 21-year-old football player who had full use of the extremity except for a slight limitation in external rotation after 6 months. This same patient later passed the Air Force physical examination and was able to participate in all major sports. A second patient of Hauser's[31] had recurrent dislocations playing volleyball. One year after repair, the patient was participating in athletics and experiencing recurrent anterior subluxation. White[95] described a repair in a 12-year-old girl who, at 3 months after surgical repair, had full, active, painless motion and full athletic activity. McAuliff[52] reported full range of motion and a return to regular activities 3 months after repair in a 54-year-old woman.

Conclusions

Isolated rupture or avulsion of the subcapularis muscle occurs infrequently. It should be suspected in cases of anterior shoulder dislocation or other upper-extremity injuries with findings of weak internal rotation and increased pain with passive external rotation.

Because of the important role of the subscapularis muscle in anterior shoulder stability and shoulder function in general, repair of rupture or avulsion is recommended. Physicians should watch for concurrent lateral capsular damage or damage to the capsulolabral complex medially.

SERRATUS ANTERIOR RUPTURES

Rupture of the serratus anterior muscle occurs infrequently. Only 12 cases are found in a review of the English-language literature. Of these 12 cases, all but two were diagnosed by clinical examination alone and with-

*References 22, 31, 56, 61, 64-66, 78, 85, 88.
†References 3, 22, 31, 64-66, 85, 96.
‡References 16, 19, 31, 52, 54, 64, 95.

*References 16, 19, 31, 52, 54, 64, 95.

out electrodiagnostic studies. One of these two cases was confirmed at surgery,[32] and the other was suspected on clinical examination and confirmed by negative electrodiagnostic studies.[59]

Anatomy

Gray's Anatomy[30] describes the serratus anterior as a muscular sheet passing backward around the thorax from an extensive costal attachment to a more limited attachment on the scapula. Its origin arises from the outer surfaces and superior borders of the upper 8, 9, or 10 ribs. Its insertion is along the medial border of the scapula. It is innervated by the long thoracic nerve. The main functions of the muscle are to draw the scapula forward and to stabilize the scapula against the thoracic wall during elevation of the upper extremity.

Etiology

Of the 12 case reports in the literature, the mechanism of injury is specified in only six. One case occurred during a football scrimmage,[25] two from falls,[25] and one each from crush injury,[25] indirect trauma,[25] and "rolling over in bed" in a rheumatoid patient.[59] As mentioned previously, only one rupture has been confirmed at surgery. This was reported by Hayes[32] in 1981 in a 25-year old carpenter. The mechanism was not given. The patient had a displaced fracture of the inferior angle of the ipsilateral scapula. During the operation, the serratus anterior and rhomboid major were detached from their scapular insertions. Clinically, the patient exhibited winging of the scapula. The muscles were repaired to their sites of avulsion. The follow-up examination showed no winging at 6 weeks and full strength with normal range of motion after 1 year. Hayes recommended electrodiagnostic studies at 3 to 6 weeks in cases where rupture cannot easily be differentiated from nerve injury. Fichet's[26] five cases were diagnosed by clinical examination alone. He reported the only sport-related injury in a 17-year-old football player. This patient was diagnosed acutely, and treatment consisted of splinting, keeping tension off the serratus muscle for a 5-week period. After 12 weeks, this patient reportedly had "entirely recovered."

Most cases of ruptures that are diagnosed late report that winging persists despite splinting and other conservative measures. Overpeck[67] thought physical therapy and support of the extremity were the most universally successful methods of treatment. However, three of his five ruptures treated in this fashion did not recover function of the serratus anterior. Gilcreest[28] believed that early recognition and treatment were necessary for a successful outcome.

Since there are only 12 cases in the literature and one operative repair, it is difficult to strongly recommend any particular treatment. A review of these cases does show that conservative treatment of a chronic rupture probably has little chance of restoring function to the extent that winging is eliminated.[25,28,59,67] Because of the role the serratus anterior muscle plays in scapular stabilization and in allowing full overhead elevation of the upper extremity, surgical repair is recommended for an acute rupture of the serratus anterior, especially in the younger, athletic population.

DELTOID RUPTURES

Rupture of the deltoid muscle is rare. Since Clemens[15] reported the first case in 1913, only four additional cases have been described. Clemens'[15] patient had a sudden force applied to the upper extremity while the patient carried a heavy rail. Davis[20] reported a case of rupture in a patient with osteomyelitis of the clavicle and associated soft-tissue suppuration about the superior shoulder. Gilcreest[28] described two cases, one associated with heavy overhead lifting and one resulting from injury sustained in an automobile accident. McEntire[53] published a report of a deltoid rupture associated with a pectoralis major tear.

Anatomy

The deltoid is described by *Gray's Anatomy*[29] as a thick, triangular muscle attached to the anterior and superior surfaces of the lateral third of the clavicle, the lateral margin and superior surface of the acromion, and the spine of the scapula. Anterior, middle, and posterior heads converge to a common tendon, which inserts into the deltoid tuberosity on the lateral humeral shaft. The deltoid gives the shoulder a rounded contour. The nerve supply is via the axillary nerve. The anterior head of the muscle provides forward elevation of the humerus while the posterior head extends the humerus. All three heads function to abduct the humerus.

Etiology and Diagnosis

With the exception of the case of rupture secondary to infection,[20] reports of rupture of the deltoid have involved a sudden force to the involved upper extremity. Pain, tenderness, and swelling are present in the area of rupture. A defect may be palpable, and there may be a visible change in shoulder contour, especially with resisted muscle contraction.[28] Abduction is also weaker than the contralateral side.

Injury to the axillary nerve may be confused with damage to the muscle itself. In this situation, lateral deltoid sensation may be altered. Electrodiagnostic studies can help if nerve injury is suspected. Although not reported in the literature, MRI may be helpful early in diagnosing muscle rupture.

Treatment

Treatment of the few cases reported in the literature has varied. Davis[20] performed surgical repair using a fascial graft in his report on a complete deltoid rupture. Excision of the most anteromedial part of the deltoid was performed by McEntire,[53] together with repair of the patient's ruptured pectoralis major. Gilcreest's[28] two patients refused surgical treatment, and the results of the nonoperative treatment are not given. Davis[20] placed his patient in a plaster abduction splint for 6 weeks followed by active range of motion. Results at 10 weeks showed active abduction against gravity to 90°. No further follow-up was reported. McEntire's[53] patient was treated postoperatively according to a protocol for pectoralis major repair, and after 9 years had full range of motion and was working as a heavy laborer.

The subject of deltoid rupture after rotator cuff repair with deltoid takedown is discussed in Chapter 7.

Conclusions

Primary rupture of the deltoid seems to be extremely rare. Because it is a very important muscle for shoulder function, repair is recommended when torn. Chapter 7 discusses repair techniques for rotator cuff repair.

CORACOBRACHIALIS RUPTURES

Rupture of the coracobrachialis muscle is rare. Review of the literature yields two case reports. Gilcreest[28] in 1939 described a case of complete muscle belly rupture. Tobin[91] in 1941 reported a case of complete rupture of the coracobrachialis and short head of the biceps. Additionally, Gilcreest[27] in 1934 commented on two cases of rupture of the short head of the biceps tendon. He did not mention the coracobrachialis in these two cases, but the muscles share a common origin.[29] As a result it is quite likely the rupture was in both muscles.

Anatomy and Etiology

In *Gray's Anatomy,*[29] the coracobrachialis is described as arising from the apex of the coracoid process of the scapula in common with the tendon of the short head of the biceps. It attaches into an impression 3 to 5 cm in length along the medial border of the humerus between the brachialis and triceps muscles. The nerve supply is the musculocutaneous nerve, which enters the muscle proximally. The actions of the coracobrachialis include arm flexion and adduction.

The mechanism of injury has been direct injury at the site of rupture in both case reports.[23,91] Gilcreest[28] described his case as the result of "direct violence"; Tobin's[91] case was secondary to a static line injury during military parachute jumping. In Gilcreest's report[27] of the short head biceps tendon ruptures, the mechanisms were not given.

Diagnosis

Tobin's report did not comment on clinical presentation. Gilcreest's patient complained of considerable impairment in arm function, but not a significant amount of pain. Although not mentioned, a palpable defect or bulge may be present. Radiographs are not mentioned in either report. MRIs may have a role in confirming the diagnosis.

Treatment

Treatment was described in Gilcreest's patient and consisted of early surgical repair of the muscle belly. According to Gilcreest, "complete recovery" was achieved. Neither treatment for Tobin's patient nor the results were mentioned.

Conclusions

Tears of the coracobrachialis with or without the short head of the biceps are rare. Diagnosis itself can be difficult. In an acute setting, repair is recommended for the overhand athlete or in a laborer requiring repetitive or forceful upper extremity use. In other patients the amount of expected or actual disability would have to be carefully weighed before operative repair can be recommended.

SUMMARY

Muscle rupture about the shoulder joint is not uncommon. The well-coordinated action of all muscle groups around the shoulder is essential to normal shoulder function, especially in the overhead athlete. A muscle rupture would obviously disrupt that coordinated action. Repair is recommended in most acute cases of tendon rupture or avulsion of tendon from bone, whereas muscle belly rupture presents a more difficult therapeutic dilemma. As in most muscle-tendon unit injuries in athletes, patients with ruptures of shoulder girdle muscles demand proper rehabilitative programs whether treatment is nonoperative or operative.

References

1. Anderson KJ, Lecocq JF: Rupture of the triceps tendon, *J Bone Joint Surg* 39A:444, 1957.
2. Andreasen AT: Avulsion fracture of lesser tuberosity of humerus, *Lancet* I:750, 1948.
3. Anzel SH et al: Disruption of muscles and tendons—an analysis of 1014 cases, *Surgery* 45:406, 1959.
4. Bach BR, Warren RF, Fronek J: Disruption of the lateral capsule of the shoulder: a cause of recurrent dislocation, *J Bone Joint Surg* 70B:274, 1988.
5. Bach BR, Warren RF, Wickiewicz TL: Triceps rupture—a case report and literature review, *Am J Sports Med* 15:285, 1987.
6. Bakalim G: Rupture of the pectoralis major muscle: a case report, *Acta Orthop Scand* 36:274, 1965.
7. Baratz M, ElAttrache N, Herndon JH: Rupture of the pectoralis major tendon: a report of 2 cases: an acute and a delayed repair, *Pittsburgh Orthop J* 1:42, 1990.
8. Berson BL: Surgical repair of pectoralis major rupture in an athlete: case report of an unusual injury in a wrestler, *Am J Sports Med* 7:348, 1979.
9. Biondi J, Bear TF: Isolated rupture of the subscapularis tendon in an arm wrestler, *Orthopedics* 11:647, 1988.
10. Bowerman JW, McDonnell EJ: Radiology of athletic injuries: baseball, *Radiology* 116:611, 1975.

11. Brumback RJ: Compartment syndrome complicating avulsion of the origin of the triceps muscle, *J Bone Joint Surg* 69A:1445, 1987.
12. Buck JE: Rupture of the sternal head of the pectoralis major, *J Bone Joint Surg* 45B:224, 1963.
13. Butters AG: Traumatic rupture of the pectoralis major, *Br Med J* 2:652, 1941.
14. Clayton ML, Thirupathi R: Rupture of the triceps tendon with olecranon bursitis—a case report with a new method of repair, *Clin Orthop* 184:83, 1984.
15. Clemens H: Traumatische hemie des m deltoideus, *Dtsch Med Wochenschr* 39:2197, 1913.
16. Collier SG, Wynn-Jones CH: Displacement of the biceps with subscapularis avulsion, *J Bone Joint Surg* 72B:145, 1990.
17. Conwell HE: Subcutaneous rupture of the biceps flexor cubiti, report of one case, *J Bone Joint Surg* 10:788, 1928.
18. Conwell HE, Alldredge RH: Ruptures and tears of muscles and tendons, *Am J Surg* 35:22, 1937.
19. Coughlin EJ, Baker DM: Management of shoulder injuries in sport, *Conn Med* 29:723, 1965.
20. Davis CB: Plastic repair of the deltoid muscle, *Surg Clin* 3:287, 1919.
21. Delport HP, Piper MS: Pectoralis major rupture in athletes, *Arch Orthop Trauma Surg* 100:135, 1982.
22. Depalma AF, Cooke Aj, Prabhakar M: The role of the subscapularis in recurrent anterior dislocations of the shoulder, *Clin Orthop* 54:35, 1967.
23. Egan TM, Hall H: Avulsion of the pectoralis major tendon in a weight lifter: repair using a barbed staple, *Can J Surg* 30:434, 1987.
24. Farrar EL, Lippert FG: Avulsion of the triceps tendon, *Clin Orthop* 161:242, 1981.
25. Fichet SM: Injury of the serratus magnus (anterior) muscle, *N Engl J Med* 203:818, 1930.
26. Gilcreest EL: Rupture of muscles and tendons—particularly subcutaneous rupture of the biceps flexor cubiti, *JAMA* 84:1819, 1925.
27. Gilcreest EL: The common syndrome of rupture, dislocation and elongation of the long head of the biceps brachii; analysis of 100 cases, *Surg Gynecol Obstet* 58:322, 1934.
28. Gilcreest EL, Albi P: Unusual lesions of muscles and tendons of the shoulder girdle and upper arm, *Surg Gynecol Obstet* 68:903, 1939.
29. Gray H: In Williams P and Warwick R, editors: *Anatomy of the human body,* Philadelphia, 1980, WB Saunders Co, pp 567-573.
30. Haldeman KO, Soto-Hall R: Injuries to muscles and tendons, *JAMA* 104:2319, 1935.
31. Hauser EDW: Avulsion of the tendon of the subscapularis muscle, *J Bone Joint Surg* 36A:139, 1954.
32. Hayes JM, Zehr DJ: Traumatic avulsion causing winging of the scapula, *J Bone Joint Surg* 63A:495, 1981.
33. Hayes WM: Rupture of the pectoralis major muscle: review of the literature and report of two cases, *J Int Coll Surg* 14:82, 1950.
34. Heckman JD, Levine MI: Traumatic closed transection of the biceps brachii in the military parachutist, *J Bone Joint Surg* 60A: 369, 1978.
35. Jens J: The role of the subscapularis muscle in recurring dislocation of the shoulder, *J Bone Joint Surg* 46B:780, 1964.
36. Jones MW, Matthews JP: Rupture of pectoralis major in weight lifters: a case report and review of the literature, *Injury* 19.219, 1988.
37. Kawashima M et al: Rupture of the pectoralis major: report of two cases, *Clin Orthop* 109:115, 1975.
38. Kingsley DM: Rupture of the pectoralis major: report of a case, *J Bone Joint Surg* 28:644, 1946.
39. Kretzler HH, Richardson AB: Rupture of the pectoralis major muscle, *Am J Sports Med* 17:453, 1989.
40. Kuniichi A, Takehiko T: Muscle belly tear of the triceps, *Am J Sports Med* 12:484, 1984.
41. Law WB: Closed incomplete rupture of pectoralis major, *Br Med J* 2:499, 1954.
42. Lee MLH: Rupture of the triceps tendon, *Br Med J* 2:197, 1960.
43. Letenneur M: Rupture sous-cutanee du muscle grand pectoral; guerison complete en quinze jours, *Gaz de Hop* 35:54, 1862.
44. Levy M, Fishel RE, Stern GM: Triceps tendon avulsion with or without fracture of the radial head—a rare injury? *J Trauma* 18:677, 1978.
45. Levy M, Goldberg I, Meir I: Fracture of the head of the radius with a tear or avulsion of the triceps tendon, *J Bone Joint Surg* 64B:70, 1982.
46. Lindenbaum BL: Delayed repair of a ruptured pectoralis major muscle, *Clin Orthop* 109:120, 1975.
47. Lotem M, Bernheim J, Conforty B: Spontaneous rupture of tendons—a complication of hemodialyzed patients treated for renal failure, *Nephron* 21:201, 1978.
48. Mackenzie DB: Avulsion of the insertion of the pectoralis major muscle, *S Afr Med J* July:147, 1981.
49. Manjarris J, Gershuni DH, Moitoza J: Rupture of the pectoralis major tendon, *J Trauma* 25:810-811, 1985.
50. Marmor L, Bechtol CO, Hall CB: Pectoralis major muscle: function of sternal portion and mechanism of rupture of normal muscle: case reports, *J Bone Joint Surg* 43A:81, 1961.
51. Mason GA: Rupture of muscle belly of biceps brachii due to direct violence, *Lancet* 2:273, 1924.
52. McAuliffe TB, Dowd GS: Avulsion of the subscapularis tendon: a case report, *J Bone Joint Surg* 69A:1454, 1987.
53. McEntire JE, Hess WE, Coleman SS: Rupture of the pectoralis major muscle: a report of eleven injuries and review of fifty-six, *J Bone Joint Surg* 54A:1040, 1972.
54. McGuinness JP: Isolated avulsion fracture of the lesser tuberosity of the humerus, *Lancet* I:508, 1939.
55. McKelvey D: Subcutaneous rupture of the pectoralis major muscle, *Br Med J* 2:611, 1928.
56. McLaughlin HL: Recurrent anterior dislocation of the shoulder, *Am J Surg* 99:628, 1960.
57. McMaster PF: Tendon and muscle ruptures: clinical and experimental studies and locations of subcutaneous ruptures, *J Bone Joint Surg* 15:705, 1933.
58. Mellen PF: Parachute static line injury with vascular compromise, *Milit Med* 154:364, 1989.
59. Meythaler JM, Reddy NM, Mitz M: Serratus anterior disruption: a complication of rheumatoid arthritis, *Arch Phys Med Rehabil* 67:770, 1986.
60. Montgomery AH: Two cases of muscle injury, *Surg Clin Chicago* 4:871, 1920.
61. Moseley HF, Overgaard B: The anterior capsular mechanism in recurrent anterior dislocation of the shoulder: morphological and clinical studies with special reference to the glenoid labrum and the glenohumeral ligaments, *J Bone Joint Surg* 44B:913, 1962.
62. Moulonguet G: Rupture spontanee du grand pectoral chez un vieillard: enorme hematome, *Mort Bull Mem Soc Anat Paris* 94:24, 1924.
63. Neer CS, Marberry TA: On the disadvantages of radical acromionectomy, *J Bone Joint Surg* 63A:416, 1981.
64. Neviaser RJ, Neviaser TJ, Neviaser JS: Concurrent rupture of the rotator cuff and anterior dislocation of the shoulder in the older patient, *J Bone Joint Surg* 70A:1308, 1988.
65. Nicola T: Anterior dislocation of the shoulder: the role of the articular capsule, *J Bone Joint Surg* 24:614, 1942.
66. Nicola T: Acute anterior dislocation of the shoulder, *J Bone Joint Surg* 31A:153, 1949.

67. Overpeck DO, Ghormley RK: Paralysis of the serratus magnus muscle, *JAMA* 114:1994, 1940.
68. Pantazopoulos W et al: Avulsion of the triceps tendon, *J Trauma* 15:827, 1975.
69. Park JY, Espiniella JL: Rupture of pectoralis major muscle: a case report and review of the literature, *J Bone Joint Surg* 52A:577, 1970.
70. Partridge: A case of rupture of the triceps cubiti, *Med Times Gazette* 1:175, 1863.
71. Patissier P: *Traite des maladies des artisans,* Paris, 1822, pp 162.
72. Penhallow DP: Report of a case of ruptured triceps due to direct violence, *NY State J Med* 91:76, 1910.
73. Preston FS, Adicoff A: Hyperparathyroidism with avulsion of three major tendons: report of a case, *N Engl J Med* 266:968, 1962.
74. Pulaski EJ, Chandlee BH: Ruptures of the pectoralis major muscle, *Surgery* 10:309, 1941.
75. Pulaski EJ, Martin GW: Rupture of the left pectoralis major muscle: report of a case, *Surgery* 25:110, 1949.
76. Purnell R: Rupture of the pectoralis major muscle: a complication, *Injury* 19:284, 1988.
77. Recht J et al: Avulsion-fracture of the subscapular muscle, *Acta Orthop Belg* 57:312, 1991.
78. Reeves B: Experiments on the tensile strength of the anterior capsular structures of the shoulder in man, *J Bone Joint Surg* 50B: 858, 1968.
79. Rocyn-Jones A: The treatment of ruptured muscles and tendons, *Lancet* 2:1186, 1925.
80. Roi GS, Respizzi S, Dworzak F: Partial rupture of the pectoralis major muscle in athletes, *Int J Sports Med* 11:85, 1990.
81. Schecter LR, Gristina AG: Surgical repair of rupture of pectoralis major muscle, *JAMA* 188:1009, 1964.
82. Scott BW, Wallace WA, Barton MAJ: Diagnosis and assessment of pectoralis major rupture by dynamometry, *J Bone Joint Surg* 74B:111, 1992.
83. Searfoss R, Tripi J, Bowers W: Triceps brachii rupture: case report, *J Trauma* 16:244, 1976.
84. Sherman OH, Snyder SJ, Fox JM: Triceps tendon avulsion in a professional body builder—a case report, *Am J Sports Med* 12: 328, 1984.
85. Singson RD, Feldman F, Bigliani L: CT arthrographic patterns in recurrent glenohumeral instability, *AJR* 149:749, 1987.
86. Smith FC: Rupture of the pectoralis major muscle: a caveat, *Injury* 19:282, 1988.
87. Smith JG: Pathological appearances of seven cases of injury of the shoulder joint with remarks, *Am J Med Sci* 16:219, 1835.
88. Symeonides PP: The significance of the subscapularis muscle in the pathogenesis of recurrent anterior dislocation of the shoulder, *J Bone Joint Surg* 54B:476, 1972.
89. Tarsney FF: Rupture and avulsion of the triceps, *Clin Orthop* 83:177, 1972.
90. Tietjen R: Closed injuries of the pectoralis major muscle, *J Trauma* 20:262, 1980.
91. Tobin WJ, Cohen LJ, and Vandover JT: Parachute injuries, *JAMA* 117:1318, 1941.
92. Urs ND, Jani DM: Surgical repair of the pectoralis major muscle: a case report, *J Trauma* 16:749, 1976.
93. Waugh RL, Hatchcock TA, Elliott JL: Ruptures of muscles and tendons, *Surgery* 25:370, 1949.
94. Weinlechner J: Ueber subcutane muskel-, sehnen- und knochenrisse, *Wien Med Blatter* 4:1561, 1881.
95. White GM, Riley LH: Isolated avulsion of the subscapularis insertion in a child: a case report, *J Bone Joint Surg* 67A:635, 1985.
96. Wolf EM: *Mitek suture anchor techniques,* presented at the Arthroscopy Association of North America specialty day, American Academy of Orthopaedic Surgeons, San Francisco, 1993.
97. Wolfe SW, Wickiewicz TL, and Cavanaugh JT: Ruptures of the pectoralis major muscle: an anatomic and clinical analysis, *Am J Sports Med* 20:587, 1992.
98. Zemen SC, Rosenfeld RT, Liscomb PR: Tears of the pectoralis major muscle, *Am J Sports Med* 7:343, 1979.

C H A P T E R 1 4

Neurovascular Disorders: Clinical Assessment and Treatment

GORDON W. NUBER
WALTER J. MCCARTHY

Athletic activity involving repetitive overhead motion produces significant stress about the shoulder. During the deceleration phase of a baseball pitch, up to 90% of the body's weight in distractive forces is generated at the glenohumeral joint. Biomechanical studies have shown angular velocities about the shoulder approaching 7000 to 9000 degrees per second and rotational torques of 17,000 kg/cm^3. The clavicle provides the only bony connection between the torso and the upper extremity. Thus these tremendous stresses must be counterbalanced by soft-tissue restraints, such as muscles, tendons, and ligaments. Although the pathology created in these soft tissues is well documented, little has been written about the stresses on the other soft-tissue elements about the shoulder, particularly the neurovascular structures. This chapter will deal with the clinical assessment and treatment of the neurovascular system within the shoulder region by first reviewing the pertinent anatomy, the various sites of compromise, and anatomic variation and then by discussing thoracic outlet syndrome, axillary thrombosis, and peripheral nerve injuries.

ANATOMY

To understand the effect of repetitive overhead motion on the neurovascular structures, the clinician must have a firm understanding of the significant anatomic structures. Fig. 14-1 is a representation of the arterial anatomy about the shoulder and the relationship to adjacent musculature. The area commonly referred to as the "thoracic outlet" is more correctly identified in anatomic terms as the *superior thoracic aperture* or *thoracic inlet.*[29] The thoracic cavity communicates with the abdomen by the inferior thoracic aperture, or thoracic outlet, which is covered by the diaphragm. In keeping with convention, the thoracic outlet relates to the area where nerves composing the brachial plexus, as well as the vessels from the innominate artery on the right and the aorta on the left, leave the chest and cervical area.[51]

The outlet is bounded posteriorly by the upper margin of the first thoracic vertebra, the superior extent of the manubria anteriorly, and the first pair of ribs and their cartilage along the sides. This area measures only about 2 inches in the sagittal plane and approximately 4 inches in the coronal plane. A canal for the exit of the vessels is formed inferiorly by the upper border of the first rib, and superiorly by the posterior inferior border of the clavicle. The subclavian artery and the brachial plexus pass between the anterior and middle scalene muscles as they exit the outlet. The anterior scalene muscle originates from the anterior tubercles of the transverse processes of the third through the sixth cervical vertebrae and inserts onto the first rib at the scalene tubercle. The middle scalene muscle originates from the posterior tubercles of the transverse processes of the first through seventh cervical vertebrae, and inserts on the first rib behind the groove for the subclavian artery.

This muscular envelope can act as the initial site of compression of the neurovascular structures in an overhead or throwing athlete. Progressing laterally, the neurovascular bundle passes beneath the coracoid tip, pos-

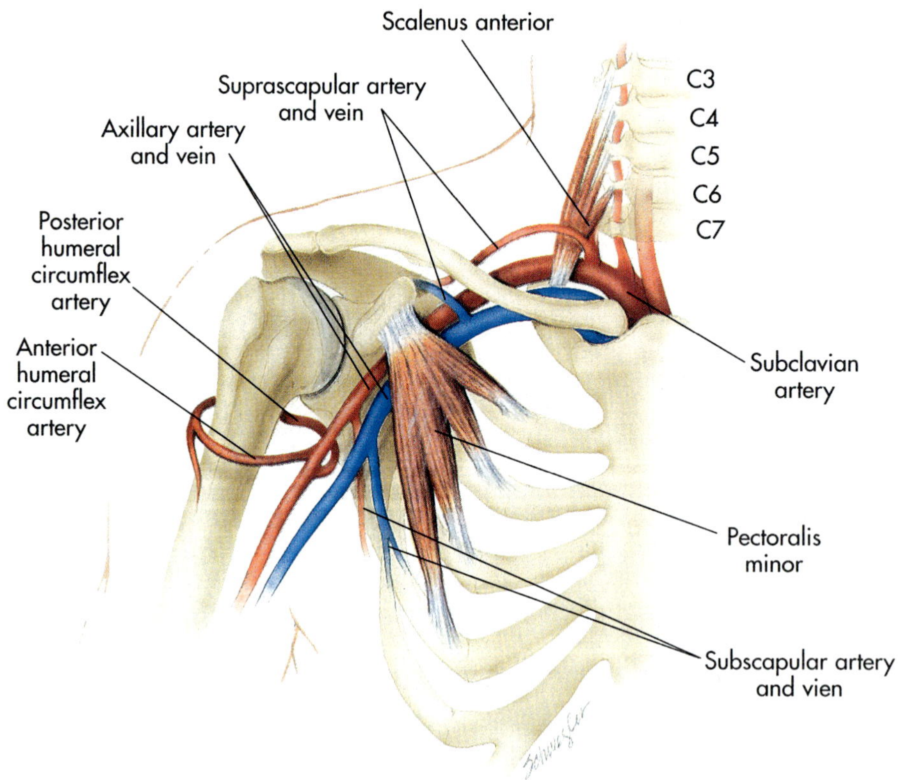

FIGURE 14-1 Arterial anatomy of the shoulder and its relationship to the adjacent musculature.

terior to the pectoralis minor muscle and anterior to the scapula and subscapularis muscle. The subclavian vein passes anterior to the anterior scalene muscle as the vein exits the thoracic cavity. The subclavian artery becomes the axillary artery after it passes the lateral border of the first rib. The axillary artery commonly has six named branches. Branches of the axillary artery include the supreme thoracic, medial to the pectoralis minor muscle; the thoracoacromial and lateral thoracic at the level of the pectoralis minor muscle; and the subscapular, anterior, and posterior humeral circumflex distal to the muscle. The thoracoacromial artery further branches into four named divisions: the acromial, clavicular, pectoral, and deltoid, which descend with the cephalic vein. The subscapular artery gives off a large branch, the circumflex scapular artery, which passes through the triangular space posteriorly. Distal to the branching circumflex scapular artery, the subscapular artery gives rise to the thoracodorsal artery.

The axillary vein begins at the lateral border of the teres major muscle, where the basilic vein joins the brachial vein. After uniting with the brachial vein, the axillary vein ascends proximally into the axilla medial to the axillary artery. It receives tributaries corresponding to the named axillary artery branches. The cephalic vein unites proximally. Proximal to the outer border of the first rib, the axillary vein becomes the subclavian vein. The subclavian vein lies anterior to the artery, separated by the anterior scalene muscle. It unites with the internal jugular vein to form the brachiocephalic vein, which unites with its contralateral vein to form the superior vena cava.

All nerves to the upper extremity arise from the brachial plexus (Fig. 14-2). The brachial plexus is formed by the ventral rami of the lower four cervical nerves (C5 to C8) and the ventral ramus of the first thoracic nerve. It may receive contributions from the fourth cervical nerve or the second thoracic, in which case it is referred to as either prefixed or postfixed in relation to the vertebral column. The ventral rami of the fifth and sixth cervical nerves unite to form the upper trunk, the seventh forms the middle trunk, and the eighth cervical and first thoracic form the lower trunk. Each trunk then divides into anterior and posterior divisions. The anterior divisions of the upper and middle trunk form the lateral cord. The anterior division of the lower trunk remains as the medial cord. The posterior divisions form the posterior cord. Each cord then divides into terminal divisions. The cords are named for their relationship to the second part of the axillary artery.

The subclavian vessels and brachial plexus traverse three narrowed straits on their way to the arm and hand. These areas also may serve as potential sites of compression with overhead activities. These sites include the interscalene triangle, the costoclavicular triangle, and the subcoracoid space. A fourth potential site of compromise can occur near the humeral head with abduction and excessive external rotation of the arm, as in the cocking phase of throwing.

A

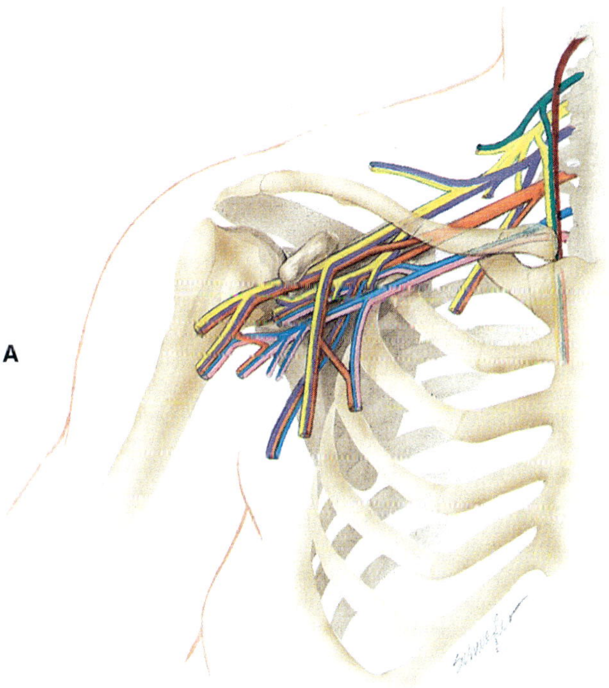

FIGURE 14-2 A, The brachial plexus.

Continued.

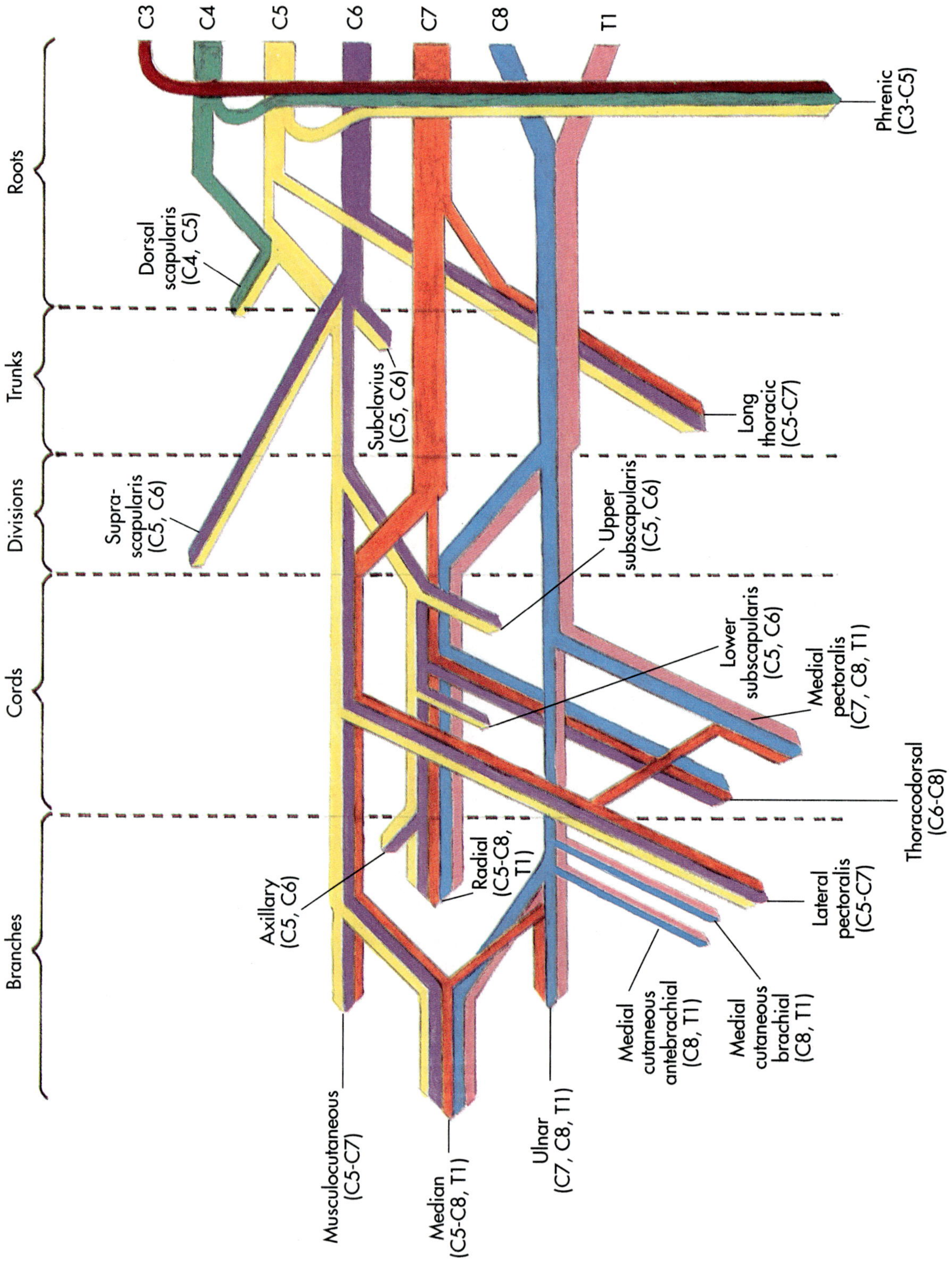

B

FIGURE 14-2—cont'd **B**, The brachial plexus.

Anatomic Variation

Anatomic variation also may predispose an athlete to neurovascular compression. The presence of a cervical rib long has been associated with thoracic outlet syndrome. The incidence of an anomalous rib is quite low (0.5%), and its pressure does not necessarily establish the diagnosis of thoracic outlet syndrome. Indeed, probably less than 10% of those with an anomalous rib develop symptoms.[54] Anomalous fibrous bands, which are more common than rib anomalies, are more likely to cause neurovascular compression. These bands, which cannot be seen on radiographic examination, may occur in association with anomalous ribs, may be related to the scalene muscles, or may be associated with the suprapleural membrane. Anomalous muscle insertions (scalene muscle) and muscular hypertrophy (pectoralis minor or scalene) have been further implicated in compression syndromes. An anomalous superficial cervical artery compressing the plexus also has been reported.[58] Another final consideration, particularly in athletes, is prior trauma, such as an old fracture of the clavicle, with callus formation causing narrowing of the costoclavicular triangle.

THORACIC OUTLET SYNDROME

Thoracic outlet syndrome can be due to either constant or intermittent compression phenomena. The mechanics of these two types of injuries will be discussed, followed by their treatment recommendations.

Compression of the neurovascular structures about the shoulder in an athlete is a rare entity but one that should not be overlooked. From 1983 to 1992, the authors have seen 16 athletes with symptoms related to compression of the subclavian or axillary arteries and their tributaries. The majority of these athletes were baseball pitchers, but others were involved in sports such as kayaking, wrestling, golf, tennis, and swimming.[47,52]

Clinical Presentation

Fatigue during the act of throwing is a common complaint. Loss of velocity during the act of pitching, particularly over a short time span such as one to three innings, also is common. Forearm pain, similar to that of ulnar neuropathy at the elbow, may be present. Most athletes complain of heaviness of the throwing arm to the point of exhaustion, and some complain of their hand becoming cold during exercise.

At times it can be difficult to differentiate those symptoms because of neurologic compression from those of an entirely vascular etiology.[42,62] Depending on the degree of compression or the site of entrapment, patients may present with a constellation of symptoms related to either a vascular or neurologic etiology. Dull pain or heaviness originates from the supraclavicular shoulder regions and may radiate down the arm. Paresthesias most typically are experienced along the inner aspect of the arm, forearm, and ulnar aspect of the hand. Numbness and tingling along the ulnar digits are common in patients with thoracic outlet syndrome. Activities that place the arm in positions of abduction and external rotation, such as the late cocking phase of throwing, are poorly tolerated. Symptoms also can be precipitated by trauma about the shoulder girdle. Pain and paresthesias may result from simply carrying heavy objects with the involved extremity or wearing a shoulder strap. The pain is typically worse at the end of the day or may wake the patient at night.

In athletes, symptoms usually are elicited relatively early because of the functional disability with overhead or throwing activities. If the symptoms are left unattended, sensory denervation may occur, with loss of pinprick and light touch along the C8 to T1 dermatomes. Thenar wasting has been reported as a late complication, with a typical thoracic outlet syndrome comprising ulnar sensory changes and median nerve motor deficit.[54]

Vasomotor changes may be found in the hand, with blanching and coldness of the digits. Discoloration of the digits may occur in the dependent position, and frank ischemia may appear in those athletes with embolization to their digital arteries.

Diagnosis

Diagnosis of a compression syndrome depends on a high index of suspicion and a thorough examination of the neck and entire upper extremity, not only checking for musculoskeletal pathology, but also checking the peripheral pulses and listening for bruits with the arm at the side and in the functional positions. The Adson maneuver is a clinical test for neurovascular compression.[2] As described by Dr. Adson, the test consists of palpating the radial pulse with the arm at the side while the seated patient takes a deep inspiration and turns his head to the affected side. Obliteration of the pulse signifies a compression at the level of the scalene muscles (scalene anticus syndrome). Wright first described the hyperabduction test for neurovascular compression.[76] This test, as noted by Tullos, actually places the arm in a position of abduction, extension, and external rotation at the shoulder, while checking the radial pulse.[40,72] This is the typical position of a pitcher during the cocking phase of throwing. Wright suggested that neurovascular compression in this position may occur at two areas: where the axillary artery passes under the coracoid process posterior to the pectoralis minor, and at a point where the artery is between the clavicle and first rib.

A variant of this test places the arm in the hyperabducted, extended, and externally rotated position while turning the head to the opposite side and noting a pulse change (Fig. 14-3). Bruits may be heard in the supraclavicular space. Symptoms, including pain and paresthe-

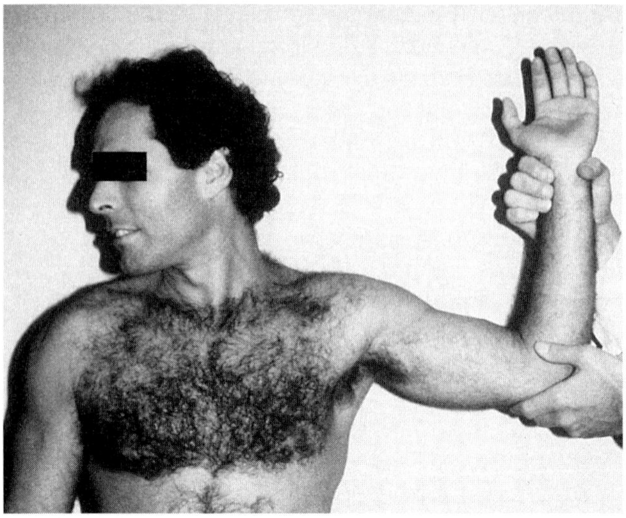

FIGURE 14-3 Testing for neurovascular compression with the arm abducted, extended, and externally rotated—the functional position.

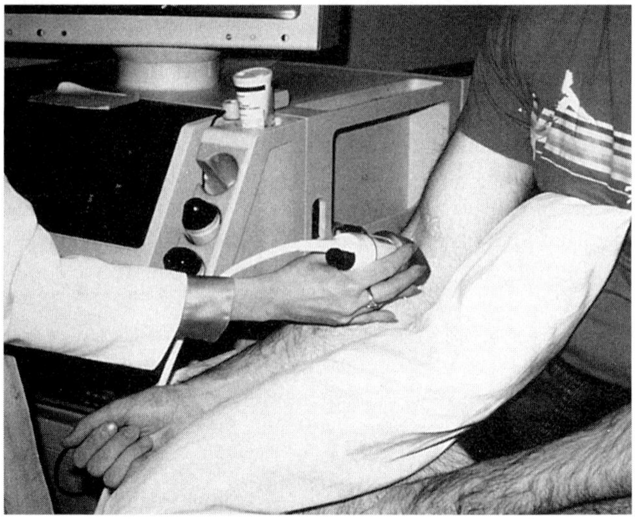

FIGURE 14-4 B-mode duplex scanning of the brachial artery.

sias, may occur if the arm is held in this position for a prolonged period. Slowly opening and closing the hand in a pumpinglike action over a few minutes also may precipitate the symptom complex.[64] A final test is the exaggerated military maneuver, in which the patient is asked to thrust the shoulders backward, take a deep inspiration and thrust the chest forward while the examiner palpates the radial pulse. This maneuver is thought to enhance compression of the axillary artery at the costoclavicular space. During any of these tests, obliteration of the pulse is considered significant. Duplication of the symptoms, along with abrupt resolution of the symptoms after assuming a relaxed position, strongly enhances the diagnosis of thoracic outlet syndrome.

Special Assessments

X-Ray

After a complete history and physical examination, the athlete should have a radiographic examination of the lower cervical and upper thoracic region to detect anomalous ribs or elongated transverse processes. These deformities also might indicate the presence of a fibrous band.

Noninvasive Vascular Tests

A vital part of the diagnostic workup of arterial occlusive disease of the upper extremity includes noninvasive vascular studies. These tests are standard procedures used to provide diagnostic vascular information and to follow patients after reconstructive arterial surgery. A Doppler flowmeter is used to determine arterial obstruction. The transcutaneous Doppler flowmeter uses sound waves generated by a piezoelectric crystal to determine changes in arterial flow. The waves generated by the flowmeter are in the low-frequency ultrasound spectrum and do not harm the local tissues. The Doppler flowmeter not only generates sound waves but also detects reflected sound waves, and can determine flow by the change in frequency of these waves. The Doppler effect is the apparent change in this frequency related to movement. The Doppler flowmeter also may be used to detect change in pressure with the arm at the side and also in functional positions.

Arteries and veins can be visualized through B-mode duplex scanning (Fig. 14-4). This method can detect luminal irregularity or compression during dynamic maneuvers.

Photoplethysmography is a test that uses infrared light transmission to determine cutaneous blood content in the capillary network. A photodetector receives the backscattered light and provides a continuous display on a strip chart recorder. The opacity of the underlying tissue changes because of changes in the blood content. This change is most affected by venous pressure, which is determined by arterial flow and venous reflux.

Nerve Conduction Velocity Test

Nerve conduction velocity tests should be performed in those patients suspected of having a true neurogenic type of thoracic outlet syndrome. The findings will include low-amplitude median nerve motor responses and ulnar nerve sensory responses, along with normal median nerve sensory function and ulnar nerve motor function.

Invasive Radiology

In those individuals determined to have arterial flow abnormalities based on physical examination and noninva-

A

B

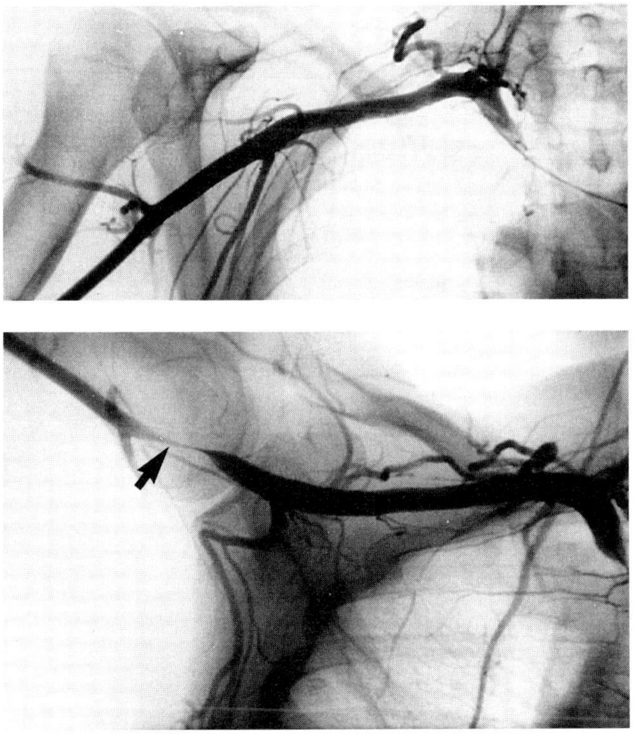

FIGURE 14-5 Arteriogram of the arm at the side **(A)** and in the functional position **(B)**. There is arterial compression at the level of the humeral head *(arrow)*.

sive testing, an arteriogram may be necessary. The arteriogram should be performed by imaging the contrast all the way to the digits, and the arm should be studied both at the side and in the functional position[66] (Figs. 14-5 and 14-6). In this manner, an obstruction to flow or aneurysm formation will be detected proximally, and the presence of distal embolization also will be detected.

Intermittent Compression Injuries

Although it is easy to understand the pathology caused by compression of neurologic structures, the effect of intermittent compression of the vascular structures is less understood. The repeated trauma caused by throwing a baseball 100 to 120 times a game may, over time, lead to changes within the intima of the arterial wall, which may then lead to the formation of a mural thrombus. In a sense, this is a form of vascular impingement. Emboli may be discharged intermittently, causing occlusion of the smaller distal arterial structures, particularly the digital vessels. Recurrent injuries may lead to complete occlusion proximally in the subclavian and axillary vessels. Poststenotic dilation of the vessel may occur, along with thrombus formation within the aneurysm and distal embolization.

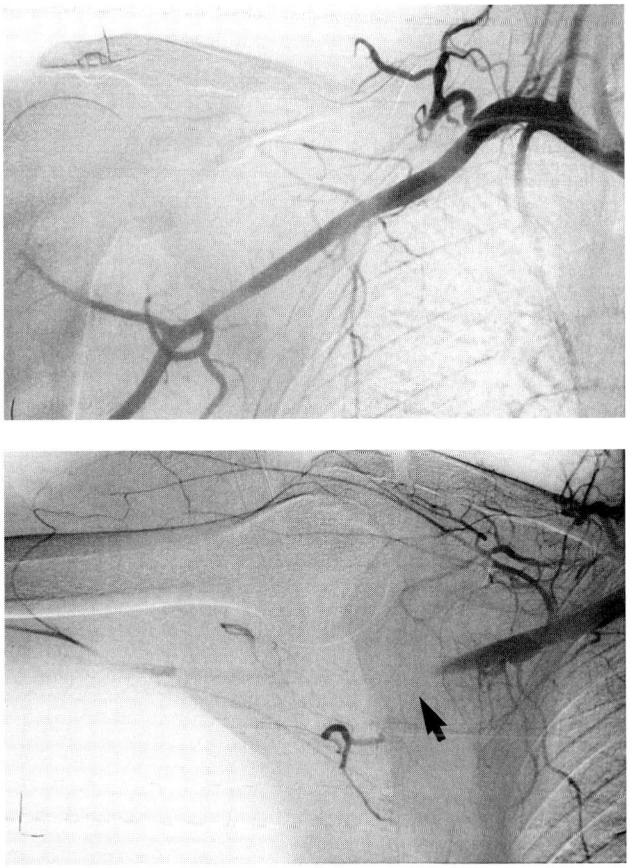

A

B

FIGURE 14-6 **A,** Arteriogram of a professional baseball player. **B,** With the arm in the functional position, the artery is completely occluded inferior to the coracoid *(arrow)*. After pectoralis minor resection, this athlete returned to a successful pitching career.

Evaluation of Vascular Occlusion

The diagnosis depends on clinical suspicion and confirmation of vascular occlusion via the noninvasive vascular studies. However, definitive confirmation of vascular occlusion lies with arteriography. Although many individuals may obliterate their radial pulse in the functional overhead position, symptoms must be recreated to establish a cause-and-effect relationship. Only if the throwing athlete's symptoms are recreated in the position of abduction, extension, and external rotation is treatment likely to be beneficial.

Progression/Complications

The late complication of a chronic vascular injury that is not detected or is left untreated is arterial thrombosis and embolization, particularly to the digital vessels. Occlusion of the digital vessels can lead to gangrenous changes or skin ulceration. If right subclavian artery thrombosis occurs, a rare but potentially devastating complication is retrograde thrombosis to the carotid artery, with embolization and right hemispheric stroke.[27]

Treatment

Conservative Treatment

Although most of the patients in the authors' series ultimately required operative intervention, an initial course of nonoperative treatment is warranted in those lacking aneurysm formation, emboli, or frank occlusion. Strukel and Garrick reported on four athletes treated with an exercise program consisting of strengthening of the shoulder girdle musculature, including the trapezius, serratus anterior, and erector spinae muscles.[70] Their program was effective in three of the four patients. None of the patients underwent arteriography, and surgical intervention was recommended in only the one patient whose symptoms persisted despite 6 weeks of conservative care.

The theory behind the exercise program is to develop the shoulder suspensory muscles so that the costoclavicular space remains patent.[36] During this time, the patient also is counseled regarding the mechanisms of injury and is advised to avoid postures and positions of the upper extremity that may lead to continued problems, and to avoid carrying bags with shoulder straps, which might lead to further compromise. Conservative therapy may be especially effective in patients with thoracic outlet syndrome who do not wish to continue athletic activity.

Surgical Treatment

Although a small percentage of athletes respond to conservative treatment, most require some form of surgical intervention to continue their sport. Surgical treatment may range from sympathectomy to thrombectomy and/or vascular reconstruction, and should be undertaken only in conjunction with a vascular surgery team. A number of professional baseball pitchers have returned to their previous level of activity after major vascular reconstruction.

As previously mentioned, arterial occlusion typically occurs at any one of four levels. After the level of occlusion is determined by arteriogram, a surgical plan is outlined. The procedure always should be performed in conjunction with a vascular surgeon. Aneurysms of a major artery, such as the subclavian artery, will require resection and venous bypass. The presence of a cervical rib with a proximal obstruction will require rib resection. Most other obstructions will respond to decompression via resection of a 2- to 3-cm segment of the anterior scalene muscle or pectoralis minor muscle, depending on the site of obstruction. Compression of the axillary artery by the humeral head (secondary to humeral hypertrophy) may respond to pectoralis minor resection.[20,38] If vascular occlusion is secondary to glenohumeral instability, a stabilization procedure is required. Branch artery compression should be released in all cases.

Quadrilateral Space Syndrome

One instance of branch artery occlusion that deserves special mention involves the posterior humeral circumflex artery. After reviewing a number of seemingly poor results after thoracic outlet surgery, Cahill and Palmer[18] termed the condition *quadrilateral space syndrome.* Blockage of the posterior humeral circumflex artery occurred with the arm in the position of abduction, extension, and external rotation. Discrete point tenderness was found over the quadrangular, or quadrilateral, space posteriorly, along with duplication of the symptoms with the arm in the functional position longer than 1 minute. Surgical decompression of the quadrangular space through a posterior scapular approach was recommended for symptomatic individuals. The authors also have seen athletes with aneurysm formation at the point of branching of the posterior humeral circumflex from the axillary artery who required aneurysm resection and venous bypass. One pitcher was noted on arteriogram to shed emboli from the aneurysm when the arm was placed in the throwing position of abduction, external rotation, and extension. This pitcher required distal bypass of an occluded ulnar and radial artery before return to throwing.

AXILLARY THROMBOSIS

Axillary Vein Thrombosis

Thrombosis of the axillary venous system was originally described by Paget and Von Schroetter.[1,5,19,46,53] It is thought to be slightly more common than arterial occlusions. Although most occlusions occur secondary to venous manipulation (such as during cannulation with a central venous catheter), spontaneous obstruction may occur after trauma or great muscular effort, known as "effort thrombosis."[17] The axillary vein lies medial to the axillary artery and may be injured or compressed at various sites along its progression. The most common site of venous compression is in the costoclavicular space.

Causes

Forced abduction of the shoulder results in compression of the vein by the subclavius muscle or costocoracoid ligament and the first rib. Stretching of the vein may result in further damage that leads to thrombosis. Other factors implicated include hyperextension of the neck at the time of injury, the military position of the shoulders, forced expiration, and the Valsalva maneuver associated with a vigorous effort. Some cases have been associated with fractures of the clavicle in athletes and the use of figure-of-eight bandages or splints in their treatment.

History

Most cases involve men and are found in the dominant extremity. A history of previous repetitive activity, strenuous effort, or trauma is noted. Symptoms usually develop within the first 24 hours after trauma.

Clinical Signs

Typically, the first sign of thrombosis is diffuse swelling and pain of the involved extremity. Swelling involves the whole extremity from shoulder to hand, and pain is described as either minor or as an aching or tight feeling. The pain is typically referred to the arm and shoulder, particularly the axilla. A thrombosed venous cord may be palpated in the axilla, and a prominent venous pattern of the entire extremity develops. A mottled cyanotic discoloration of the extremity with dependent rubor is typical. Depending on the degree of swelling, some limitation of shoulder motion also may be experienced.

Venography

Axillary vein thrombosis often is suggested by clinical signs and symptoms alone, then is confirmed with venography (Fig. 14-7). There is some concern about propagation of the thrombosis with venography. Coon and Willis, and Butsch noted cases of increased swelling after venograms.[17,19] Noninvasive venous Doppler examination also may be helpful in determining the diagnosis through a noninvasive technique. Final diagnosis, according to Adams and DeWeese, can be made only by phlebographic demonstration of occlusion of the deep venous network.[1] Acutely, the venogram demonstrates thrombosis of the vein with nonvisualization of only a short segment of vein. Later, the entire vein may nonvisualize, with demonstration of significant collateralization. Recanalization of the thrombosed segment may occur later.

Treatment

Clotting abnormalities should be suspected and ruled out. Treatment consists of elevation of the arm and bed rest. Anticoagulants are used in the acute phase to prevent propagation of the clot and promote recanalization of the vein. Prevention of pulmonary embolism is another benefit of anticoagulation therapy. Local thromboembolic therapy (streptokinase and urokinase) has been used with some success.

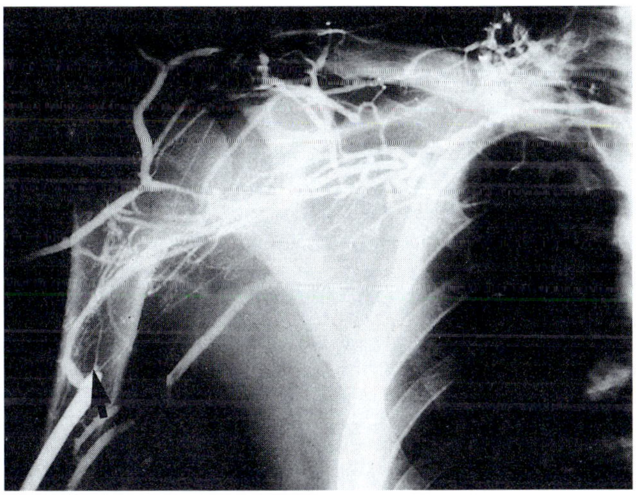

FIGURE 14-7 Venogram demonstrating axillary vein thrombosis.

Thrombolytic and Surgical Treatment

Because of residual complaints with conservative care, some authors recommend treatment with thrombolytic therapy and relief of venous compression at the costoclavicular space. This space can be enlarged by first-rib resection or scalene muscle resection and should be undertaken only by a vascular surgeon.

Complications

Complications of treatment include persistence of symptoms, including swelling and exertional claudication. The most devastating complication, pulmonary embolus, is unusual.

PERIPHERAL NERVE LESIONS

Suprascapular Nerve Lesions

Neurologic reasons for shoulder pain other than thoracic outlet syndrome include lesions of the peripheral branches of the brachial plexus. The nerve branch most frequently injured in athletes is the suprascapular nerve.

Although isolated lesions of the suprascapular nerve are rare, they have been reported in throwing athletes and those athletes exposed to repetitive trauma.* Physicians taking care of professional teams occasionally note significant infraspinatus atrophy in pitchers with seemingly little dysfunction. In baseball players who throw hard, the nerve lesion is most often localized to the spinoglenoid notch and is usually incomplete.[15] In this case, the infraspinatus is the only muscle involved, and, because of the incomplete nature of the lesion, there is usually some limited function of the muscle.

An injury to the suprascapular nerve should be suspected in any athlete who presents with atrophy of the supraspinatus muscle and the infraspinatus muscle, and weakness of abduction and external rotation.[21,22] Although rotator cuff pathology is the most typical reason for such a presentation, an injury to the suprascapular nerve may create similar findings.

Anatomy

The suprascapular nerve is a branch of the upper trunk of the brachial plexus at Erb's point. It receives branches primarily from the fifth cervical nerve root but also may receive nerve fibers from the fourth and sixth cervical roots. The nerve lies in the posterior triangle of the neck, deep to the posterior belly of the omohyoid muscle. It follows this muscle laterally and passes beneath the anterior border of the trapezius muscle to the upper bor-

*References 6, 16, 22, 25, 41, 59, 63, 68, 74, 77.

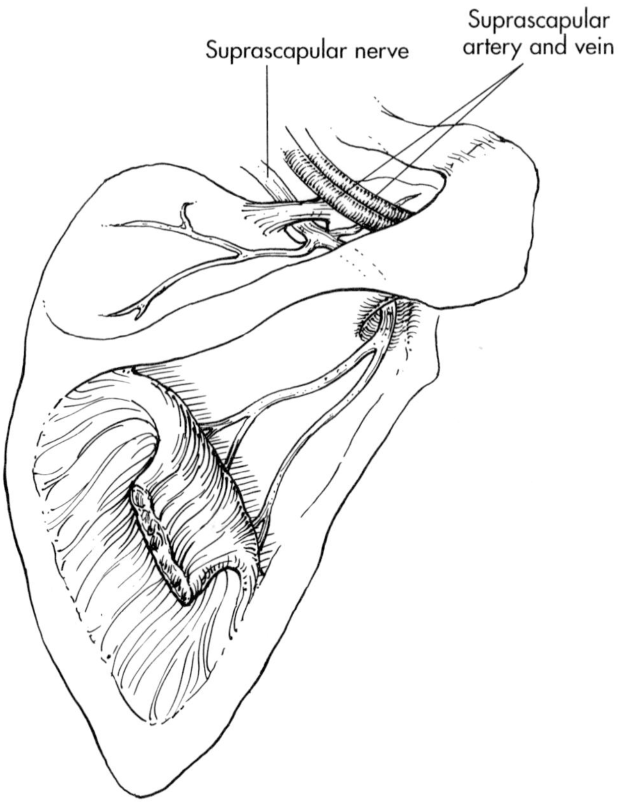

FIGURE 14-8 Anatomy of the suprascapular nerve.

der of the scapula, accompanied by the suprascapular artery and a branch of the thyrocervical trunk. The nerve passes close to the omohyoid attachment on the scapula medially and the coracoid process laterally. From here it passes through the suprascapular notch, which is converted to a foramen by the bridging transverse scapular ligament (Fig. 14-8). (In a cadaver study, Rengachary et al noted six types of suprascapular notches and postulated that the type IV, which was small and V-shaped, is most often associated with neuropathy.[60,61]) The artery and vein pass superficial to the ligament before joining the nerve within the supraspinous fossa. Multiple branches arise near the suprascapular notch. These branches provide sensory innervation to the glenohumeral and acromioclavicular joint, and a branch to the coracoacromial ligament. After passing through the notch, the nerve innervates the supraspinatus muscle. It then passes around the lateral free margin of the scapular spine (spinoglenoid notch) to innervate the infraspinatus muscle. The nerve travels obliquely approximately 2 cm from the glenoid rim, with two or three branches supplying each bundle of the bipennate infraspinatus.[67,73]

Black and Lombardo noted that in 50% of their subjects, an osteofibrous orifice is found, circumscribed by the spinoglenoid ligament, through which the nerve and vessels pass.[9] The nerve then arborizes to innervate the infraspinatus muscle. In some cases, the nerve will form an acute angle as it passes lateral to the spinoglenoid notch and then travels medially, parallel to the spine of the scapula, innervating the infraspinatus muscle.

Mechanism of Injury

During the course of the progression of the suprascapular nerve, there are a number of critical points of fixation and potential compromise. The first fixation point is at its origin from the upper trunk at Erb's point. The nerve at this point also is encased in the fascia of the scalene muscles.

The next critical area is where the suprascapular nerve passes through the suprascapular notch and around the lateral spine of the scapula. From here, it is finally fixed at its insertion to the infraspinatus muscle. Ringel et al have discussed another potential site of compromise, the supraspinous fossa in a thin individual with a well-developed supraspinatus muscle.[63] Here the nerve may be compressed between the bone and the fascia of the hypertrophic muscle.

Because of this circuitous pathway and the extreme torques and angular velocity placed on the shoulder during the act of pitching, the nerve may be subject to not only compressive forces but also tensile loads—particularly during the cocking, acceleration, and deceleration phases of throwing. The suprascapular artery also is subject to these tensile loads, and vascular damage may lead to microthrombi and secondary ischemic damage to the nerve.[22]

Injuries to the suprascapular nerve have been reported in athletes involved in weight-lifting, tennis, volleyball, and baseball pitching.[6,9,22,25] Neuropathy of the suprascapular nerve usually produces shoulder pain and weakness of abduction and external rotation. If both muscles are affected, wasting of the infraspinatus muscle will be more apparent because the infraspinatus is more superficial and the supraspinatus is covered by the trapezius (Fig. 14-9).

Injury to the suprascapular nerve via traction or direct trauma may be the most common form of injury, but injury secondary to ganglion cysts, penetrating injury, and inflammation also have been reported.[28,71] Entrapment of the nerve at the suprascapular notch or spinoglenoid notch is most often thought to contribute to injury. Drez, however, reports that these merely act as points of fixation that lead to traction injuries to the nerve, particularly with overhead activities that produce great amounts of torque, such as racquet sports or throwing.[22]

Diagnosis

Individuals suspected of suprascapular nerve injury should undergo electromyography, stimulating at Erb's point proximally and recording distally in the infraspinatus muscle. Normal mean latencies of 3.3 m/sec have been recorded. In a study of professional baseball pitchers, Ringel et al showed a progressive slowing of the

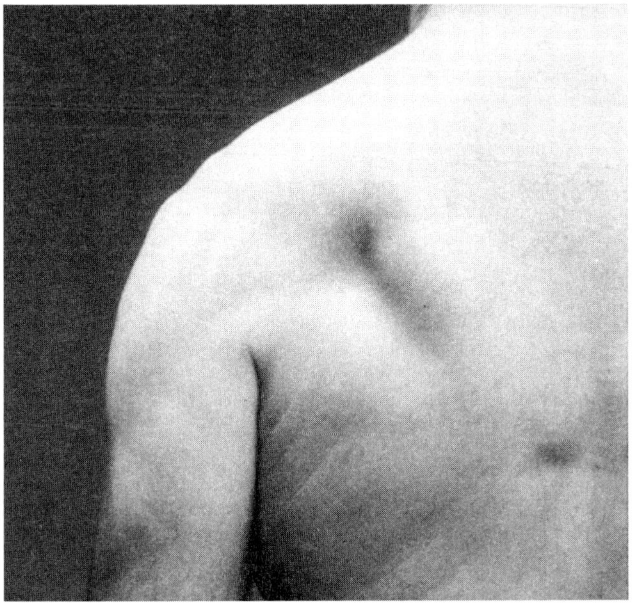

FIGURE 14-9 Marked infraspinatus atrophy in an individual with suprascapular neuropathy.

suprascapular nerve conduction as the season progressed.[63] They could not, however, show a decline in performance associated with this decrease in nerve conduction. An arthrogram or MRI to rule out rotator cuff pathology may be warranted.

Treatment

After injury of the suprascapular nerve is confirmed by electrodiagnostic testing, a plan of treatment must be formulated. Because these injuries are thought to be traction neuropraxias in most cases, a period of nonoperative treatment, including an exercise program aimed at promoting muscle balance about the shoulder, is warranted. According to Drez, this period should last 4 to 6 months, with follow-up electrodiagnostic testing to determine whether regeneration occurs.[22] In those cases where no regeneration occurs, surgical exploration of the nerve to release any area of compression or traction along with neurolysis may be warranted but in most cases fails to help with regeneration. The function of the remaining muscles should be maximized with exercise so that a balance is restored to the rotator cuff musculature. Pitchers are then able to return to a regular level of activity with minimal loss of endurance.

This treatment may be successful because in overhead athletes, the usual area of entrapment is at the spinoglenoid notch, which spares the supraspinatus muscle and usually leaves 30% to 40% of the infraspinatus innervation intact.[25] With appropriate rehabilitation, the muscle function can be maximized to provide the balance needed for pitching.

Long Thoracic Nerve Injuries

Injuries to the long thoracic nerve have been reported during several athletic activities. Tennis, golf, gymnastics, bowling, weight-lifting, soccer, hockey, archery, and shooting a rifle all have been implicated as precipitating events.* Traction to the nerves, with resultant neuropraxia, was thought to be the mechanism of injury.

The long thoracic nerve of Bell or "external respiratory nerve" originates from the anterior branches of the fifth, sixth, and seventh cranial nerves. In 8% of cases, a contribution from the eighth cervical nerve is found. The lower digitations of the serratus anterior also may receive innervation from the intercostal nerves in 20% of cases.[34,35] Branches from the fifth and sixth cervical nerves pass through the scalenus medius muscle and then unite with the branch of the seventh cervical nerve, which passes between the anterior and middle scalene. The branches form a single cord, which passes anterior to the scalenus posterior muscle. The long thoracic nerve then passes downward and laterally along the outer border of the serratus anterior muscle, giving branches to each of the digitations of muscle.

The serratus anterior is a large muscle that arises from the first through ninth ribs. It inserts on the costal medial border of the scapula. The muscle can be divided into three functional parts. The upper fibers insert into the superior angle of the scapula and stabilize the scapula during the initial stages of abduction.[65,75] The middle fibers insert along the vertebral border of the scapula and are instrumental in protraction. The lower fibers insert along the inferior angle of the scapula and function primarily as an upward rotator during abduction of the arm. As a whole, the serratus anterior maintains the medial border of the scapula against the thorax during motion of the arm, particularly in forward flexion.

Mechanism of Injury

Gregg et al proposed the most plausible explanation for injury to the long thoracic nerve to be a traction injury.[31] In their anatomic studies, this traction could occur when the head was tilted or rotated laterally away from the ipsilateral extremity while the arm was raised overhead, as might be a common maneuver in tennis or bowling. In their cadaver specimens, they found that they could easily double the length of the nerve between its point of fixation at the scalenus medius and the distal fixation at the superior serratus anterior. Stretch neuropraxia can occur with any elongation beyond a 10% increase in resting length.[11]

Other possible explanations for injury include direct trauma and compression of the nerve between the clavicle and the second rib. Based on the work of Gregg, this mechanism of injury seems unlikely. Compression of the nerve by an inflamed bursa (subscapular, accessory sub-

*References 26, 30, 31, 37, 65, 69.

scapular, subcoracoid, and supracoracoid) also has been proposed.[35,36] Foo and Swann believe that "neurologic amyotrophy" was the most likely etiology because of the high incidence of spontaneous onset unrelated to trauma.[26] Neuralgic amyotrophy is a paralytic brachial neuritis, first described by Parsonage and Tuner.[55]

Presentation

Most patients develop pain or discomfort about the shoulder related to an athletic activity. The pain may not be severe enough to motivate ceasing the activity and is frequently located in the posterior neck and scapular area. The pain is exacerbated by tilting the head away and elevating the ipsilateral arm. The pain usually lasts only 2 or 3 weeks. Shoulder weakness may occur immediately but most frequently develops over a few weeks. Also noted is a decrease in active forward elevation as the shoulder weakness progresses. An active athlete may relate a history of difficulty with overhead motions, such as serving in tennis or volleyball. The pain in the shoulder usually resolves, and the athlete then notes the progressive scapular winging. Many first note the "winging" when looking in the mirror or when told of the asymmetry by others. Some can feel the protuberance of the scapula when seated in a chair.

Diagnosis

Physical examination generally will show a decreased active elevation of the arm with weakness in abduction. The examining physician should observe for discoordinated scapulohumeral motion on the involved side. Scapular winging is most pronounced at the inferior border.[65] Winging may be provoked by having the patient do a standing push-up against the wall or resisted scapular protraction (Fig. 14-10).

Scapular winging also may be present with isolated paralysis of the trapezius muscle. This generally presents as a depression of the lateral aspect of the scapula while the arm droops down via the unsupported weight of the arm.[13,65] Winging with a dysfunctional trapezius is most pronounced with abduction to 90° and is eliminated with forward flexion.

Although diagnosis of long thoracic nerve injury should be apparent on physical examination, an electromyogram should be used to confirm the diagnosis and to follow recovery. The long thoracic nerve is readily accessible to electromyography. Stimulation is performed at Erb's point and is recorded over the fifth or sixth rib in the midaxillary line. The mean conduction velocity for the long thoracic nerve of 67 m/sec was noted by Petrera and Trojaborg.[57]

Treatment

The accepted form of treatment for scapular winging is avoidance of activities that place the nerve at risk. We also have started our patients on a protocol of active exercises that strengthen the associated scapular muscles, the trapezius, rhomboids, and levator scapulae. Gregg et al also recommend exercises to maintain shoulder motion, along with stretching of the latissimus dorsi and pectoralis minor, which may become contracted.[31] During the acute phase, there is no indication for surgery. In most series, nerve function will be recovered spontaneously within 2 years.

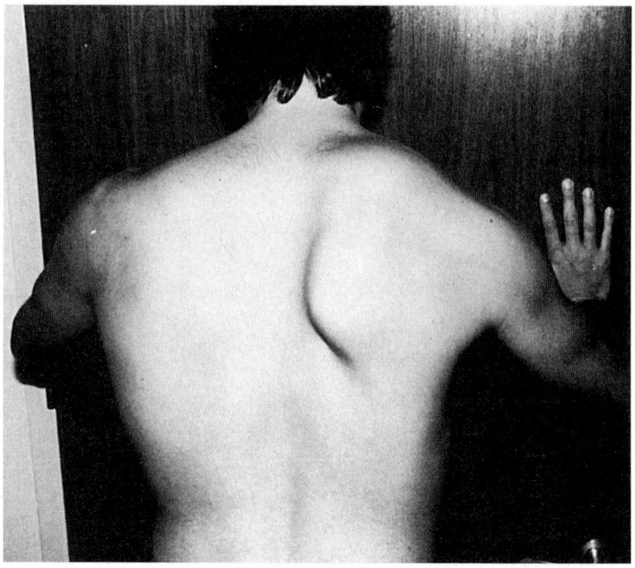

FIGURE 14-10 Winging of scapula with wall push-ups in an individual with long-thoracic-nerve injury after weight lifting.

Progression

Gregg et al recommend surgical substitution for the serratus anterior only if function does not recur within 2 years.[31] Substitutions using the pectoralis major and minor, rhomboids, and teres minor all have been described.[24,31,32] The authors have had no experience with surgical substitutions. The prognosis for patients with long thoracic nerve injuries is excellent for complete recovery without need for surgical substitutions.

The Axillary Nerve

The axillary nerve has received attention in the sports medicine literature because of fear of its possible injury during surgical procedures for glenohumeral instability, particularly the inferior capsular shift.[14,44,50] Neer and Foster reported three axillary neuropraxias in the first 40 patients on whom they performed this procedure.

Mechanism of Injury

The nerve also can be injured during an acute anterior dislocation of the shoulder.[10,56] Blunt trauma, as in boxing or motor vehicle accidents, and violent internal rotation during arm wrestling also have been implicated in the etiology of these injuries.[6,7,30,49]

The axillary nerve, formed from the fifth and sixth cervical roots, arises from the posterior cord, just inferior to the coracoid process. It passes anterior to the subscapularis muscle and winds posteriorly and inferiorly around the muscle, just medial to its musculotendinous border. Here it courses posteriorly, with the posterior humeral circumflex artery, through the quadrangular space, or what is frequently called the *quadrilateral space,* bounded by the teres major and minor muscles, the long head of the triceps, and the shaft of the humerus.[48] Hinton, in his anatomic studies, has identified muscular portions of the subscapularis muscle that insert onto the humerus inferior to the lesser tuberosity and may be a source of neural compression, particularly in a hypertrophied athlete.[33] The nerve gives off articular branches to the glenohumeral capsule, to which it closely approximates. As it passes posteriorly, the nerve divides into anterior and posterior branches, which innervate the anterior and posterior divisions of the deltoid muscle. The posterior division also gives a branch to the teres minor muscle. The posterior branch also winds around the posterior border of the deltoid and supplies sensation to an area of skin on the lateral and posterior arm. Here the nerve is known as the *upper lateral brachial cutaneous nerve.*

Axillary nerve compression may present as weakness and possibly wasting of the deltoid muscle. The authors recently saw a professional pitcher who presented with an insidious onset of significant abduction weakness and pain with abduction and external rotation of the arm. His EMG showed significant slowing of the axillary nerve, and the arteriogram demonstrated obliteration of the posterior humeral circumflex artery in the quadrangular space with the arm abducted and externally rotated. An article by Cahill and Palma identified this as quadrilateral space syndrome.[18] The authors hypothesize that any overhead athlete, such as this pitcher, may compromise this space secondary to significant hypertrophy of the muscular and bony structures about this space.

Typically, the pain is located anteriorly but is poorly localized. Discrete point tenderness is located posteriorly over the quadrangular space, and continued abduction and external rotation reproduce the symptoms.

Clinical Presentation

Tests to evaluate the radial pulse with the arm abducted and externally rotated should be performed. The professional pitcher mentioned previously had complete obliteration of the radial pulse with the arm abducted and externally rotated. Another pitcher recently developed an aneurysm of the posterior humeral circumflex artery and developed a blood clot in the aneurysm that would embolize into the axillary artery when the arm was placed in the throwing position. Arteriograms with the arm in the provocative position demonstrated the extrusion of the clot into the axillary artery as the arm was placed in the pitching position. Most patients, however, will not present with compromise of the radial pulse.

Diagnosis

The differential diagnosis should include lesions of the posterior cord of the brachial plexus, along with thoracic outlet syndrome or cervical radiculopathy. An EMG confirms the diagnosis when the motor response to the deltoid muscle is diminished. An arteriogram should be obtained if the compression at the quadrangular space is suspected. This must be performed with the arm at the side and again with the arm in the provocative position.

Treatment

Treatment of an isolated axillary nerve injury consists of initial rest followed by a program of exercises to restore strength to the deltoid muscle.[6,30] The prognosis is generally thought to be good for complete recovery of motor function and sensation over a few months. If no evidence of recovery is demonstrated, surgical exploration and neurolysis may be considered.[6]

For those found to have quadrilateral space syndrome with typical clinical findings and a positive arteriogram, Cahill and Palmer recommend decompression through a posterior approach.[18] This approach releases the deltoid posteriorly from the scapular spine, and the teres minor from its insertion on the humerus. Of 18 cases, they found dramatic relief of symptoms in 8, partial relief in 8, and 2 cases with no improvement. No mention was made of the number of athletes in this group and whether they returned to athletic activity.

A throwing athlete may require a less extensive surgical exposure and muscular dissection. The authors recommend a decompression, releasing fibrous scar from the quadrangular space, along with release of the upper border of the teres major and any anomalous subscapularis fibers that may be impinging the artery and nerve. This approach allows access to the axillary artery and its branches while eliminating the need for extensive muscular disruption during surgery. These cases are always performed in conjunction with a vascular surgeon familiar with this approach.

OTHER INJURIES SUSTAINED IN SPORTS-RELATED ACTIVITIES

Isolated paralyses of the musculocutaneous nerve or spinal accessory nerve are extremely rare injuries associated with athletics. The musculocutaneous nerve is a branch of the lateral cord of the brachial plexus, comprising primarily cervical nerve roots C5 and C6. It passes through the coracobrachialis muscle before descending between the biceps and brachialis muscles, which it innervates. After coursing between the two muscles, it penetrates the brachial fascia above the elbow, becoming the lateral cutaneous nerve of the forearm. Injuries to the nerve have been described in individuals participating in rowing, weight-lifting, football, and model-airplane flying.[12,39,45] The musculocutaneous nerve also is at risk for injury during operative procedures that require retraction or transfer of the conjoined tendon (coracobrachialis, short head biceps) or after an anterior shoulder dislocation.[4,23]

Patients with an injury to the musculocutaneous nerve present with weakness of the biceps and brachialis, along with sensory impairment along the lateral forearm. The differential diagnosis should include rupture of the distal biceps tendon, along with cervical radiculopathy of the C5 and C6 nerve roots. Diagnosis is established with an EMG stimulating at Erb's point, and recording of motor responses just distal to the midpoint of the biceps muscle belly.[49] These injuries usually resolve spontaneously with cessation of the precipitating activity.

Injuries to the spinal accessory nerve (cranial nerve XI) are extremely rare. The authors have seen two athletes, both involved in football, who sustained such an injury. The mechanism of injury is either a stretch neuropraxia or compression from blunt trauma.

The spinal accessory nerve is a purely motor nerve, innervating the trapezius muscle. (Additional innervation may arise from cervical nerves III and IV.) It exits the skull via the jugular foramen and innervates the sternocleidomastoid muscle. The nerve crosses the posterior triangle obliquely while lying on the levator scapulae. Approximately 5 cm proximal to the clavicle, it passes deep to the anterior border of the trapezius and with the cervical nerves forms a plexus.

The patient with a spinal accessory nerve injury may initially be unaware of any disability. Weakness of shoulder elevation and abduction occurs with time. Persistent ache about the shoulder is common. Drooping of the shoulder and inability to abduct without scapular winging develops. Scapular winging is enhanced by resisted abduction. Asymmetry and wasting of the trapezius are easily noted.

EMGs reveal fibrillation and positive sharp waves of the sternocleidomastoid muscle and all portions of the trapezius.[43]

Initially, treatment should be aimed at reducing the discomfort, using a sling, nonsteroidal antiinflammatory medication, and analgesics.[49] Conservative treatment is generally thought to be unsuccessful, and if the injury does not resolve, strengthening exercises generally cannot compensate for the functional loss. If recovery does not occur within the first few months after injury, exploration of the nerve and neurolysis are warranted. Bigliani et al described excellent results with lateral transfer of the levator scapulae, rhomboid minor, and rhomboid major to the spine and body of the scapulae in patients who failed to recover in 1 year.[8] Postoperatively, many of their patients were able to participate in strenuous athletic activity.

SUMMARY

Injuries to the neurovascular structures about the shoulder are rare during athletic activity. Many of these injuries occur only during isolated instances. Frequently their presence can mimic many of the more common musculotendinous injuries that occur with athletic endeavors. An awareness of these injuries and of the means of diagnosis and treatment is essential in providing proper care of an athlete. The authors hope that this chapter has helped the reader understand these lesions.

References

1. Adams JT, DeWeese JA: "Effort" thrombosis of the axillary and subclavian veins, *J Trauma* 11(11):923-930, 1971.
2. Adson AW: Surgical treatment for symptoms produced by cervical ribs and the scalenus anticus muscle, *Surg Gynecol Obstet* 85:687-700, 1947.
3. Andrews JR, Kupfermen SP, Dillman CJ: Labral tears in throwing and racquet sports, *Clin Sports Med* 10(4):901-911, 1991.
4. Bach BR et al: An unusual neurological complication of the Bristow procedure, *J Bone Joint Surg [Am]* 70A:458-460, 1988.
5. Baker CL, Thornberry R: Neurovascular syndromes. In Zarins B, Andrews JR, Carson WG, editors: *Injuries to the throwing arm,* Philadelphia, 1985, WB Saunders, pp 176-188.
6. Bateman JE: Nerve injuries about the shoulder in sports, *J Bone Joint Surg [Am]* 49A:785-792, 1967.
7. Berry H, Brill V: Axillary nerve palsy following blunt trauma to the shoulder region: a clinical and electrophysiological review, *J Neurol Neurosurg Psych* 45:1027-1032, 1982.
8. Bigliani LV, Perez-Sang JR, Wolfe IN: Treatment of trapezius paralysis, *J Bone Joint Surg [Am]* 67A:871-877, 1985.
9. Black KP, Lombardo JA: Suprascapular nerve injuries with isolated paralysis of the infraspinatus, *Sports Med* 18(3):225-228, May-June, 1990.
10. Blom S, Dhalback LO: Nerve injuries in dislocations of the shoulder joint and fractures of the neck of the humerus, *Acta Chir Scand* 35:461-466, 1970.
11. Bora FW Jr, Pleasure DE, Didizian NA: A study of nerve regeneration and neuroma formation after nerve suture by various techniques, *J Hand Surg* 1:138-143, 1976.
12. Braddon RL, Wolfe C: Musculocutaneous nerve injury after heavy exercise, *Arch Phys Med* 59:290-293, 1978.
13. Branston S: Muscle testing around the shoulder girdle: a study of the function of shoulder-blade fixators in seventeen cases of shoulder paralysis, *J Bone Joint Surg* 23:263-272, 1941.
14. Bryan WJ, Schauder K, Tullos HS: The axillary nerve and its relationship to common sports medicine shoulder procedures, *Am J Sports Med* 14:113-116, 1986.
15. Bryan WJ, Wild JJ: Isolated infraspinatus atrophy: a common cause of posterior shoulder pain and weakness in throwing athletes *Am J Sports Med* 17:130-131, 1986.
16. Brown C: Compressive, invasive referred pain to the shoulder, *Clin Orthop* 173:55-62, March, 1983.
17. Butsch JL: Subclavian thrombosis following hockey injuries, *Am J Sports Med* 11(6):448-450, 1983.
18. Cahill BR, Palmer RE: Quadrilateral space syndrome, *J Hand Surg* 8:65-69, 1983.
19. Coon WW, Willis PW: Thrombosis of axillary and subclavian veins, *Arch Surg* 94:657-663, 1967.
20. Dijkstra PF, Westra D: Angiographic features of the axillary artery by the musculus pectoralis minor and the head of the humerus in the thoracic outlet compression syndrome: case report, *Radiol Clin* 47:423-427, 1978.
21. Donovan WH, Kraft GH: Rotator cuff tear versus suprascapular nerve injury: a problem in differential diagnosis, *Arch Phys Med Rehabil* 55:424-428, 1974.

22. Drez D Jr: Suprascapular neuropathy in the differential diagnosis of rotator cuff injuries, *Am J Sports Med* 4(2):43-45, 1976.
23. Dundore DE, Delisa JA: Musculocutaneous nerve palsy: an isolated complication of surgery, *Arch Phys Med Rehabil* 55:424-428, 1974.
24. Durman DC: An operation for paralysis of the serratus anterior, *J Bone Joint Surg* 27:380-382, 1945.
25. Ferretti A, Cerullo G, Russo G: Suprascapular neuropathy in volleyball players, *J Bone Joint Surg [Am]* 69A:260-263, 1987.
26. Foo CL, Swann M: Isolated paralysis of the serratus anterior: a report of 20 cases, *J Bone Joint Surg [Br]* 65B:552-556, 1983.
27. Fields WS, Lemak NA, Ben-Manachem Y: Thoracic outlet syndrome: review and reference to stroke in a major league pitcher, *AJR* 146:809-814, 1986.
28. Ganzhorn RW et al: Suprascapular nerve entrapment, *J Bone Joint Surg [Am]* 63A:492-494, 1981.
29. Gardner E, Gray DJ, O'Rahilly R: *Anatomy: a regional study of human structure*, ed 3, Philadelphia, 1985, WB Saunders.
30. Goodman CE: Unusual nerve injuries in recreational activities, *Am J Sports Med* 11:224-227, 1983.
31. Gregg JR et al: Serratus anterior paralysis in the young athlete, *J Bone Joint Surg [Am]* 61A:825-832, 1979.
32. Harmen PH: Surgical reconstruction of the paralytic shoulder by muscle transplantation, *J Bone Joint Surg [Am]* 32A:583-595, 1950.
33. Hinton MA et al: An anatomic study of the subscapularis muscle and its humeral insertion, unpublished data.
34. Horwitz MT, Tocantins LM: An anatomical study of the role of the long thoracic nerve and the related scapular bursae in the pathogenesis of local paralysis of the serratus anterior muscle, *Anat Rec* 71:375-385, 1938.
35. Horwitz MT, Tocantins LM: Isolated paralysis of the serratus anterior (magnus) muscle, *J Bone Joint Surg [Am]* 20A:26-27, 1938.
36. Huffman JD: Electrodiagnostic techniques for and conservative treatment of thoracic outlet syndrome, *Clin Orthop* 207:21-23, 1986.
37. Johnson JTH, Kendall HO: Isolated paralysis of the serratus anterior muscle, *J Bone Joint Surg [Am]* 37A:567-574, 1955.
38. Jones HH et al: Humeral hypertrophy in response to exercise, *J Bone Joint Surg* 59A:204-208, 1977.
39. Kim SM, Goodrich JA: Isolated proximal musculocutaneous nerve palsy, *Arch Phys Med* 65:735-736, 1984.
40. King JW, Brelsford HJ, Tullos HS: Analysis of the pitching arm of the professional baseball pitcher, *Clin Orthop* 67:116-123, 1969.
41. Lang C et al: Lasionssyndrome des N suprascapularis, *Dtsch Med Wschr* 113:1349-1353, 1988.
42. Leffert RD, Gumley G: The relationship between dead arm syndrome and thoracic outlet syndrome, *Clin Orthop* 223:20-31, 1987.
43. Logigian EL et al: Stretch-induced spinal accessory nerve palsy, *Muscle Nerve* 11:146-150, 1988.
44. Loomer R, Graham B: Anatomy of the axillary nerve and its relation to inferior capsular shift, *Clin Orthop* 243:100-105, 1989.
45. Mastiglia FL: Musculocutaneous neuropathy after strenuous physical activity, *Med J Aust* 145:153-154, 1986.
46. McCarthy WJ, Vogelzang RL, Bergan JJ: Changing concepts and present day etiology of upper extremity venous thrombosis. In Bergan JJ, Yao JST, editors: *Venous disease,* Philadelphia, 1991, WB Saunders, pp 360-361.
47. McCarthy WJ et al: Upper extremity arterial injury in athletes, *J Vasc Surg* 9(2):317-327, 1989.
48. McKowen HC, Voorhies RM: Axillary nerve entrapment in the quadrilateral space, *J Neurosurg* 66:932-934, 1987.
49. Mendoza FX, Main K: Peripheral nerve injuries of the shoulder in the athlete, *Clin Sports Med* 9(2):331-342, 1990.
50. Neer CS, Foster CR: Inferior capsular shift for involuntary inferior and multidirectional instability of the shoulder, *J Bone Joint Surg [Am]* 62A:879, 1980.
51. Nichols HM: Anatomic structures of the thoracic outlet, *Clin Orthop* 207:13-20, 1986.
52. Nuber GW et al: Arterial abnormalities of the shoulder in athletes, *Am J Sports Med* 18(5):514-519, 1990.
53. Paget J: *Clinical lectures and essays,* London, 1879, Longman, Green & Co.
54. Pang D, Wessel HB: Thoracic outlet syndrome, *Neurosurgery* 22(1):105-119, 1988.
55. Parsonage MJ, Tune JWA: Neurologic amyotrophy: the shoulder-girdle syndrome, *Lancet* (1):973-978, 1948.
56. Pasila M et al: Early complications of primary shoulder dislocations, *Acta Orthop Scand* 49:266, 1978.
57. Petrera JE, Trojaborg W: Conduction studies of the long thoracic nerve in serratus anterior palsy of different etiology, *Neurology* 34:1033-1037, 1984.
58. Raaf J: Surgery for cervical rib and scalenus anticus syndrome, *J Am Med Assoc* 157:219-223, 1955.
59. Rask MR: Suprascapular nerve entrapment: a report of two cases treated with suprascapular notch resection, *Clin Orthop* 123:73-75, 1977.
60. Rengachary SS et al: Suprascapular entrapment neuropathy: a clinical anatomical and comparative study. I. Clinical study, *Neurosurgery* 5:441-446, 1979.
61. Rengachary SS et al: Suprascapular entrapment neuropathy: a clinical anatomical and comparative study. II. Anatomical study, *Neurosurgery* 5:447-451, 1979.
62. Riddell DH, Smith BM: Thoracic and vascular aspects of thoracic outlet syndrome: 1986 update, *Clin Orthop* 207:31-36, 1986.
63. Ringel SP et al: Suprascapular neuropathy in pitchers, *Am J Sports Med* 18(1):80-86, 1990.
64. Roos DB: Congenital anomalies associated with thoracic outlet syndrome; anatomy, symptoms, diagnosis and treatment, *Am J Sports Med* 132:771, 1976.
65. Schultz JS, Leonard JA: Long thoracic neuropathy from athletic activity, *Arch Phys Med Rehabil* 73:87-90, 1992.
66. Seldinger SI: Catheter placements of the needle in percutaneous arteriography, *Acta Radiol* 39:368-376, 1953.
67. Shaffer BJ et al: Infraspinatus splitting incision in posterior shoulder surgery, an anatomic and electromyographic study, unpublished data.
68. Simeone FA: Neurologic complications of closed shoulder injuries, *Orthop Clin North Am* 6(2):499-506, 1975.
69. Stanish WD, Lamb H: Isolated paralysis of the serratus anterior muscle: a weight training injury, *Am J Sports Med* 6:385-386, 1978.
70. Strukel RJ, Garrick JG: Thoracic outlet compression in athletes. A report of four cases, *Am J Sports Med* 6:35-39, 1978.
71. Thompson RC Jr, Schneider W, Kennedy T: Entrapment neuropathy of the inferior branch of the suprascapular nerve by ganglia, *Clin Orthop* 166:185-187, 1982.
72. Tullos HS et al: Unusual lesions in the pitching arm, *Clin Orthop* 88:169-182, 1972.
73. Warner JP et al: Anatomy and relationships of the suprascapular nerve: anatomical constraints to mobilization of the supraspinatus and infraspinatus muscles in the management of massive rotator-cuff tears, *J Bone Joint Surg* 74A(1):36-45, 1992.
74. Weaver HL: Isolated suprascapular nerve lesions, *Injury* 15(2):117-126, 1983.
75. Woodhead AB III: Paralysis of the serratus anterior in a world class marksman: a case study, *Am J Sports Med* 13:359-362, 1985.
76. Wright IS: The neurovascular syndrome produced by hyperabduction of the arms, *Am Heart J* 29:1-19, 1945.
77. Yoon TN, Grabois M, Guillen M: Suprascapular nerve injury following trauma to the shoulder, *Trauma* 21(8):652-655, 1981.

PART THREE

The Elbow and Forearm

CHAPTER 15

Biomechanics of the Elbow

JACQUELIN PERRY

PHILIP A. DAVIDSON

The elbow comprises three functional systems, divided according to bones, ligaments, and muscles. The bony articulations include both a hinge joint and a rotational joint. Complex medial and lateral collateral ligaments provide stability to the elbow. Muscle groups emanating principally from the medial and lateral humeral epicondyles control the wrist and fingers. Each of the three functional systems of the elbow has a unique involvement in overhead activities such as throwing, swimming, or racquet sports.

ARTICULATIONS

The elbow is a trochoginglymus joint involving three articulations with two rotational degrees of freedom. The three articulations are the humeroulnar, humeroradial, and proximal radioulnar (Fig. 15-1). Motion of the elbow occurs in two planes, flexion-extension and forearm rotation (pronation-supination).[9] The elbow and its articulations are subject to tremendous forces during overhead sports (Fig. 15-2). For example, the valgus moment across the medial elbow during the acceleration phase of pitching has been calculated at up to 94.7 N/kg by Hang et al.[15] This provides both a tensile load to the medial collateral ligament and a compressive load to the lateral column. The elbow rapidly extends during the acceleration phase. There is a potential for compressive loading of the posterior compartment of the elbow in terminal extension that requires dynamic deceleration. Rotation of the forearm and rotatory forces at the proximal radioulnar

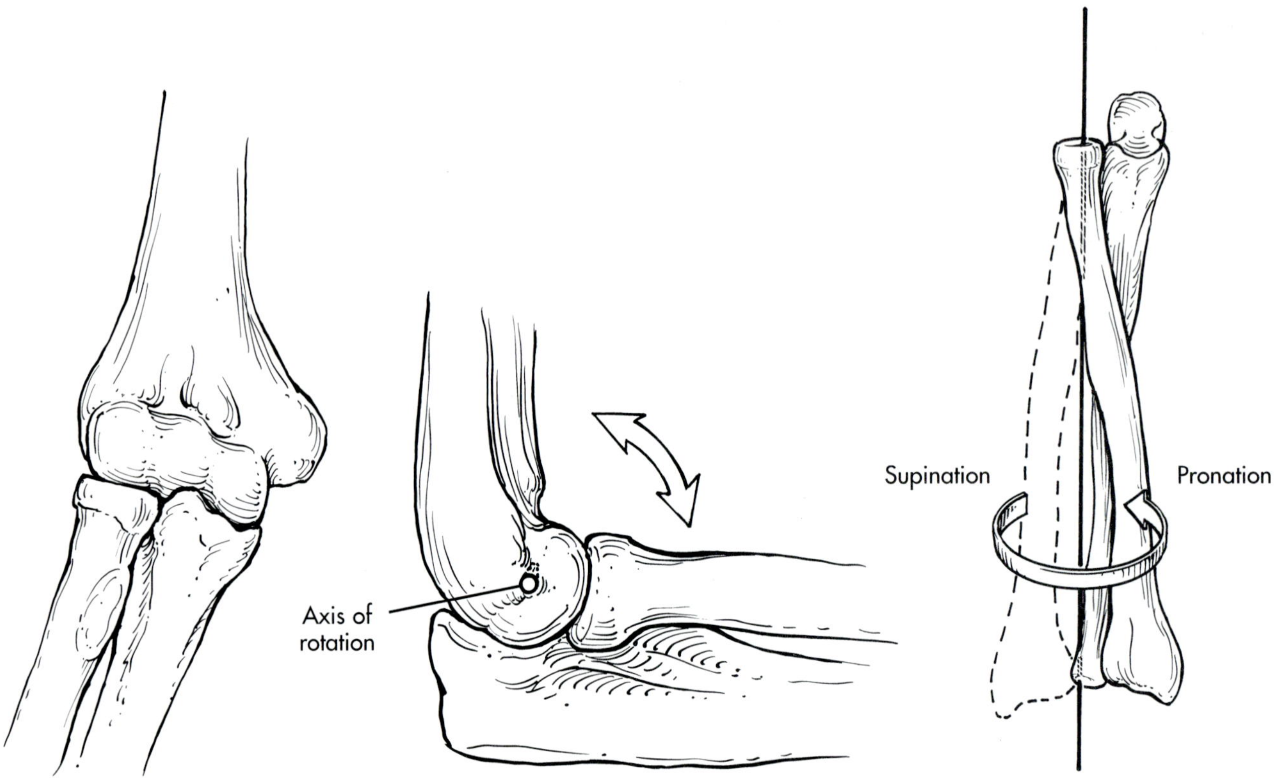

FIGURE 15-1 Bones with two planes of motion.

A

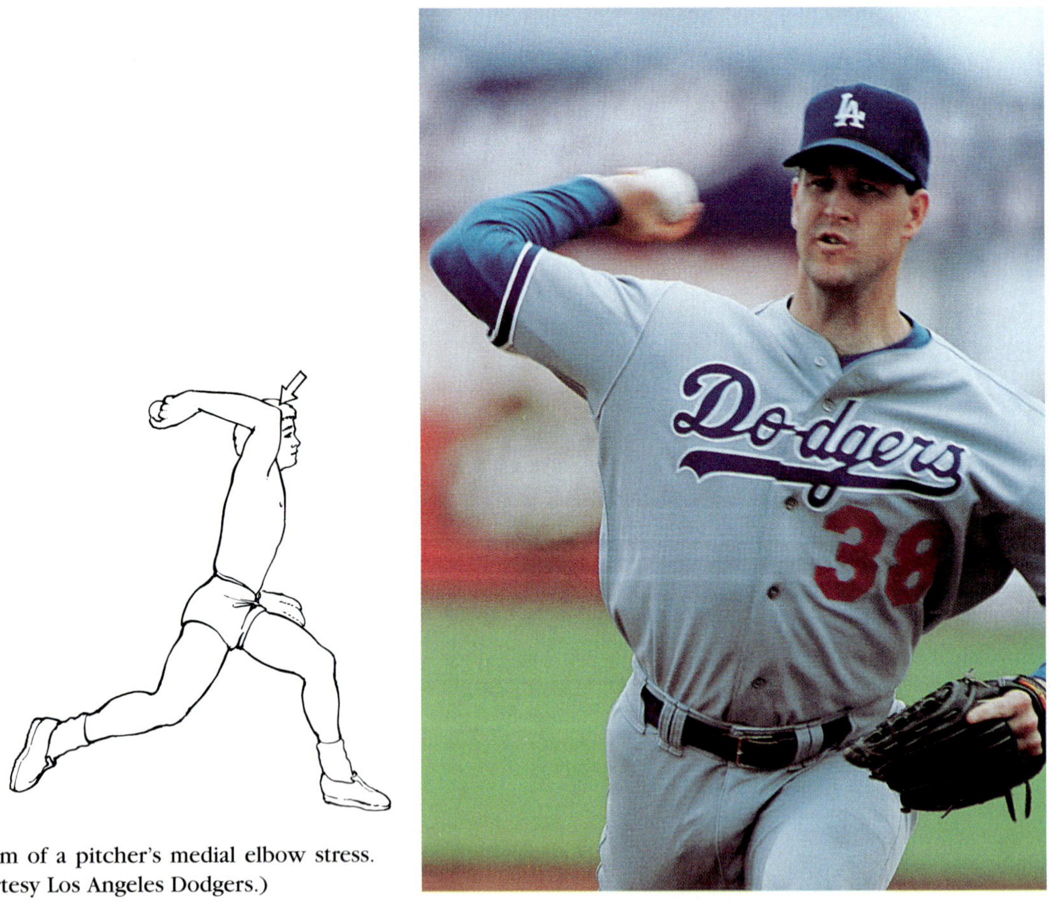

B

FIGURE 15-2 **A,** Diagram of a pitcher's medial elbow stress. **B,** Dodger pitcher. (Courtesy Los Angeles Dodgers.)

joint are used to help maintain throwing accuracy and precise delivery when throwing a ball or swinging a racquet.

Elbow Hinge

Kinematic analysis by London[23] radiographically identified a single axis of flexion. The axis passes through the center of an arc outlined by the bottom of the trochlear sulcus and the periphery of the capitellum. Relative motion of the hinge joint surfaces is of a sliding type, except at the extremes of flexion or extension, where rolling-type motion was observed.[23]

Humeroulnar Joint

Major stability is provided by the medial joint, formed by the trochlea of the humerus and the trochlear notch of the ulna. Near congruence of their biconcavoconvex articular surfaces significantly limits motion to a single plane.

The contribution of the humeroulnar joint to elbow stability was investigated by An et al.[3] They serially resected the proximal ulna, in 25% increments, evaluating the effect on four displacement, two torsional, and two axial modes. They found a proportional relationship between constraint of the humeroulnar joint in all modes and the area of remaining articulation.

Haberneck and Ortner[14] analyzed the effect of humeroulnar carrying angle and curvature of the ulnar trochlear notch on stability after elbow dislocation. They found no association between these two angles and instability.

Peak valgus mobility (averaging 5°) between the ulna and humerus is present with 20° or more of elbow flexion.[26] This physiologic laxity appears to be a function of variable tension in the anterior band of the medial collateral ligament (MCL).[31] At 20° of elbow flexion, the olecranon is disengaged from its fossa while the MCL is not maximally tense. There is also slight axial rotational mobility (3°) in this position.

Humeroradial Joint

The lateral joint within the elbow hinge is formed by the junction of the radial head and the capitellum of the humerus. The spherical shape of the capitellum and the shallow concavity of the radial head are designed to accommodate combined axial and rotational loads. This joint configuration confers little sagittal stability, because that function is performed principally by the humeroulnar articulation. Longitudinal force transmission through the radial head was evaluated by Morrey et al.[25] They found, while loading the forearm, that the greatest amount of force passed across the radiocapitellar joint when elbow flexion was at 0° to 30°. Furthermore, they noted increased loading of the radiocapitellar joint at all degrees of flexion with forearm pronation.

Inequality of the two "spools" of the distal humeral trochlea, with the medial diameter being larger, results in an oblique alignment of the joint axis relative to the long axis of the humeral shaft. The functional effect is a 10° to 15° lateral deviation of the forearm when the elbow is in full extension.[41] This is called the *carrying angle.* The functional advantage is the placement of the hand lateral to the hip when objects are carried in the dependent position. As the elbow flexes, such as during the windup phase of pitching, the lateral deviation decreases to zero at the end of the range, allowing the hand to be aligned with the shoulder.

The radial head plays a role in coronal plane stabilization because it acts as a constraint to both varus and valgus moments. Sojberg et al[33] performed isolated radial head excision, sparing the lateral collateral ligaments, to analyze varus rotatory instability. They found a 5° maximum varus displacement at 40° of elbow flexion.

The radial head contribution to valgus stability has been the focus of debate. Hotchkiss and Weiland,[16] in a serial sectioning study, evaluated valgus elbow stability at 0°, 45°, and 90° of flexion with isolated radial head resection. They found 24%, 27%, and 32% respective loss of relative stability for these three elbow positions. In a similarly performed study, Morrey and An[26] evaluated elbow specimens at 0° and 90° of elbow flexion. They reported a 33% relative contribution to valgus stability at 0° of flexion and 45% at 90°. Investigators citing the valgus-support role of the radial head advocate prosthetic replacement for comminuted fractures. A later report by these investigators[28] using modified methods suggested that, in the presence of an intact MCL, radial head resection does not appreciably change either abduction-adduction or axial rotation. The effect of radial head resection in a situation of high demand, such as that in overhead athletes, has not been analyzed.

Proximal Radioulnar Joint

The proximal and distal articulations between the ulna and radius share a single axis that allows forearm rotation. The axis for pronation/supination runs from the middle of the capitellum, through the center of the radial head, and through the base of the ulnar styloid distally.[21] At the elbow, the lateral side of the ulnar articulating surface is a concave arc (the radial notch) into which the radial head is held by a strong annular ligament. Four fifths of this osseofibrous ring is ligamentous.[40] The only motion at this joint is rotation of the radius within the ulnar notch.

ELBOW LIGAMENTS

Medial Ligaments

The medial collateral ligament (MCL) is the primary stabilizer of the medial elbow. In throwing, the maximum valgus force is encountered across the medial elbow during the cocking and acceleration phases[10] (Fig. 15-3). The elbow is between 80° and 120° of flexion during this period of maximal valgus loading.[10] The ulnohumeral articulation and anterior joint capsule, which provide two thirds of valgus elbow stability in full extension, contribute minimally to valgus support in this functionally demanding range.[26] As the motion proceeds, all the forces sequentially generated from the legs, hips, trunk, torso, and shoulder are transmitted directly through the MCL.

The MCL consists of three bands (Fig. 15-4). The prominent anterior band (oblique bundle) is the functionally significant ligamentous component resisting valgus elbow stress. The posterior and transverse bands have been ascribed limited functional significance.[27] Investigators have calculated the load to failure of the anterior band of the MCL to be approximately 260 N. This compares with palmaris longus (the most frequently used autogenous replacement graft) strength of 357 N. The anterior band has a variable morphology.[7,19] It is either cord-shaped or fan-shaped. The anterior band functions like a cam, with variably located lines of tension, depending on the degree of elbow flexion.[27,31] When the elbow is flexed, tension is present posteriorly. In full elbow extension, the anterior fibers are tense, while the more posterior fibers are slack. As the elbow flexes, the middle and posterior fiber bundles become tense in succession. The origin of the ligament is posterior to the axis of flexion and extension about the distal humerus, arising from the posterior distal aspect of the medial epicondyle.[19] Its insertion has an arc configuration along the base of the coronoid process.[31] Anatomic observations by Jordan and Jobe[19] noted that the flexor digitorum superficialis (FDS) takes partial origin from the anterior fibers of the anterior band of the MCL. Microscopic and histologic analysis by these authors demonstrated skeletal muscle of the FDS taking origin directly from the fibrous layer of the anterior band of the MCL.

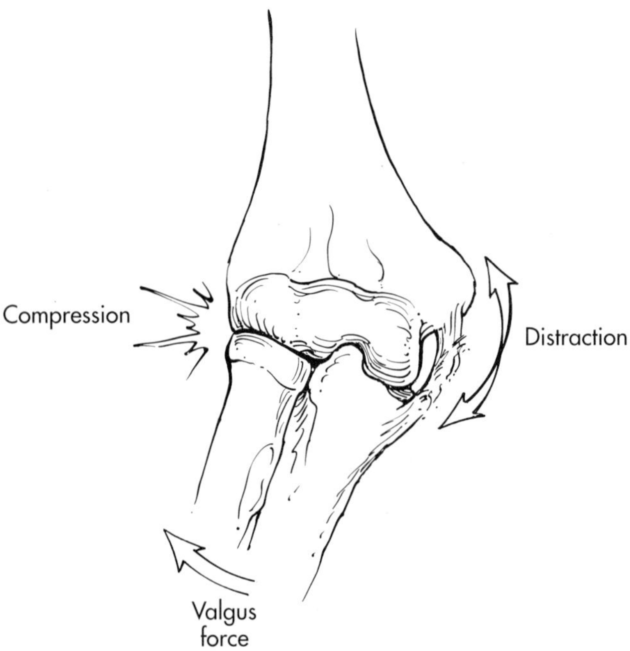

FIGURE 15-3 Coronal elbow with valgus stress. Forces: compressive, and distraction.

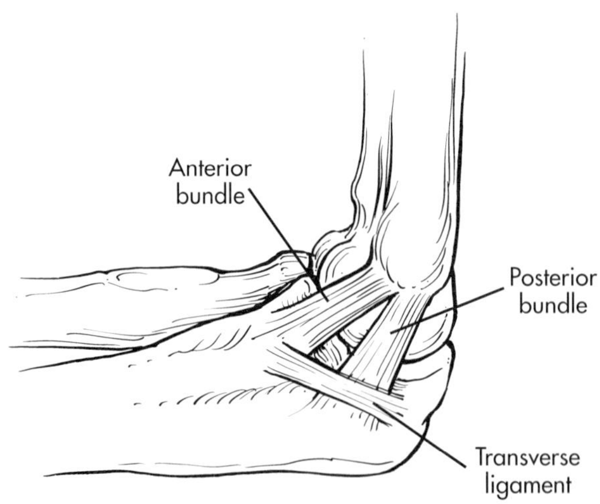

FIGURE 15-4 Medial ligament anatomy.

Sectioning studies in cadaver elbows have been performed to analyze the relative contribution of elbow structure to valgus stability. Morrey and An[26] reported that in full extension, valgus stability was equally conferred by the MCL, anterior capsule, and bony articulation. At 90° of flexion, they found the MCL provided 55% of valgus stability while the articular restraints provided the remainder. Using a modified method of analysis, Morrey et al[28] subsequently evaluated isolated MCL release, reporting an increase of 6° to 8° in valgus angulation. They further report that combined release of the anterior band of the MCL with radial head resection leads to gross elbow instability. Hotchkiss and Weiland[16] also performed serial sectioning to evaluate valgus elbow stability. They reported a minimal contribution to stability of the posterior band of the MCL, a 30% reduction in load-displacement curves for isolated radial head resection, and gross instability after isolated sectioning of the anterior band of the MCL. Sojberg[34] also reported on serially sectioned cadaver elbows. He found stability of the elbow independent of the MCL in extension beyond 20° or flexion past 120°. Between these degrees of flexion, he reported a maximum of 20.2° valgus opening and 21.0° internal rotatory instability with isolated MCL sectioning.

The role of the MCL as a primary stabilizer of the medial elbow has been indirectly confirmed by surgical studies. Josefsson et al[20,21] noted that in 15 of 15 patients undergoing surgery for dislocation of the elbow, there was a complete rupture of the anterior band of the MCL. Tullos et al[36] similarly reported that 32 of 32 patients surgically explored for elbow dislocation had a completely ruptured MCL. All patients in both of these series had clinical and radiographic evidence of valgus instability.

Lateral Ligaments

The lateral elbow is subjected to compressive, rather than distraction, forces during most of the throwing motion. Ligaments on the lateral side are somewhat variable in their morphology. The principal components of the lateral collateral ligament complex include the radial collateral ligament and the annular ligament (Fig. 15-5). The accessory collateral ligament and the lateral ulnar ligament are smaller structures that are present in variable configurations.[24] The radial collateral ligament originates on the anteroinferior aspect of the annular ligament.[19] The axis of elbow flexion passes through the common origin of the lateral collateral ligament; therefore no length change was observed with elbow flexion.[27] Sectioning studies performed by Morrey and An[26] ascribed a maximum of 14% relative varus stability to the radial collateral ligament, with only 9% at 90° elbow flexion. In their sectioning series, Sojberg et al[33] reported that the annular ligament was the primary stabilizer of the lateral elbow. They found a minimal contribution to varus stability from the lateral collateral ligament, whereas sectioning the annular ligament caused 13.7° of varus instability and 32.8° of external rotatory instability at 70° of elbow flexion.

Posterolateral rotatory instability of the elbow has been described by O'Driscoll et al.[29] They have described an entity that involved subluxation with a complex provocative maneuver. The etiology of this condition was postulated to be laxity of the ulnar part of the lateral collateral ligament, which allowed the transient rotatory subluxation to occur. The motion of posterolateral rotatory instability is pertinent in the context of preserving this ligament during surgery for lateral epicondylitis or detachment of the extensor musculature.

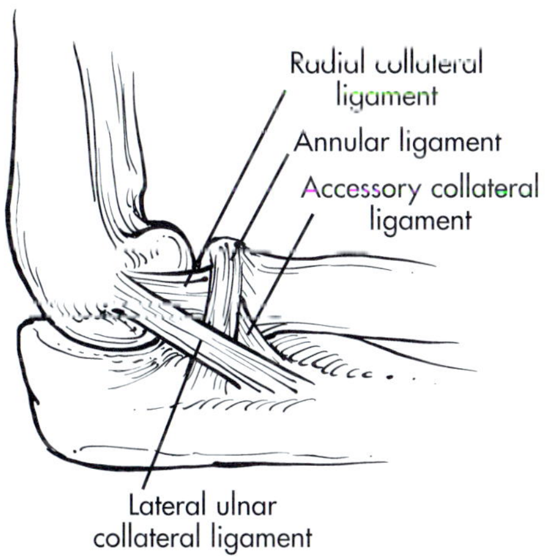

FIGURE 15-5 Lateral ligament anatomy.

ELBOW MUSCULATURE

Each of the axes of motion at the elbow has a dedicated group of controlling muscles. In addition, there is some shared function among the muscle groups. Basically, four muscle groups control the elbow joints: flexors and extensors of the hinge axis, and pronators and supinators of the proximal radioulnar joint.

Flexors

Three muscles, the biceps, brachialis, and brachioradialis, have elbow flexion as their primary function (Fig. 15-6). Only the brachialis, however, has elbow flexion as its sole action. This relates to the fact that its insertion is on the ulna, while the biceps and brachioradialis cross the radioulnar joint by inserting on the radius. The three muscles also differ in size, fiber length, and leverage.[1,2] Muscle size determines its force potential, while leverage, indicated by the muscle's moment arm length, represents the muscle's mechanical advantage. Fiber length is significant for the relative speed of motion vs. holding force.

The brachialis is the largest flexor muscle (7 cm^2) but has the shortest moment arm (1.3 cm) because of its close proximity to the joint surface. It also contains the shortest muscle fibers (9 cm). These are deep and adjacent to the joint capsule. The more superficial fibers of this bulky muscle approximate the lengths found in the biceps.

The two heads of the biceps, which are of similar size (the long, 2.5 cm^2, and the short, 2.1 cm^2), combine to form an elbow flexor approximately two thirds as large as the brachialis. Both points of origin (superior glenoid for the long head and coracoid for the short head) provide a more effective lever arm (2.3 cm) than the brachialis. Fiber length of the two heads differs slightly, but both support rapid motion (the long head is 13.6 cm, and the short head is 15.0 cm).

The brachioradialis is the smallest muscle (1.5 cm^2) in this group, but its moment arm is longest (3.7 cm). This mechanical advantage combined with its longer fiber length (16.4 cm) favors the muscle for rapid action, although its small size limits the effective force.

Based on each muscle's physical characteristics, the biceps has the greatest elbow flexion and supination capability, and it is most suitable for fast action. The effectiveness of the brachialis is about 75%, and through its shorter fibers this contributes more to stability than rapid motion. The brachioradialis is least effective.

Both forearm and elbow position modify the muscles' mechanical advantage. An found that forearm supination significantly increased the lever arm of the biceps (+35%), although there was little effect on the brachialis and brachioradialis.[2] Increasing elbow flexion, however, led to significantly greater effectiveness of all three muscles but with different magnitudes. Flexion to 50° had the greatest effect on the biceps moment arm (+80%),

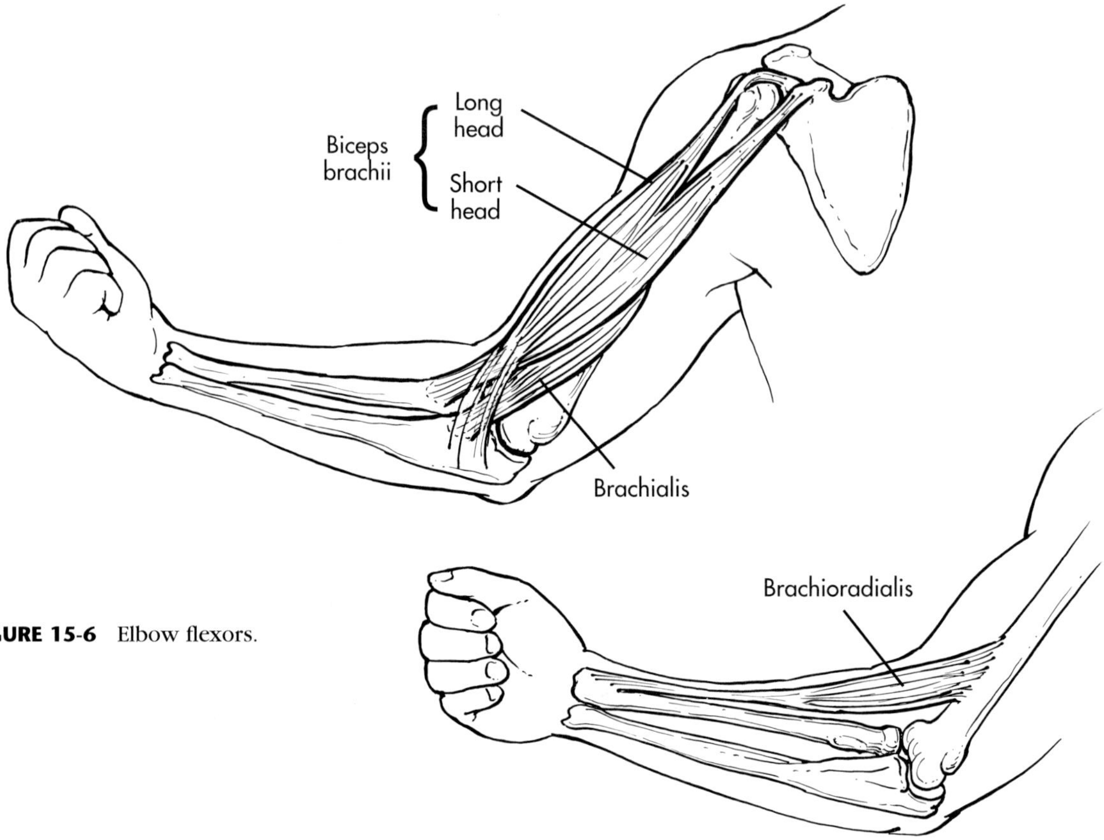

FIGURE 15-6 Elbow flexors.

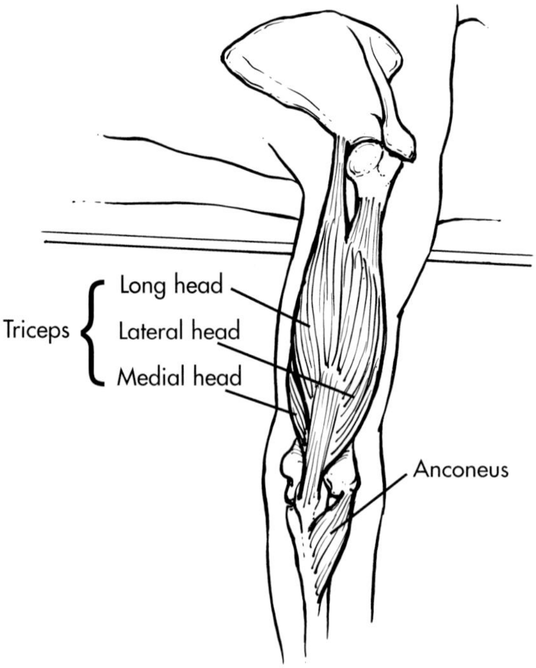

FIGURE 15-7 Triceps.

and flexion to 100° had the least effect on the brachioradialis.[2]

Supplementary flexion also is supplied by the medial and lateral epicondylar muscle groups. Most effective are the pronator teres (PT, medial) and extensor carpi radialis longus (ECRL, lateral), which originate at their respective locations on the supracondylar ridge.[30] Their flexor moment arms approximate 1.5 cm. The other muscles that originate on the epicondyles have far less flexor potential. In fact, the flexor carpi radialis (FCR) and the extensor digitorum superficialis (EDS) displayed an extensor moment with the elbow fully extended but had a flexor alignment with the elbow flexed 50°.

Extensors

The elbow hinge is extended by the triceps muscle group (Fig. 15-7). All three heads (long, lateral, and medial) as well as the small anconeus muscle insert into the ulna and thus are dedicated to elbow extension. The strength of the elbow extensor muscles is approximately 61% of the flexors.[4] Increasing elbow flexion reduced the extensor moment arm of the triceps slightly (15%) but tended to increase the mechanical advantage of the anconeus.[1]

Supplementary elbow extension by the ulnar wrist muscles (flexor carpi ulnaris [FCU] and extensor carpi ulnaris [ECU]) has been identified by An.[1] This contradicts

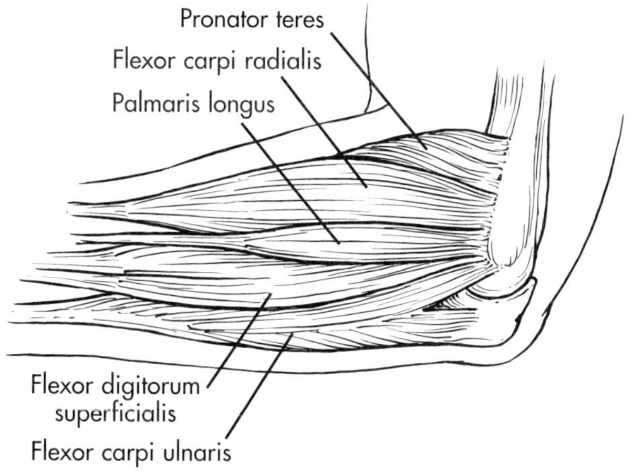

FIGURE 15-8 Medial mass: generic pictures of medial elbow muscles.

the common assumption that the whole epicondylar muscle masses are weak elbow flexors.

Pronators

Radioulnar pronation is provided by the pronator teres and to a lesser extent by the wrist/finger flexor mass. Because the pronator teres also has sufficient leverage to contribute to elbow flexion, there is no dedicated pronator muscle mass at the elbow. Distally there is the pronator quadratus.

Supinators

There are three sources of radioulnar supination control. Isolated supination is available from the small supinator muscle overlying the radial head. The strongest source of supination is the biceps brachii. In fact, this muscle's leverage for elbow flexion is best when the forearm is supinated. As was true medially, the lateral epicondylar extensors of the wrist and fingers also contribute to forearm supination. The pronator muscle group strength is about 86% of the supinator capability.[4]

Varus Torque

The muscles that cross the medial side of the elbow joint have an alignment favoring dynamic protection of the medial ligaments (MCL complex) of the elbow joint (Fig. 15-8). The centroid calculations of An[1] identify a significant moment arm (approximately 2 cm) for the pronator teres, FCU, FCR, and flexor digitorum superficialis (FDS).[1] Little difference was identified with either forearm rotation or elbow flexion.

An anatomic study performed by Davidson et al[7] evaluated the relationship of the flexor pronator muscle group to the anterior band of the MCL. These investigators found that at 90° and 120° of elbow flexion (Fig. 15-9), corresponding to the position of valgus loading, the humeral head of the flexor carpi ulnaris (FCU) covered the anterior band of the MCL. The flexor digitorum superficialis (FDS) was immediately anterior to the ligament. They noted that the FCU and FDS were optimally positioned to provide secondary valgus stability to the medial elbow.

Electromyographic analysis of medial elbow musculature showed an increase in effort (percentage maximal muscle test, percentage MMT) for all components of the flexor pronator mass as the arm progressed from the cocking to acceleration phases.[8] Evaluation of muscle function in medially unstable elbows showed paradoxically decreased percentage MMT for the FCR and PT.[12] Although the FDS and FCU were not tested, it might be expected that a similar decrease would be seen in the FDS and FCU in an unstable situation. It appears that, while providing secondary valgus support, the flexor pronator muscles are unable to compensate for an insufficient or torn MCL.

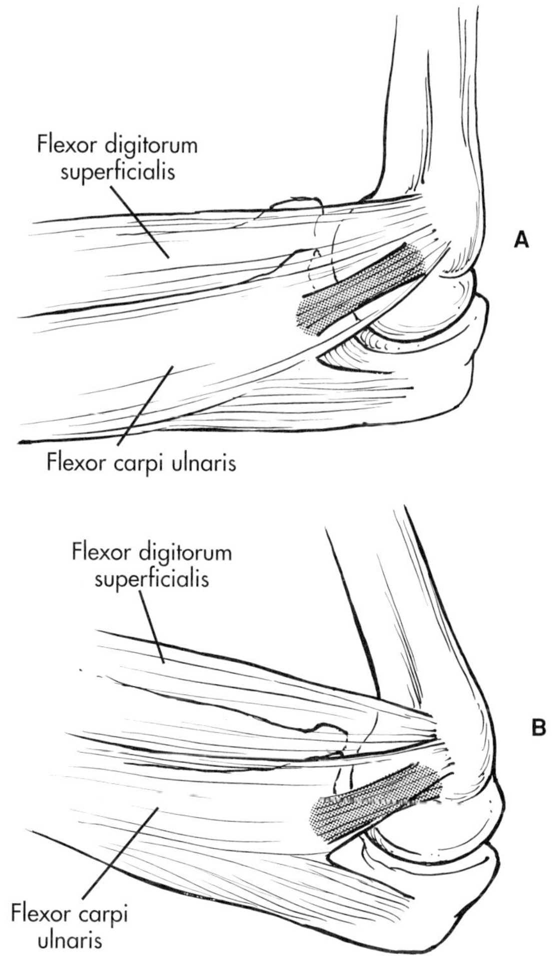

FIGURE 15-9 Medial collateral ligament at 90° **(A)** and 120° **(B)**.[7]

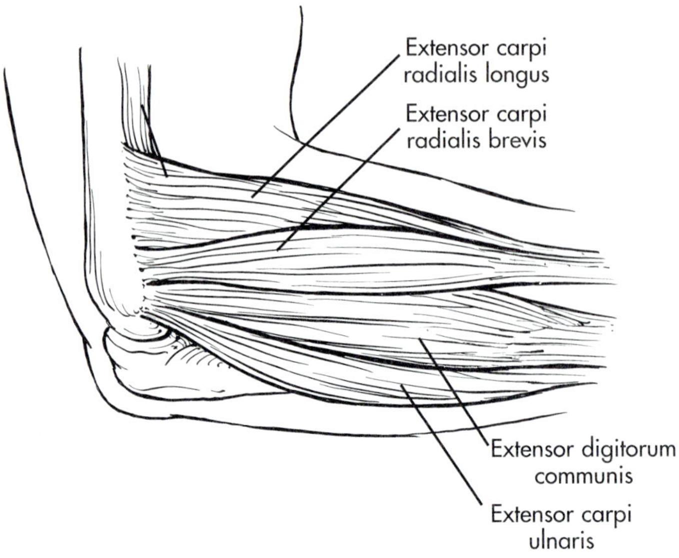

FIGURE 15-10 Lateral mass: generic pictures of lateral elbow muscles.

Valgus Torque

Muscles arising from the lateral epicondylar area of the humerus have a valgus moment arm (Fig. 15-10). For the three muscles studied (ECR, ECU, EDC), the leverage was best with the elbow fully extended. Both forearm rotation and elbow flexion reduced these muscles' potential to provide dynamic protection of the lateral ligaments.

THROWING

One of the more challenging and more studied activities for the elbow is the act of throwing or pitching. During each throw or pitch, the elbow is subject to both imposed forces and functional demands. Basically the elbow is designed for planar motion, whereas the act of throwing relies on peak rotatory power to propel the ball. This presents a major challenge to the stabilizing structures of the elbow.

Power to propel the ball is sequentially provided by derotation of the lower extremities, trunk, arm, forearm, and hand. Vigorous muscular effort mobilizes each segment in turn. To throw the ball, the player cocks the hand by sequentially rotating each body segment posteriorly. When the maximum position has been reached at all segments, the process is aggressively reversed to propel the ball forward toward its intended target.[39] As one body unit reaches its peak velocity, the next segment responds, after a momentary lag, by actively adding its own power to further increase the cumulative angular velocity available to the ball.[5] The significance of this power progression is enhanced by Toyoshima's finding that the legs and trunk provide 50% of the throw velocity.[35] The upper extremity musculature completes the throw. Because the elbow is near the end of the kinetic chain, the external forces are considerable.

Phasic Events

For the elbow, the significant phases of the pitch are late cocking, acceleration, and deceleration (Fig. 15-11). Muscle intensity and timing are selectively coordinated to control the external forces in a manner that provides optimal elbow positioning.

Late Cocking

During this phase, the elbow increases its angle of flexion from 63° to 74°,[10] yet the intensity of the primary flexor muscle action is low (average 22% MMT) and similar to the intensity that occurred in early cocking. Activity in the triceps (37% MMT) is greater than that of the flexors during this phase.[17] The stimulus for this difference lies in the dynamics of the humerus. Strong muscular action combined with the trunk's momentum rapidly externally rotates the humerus to 170° while maintaining arm elevation and retraction. In the experimental situation of a paralyzed triceps (radial nerve block) the elbow increases its flexion to 155°. Thus the function of the triceps during late cocking is to restrain the passive flexor force. The low level of flexor muscle activity maintains the optimum elbow position.

Momentum transmitted through the entire body to the forearm requires active muscular control to position the hand for the pitch or throw. The finding of greater response by the supinator (54% MMT) than the pronator teres (39% MMT)[8] may represent a difference in muscle

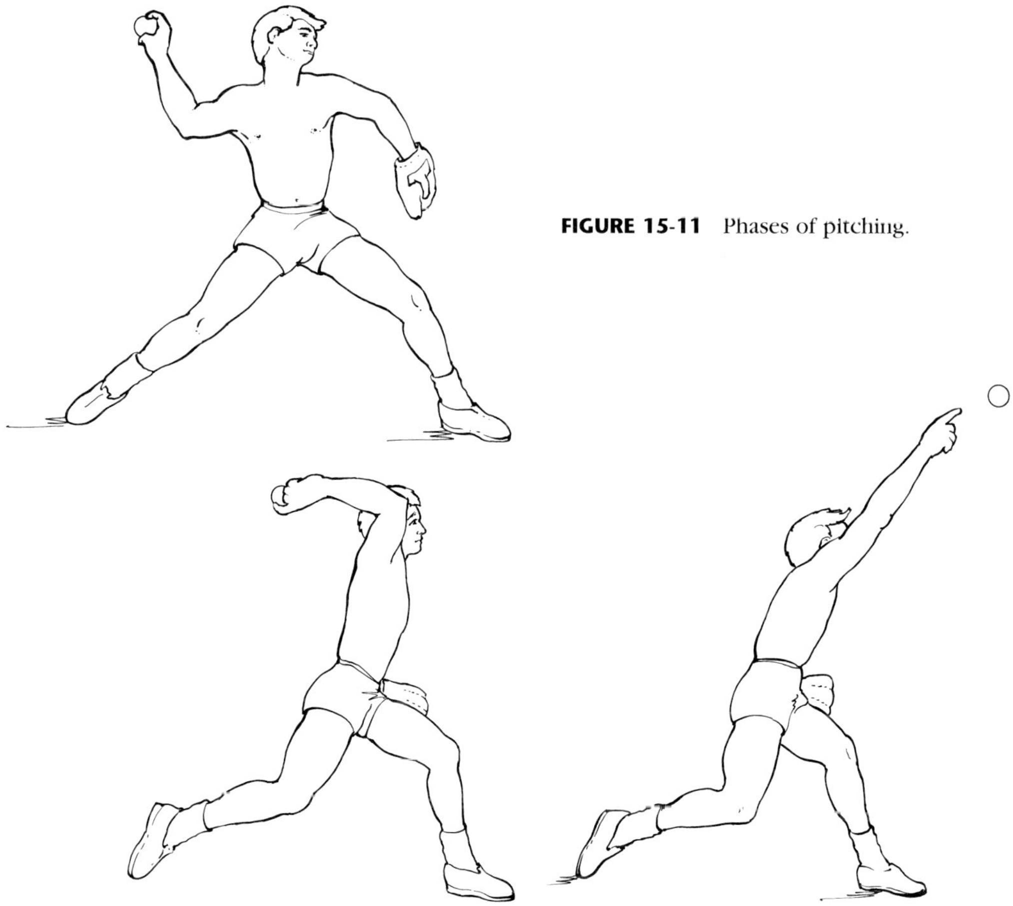

FIGURE 15-11 Phases of pitching.

size or a passive pronation torque imbalance. A curveball is associated with supination, and a straight pitch is associated with pronation.[15]

The lateral epicondylar muscle mass has the strongest level of muscle action registered during late cocking. Both radial wrist extensors (ECRB and ECRL) have a high intensity (75% and 72% MMT) at this time, while there also is moderate action in the finger extensors (EDC, 59% MMT). These levels of action are notably greater than that generated during early cocking and that continued in the later phases.

Acceleration

From its previously flexed position, the elbow rapidly extends (i.e., 70° in 40 ms).[11] At a calculated rate of 2200°/sec, the elbow reduces its flexed position to 20°.[10] Because more than 50% of pitchers have a flexion contracture,[18] this 20° may approach the joint extension limits. Strong triceps action (89% MMT) indicates this is a deliberate rather than a passive motion. The experimental radial nerve palsy, however, showed that triceps activity is not essential. During the arm's accleration phase, the muscles of the anterior wall flex and rotate the humerus. As the upper arm moves forward, inertia of the forearm induces elbow extension. With a little practice, the subject with an experimentally absent triceps could pitch at 80% of his normal velocity.[32]

The elbow also experiences a major valgus thrust during the phase of acceleration.[37] The majority of this load is borne by the MCL. As a result of both trunk and shoulder propulsive action, the angular velocity of humeral rotation is equivalent to 6100°/sec.[10] Because advancement of the humerus precedes that of the ulna and radius, a resulting torque of 100 nm for a 49 mph throw is imposed on the medial structures of the elbow.[10] Transmission of the propulsive impulse to the forearm stimulates the medial epicondylar muscle mass to participate. Protection of the medial elbow ligaments by the flexor pronator muscles was postulated by Tullos.[36] Davidson et al[7] showed that the FDS lay directly over the anterior aspect of the MCL anterior band at 30° of elbow flexion. However, by 120° of elbow flexion, the FDS moved anteriorly with respect to the MCL. As such, the FCU covered the entire anterior band of the MCL at this position. The medial collateral ligament is the primary constraint to the valgus moment.

The response of the medial epicondylar muscle group is intense. Activity of the wrist flexors (FCR and FCU) approaches 120% MMT, while the finger flexors (FDS) contract at the 80% MMT level.[8] The muscles, by actively flexing the previously extended wrist, contribute to the final stage of ball propulsion. The dual effect of passive stretch by the humeral torque and the stimulus to participate in ball propulsion may lead to flexor muscle injury in adult pitchers[22,38] and to medial epicondyle avulsion in youngsters.[11]

Another component of the medial elbow muscle mass is the pronator teres. Its high participation (85% MMT) in arm acceleration is notably higher than that of the supinator muscle action (55% MMT). Either the dynamic humeral rotation also imparts a supination thrust on the radius that requires control, or modest forearm pronation is needed for appropriate ball direction.

Deceleration

After ball release, the elbow flexes a moderate degree (50°) in response to a sharp change in muscle intensities. All three major elbow flexors reach their peak intensity, averaging 48% MMT. At the same time, the triceps rapidly reduces its activity to 54% MMT. Although these intensities are similar, there is a bias toward flexion because the elbow flexors normally are a significantly stronger muscle group than the triceps (40% differential).[4] Countering this fact is the evidence that rapid concentric contractions generate less force than comparable eccentric activity.[13] The change in the elbow's position is so rapid that a deceleration rate of 500,000°/sec has been calculated. A delay or imbalance in the triceps/elbow flexors exchange could allow posterior humeroulnar impingement, leading to traumatic osteophyte formation.

SUMMARY

The elbow is the last major joint in the vigorous kinetic chain that propels the ball during a throw. As a result of external torques and intrinsic function, the elbow structures are subject to three major stress experiences that can result in injury. Arm acceleration induces a valgus torque that imparts strain of the medial collateral ligament and potential compression at the radiohumeral joint. Medial ligament failure and impact osteoarthritis are common pathologies.[6] The medial epicondylar flexor pronator mass also is subjected to strain that may result in muscle tears.[38] Deceleration demands challenge the elbow flexor mass, which may lead to tendinitis and contracture.

References

1. An K-N et al: Muscles across the elbow joint: a biomechanical analysis, *J Biomech* 14(10):659-669, 1981.
2. An K-N, Kaufman KR, Chao EYS: Physiological considerations of muscle force through the elbow joint, *J Biomech* 22(11):1249-1256, 1989.
3. An K-N, Morrey BF, Chao EYS: The effect of partial removal of proximal ulna on elbow constraint, *Clin Orthop* 209:270-279, 1986.
4. Askew LJ et al: Isometric strength in normal individuals, *Clin Orthop* 222:261-266, 1987.
5. Atwater AE: Biomechanics of overarm throwing movements and of throwing injuries. In Hutton RS, Miller DI, editors: *Exercise Sports Science Reviews,* vol 7, Philadelphia, 1979, The Franklin Press.
6. Conway JE et al: Medial instability of the elbow in throwing athletes, *J Bone Joint Surg* 74-A(1):67-83, 1992.
7. Davidson PA et al: Functional anatomy of the flexor pronator muscle group in relationship to the medial collateral ligament of the elbow, *Am J Sports Med* 23(2):245, 1995.
8. DiGiovine NM et al: An electromyographic analysis of the upper extremity in pitching, *J Shoulder Elbow Surg* 1(1):15-25, 1992.
9. Engin AE, Chen SM: Kinematic and passive resistive properties of human elbow complex, *J Biomech Engr* 109:318-323, 1987.
10. Feltner M, Dapena J: Dynamics of the shoulder and elbow joint of the throwing arm during a baseball pitch, *Int J Sport Biomech* 2:235-259, 1986.
11. Gainor BJ et al: The throw: biomechanics and acute injury, *Am J Sports Med* 8(2):114-118, 1980.
12. Glousman RE et al: An electromyographic analysis of the elbow in normal and injured pitchers with medial collateral ligament insufficiency, *Am J Sports Med* 20(3):311-317, 1992.
13. Griffin JW: Differences in elbow flexion torque measured concentrically, eccentrically and isometrically, *Phys Ther* 67(8):1205-1212, 1987.
14. Haberneck H, Ortner F: The influence of anatomic factors in elbow joint dislocation, *Clin Orthop* 274:226-230, 1992.
15. Hang Y-S et al: Biomechanical study of the pitching elbow, *Int Orthop* 3:217-223, 1979.
16. Hotchkiss RN, Weiland AJ: Valgus stability of the elbow, *J Orthop Res* 5:372-377, 1987.
17. Jobe FW et al: An EMG analysis of the shoulder in pitching, a second report, *Am J Sports Med* 12(3):218-220, 1984.
18. Jobe FW, Nuber G: Throwing injuries of the elbow, *Clin Sports Med* 5(4):621-636, 1986.
19. Jordan SE, Jobe FW: The anatomy and histology of the collateral ligaments of the elbow, abstract presented.
20. Josefsson PO et al: Surgical versus non-surgical treatment of ligamentous injuries following dislocation of the elbow joint, *J Bone Joint Surg* 69-A(4):605-608, 1987.
21. Josefsson PO, Johnell O, Wendeberg B: Ligamentous injuries in dislocations of the elbow joint, *Clin Orthop* 221:221-225, 1987.
22. Kuroda S, Sakamaki K: Ulnar collateral tears of the elbow joint, *Clin Orthop* 208:266-271, 1986.
23. London JT: Kinematics of the elbow, *J Bone Joint Surg* 63-A(4):529-535, 1981.
24. Morrey BF: Applied anatomy and biomechanics of the elbow joint, *AAOS Instructional Course Lecture* chapter 8, vol 35, pp 59-68, 1986.
25. Morrey BF, An K-N, Stormont TJ: Force transmission through the radial head, *J Bone Joint Surg* 70A(2):250-256, 1988.
26. Morrey BF, An K-N: Articular and ligamentous contributions to the stability of the elbow, *Am J Sports Med* 11(5):315-319, 1983.
27. Morrey BF, An K-N: Functional anatomy of the ligaments of the elbow, *Clin Orthop* 201:84-90, 1985.
28. Morrey BF, Tanaka S, An K-N: Valgus stability of the elbow, *Clin Orthop* 265:187-195, 1991.
29. O'Driscoll SW, Bell DF, Morrey BF: Posterolateral rotatory instability of the elbow, *J Bone Joint Surg* 73-A(3):440-446, 1991.
30. Perry J, Dail C, Allen JR: Phasic relations of hand muscles applied to tendon transplants. Final project report PHS grant number AM-07192, National Institutes of Health, Attending Staff Association, Rancho Los Amigos, Downey, Calif, 1987.
31. Regan WD et al: Biomechanical study of ligaments around the elbow joint, *Clin Orthop* 271:170-179, 1991.
32. Roberts EM: Cinematography in biomechanical investigation. In Cooper JM, editor: *Committee on institutional cooperation symposium on biomechanics,* Indiana University, 1970, Chicago Athletic Institute, 1991.

33. Sojbjerg JO, Ovesen J, Gundorf CE: The stability of the elbow following excision of the radial head and transection of the annular ligament: an experimental study, *Arch Orthop Trauma Surg* 106: 248-250, 1987.
34. Sojbjerg JO, Ovesen JO, Nielsen S: Experimental elbow instability after transection of the medial collateral ligament, *Clin Orthop* 218:186-190, 1987.
35. Toyoshima S, Hosikawa T, Miashita M, Oguri T: Contribution of the body parts to throwing performance. In Nelson RC, Moorehouse CA, editors: *Biomechanics IV,* 1974, University Park Press, pp 169-174.
36. Tullos HS et al: Adult elbow dislocations: mechanism of instability, *AAOS Instructional Course Lecture* chapter 9, vol 35, pp 69-82, 1986.
37. Tullos HS, King JW: Throwing mechanism in sports, *Orthop Clin North Am* 4(3):709-720, 1973.
38. Vangsness CT, Jobe FW: Surgical treatment of medial epicondylitis, *J Bone Joint Surg* 73B(3):409-411, 1991.
39. Watkins RG et al: Dynamic EMG analysis of torque transfer in professional baseball pitchers, *Spine* 14(4):404-408, 1989.
40. Williams PL, Warwick R: *Gray's anatomy,* British ed 36, Philadelphia, 1908, WB Saunders, p 462.
41. Yocum LA: The diagnosis and nonoperative treatment of elbow problems in the athlete, *Clin Sports Med* 8(3):439-451, 1989.

CHAPTER 16

Surgical Anatomy of the Elbow

STEVE E. JORDAN

This chapter links the pertinent anatomy of the elbow to the surgical approaches. The surgical surface anatomy will be discussed first; then the anatomy and surgical approaches of the medial, lateral, and posterior compartments; and finally the anatomy as seen through the arthroscope.

SURFACE AND SUBCUTANEOUS ANATOMY

The three most useful surface landmarks about the elbow are the medial and lateral epicondyles and the olecranon process. With the elbow extended, these easily palpable bony prominences are colinear, and with the elbow flexed 90°, they form an inverted triangle. Anteriorly, a line between the epicondyles corresponds with the flexion crease, and when the elbow is extended, this line is 1 to 2 cm proximal to the joint line.[19] The cubital fossa (or antecubital fossa) is the triangular space just distal to the flexion crease. The apex of the cubital fossa distally is formed by the brachioradialis laterally and the tendons of the biceps and the brachialis medially.

Traversing the cubital fossa superficially is the median cubital vein, which connects the cephalic and basilic veins (Fig. 16-1). Below the medial cubital vein, the bicipital aponeurosis (lacertus fibrosus) arises from the biceps tendon and protects the underlying brachial artery and median nerve. In the days of the barber-surgeons, this aponeurosis was called the "grace a Dieu" fascia (praise be to God fascia) because it protected the artery and nerve during phlebotomy.[7] The cephalic and basilic

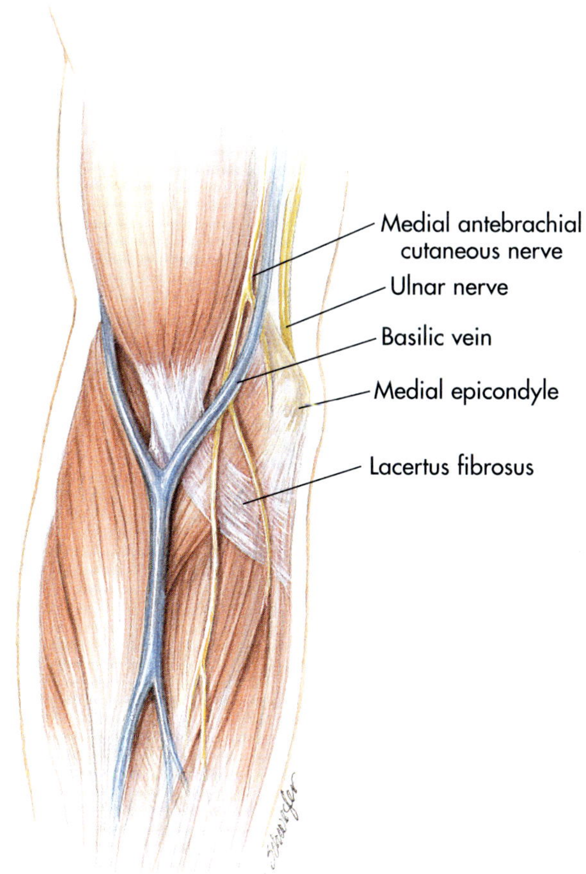

FIGURE 16-1 Superficial medial anatomy. Lacertus fibrosus, medial epicondyle, ulnar nerve, median antebrachial cutaneous nerve, basilic vein.

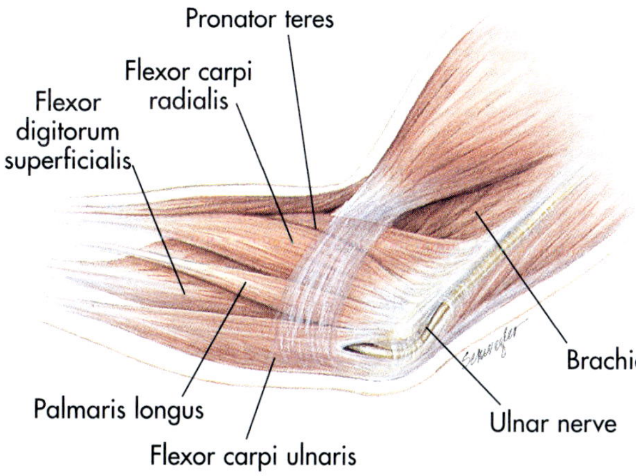

FIGURE 16-2 Medial muscular anatomy. Biceps, triceps, pronator teres, FCR, PL, FCU, FDS, FDP.

veins occupy the bicipital furrows on each side of the biceps muscle as they leave the cubital fossa proximally.

In the lateral bicipital furrow, the lateral antebrachial cutaneous nerve (the cutaneous portion of the musculocutaneous nerve) passes deep to the cephalic vein and divides at the level of the elbow joint into an anterior and posterior branch supplying cutaneous sensation to the radial half of the forearm.[9]

The medial antebrachial cutaneous nerve arises from the medial cord of the brachial plexus and with the basilic vein pierces the deep fascia midway down the arm.[9] Distally in the medial bicipital furrow, usually deep to the superficial veins, the nerve divides into an anterior and an ulnar branch. Both branches usually cross the elbow anterior to the medial epicondyle.

Posterior cutaneous sensation at the elbow and forearm is provided by the posterior antebrachial cutaneous nerve, which is a branch of the radial nerve.[9] The posterior antebrachial cutaneous nerve has branches both anterior and posterior to the lateral epicondyle. Awareness of these cutaneous nerves is vital in both open and arthroscopic surgery of the elbow.

The ulnar nerve enters the posterior compartment of the arm through the arcade of Struthers in the medial intermuscular septum approximately 8 cm proximal to the medial epicondyle.[9] The nerve follows the medial border of the triceps just posterior to the medial intermuscular septum until it enters the cubital tunnel behind the medial epicondyle.

The roof of the cubital tunnel is the arcuate ligament, which when inflamed and thickened forms the so-called Osborne lesion, entrapping the underlying nerve.[24] Laxity or absence of this ligament contributes to ulnar nerve instability.

Branches of the ulnar nerve include small sensory branches to the elbow joint that innervate the capsule.[9] The first motor branch goes to the humeral head of the flexor carpi ulnaris (FCU) and may be found arising high within the cubital tunnel. The main body of the ulnar nerve leaves the cubital tunnel between the two heads of the FCU, and the second motor branch supplies the ulnar head of the FCU. The posterior recurrent ulnar artery is deep to the ulnar nerve within the cubital tunnel.

MEDIAL

Muscular Anatomy

The medial musculature of the elbow and forearm is divided into two groups: superficial and deep (Fig. 16-2). The superficial group consists of five muscles often referred to as the flexor-pronator group. These are the pronator teres (PT), the flexor carpi radialis (FCR), the palmaris longus (PL), the flexor carpi ulnaris (FCU), and the flexor digitorum superficialis (FDS).[9] The deep layer proximally comprises the flexor digitorum profundus (FDP) and the flexor pollicis longus (FPL).[9]

The pronator teres has two heads of origin: the humeral and the ulnar. The humeral head, which is the largest and most superficial, arises just proximal to the medial epicondyle, and its inferior fibers blend with the common flexor origin. The ulnar head, which is deeper and smaller, arises from the medial side of the coronoid process of the ulna. The median nerve passes into the forearm between the two heads of the pronator teres.

The common flexor tendon, which arises from the intermuscular septum, the medial epicondyle, and the medial collateral ligament complex, is a blending of the origins of the FCR, the palmaris longus, when present, and the medial head of the FCU. The FDS has a broad medial origin with fibers arising from the medial epicondyle and the common flexor tendon, from the medial collateral ligament complex, and from the coronoid process of the ulna.[13] The lateral head of the FDS arises from the proximal radius.

The deep medial layer of muscles is rarely significant during surgery about the elbow. The FDP arises from the volar and medial surface of the proximal three fourths of the ulna, and the FPL arises from the radius distal to the bicipital tuberosity.[9]

The muscles of the medial elbow all are innervated by the median nerve, except the FCU, which is supplied by the ulnar nerve, as previously described.

Ligaments

Gross anatomic dissection of the elbow reveals four consistent components of the medial (or ulnar) collateral ligament complex (MCLC): the anterior band, the posterior band, the transverse band, and the intermediate area (Fig. 16-3).[13] The anterior band consists of two functional and qualitatively different bundles, an isometric inferior bundle, and a nonisometric superior bundle.

There are two morphologic types of isometric bundles, the more common round or cordlike bundle and a flat or ribbonlike variant found in 25% of specimens.[13] This isometric bundle of the anterior band is the primary stabilizer of the medial elbow, and this is the portion of the MCLC to which most discussions of the medial collateral ligament refer.[19]

The isometric bundle arises from the medial epicondyle, just below the common tendon, and spans the ulnotrochlear joint, inserting onto a small tubercle on the medial ulna.

The nonisometric band superiorly is taut in elbow extension and appears to function as a secondary stabilizer of the elbow when it is extended, as well as providing a broader surface for origins of the flexor pronator muscles.[13]

The functional importance of the transverse band, the intermediate band, and the posterior band of the MCLC is insignificant to this discussion; however, a thorough review can be found in the literature.[9,13,19]

Microscopic examination of the MCLC revealed three distinct layers (Fig. 16-4).[13] Perhaps the most clinically significant finding in this work was the identification of skeletal muscle fibers arising within the fibrous layer. This observation helps explain the surgical difficulty of isolating the ligamentous tissue as well as the clinical difficulty in separating the location of pathology involving these tissues.

Surgical Approaches

Classically, medial exposures to gain access to the elbow joint are not as successful as lateral exposures. Transepicondylar approaches were described[2,5,18,21] for removal of loose bodies or repair of medial articular injuries, but the morbidity associated with the osteotomy has led to decreased use of this approach over the years.

Banks and Laufman also described a posteromedial exposure of the medial capsule,[2] but this approach entailed the morbidity of mobilizing the ulnar nerve. For simple access to the elbow joint, this exposure has been replaced by arthroscopic techniques. Anteromedial exposures, such as that described by Cosentino,[6] require dissection of the cubital fossa, the median nerve, and the brachial artery and therefore have limited indications.

A medial utility approach centered over the medial epicondyle has provided satisfactory exposure for the clinical entities to be discussed in subsequent chapters of this book.

With the patient supine and the arm extended on an arm board, the medial arm and elbow are easily accessed.

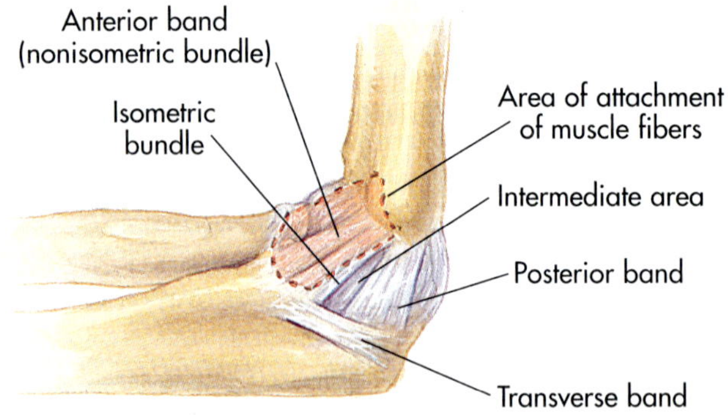

FIGURE 16-3 Medial capsuloligamentous complex. Bony anatomy, anterior band: isometric bundle, nonisometric bundle.

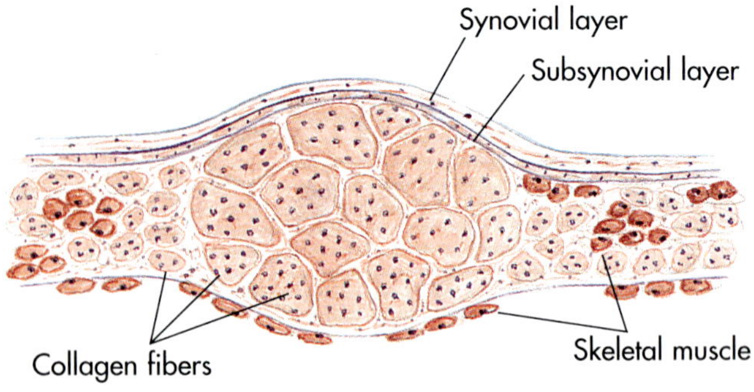

FIGURE 16-4 Histologic cross-section of medial capsuloligamentous complex. Synovial layer, subsynovial layer, fibrous layer, collagen bundles, skeletal muscle fibers.

Under tourniquet control, a curvilinear incision is centered over the anterior aspect of the medial epicondyle (Fig. 16-5, *A*). Superficial veins are cauterized if necessary, but care is taken to identify and protect the medial antebrachial cutaneous nerve branches as they are encountered.

To inspect the anterior band of the MCLC or to debride the common flexor tendon in cases of suspected MCL insufficiency or medial epicondylitis, the flexor pronator muscles are divided sharply in the direction of their fibers. When reflection of the common flexor tendon is required, as in submuscular transposition of the ulnar nerve or some techniques of MCL reconstruction, a small cuff of tendinous tissue is left attached to the epicondyle to aid in reattachment (see Fig. 16-5, *B*).

The medial utility exposure is easily extended both proximally and distally when warranted. It also allows access to the posterior compartment if dissection is continued posterior to the cubital tunnel, particularly in those cases where the ulnar nerve is transferred anteriorly.

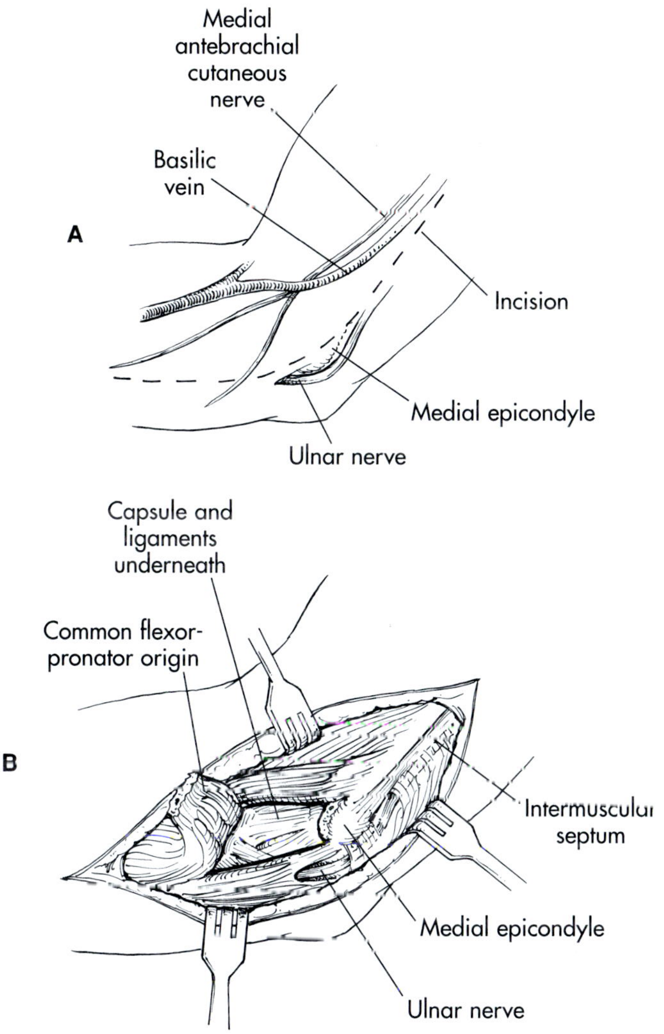

FIGURE 16-5 **A,** Medial utility approach (superficial). Skin incision, median antebrachial cutaneous nerve, ulnar nerve, muscular anatomy. **B,** Medial utility approach (deep). Skin incision, reflected common extensor origin, medial capsuloligamentous complex.

LATERAL

Muscular Anatomy

The muscles of the lateral or extensor surface of the elbow can be divided into superficial and deep groups, as were the medial muscles. The superficial group contains seven muscles. From anterior to posterior, they are the brachioradialis, the extensor carpi radialis longus (ECRL), the extensor carpi radialis brevis (ECRB), the extensor digitorum communis (EDC), the extensor digiti minimi (EDM), the extensor carpi ulnaris (ECU), and the anconeus (Fig. 16-6).[9] The deep layer contains the supinator and four muscles that rarely are clinically significant in surgery of the elbow. These four muscles are of more concern in surgery of the hand. They are the abductor pollicis longus, the extensor pollicis brevis, the extensor pollicis longus, and the extensor indicis proprius.

The brachioradialis separates the brachialis muscle and the lateral head of the triceps as it arises from the lateral intermuscular septum and the proximal two thirds of the lateral supracondylar ridge of the humerus. Proximally, the muscle protects the radial recurrent artery and the radial nerve as it emerges from the spiral groove. Distally, the brachioradialis forms the lateral border of the cubital fossa, as previously mentioned.

The extensor carpi radialis longus arises from the distal third of the lateral supracondylar ridge of the humerus and the lateral intermuscular septum just be-

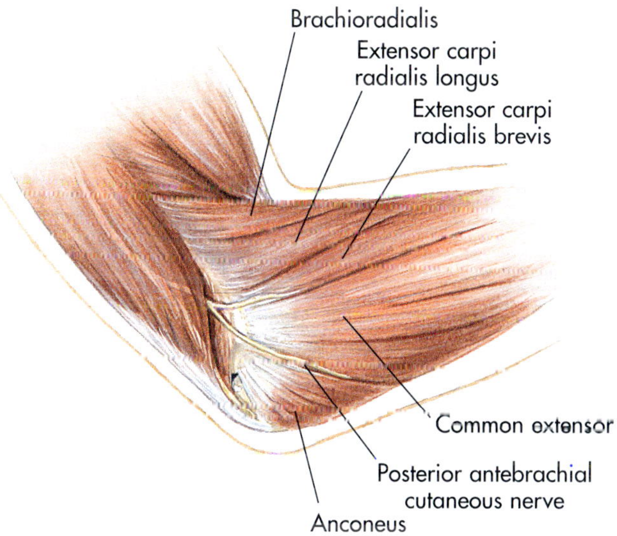

FIGURE 16-6 Lateral muscular anatomy. Anconeus, ECU, EDQ, EDC, ECR (longus and brevis), brachioradialis, brachialis, biceps, triceps, supinator.

low the brachioradialis.[9] Its most distal fibers may blend with the common extensor tendon. In this respect, the ECRL is similar to the pronator teres medially, which blends with the common flexor origin.

The extensor carpi radialis brevis arises below the ECRL in conjunction with the common extensor tendon from the lateral epicondyle, the lateral collateral ligament complex, and the surrounding intermuscular septae. This diffuse origin is significant in the clinical treatment of lateral epicondylitis, as will be described later. Proximally, the fibers of the ECRL, ECRB, and EDC are difficult to separate, and more distal dissection is required when indicated for accurate separation.

The extensor digitorum communis arises diffusely from the lateral epicondyle and the lateral collateral ligament complex just distal to the ECRB. The extensor digiti minimi blends with the medial border of the EDC and is clinically insignificant at the elbow.

The extensor carpi ulnaris (ECU) has two heads of origin. The humeral head arises in conjunction with and is the most medial of the common extensor group. The ulnar head arises from the proximal ulna and the aponeurosis covering the anconeus. The plane between the anconeus and the ulnar head of the ECU also is more easily separated distally than proximally because of this investing common fascia proximally. The anconeus is a triangular-shaped muscle that may appear to be a continuation of the lateral head of the triceps muscle. It has a broad muscular origin on the posterior aspect of the lateral epicondyle and inserts on the lateral surface of the proximal ulna.

The supinator muscle curves around the proximal radius and is most important for its relationship with the radial nerve. The radial nerve divides into its terminal branches, the superficial radial nerve and the posterior interosseous nerve, at the level of the elbow joint. The posterior interosseous nerve enters the extensor compartment after passing between the fibers of the supinator muscle, and the terminal superficial branches usually lie on the surface of the supinator. The posterior interosseous nerve is classically located within the supinator muscle three finger widths distal to the neck of the radius, as described by Henry.[11]

The muscles of the lateral elbow all are innervated by the posterior interosseous nerve, except for the brachioradialis and the ECRL, which are innervated by the radial nerve before it divides into the superficial and deep branches.

Ligaments

The lateral collateral ligament complex (LCLC) is classically composed of two components, the radial collateral ligament and the annular ligament (Fig. 16-7). The first American edition of *Gray's Anatomy* in 1870 pointed out that some of the posteriormost fibers of the radial collateral ligament insert onto the outer margin of the

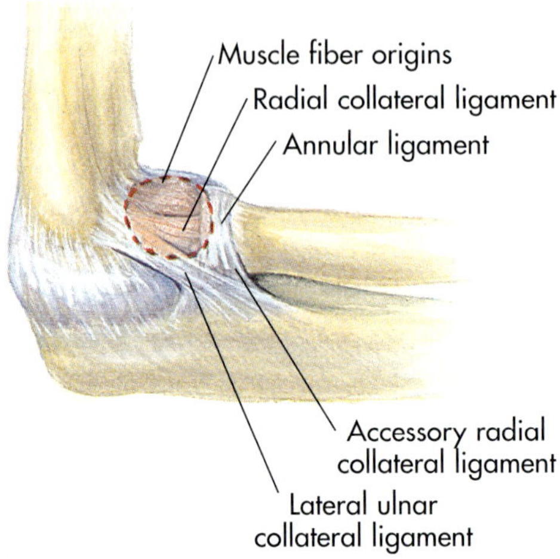

FIGURE 16-7 Lateral capsuloligamentous complex. Radial collateral ligament, annular ligament, accessory radial collateral ligament, lateral ulnar collateral ligament, muscle fiber origins.

ulna.[8] Others also have noted the thicker posterior and anterior portions of this ligament.[4,17] Recently, Morrey and An described the posterior portion of the radial collateral ligament in some cadavers as a separate entity and named it the lateral ulnar collateral ligament.[20] These authors also have established the importance of this ligament in preventing lateral elbow instability. O'Driscoll et al established its importance in preventing posterolateral rotatory instability of the elbow.[20,22] Regardless of whether the posterior border of the radial collateral ligament is seen as a separate ligament, it is believed to be vital to the stability of the lateral aspect of the elbow joint.

The annular ligament is a strong band of tissue that encircles four fifths of the radial head and serves to stabilize it within the ulnar notch. The majority of the fibers of the radial collateral ligament blend into the annular ligament. Superficial fibers of the annular ligament have been noted to attach on the ulna separately, and these fibers are the accessory lateral collateral ligament. This ligament is seen in only a small percentage of cadavers.[13,19]

The LCLC serves as a source of origin for portions of the common extensor tendon, the ECRB, and the supinator muscle, which has fibers arising from the annular ligament. Microscopic examination of the LCLC revealed muscle fibers within the outer fibrous layer of the ligament complex similar to that seen in the MCLC.[13] Similarly, clinical syndromes involving the lateral aspect of the elbow, such as lateral epicondylitis, may involve ligamentous fibers as well as muscular or tendinous tissue.

Surgical Approaches

The lateral elbow can be exposed through either lateral or posterolateral incisions. The lateral approaches ex-

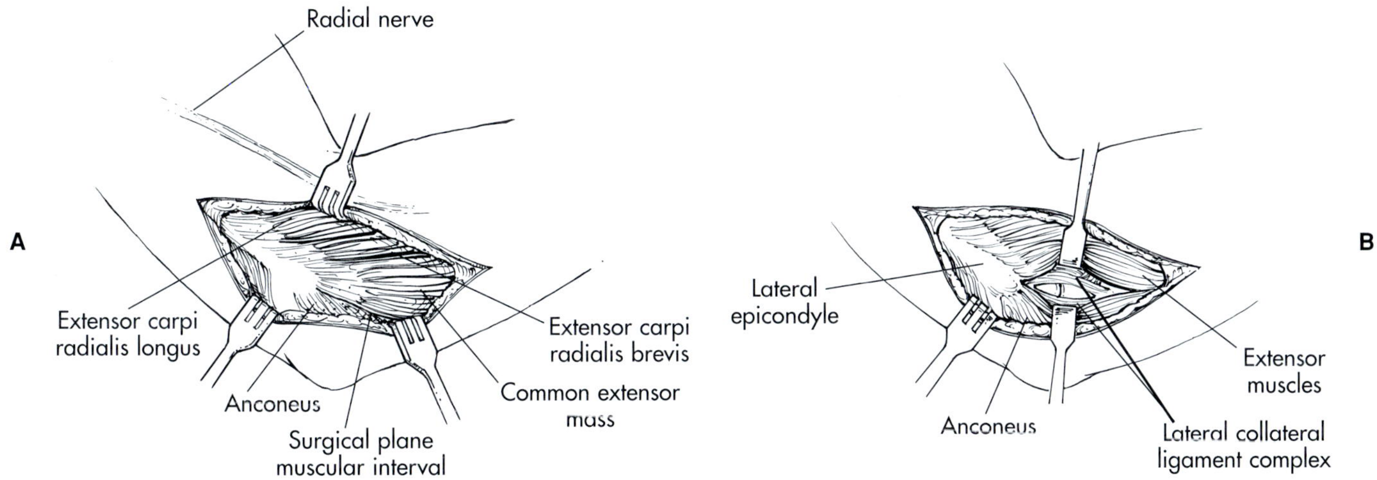

FIGURE 16-8 **A,** Lateral Kocher utility approach (superficial). Skin incision, muscular anatomy, supinator muscle, radial nerve, lateral capsuloligamentous complex. **B,** Lateral Kocher utility approach (deep). Muscular interval, arthrotomy, LCLC, radial head, capitellum, supinator, radial nerve.

ploit one of three planes to reach the joint. The first, described by Kaplan,[14] is between the common extensor and the ECRL and ECRB. As noted previously, the plane between the common extensor and the ECRB must be developed distally because the muscles blend at a common origin. The second approach is a transepicondylar approach that, similar to the medial transepicondylar approach, is rarely indicated today. The third lateral plane is between the ECU and the anconeus, as described by Kocher[15] (Fig. 16-8, *A*). This approach is the one most favored today.

The posterolateral approaches of Boyd[3] and Pankovich[25] both require dissection of the anconeus from the ulna. Although these two approaches allow safe exposure of the supinator muscle and the underlying proximal radius, they place the important posterior fibers of the radial collateral ligament in jeopardy. When using the lateral approaches of Kocher or Kaplan, the surgeon must carefully repair the components of the LCLC to avoid destabilizing the elbow.

The approach favored for revision of the lateral epicondyle, repair or reconstruction of the lateral collateral ligament, and lateral arthrotomy is the lateral approach of Kocher (Fig. 16-8). With the patient supine, the arm is placed in a pronated position on an arm board. A curvilinear incision is centered over the lateral epicondyle. Superficial dissection is performed to isolate and protect sensory nerve branches and identify the underlying muscle and fascial planes. Depending on the procedure, the appropriate deep dissection may be performed (Fig. 16-8, *B*). For exposure of the LCLC and the radiocapitellar joint, the plane between the anconeus and the ECU is developed. Deep dissections vary depending on the pathology present.

POSTERIOR

Muscular Anatomy

The triceps is the only muscle of the posterior compartment of the elbow. The tendon of the triceps consists of two aponeurotic lamellae that converge distally and insert primarily on the olecranon process. Laterally, a portion of the triceps tendon fans out to insert on the fascia of the anconeus and the lateral ulna. The ulnar nerve and the cubital tunnel border the triceps medially.

Surgical Approaches

Posterior surgical approaches to the elbow can be divided into four categories: triceps splitting, triceps reflection, transosseous, and extensile continuations of posteromedial or posterolateral exposures.[11,15,19,21]

The approach used (Fig. 16-9) depends on the clinical indications for surgery. For direct open access to the posterior compartment, a limited triceps splitting incision is used. In situations that require wide exposures of the joint, either a wide stripping of the triceps or an olecranon osteotomy can be used. All posterior incisions should be made with care not to cross the tip of the olecranon to prevent painful scarring. Most procedures in the posterior compartment can be performed through either a medial or lateral incision.

ARTHROSCOPIC ANATOMY

The indications and efficacy for elbow arthroscopy have been well established.[1,10,12,17,19] This section reviews the pertinent anatomy of the elbow relative to the six most common arthroscopic portals. Later chapters in this book outline and discuss the various applications and techniques for arthroscopy of the elbow.

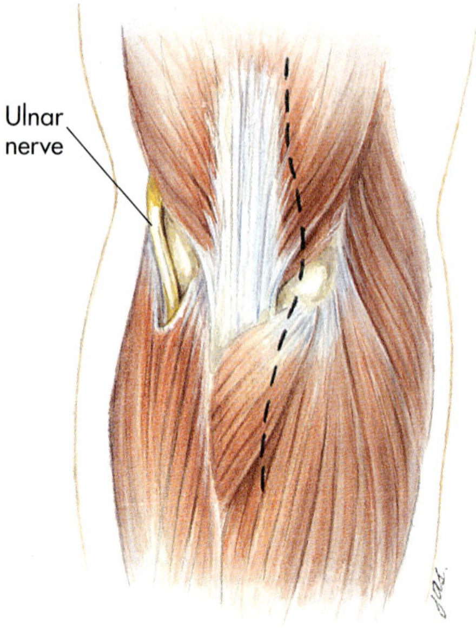

FIGURE 16-9 Posterior incision. Skin incision, triceps muscle, ulnar nerve, anconeus.

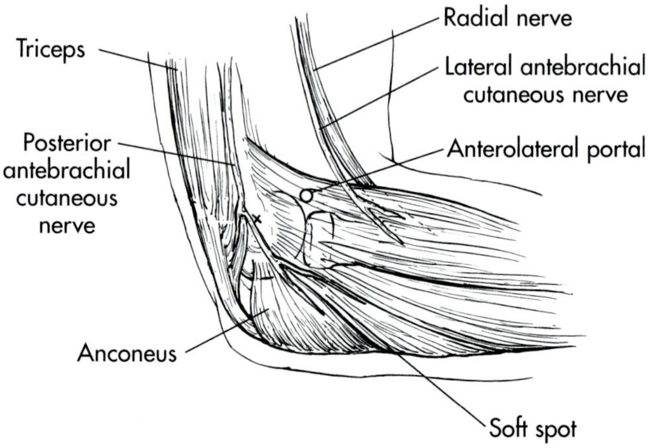

FIGURE 16-10 Lateral arthroscopic portals. Lateral antebrachial cutaneous nerve, posterior antebrachial cutaneous nerve, bony anatomy, anterolateral portal, soft-spot portal, posterolateral portal.

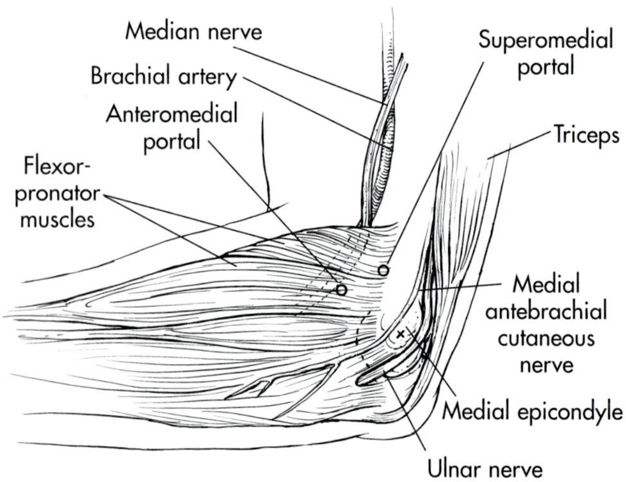

FIGURE 16-11 Medial arthroscopic portals. Medial antebrachial cutaneous nerve, medial nerve, ulnar nerve, brachial artery, bony anatomy, anteromedial portal, superomedial portal.

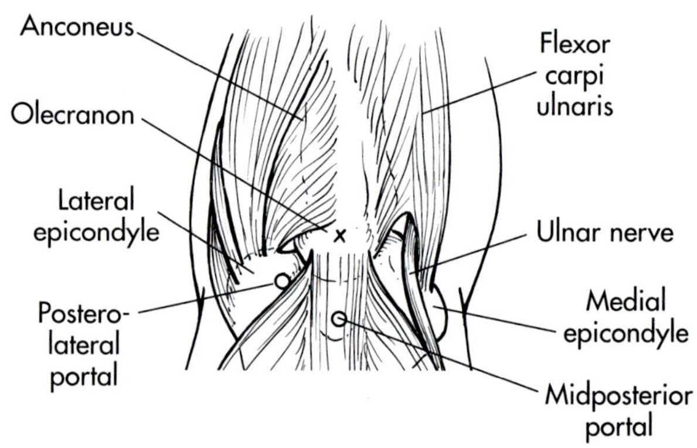

FIGURE 16-12 Posterior arthroscopic portals. Ulnar nerve, triceps muscle and tendon, bony anatomy, posterolateral portals, posterior portals.

There are six routine portals for arthroscopy of the elbow: two medial portals, two lateral portals, and two posterior portals (Figs. 16-10 to 16-12). Depending on the surgeon's choice, the patient's positioning, and the location of pathology, any of the six portals may be used for initial visualization. Medial portals may be established inside-out from lateral portals via the Wissinger rod technique, and vice versa. Posterior portals are established directly.

Patient positioning for elbow arthroscopy may be supine, lateral decubitus, or prone. Recently, the prone position has been used, at first for patients with primarily posterior elbow pathology, and lately for anterior compartment pathology as well. These positions have been well described previously.[18] A good transition position for surgeons who are more comfortable with supine positioning but who desire easier access to the posterior compartment is the lateral position. For this technique, the patient is secured in a lateral decubitus position with a bean bag. The arm is then sterilely prepared, draped, and supported in 90° of abduction on an angled arm rest with the anterior elbow free.

Arthroscopy of the elbow should begin with careful marking of the bony landmark before distension. The joint should be distended with 15 to 20 ml of saline solution and with the elbow flexed 80° to 90°.[23] Proper joint positioning and distension before instrumentation increases the margin of safety for the neurovascular structures.[16] The usual portal for distension is the direct midlateral or soft-spot portal (see Fig. 16-10). The needle penetrates skin, the anconeus muscle, and joint capsule before entering the joint. All of the arthroscopic portals to be discussed can be used with each of the three patient positions mentioned previously.

Medial Portals

The two medial portals are the anteromedial portal and the superomedial portal (see Fig. 16-11). The anteromedial portal is 2 cm distal and 2 cm anterior to the medial epicondyle. The instrumentation cannulas pass between the flexor carpi radialis and the flexor digitorum superficialis and through the deep portion of the pronator teres before entering the joint.[16]

Whether the portal is established directly or with the Wissinger rod technique via the anterolateral portal, proper technique in establishing the anteromedial portal is essential to avoid neurovascular injury.[16] The medial antebrachial cutaneous nerve was within 1 mm of the arthroscopic sheath in three of five cadavers, and the brachial artery and median nerve were a mean distance of 9 mm and 4 mm respectively from the sheaths in this same study.[16] These latter measurements improved approximately 1 cm with joint distension.[16] The lateral and prone positions improve this margin of safety by allowing gravity to further displace the neurovascular structures from the trocar sheaths.

The superomedial portal (or proximal medial portal) as described by Poehling et al[26] is the preferred beginning portal when using the prone and lateral positions (see Fig. 16-10). The entry point is 2 cm proximal to the medial epicondyle. Proper technique again is essential to avoid injury to the neurovascular structures. The trocar is directed anterior to the intermuscular septum to avoid injury to the ulnar nerve and is aimed toward the radial head. By maintaining contact with the anterior humerus, the surgeon avoids the median nerve and brachial artery (which lie directly anterior).

Lateral Portals

The two lateral portals are the direct midlateral portal (or soft spot) and the anterolateral portal (see Fig. 16-11). The direct lateral portal, as mentioned previously, is used primarily for initial joint distension. It is located in the lateral soft spot between the lateral epicondyle, the radial head, and the tip of the olecranon. The risk to neurovascular structures with this portal is negligible.

The anterolateral portal has been the traditional portal used for initial viewing of the anterior compartment. Although it is being replaced as the initial portal by the superomedial portal, it is still an important portal, especially for viewing the anterior medial compartment. The anterolateral portal is located 2 cm distal and 1 cm anterior to the lateral epicondyle and lies directly over the radiocapitellar joint. The lateral antebrachial cutaneous nerve and the radial nerve are the structures at greatest risk when using this portal. The cannula penetrates the skin just anterior to the radial head and passes through the extensor carpi radialis brevis and the deep portion of the supinator muscle below the radial nerve before entering the joint.[16] The cutaneous nerve is within 1 to 3 mm of the trocar, and the radial nerve is within 10 to 12 mm with the joint distended and the elbow flexed.[16]

Posterior Portals

The two posterior portals are the direct posterior and the posterolateral portals (see Fig. 16-12). The direct posterior portal is placed approximately 3 cm proximal to the tip of the olecranon. The fibers of the triceps are split with care taken to avoid directing the cannula too far medial, because this would risk injury to the ulnar nerve.

The posterolateral portal is made just lateral to the triceps tendon (approximately 2 cm lateral to the direct posterior portal). The authors have found advantages in making the posterolateral portal approximately 1 to 2 cm proximal to the tip of the olecranon when the posterolateral portal is used in conjunction with a direct posterior portal placed 3 cm from the tip. This staggered positioning aids in triangulation, especially in smaller patients. The neurovascular structures at risk include the posterior cutaneous nerves if portals are made improperly and the ulnar nerve if the cannula is directed too far medially.

SUMMARY

The anatomy and approaches described in this chapter provide a foundation for understanding the clinical conditions and surgical techniques of the elbow to be described in subsequent chapters of this book. However, as Leonardo Da Vinci the anatomist taught, there is no limit to the powers of observation, and the reader is encouraged to continue to note the many anatomic variations and subtleties that continue to make the practice of surgery an art form.

References

1. Andrews JR, Carson WG: Arthroscopy of the elbow, *Arthroscopy* 1:97, 1985.
2. Banks SW, Laufman H: *An atlas of surgical exposures of the extremities,* Philadelphia, 1953, WB Saunders.

3. Boyd HB: Surgical exposure of the ulna and proximal third of the radius through one incision, *Surg Gynecol Obstet* 71:86, 1940.
4. Brash JC: *Cunningham's textbook of anatomy,* ed 9, New York, 1951, Oxford University Press.
5. Campbell WC: Incision for exposure of the elbow joint, *Am J Surg* 15:65, 1932.
6. Consentino R: *Atlas of anatomy and surgical approaches in orthopaedic surgery,* Springfield, Ill, 1960, Charles C Thomas.
7. Ellis H: *Clinical anatomy,* London, 1977, Blackwell Scientific Publications.
8. Gray H: *Anatomy, descriptive and surgical,* Philadelphia, 1870, Henry C. Lea.
9. Gray H: *Anatomy of the human body,* ed 29, Philadelphia, 1973, Lea & Febiger.
10. Guhl JF: Arthroscopy and arthroscopic surgery of the elbow, *Orthopaedics* 8:290, 1985.
11. Henry AK: *Extensile exposure,* ed 2, New York, 1973, Churchill Livingstone.
12. Johnson LL: *Diagnostic and surgical arthroscopy,* St Louis, 1981, Mosby.
13. Jordan SE, Jobe FW: *Anatomy and histology of the collateral ligaments of the elbow,* American Shoulder and Elbow Surgeons Seventh Open Meeting, San Francisco, 1993.
14. Kaplan EB: Surgical approaches to the proximal end of the radius and its use in fractures of the head and neck of the radius, *J Bone Joint Surg* 23:86, 1941.
15. Kocher T: *Textbook of operative surgery,* ed 3, London, 1911, A & C Black.
16. Lynch GJ et al: Neurovascular anatomy and elbow arthroscopy: inherent risks, *J Arthros Rel Surg* 2:191, 1986.
17. Martin BF: The annular ligament of the superior radioulnar joint, *J Anat* 52:473, 1958.
18. Molesworth WHL: Operation for complete exposure of the elbow joint, *Br J Surg* 18:303, 1930.
19. Morrey BF: *The elbow and its disorders,* Philadelphia, 1985, WB Saunders.
20. Morrey BF, An KN: Functional anatomy of the ligaments of the elbow, *Clin Orthop* 201:84-90, 1985.
21. Muller ME, Allgower M, Willenegger H: *Manual of internal fixation: technique recommended by the AO-Group,* New York, 1970, Springer-Verlag.
22. O'Driscoll SW, Bell DF, Morrey BF: Posterolateral rotatory instability of the elbow, *J Bone Joint Surg* 73A:440, 1991.
23. O'Driscoll SW, Morrey BF, An KN: Intra-articular pressure and capacity of the elbow, *J Arthros Rel Surg* 6:100, 1990.
24. Osborne GV: The surgical treatment of tardy ulnar neuritis, *J Bone Joint Surg* 39B:782, 1957.
25. Pankovitch AM: Anconeus approach to the elbow joint and the proximal part of the radius and ulna, *J Bone Joint Surg* 59A:124, 1972.
26. Poehling GG et al: Elbow arthroscopy: a new technique, *Arthroscopy* 5:222, 1989.

CHAPTER 17

Ligamentous and Posterior Compartment Injuries

RONALD S. KVITNE
FRANK W. JOBE

The elbow joint is susceptible to a variety of injuries as a result of either acute traumatic events or chronic repetitive overuse.[3,13,43,48] In athletes the incidence of injury seems to directly relate to the duration of exposure and to the intensity of their athletic participation.[1] Although sudden traumatic injuries are common, most symptomatic conditions unique to the elbow result from chronic, excessive, repetitive stress. These injuries may be classified according to their mechanism of injury: type 1—tension overload of the medial structures, type 2—compression injuries of the lateral structures, type 3—extension overload within the posterior compartment, type 4—a combination of these injuries, and type 5—laxity of the ulnar part of the lateral collateral ligament resulting in posterolateral rotatory instability of the elbow.[32,44] To successfully manage the injuries that may be encountered, a thorough understanding of the pertinent regional anatomy, the pathophysiology, and the relationship between elbow motion and stability are essential.

ANATOMY

The medial collateral ligament (ulnar collateral ligament complex) consists of an anterior, posterior, and transverse band (Fig. 17-1). The anterior band is composed of two distict bundles (see Chapter 16). The anterior band, which inserts onto the medial aspect of the coronoid process of the ulna, is functionally the most important constraint in resisting valgus stress of the elbow. Its humeral origin is eccentrically located with respect to the axis of elbow flexion and extension, thus providing

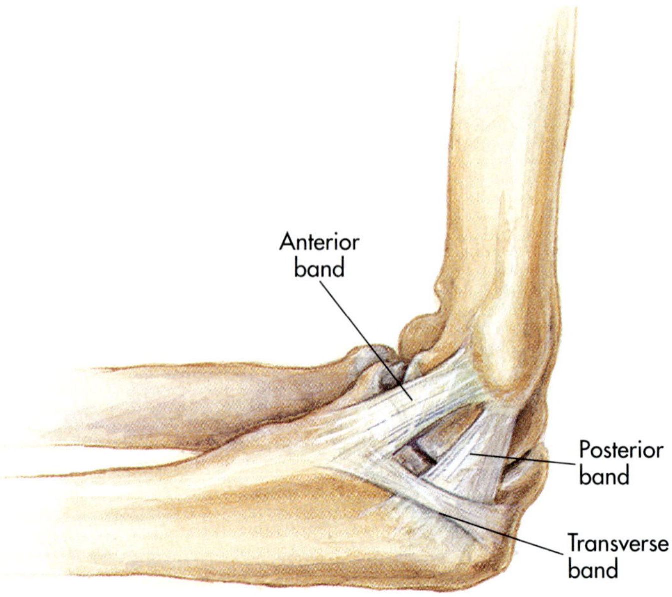

FIGURE 17-1 Medial collateral ligament (medial ulnar collateral ligament complex) consisting of the anterior band, posterior band, and transverse band.

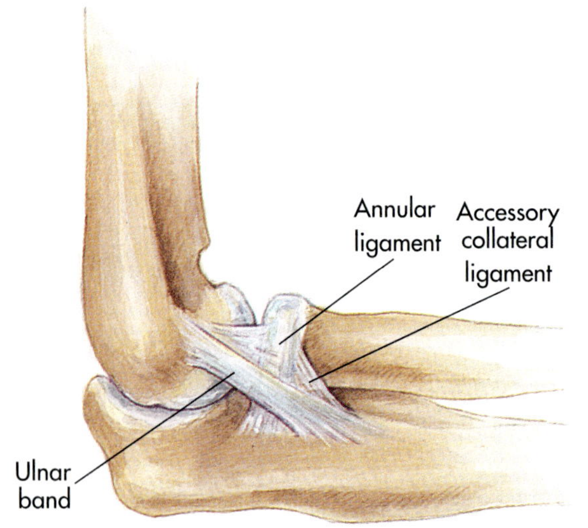

FIGURE 17-2 Lateral collateral ligament complex (lateral ulnar collateral ligament complex) composed of the annular ligament, ulnar band of the lateral collateral ligament, and accessory collateral ligament.

stability throughout a full range of elbow motion.[42] The weaker posterior band is fan-shaped and inserts onto the medial and posterior aspect of the olecranon, providing stability primarily beyond 90° of elbow flexion. The transverse ligament does not cross the ulnar-humeral joint but exists as a thickening of the caudalmost portion of the joint capsule to expand the greater sigmoid notch.

The lateral collateral ligament complex is less consistent and not as well understood as the medial collateral ligament.[33] The annular part of the lateral collateral ligament originates from the lateral epicondyle and blends with the fibers of the annular ligament (Fig. 17-2). The ulnar band of the lateral collateral ligament originates from the anteroinferior portion of the lateral epicondyle, crosses the radial-capitellar joint (superficial to the annular ligament), and inserts onto the tubercle of the supinator crest (crista musculi supinatoris). Additionally, there is a fan-shaped portion that inserts onto the ulna proximal to the supinator crest.

INJURY PATTERNS AND THEIR PATHOPHYSIOLOGY

Many laboratory investigations have shown that elbow stability is maintained by its bony configuration, the joint capsule, the medial and lateral collateral ligaments, and the surrounding musculature. According to Morrey and An, valgus stability is derived equally from the medial collateral ligament, the anterior joint capsule, and the bony articulation of the radiocapitellar joint when the elbow is in full extension.[27] With elbow flexion approaching 90°, the anterior bundle of the medial collateral ligament serves as the primary constraint of the elbow joint in resisting valgus stress. Morrey, Tanaka, and An have shown experimentally that removal of the radial head or release of the posterior portion of the medial collateral ligament in an otherwise intact elbow joint does not lead to increased valgus instability. However, release of the anterior portion of the medial collateral ligament leads to moderate valgus laxity, even when the radial head is present. Finally, gross valgus instability is observed when the radial head has been excised and the entire medial collateral ligament has been removed.[28] Therefore under most clinical circumstances, the medial collateral ligament (anterior bundle) is the primary stabilizer in resisting valgus stress.[42,46] The radial head is a secondary stabilizer that resists valgus and rotatory stress and is significant only when the anterior bundle of the medial collateral ligament is absent.

Stability of the elbow joint in resisting varus stress is provided primarily by the bony architecture, the anterior joint capsule, and the lateral collateral ligament complex. The ulnar band of the lateral collateral ligament is the major stabilizer in resisting both varus stress and posterolateral rotatory stress across the elbow joint. These patterns of instability, although uncommon, are usually the result of an acute traumatic event (hyperextension injury or elbow dislocation) or, rarely, occur after a surgical release for refractory lateral epicondylitis. The development of ligamentous laxity of the lateral collateral ligament complex may allow transient rotatory subluxation of the ulnohumeral joint with a secondary subluxation or dislocation of the radiohumeral joint. With this particular type of instability, however, the annular ligament remains intact, and thus the proximal radioulnar articulation is not disturbed. Symptoms of pain, catching, snapping, or instability may result as the radial head sub-

BOX 17-1
SEQUELAE OF CHRONIC, EXCESSIVE REPETITIVE STRESS

A. Medial tension overload injuries
   1. Musculotendinous involvement
      a. Medial epicondylitis; muscle/tendon rupture
   2. Bony involvement
      a. Avulsion of medial epicondyle
   3. Ligamentous and capsular involvement
      a. Medial ulnar traction spur formation
      b. Hypertrophy, attenuation, or rupture of the medial collateral ligament
      c. Calcium deposition within the medial collateral ligament
B. Lateral compression injuries
   1. Soft-tissue involvement
      a. Synovitis
   2. Bony involvement
      a. Osteochondral fracture of the capitellum
      b. Osteochondritis dissecans
      c. Traumatic osteoarthritis
C. Extension overload injuries
   1. Musculotendinous involvement
      a. Triceps muscle strain
   2. Bony involvement
      a. Avulsion of the tip of the olecranon
      b. Hypertrophic spur formation—olecranon tip, medial olecranon, or olecranon fossa hyperostosis
      c. Stress fracture—olecranon
      d. Osteochondral loose-body formation
D. Posterolateral rotatory instability

Modified from Slocum DB: *Texas Med* 64:48, 1968.

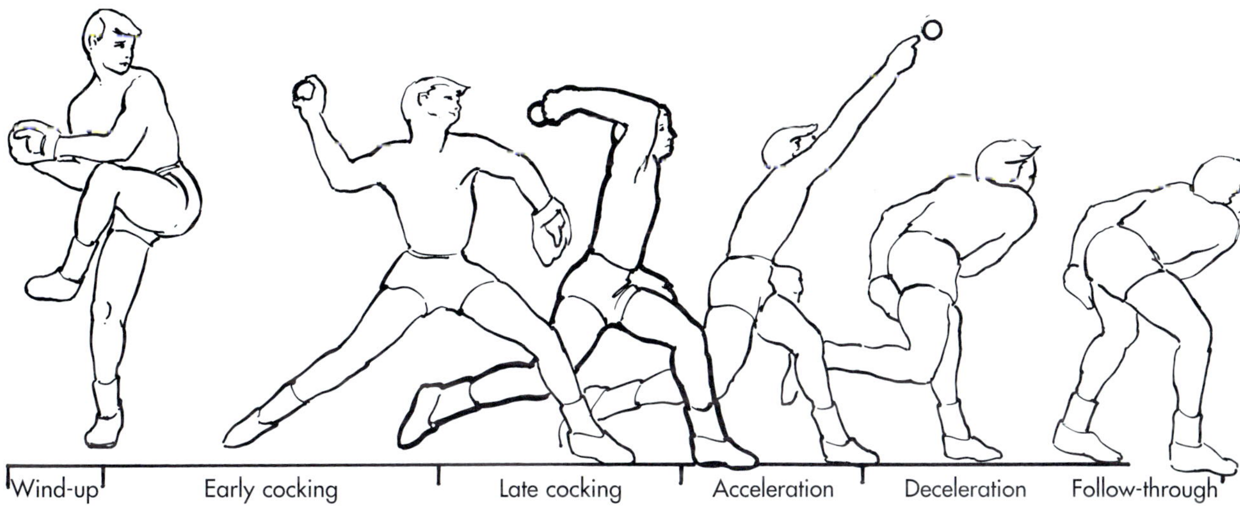

FIGURE 17-3 The throwing motion: wind-up, early cocking, late cocking, acceleration, deceleration, and follow-through.

luxates or dislocates posteriorly with an associated rotatory subluxation of the ulnohumeral joint.

However, the most common symptomatic conditions affecting the elbow joint are the sequelae of chronic, excessive repetitive stress (Box 17-1). Overhead or throwing athletes generate tremendous forces, which are transmitted to the stabilizing mechanisms about the medial aspect of the elbow joint. With minor modifications, similar types of forces are generated in a number of other athletic activities. These include the throwing motion in football and javelin,[26] as well as the overhead motion in racquet sports and swimming activities. A closer look at the pitching motion in baseball provides valuable details about the pathophysiology associated with any overhead throwing motion[2,3,19,20,49] (Fig. 17-3). During the late cocking phase of the throwing motion, the shoulder is abducted approximately 90°, the elbow is flexed approximately 90° to 120°, and the humerus is maximally externally rotated. The acceleration phase is marked by internal humeral rotation and rapid extension of the elbow over 40 to 50 ms (0.05 second), which generate tremendous valgus forces about the medial aspect of the elbow joint.[14,38] These stresses are transmitted primarily to the medial collateral ligament complex, the flexor carpi ulnaris, and, to a lesser extent, the medial flexor-pronator musculature. Initially these forces are well tolerated in athletes exhibiting proper throwing mechanics, conditioning, and warm-up. However, poor throwing mechanics, inflexibility, or fatigue can have a cumulative effect that leads to muscle strain, allowing further stress to be transmitted to the medial collateral ligament. If these forces are applied at a rate that exceeds that of tissue repair, progressive microscopic damage can occur. Initially, this damage appears as edema and inflammation within the medial collateral ligament. Pain, tenderness, and swelling about the medial aspect of the elbow joint may then arise. With continued throwing, additional stress may result in attenuation of the ligament or degeneration of the ligament fibers themselves. Ultimately, calcification or ossification within the ligament may occur. The stress riser effect from this intraligamentous scar tissue may allow further attenuation of the entire capsuloligamentous complex, leading to instability.[19,48,49] On occasion the ligament can become avulsed from its ulnar insertion, or, more commonly, it can rupture in its midsubstance. Rarely it can become detached from the medial epicondylar origin.[11,19,26]

Over time these injuries affecting the medial aspect of the elbow joint (medial tension overload) may render the joint susceptible to further injury. For example, while tremendous tensile forces are being generated about the medial aspect of the elbow joint during overhead or throwing activities, equally strong compressive forces are being created about the lateral (lateral compression injuries) and posterior (extension overload injuries) compartments* (Fig. 17-4). As with medial injuries, those within the radiocapitellar joint laterally may be because of a single traumatic event, although they more often result from chronic overuse. Repetitive, excessive force transmitted to the lateral aspect of the elbow joint may produce synovitis, osteochondral injury (osteochondritis dissecans, osteochondral fracture), or traumatic degenerative arthritis. These lateral compression injuries may occur with or without coexisting tension overload on the medial aspect of the elbow joint.

Finally, during the deceleration and follow-through phases of the throwing motion, all excess kinetic energy is dissipated as the elbow reaches full extension. As seen with medial tension overload and lateral compression injuries, extension injuries within the posterior compartment of the elbow may result from an acute injury or from chronic, repetitive elbow extension. These injuries may include triceps muscle strain, avulsion of the tip of the olecranon process, hypertrophic olecranon spur formation, medial joint laxity with posterior medial impingement, posteromedial osteophyte formation, stress fracture of the olecranon, loose-body formation, and posterior compartment impingement with scar tissue and osteophyte formation encroaching on the olecranon fossa.† Again, these injuries may be seen with or without an associated medial tension overload injury. Although in the overhand athlete, this relationship is quite common.

Any of these conditions can, over time, significantly affect athletic performance, making nonoperative (rehabilitative) or surgical intervention necessary.

*References 2, 3, 6, 7, 12, 37, 44.

†References 2, 3, 6, 12, 17, 22, 26, 31, 50.

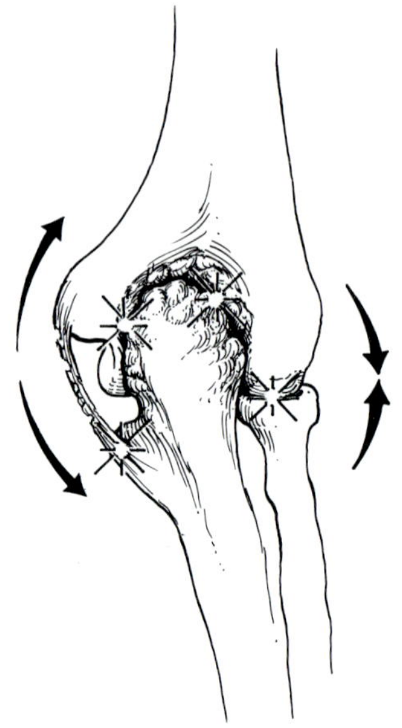

FIGURE 17-4 Overuse stresses around the elbow joint. This shows medial tension (traction) overload, lateral compression, and extension overload within the posterior compartment.

CLINICAL PRESENTATION AND DIAGNOSIS

The diagnosis of elbow instability is based on the athlete's history, physical findings, and radiographic studies. Affected patients often have a history of repetitive overhead or throwing activities. Patients who are developing medial tension overload may experience pain localized about the medial aspect of the elbow, particularly during the late cocking and acceleration phases of the overhead throwing motion. The pain typically has a gradual onset that is exacerbated with overhead activities. Throwing athletes may complain of pain after a period of "heavy throwing," or they may develop the inability to throw beyond 50% to 75% of normal effort on successive attempts. On occasion, an athlete may experience a sudden "pop" or develop sharp pain along the medial aspect of the elbow joint as the medial collateral ligament ruptures or the medial epicondyle fractures acutely.[52] The athlete is unable to continue throwing overhead after such a traumatic event.

Depending on the amount of inflammation within the medial soft tissues, patients may exhibit tenderness over the medial flexor-pronator muscles, over the medial collateral ligament, or along the medial joint line (ulnar-trochlear joint). Patients with medial epicondylitis may exhibit pain within the muscle origin with resisted wrist palmar flexion, with resisted forearm pronation, and with maximum finger flexion such as when making a tight fist. A significant number of patients with chronic elbow instability also experience ulnar nerve symptoms. These symptoms result from extensive inflammation about the medial collateral ligament, medial epicondylar muscle origins, cubital tunnel, and ulnar nerve. Patients may re-

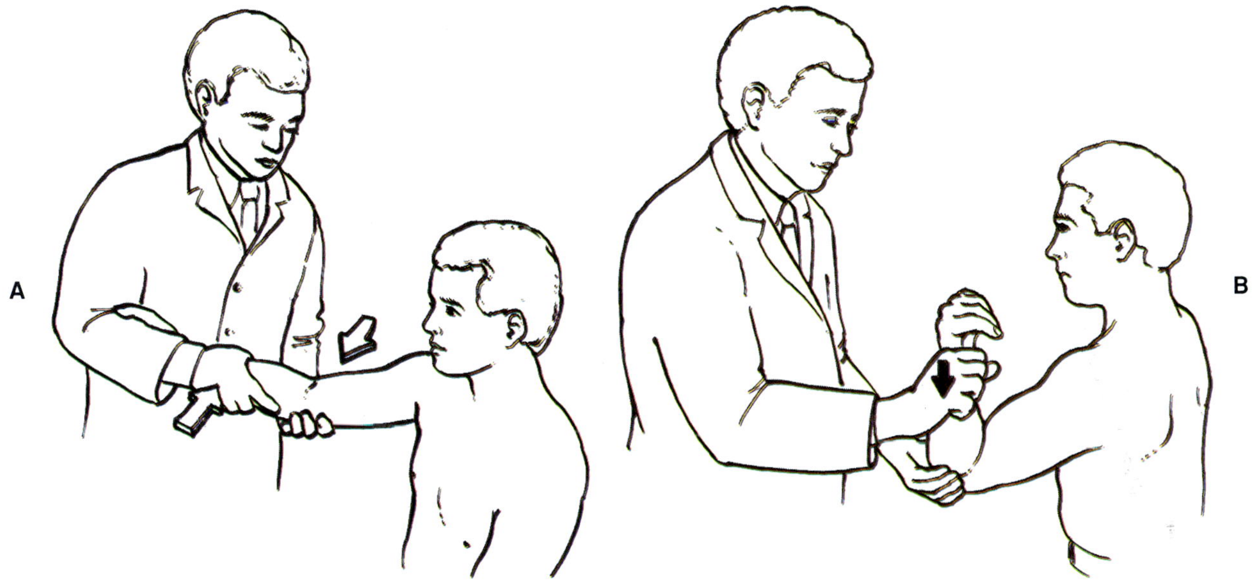

FIGURE 17-5 **A,** Stability testing of the elbow. Valgus stress testing of the elbow joint to test the anterior bundle of the anterior band of the MCL. **B,** To test the posterior bundle of the anterior band, the milking maneuver, O'Brien (personal communication), is especially helpful. This is done with the elbow flexed beyond 90° and placed in valgus stress.

port radiation of pain or paresthesias along the ulnar aspect of the forearm, hand, or ulnar digits. On examination, may also show a positive Tinel's sign.

Elbow instability findings are often subtle, making examination difficult (Fig. 17-5). Testing for valgus instability is best performed with the athlete seated and the patient's hand and wrist held securely between the examiner's elbow and trunk. The examiner firmly grasps the patient's elbow and proximal forearm while simultaneously palpating the ulnar collateral ligament along the medial joint line. Varus and valgus stress can then be applied to determine end-point laxity.[19,30] It is important to flex the elbow beyond 25° to unlock the olecranon from its fossa. Compare the athlete's contralateral elbow to differentiate physiologic laxity from pathologic instability.

In addition to the signs and symptoms of medial tension overload, patients also suffering from lateral compression injuries may exhibit swelling, tenderness, or palpable crepitus laterally around the radiocapitellar joint.[25]

Whether associated with the repetitive stresses of the acceleration phase or with the follow-through phase of the throwing motion, patients with extension overload injuries may exhibit tenderness around the posterior compartment or distal triceps/extensor mechanism. Decreased elbow range of motion (loss of extension) and pain with valgus stress testing and/or pain at the extreme ranges of elbow extension may also be present.[2,3,6,7]

Varus instability and recurrent posterolateral rotatory instability of the elbow joint have previously been unrecognized clinical conditions.[16,36,47] Recent descriptions of these instability patterns by Morrey et al have aided in diagnosis and treatment.[29,32,35] Posterolateral rotatory instability may result from an acute injury to or developmental laxity of the ulnar part of the lateral collateral ligament (radial collateral ligament). This may then allow transient rotatory subluxation of the ulnohumeral joint and a secondary subluxation or dislocation of the radiohumeral joint. However, because the annular ligament remains intact, the radioulnar joint is undisturbed.

Patients with recurrent posterolateral rotatory instability of the elbow may complain of pain, tenderness, catching, snapping, or gross instability of the elbow joint. Although this instability pattern may be seen without any history of significant trauma, this condition usually follows a significant injury to the elbow joint such as elbow dislocation, hyperextension injury, or an acute varus stress applied to the elbow joint in a position of elbow extension and forearm pronation. This entity has also been reported in patients who underwent common extensor release for refractory lateral epicondylitis. During the physical examination, these patients may exhibit tenderness over the lateral aspect of the elbow joint, decreased elbow range of motion (elbow flexion contracture), and, occasionally, signs of ulnar nerve irritability.

Patients with varus instability may show gross laxity to varus stress testing. However, most patients have merely a "sense" of instability with varus stress testing. O'Driscoll et al noted that patients with posterolateral rotatory instability of the elbow joint may be identified with the lateral pivot-shift test.[32] This test involves flexion of the elbow from an extended position and supination of the forearm while a valgus stress and axial load are applied (Fig. 17-6). This maneuver subluxates or dislocates the radial head posteriorly with rotatory subluxation of the ulnohumeral joint. When the lateral pivot-shift test is positive, there is a palpable and visible re-

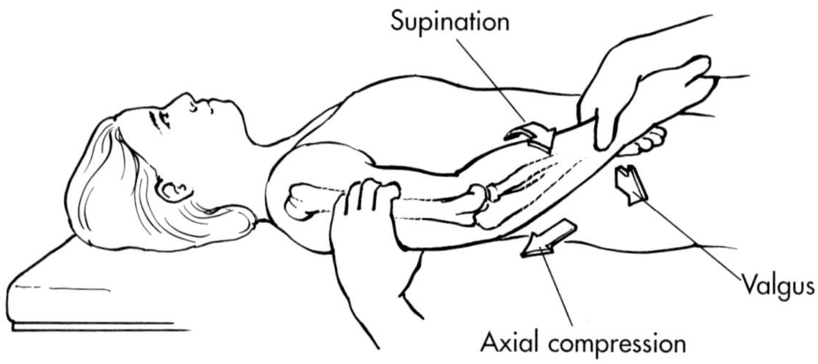

FIGURE 17-6 Stability testing for posterolateral rotatory instability of the elbow. With the patient lying supine, the elbow flexed 20° to 30° and the forearm supinated, a valgus moment and axial stress across the elbow cause a visual posterolateral subluxation. As the elbow is brought into further flexion, the posterolateral subluxation is reduced.

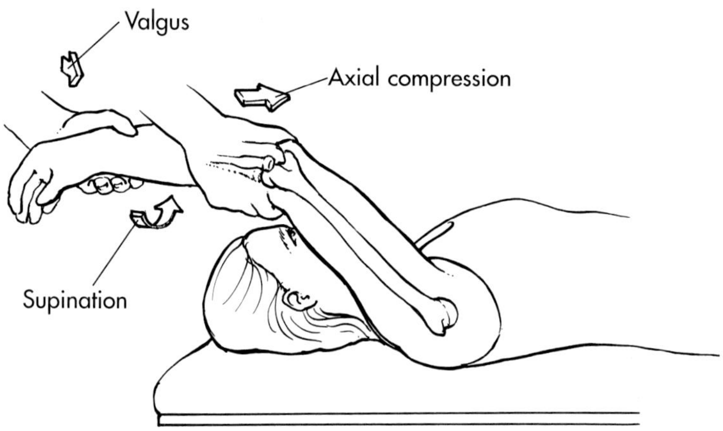

FIGURE 17-7 Stability testing for posterolateral rotatory instability with the arm in the overhead position. With the elbow flexed 20° to 30° and the forearm supinated, axial compression and valgus stress produce a posterolateral subluxation that can be reduced as the elbow is flexed beyond 30°.

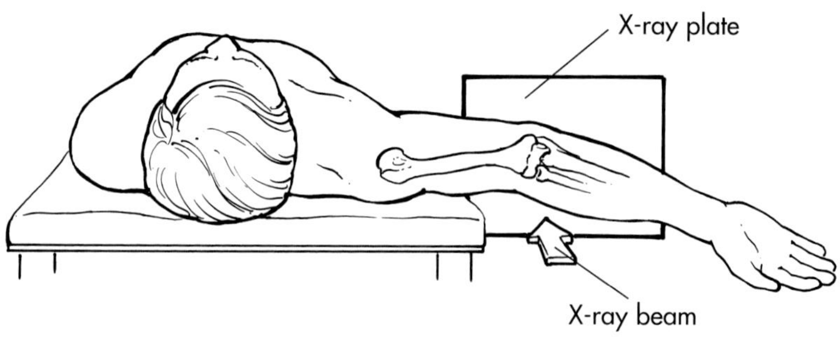

FIGURE 17-8 Stress evaluation of medial collateral ligament. The elbow is flexed 25° to unlock ulnohumeral joint.

duction of the radiohumeral joint together with the ulnohumeral joint when the elbow is flexed beyond approximately 40°. This provocative maneuver may be performed with the patient awake and lying supine with the arm held at the side. However, best results are obtained when the patient is examined lying supine while under general anesthesia and with the involved extremity placed in an overhead position (Fig. 17-7).

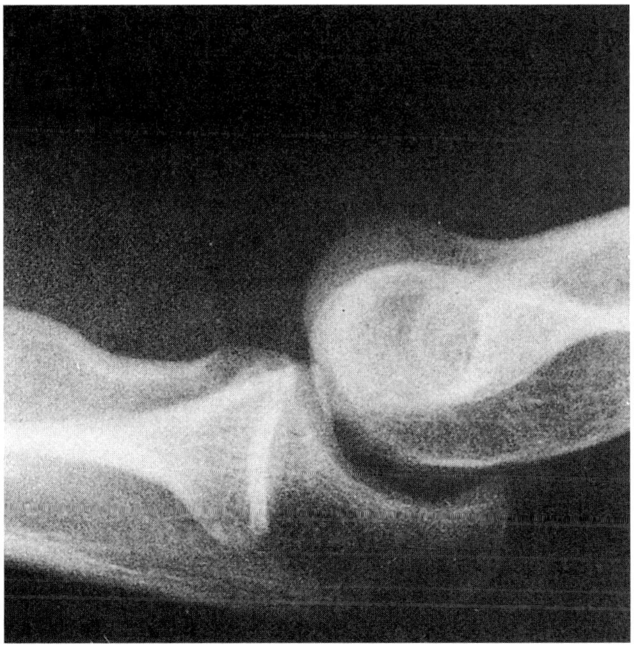

FIGURE 17-9 Lateral radiograph demonstrating posterolateral rotatory instability.

Special Assessments

Radiographs taken during stability testing and compared with those of the contralateral elbow can often document excessive laxity of the elbow, even when the clinical findings are equivocal. In patients with medial collateral ligament instability, valgus stress testing can be used to assess and objectively document the degree of elbow instability (Fig. 17-8). Patients with lateral collateral ligament instability may also be diagnosed radiographically with use of fluoroscopy or plain radiographs.[8,42] Posterolateral rotatory instability is characterized by posterolateral dislocation of the radial head in conjunction with widening of the ulnohumeral articulation as the ulna rotates away from the trochlea (Fig. 17-9). Plain radiographs, bone scans, computed tomography (CT), and magnetic resonance imaging (MRI) may also be used in evaluating patients with medial tension overload injuries, lateral compression injuries, and extension overload injuries (Figs. 17-10 to 17-12). In addition, MRI has become particularly useful in assessing the elbow for ligamentous abnormalities in both acute and chronic conditions (Fig. 17-13). The authors recently completed an investigation of the efficacy of MRI as a diagnostic tool for medial collateral ligament injuries. The MR images of MCL-deficient elbows and MR images of asymptomatic, normal elbows of professional baseball players were compared and correlated with operative findings. The results demonstrated that, although

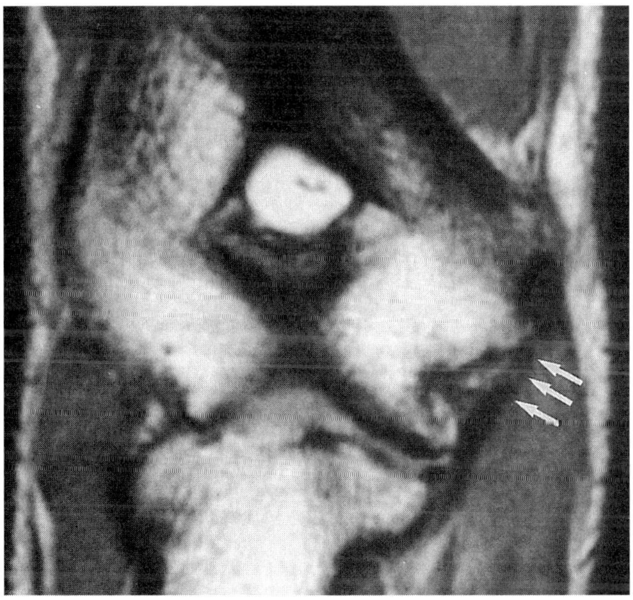

FIGURE 17-10 Medial tension overload injury. MRI of an elbow with chronic disruption *(arrows)* of ulnar collateral ligament, coronal image.

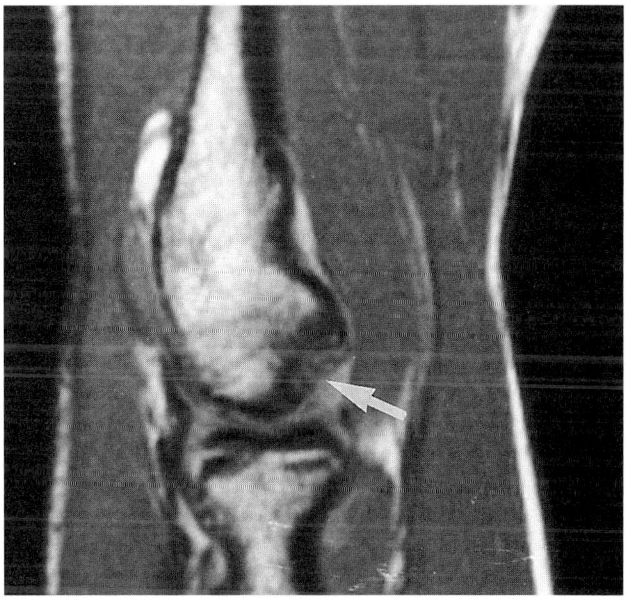

FIGURE 17-11 Lateral compression injury. MRI of an elbow with osteochondral lesion of capitellum *(arrow)*, sagittal image.

MRI does not replace a carefully obtained history, physical examination, or stress radiographs, MRI proved to be a valuable adjunctive diagnostic tool that clearly delineates ligament ossification, avulsion, or midsubstance tears.

NONSURGICAL TREATMENT

When the diagnosis has been established, a specific treatment program can be initiated. Since most elbow injuries in overhead athletes result from chronic, repetitive microtrauma, an aggressive but conservative treatment pro-

A 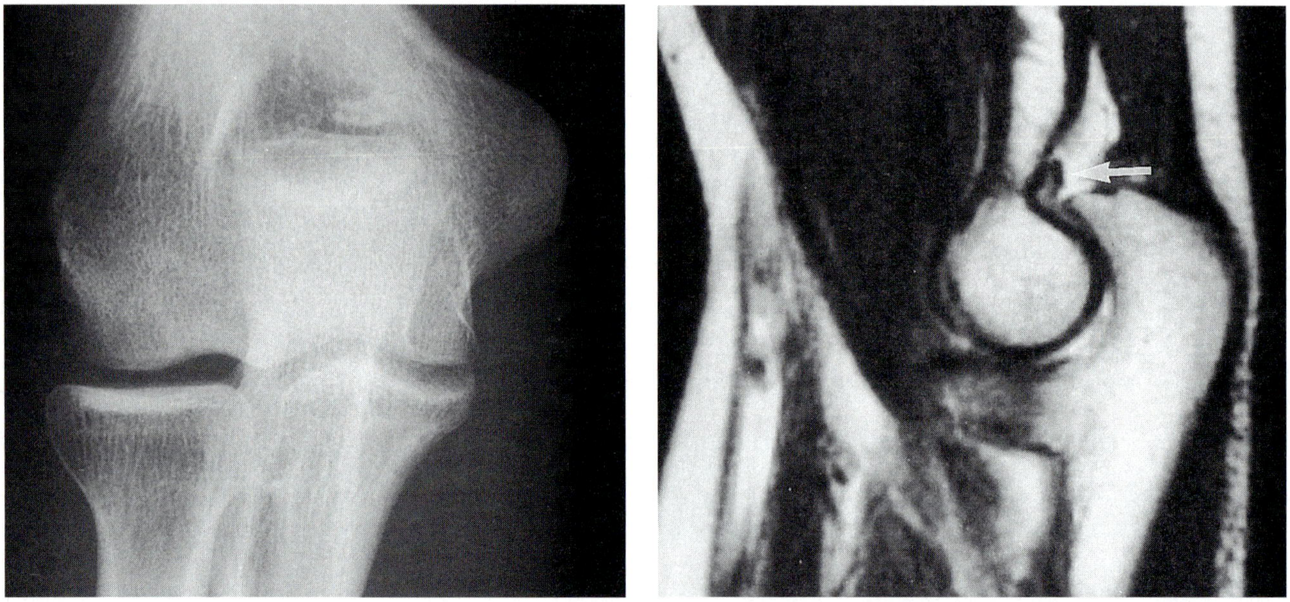 B

FIGURE 17-12 **A,** Extension overload injury. Plain x-ray image, anteroposterior view with osteophytic enlargement of the olecranon process and loose-body formation within the posterior compartment. **B,** MRI of the same patient, sagittal image revealing loose body within olecranon fossa *(arrow).*

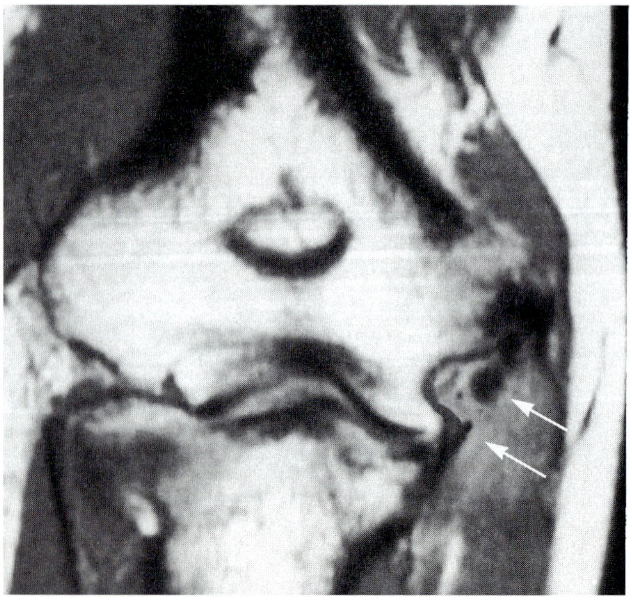

FIGURE 17-13 MRI of an acute avulsion *(arrows)* of the medial collateral ligament, coronal image, T1 signal.

gram is recommended. An initial period of relative rest (avoiding the offending activity) in conjunction with cryotherapy, contrast baths, and other physical therapy modalities applied to the affected area may reduce inflammation and pain in symptomatic patients. The use of nonsteroidal oral antiinflammatory medications is also beneficial. However, corticosteroid injections are generally not recommended in treating ligamentous injuries about the elbow. After swelling and pain have subsided, a supervised flexibility and strengthening program for all of the muscles around the elbow is essential in restoring the muscle tone and endurance needed to provide dynamic support to the elbow joint. Strengthening exercises can be performed isometrically, isotonically, or isokinetically.

Patients showing little or no improvement after 3 to 6 months of treatment, surgical intervention should be considered. Muscle ruptures/avulsions need immediate surgery.

OPERATIVE TREATMENT, POSTOPERATIVE CARE, AND REHABILITATION

Medial Tension Overload Injuries

Medial Ulnar Collateral Ligament Ruptures with Valgus Instability

Definitive surgical treatment is necessary for athletes with an acute complete disruption of the ulnar collateral ligament or patients with chronic pain and instability who show little or no improvement with conservative management.[8,11,19,21] In the presence of acute or chronic symptomatic laxity, the goal of surgery is to reestablish stability of the elbow to resist valgus stress. In the rare instances of an acute avulsion of the ulnar collateral ligament from its proximal humeral attachment, primary repair may be achieved. However, as is frequently the case, the attenuation, scarring, or disruption of the medial collateral ligament is such that primary repair is unreasonable and reconstruction with an autogenous graft becomes necessary. Viable graft sources include the ipsilateral or contralateral palmaris longus tendon, the plantaris tendon, a 3- to 5-mm medial strip of Achilles tendon, or an extensor tendon from one of the lesser toes.

Surgical Technique

In an effort to avoid intraoperative or postoperative complications associated with anterior transposition of the ulnar nerve the previously published operative technique has recently been modified.[21] These changes involve reconstruction of the medial collateral ligament without transposition of the ulnar nerve. In doing so, the risk of nerve injury secondary to segmental devascularization, intraoperative traction or compression, and scarring within the submuscular portion is avoided.

Under tourniquet control an incision is made over the medial epicondyle extending both proximally and distally 3 to 5 cm. Extreme care is taken to protect the ulnar nerve and the branches of the medial antebrachial cutaneous nerve throughout the procedure. The flexor-pronator muscle origin on the medial epicondyle is preserved as the muscle is split horizontally (Fig. 17-14), and the muscle fibers are retracted anteriorly and posteriorly, exposing the medial collateral ligament. Close inspection of the ulnar collateral ligament (especially the anterior bundle) may reveal soft-tissue calcification and degeneration, attenuation, or complete disruption of the liga-

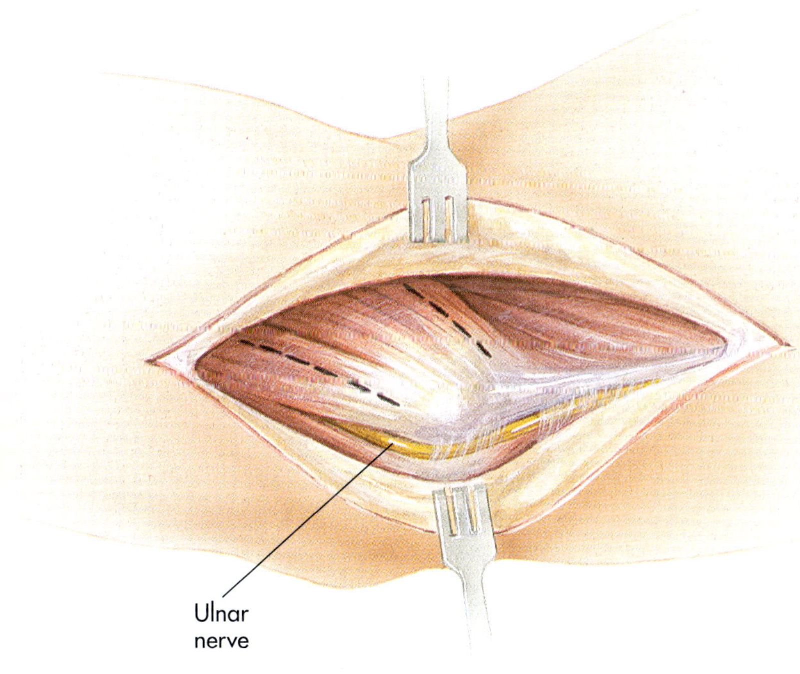

FIGURE 17-14 Flexor-pronator muscle origin on medial epicondyle. The dotted line indicates the incision through the flexor-pronator muscle origin.

ment. A longitudinal incision made through the ligament itself allows inspection of the underlying joint. Synovitis, osteochondral loose bodies, osteophytes, or degenerative changes may be identified and treated at this time. Posterior compartment impingement, if present clinically and verified radiographically, may also be addressed at this time with careful dissection (posterior to the ulnar nerve) into the posterior compartment, allowing inspection and débridement of the olecranon process and olecranon fossa.

Next, bone tunnels, through which the graft is placed, are created within the medial epicondyle and proximal ulna with a 3.2-mm drill. The convergent drill holes placed in the proximal ulna are oriented vertically and placed at the level of the coronoid tubercle (Fig. 17-15). The drill holes within the medial epicondyle are placed at the level of the anatomic origin of the anterior bundle, midway between the base and the tip of the medial epicondylar prominence. The holes are drilled in such a way as to create a single entrance hole anteriorly, which then diverges anterosuperiorly and posterosuperiorly to avoid penetration of the posterior cortex and possible injury to the ulnar nerve within the cubital tunnel. Tunnels drilled in this manner allow the graft to be placed so it remains isometric throughout a full range of elbow motion.

The flexor-pronator muscle is then split just proximal to the medial epicondyle in a longitudinal fashion to facilitate placement of the anterosuperior and posterosuperior drill holes at their correct positions, as well as passage of the graft in a figure-of-eight fashion using the flexible suture passer.

At this point, attention turns toward harvesting a suitable autogenous tendon for graft. The palmaris longus tendon can be obtained from either upper extremity without sacrificing strength, power, or endurance; therefore it is usually harvested from the ipsilateral extremity. (It is essential to document the presence of this tendon before surgery). The palmaris longus tendon is harvested by creating a 2-cm transverse skin incision within the distal flexor crease of the wrist. The median nerve and its palmar cutaneous branch are protected as the tendon is isolated at its insertion into the palmar fascia. Additional transverse skin incisions are made 7.5 to 15 cm proximal to the wrist, exposing the entire length of the palmaris longus proximally (Fig. 17-16). With tension applied distally, the muscle is divided at its musculotendinous junction and brought out through the distal skin incision, where it is detached from its insertion. Approximately 15 to 17 cm of tendon length is necessary for reconstruction of the medial collateral ligament. These incisions are then irrigated and routinely closed.

A single #1 nonabsorbable, braided suture is then placed through the ends of this free-tendon graft, and a flexible suture passer is used to thread the tendon through the bone tunnels within the proximal ulna and medial epicondyle, creating a figure-of-eight configuration (Figs. 17-17 to 17-19). With the elbow then held in

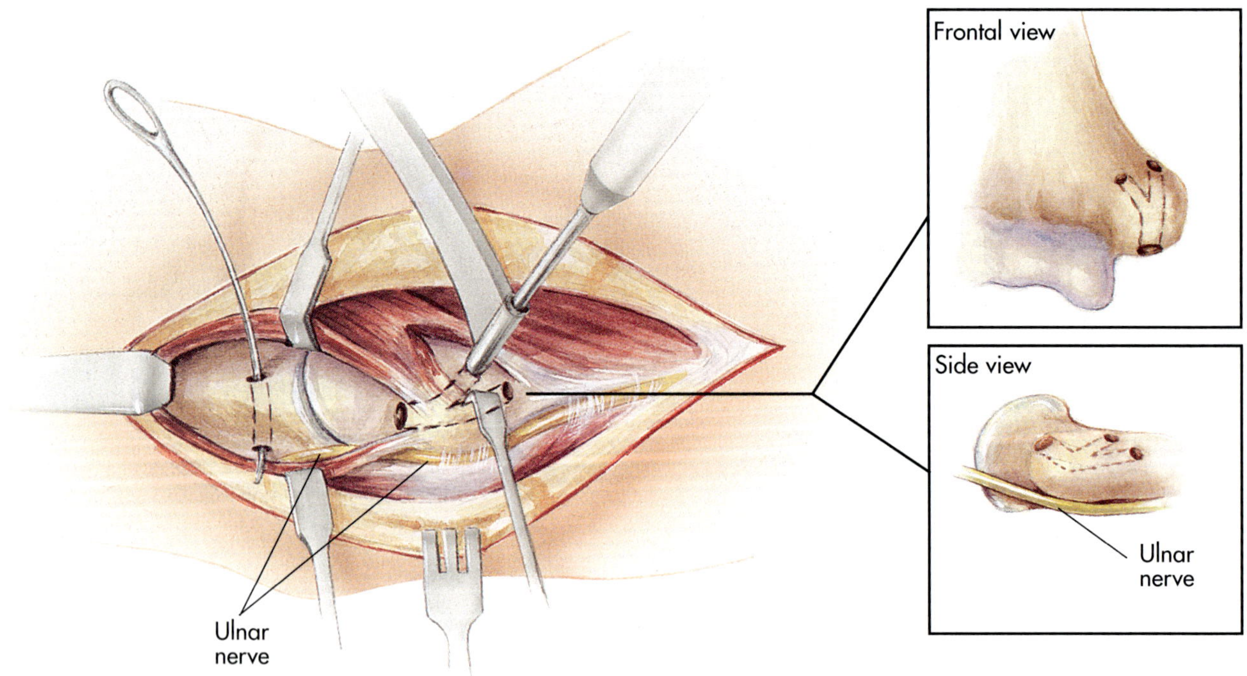

FIGURE 17-15 Bone tunnels placed within proximal ulna and medial epicondyle. *(Inset),* Divergent tunnels created within medial epicondyle to avoid penetration of posterior cortex and injury to ulnar nerve within cubital tunnel (frontal and side views). Be careful to place the tunnel closer to the tip of the medial epicodyle rather than at the base.

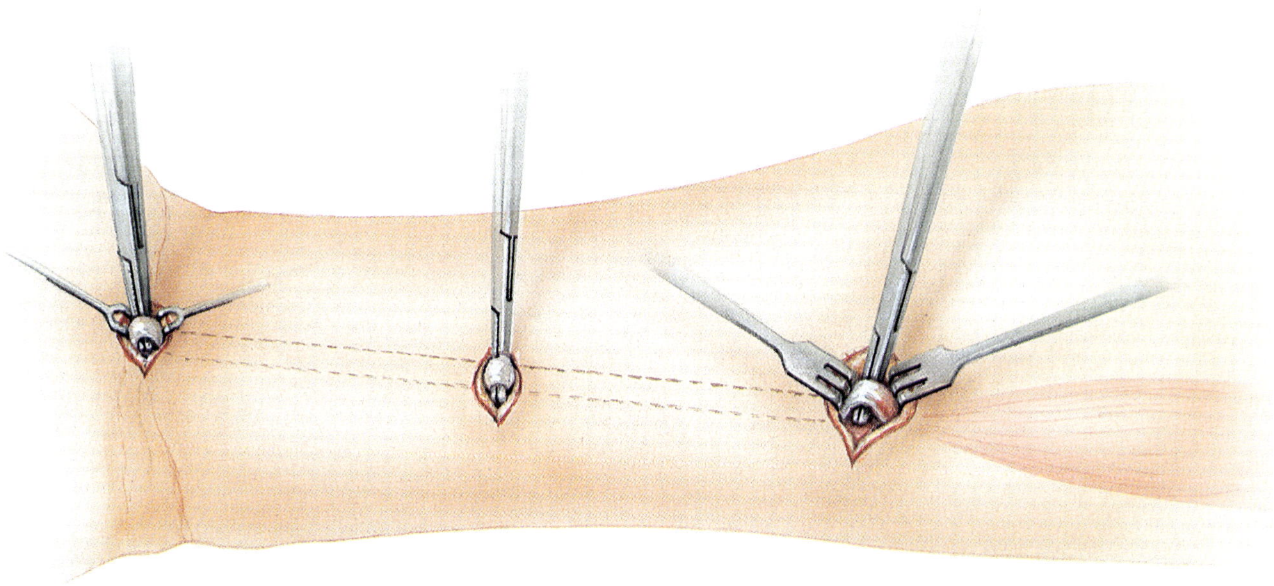

FIGURE 17-16 Exposure/harvesting of palmaris longus tendon.

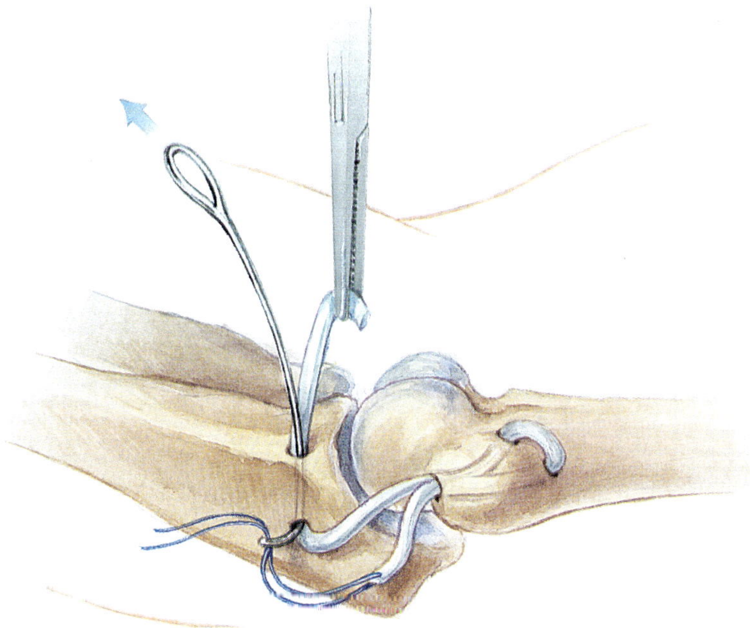

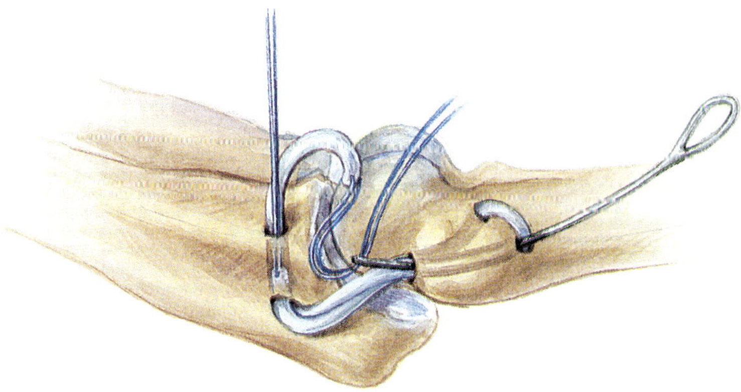

FIGURES 17-17 and **17-18** Passage of autogenous tendon graft through drill holes in figure-of-eight fashion.

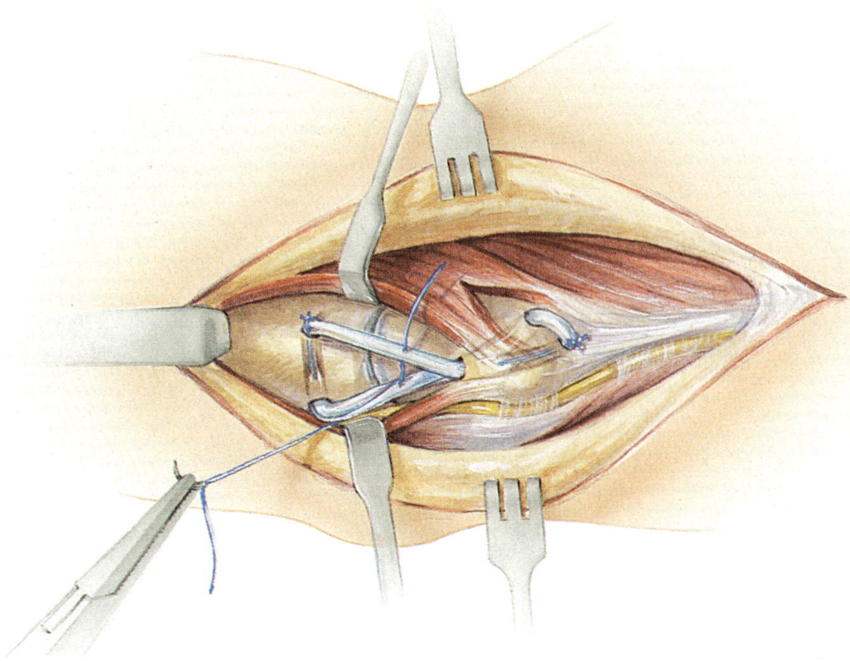

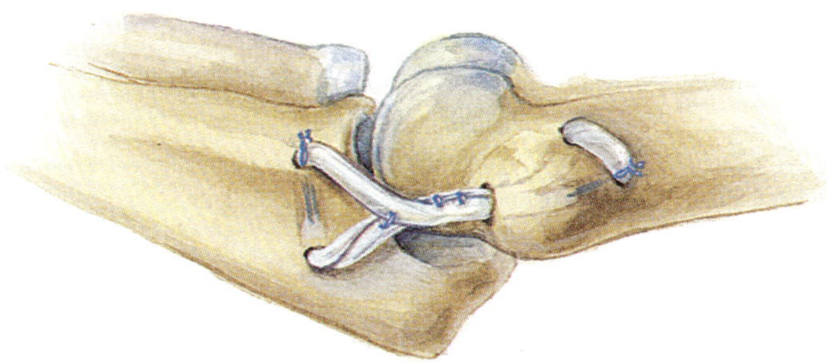

FIGURES 17-19 and **17-20** Suture fixation of autogenous tendon graft.

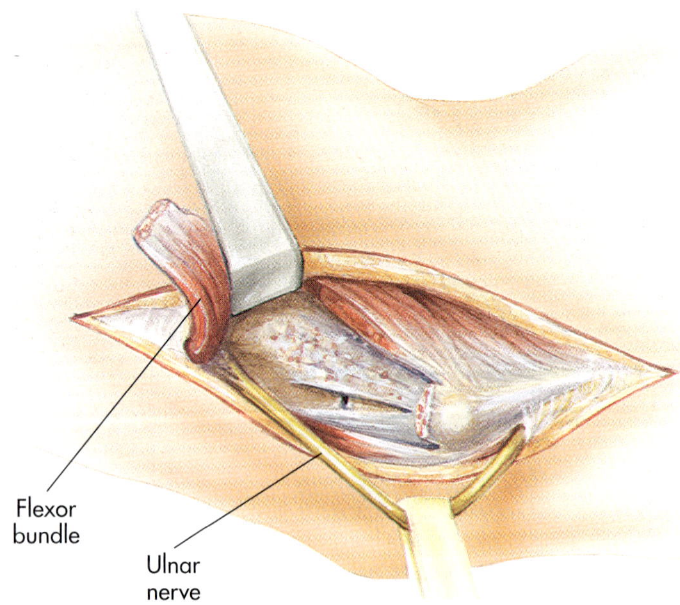

FIGURE 17-21 Flexor-pronator bundle retracted distally, exposing underlying medial collateral ligament.

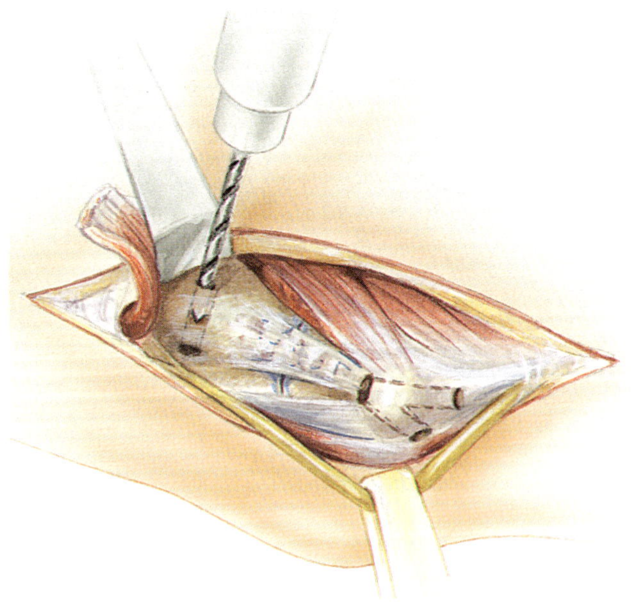

FIGURE 17-22 Bone tunnels within proximal ulna and medial epidcondyle with ulnar nerve dissected and gently retracted.

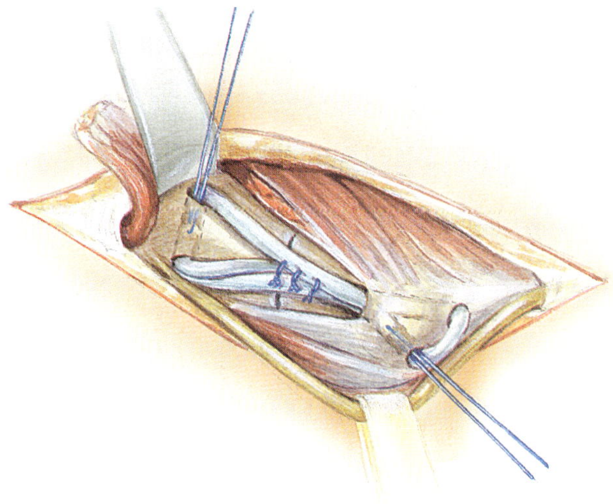

FIGURE 17-23 Figure-of-eight configuration of autogenous tendon graft with suture fixation.

neutral varus-valgus position and 45° of elbow flexion, the graft is pulled taut and sutured to itself with additional #1 nonabsorbable sutures (Fig. 17-20). Additional sutures are used to reattach any remnants of the original medial collateral ligament to the autogenous graft, thereby providing additional soft-tissue support. The elbow is then brought through a full passive range of motion to verify the isometry and stability of the ligament reconstruction.

The tourniquet is then released, hemostasis is achieved with electrocautery, and the wound is closed over a surgical drain. A long arm posterior plaster splint is used to immobilize the elbow in 90° of elbow flexion and neutral forearm rotation, leaving the hand and wrist free.

Medial Ulnar Collateral Ligament Injuries with Valgus Instability and Chronic Ulnar Neuritis

Patients with medial elbow instability (medial tension overload), who also have chronic ulnar nerve symptoms, benefit from anterior transposition of the ulnar nerve in conjunction with medial collateral ligament reconstruction. This is performed with a slight modification of the preceding technique. The ulnar collateral ligament is exposed by incising the common flexor-pronator bundle at its origin on the medial epicondyle. The flexor-pronator bundle is elevated and reflected distally from the medial epicondyle, leaving behind a fringe of the bundle's tendinous origin to facilitate its later reattachment (Fig. 17-21).

Next, the ulnar nerve is dissected and mobilized proximally to the level of the arcade of Struthers. A small, 2- to 3-cm portion of the medial intermuscular septum is also removed proximally to prevent tethering of the ulnar nerve as it is transposed anteriorly. Distal mobilization of the ulnar nerve involves carefully splitting of the intermuscular septum between the ulnar and humeral heads of the flexor carpi ulnaris 2.5 cm distal to the medial epicondyle. After mobilization, the ulnar nerve can be retracted out of harm's way with a 6.4-mm Penrose drain.

Converging drill holes within the proximal ulna are then created, as previously described, at the level of the coronoid tubercle. The tunnels within the medial epicondyle are again drilled in a diverging manner with a single entrance hole anteriorly and two exit holes posteriorly (Fig. 17-22).

The graft is then passed in a figure-of-eight fashion through the drill holes with a flexible suture passer. When the graft is in position, tension along the proximal and distal graft margins takes up any excess slack of the graft across the medial joint line, and this graft is sutured into position as previously described (Fig. 17-23).

Anterior transposition of the ulnar nerve is then carried out by positioning the nerve anterior to the medial epicondyle and submuscularly beneath the flexor-pronator bundle. A portion of the intermuscular septum and muscle fibers of the flexor-pronator group is also resected to prevent tethering or impingement on the nerve as the muscle is reattached to the medial epicondyle (Fig. 17-24). Wound closure, postoperative immobilization, and rehabilitation then are performed in a similar fashion to patients without ulnar nerve transposition.

Postoperative rehabilitation begins immediately in the postoperative period with the patient gently squeezing a soft sponge or rubber ball on the same day of surgery. The splint is removed 7 to 10 days after surgery, and active elbow and shoulder range-of-motion exercises are begun. Within 4 weeks of surgery, isometric, isotonic, and progressive resistive strengthening exercises may be initiated, thereby concentrating on elbow flexion and extension, as well as with forearm pronation and supination. In addition, rotator cuff muscle stretching and strengthening exercises must also be maintained to avoid developing a stiff shoulder. At 4 months after surgery, elbow range of motion and strength have usually returned to normal, and incorporation of the graft is sufficient to allow the athlete to begin a progressive throwing program. After 7 months, throwers can begin increasing the distance and velocity to approximately 50% of full speed; and pitchers can begin throwing from the mound at approximately 75% of normal speed. As strength, power, and endurance of the elbow and shoulder muscles improve over the next few months, usually within 12 to 18 months after surgery, performance becomes maxi-

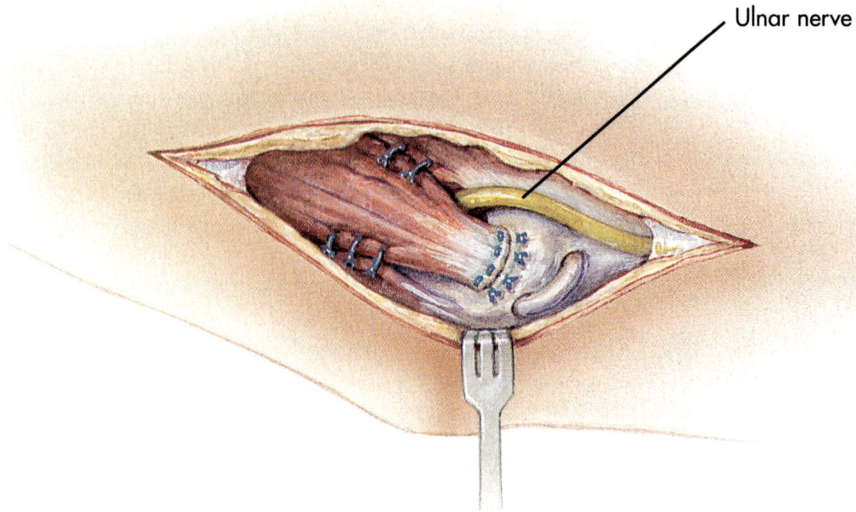

FIGURE 17-24 Submuscular transposition of ulnar nerve beneath flexor-pronator bundle.

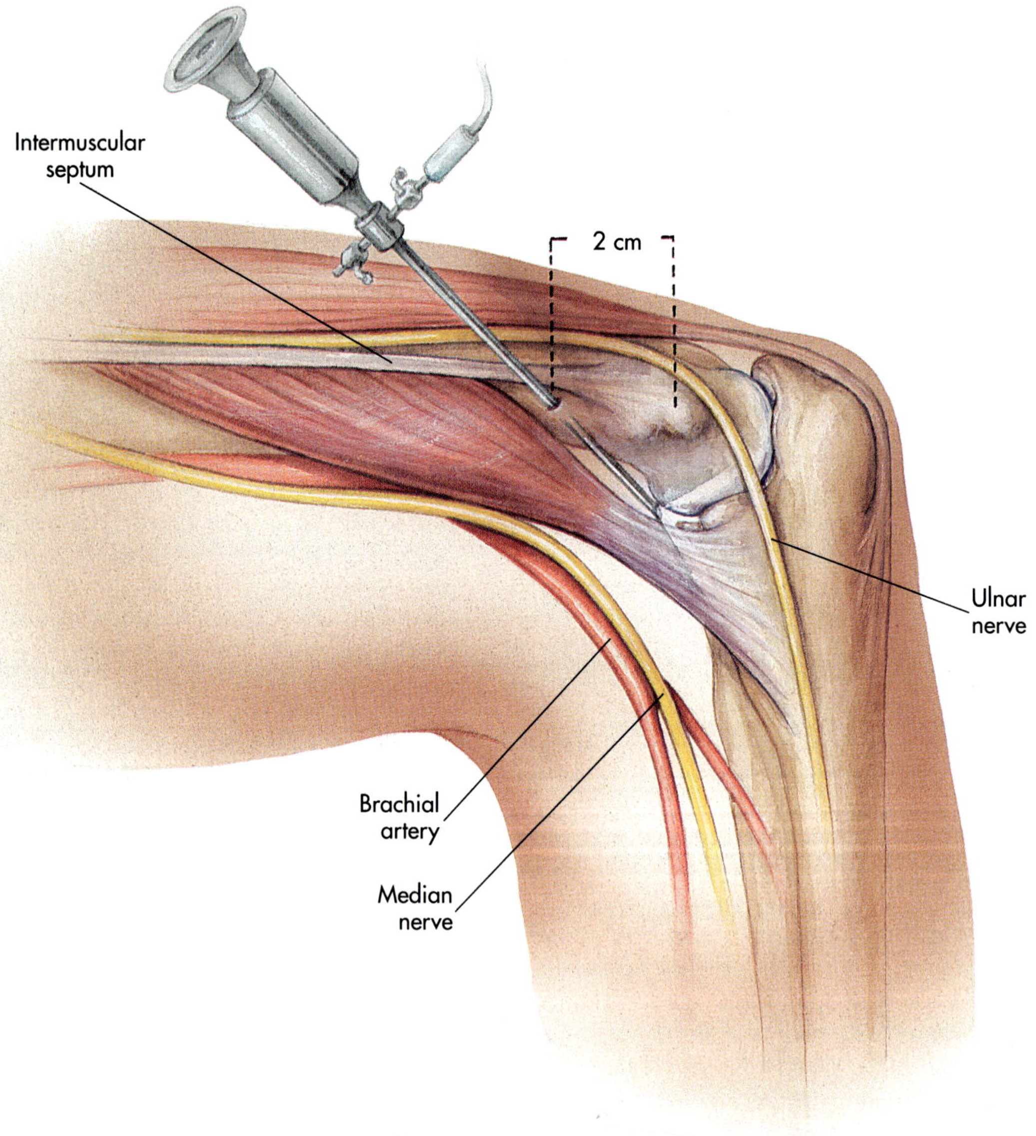

FIGURE 17-25 Proximal medial arthroscopic portal (prone patient positioning) with placement of portal 2 cm proximal to medial epicondyle, just anterior to the medial intermuscular septum.

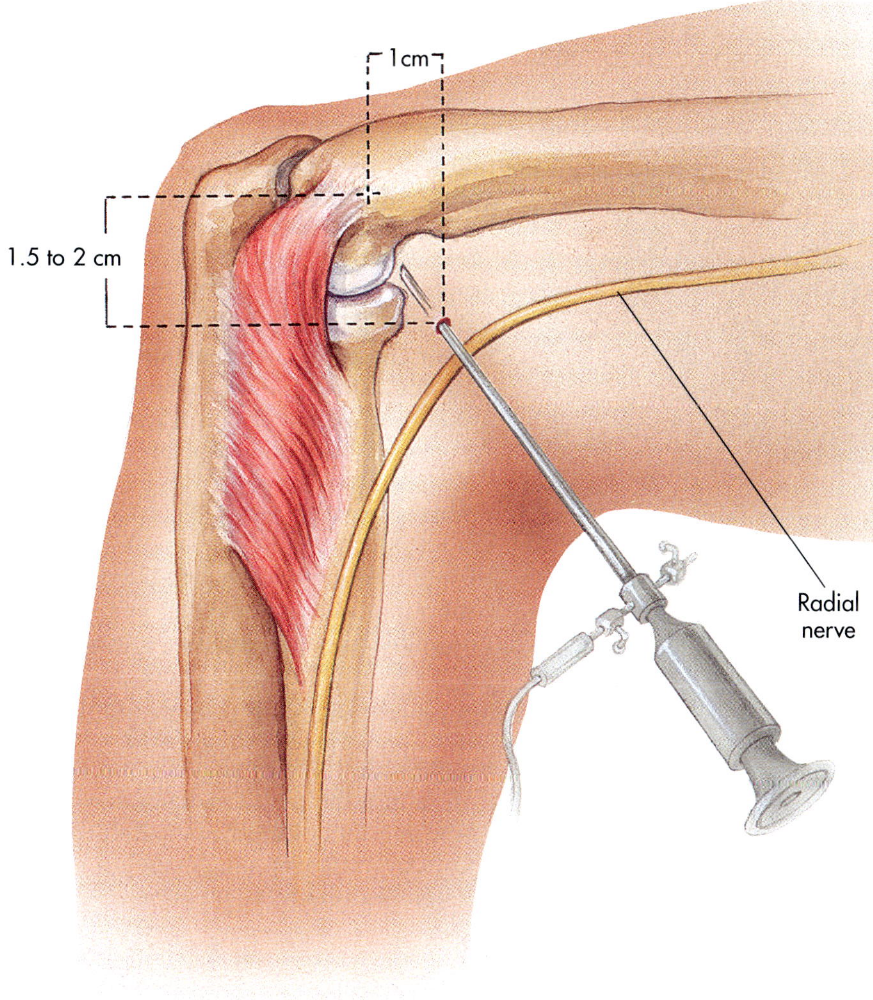

FIGURE 17-26 Anterolateral arthroscopic portal (prone patient positioning) with placement of portal 2 cm distal and 1 cm anterior to the lateral epicondyle.

mized as the athlete returns to the preinjury competitive level of throwing.

Lateral Compression Injuries

Definitive surgical treatment of lateral compression injuries (i.e., osteochondritis dissecans, loose bodies, or osteochondral defects within the elbow joint) can be performed through conventional open or arthroscopic techniques.[18,25,39,41] However, advances in arthroscopic surgical technique have allowed improved visualization, decreased morbidity, and a reduced risk of complications in the assessment and treatment of these lesions.[4,10,15,34,45] Use of proper arthroscopic portals, maintenance of maximum elbow distension, and careful attention to detail help minimize the risk of major neurovascular complications.[51] Although patient positioning during arthroscopy of the elbow joint is subject to surgeon preference,[40] the basic principles remain the same—bony landmarks are outlined before beginning the surgical procedure; the elbow joint is distended maximally to displace the neurovascular structures away from the intended arthroscopic portal sites; and the elbow is maintained in a relaxed position (90° of elbow flexion) to relax the neurovascular structures, further reducing the risk of neurovascular compromise.[24] Standard arthroscopic portals are created, beginning with the proximal medial portal[5] (Fig. 17-25) and using the Wissinger rod to create an accessory anterolateral portal[23] (Fig. 17-26). Additional midlateral and posterior arthroscopic portals can be created as necessary to allow complete visualization of the entire elbow joint and surgical treatment of the pathology encountered (Fig. 17-27). Postoperatively, the joint is thoroughly irrigated and drained to remove all debris. Each portal is closed with sutures, and a well-padded gentle compression dressing is applied. The injection of local anesthetics into the elbow joint or around the arthroscopic portals is discouraged because these anesthetics may create a temporary nerve block that interfers with the immediate postoperative neurovascular assessment.

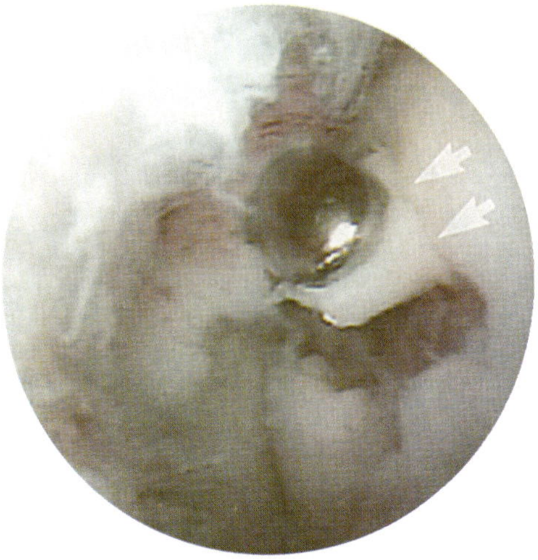

FIGURE 17-27 Arthroscopic débridement of osteochondral defect *(arrows)* in capitellum (lateral compression injury).

Active elbow range-of-motion exercises are initiated as soon as pain and swelling subside. The strengthening exercises are then begun and progressed as tolerated until full elbow and shoulder motion, strength, and endurance have been regained.[9]

Posterior Extension Overload Injuries

Recent advancements in arthroscopic surgical techniques continue to expand the list of conditions that are amenable to arthroscopic elbow surgery. Injuries associated with valgus extension overload or chronic extension overload within the posterior compartment of the elbow include olecranon spur formation, posteromedial osteophyte formation, loose body formation, posterior compartment impingement, and scar tissue or osteophyte formation encroaching on the olecranon fossa.[4,10,15,34,39]

After the induction of general anesthesia, the patient is positioned in either the lateral decubitus position or the prone position. Either of these positions allows access to both the anterior and posterior compartments of the elbow joint. More important, however, they eliminate the awkwardness associated with the supine position and overhead suspension, where the arm tends to "swing like a pendulum."[5,40] In addition, these positions facilitate surgery within the posterior compartment of the elbow joint as they eliminate operating "uphill," and further patient positioning or draping is unnecessary should an arthrotomy be required.

After the successful induction of general anesthesia and proper positioning of the patient's involved extremity, the bony landmarks and surface anatomy are outlined with a marking pen at the start of the procedure. This reduces the risk of neurovascular compromise during the procedure when large amounts of fluid may extravasate from the elbow joint into the soft tissues, obscuring these bony landmarks. Using these bony landmarks for reference, standard anterior arthroscopic portals are created, which allow access to both the anterior and posterior compartments. Arthroscopic treatment for posterior compartment impingement, osteophyte formation within the olecranon fossa, hypertrophic spur formation about the olecranon tip, or loose bodies within the posterior compartment can be provided arthroscopically using standard posterior arthroscopic portals for arthroscopic visualization and instrumentation. After débridement of the olecranon fossa, the posterior compartment is evaluated for signs of hypertrophic spur formation and impingement. A 5.5-mm burr is used to resect humeral osteophytes encroaching on the olecranon fossa (Fig. 17-28). Using an osteotome and mallet, hypertrophic olecranon spurs may likewise be resected, eliminating the bony impingement posteromedially[2,3,50] (Fig. 17-29). Final irrigation and drainage of the entire elbow joint ensure the removal of all debris and loose bodies. Routine wound closure is then performed with the application of a well-padded, gentle, sterile compression dressing. Postoperatively, active range-of-motion exercises of the elbow and shoulder joints should begin within the first 5 to 7 days. Strengthening exercises are progressed as tolerated. Within 8 to 12 weeks a progressive throwing program is permitted, with a return to athletic activities achieved at approximately 3 to 6 months after surgery.[9]

Posterolateral Rotatory Instability

The patient lies in a supine position, and a pneumatic tourniquet is placed on the upper arm for hemostasis. The elbow is approached through a modified lateral Kocher incision. The dissection is carried down to the level of the common extensor origin. The tendon is then reflected anteriorly from the lateral epicondyle through subperiosteal dissection, to expose the origin of the radial collateral ligament complex. Distal dissection is achieved by reflecting the anconeus muscle posteriorly, and the extensor carpi ulnaris muscle anteriorly. Intraoperative findings may reveal a lax ulnar band of the lateral radial collateral ligament, proximal to the annular ligament. The lateral pivot-shift maneuver demonstrates subluxation of the radial humeral and ulnar humeral joints, as well as attenuation of the capsule. An arthrotomy incision is created at the level of the radiocapitellar and ulnar humeral joints, which allows intraarticular inspection. Loose bodies, synovitis, and osteochondral lesions may then be treated. Plication sutures are then placed within the anterior and posterior aspects of the joint capsule and are tied at the completion of the procedure (Fig. 17-30). If the radial or ulnar portions of the radial

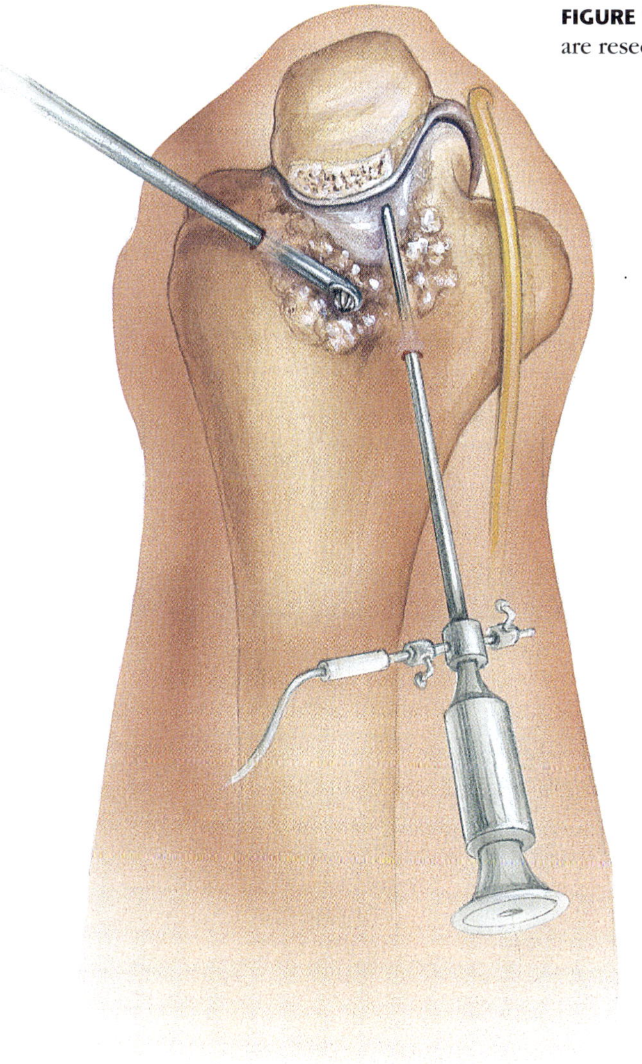

FIGURE 17-28 Posterior humeral osteophytes surrounding olecranon fossa are resected with high-speed burr (patient positioning: prone).

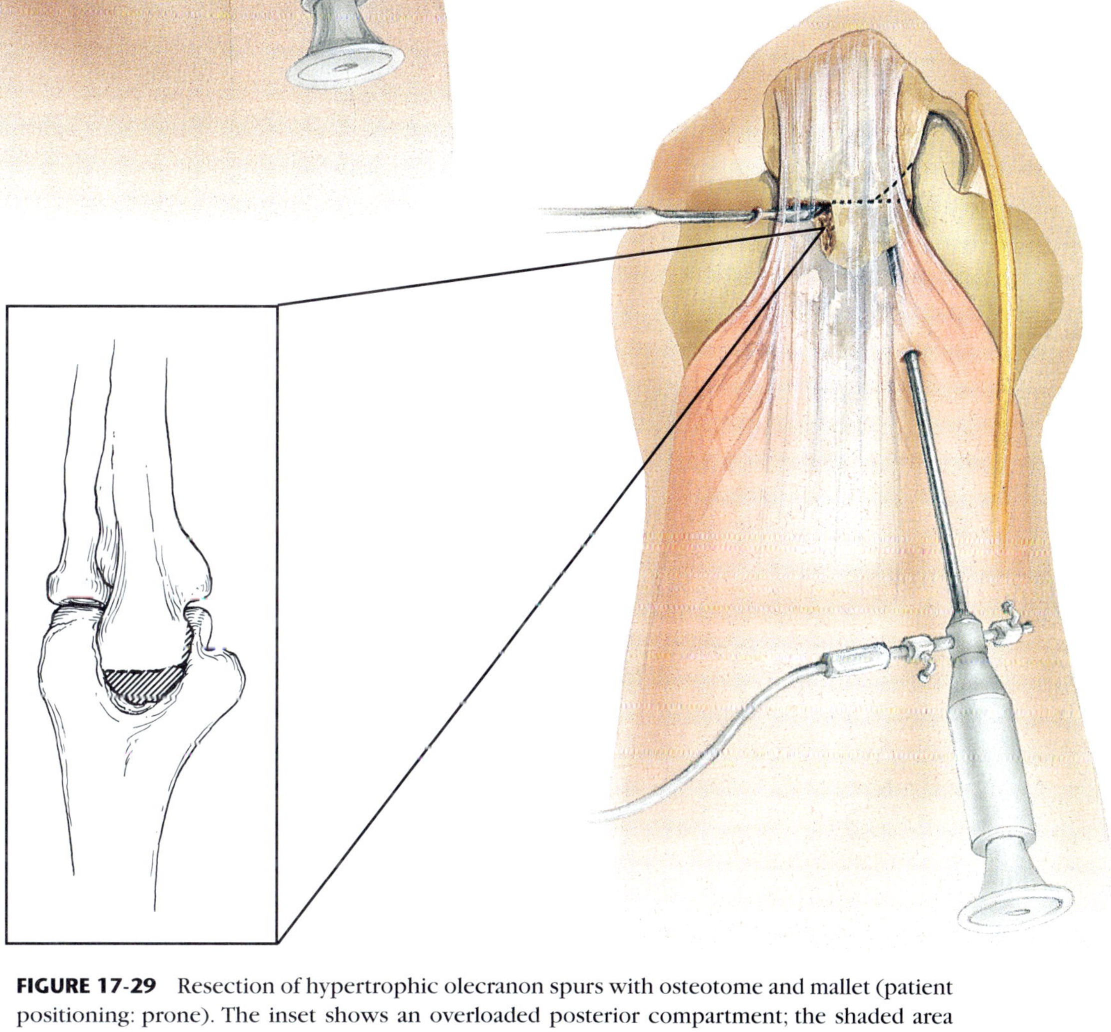

FIGURE 17-29 Resection of hypertrophic olecranon spurs with osteotome and mallet (patient positioning: prone). The inset shows an overloaded posterior compartment; the shaded area represents posteromedial bony impingement that is to be resected arthroscopically.

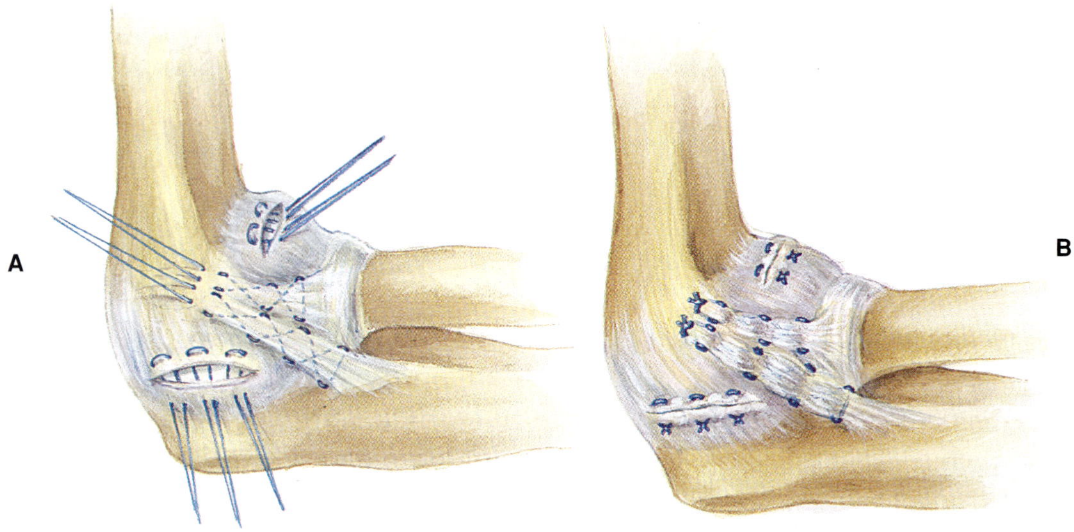

FIGURE 17-30 **A,** Plication sutures placed within the anterior and posterior aspects of the joint capsule, as well as the radial part of the lateral collateral ligament and the ulnar band of the lateral ulnar collateral ligament (LUCL). **B,** Advancement and imbrication of the radial part of the lateral collateral ligament and the ulnar part of the lateral ulnar collateral ligament complex.

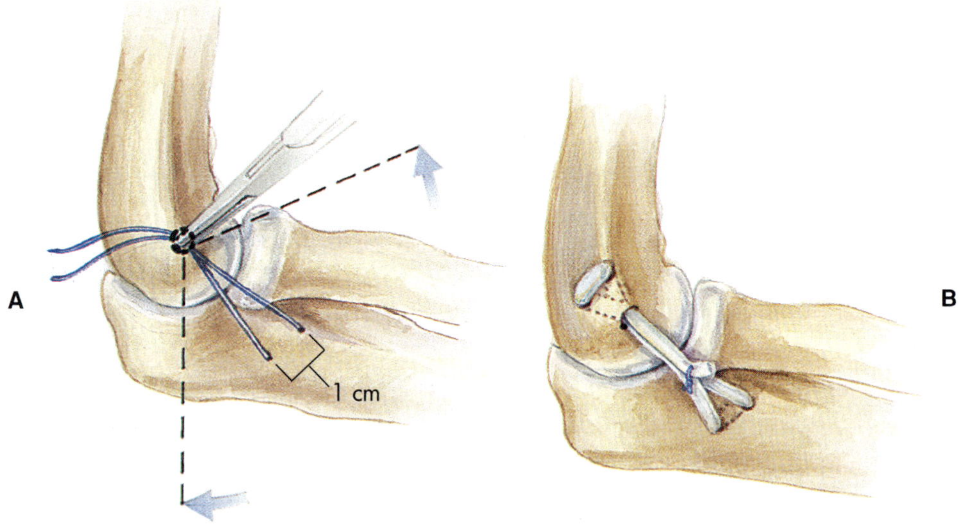

FIGURE 17-31 **A,** Converging drill holes within the tubercle of the supinator crest. The suture is passed through a tunnel within the proximal ulna, is held with a clamp, and then used to determine isometric point on the lateral humeral epicondyle as the elbow is passively flexed and extended. **B,** Divergent bone tunnels at humeral origin of the ulnar band of the radial collateral ligament (LUCL) with autogenous tendon graft placed in figure-of-eight fashion.

collateral ligament complex appear intact but are merely attenuated or detached from the epicondylar origin, primary suture repair and plication may be undertaken. Using Bunnell suture technique, both ulnar and radial components of the radial collateral ligament complex are advanced and anchored through drill holes placed at the anatomic humeral epicondylar origin.

If the radial collateral ligament complex is damaged or attenuated extensively, reconstruction of the ulnar portion of the radial collateral ligament is undertaken with an autogenous free graft (palmaris longus tendon, plantaris tendon, or a 3- to 5-mm medial strip of Achilles tendon). As with medial collateral ligament reconstructions, the tendon is passed through osseous tunnels. On the lateral aspect of the elbow, however, these are created at the level of the supinator crest on the proximal ulna and at the isometric point on the lateral humeral epicondyle. Converging drill holes are created with a 3.2-mm drill bit within the tubercle of the supinator crest. An entrance tunnel is then made at the isometric anatomic humeral origin, creating divergent bone tunnels (Fig. 17-31, *A*). The graft is then passed through these osseous tunnels with a flexible suture passer. The elbow is placed in 30° of flexion with full forearm pronation. As tension is applied to the distal and proximal aspects of the graft, #1 nonabsorbable sutures are used to anchor the tendon to itself and to the surrounding soft tissues (Fig. 17-31, *B*). The elbow is then brought through a full range of motion as the graft is observed for isometry and evaluated for stability. The anconeus and extensor carpi ulnaris muscles are reapproximated with absorbable sutures, and the common extensor origin and extensor carpi radialis longus muscles are reattached likewise. The subcutaneous tissue and skin are closed over a surgical drain, and the extremity is immobilized in a posterior splint for 2 to 4 weeks with the elbow maintained in a position of 90° flexion and full forearm pronation. A postoperative hinged splint is then applied for an additional 4 to 6 weeks. Elbow range-of-motion and muscle-strengthening exercises are begun as tolerated while maintaining rotator cuff muscle flexibility and strength. Within 6 to 8 months after surgery, motion, strength, and endurance have usually recovered sufficiently to resume athletic activities.

SUMMARY

As is true of the shoulder, the elbow joint is at considerable risk for developing a number of injuries as a result of a single traumatic event, or more likely, as a result of chronic repetitive overuse.[20] In overhead activities, the elbow is particularly vulnerable to medial tension overload injuries because of the tremendous valgus stresses applied to the joint. Over time, excessive, repetitive stress may also lead to compression injuries of the lateral structures, extension overload injuries within the posterior compartment, or a combination of these injury patterns. Finally, patients may also suffer from posterolateral rotatory instability of the elbow, which is an entirely separate and distinct clinical entity arising from an injury and subsequent laxity of the ulnar part of the lateral collateral ligament.

Fortunately, most symptomatic conditions unique to the elbow, regardless of etiology, respond to an initial trial of aggressive, nonoperative treatment. For patients with refractory symptoms, despite at least 3 to 6 months of conservative management, surgical intervention may be necessary.[17]

Open ligamentous repair or reconstruction has been shown to reliably and predictably reestablish stability in patients with valgus instability caused by medial collateral ligament laxity or posterolateral rotatory instability caused by laxity of the lateral collateral ligament.

Refinements in arthroscopic surgical technique have allowed improved visualization, decreased morbidity, and a reduced risk of complications in the assessment and treatment of compression injuries of the lateral compartment and most extension overload injuries within the posterior compartment.

Future modifications of existing open or arthroscopic surgical techniques and improvements in rehabilitation programs will return future athletes more predictably and reliably to their prior competitive level. Hopefully, continued research in the anatomy, basic biomechanics, and pathophysiology associated with overhead activities may someday prevent most, if not all, of these repetitive, overuse elbow injuries.

References

1. Albright JA et al: Clinical study of baseball pitchers: correlation of injury of the throwing arm with method of delivery, *Am J Sports Med* 6(1):15, 1978.
2. Andrews JR: Bony injuries about the elbow in the throwing athlete, *Instr Course Lect* 34:323, 1985.
3. Andrews JR, Craven WM: Lesions of the posterior compartment of the elbow, *Clin Sports Med* 10(3):637, 1991.
4. Andrews JR, Pierre RK, Carson WG Jr: Arthroscopy of the elbow, *Clin Sports Med* 5(4):653, 1986.
5. Baker CL, Shalvoy RM: The prone position for elbow arthroscopy, *Clin Sports Med* 10(3):623, 1991.
6. Barnes DA, Tullos HS: An analysis of 100 symptomatic baseball players, *Am J Sports Med* 6(2):62, 1978.
7. Bennett GE: Elbow and shoulder lesions of baseball players, *Am J Surg* 98:484, 1959.
8. Bennett JB, Green MS, Tullos HS: Surgical management of chronic medial elbow instability, *Clin Orthop* 278:62, 1992.
9. Blackburn TA Jr: Rehabilitation of the shoulder and elbow after arthroscopy, *Clin Sports Med* 6(3):587, 1987.
10. Carson WG Jr, Meyers JF: Diagnostic arthroscopy of the elbow: surgical technique and arthroscopic and portal anatomy. In McGinty JB et al, editors: *Operative arthroscopy,* New York, 1991, Raven Press.
11. Conway JE et al: Medial instability of the elbow in the throwing athlete, *J Bone Joint Surg* 74A:67, 1992.
12. DeHaven KE, Evarts CM: Throwing injuries of the elbow in athletes, *Orthop Clin* 4(3):801, 1973.
13. Del Pizzo W, Jobe FW, Norwood L: Ulnar nerve entrapment syndrome in baseball players, *Am J Sports Med* 5(5):182, 1977.
14. Gainor BJ et al: The throw: biomechanics and acute injury, *Am J Sports Med* 8(2):114, 1980.
15. Guhl JR: Arthroscopy and arthroscopic surgery of the elbow, *Orthopaedics* 8(10):1290, 1985.
16. Hassman G, Neer CS: Recurrent dislocation of the elbow, *J Bone Joint Surg* 54A:1080, 1975.
17. Indelicato PA et al: Correctable elbow lesions in professional baseball players: a review of 25 cases, *Am J Sports Med* 7(1):72, 1979.
18. Jackson DJ, Silvino N, Reinman P: Osteochondritis in the female gymnast's elbow, *Arthroscopy* 5(2):129, 1989.
19. Jobe FW, Kvitne RS: Elbow instability in the athlete, *Instr Course Lect* XL:17, 1991.
20. Jobe FW, Nuber G: Throwing injuries of the elbow, *Clin Sports Med* 5(4):621, 1986.

21. Jobe FW, Stark H, Lombardo SJ: Reconstruction of the ulnar collateral ligament in athletes, *J Bone Joint Surg* 68A:1158, 1986.
22. King JW, Brelsford HJ, Tullos HS: Analysis of the pitching arm of the professional baseball pitcher, *Clin Orthop* 67:116, 1969.
23. Lindenfeld TN: Medial approach in elbow arthroscopy, *Am J Sports Med* 18(4):413, 1990.
24. Lynch GJ et al: Neurovascular anatomy and elbow arthroscopy: inherent risks, *Arthroscopy* 2(3):191, 1986.
25. McManama GB Jr et al: The surgical treatment of osteochondritis of the capitellum, *Am J Sports Med* 13(1):11, 1985.
26. Miller JE: Javelin thrower's elbow, *J Bone Joint Surg* 42B:788, 1960.
27. Morrey BF, An KN: Articular and ligamentous contributions to the stability of the elbow joint, *Am J Sports Med* 11(5):315, 1983.
28. Morrey BF, Tanaka S, An KN: Valgus stability of the elbow: a definition of primary and secondary constraints, *Clin Orthop* 265:187, 1989.
29. Nestor BJ, O'Driscoll SW, Morrey BF: Ligamentous reconstruction for posterolateral rotatory instability of the elbow, *J Bone Joint Surg* 74A:1235, 1992.
30. Norwood LA, Shook JA, Andrews JR: Acute medial elbow ruptures, *Am J Sports Med* 9(1):16, 1981.
31. Nuber GW, Diment MT: Olecranon stress fractures in throwers: a report of two cases and a review of the literature, *Clin Orthop* 278:58, 1992.
32. O'Driscoll SW, Bell DF, Morrey BF: Posterolateral rotatory instability of the elbow, *J Bone Joint Surg* 73A:440, 1991.
33. O'Driscoll SW et al: Anatomy of the ulnar part of the lateral collateral ligament of the elbow, *Clin Anat* 5:296, 1992.
34. O'Driscoll SW, Morrey BF: Arthroscopy of the elbow, *J Bone Joint Surg* 74A:84, 1992.
35. O'Driscoll SW et al: Posterolateral rotatory instability of the elbow: a kinematic and biomechanical analysis, *Orthop Trans Res Soc* 15:6, 1990.
36. Osborne G, Cotterill P: Recurrent dislocation of the elbow, *J Bone Joint Surg* 48B:340, 1966.
37. Pappas AM: Elbow problems associated with baseball during childhood and adolescence, *Clin Orthop* 164:30, 1982.
38. Pappas AM, Zawacki RM, Sullivan TJ: Biomechanics of baseball pitching: a preliminary report, *Am J Sports Med* 13(4):216, 1985.
39. Parisien JS: Arthroscopic surgery of the elbow, *Bull Hosp Joint Dis Orthop Inst* 48(2):149, 1988.
40. Poehling GG et al: Elbow arthroscopy: a new technique, *Arthroscopy* 5(3):222, 1989.
41. Ruch DS, Poehling GG: Arthroscopic treatment of Panner's disease, *Clin Sports Med* 10(3):629, 1991.
42. Schwab GH et al: Biomechanics of elbow instability: the role of the medial collateral ligament, *Clin Orthop* 146:42, 1980.
43. Slager RF: From little league to big league, the weak spot is the arm, *Am J Sports Med* 5(2):37, 1977.
44. Slocum DB: Classification of elbow injuries from baseball pitching, *Texas Med* 64:48, 1968.
45. Small NC: Complications in arthroscopy: the knee and other joints, *Arthroscopy* 2(4):253, 1986.
46. Sojbjerg JO, Ovesen J, Nielsen S: Experimental elbow instability after transection of the medial collateral ligament, *Clin Orthop* 218:186, 1986.
47. Symeonides PP et al: Recurrent dislocation of the elbow, *J Bone Joint Surg* 57A:1084, 1975.
48. Tullos HS et al: Unusual lesions of the pitching arm, *Clin Orthop* 88:169, 1972.
49. Tullos HS, King JW: Throwing mechanism in sports, *Orthop Clin North Am* 4(3):709, 1973.
50. Wilson FD et al: Valgus extension overload in the pitching elbow, *Am J Sports Med* 11(2):83, 1983.
51. Woods GW: Elbow arthroscopy, *Clin Sports Med* 6(3):557, 1987.
52. Woods GW, Tullos HS: Elbow instability and medial epicondyle fractures, *Am J Sports Med* 5(1):23, 1977.

CHAPTER 18

Lateral and Medial Epicondylitis of the Elbow

MICHAEL G. CICCOTTI
STEPHEN J. LOMBARDO

From an austere initial description as "lawn tennis arm,"[34] a vast array of detailed diagnostic and therapeutic treatises on epicondylitis of the elbow has emerged. Morris' cornerstone correspondence in 1882[34] focused on medial epicondylitis as caused by the lawn tennis backstroke. Subsequent works have greatly expanded both the location and etiology of epicondylitis. The lateral elbow has become the most common site of occurrence, and many sports activities other than tennis, as well as occupational activities, have been identified as causes. Countless treatment regimens have been prescribed, all of which leave the physician with a perplexing array of options. The most successful treatment for epicondylitis of the elbow is derived from a thorough understanding of the inherent anatomy, biomechanics, pathology, presentation, and therapeutics.

LATERAL EPICONDYLITIS

Anatomy

The musculotendinous anatomy of the elbow's lateral epicondyle consists of the common extensor origin (Fig. 18-1). This includes the extensor carpi radialis longus, extensor carpi radialis brevis, extensor digitorum communis, and extensor carpi ulnaris. The extensor carpi radialis longus arises from the distal third of the lateral supracondylar ridge and also in part from the distal portion of the upper arm's lateral intermuscular septum. The extensor carpi radialis brevis lies beneath the extensor longus muscle. Its complex origin includes the common extensor tendon at the lateral epicondyle, the lateral collateral and annular ligaments, the investing fascia, and the intermuscular septum, both proximal and distal to the elbow joint. The extensor digitorum communis and extensor carpi ulnaris arise from the anterolateral aspect of the common tendon of the lateral epicondyle.

Biomechanics

The normal biomechanics of the lateral epicondylar structures have been most thoroughly described during the tennis stroke. Morris et al[35] described four phases of the groundstrokes (forehand and backhand), which are the following:

Phase 1 (preparation)—This phase begins with the initiation of backward racquet motion and ends with the start of forward racquet motion.

Phase 2 (acceleration)—This phase begins with forward racquet motion and ends with ball contact (Fig. 18-2).

Phase 3 and phase 4 (follow through)—This phase begins at ball contact and ends with the completion of the stroke. Phase 3, or early follow-through, consists of the initial 25% of this phase: phase 4, or late follow-through, includes the final 75% of this phase.

These authors evaluated the muscle activity about the elbow during tennis strokes in nine healthy professional and college-level players using indwelling electromyography. They noted the highest muscle activity during the groundstrokes in those muscles stabilizing the wrist, specifically the extensor carpi radialis brevis, extensor carpi radialis longus, and extensor digitorum communis. The extensor carpi radialis brevis was noted to have the highest activity of all muscles tested; this peak occurred during the acceleration and early follow-through phases. The authors suggested that these muscles provide optimal stability by positioning the wrist in extension and radial deviation during these phases of the groundstrokes. Leach[31] has suggested that repetitive concentric loading of these muscles as they maintain tension to stabilize the wrist may lead to chronic overload and subsequent symptoms of lateral epicondylitis. The specific biomechanics identified in the groundstrokes of tennis may theoretically be extrapolated to the various other activities that lead to this entity.

Epidemiology/Etiology

Morris' report of 1882[34] identified tennis as the causative factor for epicondylitis and thus initiated the acceptance of the term *tennis elbow* for this syndrome. This initial implication of racquet sports as the primary etiology has led to a plethora of literature reviewing the epidemiologic and etiologic factors in tennis and its associated lateral epicondylitis. Consequently, lateral epicondylitis has been most thoroughly defined in the context of tennis play. Various authors[42,47,48] have estimated that 10% to 50% of people who engage in tennis regularly will at some point during their careers experience symptoms of tennis elbow. A review of 200 club tennis players over the age of 30 noted a 50% incidence of symptoms compatible with tennis elbow.[47] Half of the players experi-

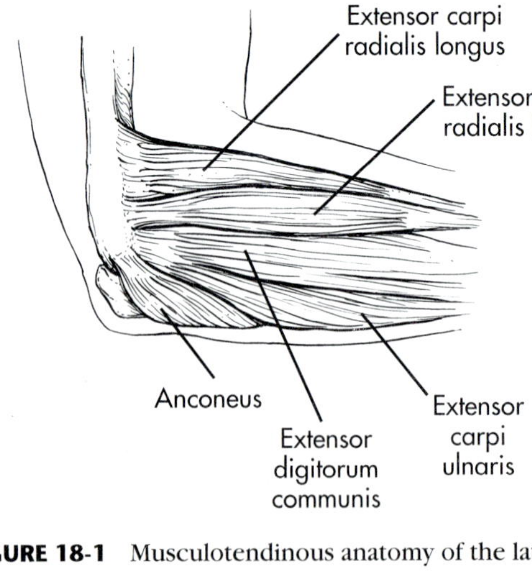

FIGURE 18-1 Musculotendinous anatomy of the lateral elbow.

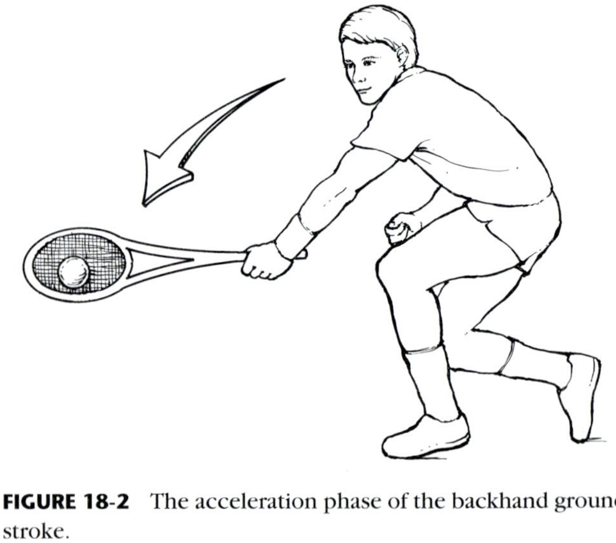

FIGURE 18-2 The acceleration phase of the backhand groundstroke.

enced minor symptoms with a duration of less than 6 months, and the remainder had major symptoms lasting an average of 2.5 years. Gruchow and Pelletier[21] in 1979 noted an association between playing time and the incidence of tennis elbow in the club player. In players with over 2 hours of racquet time per week, the risk of developing symptoms consistent with tennis elbow was 2 to 3.5 times greater than those playing tennis less than 2 times per week. They also noted a significant correlation between the prevalence of lateral epicondylitis and player age. Those players over the age of 40 years had a fourfold increased occurrence in males and a twofold increase in females. Nirschl[41] and Berhung[3] have implicated several specific factors of technique, equipment, and playing surface in lateral epicondylitis. Club players developing tennis elbow displayed a higher incidence of poor stroke mechanics, such as leading with a flexed elbow, rather than the body or shoulder, and striking the ball off center on the racquet, both of which impart greater loads to the wrist extensors. Kelley[29] also identified these poor techniques in an electromyographic and cinematographic comparison of healthy tennis players and tennis players having a history of lateral epicondylitis. He noted the occurrence of a leading elbow, forearm pronation, and off center ball contact in the injured players, all of which necessitated significantly increased wrist extensor activity to compensate for the aberrant technique. Improper grip size, racquet weight, and racquet stringing generate higher loads in the lateral elbow muscle tendon unit and, as such, also have been noted in those players affected. Additionally, the more frequent use of harder court surfaces by these affected players has been postulated by Nirschl[41] to impart greater momentum on the ball, with subsequently increases force transmission through the racquet to the extensor mass of the forearm.

Tennis as the primary etiology of this syndrome, however, actually may be a misconception, because several large reviews have noted its occurrence more commonly in other activities.[12,31] In his review of 339 patients with lateral epicondylitis, Coonrad[12] documented the incidence of tennis participation to be less than 5%. Many other sports, including baseball,[2] javelin throwing,[33] swimming, and fencing, also have been identified as etiologies.[41] Occupational activities that require forceful or repetitive forearm use, such as carpentry, plumbing, and meat cutting, also have led to the occurrence of this syndrome.[41]

Lateral epicondylitis typically occurs in the fourth and fifth decades,[3,6,38,47,48] although it has been identified in patients ranging from 12 to 80 years.[41] The male-to-female prevalence appears equal,[3,41] but arm dominance seems to be a determinant. For example, Bernhung[3] and Nirschl[38] have noted that more than 75% of patients in their reviews exhibited symptoms in the elbow of their dominant arm.

Pathophysiology

Since the earliest description of lateral epicondylitis, an abundance of literature has been devoted to its precise pathophysiology, resulting in a wide spectrum of proposed theories. Traumatic periostitis with partial detachment of the common extensor from repeated wrist extension and forearm supination was advocated by Runge[51] in the late 1800s. Hansson[23] extended this theory by suggesting that the periosteal avulsion resulted in a myositis of the extensors attached to the lateral epicondyle. Garden[14] proposed further that the specific muscle implicated in the periostitis was the extensor carpi radialis brevis. Osgood[44] in 1922 suggested that inflammation of an extraarticular, radial humeral bursa was the primary cause. An inflamed synovial fringe was described by Trethowan[55] and Ogilvie[43] in 1929. They thought that the synovium was compressed between the radial head and capitellum, leading to the inflammation. Fibrositis of the annular ligament resulting from trauma was initially described by Stack[54] in 1949. Bosworth[5] championed this as the primary etiology, proposing that trauma to the annular ligament was due to eccentric stress generated by the repeated rotation of an asymmetric radial head. Radial nerve entrapment was suggested by Kaplan[28] in 1959 as an etiology for this entity. He proposed that compression of the articular branches of the radial nerve could occur at one of four different levels in the radial tunnel: (1) from a fibrous band anterior to the radial head at the entrance of the radial tunnel, (2) from the recurrent branch of the radial artery just distal to this point, (3) from the distal tendinous margin of the extensor carpi radialis brevis, or (4) from the margin of the supinator at the arcade of Frohse. Chondromalacia of the radiocapitellar joint was proposed as a primary etiology by Newman and Goodfellow[37] in 1979. These authors suggested that with the progression of articular changes, osteocartilaginous loose bodies may form and subsequent synovitis and periarticular soft-tissue inflammation may develop.

The current consensus based on clinical and surgical evidence suggests that lateral epicondylitis is initiated as a microtear, most often within the origin of the extensor carpi radialis brevis. This process may originate in the extensor communis tendon as well. Nirschl[38] has proposed that with repetitive trauma, this process of microtearing results in mucoid degeneration and subsequent reactive granulation within the tendinous origin of the extensor carpi radialis brevis and/or extensor digitorum communis. These pathologic alterations within the extensor carpi radialis brevis, which are contiguous with the lateral collateral ligaments, the annular ligament, the joint capsule, and the bursa, help to condense the variety of previously proposed pathophysiologic theories.

In his classic study of 1964, Goldie[19] was the first to describe evidence of pathology within the tendinous insertions on the lateral epicondyle. He demonstrated that the reactive granulation tissue that replaces the tendon of the extensor carpi radialis brevis contains large numbers of free nerve endings and, as such, may lead to the pain produced with tension or compression. In a subsequent article, Nirschl[38] thoroughly described the pathologic changes of lateral epicondylitis. The tendon usually contains a grayish, homogeneous, edematous, and friable tissue that Nirschl cogently described as a "thick, unhappy, gray tendon, weeping with edema."[41] Tendon fibers may appear fibrillated with an apparent sinus tract extending from the elbow joint. In his series of 88 surgically treated elbows, 97% demonstrated varying degrees of this gross pathologic tissue at the origin of the extensor carpi radialis brevis tendon. Of those with macroscopic pathology within the extensor carpi radialis brevis, 35% also demonstrated gross tendon rupture.[38] Nirschl has described a characteristic microscopic "angiofibroblastic hyperplasia"[38] of the involved tissue. The normal parallel orientation of collagen fibers is disrupted by an invasion of fibroblasts and vascular granulation-like tissues. The adjacent portions of the tendon have a hypercellular, degenerated, and microfragmented appearance with a paucity of inflammatory cells. He suggested that the degree of angiofibroblastic infiltration appears to correlate with the duration of symptoms.[41] Regan,[49] in his 1990 histologic study, confirmed the findings of Nirschl; he clearly demonstrated a significant vascular and fibrous proliferation as well as a lack of acute or chronic inflammatory components within the surgical specimens.

Diagnosis

Lateral epicondylitis is characterized by pain at the lateral epicondyle that often radiates into the forearm. It also may be associated with a sense of wrist and finger weakness with grasping. The pain may occur acutely, but more typically is insidious in its onset with gradually increasing symptoms. A history of repetitive activity or overuse often can be elicited, but in some instances no predisposing activity can be determined. As symptoms progress, even generic activities such as shaking hands, picking up a bottle, or carrying a briefcase may cause severe pain at the elbow. In tennis, pain in the lateral aspect of the elbow usually occurs at the point of ball contact during the groundstrokes and is more often noted with the backhand than the forehand strokes.

Examination reveals tenderness at the conjoined tendon origin, usually precisely localized to the extensor carpi radialis brevis portion. The area of maximal tenderness lies 2 to 5 mm distal and anterior to the midpoint of the lateral epicondyle. Grasping or pinching with the wrist in extension, the so-called "coffee cup" test,[12] usually reproduces the pain. Resisted wrist and finger extension with the elbow in full extension will intensify the pain. Resisted long finger extension often elicits the most severe pain. Range of motion of the elbow and wrist is usually complete, but in some instances of long-standing lateral epicondylitis, a loss of 5° to 10° of active elbow extension, active wrist extension, and passive wrist flexion may be present. An elbow joint effusion is rarely seen initially, but Coonrad[12] has noted its occurrence with more chronic lateral epicondylitis, usually with a duration of 6 to 9 months. Sensation typically is normal in the extremity, but wrist extensor weakness secondary to pain may be detected. In patients with prolonged symptoms, measurable muscle atrophy may be present. In some instances, a more localized loss of tissue substance may be palpated distal and anterior to the lateral epicondyle, which may represent a partial or complete rupture, most commonly of the extensor carpi radialis brevis.

Radiographs of the affected elbow usually are normal, but 22% to 25% may show calcification within the soft tissues about the lateral epicondyle.[7,19,31] Leach[31] has suggested that the occurrence of this calcification has no prognostic implication and that with treatment the calcification actually may dissipate. The use of other radiographic modalities, such as ultrasonography or magnetic resonance imaging, does not seem to improve the diagnostic or therapeutic decision-making for primary lateral epicondylitis. Care must be taken in evaluating the patient with lateral elbow pain because abnormalities unrelated to true lateral epicondylitis may be present. The most common entities in the differential diagnosis include cervical disease, radial nerve compression at the elbow, and intraarticular elbow disease.

A thorough evaluation of the neck and the entire upper extremity is prudent in patients with lateral elbow pain. Gunn and Milbrandt[22] have suggested that lateral epicondylar pain may be secondary to cervical radiculopathy. These authors have reported satisfactory results in 53 patients with recalcitrant lateral elbow pain who subsequently had their treatment directed to their cervical arthritis. They have recommended clinical, radiographic, and possibly electrodiagnostic evaluations of the cervical spine, especially in patients with lateral epicondylar pain unresponsive to local measures and with concomitant cervical arthrosis. Nirschl[41] has pointed out, however, that true lateral epicondylitis most frequently occurs during the fourth and fifth decades, when radiographic evidence of cervical arthrosis is, most likely, merely coincidental.

Entrapment of branches of the radial nerve within the radial tunnel may produce symptoms that mimic those caused by lateral epicondylitis. Roles and Maudsley[50] have proposed that compression neuropathy of the radial nerve may lead to resistant lateral elbow pain. They have suggested that electrodiagnostic studies of the radial nerve are helpful in the evaluation of radial tunnel compression syndrome if polyphasic wave potentials are present; conduction velocities, however, usually are normal. Nirschl[39] and Van Rossum[58] have reported normal electromyographic and nerve conduction studies in patients with true lateral epicondylitis.

Individuals who participate in activities that impart high torque, shear, or compressive forces on the elbow are vulnerable to developing intraarticular pathology. This pathology may take the form of traumatic arthritis and osteocartilaginous loose bodies, most often laterally but also medially and posteriorly.[26,42,60] These patients may complain of lateral elbow pain similar to lateral epicondylitis but most often will exhibit evidence of intraarticular damage on radiographic studies.

Treatment

Nonsurgical

The volumes of orthopedic literature addressing lateral elbow epicondylitis illustrate the success of nonoperative treatment for this entity. Essential to the success of conservative management, however, is an understanding of its basic principles. Relief of initial pain and inflammation followed by promotion of tissue healing with guided rehabilitation of the elbow has been emphasized by a variety of authors.[11,12,31,41]

Relief of pain and inflammation is the primary goal of the first phase of nonsurgical treatment. Avoidance of the offending activity is required initially, but any other activities that aggravate the condition also should be avoided. Competitive athletes who have acute pain with their sport must stop until symptoms resolve during daily activities. If playing produces only minimal pain that does not increase, however, then monitored sport participation may be continued during treatment. The transient local vasoconstrictive and analgesic effects of ice have been documented by a variety of authors. Oral antiinflammatory medication should be initiated for 10 to 14 days if the patient's overall medical condition allows. No particular nonsteroidal antiinflammatory agent has been shown most efficacious for epicondylitis, but a course of 2 to 3 weeks, followed by a period of abstinence from the medication, generally is suggested. If pain recurs, the regimen is reinstituted for an additional 2 to 3 weeks. If the patient does not respond to these initial therapeutic measures, a corticosteroid injection has been proposed by several authors.* The choice and dose of steroid preparation, however, have remained arbitrary because few comprehensive comparisons of commonly used agents have been performed. Most authors suggest that the steroid compound be mixed with a local anesthetic. Care should be taken to instill the mixture deep to the extensor carpi radialis brevis, anterior and distal to the lateral epicondyle, and into the fatty subaponeurotic recess (Fig. 18-3). Injection of the mixture superficially may result in subcutaneous atrophy,[9,40] and intratendinous injection may lead to permanent changes within the tendon ultrastructure.[40,57] In light of these potential deleterious effects, a maximum of two to three injections at any one site is recommended. Several short-term studies evaluating the use of steroid injections have noted pain relief in 55% to 89% of patients, but recurrence in 18% to 54% of these patients with initial relief.[10,36] The physical therapy modalities of ultrasound and high-voltage galvanic stimulation have been used with variable success. Binder[4] noted a lower initial response using ultrasound as opposed to steroid injection, but a lower recurrence rate in patients responding to the ultrasound. Nirschl[41] recommended four to six sessions of galvanic stimulation during the initial 2- to 3-week treatment period.

*References 4, 6, 30, 31, 41, 46.

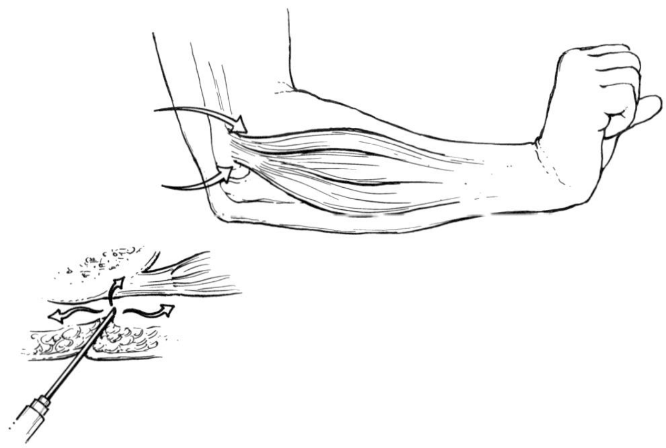

FIGURE 18-3 Site of corticosteroid injection for lateral epicondylitis.

Upon relief of initial pain and inflammation, the second phase of nonsurgical treatment is begun. This phase emphasizes continued tissue healing through avoidance of the abusive aspects of the causative activity and through guided rehabilitation. Distinction is made between complete rest, which may be necessary in chronic or recalcitrant cases, and modified function with continued activity. Formal immobilization is not effective in controlling the pain after activity is resumed, but rather immobilization leads to disuse atrophy of the surrounding tissues, further compromising rehabilitation. In the majority of cases, patients may continue their sport or work, but with alterations in technique or equipment.

A careful history and close observation are essential to detect aberrant patient technique that may lead to epicondylitis. Certainly the physician is an important part of this surveillance, but observers knowledgeable in the sport or occupational activity also are essential. In tennis, certain technique modifications will diminish stress at the lateral epicondyle. Hitting the ball in front of the body with the wrist and elbow extended allows the trunk and upper arm to provide the majority of stroke power, rather than the wrist extensors solely. The two-handed backhand allows force to be divided between both upper extremities and thus greatly diminishes force at the leading lateral epicondyle. Off-center contact has been noted consistently in injured players[29] and is thought to increase mechanical loads at the lateral epicondyle by generating additional rotatory forces.[41]

Proper equipment, especially in the racquet sports, is essential to promoting and maintaining ideal tissue health. Various authors[3,41,42] have recommended that proper racquet grip size be determined by measuring from the proximal palmar crease to the tip of the ring finger along its radial border (Fig. 18-4). Lighter racquets, although providing less momentum, allow ease of positioning for impact. Frames of low-vibration materials, such as graphite and epoxies, dampen impact forces imparted on the extensor origin. Less tightly strung racquets, higher string count per unit area, and slower surfaces such as clay courts, although decreasing ball speed, will diminish the loads transmitted to the elbow.

Counterforce bracing was introduced by Ilfeld[25] in 1965 and further promoted by Froimson[13] in 1971. Theoretically, this type of brace inhibits full muscular expansion and thus decreases the force experienced by sensitive or injured muscular tissue proximal to the band. The brace is applied firmly around the forearm just distal to the elbow and over the extensor mass. Groppel and Nirschl[20] demonstrated with three-dimensional cinematography and surface electromyography that lower extensor muscle activity and elbow angular acceleration were produced with the use of counterforce bracing during the tennis serve and one-handed backhand. Snyder-Mackler,[52] employing the more sensitive indwelling EMG technique, noted significantly reduced muscle activity in the extensor carpi radialis brevis and extensor digitorum communis of healthy subjects during maximum voluntary isometric contraction while using an air-bladder type counterforce brace. Leach[31] suggested that such bracing may be most appropriate for patients with mild epicondylitis or acute symptoms responding to nonoperative treatment.

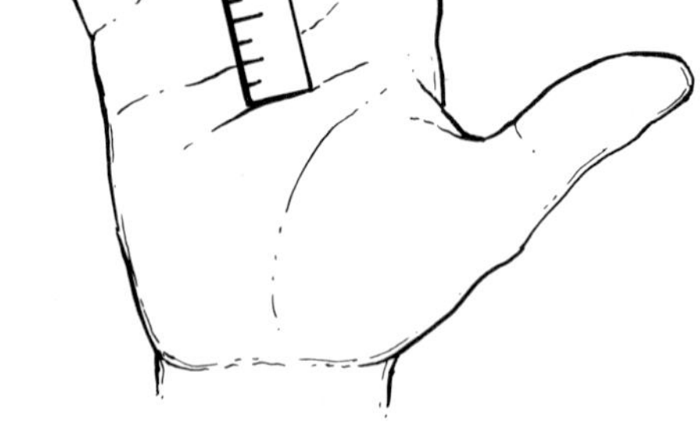

FIGURE 18-4 Determining the proper racquet grip size.

The second phase of nonsurgical treatment also includes guided rehabilitation of the elbow as well as the remainder of the involved extremity. Counterforce bracing may be used during the early rehabilitation, and if pain recurs, the components of the initial phase can be reimplemented. The rehabilitative program begins with wrist extensor stretching and progressive isometric exercises. These exercises initially may be performed with the elbow flexed to minimize pain and then, as the symptoms allow, the exercises are performed with the elbow in full extension. As strength, endurance, and flexibility improve, eccentric and concentric resistive exercises are performed. When the patient is capable of sprint repetitions to fatigue without significant elbow symptoms, a sport or job simulation is staged to assess ability to return. If the simulation is successfully completed, the patient is encouraged to return to normal activity and to gradually increase the duration and intensity of exposure. Continued proper stretching, strengthening, and warm-up will help to prevent the recurrence of symptoms on return to the sport or activity.

Although most authors admit that the majority of patients with lateral epicondylitis respond to nonoperative care, few studies have examined the long-term outcome of nonsurgical treatment. Various authors[31,38,41] have suggested that 5% to 15% of patients will suffer a recurrence of symptoms, but the majority of these patients will not have been fully rehabilitated or will have prematurely discontinued preventive measures. Binder[4] reviewed 125 patients with lateral epicondylitis who were followed between 1 and 5 years. Sixty were studied prospectively, and the remainder were studied retrospectively. At discharge, 10% of the patients remained symptomatic to some degree, 26% had recurrence of symptoms, and more than 40% noted prolonged minor discomfort that affected some aspect of their activities. His findings suggest that the previously documented rates of 85% to 90% for successful nonoperative treatment may be somewhat optimistic, and that persistent or recurrent symptoms may occur more frequently.

Surgical

History

The indications for surgical treatment of lateral epicondylitis include persistent, debilitating pain at the lateral epicondyle in spite of a well-managed nonoperative program spanning at least 6 months, and the exclusion of other pathologic etiologies for the pain. Various studies[6,18,45] have suggested that 3% to 8% of patients with lateral epicondylitis will require operative intervention for resistant symptoms. The history of surgical treatment for lateral epicondylitis spans nearly three quarters of a century and includes a host of variously popular techniques. In general, four main approaches have been employed: (1) extraarticular procedures that involve tenotomy of the common extensor origin, (2) intraarticular procedures that excise the synovial fringe and a portion of the orbicular ligament, (3) extraarticular procedures that lengthen the extensor carpi radialis brevis tendon distally, and (4) extraarticular procedures that excise the pathologic tendon and then reattach the origin.

Reviewing treatments in chronological order, Hohmann[24] initiated the surgical treatment of tennis elbow in 1926 when he described release of the extensor aponeurosis at the level of the lateral epicondyle (Fig. 18-5). Modifications of this extraarticular, tension-relieving technique have ranged from open fasciotomy as described by Spencer[53] in 1953 to percutaneous release as presented by Baumgard[1] in 1982. The proponents of this technique suggest that proximal release reduces tension at the extensor tendon origin with low morbidity and early recovery. These authors[1,18,45,53] have documented 86% to 91% good or excellent results on long-term follow-up. However, the lack of objective strength assessments in these studies has perpetuated the concern over diminished postoperative strength leading to disability in more active individuals such as athletes or laborers.

Bosworth[5] in 1955 reported on several variations of an intraarticular technique that included a release of the orbicular ligament at the radial head. One subset of patients in his series also underwent a release of the extensor aponeurosis (Fig. 18-6); this specific technique was deemed "curative" by the author. With release of the extensor aponeurosis and removal of the orbicular ligament, the origin of the extensor brevis undoubtedly was debrided or removed.

In 1961, Garden[14] presented an alternative extraarticular method of reducing tension at the extensor carpi radialis brevis origin. He asserted that pain resulted from a periosteal tear at the origin of the extensor carpi radialis brevis where an intimate anatomic relationship to the orbicular ligament occurred. He warned, however, against the high morbidity of the Bosworth technique with annular ligament resection. Alternatively, he proposed an open Z-plasty lengthening at the extensor carpi radialis brevis' distal musculotendinous junction (Fig. 18-7). In 44 cases treated by this technique, all patients obtained complete pain relief. Garden assessed grip strength by using dynamometer evaluation and concluded that neither wrist dorsiflexion power nor grip efficiency was diminished. On critical review of the data, however, 40% were noted to have residual strength deficits at follow-up. Carroll[8] in 1968 evaluated the Garden technique in 16 patients. He noted only 3 with immediate pain relief and no recurrence of symptoms; 8 patients had only partial relief; the remaining 5 patients experienced no relief at all.

Considering the experiences of these predecessors, the authors suggest an extraarticular technique, as used

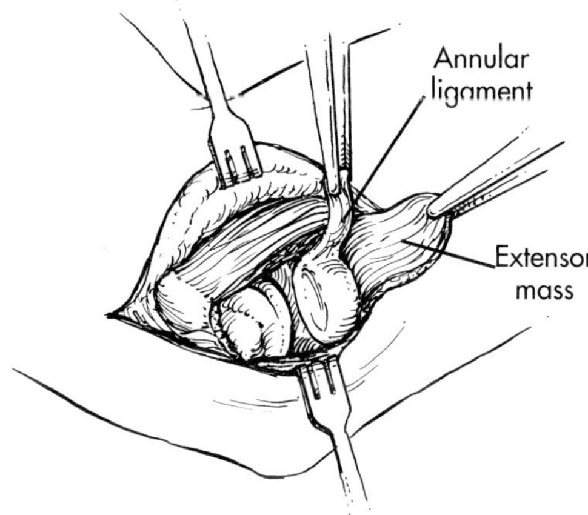

FIGURE 18-6 Intraarticular technique with excision of the synovial fringe and a portion of the orbicular ligament.

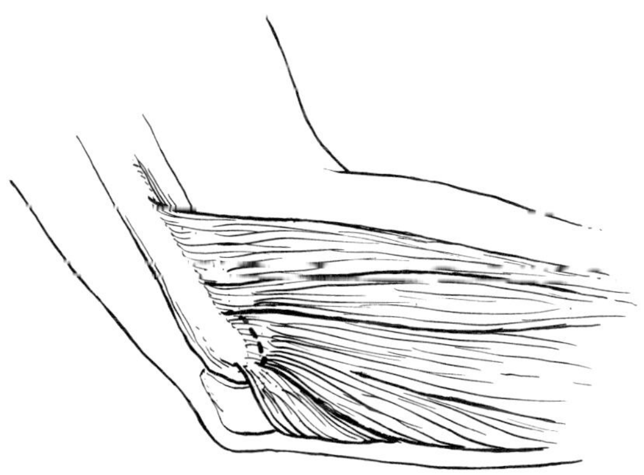

FIGURE 18-5 Extraarticular technique with tenotomy of the common extensor origin.

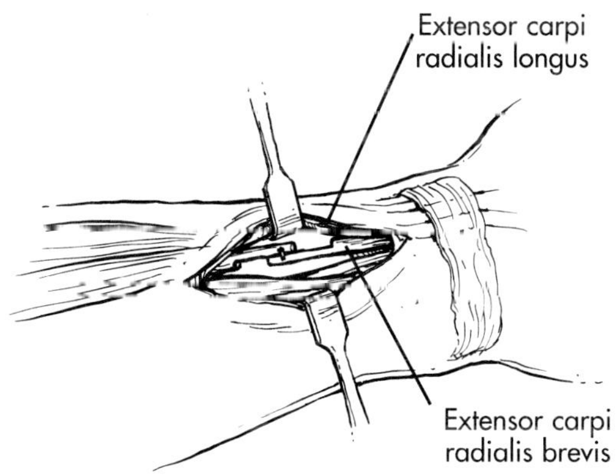

FIGURE 18-7 Extraarticular technique with distal lengthening of the extensor brevis tendon.

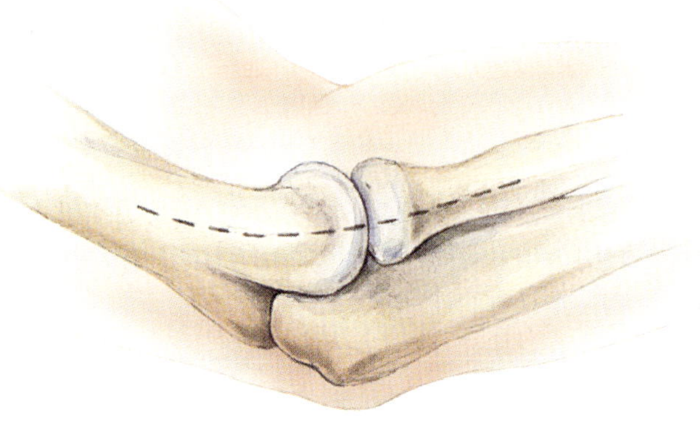

FIGURE 18-8 Skin incision overlying the lateral epicondyle.

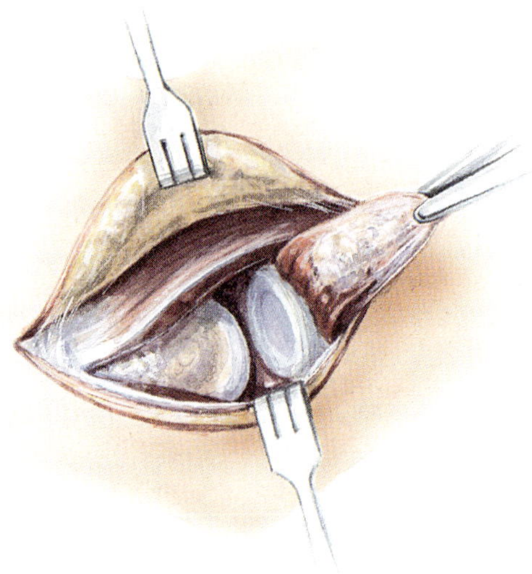

FIGURE 18-9 Distal reflection of the extensor mechanism, exposing the lateral compartment of the elbow.

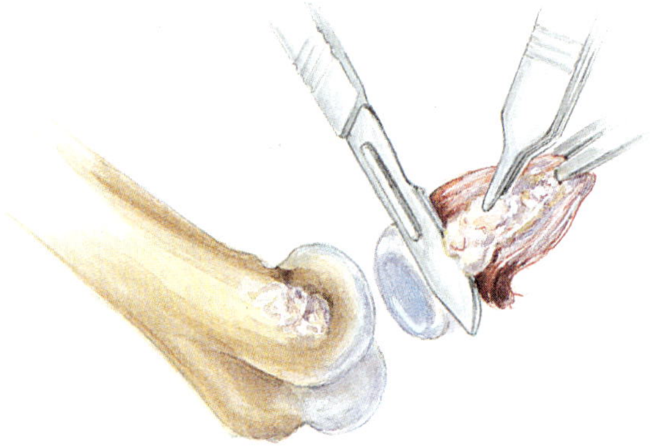

FIGURE 18-10 Débridement of pathologic tissue from the underside of the extensor mechanism.

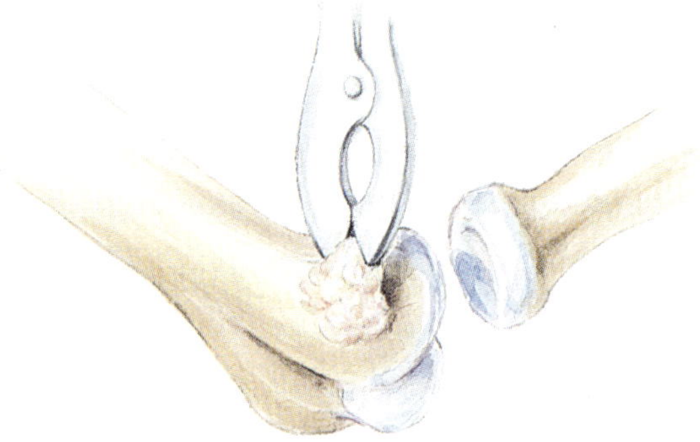

FIGURE 18-11 Decortication of the lateral epicondyle.

at the Kerlan-Jobe Orthopaedic Clinic, that excises the pathologic portion of the extensor tendon origin, repairs the defect, and reattaches the origin to the epicondyle.

Technique

Positioning

The patient is placed supine with the arm supported by an arm board. A tourniquet is applied to the upper arm, and the limb is then draped freely to allow ease of elbow and arm positioning.

Approach

An 8- to 10-cm incision centered over the lateral epicondyle is made in line with the upper arm and forearm (Fig. 18-8). Anterior and posterior subcutaneous flaps are developed with care to avoid any branches of the lateral cutaneous nerves.

Exposure and Débridement of Extensor Mechanism

The common extensor tendon then is completely delineated. The deep antebrachial fascia is incised over the lateral epicondyle, and the incision is continued distally toward the radiocapitellar articulation, exposing the fibrous common extensor origin and the extent of the lateral epicondyle. A sinus tract extending from the joint to the point of tendon damage often is noted. The common extensor tendon is then sharply detached subperiosteally from the epicondyle and reflected distally to expose the lateral compartment of the elbow (Fig. 18-9). The undersurface of the extensor mechanism is inspected for granulation tissue or tears. Most often a fibrinous tissue replacing the normal tendon is identified, but in approximately 35% a discrete tear of the extensor

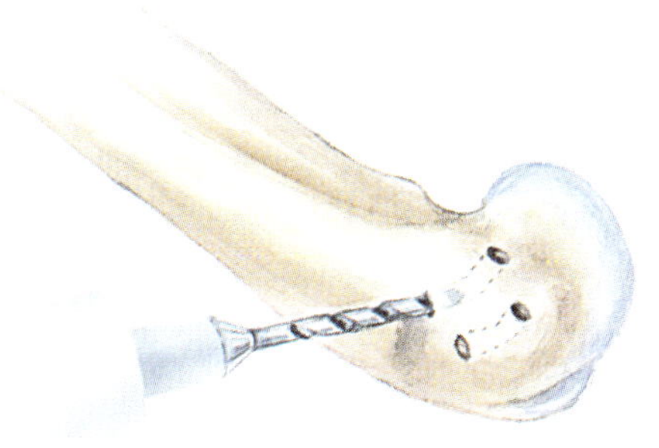

FIGURE 18-12 Drilling of V-shaped tunnels within the lateral epicondyle.

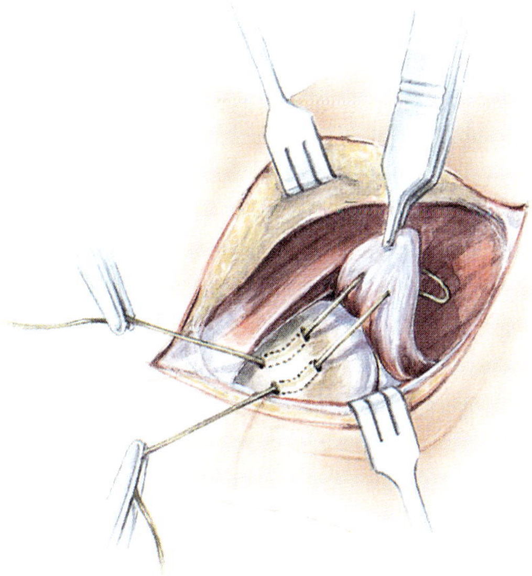

FIGURE 18-13 Reattachment of the extensor mechanism to the lateral epicondyle.

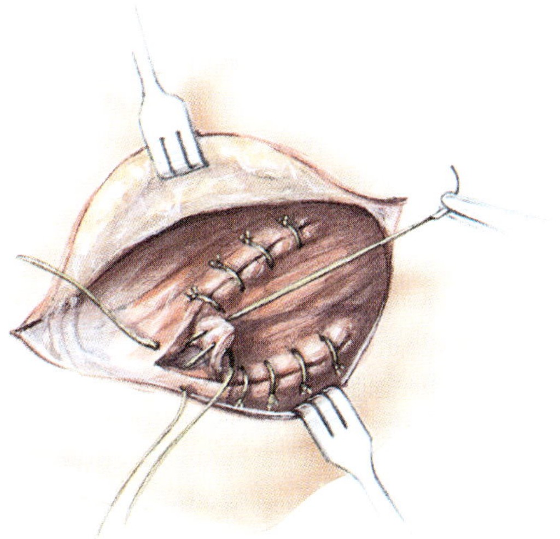

FIGURE 18-14 Side-to-side repair of the extensor tendon mechanism.

carpi radialis brevis is noted.[41] The radiocapitellar joint and synovium also are inspected for pathology. The degenerated portion of tendon, any granulation tissue, and fibrillated edges are sharply excised (Fig. 18-10). Most often this occurs on the undersurface of the extensor brevis, but in more severe cases it may extend to the extensor longus or extensor communis. The lateral epicondyle then is rongeured to provide a bleeding surface for extensor reattachment (Fig. 18-11). Care is taken not to excise too much bone, which may change the contour of the epicondyle and thus alter the resting length of the extensor muscles.

Repair of Extensor Mechanism

A 5/64-inch drill is used to create two parallel V-shaped tunnels directed anteroposteriorly in the lateral epicondyle (Fig. 18-12). A heavy suture is passed from posterior to anterior through the proximal tunnel, then through the extensor origin in a horizontal mattress fashion, and finally back anterior to posterior through the distal tunnel (Fig. 18-13). This provides optimal fixation and eliminates potential dead space between the tendon and the lateral epicondyle. A side-to-side repair of the extensor tendon mechanism is completed with simple interrupted absorbable sutures (Fig. 18-14).

Closure

The subcutaneous tissues are reapproximated with #3 absorbable sutures, and the skin is closed with a running subcuticular stitch. A molded posterior plaster splint is applied with the elbow in 90° of flexion and the forearm in neutral rotation, leaving the wrist and hand free.

Alternative Technique

Several authors[11,15,31,38] have described variations of this technique that involve a more limited extensor mechanism exposure. The origin of the extensor carpi radialis brevis is identified and split longitudinally (Fig. 18-15, *A*). The area of pathology is carefully identified and then sharply débrided (Fig. 18-15, *B*). Glousman[15] has recommended that a V-shaped tunnel be drilled perpendicular to the long axis of the extended arm (Fig. 18-15, *C*) and the extensor tendon be firmly attached to the lateral epicondyle with a nonabsorbable suture through the tunnel (Fig. 18-15, *D*). Coonrad,[11] Leach,[31] and Nirschl[38] have suggested that a side-to-side repair of the incised extensor be performed (Fig. 18-15, *E*). Regardless of the

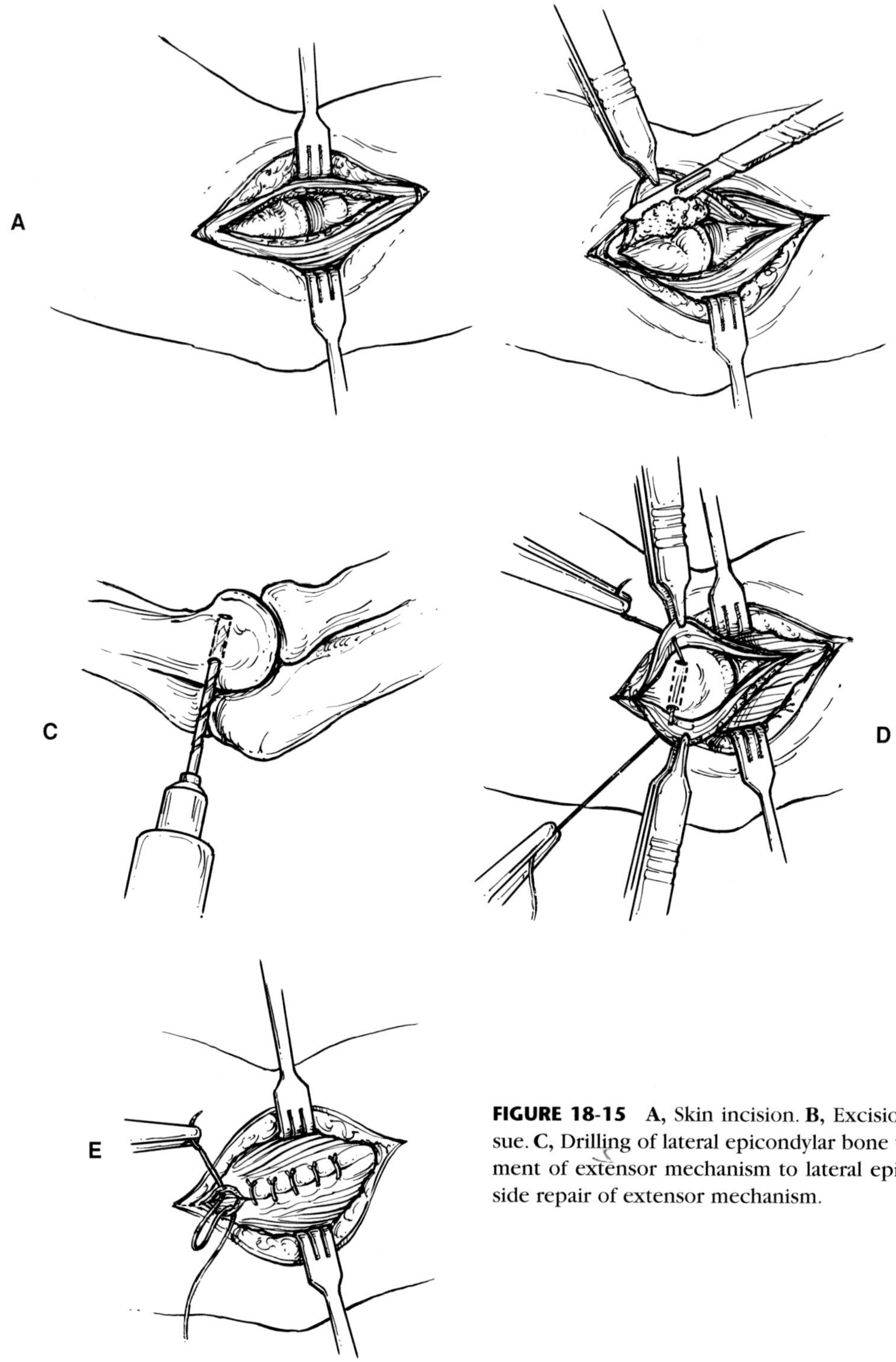

FIGURE 18-15 **A,** Skin incision. **B,** Excision of pathologic tissue. **C,** Drilling of lateral epicondylar bone tunnel. **D,** Reattachment of extensor mechanism to lateral epicondyle. **E,** Side-to-side repair of extensor mechanism.

amount of extensor mechanism exposed, care must be taken to meticulously examine the extensor tendon and thoroughly débride all pathologic tissue.

Postoperative Regimen

A posterior splint is maintained for 7 to 10 days. The splint and skin sutures then are removed, and the patient is begun on a progressive mobilization program. Gentle passive and active elbow, wrist, and hand range of motion is encouraged, but lifting and resisted wrist and finger dorsiflexion are avoided.

Light resisted isometric exercises are begun by 4 weeks, and progressive strengthening, including isotonic exercises, is initiated by 6 weeks. The patient returns to lifting activities or athletics by the third or fourth month. As activities begin, a body-conditioning program is conducted, as well as continued elbow-strengthening and endurance exercises.

Surgical Results

Many authors have reported favorable results with the aforementioned technique of extraarticular extensor débridement and repair. Nirschl,[38,41] Coonrad,[11,12] and Leach[31] noted 85% to 90% of patients returning to full activity without pain. Approximately 10% to 12%, however, were noted to have improvement but with some pain during aggressive activity. In approximately 2% to 3%, no appreciable improvement was obtained. In patients with persistent symptoms, the other previously mentioned etiologies of lateral elbow pain were pursued. Nirschl noted the maintenance of strength with dynamometer testing by 1 year in all those patients tested. At the Kerlan-Jobe Orthopaedic Clinic, 1200 patients with a diagnosis of lateral epicondylitis were treated over a 10-year period. Of these, 60 patients subsequently underwent extensor débridement and repair for persistent symptoms unresponsive to nonoperative treatment. Of these 60, 39 were seen in long-term follow-up. Of these 39 patients, 94% felt dramatic improvement in symptoms. Objectively, 36% had limitations with heavy lifting, 15% had grip dynamometer deficits, and 100% had some degree of isokinetic deficit. These authors have noted that the excellent subjective results after surgical treatment do not necessarily correlate with the objective findings of persistent weakness. With surgical treatment of lateral epicondylitis, patient satisfaction is extremely high, but residual strength deficits are concerns, especially in the heavy laborer or competitive athlete (unpublished data, Centinela Hospital Medical Center).

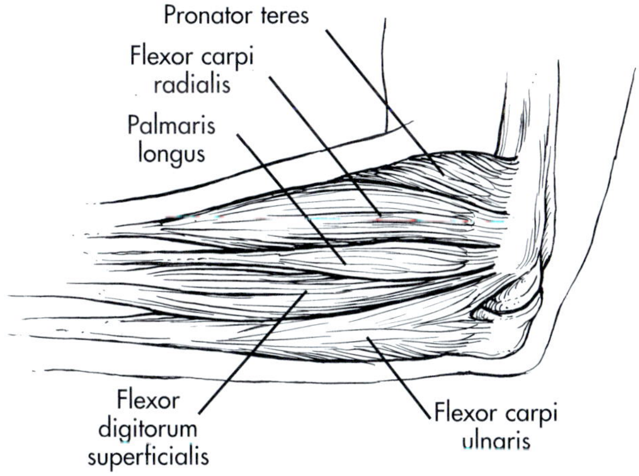

FIGURE 18-16 Musculotendinous anatomy of the medial elbow.

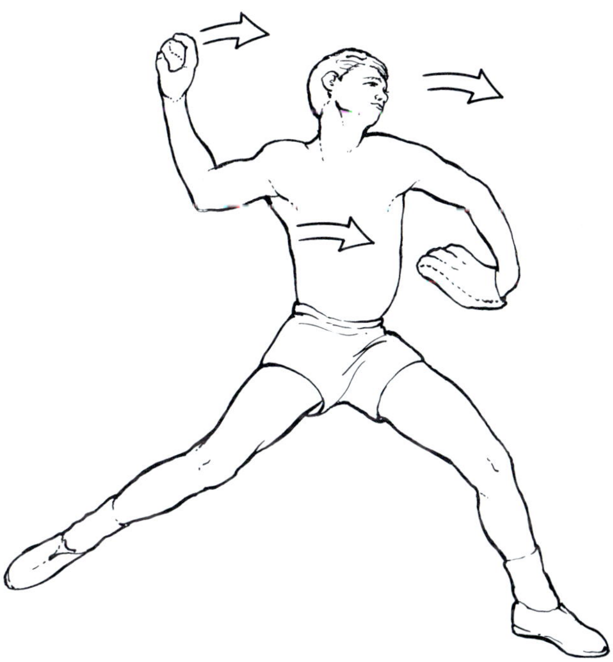

FIGURE 18-17 The acceleration phase of throwing.

MEDIAL EPICONDYLITIS

Anatomy

The musculotendinous anatomy of the medial epicondyle includes the flexor pronator muscle mass origin (Fig. 18-16). From proximal to distal, this includes the pronator teres, the flexor carpi radialis, the palmaris longus, the flexor digitorum superficialis, and the flexor carpi ulnaris. The pronator teres and flexor carpi radialis arise from the medial supracondylar ridge. The palmaris longus originates from the anterior midportion of the medial epicondyle. The flexor carpi ulnaris arises from beneath the palmaris longus fascia at the anterior base of the epicondyle. The flexor carpi ulnaris has two heads of origin, one from the most anterior distal aspect of the medial epicondyle, and the other from the medial aspect of the ulna.

Biomechanics

The biomechanics of the medial elbow have been most thoroughly defined by study of the throwing mechanism. Various authors[2,27,56] have described the phases of windup, cocking, acceleration, deceleration, and follow-through. It is primarily during the acceleration phase (Fig. 18-17), which extends from the point at which forward velocity of the ball is essentially zero to ball release, that peak angular velocity and valgus forces exceeding the tensile strength of the medial musculotendinous and ligamentous structures may be produced. As this phase begins, anterior momentum is transferred from the trunk to the arm. The humerus is internally rotated and adducted, creating torque at the elbow. At the midpoint of this phase, the rate of humeral adduction is slowed by the teres minor, infraspinatus, and supraspinatus, transferring momentum to the forearm and thereby accelerating the ball. Centrifugal forces on the ball and the forearm extend the elbow, creating the combination of medial tensile, lateral compressive, and resultant shear forces. These forces are transmitted initially to the flexor pronator musculature originating at the medial epicondyle and subsequently to the deeper medial collateral ligament.

Morris,[35] in his electromyographic evaluation of the tennis serve, corroborated the biomechanical theories of the baseball pitch. He noted that the highest muscle activity occurred during the acceleration phase and was seen in the pronator teres of the flexor pronator mass. He suggested that during this phase, the pronator is providing optimal forearm positioning while transferring momentum and power to the ball. Whether it be during a baseball pitch or a tennis serve, tremendous medial elbow forces are generated by the overhead mechanism.

Epidemiology/Etiology

Medial epicondylitis is a much rarer entity than its lateral counterpart, occurring at a ratio of 1:7 to 1:20,[11,31] and as such, it has received much less literary review. Medial epicondylitis similarly seems to occur within the fourth and fifth decades,[31] with an apparently equal male-to-female prevalence[31] and with a variety of sports and occupational activities.[2,31,33] Morris' original description[34] framed lawn tennis as the primary cause but also eluded to sculling as a possible etiology. Since then, many other activities that create a valgus stress across the elbow have been implicated.[31,33,41]

Pathophysiology

Much less controversy has shrouded the pathophysiology of medial epicondylitis than lateral epicondylitis. Most authors[27,31,41,60] suggest that valgus forces at the elbow create stress in the flexor pronator origin as well as the medial collateral ligament. The throwing athlete repetitively generates these forces with practice and competition. With proper mechanics, conditioning, and warm-up, most competitive athletes can tolerate the tremendous forces created by the throwing mechanism. Improper technique, poor conditioning, inadequate warm-up, and fatigue all can lead to inflammation of the flexor pronator mass. Nirschl,[41] Leach,[31] and Coonrad[11] have identified the pronator teres and flexor carpi radialis as the most common sites of these pathologic changes. Nirschl[41] suggests that vascular compromise, an altered nutritional state, and tissue overload result initially in the microscopic histologic changes of angiofibroblastic hyperplasia, and ultimately in macroscopic tissue disruption. Vangsness and Jobe[59] noted macroscopic tearing of the flexor pronator origin in 100% of their patients undergoing surgical treatment for recalcitrant medial epicondylitis.

Pathologic changes within the flexor pronator mass undoubtedly detract from its proper biomechanical function and thereby allow added stress to be transmitted to the medial collateral complex. Glousman[16] in 1992 used cinematography and indwelling electromyography to examine elbow muscle activity in pitchers with normal elbows and pitchers with medial collateral ligament injuries. He noted less pronator teres and flexor carpi radialis activity during the late cocking and acceleration phases in the subjects with collateral ligament injuries. He proposed that flexor pronator injury, as possibly reflected by its diminished, asynchronous EMG response, may lead to progressive medial ligamentous injury. Glousman and other authors[31,41] have proposed that these pathologic changes in the flexor pronator mass and medial ligaments may lead to a cascade of pathologic changes, including ulnar traction neuropathy, radiocapitellar joint overload, and posteromedial olecranon impingement.

Diagnosis

Medial epicondylitis is characterized by pain along the medial elbow that is worsened by resisted forearm pronation or wrist flexion. As with lateral epicondylitis, the medial pain may occur acutely but more often is insidious in onset. Patients also may complain of vague tingling in the ring and little fingers if ulnar nerve irritation has occurred.

Examination demonstrates tenderness over the flexor pronator origin. The tenderness usually is radial to the medial epicondyle and most often is over the pronator teres and flexor carpi radialis. Resisted wrist flexion and forearm pronation exacerbate the pain. Range of motion of the elbow and wrist is usually full. Normal strength and sensation typically are noted in the extremity. If the patient has concomitant ulnar neuropathy, however, varying degrees of diminished sensibility in the ring and little fingers as well as a positive Tinel's sign at the elbow may be present.

Radiographically, plain x-rays of the elbow often are normal. Throwing athletes, however, may have medial ulnar traction spurs and calcification within the medial ligament that are associated with chronic ligament strain.

When evaluating the patient with suspected medial epicondylitis, the clinician must consider primary ligamentous instability or primary ulnar neuropathy in the differential diagnosis. Both these entities undoubtedly will produce medial elbow pain. Medial elbow ligamentous instability produces pain during the acceleration phase of throwing. Tenderness occurs most often over the ulnar insertion of the medial collateral ligament and is exacerbated by valgus stress. If the patient's symptoms are due solely to medial epicondylitis, applying valgus stress with the wrist flexed and forearm pronated will not produce either pain or laxity.

The patient with long-standing primary ulnar neuritis often will complain of posteromedial elbow pain and symptoms extending into the forearm and hand.[17] Examination typically reveals tenderness directly along the ulnar nerve, especially within the cubital tunnel and along its course between the heads of the flexor carpi ulnaris. The elbow flexion test may help confirm the diagnosis of ulnar neuropathy within the cubital tunnel. This test involves maximally flexing the elbow and extending the wrist for 3 minutes. If this test is positive, the patient will feel pain, numbness, and tingling along the ulnar nerve distribution. Electrodiagnostic tests are helpful when positive, but a normal test does not rule out neuritis. Nirschl[41] has reported ulnar neurapraxia in 60% of patients with symptoms of medial epicondylar origin, but Coonrad[11] believes ulnar neuropathy associated with medial epicondylitis is much less common. Appropriate diagnosis of medial elbow pain obviously is essential to successful treatment.

Treatment

Nonsurgical

The basic principles of nonoperative treatment for lateral epicondylitis apply to medial elbow musculotendinous pathology as well. Relief of initial pain and inflammation, or phase 1, similarly consists of rest from the offending activity. The use of nonsteroidal antiinflammatories, galvanic stimulation, and possibly corticosteroid injection may provide adjuvant benefit. Phase 2, as with lateral epicondylitis, emphasizes continued tissue healing through the avoidance of the abusive aspects of the causative activity and through guided rehabilitation. Technique enhancement, equipment modification, and counterforce bracing also are important at this point. The rehabilitative program begins with wrist flexor and forearm pronator stretching and progressive isometric exercises. As flexibility, strength, and endurance improve, eccentric and concentric resistive exercises are included. As with lateral epicondylitis, when the patient can perform repetition to fatigue without significant medial pain, a sport or job simulation is performed. With successful completion of the simulation, return to normal activity is allowed. The duration and intensity of exposure are gradually increased on return. The majority of authors[11,31,41,59] note that medial epicondylitis most often responds successfully to such a nonsurgical regimen.

Surgical

History

The indications for surgical treatment of medial epicondylitis include persistent pain at the medial elbow unresponsive to a well-managed nonoperative program for at least 6 to 12 months and exclusion of any other pathologic causes for the pain.

There is little historical information on the surgical treatment of medial epicondylitis. Coonrad[12] in 1973 described resection of the degenerated or torn tissue with subsequent reapproximation of the remaining healthy tendon in 39 patients with either lateral or medial epicondylitis. Baumgard[1] in 1982 suggested the percutaneous release of epicondylar muscles for medial epicondylitis. Nirschl[41] in 1985 proposed longitudinal and elliptic excision of the reactive fibrous tissue in the flexor pronator mass with care to preserve the origin's integrity. The same basic principles of resection of all pathologic tissue and firm reattachment of the flexor pronator mass were reiterated by Vangsness and Jobe[59] in 1991.

Technique

Positioning

The patient is placed supine with the arm resting on an arm board. A tourniquet is employed, and the limb is draped free for ease of positioning.

Approach/Exposure

An 8- to 10-cm incision is centered over the medial epicondyle paralleling the longitudinal axes of the upper arm and forearm (Fig. 18-18). The cutaneous nerves are identified and protected, and the position and status of the ulnar nerve are confirmed. The common flexor origin is incised sharply and reflected with care not to violate the medial collateral ligament. The pathologic tissue is identified on the undersurface of the flexor pronator mass, most often the pronator teres and flexor carpi radialis, and excised (Fig. 18-19).

Repair of Flexor Pronator Mechanism

The underlying medial epicondyle is debrided of soft tissue, and multiple small holes are drilled to create a vascular bed. The common flexor pronator origin is then

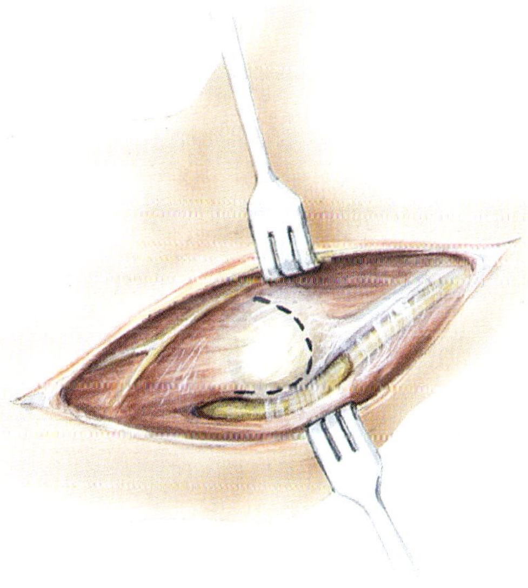

FIGURE 18-18 Skin incision overlying the medial epicondyle with exposed cutaneous and ulnar nerves; intended incision of common flexor pronator mass.

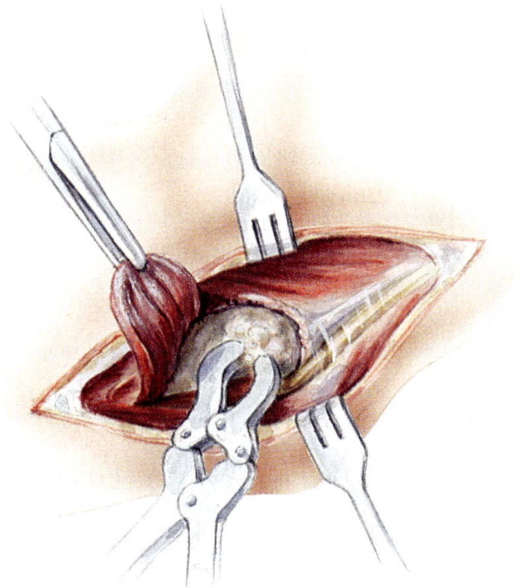

FIGURE 18-19 Distal reflection of the common flexor pronator origin with excision of pathologic tissue.

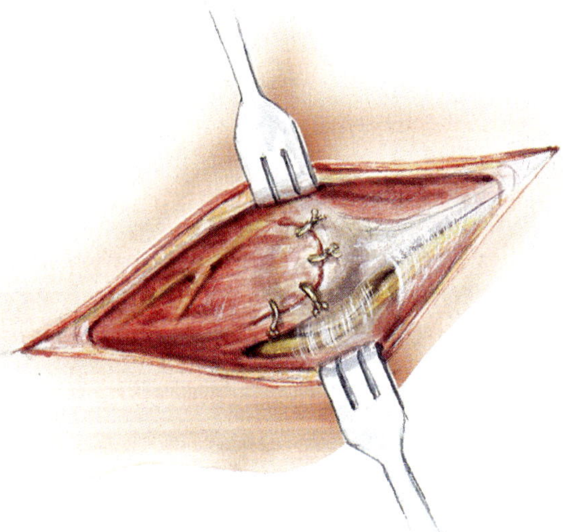

FIGURE 18-20 Reattachment of the common flexor pronator origin to the medial epicondyle.

reattached to this bleeding surface with interrupted absorbable sutures (Fig. 18-20). Care is taken to preserve the normal resting length of the forearm muscles.

Closure

The subcutaneous tissues are reapproximated with #3 absorbable sutures, and the skin is closed with a running subcuticular stitch. A molded posterior plaster splint is then applied with the elbow at 90° of flexion, the forearm in neutral rotation, and the wrist and hand free.

Postoperative Regimen

Sponge-squeezing exercises and wrist and hand range-of-motion exercises are initiated immediately. The splint and skin sutures are removed at 7 to 10 days after surgery. Gentle passive and active elbow, wrist, and hand range of motion are encouraged. Resisted wrist flexion and pronation exercises are initiated at 4 to 6 weeks, followed by a progressive strengthening program. Return to activity is generally attained by the fourth postoperative month.

Surgical Results

Coonrad's 1973 review of epicondylitis[12] addressed both lateral and medial pathology. The results of both entities were presented together, and so selective analysis of patients with medial epicondylitis is not possible. The author reported, however, satisfactory results with return to preoperative activities in all patients undergoing surgery.

Baumgard's 1982 report[1] also described the results for both lateral and medial epicondylitis after percutaneous release. The author performed the medial procedure on six patients; the results of five were rated as excellent and one was unsatisfactory. This one unsatisfactory result was related to a persistent anterior muscle band that required rerelease.

Vangsness and Jobe's review of 35 patients with recalcitrant medial epicondylitis[59] treated surgically revealed that subjective elbow function improved from 38% to 98% of normal. Excellent or good results were obtained in 97%, and 86% of patients had no limitation in the use of the elbow. Isokinetic and grip strength testing in 16 patients revealed no significant difference between operated and unoperated elbows. Of the 35, 14% had significant preoperative ulnar nerve symptoms with subluxation or scarring that required concomitant anterior transposition. All of the 20 athletically active patients returned to their sport. The authors concluded that surgical treatment of recalcitrant medial epicondylitis is efficacious in relieving pain, restoring strength, and allowing return to previous activities.

SUMMARY

Although named in a simple correspondence in the pages of *Lancet* in 1882, epicondylitis of the elbow has since prompted the minds and pens of many researchers. This has resulted in a plethora of descriptive, diagnostic, and therapeutic reports detailing every aspect of this entity. For example, researchers have reported that epicondylitis may result not only from sport but also from occupational activities, that its diagnosis may be confused with a variety of other elbow pathologic entities, and that in the majority of patients it will respond to nonoperative treatment. Yet, in spite of this dramatically increased knowledge, diagnostic and therapeutic dilemmas continue. So, it is only with a thorough understanding of lateral and medial epicondylitis of the elbow that the physician may provide the most effective treatment regimen, as was the hope of those who first described it: "I trust we shall get some advice which will enable us to effect a speedy cure to this, to say the least, very inconvenient affection, 'tennis elbow.' "[32]

References

1. Baumgard SH, Schwartz DR: Percutaneous release of the epicondylar muscles for humeral epicondylitis, *Am J Sports Med* 10(4):233-236, 1982.
2. Bennett GE: Elbow and shoulder lesions of baseball players, *Am J Surg* 98:484-492, 1959.
3. Bernhang AM, Dehner W, Fogarty C: Tennis elbow: a biomechanical approach, *J Sports Med* 2:235-260, 1974.
4. Binder AI, Hazleman BL: Lateral humeral epicondylitis—a study of natural history and the effect of conservative therapy, *Br J Rheumatol* 22:73-76, 1983.
5. Bosworth DM: The role of the orbicular ligament in tennis elbow, *J Bone Joint Surg* 37A:527-533, 1955.
6. Boyd HB, McLeod AC: Tennis elbow, *J Bone Joint Surg* 55A(6): 1183-1187, 1973.
7. Carp L: Tennis elbow caused by radiohumeral bursitis, *Arch Surg* 24:905-909, 1932.
8. Carroll RE, Jorgensen EC: Evaluation of the garden procedure for lateral epicondylitis, *Clin Orthop* 60:201-204, Sept-Oct, 1968.
9. Cassidy J, Bole G: Cutaneous atrophy secondary to intra-articular corticosteroid administration, *Ann Intern Med* 65:1008-1017, 1966.
10. Clarke A, Woodland J: Comparison of two steroid preparations used to treat tennis elbow using the hypospray, *Rheumatol Rehabil* 14:47-49, 1979.
11. Coonrad RW: Tendonopathies at the elbow, *AAOS Instr Course Lect* XL:25-32, 1991.
12. Coonrad RW, Hooper WR: Tennis elbow: its course, natural history, conservative and surgical management, *J Bone Joint Surg* 55-A(6):1177-1182, 1973.
13. Froimson AI: Treatment of tennis elbow with forearm support band, *J Bone Joint Surg* 53A:183-184, 1971.
14. Garden RS: Tennis elbow, *J Bone Joint Surg* 43B:100-106, 1961.
15. Glousman RE: Surgical treatment of lateral epicondylitis (tennis elbow), *Tech Orthop* 6(1):33-38, 1991.
16. Glousman RE et al: An electromyographic analysis of the elbow in normal and injured pitchers with medial collateral ligament insufficiency, *Am J Sports Med* 20(3):311-317, 1992.
17. Glousman RE: Ulnar nerve problems in the athlete's elbow, *Clin Sports Med* 9(2):365-377, 1990.
18. Goldberg EJ, Abraham E, Siegel I: The surgical treatment of chronic lateral humeral epicondylitis by common extensor release, *Clin Orthop* 233:208-212, 1983.
19. Goldie I: Epicondylitis lateralis humeri: a pathologic study, *Acta Chir Scand* (suppl) 34:339-344, 1964.

20. Groppel JL, Nirschl RP: A mechanical and electromyographical analysis of the effects of various joint counterforce braces on the tennis player, *Am J Sports Med* 14(3):195-200, 1986.
21. Gruchow HW, Pelletier D: An epidemiologic study of tennis elbow: incidence, recurrence, and effectiveness of prevention strategies, *Am J Sports Med* 7(4):234-242, 1979.
22. Gunn CC, Milbrandt WE: Tennis elbow and the cervical spine, *Can Med Assoc J* 114:803-809, 1976.
23. Hansson KG, Horwich ID: Epicondylitis humeri, *JAMA* 94:1557-1561, 1930.
24. Hohmann G: Uber den tennisellboggen. Verhand lungen der deutschen orthopaedischen gesselschaft, *Kong* 21:349-353, 1926.
25. Ilfeld FW, Field SM: Treatment of tennis elbow: use of special brace, *JAMA* 195(2):67, 1966.
26. Indelicato PA et al: Correctable elbow lesions in professional baseball players: a review of 25 cases, *Am J Sports Med* 7(1):72-77, 1979.
27. Jobe FW, Kvitne RS: Elbow instability in the athlete, *AAOS Instr Course Lect* XL:17-23, 1991.
28. Kaplan EB: Treatment of tennis elbow (epicondylitis) by denervation, *J Bone Joint Surg* 41-A:147-151, 1959.
29. Kelley J et al: EMG and cinematographic analysis of elbow function in tennis players with lateral epicondylitis, *Am J Sports Med* 22(3):359-363, 1994.
30. Kerlan RK, Glousman RE: Injections and techniques in athletic medicine, *Clin Sports Med* (8):541-560, 1989.
31. Leach RE, Miller JK: Lateral and medial epicondylitis of the elbow, *Clin Sports Med* 6(2):259-272, 1987.
32. Major HP: Lawn tennis elbow, *Br Med J* 2:557, 1883.
33. Miller JE: Javelin thrower's elbow, *J Bone Joint Surg* 42B:788-792, 1960.
34. Morris H: The rider's sprain, *Lancet* 2:133-134, 1882.
35. Morris M et al: Electromyographic analysis of elbow function in tennis players, *Am J Sports Med* 17(2):241-247, 1989.
36. Nevelos AB: The treatment of tennis elbow with triamcinolone acetonide, *Curr Med Res Opin* (6):507-509, 1980.
37. Newman JH, Goodfellow JW: Fibrillation of the head of the radius as one cause of tennis elbow, *Br Med J* 2:328-330, 1975.
38. Nirschl RP, Pettrone FA: Tennis elbow. The surgical treatment of lateral epicondylitis, *J Bone Joint Surg* 61A(6):832-839, 1979.
39. Nirschl RP: Correspondence, *J Bone Joint Surg* 62A:314, 1980.
40. Nirschl RP, Sobel J: Conservative treatment of tennis elbow, *Phys Sports Med* 9:42-49, 1981.
41. Nirschl RP: Muscle and tendon trauma; tennis elbow, the elbow and its disorder. In Morrey BF, editor: *The elbow and its disorders,* Philadelphia, 1985, WB Saunders, pp 481-496.
42. Nirschl RP: Tennis elbow. *Orthop Clin North Am* 4(3):787-800, 1973.
43. Ogilvie WH: Discussion on minor injuries of the elbow, *Joint Proc Royal Soc Med* 23:306-322, 1929.
44. Osgood RB: Radiohumeral bursitis, epicondylitis, epicondylalgia (tennis elbow): a personal experience, *Arch Surg* 4:420-433, 1922.
45. Posch JN, Goldberg VM, Larrey R: Extensor fasciotomy for tennis elbow: a long term follow-up study, *Clin Orthop* 135:179-182, 1978.
46. Price R et al: Local injection treatment of tennis elbow—hydrocortisone triamcinolone and lignocaine compared, *Br J Rheumatol* 30:39-44, 1991.
47. Priest JD, Braden V, Gerberich JG: The elbow and tennis (part I), *Phys Sports Med* 8(4):80-87, 1980.
48. Priest JD, Braden V, Gerberich JG: The elbow and tennis (part II), *Phys Sports Med* 8(5):77-83, 1980.
49. Regan W et al: *Microscopic histopathology of lateral epicondylitis.* Presented at the 57th Annual Meeting of the American Academy of Orthopaedic Surgeons, New Orleans, Feb 8-13, 1990.
50. Roles NC, Maudsley RH: Radial tunnel syndrome: resistant tennis elbow as a nerve entrapment, *J Bone Joint Surg* 54:499-508, 1972.
51. Runge F: Zur genese und behandlung des schriebek-rampfes, *Berliner Klin Wchnschr* 10:245-248, 1873.
52. Snyder-Macker L, Epler M: Effect of standard and aircast tennis elbow bands on integrated electromyography of forearm extensor musculature proximal to the bands, *Am J Sports Med* 17(2):278-281, 1989.
53. Spencer GE, Herndon CH: Surgical treatment of epicondylitis, *J Bone Joint Surg* 35-A:421-424, 1953.
54. Stack JK: Acute and chronic bursitis in the region of the elbow joint, *Surg Clin North Am* 29:155-162, 1949.
55. Trethowan WH: Tennis elbow, *Br Med J* 2:1218-1224, 1929.
56. Tullos HS, King JW: Throwing mechanism in sports, *Orthop Clin North Am* 4:709-720, 1973.
57. Unverferth LJ, Olix ML: The effect of local steroid injection on tendon, *J Sports Med* 1(4):31-37, 1973.
58. Van Rossum et al: Tennis elbow—a radial tunnel syndrome, *J Bone Joint Surg* 60-B:197-198, 1978.
59. Vangsness CT, Jobe FW: Surgical treatment of medial epicondylitis, *J Bone Joint Surg* 73B(3):409-411, 1991.
60. Woods GW, Tullos HS, King JW: The throwing arm—elbow joint injuries, *J Sports Med* 1(4):43-52, 1973.

CHAPTER 19

Fractures and Dislocations of the Elbow

ROBERT W. CHANDLER
JERRY L. BARRON

Athletes are not prone to unusual types of fractures other than stress fractures,* so the sports-medicine physician must have a good working knowledge of the overall range and depth of fractures and dislocations about the elbow. The purpose of this chapter is to present a condensed version of the voluminous material on these injuries to aid orthopedists treating athletes with such injuries.

Fractures and dislocations of the elbow result from moderately high-energy trauma. Commonly, injury forces

*References 58, 67, 80, 89, 94, 97.

are indirect, having been transmitted through the extremity in a fall, and are the result of leverage applied in various directions as the forearm and hand twist, rotate, and/or bend relative to the arm and torso. More willful activity may contribute direct forces producing significant injury, such as in contact sports. It is important to consider the possibility that the injury mechanism has caused associated injuries elsewhere, specifically, the soft-tissue component, which may have a more profound influence on recovery than does the obvious bone injury.[60,91]

Motion loss of the elbow may be disabling, particularly for athletic individuals, so initial treatment must consider the aggressive rehabilitation necessary to restore adequate function.[34,66] Active people come with high expectations and will judge their recovery on a comparison with normal function, in spite of the severity of the injury.

Stable bone injuries must be moved rapidly or operatively stabilized to be moved rapidly. After anatomic restoration of bone, loss of function after elbow trauma occurs primarily because of these soft-tissue injuries: capsular thickening with loss of compliance, capsular contracture, adhesions between the capsule and the articular cartilage, and muscular fibrosis and contracture.

The soft-tissue constraints of the elbow have been studied in both their normal and pathologic states.* Fig. 19-1 illustrates the capsule and capsular ligaments. Treatment of fractures around the elbow should take into account the soft-tissue and bony injuries.

*References 26,27,36,59-62,90,91.

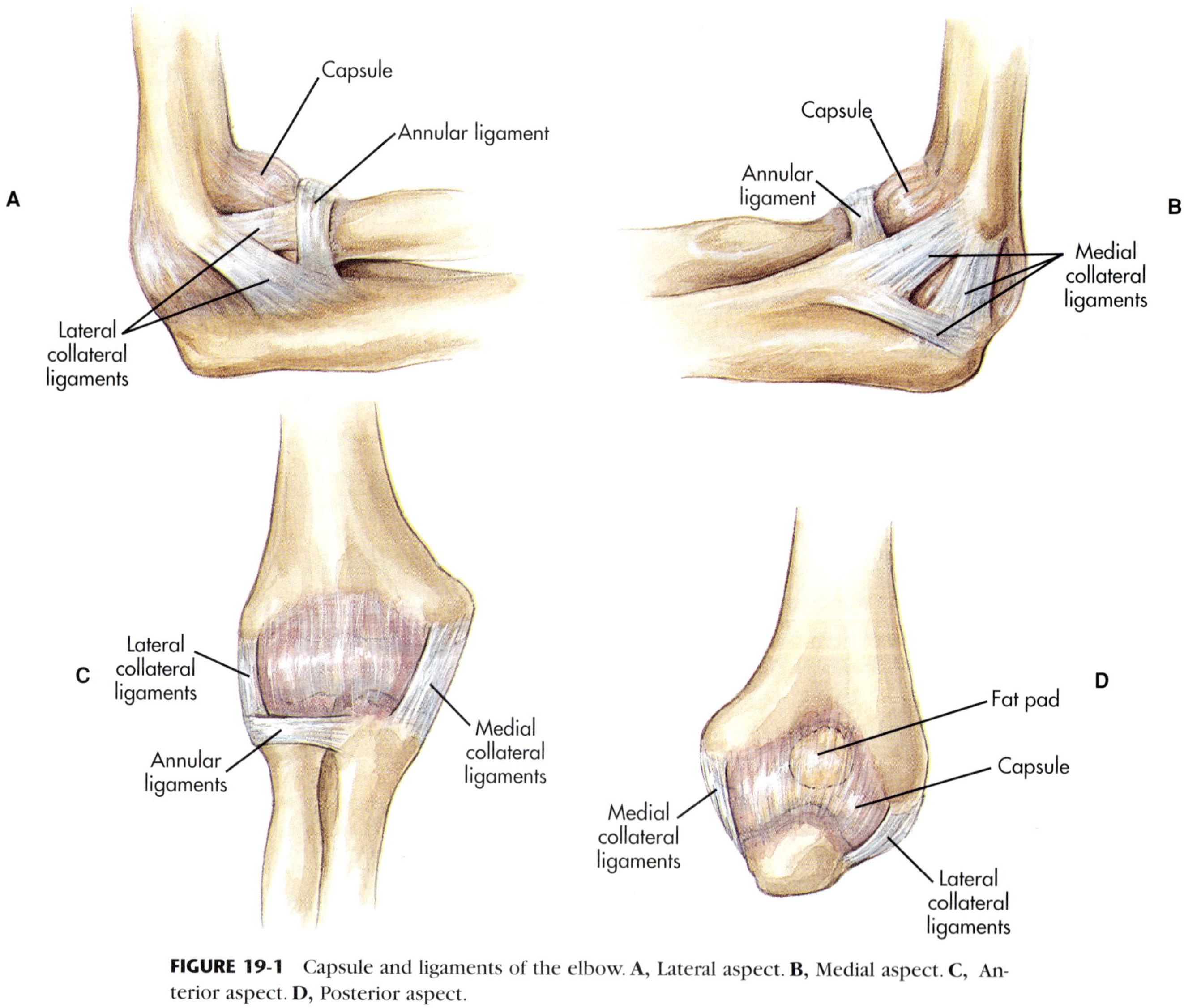

FIGURE 19-1 Capsule and ligaments of the elbow. **A,** Lateral aspect. **B,** Medial aspect. **C,** Anterior aspect. **D,** Posterior aspect.

EVALUATION

Swelling, pain, guarding, reduced motion, point tenderness, and deformity should be assessed and noted on examination. A neurovascular assessment should be performed immediately and should be repeated subsequently to detect the rare but devastating problems of nerve palsy, vascular disruption, and compartment syndrome. The state of the arm after trauma is dynamic and may progress from a benign condition to an emergency. Fig. 19-2 presents a flow chart for initial and subsequent assessments.

Significant swelling of the antecubital fossa may be present. If the patient is examined early, the bony prominence about the elbow can be palpated. Disruption of the isosceles triangle formed by the olecranon and epicondyle indicates dislocation or fracture. Tenderness over the lateral elbow associated with pain radiating down the radial aspect of the forearm is presumptive evidence of a radial head fracture.

Physical examinations must be supplemented with anteroposterior, lateral, and condylar view radiographs. Tomography, planar or computed, is necessary in some instances to clarify anatomic vagaries in complex fractures, whereas magnetic resonance imaging helps in detecting occult trauma, such as a stress fracture of the olecranon.

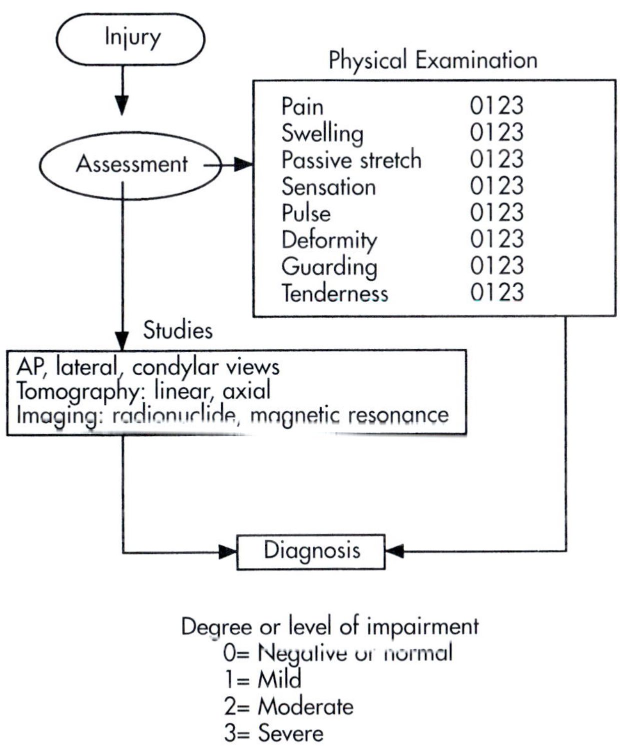

FIGURE 19-2 Clinical assessment flow chart. Initial stages of patient management after elbow fracture identify and grade the soft-tissue components of the injury as well as the bony ones. A graded scale of severity is useful in sequential observations, particularly with compartment syndrome and neurovascular injuries.

Treatment

When the diagnosis has been clearly established, treatment is considered. Rapid mobilization to attain the highest functional level is the key objective of treatment and should guide decision-making.[34,66] Ideally, fracture healing and rehabilitation occur simultaneously (Fig. 19-3). Conservative care will yield good results for many injuries, but surgery must be considered first in displaced fractures.

Early surgery is preferable to later surgery, but the surgeon must balance urgency with his or her skill level and the readiness of the surgical team. The surgeon first must adequately comprehend complex fractures, then prepare an operative plan, select a proper incision, and assemble the proper tools and personnel.[49] Only after these requirements are satisfied should surgery proceed.

OPERATIVE APPROACHES

Access to the elbow from every direction is necessary to treat the wide range of injuries occurring in the region (Box 19-1). It is essential to master the neurovascular anatomy of the region to avoid ruinous complications. Soft-tissue handling must be delicate, and frequent irrigation with Ringer's lactate solution will help preserve tissue viability.

Posterior

Indications

A posterior approach allows for visualization of the entire posterior aspect of the distal humerus from the mid-distal-third junction of the diaphysis to the chondral surfaces of the joint. Three variations are possible: (1) reflection of the triceps tendon insertion (pure soft tissue), (2) reflection of the triceps tendon with a bone pedicle but without violation of the ulnar humeral joint (extraarticular osteotomy), and (3) olecranon osteotomy through the elbow joint (intraarticular osteotomy).

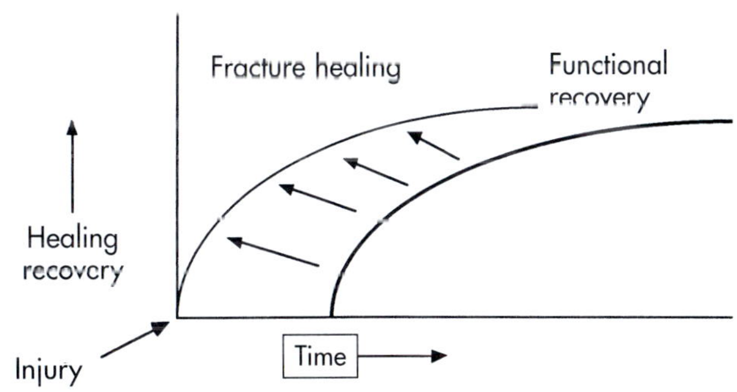

FIGURE 19-3 Fracture healing and rehabilitation. The process of fracture healing is more rapid than the process of functional recovery. Ultimate functional recovery is greater when the two processes are simultaneous rather than sequential. Synchronous fracture healing and recovery of function are possible with stable fractures or fractures made stable.

BOX 19-1

OPERATIVE APPROACH AND FRACTURE PATTERNS

Posterior Approach

Extraosseous
- Olecranon
- Coronoid
- Humerus: A3

Extraarticular olecranon osteotomy
- Humerus: A2, A3, B1, C1

Intraarticular olecranon osteotomy
- Humerus: B2, B3, C2, C3

Lateral Approach

Kocher
- Humerus: A1, B3
- Radius: type II
- Arthrofibrosis

Modified Kocher
- Radius: type III

Medial Approach

Humerus: A1

Anterior Approach

Coronoid
Myositis

Morrey has recommended avoiding intraarticular osteotomies to avoid nonunion (5%) and intraarticular adhesions.[60] However, intraarticular osteotomy is necessary in cases of severe articular fragmentation. The nonarticular approaches are adequate for the remainder of fractures requiring posterior exposure. The authors prefer the bone pedicle technique because it uses tension band wiring that is secure enough for immediate motion.[22]

Technique

The patient is placed prone or in the half-lateral position with the fractured extremity draped free. A sterile tourniquet is used for most fractures. The skin incision is over the subcutaneous border of the ulna and extended proximally parallel to the long axis of the humerus. A short proximal extension is needed for olecranon fractures.

Olecranon osteotomies must be preceded by the exposure of the ulnar nerve and release of the ulnar nerve from the arcade of Frohse to the branch of the flexor carpi ulnaris. The nerve should be protected during the procedure and transferred anteriorly and subcutaneously at the end of the procedure. Submuscular transposition risks entrapment in scarring in already traumatized muscle.

Skin flaps are well vascularized but must be respected as the barrier to infection. Gentle handling of the soft tissue is essential. Desiccation must be prevented by frequent irrigation. Soft-tissue attachments to bone must be preserved. At the same time, adequate visualization is mandatory. All fixation, including the olecranon osteotomy, must be solid to allow for motion in the first few days after surgery. Tension band fixation with Kirschner wires and a wire loop will apply to all osteotomies, and lag fixation with a 6.5- to 7.0-mm cancellous screw will provide very secure fixation for most osteotomies.

Lateral

Indications

Fragments of bone can be removed from the joint, including radial head fragments, from the lateral approach. Lateral condyle fractures and some capitellar fractures also are accessible. Repairable radial head fractures can be internally fixed through this aperture. The extensor group can be reflected with a bone pedicle from the lateral humerus to provide additional visualization. The bone pedicle is reattached with a small lag screw.

Technique

The patient can be positioned either prone or supine. The prone position allows for better orientation for capitellar fractures without trochlear involvement but requires more setup time and potentially compromises ventilation.

The interval between the anconeus and the extensor carpi ulnaris is opened down to the capsule, which is opened in line with the skin. A generous incision allows for visualization of the entire radiocapitellar joint without risk to the radial nerve as long as the incision is not extended distal to the annular ligament or proximal to the brachioradialis. Proximal extension divides the interval between the triceps posteriorly and the brachioradialis and extensor group anteriorly.

Medial

Indications

Medial epicondylar fractures, with either acute or chronic instability, are best approached medially. This approach is used for decompression of the ulnar nerve and anterior transfer.

Technique

The surgeon must be aware of the location of the ulnar nerve but need not dissect the nerve unless ligament reconstruction is being performed. External rotation of the shoulder must be adequate for good visualization of medial epicondylar fractures; otherwise a half-lateral or prone position is advisable.

Anterior

Indications

Classic myositis can be excised through an anterior approach. The anterior capsule also is accessible for exci-

A

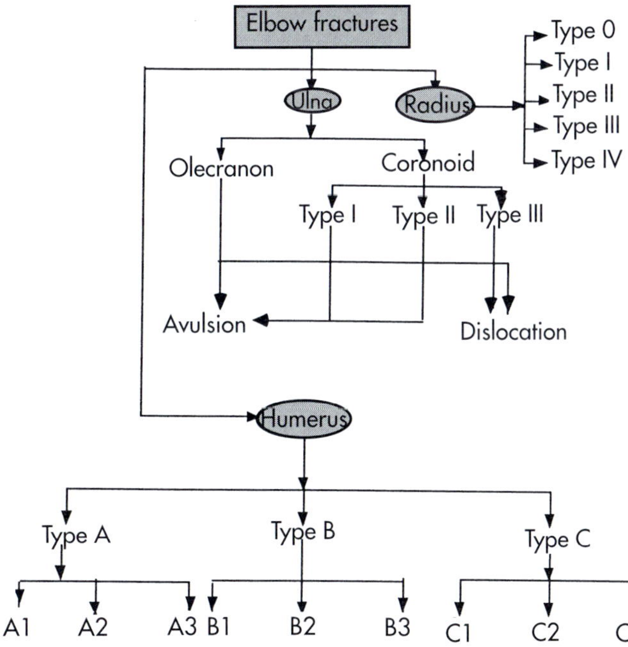

FIGURE 19-4 **A,** Combined classification of fractures about the elbow: distal humerus, proximal radius, and proximal ulna. *Continued.*

sion in cases of severe capsular adhesions. This approach may be useful in cases of coronoid fracture that are not accessible from a posterior approach. Anterior capsulectomy with lengthening of the brachialis tendon is possible with this approach.

Technique

An incision is initiated proximal to the flexion crease of the elbow, extends longitudinally to the antecubital fossa, curves medially, and then extends distally down the lateral border of the forearm. After the surgeon divides the cubital fascia and the lacertus fibrosus, the median nerve, brachial artery, brachialis, and biceps tendons are visualized. Access to the anterior capsule is gained by splitting the brachialis muscle.

FRACTURES

Distal Humerus

Elbow fractures are known according to eponym, anatomic location, and systematic cataloging (Fig. 19-4, *A*). Recent efforts have contributed newer classifications that illustrate changing perceptions and deeper insights into these complex injuries.[54] A classification system has merit for several reasons: It adequately describes variations in morphology, it suggests a type of treatment, it has prognostic significance, and finally, it can be remembered from month to month (Fig. 19-4, *B*). The classification system developed by the Arbeitsgemeinschaft für Osteosynthesefragen (AO/ASIF) is most consistent with these objectives.[64] The AO classification takes into account comminution and therefore takes the severity of the fracture into account (Fig. 19-5).

A-type distal humerus fractures are metaphyseal and consist of three subclasses. A1 fractures are avulsion fractures of purely metaphyseal bone, A2 fractures are simple, complete metaphyseal fractures, and A3 fractures are similar to A2 but comminuted (Fig. 19-6). The B-series fractures are intraarticular fractures, with B1 involving the lateral column, B2 the medial column, and B3 the anterior aspect of the joint portion of the humerus (Fig. 19-7). The C-series fractures consist of bicolumnar intraarticular fractures with three grades of comminution (Fig. 19-8).

A-Series Fractures: Treatment and Results

A-series fractures (supracondylar fractures) are extraarticular. They are rare in adults and occur in children.[31,33,83] There are three subgroups of this fracture:

A1—apophyseal avulsion
A2—simple metaphyseal
A3—comminuted metaphyseal

A1 injuries are avulsion fractures and typically involve the medial epicondyle of adolescents or children.[41] The medial epicondyle is avulsed from the humerus during a posterior elbow dislocation. Occasionally, the epicondylar fragment may become incarcerated within the joint when the elbow is reduced.[41] This fracture almost always is associated with dislocation of the elbow when it occurs in an adult.[81] Indications for open reduction and internal fixation include entrapment of the ulnar nerve within the joint, incarcerated epicondylar frag-

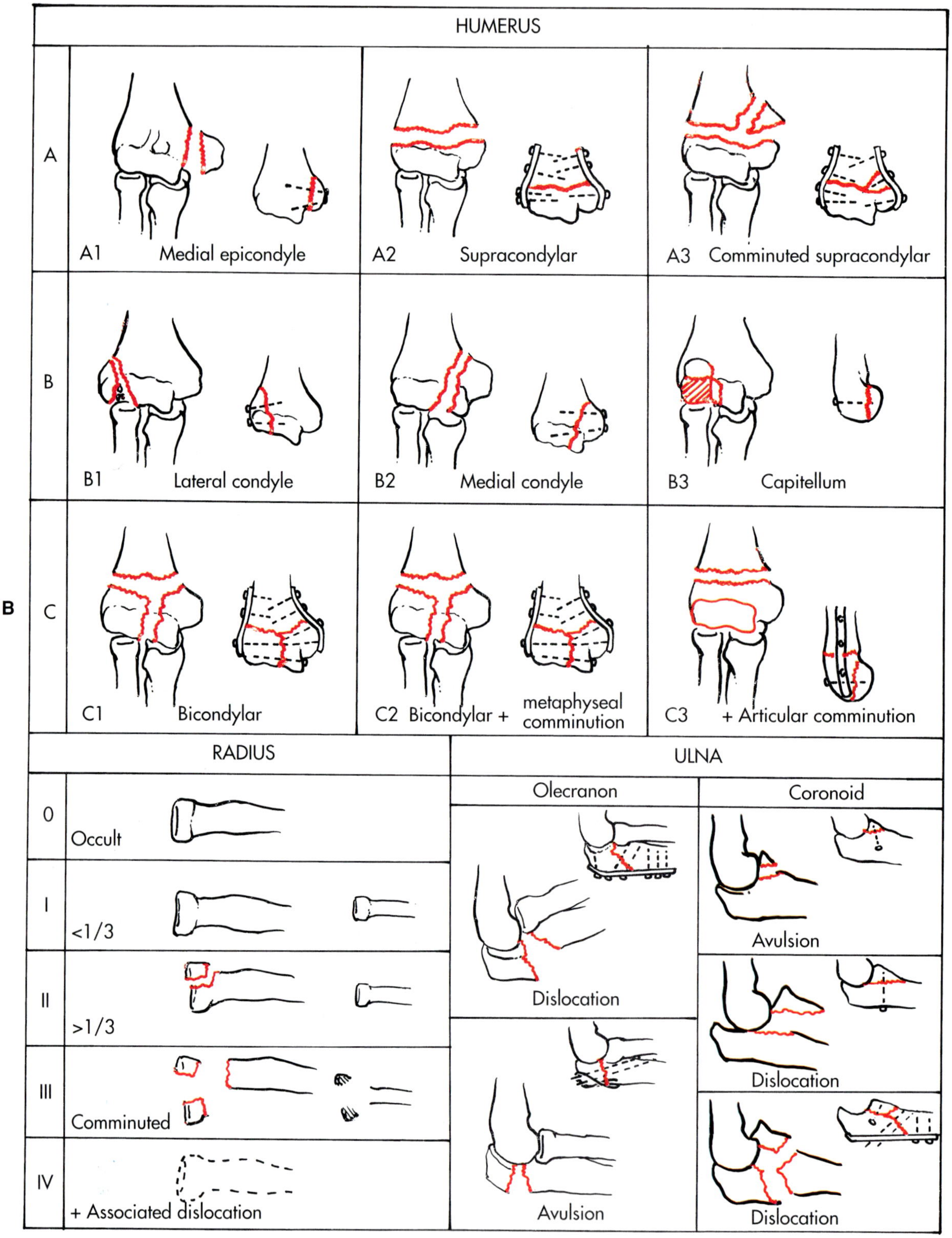

FIGURE 19-4—cont'd **B,** the spectrum of fractures about the elbow along with the treatments by internal fixation.

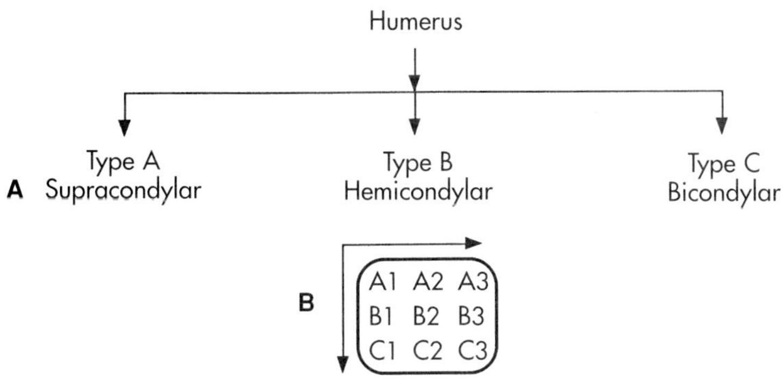

FIGURE 19-5 **A,** AO/ASIF classifications of distal humerus fractures. **B,** Severity and prognosis matrix. The AO/ASIF classification orders injuries according to morphology as well as severity.

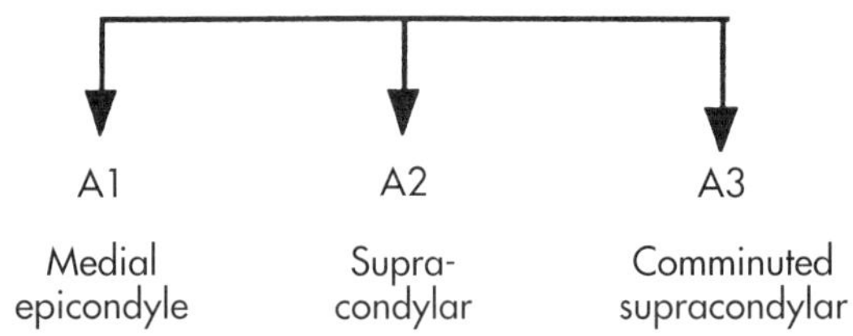

FIGURE 19-6 A fractures comprise three subgroups (see text).

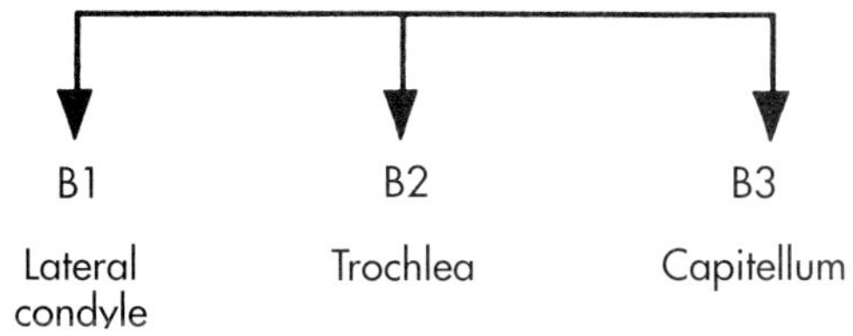

FIGURE 19-7 Anatomic and morphologic correlates in the B fracture group are shown.

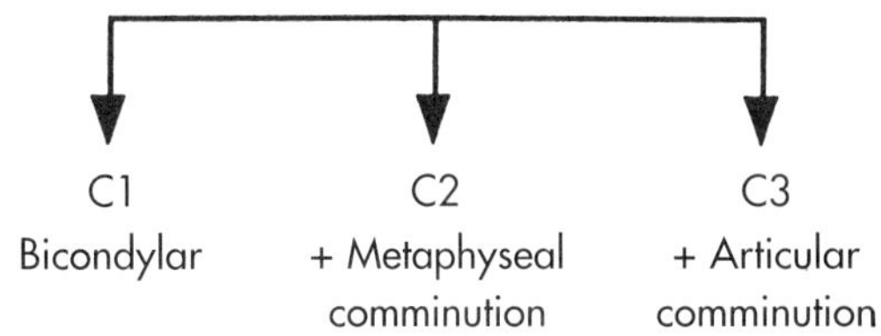

FIGURE 19-8 C fractures with increasing comminution.

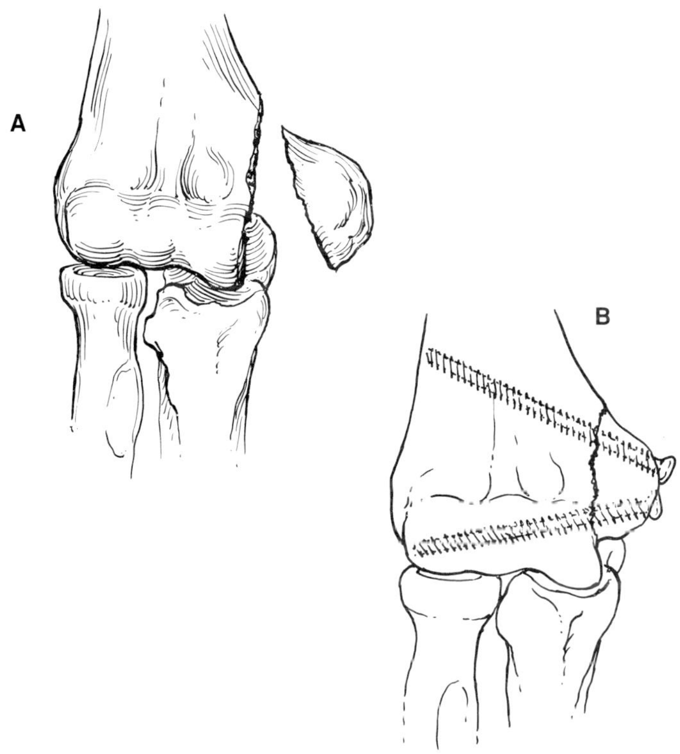

FIGURE 19-9 An A1 fracture fixed with two screws. Overdrilling the near fragment produces maximal purchase from the fully threaded screws. Proximal bone is cortical, making the 3.5-mm cortex screw the ideal screw. Distal bone is cancellous, making the 4.0-mm fully threaded screw the ideal choice. An acceptable alternative is to use the distally threaded 4.0 screw in the cancellous bone.

ment within the joint, and displacement of more than 5 mm[16] (Fig. 19-9). As with all injuries about the elbow, early resumption of motion is essential for recovery of elbow function.

A2 and A3 fractures in the supracondylar area involve both the medial and lateral columns and have been described as extension or flexion types, depending on displacement of the distal fragment (posterior is an extension type; and anterior is a flexion type).[9] Extension supracondylar fractures are much more common; flexion fractures account for only 2% to 4% of supracondylar fractures.[82] The A2 and A3 fractures are caused by a fall on the outstretched hand with the elbow extended or, occasionally, by a direct blow (flexion type).

Closed functional treatment is not often possible but could be considered for some nondisplaced A2 and A3 fractures that are stable enough to be moved without displacement. Operative treatment is recommended for fractures that are displaced and should be considered even in nondisplaced fractures so that rehabilitation will not be delayed (Fig. 19-10).

Horne reported good results in 4 patients treated with open reduction and internal fixation, but 3 of 12 treated by casting had poor results caused by displacement.[31] Similarly, Aitken and Rorabeck reported satisfactory outcomes in all six supracondylar fractures, two with surgery and four with casting, but cautioned that motion should be initiated within 6 weeks[2] (Fig. 19-11).

Transcondylar fractures have been indexed separately from the supracondylar fractures by some authors. Supracondylar and transcondylar fractures are both extraarticular. Bryan et al have considered transcondylar fractures as an entity separate from supracondylar fractures because the distal fragment is small and makes operative treatment more difficult.[9] Like supracondylar fractures, transcondylar fractures also have been subdivided into flexion and extension types. The mechanism of injury and treatment of transcondylar fractures are similar to those of the supracondylar fractures.

B-Series Fractures: Treatment and Results

B-series fractures are intraarticular, single-condyle fractures of the distal humerus (see Fig. 19-7). They are separated into groups based on the fracture plane's direction (frontal, sagittal) and which condyle is involved. These fractures are grouped as B1, lateral condyle (sagittal plane); B2, medial condyle (sagittal plane); and B3, in which a portion of the articular surface separated from the remainder of the joint (frontal plane). B-series fractures are more common in children than adults.[15,77] B1 fractures are more common than B2 fractures.[15]

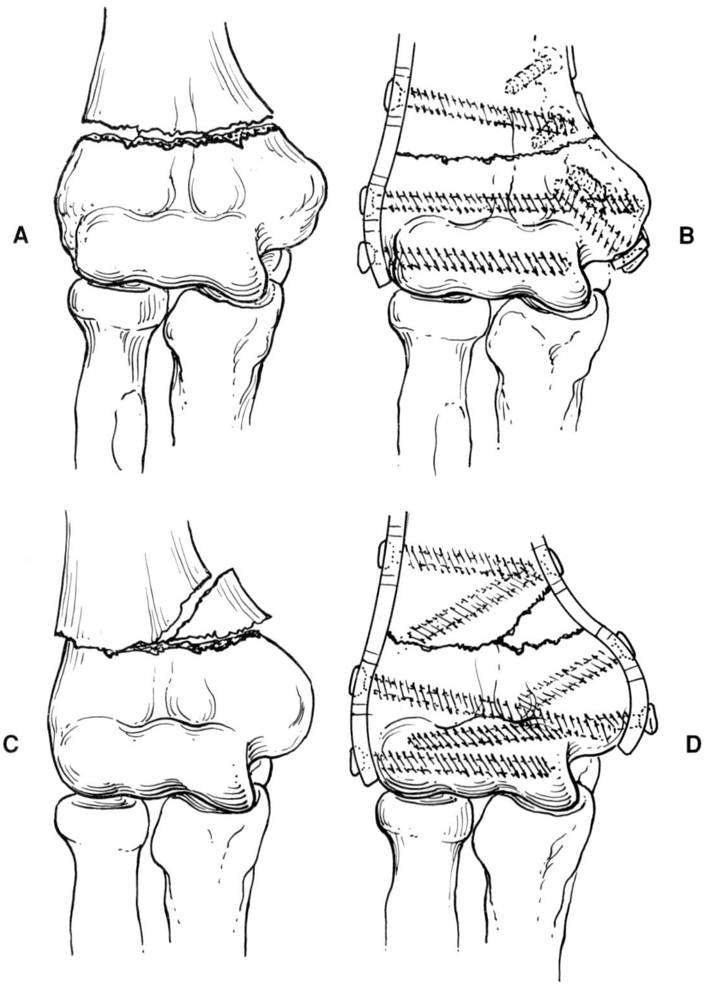

FIGURE 19-10 **A,** A supracondylar or A2 fracture with suggested internal fixation. **B,** The fracture is reduced and stabilized with provisional fixation, and the 3.5-mm reconstruction plates are contoured to fit the distal humerus. The lateral plate contours well to both the posterior and lateral surfaces, and the medial plate usually fits best on the posterior surface. Distally, fully threaded 4.0 cancellous screws anchor the plates to the bone, and the plates are simultaneously tensioned proximally. **C** and **D,** A comminuted supracondylar or A3 fracture is treated much like the A2 fracture, with the added complexity of having to fix additional fragments. Small secondary fragments can wedge into place as the plates are tensioned, but large pieces may require additional lag screw fixation.

B1 and B2 condylar fractures result from avulsion forces delivered through the collateral ligaments as the extended elbow is abducted or adducted.[56] Direct trauma to this area also may result in fracture. The lateral trochlear ridge of the humerus is the key to elbow stability in condylar fractures and separates simple fractures from fracture dislocations. Milch classified condylar fractures as type I and type II fractures (AO B1 and B2 fractures).[56] If the lateral trochlear ridge is part of the unstable fragment, the elbow will become unstable (Milch type II).

Rarely incomplete and nondisplaced condylar fractures can be treated by brief immobilization followed by aggressive rehabilitation. Operative treatment is recommended for displaced condylar fractures and should include joint débridement[16] (Fig. 19-12).

Most B1 fractures may be adequately exposed through a simple lateral approach. A lag screw technique usually suffices unless the fragment is large, in which case a small plate must be used as a buttress. A large fragment with articular involvement is best approached posteriorly to allow for assembly of the comminuted joint.

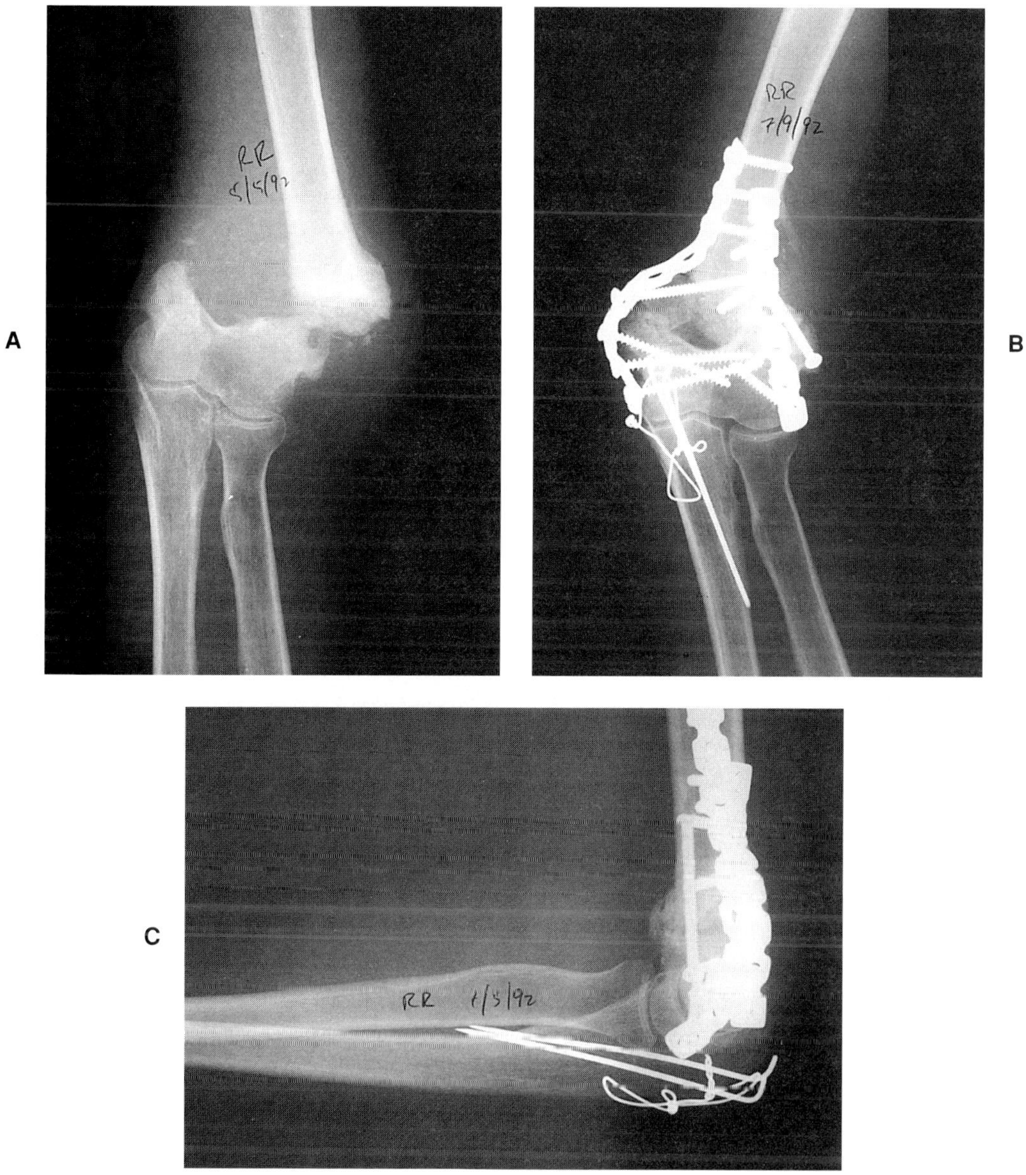

FIGURE 19-11 An aseptic lax defect pseudarthrosis of an A2 fracture treated with tricorticate autogenous iliac crest interposition bone graft (**A**) and dual 3.5-mm reconstruction plates (**B** and **C**). The patient rode in the Kentucky Derby the next year.

A

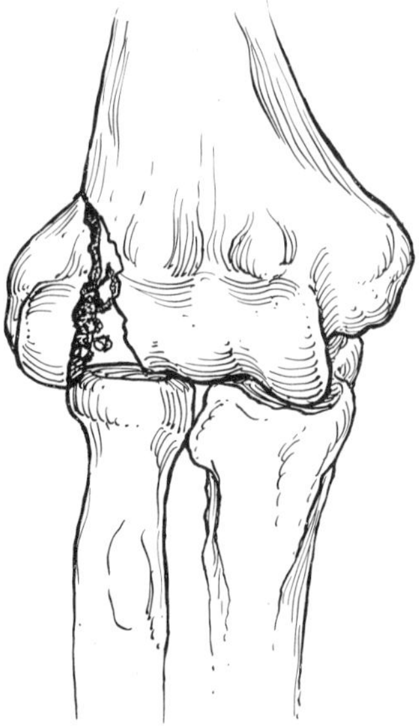

B

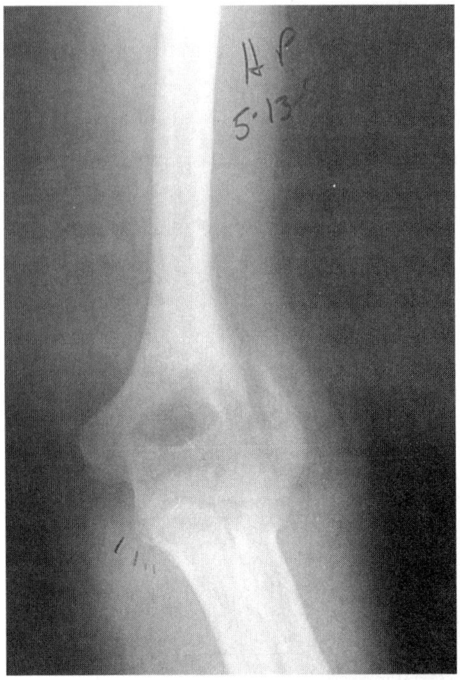

C

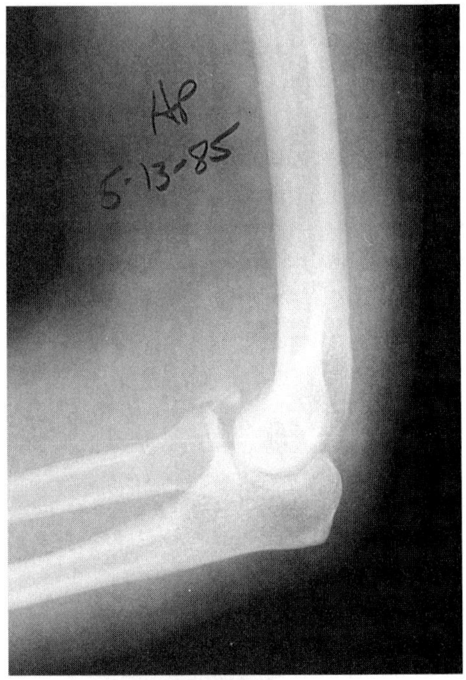

D

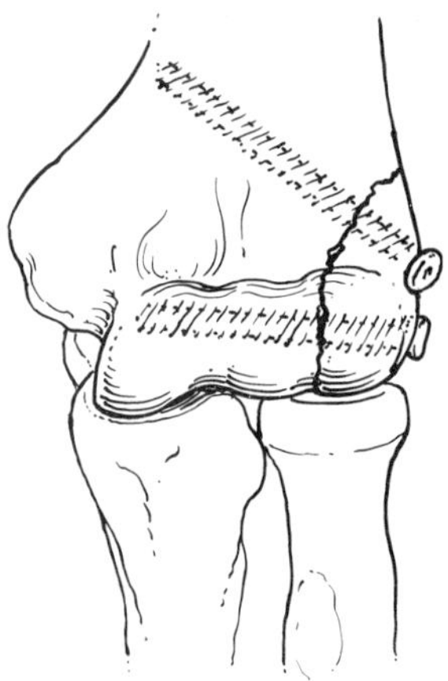

E

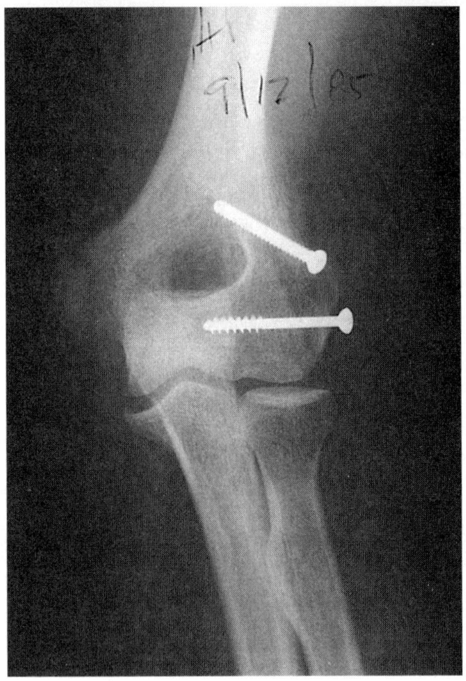

F

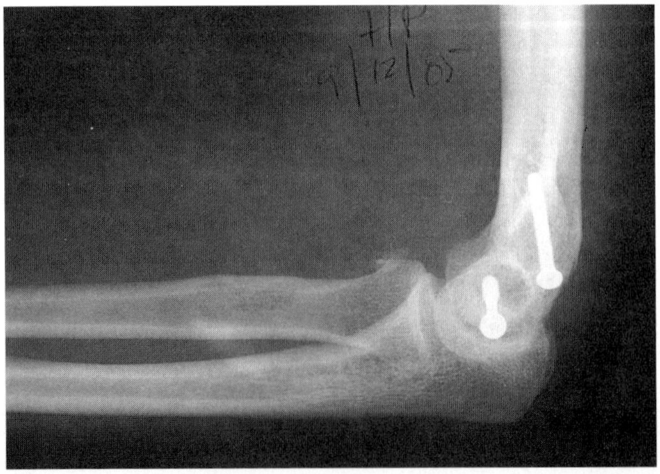

FIGURE 19-12 These illustrations show three grades of lateral condyle fractures. **A,** The B1 fracture. **B** and **C,** Radiographs of the lateral condyle fracture with associated comminution. **D** through **F,** Schematic illustration of internal fixation of the lateral condyle with a fully threaded 3.5-mm cortical lag screw proximally and a fully threaded 4.0-mm cancellous lag screw distally. The clinical case in **E** and **F** shows the partially threaded shaft of the cancellous screw distally.

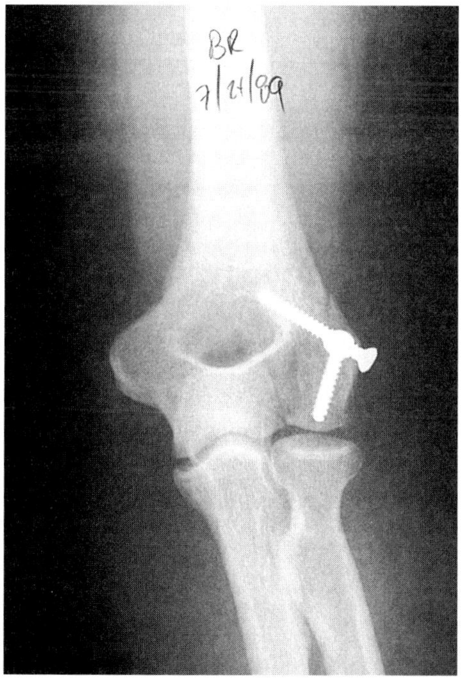

G

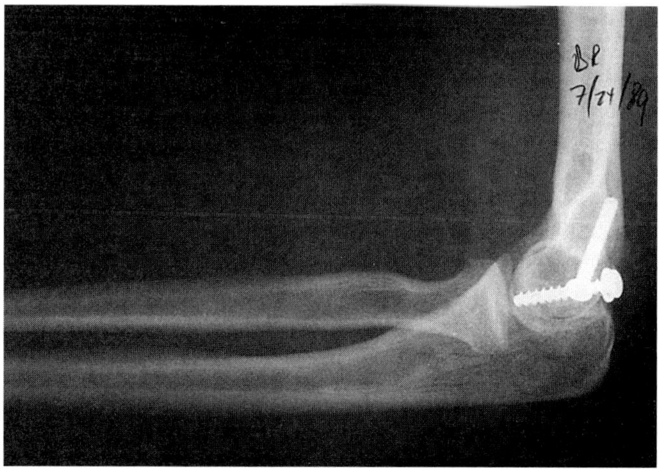

H

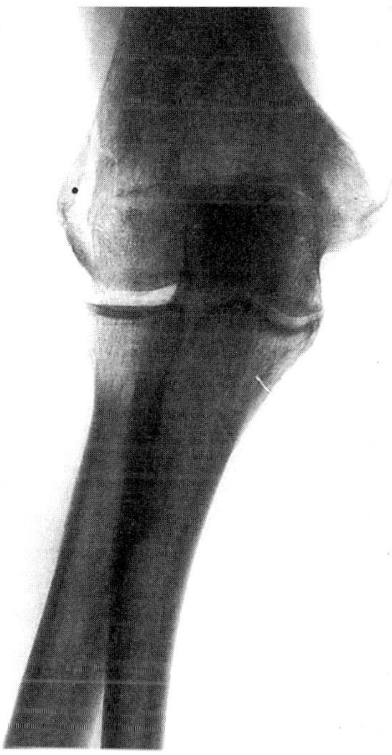

I

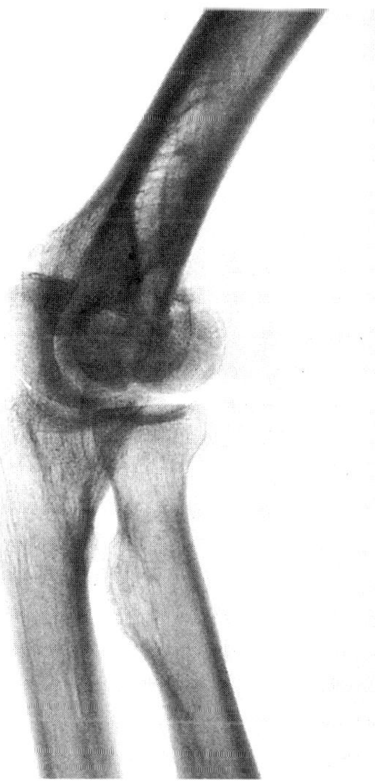

J

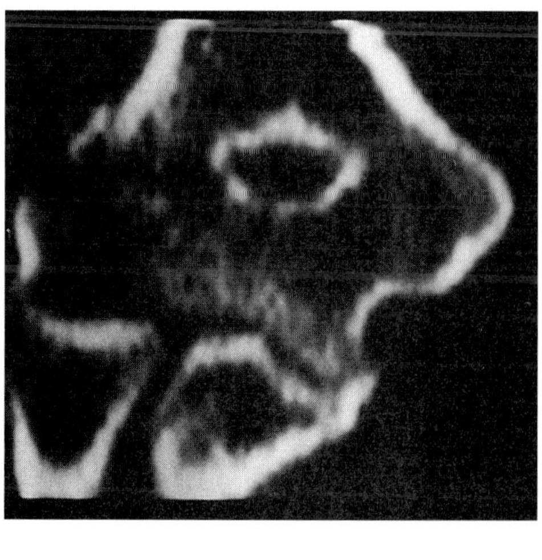

K

FIGURE 19-12—cont'd **G** and **H**, The entire lateral condyle and capitellum are involved but are still amenable to fixation with lag screws only. **I** and **J**, In a third case, conventional radiographs show that an apparently simple lateral condyle fracture is much more complex, as shown on CT (**K**). *Continued.*

L

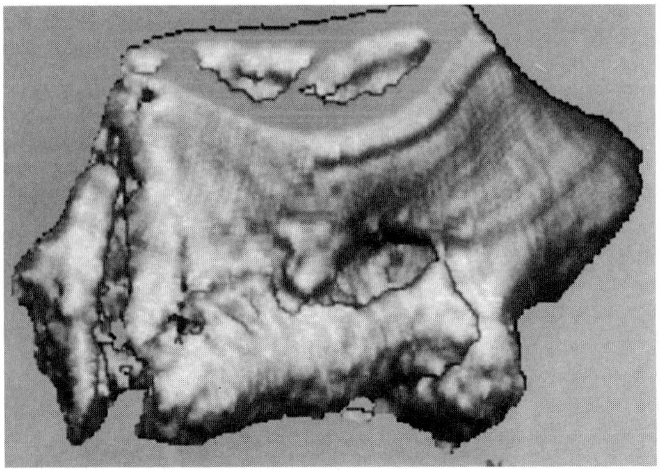

M

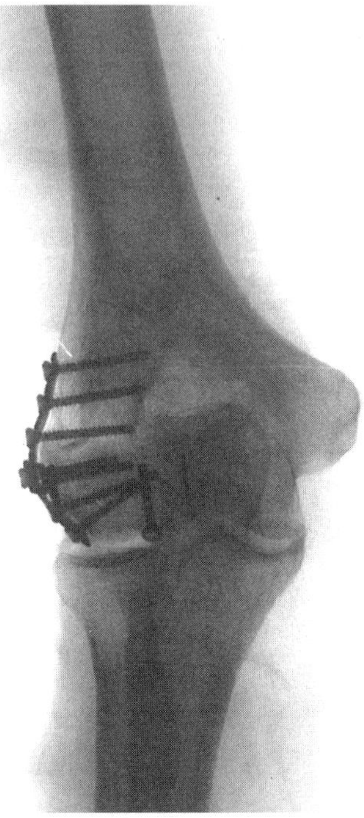

N

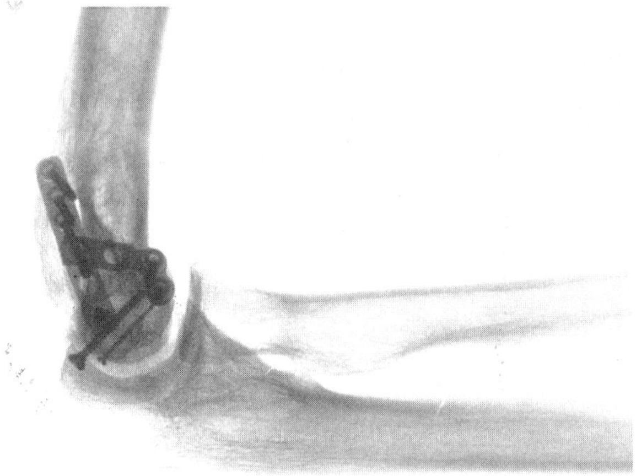

FIGURE 19-12—cont'd L, CT with three-dimensional representation. More extensive surgery is required to reconstruct the trochlear component then fully stabilize the lateral condylar elements with two one-quarter tubular plates, **M** and **N.**

A

B

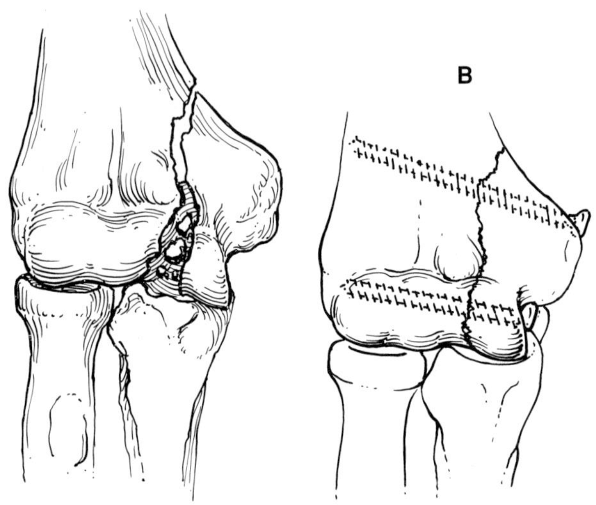

FIGURE 19-13 Illustration and reconstruction of the B2 fracture. An extraarticular transolecranon approach gives the surgeon adequate exposure for reduction and fixation with lag screws only or, for extra stability, a short 3.5-mm reconstruction plate to reconstruct the proximal cortex.

Medial condylar fractures are best approached through an intraarticular transolecranon incision with transposition of the ulnar nerve. A pure metaphyseal fracture may be assembled with lag screws only, whereas a similar fracture with diaphyseal extension may require plate support (Fig. 19-13).

B3-series fractures occur in the coronal plane and involve the distal humeral articular surface (capitellar fractures). Capitellar fractures account for 0.5% to 1% of elbow injuries.[15,76] Variable amounts of the capitellum and trochlea may be included. These are three variations: (1) type I whole capitellum or complete (Hahn-Steinthal),[29,84] (2) type II or osteochondral fracture with minimal bone attached (Kocher-Lorenz),[42,46] and (3) capitellum with variable extension into the trochlea. Type I fractures are more common than type II fractures.

Capitellar fractures are caused by forces acting through the radial head that shear off the capitellum.[41] Axial load of the radial head is required to fracture the capitellum, and the flexion-extension position determines whether the fragment is displaced anteriorly or posteriorly.[3,41] Extension of the elbow causes the fragment to displace anteriorly in type I fractures blocking flexion (Fig. 19-14). Flexion tends to displace the fragment posteriorly with type II fractures. Type II fractures actually may represent osteochondritis dissecans with a portion of the fragment displaced posteriorly.[43]

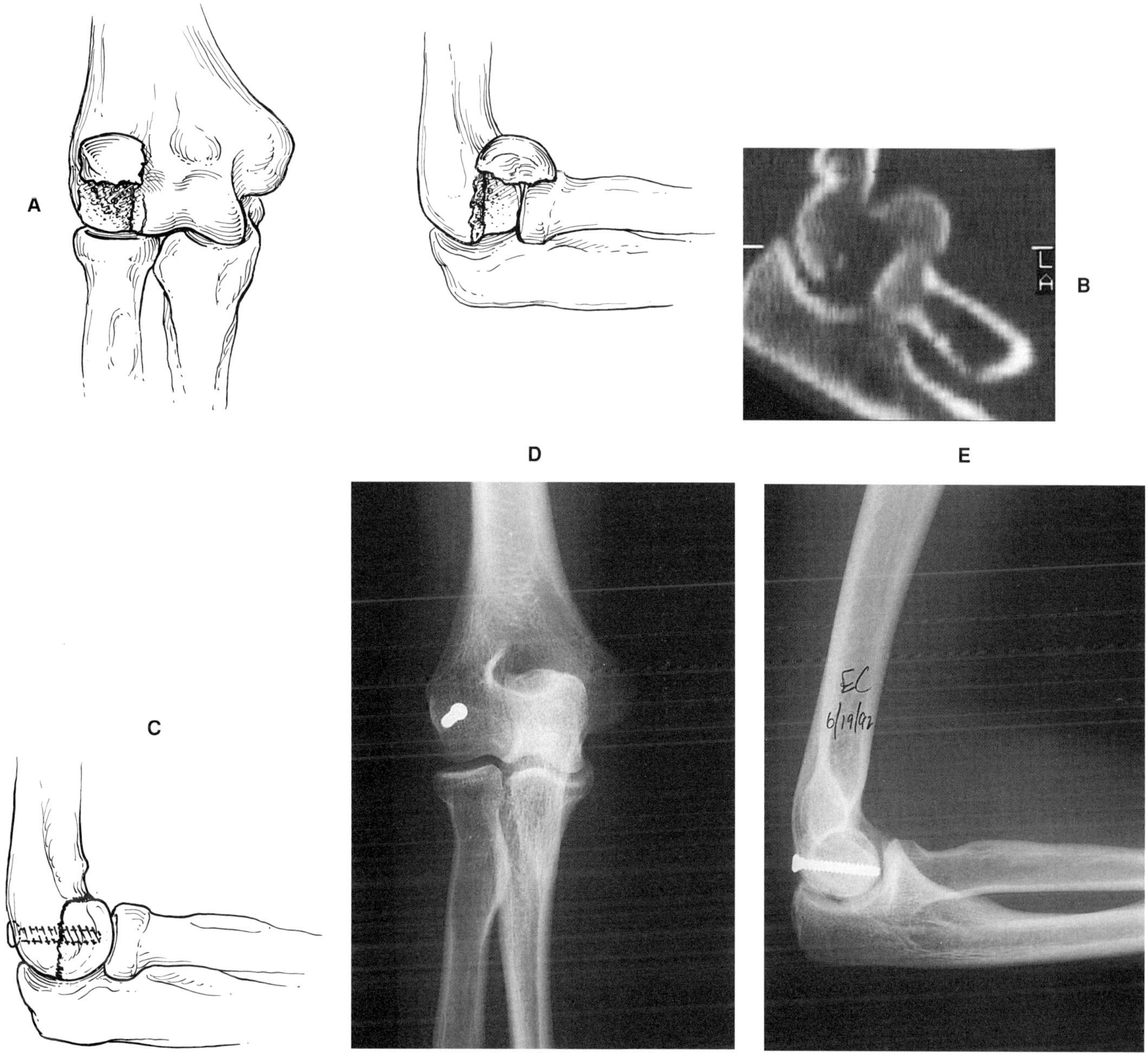

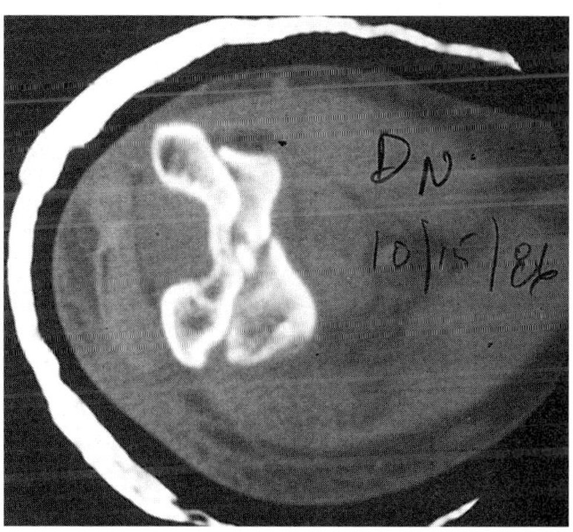

FIGURE 19-14 **A,** Front and side view of one type of capitellar fracture, in which the displacement is cephalad and anterior 90°. **B,** A clinical case demonstrating successful application of the technique of rigid fixation and immediate mobilization in a professional volleyball player who returned to her prior level of competition. Computerized tomographic image showing marked displacement of the capitellum. **C,** Possible internal fixation for the fracture illustrated in **A** and **B.** A fully threaded 4.0-mm cancellous screw is placed from posterior to anterior through a lateral approach. The near side is overdrilled to 4.0-mm. **D, E,** and **F,** A more complicated variation of capitellar fracture with involvement of the entire anterior cartilage bearing element of the distal humerus, as shown on the computerized axial tomographic image. Both the capitellum and trochlea are displaced. *Continued.*

G

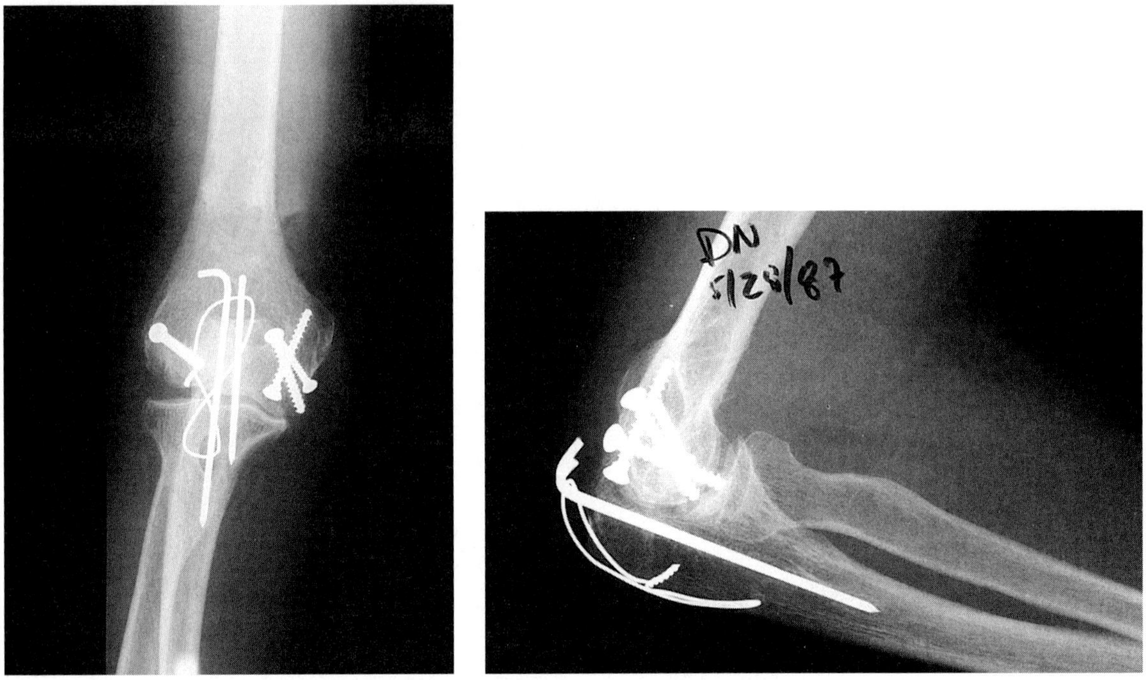

H

FIGURE 19-14—cont'd **G** and **H,** Multiple lag screws were necessary to stabilize the fracture shown in **F.** Note that a posterior intraarticular transolecranon approach was necessary to accomplish the reconstruction.

Treatment options include closed reduction, open reduction with or without internal fixation, and excision of the fragment.[3,14,21,43] Good and poor results have been reported with all methods. Alvarez reviewed 163 cases reported in the literature and concluded that early excision of even a large capitellar fragment gave the best overall results. The excision group contained 84 patients, with 66 (79%) obtaining a good or excellent result, as compared with 51% good or excellent results in the group treated with open reduction.[3]

More recent series, such as that of Collet, have recommended open reduction and internal fixation, depending on the size of the fragments, the amount of comminution, and the skill of the surgeon.[14] Newer fixation techniques, such as small fragment lag screws and the Herbert screw, allow stable fixation with anatomic reduction and early range of motion. Complex capitellar-trochlear fractures require an intraarticular transolecranon approach, whereas capitellar fractures can be repaired through a lateral incision. Gentle repositioning is followed by lag screw fixation. Open reduction and internal fixation is recommended in a young athletic population unless comminution or small fragment size mandates excision.

C-Series Fractures: Treatment and Results

C-series fractures of the distal humerus involve the entire articular surface and are at high risk of poor outcome despite treatment method.[2,12,40,75] They are classified according to the degree of articular involvement and comminution of the metaphysis. C1 fractures are simple fractures of the articular surface with a transverse or oblique metaphyseal component. C2 fractures are simple fractures of the surface with metaphyseal comminution. C3 fractures are multifragmentary injuries of the articular surface with or without metaphyseal comminution. The intercondylar portion of the fracture is created by the proximal ulna, which acts like a wedge, splitting the articular surface during a fall on the outstretched arm with the elbow either flexed or extended.[6]

Early treatment methods, including cast immobilization, traction, and limited internal fixation, have resulted in poor results secondary to loss of motion.[22,40,98] More recently, dual-plate fixation has resulted in better stability and improved range of motion. Nonoperative care should be the exception rather than the rule for C-series fractures, but considerable experience and excellent technique are required for these very demanding injuries.

A posterior approach is necessary to adequately expose both columns. The joint must be reassembled with effective lag screw fixation using screws of 3.5 to 4.0 mm diameter. Small comminution often is present, and the clinician may treat it by removing loose pieces and retaining those with intact soft tissues and/or cartilage. Bone graft may be necessary to fill defects. The medial and lateral columns are reconstructed with neutraliza-

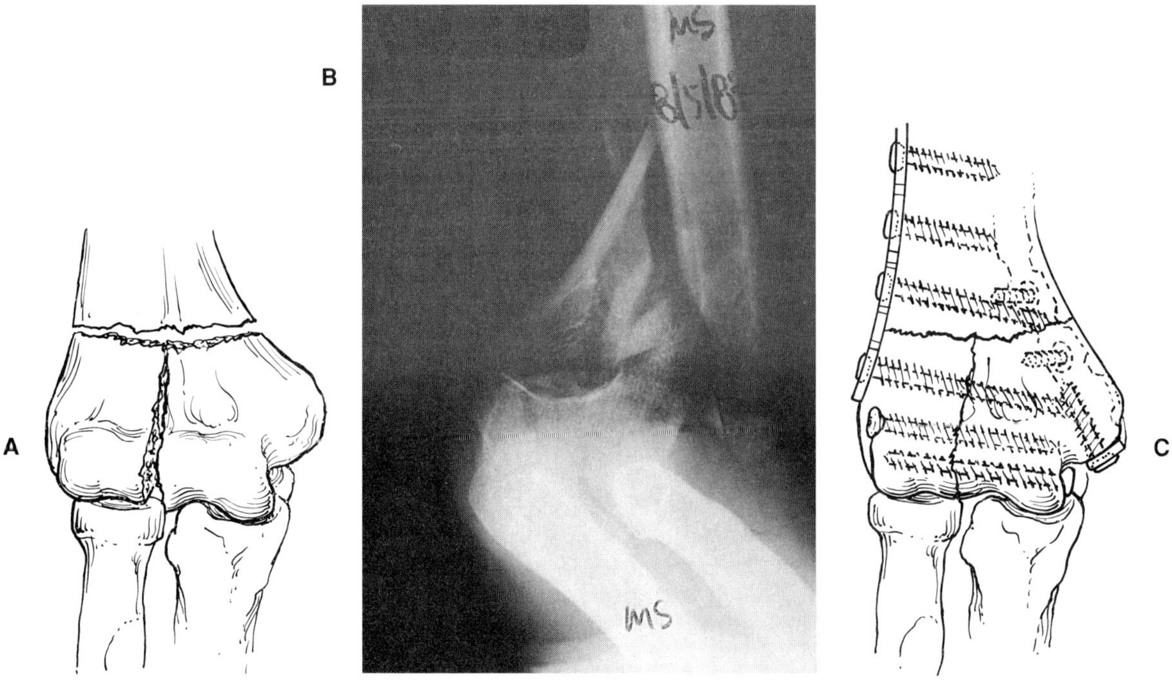

FIGURE 19-15 **A,** The classical T-condylar fracture of the distal humerus. **B,** Preoperative AP radiograph. **C,** Fixation of the fracture. The joint component is reassembled with 4.0- mm cancellous lag screws, creating a two-part supracondylar fracture that is fixed with two 3.5-mm reconstruction plates, as described for A2 and A3 fractures (see Figs. 19-10 and 19-11).

Continued.

tion or bridge plates using lag screws whenever possible (Fig. 19-15).

Reconstruction plates of 3.5 mm are well suited for this application because of their malleability in all planes. Different fracture configurations may require slightly different plate locations, and these plates may be effectively applied to any surface of the bone. Axial compression can be applied through the plate if the fracture surfaces are flat and not too comminuted.

Results with C-series fractures have varied with the mix of cases and the technique used. Table 19-1 presents range-of-motion data as a function of fixation type. Jeshrani obtained greater than 100° ranges of motion in 16 of 21[35] cases, and Jupiter et al obtained greater than 100° in 11 of 14 cases using dual plates.[40] Zagorski compared operative with nonoperative treatment of these fractures and recommended dual-plate fixation with range of motion.[98] Poor results were associated with poor internal fixation technique and prolonged postoperative immobilization.

Proximal Radius

Radial head fractures, representing 20% of all elbow trauma, are caused by indirect trauma, most often a fall on an outstretched hand. Maximum force is exerted on the radial head with the elbow extended and the forearm pronated.[4,63] More violent injuries cause dislocation of the elbow with or without associated radial fractures.

The radiocapitellar view, as described by Greenspan and Normal, may help in some cases in addition to plain radiographs to better evaluate the displacement and comminution of radial head fractures.[28] The wrist should be examined for tenderness and instability caused by the presence of concurrent distal injuries. Aspiration of the elbow joint and injection with local anesthetic help to evaluate motion and ligamentous stability.[20,30]

Classification

The classification proposed by Mason and later expanded by Johnston is most widely used[37,48] (Fig. 19-16). Mason's classification is easy to remember and applies to most fractures based on plain radiographs of the elbow, not the mechanism of injury.

Johnston demonstrated associated ligamentous and capsular injury to the elbow with radial head fractures by positive arthrograms.[37] Positive arthrograms for ligamentous or capsular injury were found in 4% of type I, 22% of type II, and 85% of type III radial head fractures.

Type I fractures are impact injuries with displacements of less than 2 to 3 mm. Type II are displaced fractures involving up to one third of the radial head. Type III fractures involve more than one third of the head and are displaced variable amounts.

Types 0 and IV are new additions to the classification system. The type 0 fracture is not visible by conventional radiographic technique but is diagnosable with MRI or

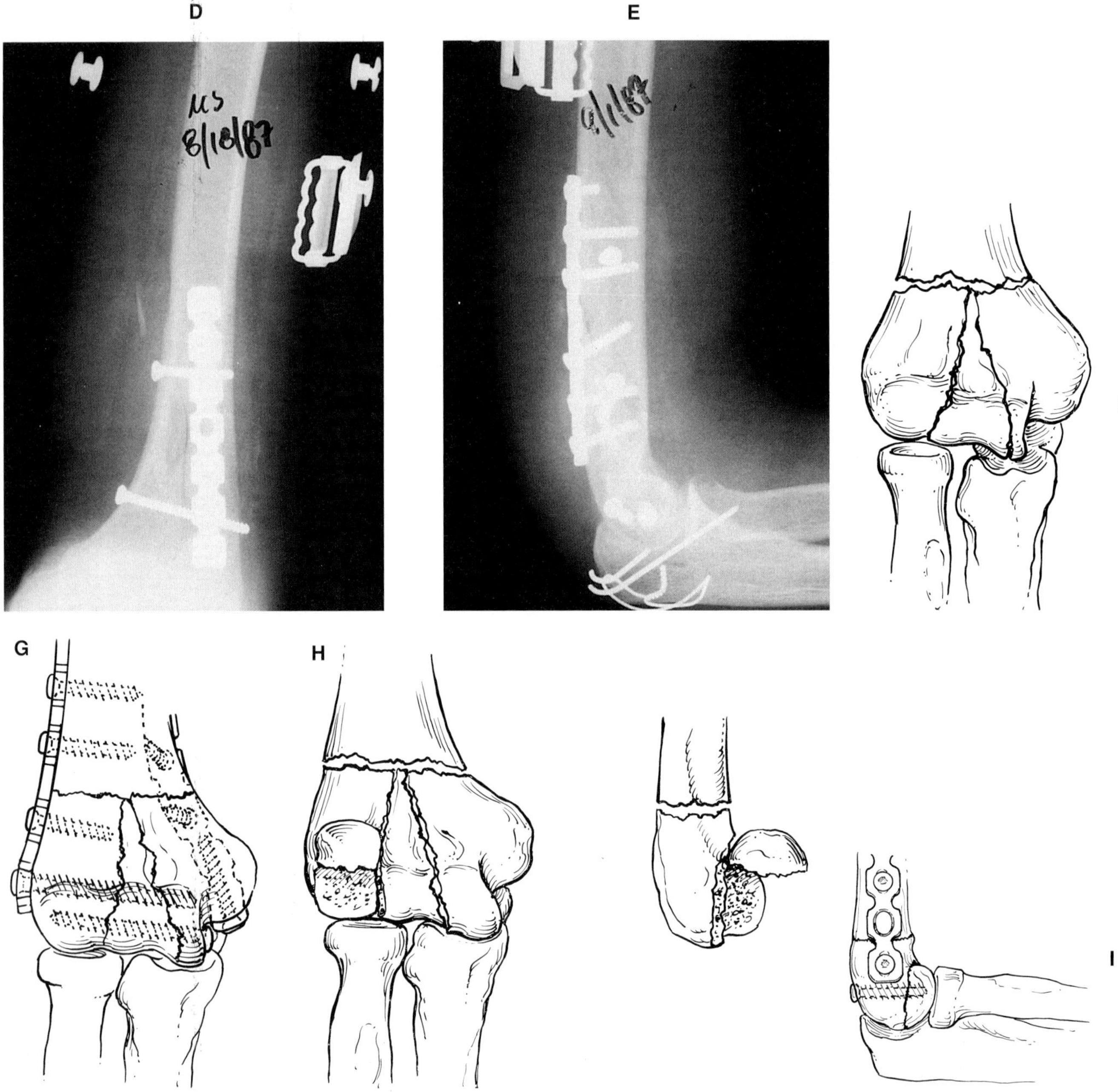

FIGURE 19-15—cont'd **D** and **E,** The fracture shown in **B** has been reassembled with a single 3.5-mm reconstruction plate and lag screws. The large cortical fragment medially acted like a plate when fixed with lag screws. The lateral plate neutralized torsion and bending forces proximal to the level of this large cortical fragment. **F** and **G,** A C3 fracture has intraarticular comminution but is stabilized by the same principles as used with the C1 fracture. **H** and **I,** Further complexity is added in the form of coronal fracture lines, such as the capitellar lesion. Supplementary lag screw fixation is required in such cases.

TABLE 19-1
Fixation in Distal Humerus Fractures

Technique	Study	Motion
Screws, pins, or wires	Riseborough and Radin[75]	<55° in 4 of 7
	Bryan[6]	
	Bickel[22]	<90° in 14 of 28
	Niemann[61]	<90° in 9 of 14
	Horne[31]	<90° in 9 of 20
	Lansinger and Mare[44]	FC >30° or F <115° in 15 of 23
	Jupiter[10]	ROM not >80° in 2 of 4
Single plates	Horne[31]	FC >30° or F <90° in 4 of 7
	Jupiter[40]	ROM not > 80° in 2 of 6
Dual screw Single plates Double plates	Jeshrani[35]	ROM not >100° in 16 of 21
Double plates	Jupiter[40]	ROM >100° in 11 of 14
	Gabel[22]	ROM >100° in 8 of 10

FC, flexion contracture; *F,* flexion; *ROM,* flexion-extension range of motion.

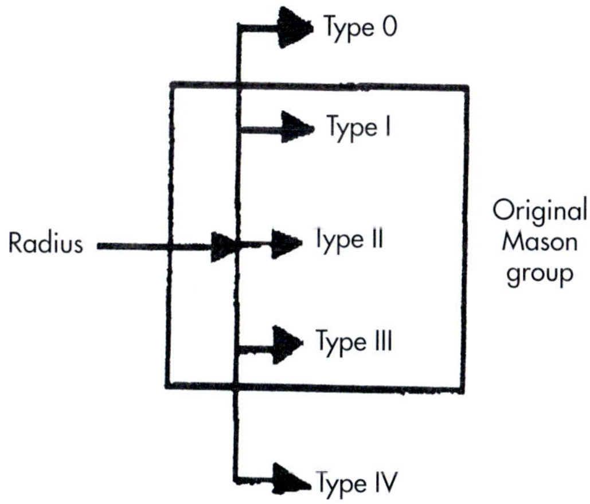

FIGURE 19-16 Modified Mason-Johnson classification of radial head fractures.

bone scan. Type 0 fractures may be presumed based on clinical examination and possibly a positive fat-pad sign on plain radiographs. Johnston has defined a type IV that is a radial head fracture (type 0, I, II, or III) associated with an elbow dislocation.[63] Radial head fractures complicate 5% to 10% of all elbow dislocations.[30]

A fracture of the radial neck should be considered separately from radial head fractures because treatment is almost always nonoperative unless there is displacement in addition to angulation. Such fractures should be treated according to the patient's range of motion rather than radiographic criteria.

Treatment

Outcome after radial head fracture is highly variable. Chronic instability is rare, but stiffness is common. Residual loss of motion has been associated with age greater than 50 years and immobilization longer than 2 weeks.[70] Extension may be lost even with immediate range-of-motion exercises.

Type 0, I

Nondisplaced fractures and fractures with less than 2 to 3 mm of depression and/or displacement (type O, I) are best treated nonoperatively with a removable splint for no longer than 7 days. Immediate motion is encouraged because the major sequela of nonoperatively treated radial head fractures is loss of extension, not pain.[20,25] Gaston and Johnston reported no poor results out of 134 patients with type I fractures treated with early range of motion.[25] Mason, however, reported that one third of his patients lost an average of 7° of extension.[48] Secondary displacement of type O, I fractures has been described but is extremely rare and should not guide treatment.[1,16a,57]

Type II, III

Treatment of displaced radial head fractures has included nonoperative treatment,[25,57] early[13] and late excision[7] of the radial head with or without radial head implants, and open reduction and internal fixation.[10,68,78] From a practical point of view, it is necessary to segregate displaced radial head fractures that can be adequately fixed internally from those that require excision or may simply be treated with immediate motion. In spite of recent attempts to devise more detailed classifications, no completely satisfactory, all-inclusive system is available. Judgment is necessary to identify operative cases from those best left alone.

Nonoperative Care

Miller et al showed good results in 77% of 40 patients with isolated type II fractures at an average of 9.6 years after nonoperative treatment.[56] No correlation between size, depression, and comminution of the fragment with the end result was found. Wesley also reported on isolated type II fractures treated for only 1 to 2 weeks in a posterior splint, with 49 of 50 having good or excellent results.[95]

Internal Fixation

Open reduction and internal fixation (ORIF) of the large-fragment displaced radial head fracture has been recommended. Internal fixation is warranted in some type II and type III fractures.[10,11,92] In the case of the type

II fracture, ORIF is an alternative to conservative care and must be considered as a primary treatment. In cases where the joint surface is depressed more than 2 mm, surgery may yield superior results.

Shumeli,[78] Odenheimer,[68] and others[10,92] have demonstrated successful open reduction and internal fixation of radial head fractures because the problems of early and late excision of the radial head were avoided and early mobilization was initiated. A prerequisite to success for open reduction and internal fixation is restoration of anatomy and rigid stabilization. If motion cannot be started immediately after surgery, operative trauma is additive with the trauma of injury and will make the result worse than closed treatment.

Techniques of internal fixation of radial head fractures are very demanding and precise. Lag screw fixation, using 2.7-mm and 2.0-mm screws, is possible in some cases (Fig. 19-17). Use of a Herbert differential-pitch bone screw for displaced radial head fractures also has been advocated.[10] Fracture fragments must be moved very carefully into their proper positions. Small Kirschner wires are placed across the fragments at locations that avoid interference with later screw placement. Implants should be placed below the articular cartilage when possible. The lateral portion of the radial head does not articulate with the ulna and may be an optimum position for placement of hardware.

Excision

When the entire radial head is fragmented (type III) and the fragments are displaced more than 3 to 4 mm, early excision of the head is recommended. Open reduction and internal fixation is an alternative to excision as discussed by Vierhout.[92] In most cases, excision will be indicated by wide displacement of the fragments or the inability to rigidly stabilize the multiple pieces. Complete removal of the fragments is confirmed by assembly of the fragments after removal and intraoperative radiographs (Fig. 19-18).

After radial head excision, elbow stability should be assessed and will fall into one of three levels:

Level I:

- The elbow is stable in all positions after the capsule is closed.
- Motion will be possible within the first 2 weeks without special precautions.

Level II:

- Elbows are stable in flexion, usually to 40°.
- Immediate motion is possible with use of a flexion dropout splint for 2 to 3 weeks.

Level III:

- Elbows are highly unstable and present a need for one of the following:
  1. Transfixation of the radiocapitellar joint with a Steinmann pin for 3 weeks
  2. Casting in flexion for 3 weeks
  3. Collateral ligament reconstruction

A

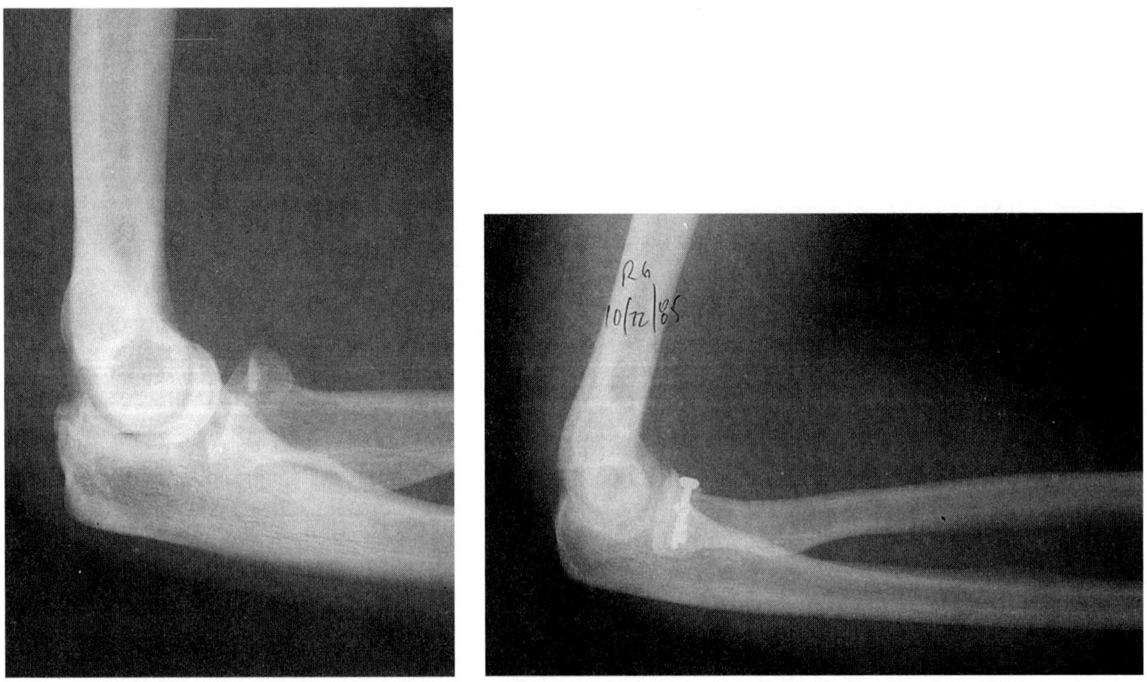

B

FIGURE 19-17 Comminuted displaced radial head fracture treated with operative reconstruction with 2.7-mm lag screws.

Transfixation with subsequent mobilization is the best course for most such injuries. Some authors have advised strongly against radial head excision in cases of instability, but such advice seems to ignore the problems arising from displaced intraarticular fragments.

Radin and others[71] have recommended early excision of the radial head with displaced fractures. Coleman et al[13] found satisfactory clinical results in 17 patients after radial head excision who had mild pain with minimal loss of motion and strength. All of these elbows radiographically demonstrated arthritis, cubitus valgus, and positive ulnar variance. Comparisons of early and late total excision have found late excision less satisfactory.

Adler[1] and Conn[15] found that early excision was not superior to delayed excision. Broberg[7] reported good results in 21 patients with delayed excision after failure of closed management in type II and type III radial head fractures. Delayed excision was justified in fractures with associated dislocations of the elbow that could be rendered unstable with immediate radial head excision.

Despite these good results with radial head excision, Mikic reported 50% fair or poor results in 60 patients with isolated radial head fractures who underwent total radial head excision at an average of 6½ years before the study.[55] Of these 60 patients, 43% had pain, 52% had osteoarthritis, 30% had valgus deformity, and 60% had loss of motion. They recommended that radial head excision be limited.

Tables 19-2 and 19-3 summarize results of excision reported in the orthopedic literature. Overall, 15% of 278 patients reported pain, and 53% had radiographic evidence of proximal radial migration. Clearly excision is to be avoided in an athletic patient if at all possible.

Replacement

Silicone prostheses[86] to prevent proximal migration and subsequent wrist pain are not routinely recommended because of the possibility of mechanical failure of the replacement.[50] Pribyl et al,[69] in a biomechanical study involving fresh cadaveric elbows, tested the ability of the Silastic radial head replacement to resist valgus stress at the elbow. Their study showed that an intact radial head provides 20% of the resistance to valgus stress in full extension. The Silastic prosthesis provided very little support against valgus stress, improving the stiffness of the elbow by only 5% when compared with radial head excision alone. They attributed this to the low mod-

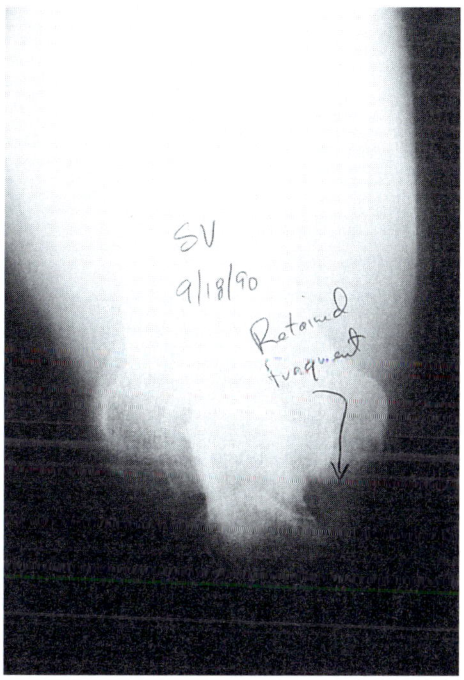

FIGURE 19-18 A type III radial head fracture was treated with excision but without complete removal of loose fragments. A retained head piece fused to the distal humerus and contributed to a blockage of extension; later excision and arthrolysis restore motion.

TABLE 19-2
Proximal Migration of the Radius after Excision of the Radial Head

	Upward Migration of the Radius		
Study	**Cases**	**Number**	**Percent**
Carstam[11]	35	27	77
McDougal and White[51]	44	25	57
Dickson[16a]	45	16	36
Taylor and O'Connor[87]	58	17	64
Radin and Riseborough[71]	36	14	39
Mikic and Vukadinovic[55]	60	28	46
TOTAL	278	147	53

TABLE 19-3
Elbow Pain after Radial Head Excision

Study	**Pain Number**	**Percent**
Carstam[11]	5	14
McDougal and White[51]	12	27
Dickson[16a]	7	16
Taylor and O'Connor[87]	29	50
Radin and Riseborough[71]	3	8
Mikic and Vukadinovic[55]	15	25
TOTAL	71	15

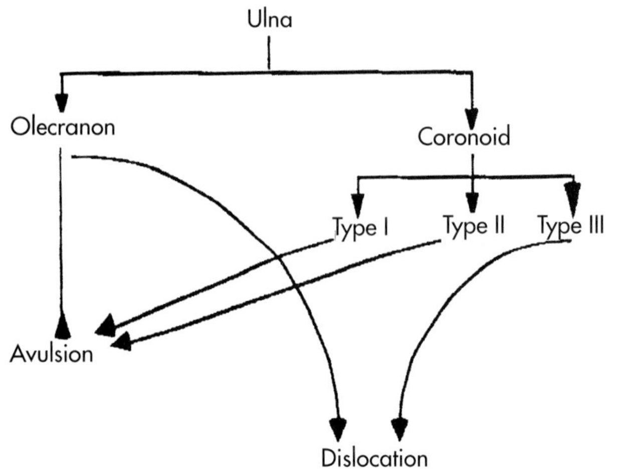

FIGURE 19-19 Proximal ulna fractures. Olecranon and coronoid fractures are either avulsion type or fracture-dislocation type.

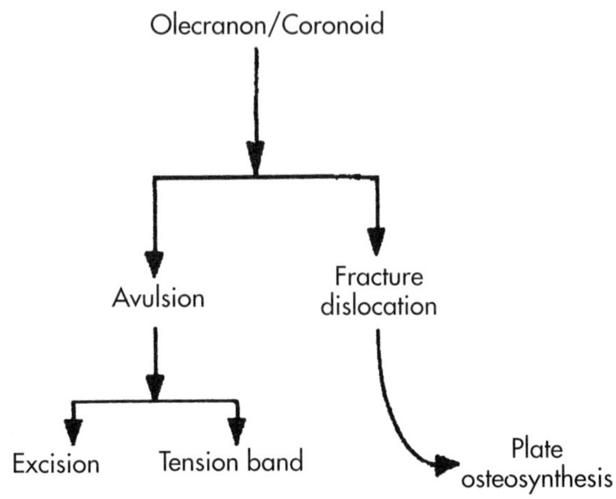

FIGURE 19-20 Treatment of proximal ulna fractures. A tension band device works well for avulsion-type fractures, but lag screw and/or plate osteosynthesis is required for fracture-dislocation–type injuries.

ulus of elasticity of the Silastic implant and correlated these findings with other clinical studies that showed no difference between excision of the radial head and Silastic radial head replacement.

Hotchkiss and Weiland[32] also found in 30 human cadaver elbows that silicone radial head replacement in the presence of an intact medial collateral ligament did not significantly improve the stability. Dislocation of the distal radial ulnar joint in association with a fracture of the radial head, otherwise known as an Essex-Lopresti fracture (total dislocation of the radius), may be the only indication for prosthetic replacement.[18,19,51]

Type IV

Type IV lesions consist of an elbow dislocation with associated radial head fracture. The morphology of the radial head fracture varies and can be any one of the three types. Management of such injuries is determined by the type of radial head fracture. Radial head replacement is indicated in Essex-Lopresti injuries but should be avoided otherwise.

Proximal Ulna

Classification

The articular portion of the proximal ulna consists of the olecranon process and the coronoid process. Both are important for joint stability and tendon insertion. Fractures involving either the olecranon or the coronoid process occur in two generic types. The first type consists of an avulsion of the process itself without a violation of the stability of the joint. The second type is a fracture-dislocation. The size of the coronoid/olecranon is greater in the second lesion, and the remaining portion of the joint is dislocated or subluxated (Fig. 19-19). Treatment of the two types is radically different (Fig. 19-20).

Olecranon Fractures

The classification of proximal ulna fractures has been based on the amount of bone necessary for joint stability, but no system has been universally accepted. Even though clinical[18] experience has shown that up to 80% of the olecranon can be excised without resulting in instability, approximately 50% of the olecranon process is necessary for ulnar humeral stability.[52] Biomechanical studies by An and Morrey have shown that the proximal half of the ulna articulation contributes to ulnar humeral stability proportionately, with stability decreasing as the excised portion increases.[5]

Coronoid Fractures

Regan and Morrey have proposed a classification system for fractures of the coronoid process based on plain radiographs.[73] Type I fractures are avulsions of the tip of the coronoid process (Fig. 19-21). Type II fractures consist of single or comminuted fragments involving 50% or less of the process. Fractures involving less than one half of the coronoid process or olecranon process (sparing the collateral ligament attachments) leave the elbow stable and represent avulsion injury involving the brachialis (coronoid) or triceps muscle (olecranon). The coronoid process provides attachments for the anterior portion of the medial collateral ligament and the middle one half of the anterior capsule.

Type III fractures are single or comminuted fragments involving more than 50% of the coronoid process. Type III fractures were further subclassified based on an associated elbow dislocation (type A, with, and B, without,

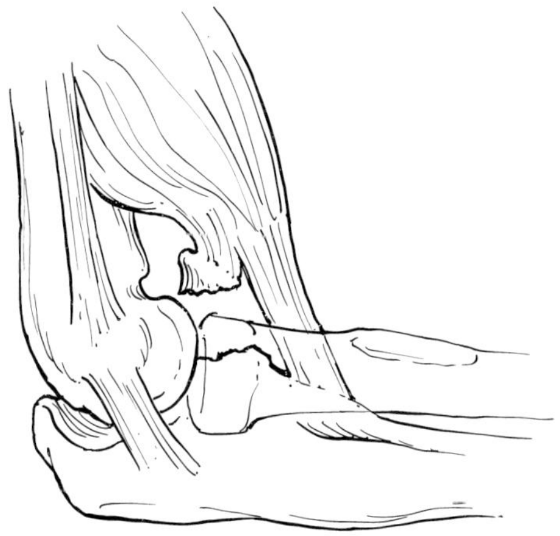

FIGURE 19-21 Avulsion-type coronoid fracture representing partial brachialis rupture. Nonoperative care should be selected in most cases.

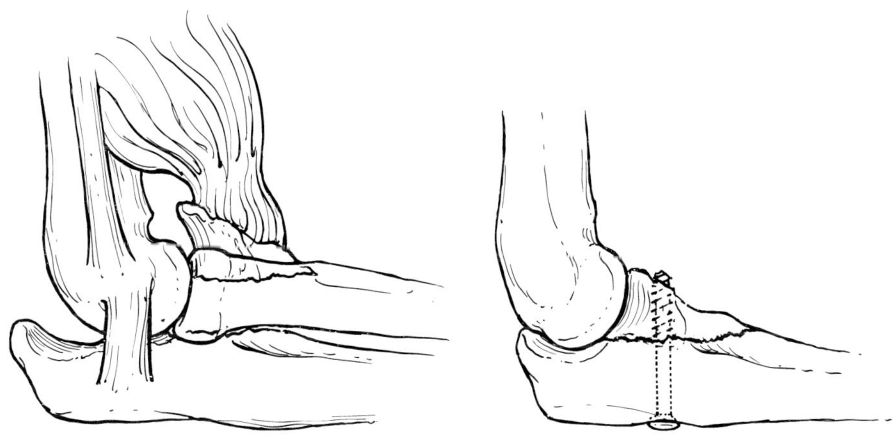

FIGURE 19-22 A large coronoid fragment contains a major portion of the joint, resulting in subluxation of the elbow unless the fragment is anatomically reduced and rigidly stabilized. One or two 3.5-mm cortical lag screws will hold the fracture well enough for the elbow to be gently moved in the first 10 days after surgery.

dislocation).[73] Displaced fractures involving more than 50% of the coronoid process may be associated with elbow joint instability caused by compromised function of the medial collateral ligament (Fig. 19-22).

Treatment and Results

Olecranon—Avulsion

The olecranon process and the coronoid process form the greater sigmoid notch of the ulna, which articulates with the trochlea of the distal humerus. The olecranon process is subcutaneous with little soft-tissue covering and is very susceptible to fracture from direct trauma. Occasionally, the olecranon is fractured indirectly by falling on an outstretched hand with the elbow flexed as the triceps contracts to avulse a portion of the olecranon. Occasionally, the fracture is minimally displaced or nondisplaced when the triceps aponeurosis remains intact. Incomplete fractures can be treated with a brief period of splintage followed by rehabilitation.

Wadsworth used an olecranon screw and washer when a single displaced fragment was present.[93] McKeever and Buck concluded that extensively comminuted fractures of the olecranon should be treated by excision and repair of the triceps tendon.[18] They also recommended excision of the fracture fragment in elderly people. Wesley treated 25 fractures of the olecranon process with no failures using a Zuelzer hook-plate, originally designed to treat fractures of the medial malleolus.[96]

Retig compared excision with internal fixation and found no difference in range of motion.[74] Of the patients with internal fixation, 15% required reoperation. More recently, Gartsman et al reviewed 107 patients who underwent surgical treatment for isolated olecranon fractures, with half of the patients being treated with primary excision and the remaining half with open reduction and internal fixation.[24] At follow-up, the two groups were similar with regard to residual pain, function, range of motion, and elbow stability. In the ORIF group, however, the complication rate was 23%, compared with 4% in the group that underwent excision. An additional 23% of those patients treated with open reduction and internal fixation required a second operation for hardware removal. Comparison of mechanical testing between groups revealed no significant difference in triceps strength.

Maeko reported on complications of tension band wiring of olecranon fractures in 20 patients.[47] The most common complication was prominence of the Kirschner wires secondary to incomplete seating of the bend of the proximal tips of the wires into the olecranon process. Complications in this group included loss of reduction in 2 elbows and the need for removal of the prominent Kirschner wires at 2 to 6 months after surgery in 12 patients. Overall, there were good functional results in 16 patients (76%).

In an athletic population, excision of all but a small fragment should be avoided if at all possible. Excision in patients with limited activities may be equivalent to internal fixation, but in individuals who continually press limits of endurance and strength, preservation of bony anatomy is recommended.

The tension band technique is exacting and must be performed with compulsive attention to detail. Technical points must be clearly understood. Seating the transfixing Kirschner wires in the ulnar cortex distal to the coronoid process is essential to anchor the tensioning wire. Intramedullary placement of pins is not secure. With continuous cycling during the healing process, intramedullary pins will tend to loosen or back out.

The wire used for the tensioning loop should be positioned immediately adjacent to the bone of the olecranon where the Kirschner wire enters without any soft tissue interposed. During tightening of the wire loop, the elbow should be gently flexed and extended to remove any slack in the system. When tensioning has been completed, the Kirschner wires are cut, bent over the wire loop, and driven into the olecranon tip through the triceps tendon (Fig. 19-23). Removal of metal after union is strongly recommended.

Olecranon—Dislocation

Large olecranon process fractures are bony components of ulnar-humeral instability patterns and must be internally fixed in a rigid manner. Plate osteosynthesis is necessary for olecranon fractures associated with ulnar-humeral instability to neutralize large forces that tend to displace the forearm anteriorly. The use of a tension band in such cases will not prevent anterior subluxation of the forearm. A plate is necessary to reconstitute the posterior cortex, and lag screws are used to fix an associated coronoid process fracture to the ulnar shaft (Fig. 19-24). Autogenous iliac crest graft or bone substitute should be available in cases of comminution. Motion must be initiated within the first 1 to 2 weeks after injury.

Coronoid Process Fractures

Two mechanisms of coronoid fracture have been recognized.[73] Isolated fractures occur by avulsion of bone by the brachialis muscle when the elbow is hyperextended. More significant injuries occur when the coronoid process is sheared off by the trochlea during posterior elbow dislocation (Fig. 19-25). Because the coronoid process provides attachment for the anterior portion of the medial collateral ligament and middle one half of the capsule, large coronoid fractures must be rigidly fixed to restore joint integrity and stability.

Regan and Morrey have reported the largest series of coronoid fractures. Type I and II fractures were immobilized for an average of 13 to 20 days, with satisfactory re-

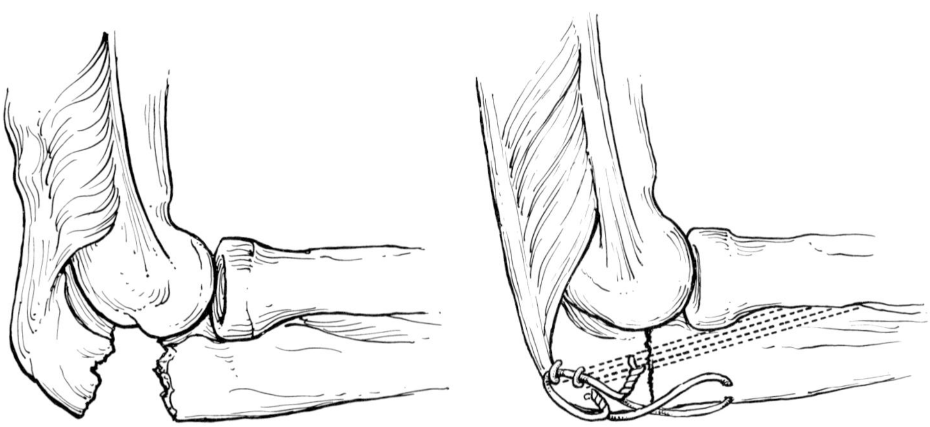

FIGURE 19-23 The extensor mechanism is disrupted by the avulsion-type olecranon fracture. Repair with a tension band is appropriate. Some fractures also may be stabilized with a plate and screws.

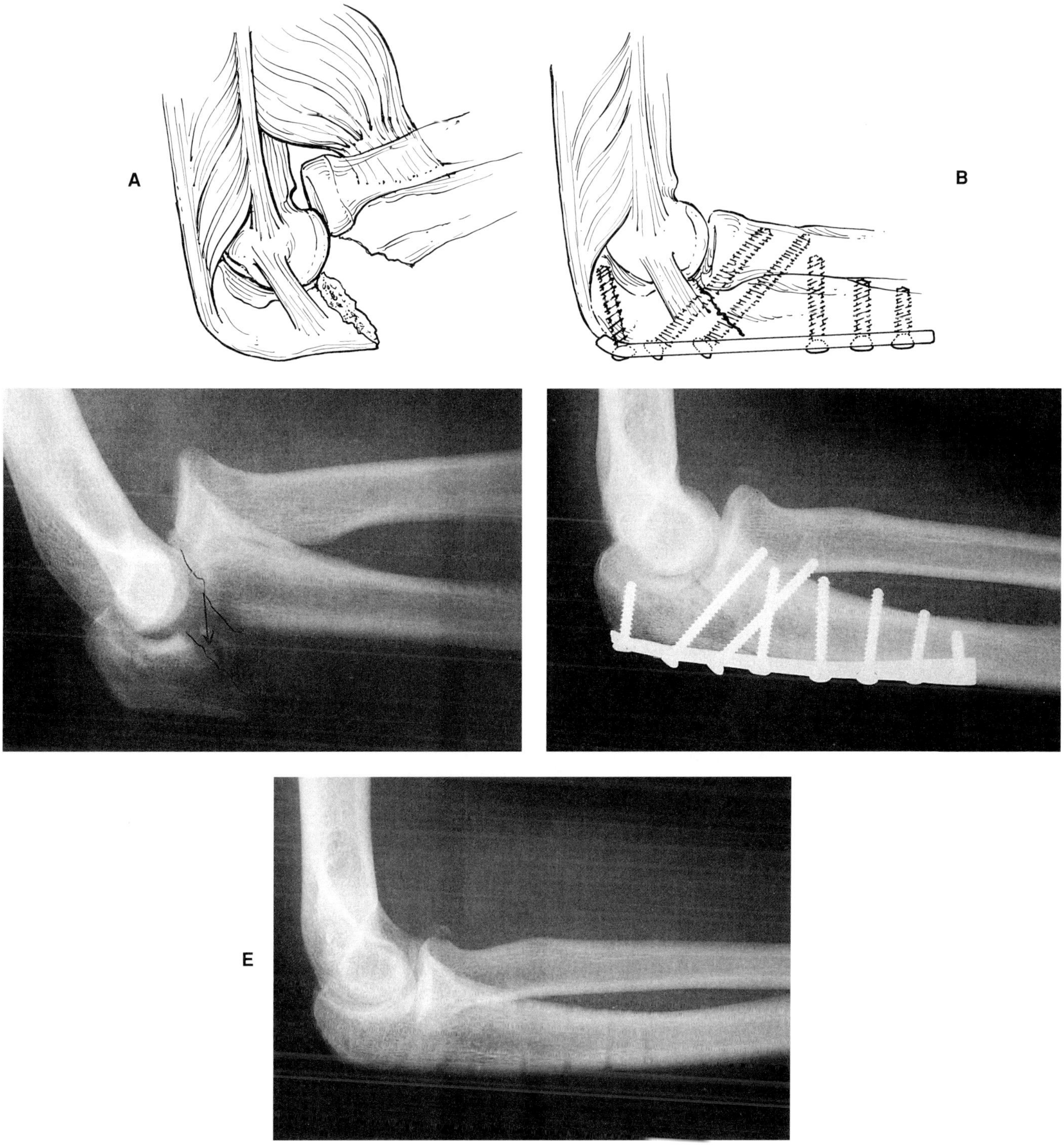

FIGURE 19-24 **A** and **B,** The forearm and the flexor group are unstable in the fracture-dislocation type of olecranon fracture. Dislocation of the radial head from the capitellum is evident. Note that the radial head and coronoid remain linked. **C** through **E,** If the fracture is oblique, lag screws through a plate provide an optimal construct. Excellent purchase from two 3.5-mm cortical lag screws reduces the requirements for plate rigidity so that only a one-third tubular plate is adequate. In other instances, a thicker plate (3.5-mm reconstruction plate, semitubular plate, or 3.5-mm LC-DC plate) may be necessary.

A B C D

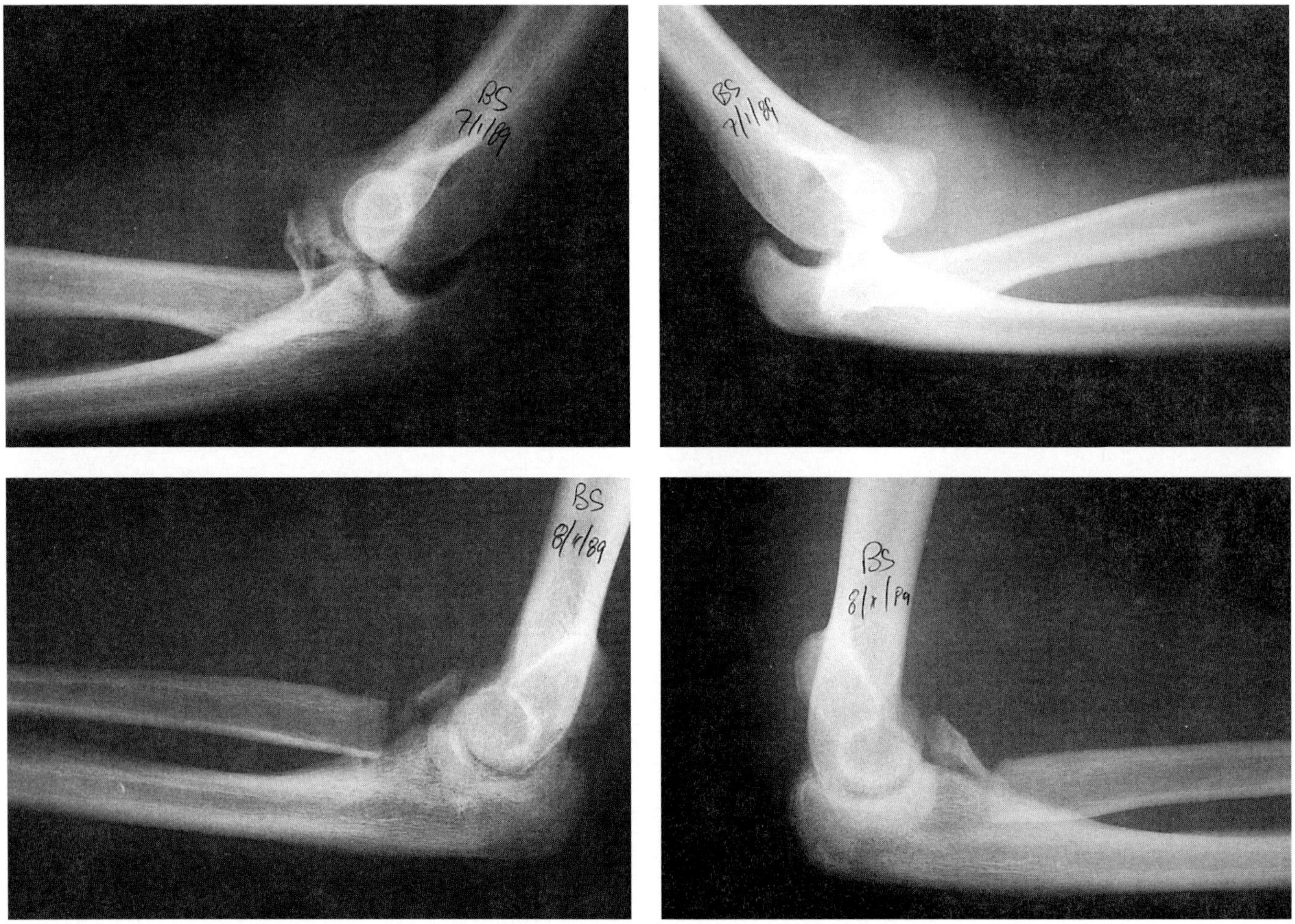

FIGURE 19-25 **A** and **B,** Bilateral fracture-dislocation with associated type III radial head fractures and type I coronoid fractures. **C** and **D,** Treatment consisted of radial head excision and capsular repair, followed by motion with restricted extension initially.

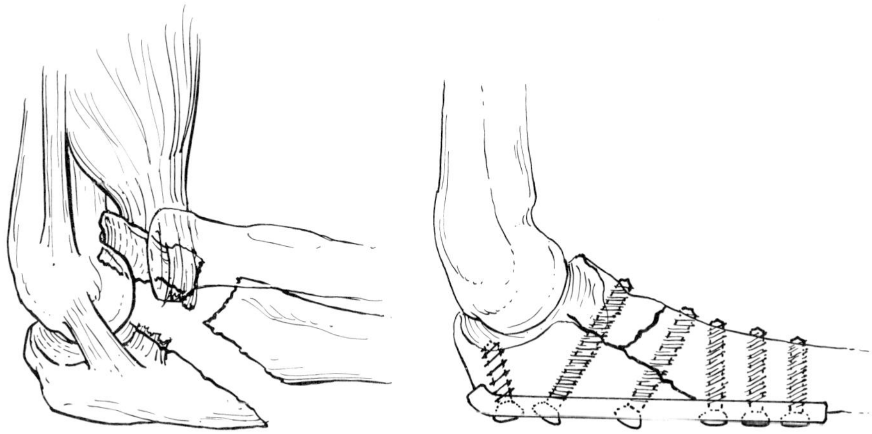

FIGURE 19-26 **A,** A type III coronoid fracture with associated unstable ulnar-shaft fracture is shown. **B,** Anatomic reconstruction of the joint surface and of the ulnar shaft is essential. Interfragmentary lag screws placed through the plate stabilize the joint. The plate then can be tensioned from a distal cortical site, the second lag screw is placed, and finally, three cortical neutralization screws are placed.

sults in 91%.[73] Open reduction and internal fixation was performed on only three elbows. Type III fractures were associated with poor results in all but 20% of patients. Complete stabilization of all components of these complex injuries is necessary.

One troublesome fracture pattern consists of an olecranon avulsion fracture associated with a coronoid fracture dislocation. The radial head may either be fractured or dislocated (Fig. 19-26). If the radial head is intact or fixable, it should be retained; otherwise it is excised. The coronoid must be rigidly fixed to the distal shaft and the olecranon. All three fragments are then plated (Fig. 19-27). Failure to follow these steps will result in pain and limited motion (Fig. 19-28).

Elbow Dislocation

Elbow dislocations account for 11% to 28% of all elbow injuries and 20% of all dislocations[15,45] (Fig. 19-29). Only dislocation of the glenohumeral joint is more frequent. Associated skeletal injuries such as radial head fractures and avulsion injuries of the coronoid process may occur. Median or ulnar nerve damage has been reported with these injuries.[70]

Stimson's classification of elbow dislocations describes the relationship of the radius and ulna to the distal humerus and to each other.[85] The radius and ulna usually dislocate together, either posteriorly, medially, laterally, or anterior to the distal humerus. Divergent dislocation of the radius and ulna, as well as isolated radial and ulnar dislocations, are very rare. Posterolateral dislocations account for up to 90% of elbow dislocations.[45]

Posterior dislocations take place during a fall on the outstretched hand with hyperextension of the elbow. The olecranon impinges on the olecranon fossa, acting as a lever to disrupt the capsule and either tear the brachialis muscle or avulse the coronoid process. Further hyperextension disrupts the collateral ligaments and occasionally fractures the radial head. Unlike the supracondylar humerus fracture, the triangular landmarks of the olecranon and the medial and lateral epicondyles are disrupted with elbow dislocation. On examination, the antecubital fossa appears full and the forearm shortened. Anteroposterior and lateral x-rays usually are sufficient to diagnose elbow dislocations, although additional views may be required to further assess associated fractures.

Elbow dislocations can be reduced closed under intravenous sedation or regional anesthetic. Gentle traction on the forearm with countertraction on the arm is applied along with downward pressure on the forearm to disengage the coronoid process from the olecranon fossa. Hyperextension should be avoided to prevent fracture of the coronoid process or further soft-tissue injury to the brachialis muscle.

After reduction, the elbow should be flexed and extended through a range of motion to verify that reduction has been obtained and that the joint is stable without mechanical block. Stability of the elbow next is determined by assessing the amount of extension possible without redislocation. Repeat neurovascular examination of the extremity is important after reduction. Repeat radiographs must be interpreted critically to evaluate the reduction and define associated fractures. Additional diagnostic measures such as tomograms or computerized axial tomograms are indicated if any uncertainty exists about the existence of additional fractures or persistent dislocation.

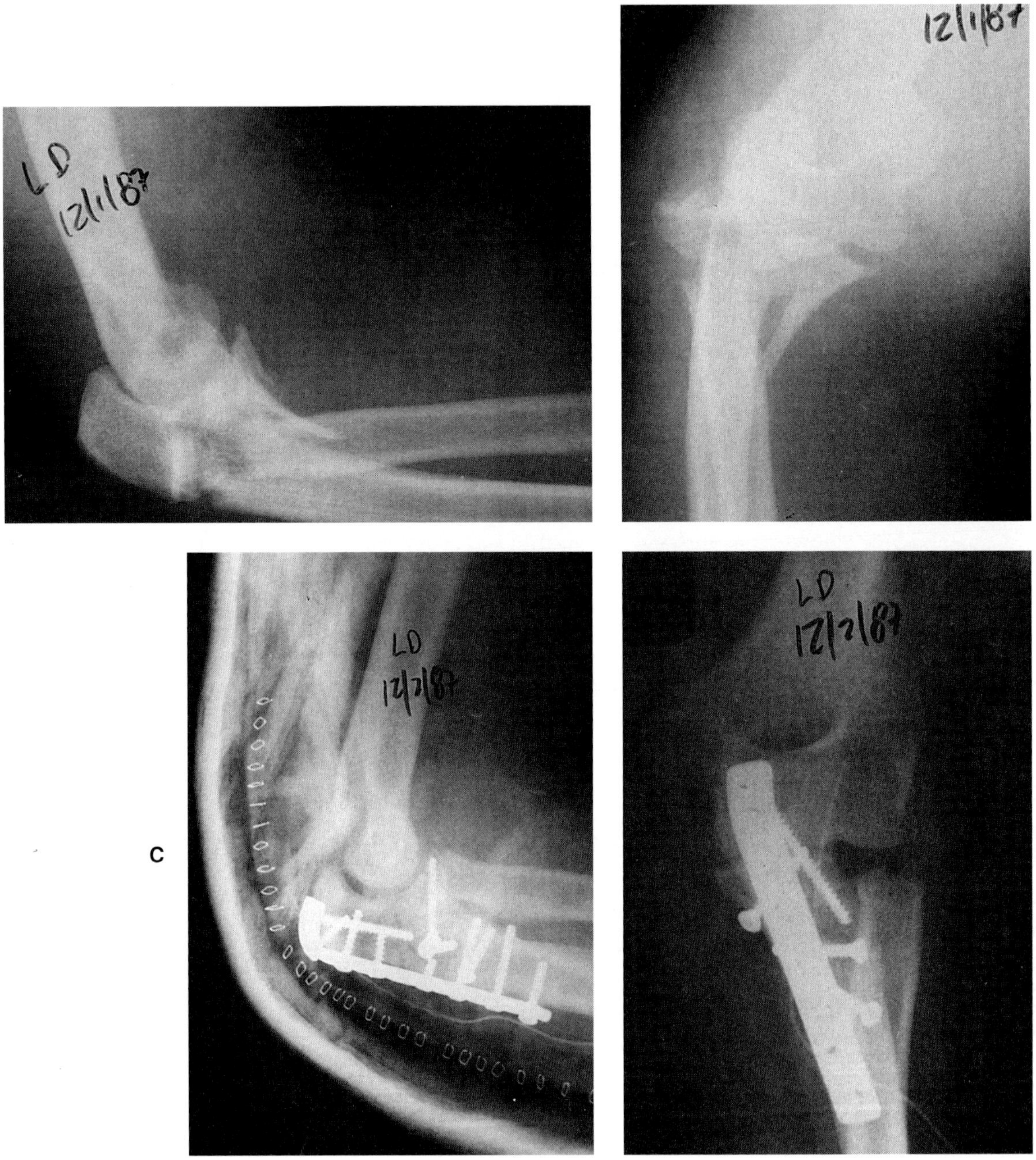

A B C D

FIGURE 19-27 **A** and **B,** A fracture-dislocation-type olecranon lesion and coronoid combined with a type III radial head fracture. **C** and **D,** The coronoid was fixed to the ulnar diaphysis with cortical lag screws. A 3.5-mm DC plate with tension loading restored the posterior cortex and compressed the olecranon into the coronoid/shaft component. The radial head was excised.

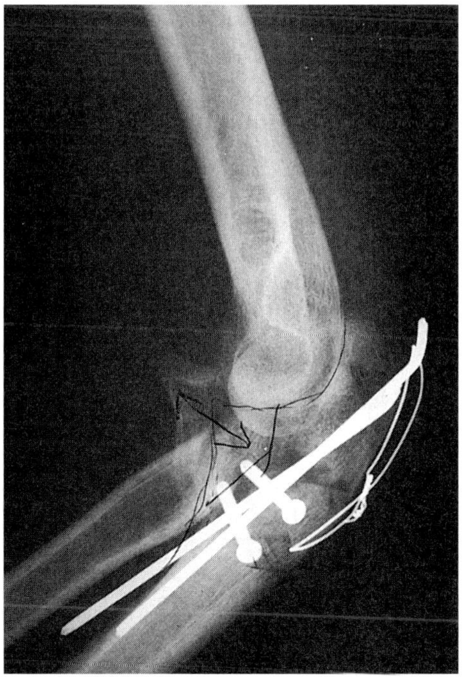

FIGURE 19-28 The coronoid fragment has not been reduced. A tension band with Kirschner wires and a wire loop is improper treatment for this type of injury and does not control the instability well enough. Secondary reconstruction was necessary in this patient.

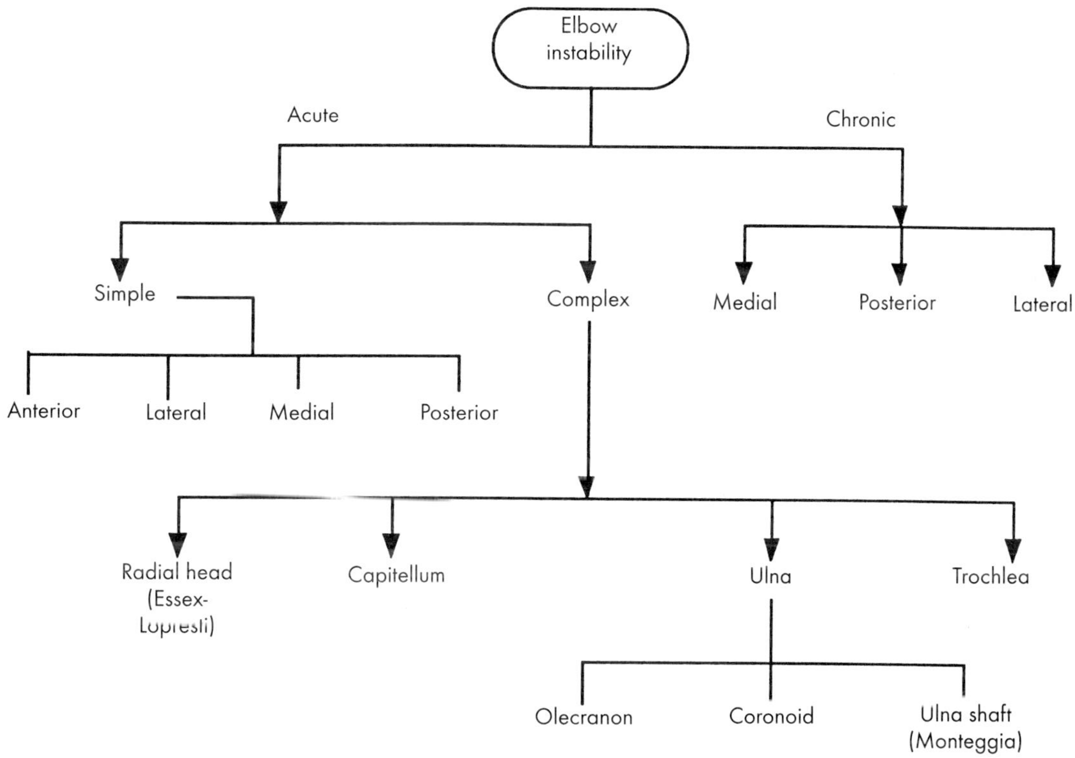

FIGURE 19-29 Elbow instabilities: acute and chronic. Acute instability without bone involvement is listed as simple. Complex acute instability combines ligamentous instability with joint fractures. Chronic instability is rare.

Open reduction is preferred over repeated attempts at unsuccessful closed reduction. Open reduction is required in approximately 11% (12 of 110) of elbow dislocations[45] (Fig. 19-30). Some authors have recommended open reduction and repair of the capsule-ligament lesion routinely, but most have presented good results with closed reduction and early range of motion for simple elbow dislocations.[17,38]

Josefsson et al compared surgical with nonsurgical treatment of ligamentous injuries after elbow dislocation in a prospectively randomized study.[39] Complete rupture or avulsion of both the medial and lateral collateral ligaments was documented. No statistically significant differences between the surgically repaired group and the nonsurgical group in terms of motion, strength, and recurrent instability were noted. Therefore closed management is recommended for all but the unusual case, even, and perhaps particularly, in cases involving an athlete.

Immobilization longer than 1 week is associated with increasing severity of stiffness, according to the work of Protzman and separately Mehlhoff[53,70] (Fig. 19-31). Both studies concluded that immobilization was strongly associated with an unsatisfactory result. Active range of motion was recommended in the first 1 to 2 weeks after injury. Recurrent or chronic instability does occur but is not common. Nevertheless, elbow stability should be monitored closely in the first few weeks after injury as rehabilitation proceeds.

Complications after elbow dislocation include loss of motion, myositis ossificans, usually involving the brachialis muscle, and calcification of the collateral ligaments.[17,23,53,70,88] Osteochondral or chondral injury also has been reported, which can lead to the production of loose bodies or subsequent painful traumatic arthritis.[17,26]

Fracture Dislocation

Fracture-dislocations of the elbow are not uncommon, as radial head fractures complicate approximately 5% to 10% of all elbow dislocations.[65] This combination of a fracture and dislocation carries a worse prognosis than a fracture or dislocation alone with an increased incidence of recurrent dislocation, loss of motion, and heterotopic bone formation (see Fig. 19-25).[8] Management of fracture-dislocations begins with reduction of the dislocation then proceeds with treatment of the associated fracture. The period of immobilization in these injuries is determined by the type and severity of the fracture and whether it can be treated with stable internal fixation.

Stress Fractures

Waris first described an olecranon stress fracture in 1946 when he reported on a transverse fracture of the olecranon in a javelin thrower.[94] Others subsequently described olecranon tip fractures.[58] Slocum suggested such fractures were caused by posterior impingement and are not true stress fractures as described by Waris.[80] Recent

A

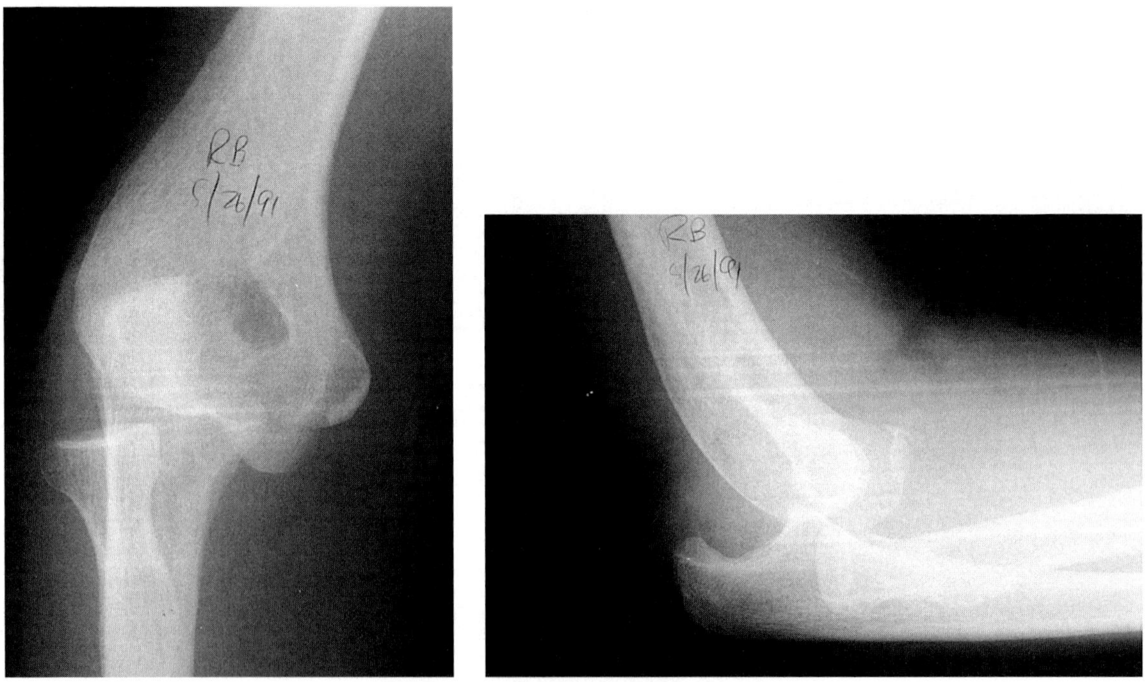

B

FIGURE 19-30 **A** and **B**, Radiographs of an acute posterior dislocation of the elbow.

C

D

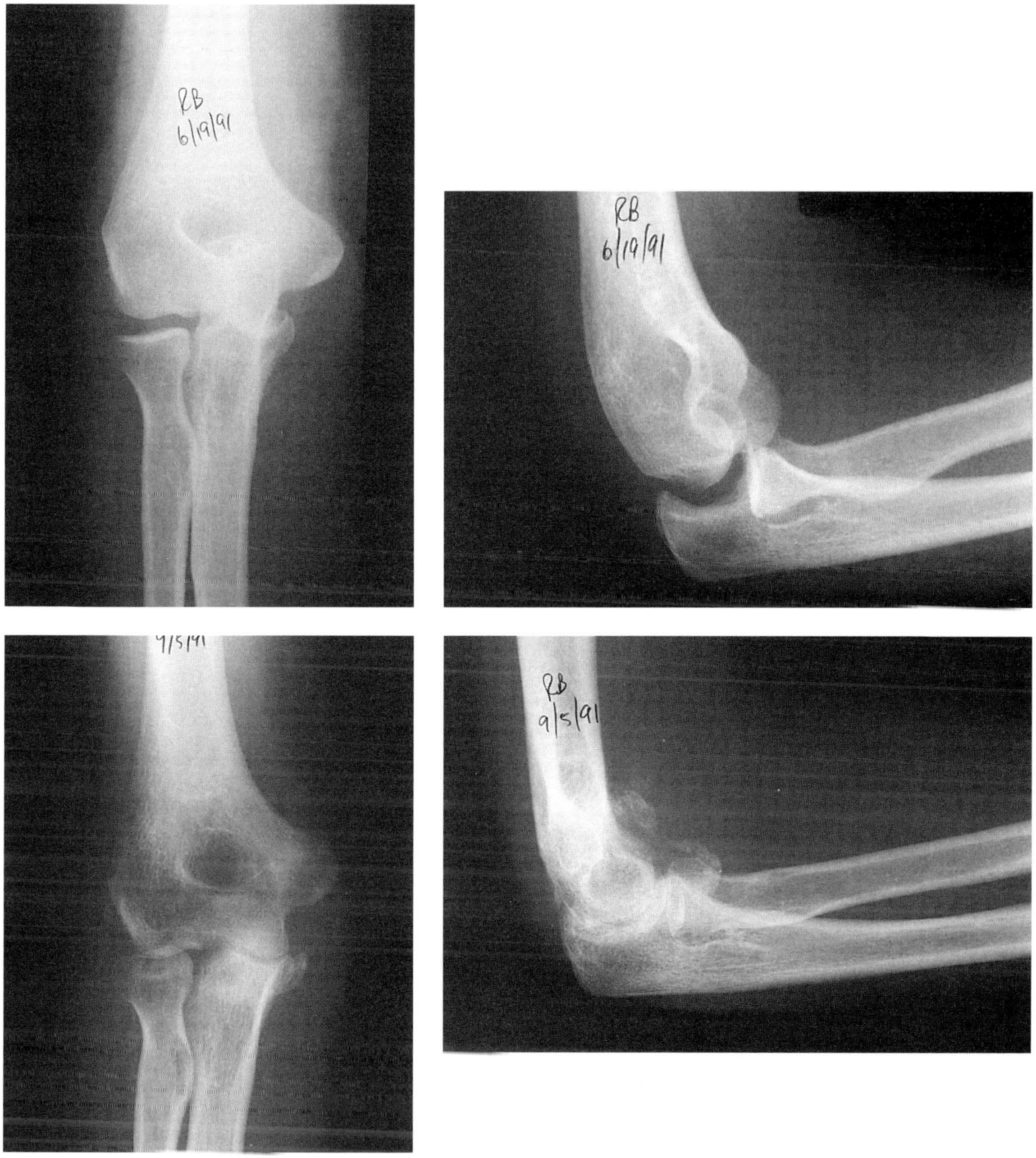

E

F

FIGURE 19-30—cont'd C and D, A closed reduction was performed, but the joint space was widened and the forearm was not reduced. Open reduction was attempted first through a lateral approach without success. At the same operation, a medial approach was made, and the humerus was found herniated through and incarcerated by the medial collateral ligament. **E** and **F**, Final radiographs 3½ months after injury show proper alignment. Capsular ossification did not prevent successful recovery of motion.

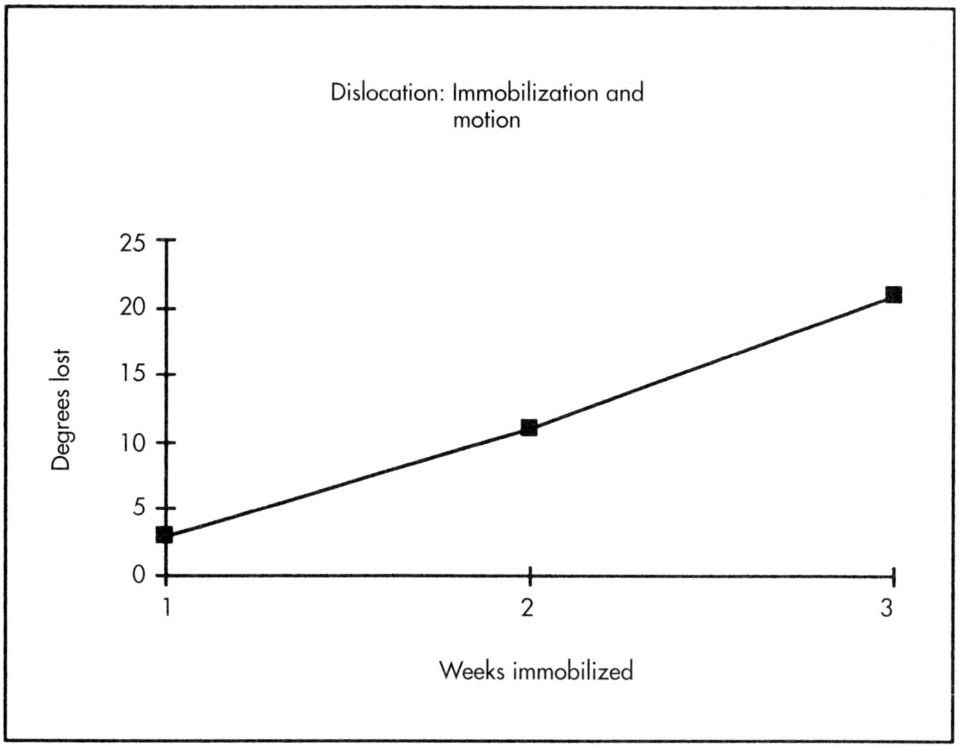

Protzman	Number	Weeks immobilization	Motion lost
	27	1	3
	13	2	11
	7	3	21
Totals	47		8

FIGURE 19-31 The association between duration of immobilization and elbow stiffness is shown by plotting data from Protzman.[70] The longer the period of immobilization, the greater the stiffness.

A

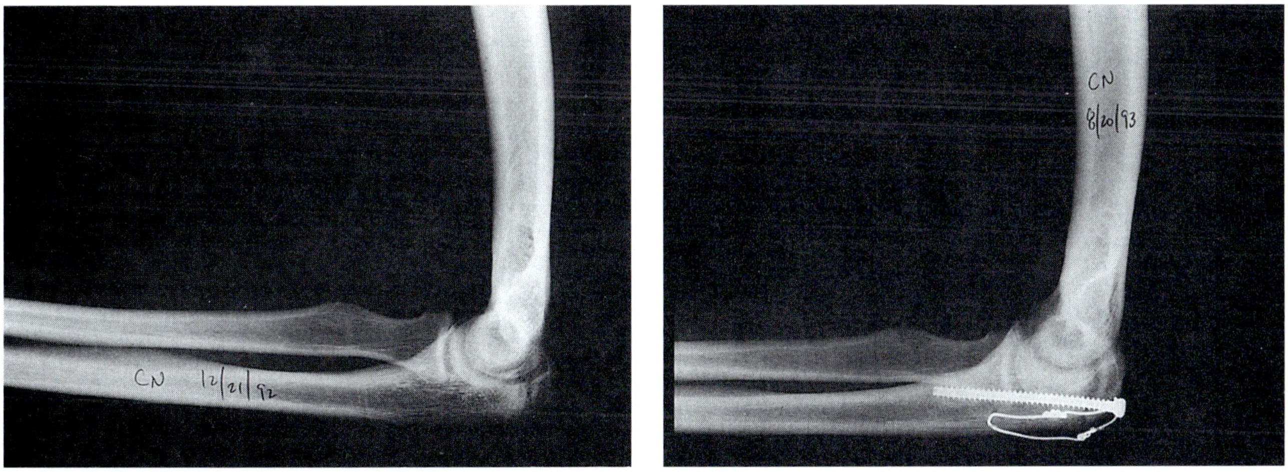

B

C

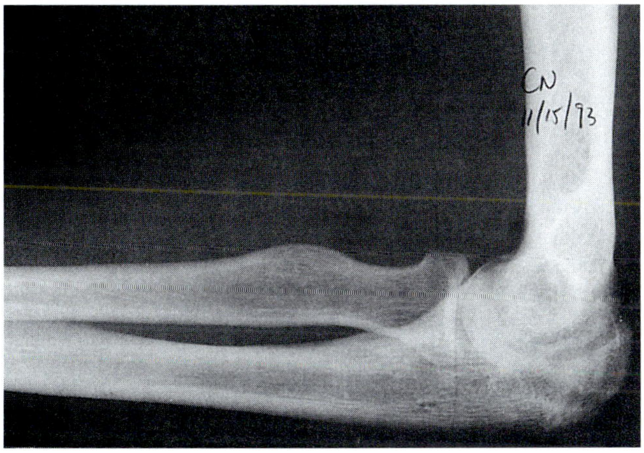

FIGURE 19-32 Chronic pain in a high-school pitcher's elbow was diagnosed as a nonunion of a stress fracture based on radiograph **A** and a bone scan showing increased uptake in the olecranon. **B,** A tension band system with cortical lag screw and loop or wire was used along with autogenous iliac cancellous bone to stabilize the pseudarthrosis. **C,** The hardware was removed 3 months later, and the patient returned to competition.

articles have reported stress fractures in adolescents and adults associated with throwing sports, baseball, or javelin.[67,89,97]

Operative and nonoperative alternatives for treatment of these injuries are justifiable. Reported cases often have been successfully treated with tension-band wiring and/or bone grafting. Tension bands neutralize high-tension forces on the posterior cortex and reduce the strain within the bone from the pull of the triceps. Bone graft may be added in delayed cases

Although the authors favor treatment with compression fixation for strain reduction and bone induction with autogenous graft (Fig. 19-32), Neuber and Dimet reported on two professional baseball pitchers with transverse olecranon fractures who were treated successfully with immobilization and elimination of throwing.[67] Both baseball pitchers resumed their previous level of throwing at approximately 5 to 6 months with healing of the fracture.

SUMMARY

As shown earlier, Fig. 19-4 A and B presents a composite of the various fracture classifications and the recommended operative treatment for each type. Anatomic position, rigid fixation, and aggressive rehabilitation are highly desirable with this set of injuries, particularly in an athletic population because of the rapid development of soft-tissue contracture and intraarticular adhesions. Careful operative planning combined with exacting technique and well-supervised rehabilitation will give the best result.

References

1. Adler JB, Shaftan GW: Radial head fractures, is excision necessary? *J Trauma* 4:115-136, 1964.
2. Aitken GK, Rorabeck CH: Distal humeral fractures in the adult, *Clin Orthop* 207:191-197, 1986.
3. Alvarez E et al: Fractures of the capitellum humeri, *J Bone Joint Surg* 57A:1093-1096, 1975.
4. An KN, Morrey BF: Biomechanics of the elbow. In Morrey BF, editor: *The elbow and its disorders,* Philadelphia, 1985, WB Saunders.
5. An KN, Morrey BF, Chad E: The effect of partial removal of proximal ulna on elbow constraint, *Clin Orthop* 209:270-279, 1986.
6. Bickel WE, Perry RE: Comminuted fractures of the distal humerus, *JAMA* 184:552-557, 1963.
7. Broberg MA, Morrey BF: Results of delayed excision of the radial head after fracture, *J Bone Joint Surg* 68A:669-674, 1986.
8. Broberg MA, Morrey BF: Results of treatment of fracture dislocations of the elbow, *Clin Orthop* 216:109-119, 1987.
9. Bryan RS: Fractures about the elbow in adults, *AAOS Instr Course Lect* 30:200-223, 1981.

10. Bunker TD, Newmon JH: The Herbert differential pitch bone screw in displaced radial head fractures, *Injury* 16:621-624, 1985.
11. Carstam Nils: Operative treatment of fracture of the head and neck of the radius, *Acta Orthop Scand* 19:502-526, 1951.
12. Cassebaum WH: Operative treatment of T- and Y-fractures of the lower end of the humerus, *Am J Surg* 83:265-270, 1952.
13. Coleman DA, Blair WF, Shurr D: Resection of the radial head for fracture of the radial head, *J Bone Joint Surg* 69A:385-392, 1987.
14. Collert S: Surgical management of fracture of the capitellum humeri, *Acta Orthop Scand* 48:603-606, 1977.
15. Conn J, Wade PA: Injuries of the elbow (a ten-year review), *J Trauma* 1:248-268, 1961.
16. Delee JC, Green DP, Wilkins KE: Fractures and dislocations of the elbow. In Rockwood C, Green DP, editors: *Fractures and dislocations,* Philadelphia, 1985, JB Lippincott, pp 559-652.
16a. Dickson I: Fractures of the upper end of the radius and ulna, *Surg Gynecol Obstet* 88:69, 1949.
17. Durgi M et al: The operative treatment of elbow dislocation in the adult, *J Bone Joint Surg* 61A:239-244, 1979.
18. Edward GS, Jupiter JB: Radial head fractures with acute distal radioulnar dislocation, *Clin Orthop* 234:61-69, 1988.
19. Essex-Lopresti P: Fractures of the radial head with distal radio-ulnar dislocation: report of two cases, *J Bone Joint Surg* 33B:244-247, 1951.
20. Fleetcroft JP: Fractures of the radial head: early aspiration and mobilization, *J Bone Joint Surg* 66B:141-142, 1984.
21. Fowles JV, Kassab MT: Fracture of the capitellum humeri: treatment by excision, *J Bone Joint Surg* 56A:794-798, 1974.
22. Gabel GT et al: Intra-articular fractures of the distal humerus in the adult, *Clin Orthop* 216:99-108, 1987.
23. Garland DE, Hanscom DA, Keenon MA: Resection of heterotopic ossification in the adult with head trauma, *J Bone Joint Surg* 67A:1261-1269, 1985.
24. Gartman GM, Sculco TP, Otis JC: Operative treatment of olecranon fractures: excision or open reduction with internal fixation, *J Bone Joint Surg* 63A:1396-1401, 1985.
25. Gaston SR, Smith FM, Baab OD: Adult injuries of the radial head and neck: importance of time element in treatment, *Am J Surg* 78A:631-635, 1949.
26. Grant IR, Miller JH: Osteochondral fracture of the trochlea associated with fracture-dislocation of the elbow, *Injury* 6:257-260, 1975.
27. Green DP, McCoy H: Turnbuckle orthotic correction of elbow flexion contractures after acute injuries, *J Bone Joint Surg* 61A:1092-1095, 1970.
28. Greenspan A, Norman A: The radial head capitellar view: useful technique in elbow trauma, *AJR* 8:1186-1190, 1982.
29. Hahn NF: Fall von eine besonderes Varietat der Fracturen des Ellenbogens, *Zeitschrift Wundartze und Gerburtshelfe* 6:185-189, 1853.
30. Holdworth BJ, Clement DA, Rothwell PN: Fractures of the radial head—the benefit of aspiration: a prospective controlled trial, *Injury* 18:44-47, 1987.
31. Horne G: Supracondylar fractures of the humerus in adults, *J Trauma* 20(1):71, 1980.
32. Hotchkiss RN, Weiland AJ: Valgus stability of the elbow, *Orthop Trans* 10:224, 1986.
33. Hoyer A: Treatment of supracondylar fracture of the humerus by skeletal traction in an abduction splint, *J Bone Joint Surg* 34A:623-637, 1952.
34. Inglis AE: The rehabilitation of the elbow after injury, *Instr Course Lect* XL:45-49, 1991.
35. Jeshrani MK, Bencivenga A: The management of intraarticular fractures at the lower end of the humerus, *East Afr Med J* 55(8):393, 1978.
36. Johansson O: Capsular and ligament injuries of the elbow joint, *Acta Chir Scand Suppl* 287, 1962.
37. Johnston GW: Follow-up of one hundred cases fracture of head of the radius with a review of the literature, *Ulster Med J* 31:51-56, 1962.
38. Josefsson PO et al: Long-term sequelae of simple dislocations of the elbow, *J Bone Joint Surg* 66A:927-930, 1984.
39. Josefsson PO et al: Surgical versus non-surgical treatment of ligamentous injuries following dislocation of the elbow joint, *J Bone Joint Surg* 69A:605-608, 1987.
40. Jupiter JB et al: Intercondylar fractures of the humerus, *J Bone Joint Surg* 67A:226-239, 1985.
41. Keon-Cohen BT: Fractures at the elbow, *J Bone Joint Surg* 48A:1623-1639, 1966.
42. Kocher R: *Beitrage zur Kenntniss einiger tisch wichtiger Frackturformen,* Basel, Switzerland, 1896, Sallman.
43. Koppis M: Uber eigernartige Knorpelverletzungen om capitulum humeri und devn Bezeihunger Zur Entstehung der freien Ellbogenbelenkhorper, *Deutsche Zeitschr F Chir* 142:182-216, 1917.
44. Lansinger O, Mare K: Fracture of the capitulum humeri, *Acta Orthop Scand* 100:37, 1982.
45. Linscheid RL, Wheeler DK: Elbow dislocations, *JAMA* 194:1171-1176, 1965.
46. Lorenz H: Zur Kenntniss der Fractura humeri (eminentiae capitatae), *Deutsche Zeitschr F Chir* 78:531-545, 1905.
47. Maeko D, Szabo RM: Complications of tension-band wiring of olecranon fractures, *J Bone Joint Surg* 67A:1396-1401, 1985.
48. Mason M: Some observations on fractures of the head of the radius with a review of one hundred cases, *Br J Surg* 42:123-132, 1954.
49. Mast J, Jakob R, Ganz R: *Planning and reduction technique in fracture surgery,* Berlin, 1989, Springer-Verlag.
50. Mayhall WST, Tiley FT, Paluska DJ: Fractures of Silastic radial head prosthesis, *J Bone Joint Surg* 63A:459-460, 1981.
51. McDougal A, White J: Subluxation of the inferior radioulnar joint complicating fracture of the radial head, *J Bone Joint Surg* 35B:278, 1957.
52. McKeever FM, Buck RM: Fracture of the olecranon process of the ulna, *JAMA* 135:1-5, 1947.
53. Mehlhoff TL et al: Simple dislocation of the elbow in the adult, *J Bone Joint Surg* 70A:244-249, 1988.
54. Mehni D, Jupiter JB: *Skeletal trauma,* vol 2. In Browner BD et al, editors: Philadelphia, 1992, WB Saunders, p 1151.
55. Mikic ZD, Vukadinovic SM: Late results in fractures of radial head treated by excision, *Clin Orthop* 181:220-228, 1983.
56. Milch H: Fractures and fracture dislocations of the humeral condyles, *J Trauma* 4:592-607, 1964.
57. Miller GK, Drennan DB, Maylahn DJ: Treatment of displaced segmental radial head fractures, *J Bone Joint Surg* 63A:712-717, 1981.
58. Miller JE: Javelin thrower's elbow, *J Bone Joint Surg* 42B:788, 1960.
59. Morrey BF: Anatomy and kinematics of the elbow, *Instr Course Lect* XI:11-16, 1991.
60. Morrey BF: Posttraumatic stiffness: distraction arthroplasty, *Orthopaedics* 15:863-869, 1992.
61. Morrey BF, An KN: Articular and ligamentous contributions to the stability of the elbow joint, *Am J Sports Med* 11:315-319, 1983.
62. Morrey BF, An KN: Functional anatomy of the ligaments of the elbow, *Clin Orthop* 201:84-90, 1985.
63. Morrey BF, An KN, Stormont TJ: Force transmission through the radial head, *J Bone Joint Surg* 70A:250-256, 1988.
64. Mueller ME et al: *Manual of internal fixation,* ed 3, New York, 1992, Springer-Verlag.
65. Neviaser JS, Wickstrom JK: Dislocation of the elbow: a retrospective study of 115 patients, *South Med J* 70:172-173, 1977.
66. Nirschl RP, Morrey BF: Rehabilitation. In Morrey BF, editor: *The elbow and its disorders,* Philadelphia, 1985, WB Saunders, pp 147-152.
67. Nuber GW, Dimets MT: Olecranon stress fractures in throwers, *Clin Orthop* 278:58-61, 1992.

68. Odenheimer K, Harvey JP: Internal fixation of fracture of the head of the radius, *J Bone Joint Surg* 61A:785-787, 1979.
69. Pribyl CR: The effect of the radial head and prosthetic radial head replacement on resisting valgus stress at the elbow, *Orthopaedics* 9:723-726, 1986.
70. Protzman RR: Dislocation of the elbow joint, *J Bone Joint Surg* 60A:539-541, 1980.
71. Radin EL, Riseborough EJ: Fractures of the radial head: a review of eighty-eight cases and analysis of the indications for excision of the radial head and non-operative treatment, *J Bone Joint Surg* 48A:1055-1061, 1966.
72. Reference deleted in proofs.
73. Regan W, Morrey B: Fractures of the coronoid process of the ulna, *J Bone Joint Surg* 71A:1348-1354, 1989.
74. Rettig AC, Waugh TR, Evanski PM: Fracture of the olecranon: a problem of management, *J Trauma* 19:23-28, 1979.
75. Riseborough EJ, Radin EL: Intercondylar T-fractures of the humerus in the adult (a comparison of operative and nonoperative treatment in twenty-nine cases), *J Bone Joint Surg* 51A: 130-141, 1969.
76. Robertson FC, Bogart FB: Fracture of the capitellum and trochlea, combined with fractures of the external humeral condyle, *J Bone Joint Surg* 15:206-213, 1933.
77. Scharplatz D, Allgoewer M: Fracture-dislocation of the elbow, *Injury* 7:143-159, 1976.
78. Shmueli G, Herold HZ: Compression screwing of displaced fractures of the head of the radius, *J Bone Joint Surg* 63B:535-538, 1981.
79. Simpson LA, Richards RR: Internal fixation of a capitellar fracture using Herbert screws, *Clin Orthop* 209:166-169, 1986.
80. Slocum DB: Classification of elbow injuries from baseball pitching, *Tex Med* 64:48, 1968.
81. Smith FM: Medical epicondyle injuries, *JAMA* 142:396-402, 1950.
82. Smith FM: *Surgery of the elbow,* ed 2, Philadelphia, 1972, WB Saunders.
83. Speed K: *Textbook of fractures and dislocation,* Philadelphia, 1935, Lea & Febiger.
84. Steinthal D: Die isolierte Fraktur der Eminentia capitata in Ellenbogengelenk, Centrallb, *f Chirurgi* 15:17-20, 1898.
85. Stimson LA: *A treatise on fractures,* Philadelphia, 1890, Henry C Lea's Son.
86. Swanson AB, Jaeger SH, Rochelle DL: Comminuted fractures of the radial head: the role of silicone-implant replacement arthroplasty, *J Bone Joint Surg* 63A:1039-1049, 1981.
87. Taylor TKF, O'Connor BT: The effect upon the inferior radio-ulnar joint of excision of the head of the radius in adults, *J Bone Joint Surg* 46B:83, 1967.
88. Thompson HC, Garcia A: Myositis ossificans: aftermath of elbow injuries, *Clin Orthop* 50:129-134, 1967.
89. Torg JS, Moyer RA: Nonunion of a stress fracture through the olecranon epiphyseal plate observed in an adolescent baseball pitcher, *J Bone Joint Surg* 59A:264-265, 1977.
90. Tullos HS et al: Factors influencing elbow instability, *Instr Course Lect* XXX:185-189, 1981.
91. Urbaniak JR et al: Correction of post-traumatic flexor contracture of the elbow by anterior capsulotomy, *J Bone Joint Surg* 67A: 1160-1165, 1985.
92. Vierhout RJ, Ostvogel HJM, Van Vroonhover JMV: Internal fixation of the head of the radius, *Neth J Surg* 35(1):13, 1983.
93. Wadsworth TG: Screw fixation of the olecranon after fracture or osteotomy, *Clin Orthop* 119:197-201, 1976.
94. Waris W: Elbow injuries of javelin throwers, *Acta Chir Scand* 93:563, 1946.
95. Weseley MS, Barenfeld PA, Eisenstein AL: Closed treatment of isolated radial head fractures, *J Trauma* 23A:36-39, 1983.
96. Weseley MS, Barenfeld PA, Eisenstein AL: The use of Zuelzer hook plate in fixation of olecranon fractures, *J Bone Joint Surg* 58A:859-863, 1976.
97. Wilkerson RD, Johns JC: Nonunion of an olecranon stress fracture in an adolescent gymnast, *Am J Sports Med* 18:432-434, 1990.
98. Zagorski JB et al: Intra-articular fractures of the distal humeral condyles, *Clin Orthop* 202:197-204, 1986.

CHAPTER 20

Long-Bone Fractures of the Upper Extremity

ROBERT W. CHANDLER

FOREARM FRACTURES

Incidence and Initial Evaluation

Patients with upper-extremity long-bone fractures present with a history of physical injury, often of a severe nature. A large series of 664 forearm fractures in 415 patients reported from multiple centers in Germany reported road accidents as the cause of fracture in 55%.[71] Additional statistics from their review showed a third of the fractures were compound, indicating the high energy of the trauma. Similar statistics were reported by Chapman from the United States.[14] Table 20-1 compares these series.

Diagnosis of forearm fracture considers the history of injury, location of pain and tenderness, condition of the skin, and neurologic and vascular status. Conventional orthogonal radiographs are sometimes difficult to obtain with adequate clarity in the acute setting but will suffice for all but the most complicated fractures. Clear visual-

TABLE 20-1
Comparison of Series Reporting Long-Bone Fractures

Number of fractures	664 in 415 patients (Weller)	129 in 88 patients (Chapman)
Open fractures	223 (34% of fractures)	49 (38% of fractures)
Both bones	249 (60% of patients)	42 (48% of patients)
Solitary ulna	92 (22% of fractures)	27 (31% of fractures)
Solitary radius	74 (18% of fractures)	18 (20% of fractures)
Monteggia fracture	41 (6% of fractures)	10 (11% of fractures)
Galeazzi fracture	18 (2.7% of fractures)	14 (16% of fractures)
Associated humerus or metacarpal	10%	

ization of the wrist and elbow joints is mandatory. Stress fractures are typified by chronic physical activity such as throwing, rowing, and lifting, yet may present with negative x-rays and require a bone scan, tomography, or magnetic resonance imaging for verification.

Classification

Complicated classification is not of great clinical value in this region of the skeleton. In 1983, Johner and Wruhs presented a series of tibial shaft fractures for which they devised a classification system that is adaptable for any shaft fracture including the forearm.[34] A fractures are spiral (A1), oblique (A2), or transverse (A3) without comminution. B fractures are fractures with butterfly fragments produced by torsion (B1), low-speed bending (B2), or high-speed bending (B3). Finally, C fractures are comminuted and include high-speed torsion (C1), four-point bending (C2), and crushing (C3).

Other than the degree of comminution and the grading of soft-tissue injury, fractures may be categorized as single-bone, radius or ulna, both bones, fracture dislocation, and complex. Care is necessary to differentiate isolated radius or ulna fractures from their fracture-dislocation counterparts. Beware of an apparent isolated radius or ulna fracture produced not by a direct blow but by a fall because it is more likely a nondisplaced fracture-dislocation (Figs. 20-1 and 20-2).

Monteggia fracture dislocation is defined as an ulna-shaft fracture with associated dislocation of the radial head. Bado has defined morphologic variants of this injury[4] (Box 20-1). The more complex and difficult variants of the Monteggia fracture dislocation involve the elbow joint and are discussed in the chapter on elbow fractures.

A radial shaft fracture with associated disruption of the distal radioulnar joint is a *Galeazzi fracture dislocation.* In a Galeazzi fracture, most often the radius fractures in the distal diaphysis, but variants do occur. Moore, having studied this lesion in the laboratory, defined four reliable radiographic signs of rupture of the capsule and ligaments of the distal radioulnar joint[42]:

BOX 20-1
BADO'S VARIANTS OF THE MONTEGGIA FRACTURE

Type I: Anterior angulation of the ulna with anterior dislocation of the radial head
Type II: Posterior angulation of the ulnar shaft with associated posterior dislocation of the radial head
Type III: Fracture of the proximal ulnar metaphysis with lateral dislocation of the radial head
Type IV: Anterior dislocation of the radial head with associated fractures of both forearm shaft bones

1. Fracture of the ulnar styloid at its base
2. Widening of the joint space of the distal radioulnar joint on an AP radiograph
3. Dislocation of the radioulnar joint on a lateral projection
4. More than 5 mm of shortening

Curr and Coe, in a case report in 1946, described an injury to both joint elements of the radius.[15] Five years later, Essex-Lopresti reported two cases of the condition that now bears his name.[24] The major problem with the Essex-Lopresti fracture dislocation lies in its recognition. Morrey and Trousdale have refined the description of the Essex-Lopresti injury, as the following[65]:

Concomitant injuries of the lateral compartment of the radiohumeral joint and ipsilateral radiocarpal joint:

1. Elbow component
   a. Fracture of the radial head with and without elbow dislocation
   b. Fracture of the radial head and capitellum
   c. Monteggia fracture
   d. Dislocation of the elbow with capitellum fracture
2. Wrist component
   a. Galeazzi fracture
   b. Ligamentous injury

Such injuries may be hard to recognize because they

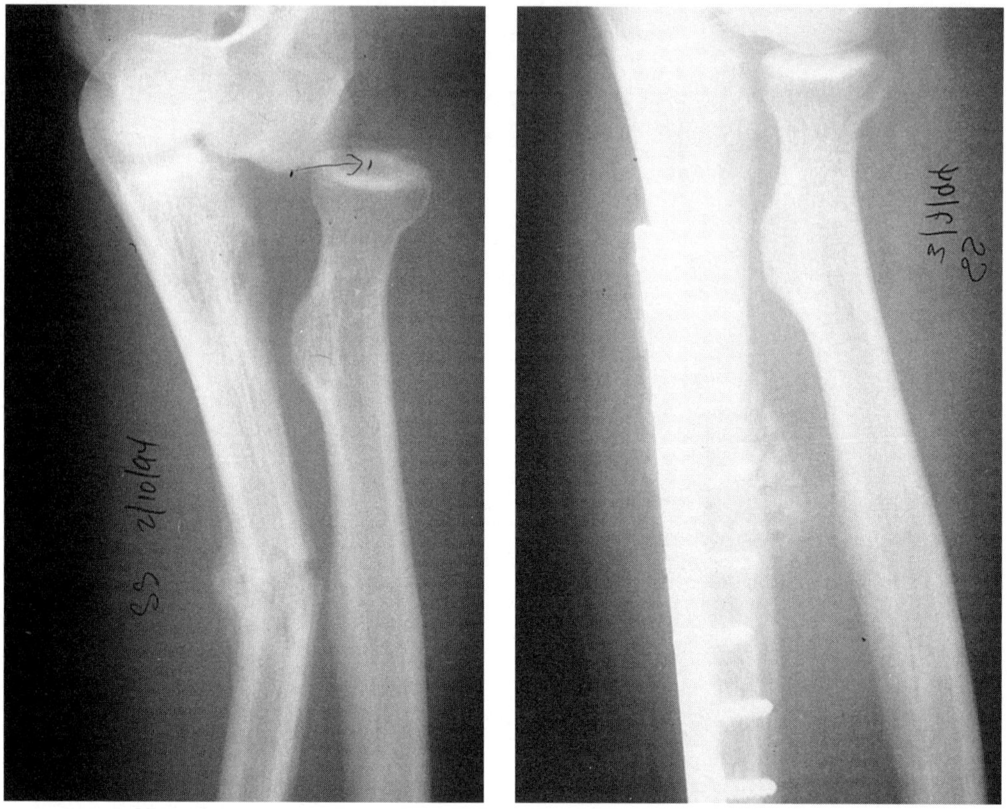

FIGURE 20-1 Displaced ulnar shaft with associated radial head fracture mistaken initially for an isolated shaft fracture.

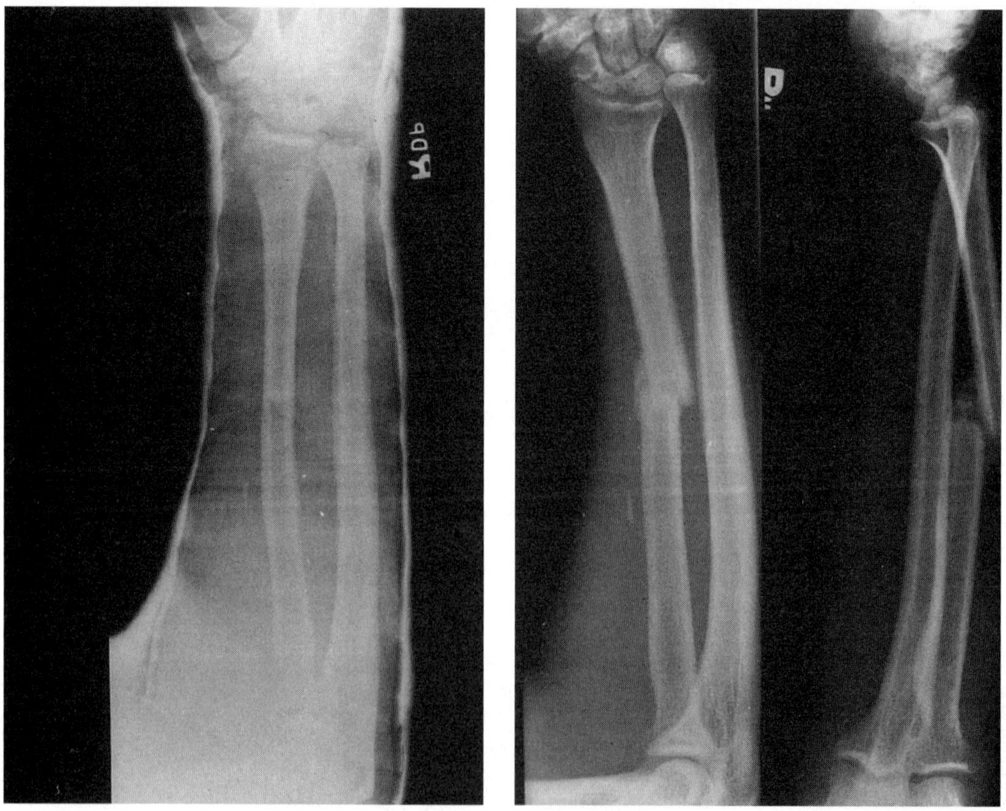

FIGURE 20-2 An apparently stable fracture of the radial shaft shows its true nature with secondary displacement during nonoperative fracture brace treatment.

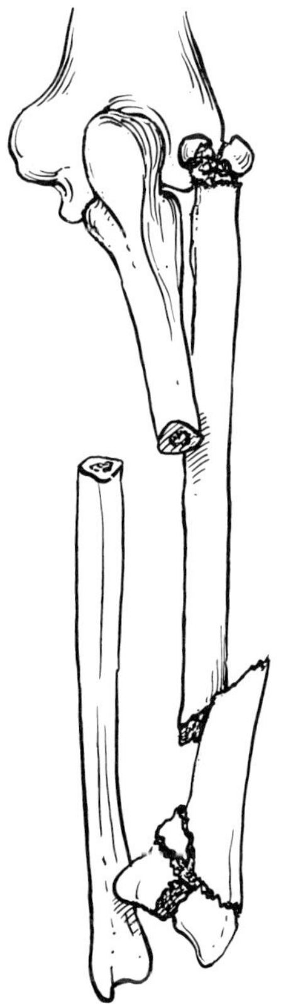

FIGURE 20-3 A complex injury consists of elements of other named lesions.

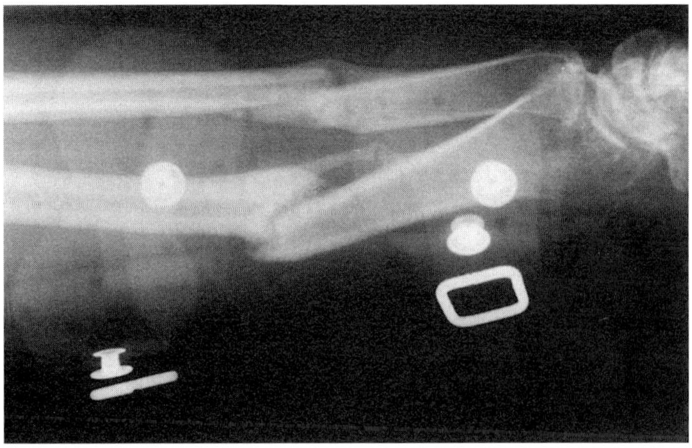

FIGURE 20-4 A failed attempt at conservative care resulted in function limited malunion.

seldom occur as an isolated problem. High-energy trauma may be involved, thus other more serious and potentially life-threatening aspects may tend to receive attention first.

A complex injury in the forearm is a manifestation of severe trauma and may be defined as a forearm fracture combined with the following:

1. More than one category in the same segment (Fig. 20-3)
   a. Galeazzi + Monteggia = Montazii
   b. Essex-Lopresti + Galeazzi + Monteggia = Essex-Montazzi
   c. Colles + Essex-Montazzi = Essex-Coll-Montazzi
   d. Barton + Essex-Montazzi = Essex-Bartomontazzi
2. More than one ipsilateral limb segment involved
   a. Contiguous (e.g., floating elbow, floating wrist, or forearm fracture combined with unnamed associated joint injury)
   b. Noncontiguous (e.g., forearm fracture + shoulder)

Treatment

Skeletal Stabilization Methods

Intramedullary devices for forearm fractures continue to attract interest even though history has recorded less desirable results than with plate osteosynthesis. Even though large series of forearm fractures include some cases treated with intramedullary devices for special circumstances, these devices have not yet become standard treatment after they were abandoned by past generations of fracture surgeons. Forearm bones present formidable obstacles for intramedullary treatment:

1. Small-diameter canals (3 mm in places)
2. Dorsal bow of the radius
3. Tapering sigmoid canal of the ulna

The standard of care for forearm fractures and fracture dislocations with few exceptions is plate osteosynthesis (Fig. 20-4). AO/ASIF plate methods are strongly recommended.[43] Shatzker and Tile[54] wrote the following plea for internal fixation in a recent text:

> The natural history of the forearm fracture, under almost all circumstances, is so uncertain when treated by means other than anatomical open reduction, stable internal fixation with plates, and early motion of the extremity, that this treatment can be recommended in almost all cases described below.
>
> 1. Fractures of both bones
> 2. Fractures of one bone
> 3. Open fracture of the forearm

External fixators have rare indications in severe open situations. Müller et al[43] have given indications for external fixation in the forearm:

> Primary use of the external fixator has proved useful in two situations:
>
> 1. Combined shaft and comminuted distal radius fractures
> 2. Compound fractures with defects

Added to these indications are stabilization in cases of infection when internal fixation is unstable, in acute open cases when contamination and/or devascularization is severe, or when plating is best avoided because of swollen soft tissues.[39] Initial application of external fixation always requires a second stage of management,

A

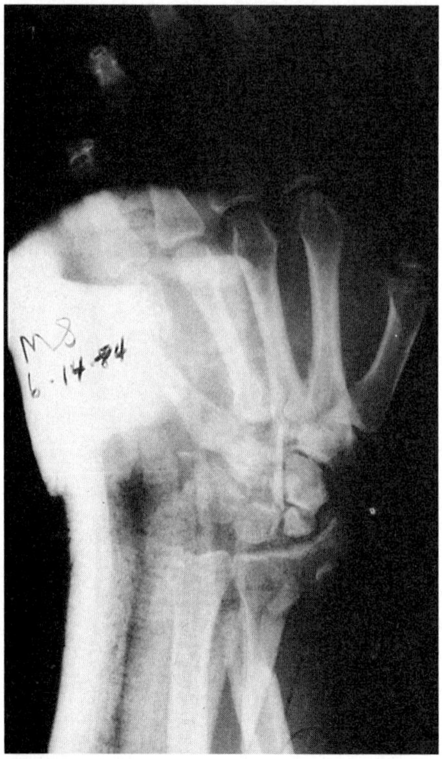

B

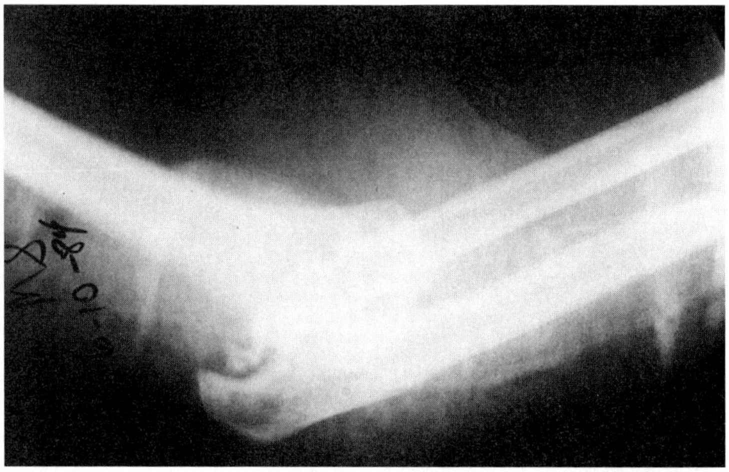

C

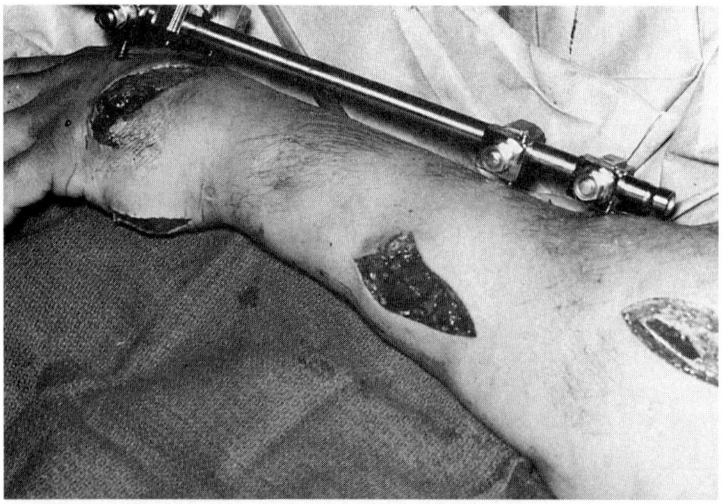

D

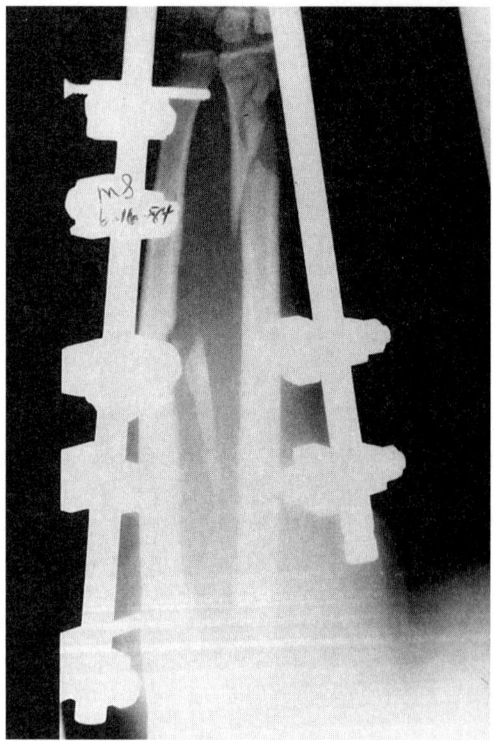

E

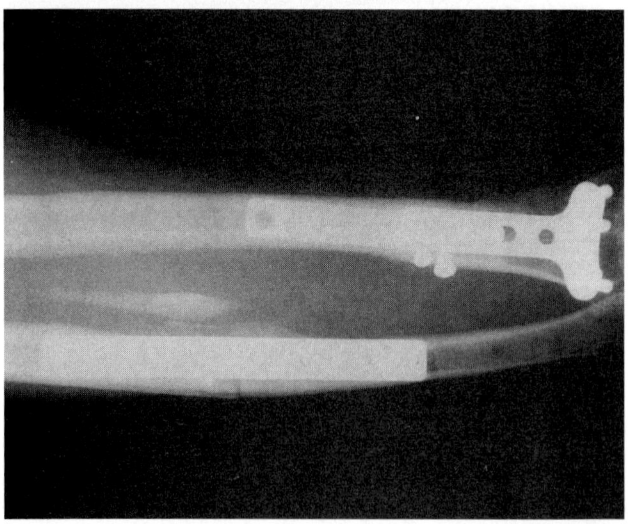

FIGURE 20-5 **A** and **B**, Initial plate osteosynthesis was rejected in favor of external fixation because of the degree of soft-tissue swelling and the presence of bacteria on Gram stain. **C** and **D**, External fixation using AO/ASIF 4.5-mm screws mounted on tubular rods stabilized both the radius and the ulna. **E**, With soft-tissue healing, frames were replaced with plates and bone graft.

such as internal fixation, bracing, or casting. Fig. 20-5 illustrates a case of initial external fixation followed by internal fixation with staged reconstruction after open fracture with associated wound colonization.

Soft-Tissue Considerations

Open Fractures

Plating of acute open fractures is indicated after surgical cleansing in all but the most contaminated wounds and devascularized bone.[22,35,40] Representative of the studies reporting the relative safety of this approach is that of Moed et al, who reviewed 57 cases of open fracture treated acutely with plate fixation.[40] They had nonunion in 6 of 57 cases (10.5%), infection in 2 of 57 (3.5%), and overall excellent results in 85%. All open fractures require the utmost care to remove nonviable tissues, preserve circulation, and provide effective prophylaxis against bacterial contamination. Open wound management is preferable to primary closure.

Compound wounds are left open initially, and at the time of secondary irrigation and débridement may be closed or may be gradually closed using rubber bands fixed to the skin edges with staples. Gradual skin tensioning with rubber bands combined with artificial skin is a good method of management until the swelling has resolved sufficiently for delayed primary closure. Delayed primary closure is preferable to split-thickness skin grafting, which contracts and leaves more scarring than delayed primary closure.

Closed Fractures

Periosteum and the soft-tissue envelope of bone are vital to revascularization of the cortex after fracture has disrupted the normal circulation by disruption of the nutrient vessel.[47-49] One of the main goals of internal-fixation operations must be preservation of soft tissues. Reduction by distraction and limited manipulation reduce trauma, preserve vascularity, and enhance healing while decreasing infection, compared with direct methods.[39] A wide array of useful instruments are available for exposure, manipulation, and temporary holding of bone fragments. Distractors, spreaders, and bone-holding clamps make the job of fracture realignment much easier.

Bone Graft

Traditionally, bone graft has been used when more than one third of the circumference of the bone at the level of the fracture is comminuted. This practice recently was questioned.[56] Large viable fragments participate in the healing response, making autologous graft unnecessary. A fracture with bone loss and comminution producing dysvascular fragments remains a good indication for autogenous cancellous graft, as is the true bone defect.

Operative Approaches

Only a few operative approaches to the forearm are necessary to accomplish reduction and fixation. The anterior, or Henry, approach (Fig. 20-6) is our preferred ap-

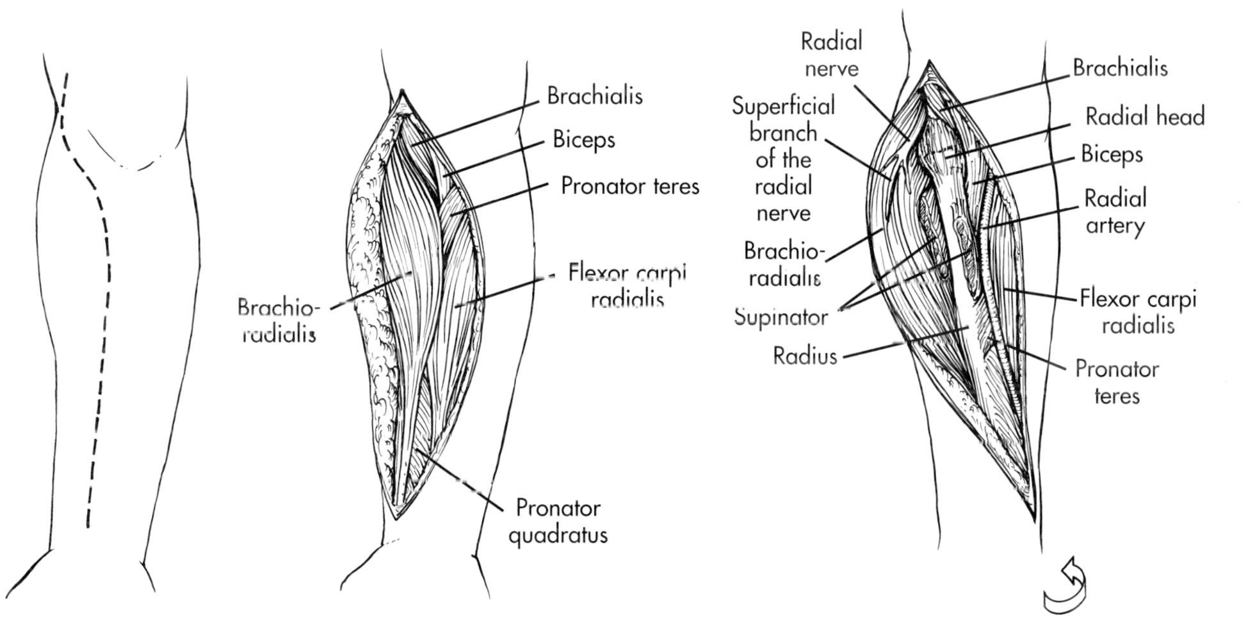

FIGURE 20-6 The anterior approach of Henry allows access to the entire radial shaft and may serve as the approach for fixations of the radial shaft. Platings of the proximal third must be applied to the dorsoradial aspect of the bone. Supination during plate application presents the proper surface of the bone.

proach because it exposes the entire radial shaft through an internervous plane with less risk of injury to the radial nerve. The posterior approach presents the dorsoradial aspect of the radius, the ideal surface for plating of the proximal half, more readily than the anterior approach, in which the forearm must be pronated for access to the proper (dorsoradial) surface but also exposes the terminal arborization of the radial nerve.[31] The ulna is accessible through a subcutaneous approach with plate placement on the dorsal aspect of the bone.

Plate selection is determined by the size of the bone and the length of the fracture.[43,44] Most bones can be adequately stabilized with 3.5-mm dynamic compression plate (DCP), or the limited contact dynamic compression plate (LC-DCP).* The minimum length should be seven holes, which allows for seven cortices above and below the fracture as well as a lag screw across the fracture. Occasionally, a large bone should have a 4.5-mm DCP or LC-DCP. The author prefers the limited-contact titanium plates because of ease of use, greater choice of screw orientation, more uniform material strain, and decreased cortical contact. One-third tubular (3.5-mm curved) plates are not appropriate for most forearm fractures.

Optimizing the mechanical function of the plate will improve union. Plates may have different functions, which are determined by application technique rather than type of plate.[43] When the fracture is fixed with a lag screw either through the plate or outside of the plate, the plate then functions to reduce bending and twisting motions and thereby protects the lag screw. The lag screw provides interfragmentary compression, and the plate is referred to as a *neutralization plate.*

When the fracture will not accept a lag screw but the fracture may be compressed with the external plate tensioner or through use of the spherical gliding principle of the dynamic compression plate, then the plate is referred to as a compression plate. The compression provided is axial in direction. Transverse fractures are suitable for axial compression alone, and short oblique fractures may have both axial and interfragmentary compression after insertion of a lag screw through the plate. Prebending the plate will result in more even compression across the fracture.

A tension band function is present when the plate has been applied to the convex surface of a curved bone and requires interfragmentary compression and cortical contact on the concave side of the fracture. The tension band converts tension forces on the convex surface into even compressive load across the plane of the fracture. Under physiologic cyclic loading, the plate functions as a dynamic tension band.

Finally, comminution sometimes makes interfragmentary, axial, and tension band plating impossible. A plate applied to such a fracture acts to maintain alignment without compression (splintage) and with various-size gaps depending on the degree of comminution. A plate applied in this manner is referred to as a bridge plate or gap plate.

If a comminuted fragment has vascularity, the vascularity should be preserved and the fragment left out of the mechanical construct if fixing the fragment into the construct would devascularize the fragment. Some suggestions for plate fixation in the forearm are offered in Box 20-2.

BOX 20-2

RECOMMENDED OPERATIVE TREATMENT TIPS FOR PLATE FIXATION

- Provisionally fix the easier of the two.
- Make liberal use of distraction methods.
- Preserve soft-tissue attachments.
- Always leave the fascia open; sometimes leave the skin open over the radius if closure would be tight.

Specific Injuries and Treatment

Single-Bone Fractures

Nondisplaced fractures of the radial and ulnar shaft have been satisfactorily treated with a brief period of arm-to-hand casting followed by a functional fracture brace, as described by Sarmiento.[52] The ideal fracture for nonoperative management occurs in the middle third of the ulnar shaft, is closed, has less than 10° of angulation, has little or no displacement, and was the result of a direct blow.[63]

Casting from the metacarpal joints to the upper arm for 7 to 14 days is followed by application of a forearm fracture orthosis commonly made from plastic materials of various sorts with Velcro enclosures. The patient begins a gradual active-motion program and in most cases will have regained normal motion by the time of fracture union at 10 to 12 weeks. Ulnar or radial shaft fractures that resulted from a fall should not be treated this way. Occult joint injury will lead to secondary displacement.

Displacement and/or angulation of isolated forearm shaft fractures should be treated with plate osteosynthesis, following ASIF recommendations.

Both-Bone Fractures

Angular malreduction has an adverse effect on forearm rotation, as shown in both laboratory testing and clinical work. Tarr et al found that when both bones of the forearm were angulated with a combined deformity of 10°

*References 14, 39, 40, 43, 54, 71.

a loss of pronation-supination of 12.5% ± 4.5% occurred with distal third fractures, and 6.0% ± 5.7% with middle third fractures.[63] Supination losses were more severe with deformities in the middle third. Schemitsch et al found in a clinical study that recreation of the normal radial bow helped determine functional outcome.[55] Restoration of grip strength and forearm rotation was strongly correlated with radial bow restoration.

Good results have been obtained by following AO/ASIF methods, as shown by statistics from a collective review of 664 forearm fractures in 415 patients.[71] Full elbow flexion was achieved in 90%, full extension in 88%, full pronation in 80%, and supination in 82%. Overall, 87% had satisfactory or better results. In this country, Chapman reported good to satisfactory outcome in 92% of 87 patients with 129 diaphyseal fractures.[14]

Fracture Dislocations

Galeazzi Fractures

Anatomic reduction of the fracture typically reduces the distal radial ulna dislocation. Both volar and dorsal incarcerated distal ulna variations that require open reduction have been described. Joint transfixion of the distal joint for 3 to 6 weeks is necessary with severe instability, but typical stable reduction of the distal joint makes immobilization for more than 1 to 4 weeks unnecessary.

Moore et al reported on 84 patients with 129 Galeazzi fractures out of 1236 fractures of the forearm treated in a 5-year period.[42] Of the 84, 36 were followed 1.5 to 7 years after open reduction and plate osteosynthesis.[42] Anatomic reduction was achieved in 97% of the 84, but 39% had complications. Seven had injuries to the sensory or interosseous branch of the radial nerve, two had infections, two had nonunions, two had refracture after plate removal, and one had 5-mm shortening of the radius. Grip strength averaged 71% of normal. Strength loss was associated with loss of motion. Of the 36 followed, 33 lost less than 20° of wrist motion or 25° of forearm rotation.

Monteggia Fractures

Monteggia fracture dislocations are a family of injuries that vary from simple to complex. Open anatomic reduction and internal fixation in most cases reestablishes normal anatomic relationships of the radiohumeral joint.[6,11,16] In late cases and cases in which the radial head is not returned to its normal position with reduction of the ulna, open reduction of the radial head through a separate lateral approach is indicated. Arthrotomy and radial head reconstruction or excision are rarely needed. Routine arthrotomy to débride the joint has been advised for posterior lesions caused by associated radial head fragmentation. Overall, satisfactory or better results have been obtained in 73% of such injuries[71] (Table 20-2).

TABLE 20-2

Function after Plate Fixation of Monteggia Fractures, $n = 55$[71]

	Deficit in Flexion-Extension (in Degrees)	Deficit in Pronation-Supination (in Degrees)
0°	19	17
5°-30°	22	14
35°-50°	4	6
>50°	10	18

Essex Lopresti Fractures

Reconstruction of the radial head fracture or replacement with a spacer is necessary to stabilize the interosseous membrane and the distal joint. Later removal of the spacer may be necessary because none have been shown to hold up over the long term.

Trousdale reported 20 cases aged 8 to 74 with follow-up ranging from 4 months to 27 years.[65] Delayed diagnosis of the wrist injury was characteristic, averaging 7 months in 15 patients. These 15 had radial head excision with resulting severe pain at the distal radioulnar joint. Only 3 of these patients had satisfactory results. The wrist injury was diagnosed at the time of injury in 5 patients, and the radial head was preserved or replaced, with 4 of 5 having a satisfactory result. Late reconstruction consisting of ulnar shortening and fascial arthroplasty of the radiocapitellar joint may offer some relief.

Complex Fractures

Combination injuries consisting of variations on the aforementioned groupings require the same aggressive approach to maximize outcome.[23] Axial realignment, care of the soft tissues, and staged reconstruction help maximize outcome.

Complications and Associated Problems

Nonunion

Nonunion after diaphyseal fractures of the forearm occurs in approximately 1% to 13% of cases.* In an article in 1988, Louis Anderson identified risk factors associated with nonunion as: open fracture, extensive comminution, devascularization, infection, distraction, and inadequate fixation.[3]

Treatment of nonunion has included electrical stimulation, bone grafting, and repeat osteosynthesis.[29,59,70] Heppenstall reported union in 80% of 50 cases after 3 months of direct-current stimulation.[29] Unfortunately, electrical stimulation requires immobilization. Furthermore, malposition of the fracture is not improved.

In his classic monograph, Weber reported on 46 forearm bone nonunions in 41 patients, including 3 with infections.[70] All fractures eventually healed. Of the 46, 42

*References 3, 13, 14, 16, 29, 42, 57, 62, 71.

fractures had one operation, 2 had two operations, and 1 had three procedures. Plates were used in 38 operations, and autologous grafts were used in half. Five cases had graft alone, and three cases were treated with an Oberholzer nail, lag screw, or tension band plus compression screw. Recently, percutaneous bone graft has been successfully applied when stable fixation was present.[25,59]

Cross Union

The incidence of radioulnar synostosis averages 2.6%, with a range of 1% to 11%.* Risk factors for development of these challenging problems include location in the proximal third, both bones fractured at the same level, Boyd approach, severe soft-tissue trauma, and delay in treatment.

There is no consensus for treatment of cross unions. Vince reported on resection of cross unions in 17 patients.[69] Three out of 4 recurred when the synostosis was in the distal third, none of 10 recurred with middle third lesions, and 2 of 3 recurred with lesions on the proximal third. Abrams combined excision with low-dose radiation successfully in 2 cases.[29] Breit excised the synostosis and interposed muscle successfully in 1 case.[12] We have resected 3 proximal cross unions without recurrence by combining resection with immediate rehabilitation.

Infection

Infection occurs in 2% to 9% of operated forearm fractures.† Débridement, antibiotics, bone stability, and bone induction are key elements to success in obtaining union and controlling or eradicating infection.[32]

Refracture

Any time plates are used, refracture is a concern. The incidence of fractures in forearms with the plates in plated retained ranges from 1% to 3%.[4,19,30,67] Fracture after plate removal is more of a problem: Moore had a refracture rate of 2 of 11, or 18%; Chapman had 2 of 34, or 6%; Hidaka had 7 of 32, or 22%; Deluca had 9 of 37, or 24%; and Weller reported a low of 1.5%. Compiling all these figures gives an overall refracture incidence of 20 of 114, or 17%.[14,19,30,42,71]

Risk factors associated with refracture include: removal less than a year after insertion, use of a 4.5-mm plate rather than the 3.5-mm plate, presence of lag screws in comminuted fragments, and incomplete union. We do not remove plates unless there is a specific problem, particularly in athletes.

FRACTURES OF THE HUMERAL SHAFT

Evaluation

Fractures of the humeral shaft are easily diagnosed on examination. Localized pain and swelling are the hallmarks

*References 1, 7, 12, 62, 64, 69.
†References 2, 14, 20, 42, 62, 71.

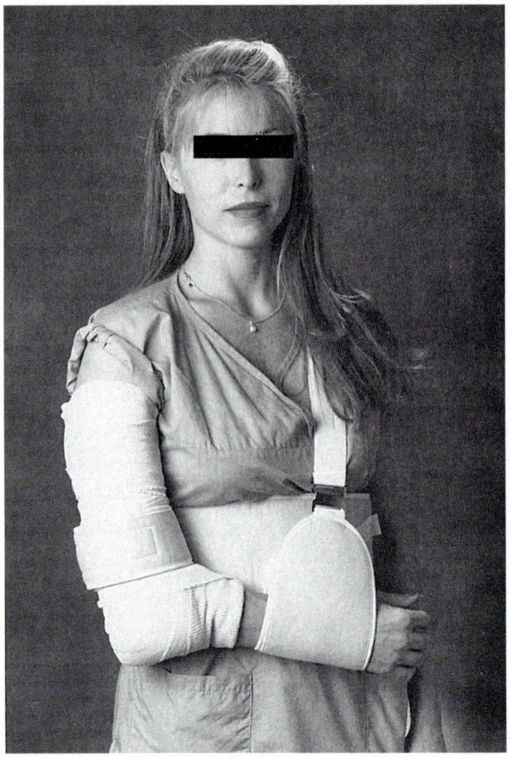

FIGURE 20-7 Initial care of humeral shaft fractures is directed at making the patient comfortable by using a plaster sugar-tong splint and shoulder immobilizer.

of these fractures. Pseudoparalysis with paroxysmal spasms makes the fracture obvious in most cases. Occasionally, the arm hangs flaccidly.[60] Neurologic and vascular injuries do occur, particularly to the radial nerve. Initial examination should record pertinent findings.

Anteroposterior and lateral radiographs (transthoracic views for proximal to middle-third fractures), are adequate in most cases but must include the joints above and below the fracture.[5] Care must be taken to diagnose associated injuries, such as head injuries, pulmonary contusion, adult respiratory distress syndrome, and head injury. Treatment of these injuries has priority, and, furthermore, the indications for conservative versus nonoperative treatment depend more on associated injury than on the type of humerus fracture itself.[8]

Classification

Humerus-shaft fractures should be described according to location, comminution, displacement, and angulation. Location and alignment are considered in determining fracture treatment, but elegant classification systems have not proven useful in this area.

Treatment

Nonoperative

Nonoperative care is appropriate for most fractures of the humeral shaft. Athletic activities alone do not constitute an indication for operative treatment. Sarmiento has

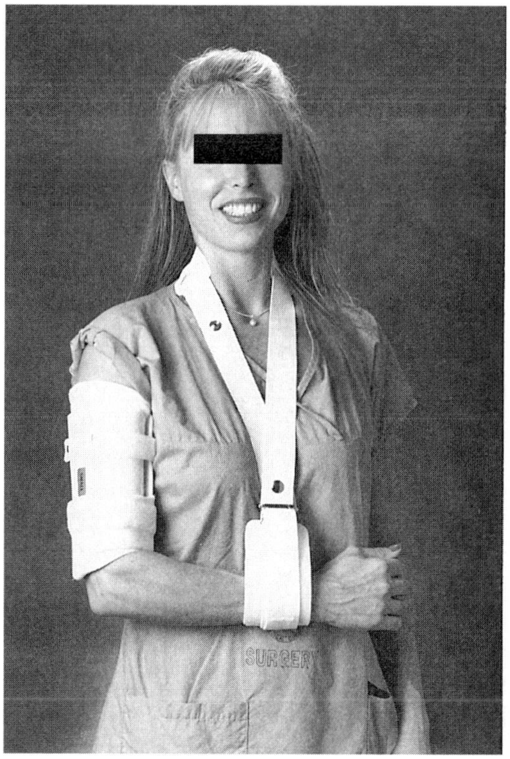

FIGURE 20-8 A functional fracture brace is applied when the patient becomes more comfortable. The brace should be "comfortably snug," as determined by the patient. The arm should hang free, unaffected by the collar and cuff.

designed a treatment program to mobilize adjacent joints and the entire extremity during the healing process.[53] Closed functional treatment has won wide approval and is the standard of care for closed management of the humeral shaft.*

Initial care consists of splintage, preferably with plaster coaptation or sugar-tong splints and a Velpeau bandage. Prefabricated shoulder immobilizers also work well when they are available (Fig. 20-7). Most patients will be ready for fracture brace application sometime in the first 1 to 3 weeks after injury. Either a custom brace made of thermoplastic materials or one prefabricated of synthetic polymer may be used[53] (Fig. 20-8). The brace provides compression and stability while gravity realigns the fracture.[45] Concern over fracture alignment should not be great at this time. After it is in the brace, the forearm must hang free, preferably with an elastic collar and cuff, for the fracture to realign.

Gravity causes a natural tendency toward varus malalignment.[58] Deformities of 10 degrees or more are not common, but this possibility should be discussed with the patient. Slight varus deformity is hardly visible and well tolerated (Fig. 20-9). Closed manipulation is not indicated. If acceptable fracture realignment does not occur, operative treatment may be necessary.

*References 21, 28, 36-38, 41, 46, 53, 61, 66.

A

B

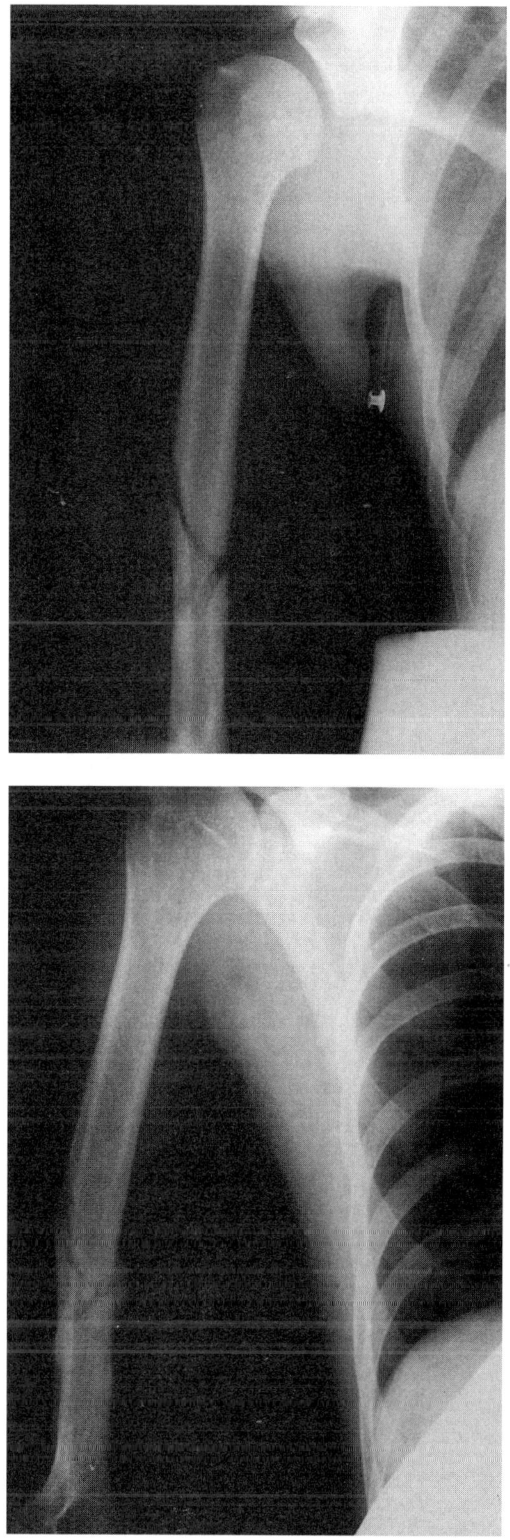

FIGURE 20-9 **A,** Initial AP radiograph of a spiral distal shaft fracture caused by throwing a baseball. **B,** Union at 10 weeks with slight marks.

Immediately after the injury, the patient must be encouraged to begin vigorous range-of-motion exercise of the fingers and wrist. Elbow motion begins after approximately 2 to 4 weeks. Shoulder flexion, abduction, and extension are possible for most individuals at 6 weeks, and torsional motions are added at 2 months or more. Radiographic consolidation, decreasing pain, fracture stability, and synchronous motion of the upper and lower fragments are favorable signs of healing. Healing is complete in well over 90% of patients by 10 weeks.[53] Strengthening exercises are initiated at this point, and supervised recovery is finished in 1 or 2 additional months. Throwing should not be allowed for 9 to 12 months.

Operative

Unacceptable deformity and uncontrollable instability are excellent reasons for internal fixation of acute humeral-shaft fractures. Internal fixation is particularly helpful in management of patients with additional injuries. Bleeker et al recommended brace treatment for patients with isolated injuries (injury severity score [ISS] equal to 4), traction then bracing for the moderately injured (ISS less than 18), and open reduction and internal fixation for the severely injured (ISS greater than or equal to 180).[8] Multiple fractures in the same extremity also are a strong indication for internal fixation.[50,68]

The necessity for internal fixation of open fractures, or fractures with associated nerve and arterial pathology, is relative. Internal fixation that stabilizes the fracture adequately without causing further injury helps to protect the vascular or nerve repair. Fractures associated with extensive contamination, bone loss, or complex soft-tissue injury may best be treated with external fixation.[72]

Plates

Mastery of the principles of plate fixation allows the orthopedist to obtain excellent results with plate osteosynthesis if necessary.[44] Using these prin-ciples and implants, Heim et al reported that 83% of 102 patients had full functional recovery at 1 year.[27] Two patients had postoperative radial nerve palsies but recovered. Five mechanical failures were due to technical inadequacies. There were four infections and two nonunions.

Satisfactory plating requires adequate exposure

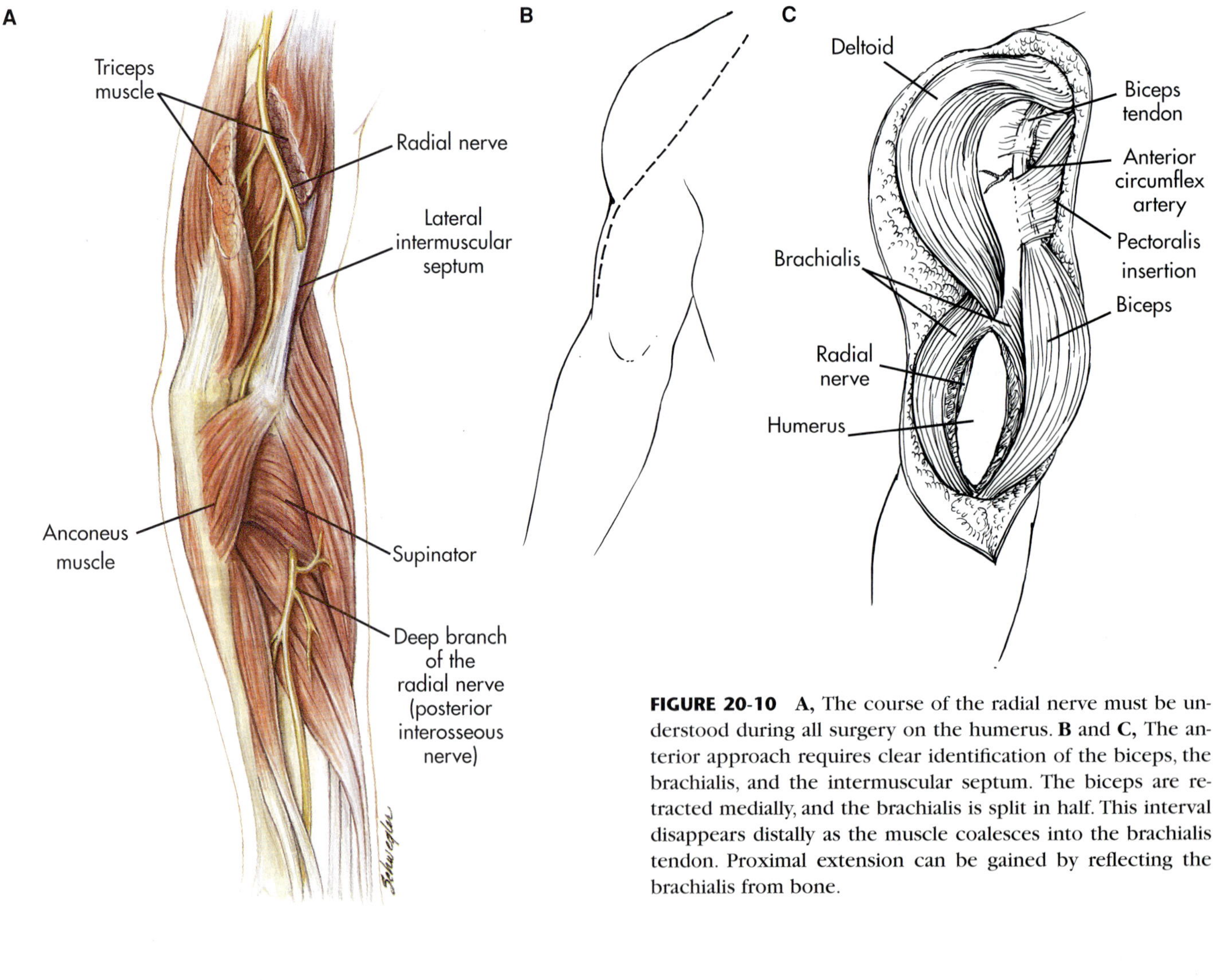

FIGURE 20-10 **A,** The course of the radial nerve must be understood during all surgery on the humerus. **B** and **C,** The anterior approach requires clear identification of the biceps, the brachialis, and the intermuscular septum. The biceps are retracted medially, and the brachialis is split in half. This interval disappears distally as the muscle coalesces into the brachialis tendon. Proximal extension can be gained by reflecting the brachialis from bone.

through a posterior approach for distal-third fractures and through an anterolateral approach for fractures in the mid to proximal thirds (Fig. 20-10). Careful exposure of the radial nerve is recommended for fractures in the distal half. The anterolateral incision protects the nerve by splitting the brachialis muscle and using the lateral half for padding. Dissection, if necessary, is then subperiosteal. The posterior approach will cross the path of the radial nerve in the musculospiral groove, and the nerve must be protected (Fig. 20-11).

Proper plate selection is essential. The 4.5-mm broad DC or LC-DC plate is advisable, with fixation above and below the fracture with six solid cortical screws. Using only lag screws should be avoided. Lag screws with a compression plate or neutralization plate are ideal. If comminution is present, autogenous bone graft is recommended.[44] Distal shaft fractures may not accommodate a single large plate. In these cases, two reconstruction plates are recommended.

Nails

The success of femoral and, later, tibial intramedullary nailing has stimulated interest in intramedullary techniques for the humerus.[17,26,33,51] Unfortunately, the humerus has some features that make it less amenable to nailing: small canal diameter, unknown canal architecture, and large torsional forces acting on the fracture. The radial nerve lies closer to the bone than does any comparable nerve relative to the tibial or femoral shaft. Finally, the entry portals may cause impingement at the shoulder or supracondylar fracture at the elbow[33] (Fig. 20-12).

In spite of the potential difficulties, humeral medullary nailing is successful in the majority of acute cases and may be less invasive than plating for comminuted fractures[33] (Fig. 20-13). The radial nerve is vulnerable at multiple locations over its course, particularly where it lies directly on the bone in the middle third. Open reduction is preferable to forceful manipulation in difficult cases. Our preference is for nails with locking options placed without preparatory reaming. Cerclage with 1.0-mm or 1.2-mm wire may be added if vascularity to comminuted fragments can be maintained (Fig. 20-14).

Nonunion

Successful pseudarthrosis repair has been reported with newer nail designs. Plating may be more reliable because it provides superior control of torsional forces.[73] The disadvantage with plating is the extensive operation that is necessary. At the least, an eight-hole 4.5-mm broad plate is necessary, and incisions spanning from shoulder to elbow are required (Fig. 20-15). Plates must be fixed with four screws with good purchase on each side of the fracture, with each screw having purchase in two cortices.

Radial Nerve Injury

Radial nerve lesions are associated with humeral-shaft fractures in 32 of 211 or 15% of cases.[18,61] Exploration of the nerve in closed fractures has not been useful in accelerating recovery of nerve function.[9,10,18,61] Open fractures and cases in which there has been no return of radial nerve function are different and warrant nerve repair if lacerations are encountered.

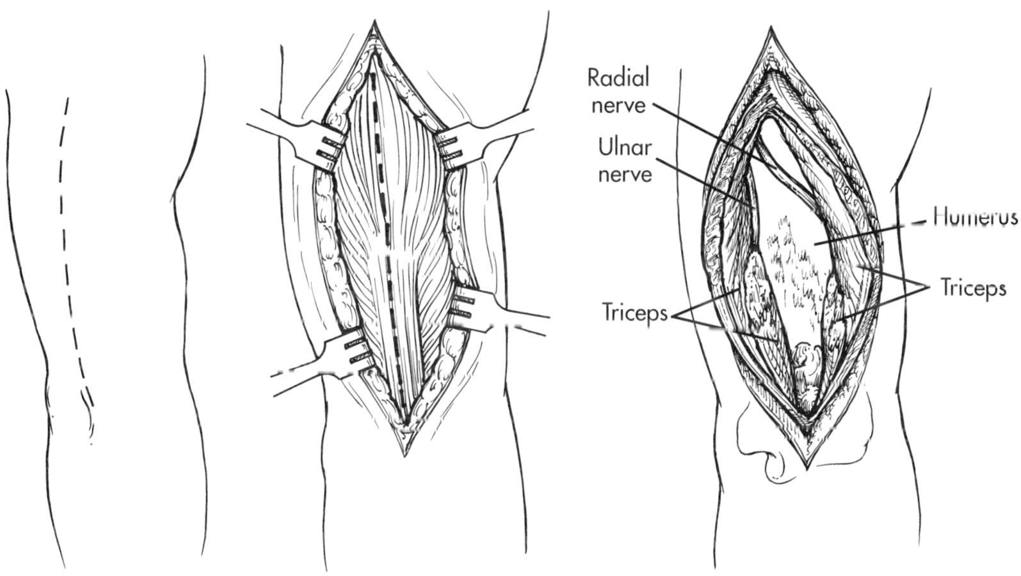

FIGURE 20-11 The posterior approach is a triceps-splitting incision. The radial nerve tranverses the field in the middle third and must be identified and protected. The ulnar and median nerves are also at risk.

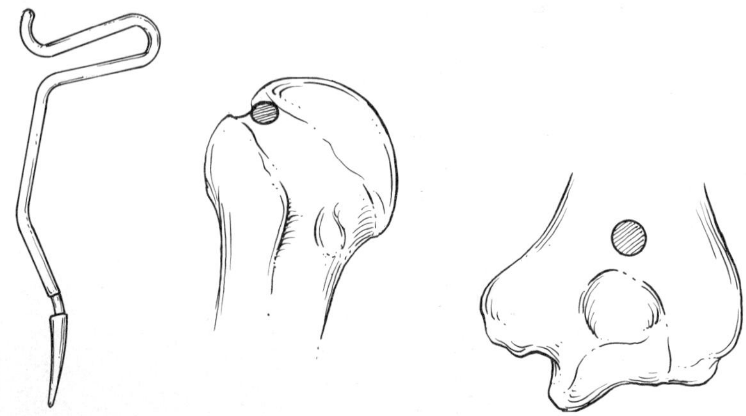

FIGURE 20-12 The awl and medullary access portals are located proximally beneath the supraspinatus tendon at the junction of the articular cartilage and greater tuberosity and distally just above the olecranon fossa.

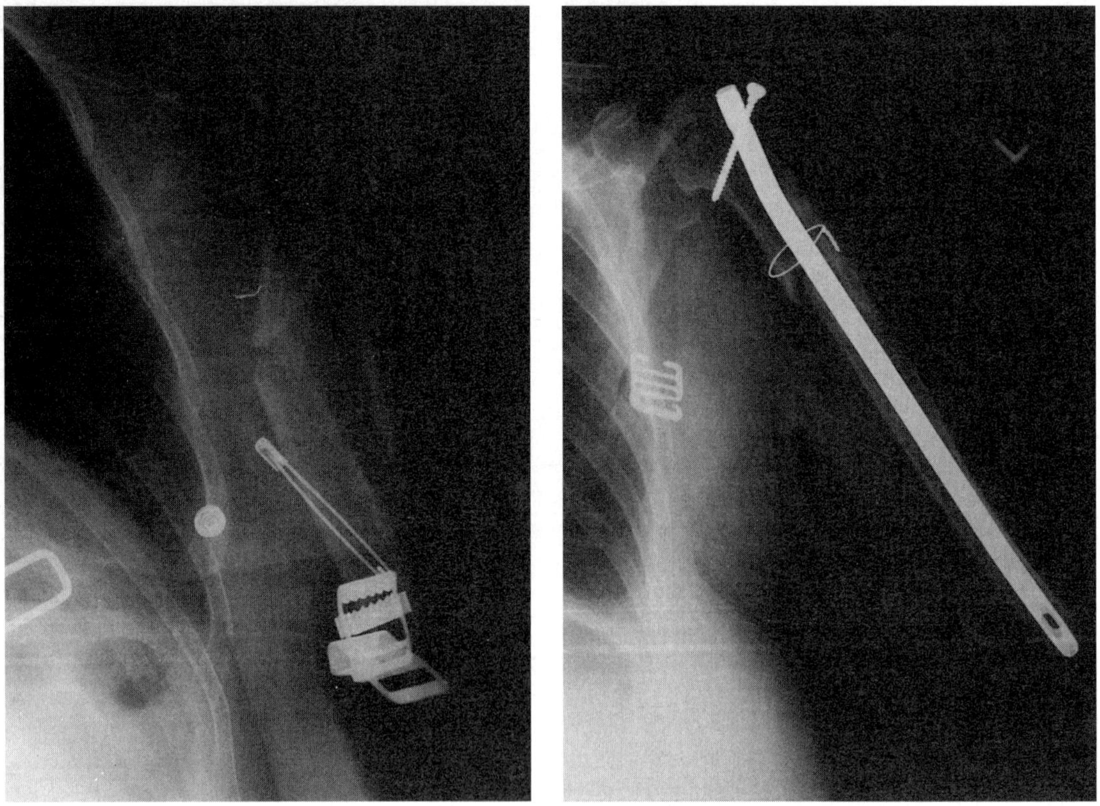

FIGURE 20-13 An intramedullary device is applicable to unstable comminuted shaft fractures in which plating would require an extensive approach.

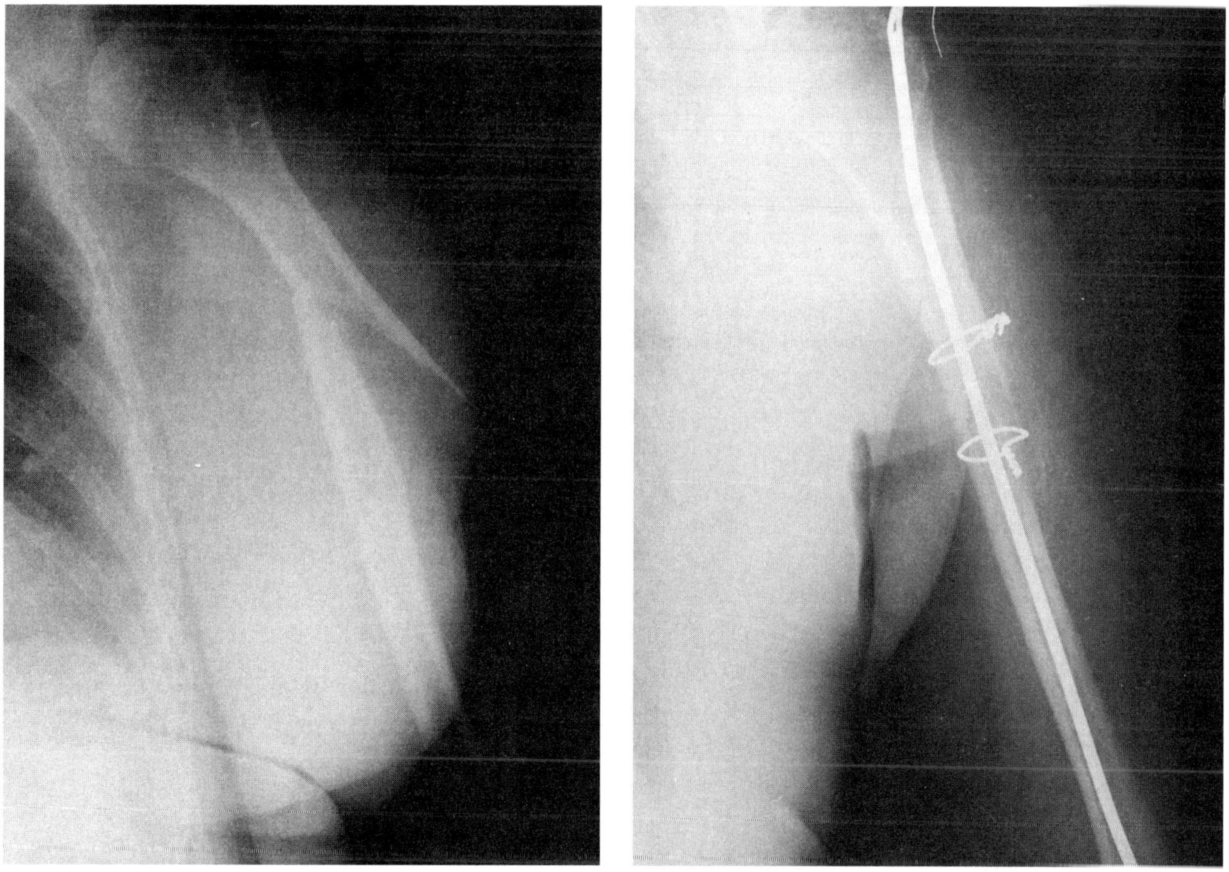

FIGURE 20-14 A single Enders pin and cerclage were used because this woman had a tiny medullary canal.

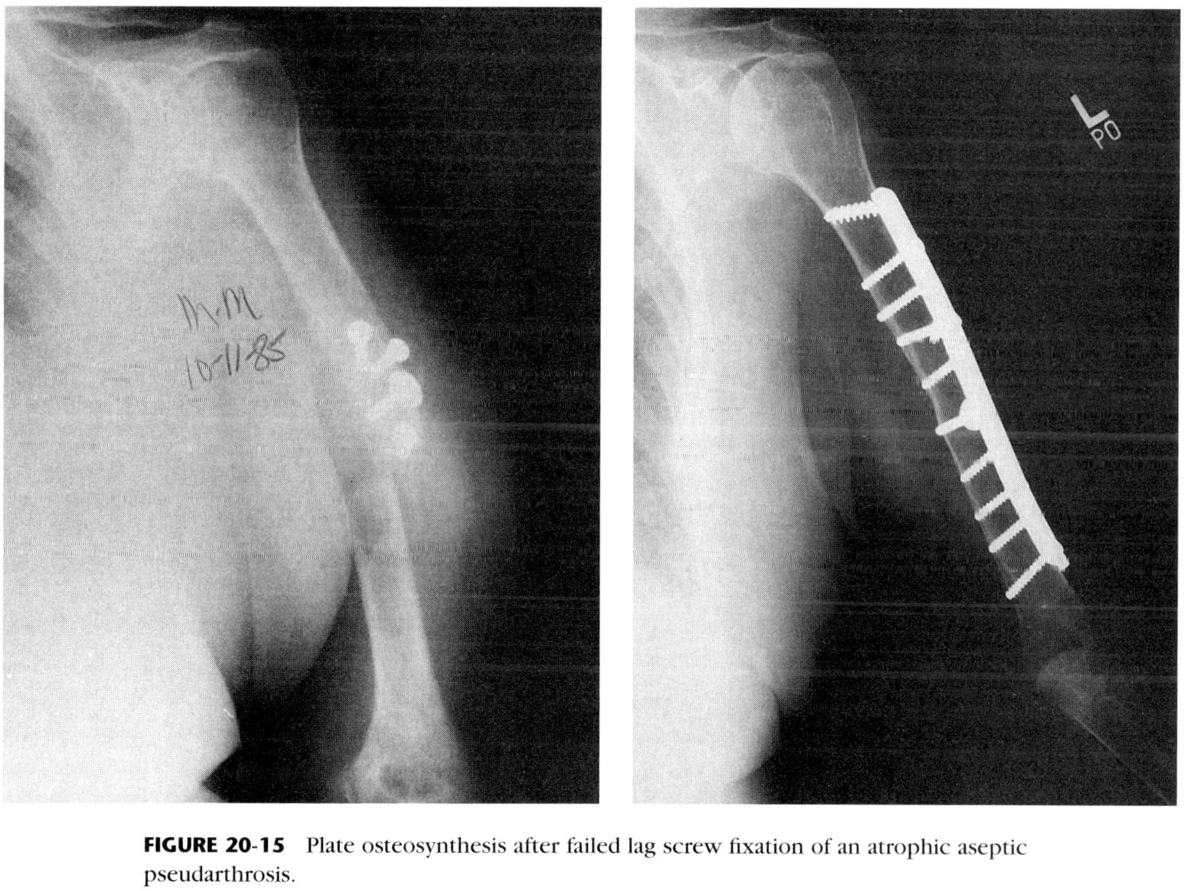

FIGURE 20-15 Plate osteosynthesis after failed lag screw fixation of an atrophic aseptic pseudarthrosis.

References

1. Abrams RA et al: Treatment of posttraumatic radioulnar synostosis with excision and low-dose radiation, *J Hand Surg (Am)* 18(4): 703-707, 1993.
2. Anderson LD et al: Compression-plate fixation in acute diaphyseal fractures of the radius and ulna, *J Bone Joint Surg (Am)* 57(3): 287, 1975.
3. Anderson LD, Meyer FN: Nonunion of the diaphysis of the radius and ulna, *Instr Course Lect* 37:157-159, 1988.
4. Bado JL: The Monteggia lesion, *Clin Orthop* 50:71-86, 1967.
5. Barquet A et al: Dislocation of the shoulder with fracture of the ipsilateral shaft of the humerus, *Injury* 16(5):300-302, 1985.
6. Barquet A, Caresani J: Fracture of the shaft of ulna and radius with associated dislocation of the radial head, *Injury* 12(6):471-476, 1981.
7. Bauer G, Arand M, Mutschler W: Post-traumatic radioulnar synostosis after forearm fracture osteosynthesis, *Arch Orthop Trauma Surg* 110(3):142-145, 1991.
8. Bleeker WA, Nijsten MW, ten Duis HJ: Treatment of humeral shaft fractures related to associated injuries: a retrospective study of 237 patients, *Acta Orthop Scand* 62(2):148-153, 1991.
9. Bostman O et al: Immediate radial nerve palsy complicating fracture of the shaft of the humerus: when is early exploration justified? *Injury* 16(7):499-502, 1985.
10. Bostman O et al: Radial palsy in shaft fracture of the humerus, *Acta Orthop Scand* 57(4):316-319, 1986.
11. Boyd HB, Boals JC: The Monteggia lesion: a review of 159 cases, *Clin Orthop* 66:94-100, 1969.
12. Breit R: Post-traumatic radioulnar synostosis, *Clin Orthop* 174:149-152, 1983.
13. Cai RB: Analysis of 81 cases of nonunion of forearm fracture, *Chin Med J* 96(1):29-32, 1983.
14. Chapman MW, Gordon JE, Zissimos AG: Compression-plate fixation of acute fractures of the diaphysis of the radius and ulna, *J Bone Joint Surg* 71-A(2):159-169, 1989.
15. Curr, Coe: *Br J Surg* 34:74-77, 1946.
16. Curtis R Jr, Corley F Jr: Fractures and dislocations of the forearm, *Clin Sports Med* 5(4):663-680, 1986.
17. Dalton JE et al: A biomechanical comparison of intramedullary nailing systems for the humerus, *J Orthop Trauma* 7(4):367-374, 1993.
18. Dameron T Jr, Grubb SA: Humeral shaft fractures in adults, *South Med J* 74(12):1461-1467, 1981.
19. Deluca PA, Lindsey RW, Ruwe PA: Refracture of bones of the forearm after removal of compression plates, *J Bone Joint Surg* 70-A(9):1372-1376, 1988.
20. Dodge HS, Cady GW: Treatment of fractures of the radius and ulna with compression plates, *J Bone Joint Surg (Am)* 54(6):1167-1176, 1972.
21. Dufour O et al: Functional treatment of recent fractures of the humeral shaft using the Sarmiento method—Traitement fonctionnel des fractures recentes d par la methode de Sarmiento, *Rev Chir Orthop* 75(5):292-300, 1989.
22. Duncan R et al: Immediate internal fixation of open fractures of the diaphysis of the forearm, *J Orthop Trauma* 6(1):25-31, 1992.
23. Elstrom JA, Pankovich AM, Egwele R: Extra-articular low-velocity gunshot fractures of the radius and ulna, *J Bone Joint Surg (Am)* 60(3):335-341, 1978.
24. Essex-Lopresti: Fractures of the radial head with distal radioulnar dislocation, *J Bone Joint Surg* 33-B: 244, 1951.
25. Garg NK, Gaur S, Sharma S: Percutaneous autogenous bone marrow grafting in 20 cases of ununited fracture, *Acta Orthop Scand* 64(6):671-672, 1993.
26. Habernek H, Orthner E: A locking nail for fractures of the humerus, *J Bone Joint Surg (Br)* 73(4):651-653, 1991.
27. Heim D et al: Can humerus shaft fractures be treated with osteosynthesis? *Helv Chir Acta* 58(5):673-678, 1992.
28. Helmreich M: Sarmiento functional treatment of humeral shaft fractures, *Unfallchirung* 90(11):502-507, 1987.
29. Heppenstall RB et al: Clinical and roentgenographic evaluation of nonunion of the forearm in relation to treatment with DC electrical stimulation, *J Trauma* 23(8):740-744, 1983.
30. Hidaka S, Gustilo RB: Refracture of bones of the forearm after plate removal, *J Bone Joint Surg* 66-A(8):1241-1243, 1984.
31. Hoppenfeld S, deBoer P: Surgical exposures in orthopaedics: the anatomic approach, New York, 1984, JB Lippincott.
32. Horster G, Hierholzer G, Bohm E: Morphologic and clinical aspects in the treatment of infected shaft pseudarthrosis, *Z Orthop* 121(2):128-136, 1983.
33. Ingman AM, Waters DA: Locked intramedullary nailing of humeral shaft fractures: implant design, surgical technique, and clinical results, *J Bone Joint Surg (Br)* 76(1):23-29, 1994.
34. Johner R, Wruhs O: Classification of tibial shaft fractures and correlation with results after internal fixation, Clin Orthop 178:7-25, 1983.
35. Jones JA: Immediate internal fixation of high-energy open forearm fractures, *J Orthop Trauma* 5(3):272-279, 1991.
36. Kulenkampff HA, Rustemeier M: Clinical experiences in the treatment of humeral shaft fractures with the Sarmiento brace, *Unfallchirung* 14:191, 1988.
37. Langenberg R: Sarmiento functional treatment of humeral shaft fractures. Results and experiences—Funktionelle Behandlung von Humerusschaftfrakturen n Ergebnisse und Erfahrungen, *Zentralbl Chir* 112(20):1271-1277, 1987.
38. Lehmann A: Functional treatment of humerus shaft fractures using the Sarmiento method, *Schweiz Z Sportmed* 30(2):53-56, 1982.
39. Mast J, Jakob R, Ganz R: *Planning and reduction technique in fracture surgery,* New York, 1989, Springer-Verlag.
40. Moed B et al: Immediate internal fixation of open fractures of the diaphysis of the forearm, *J Bone Joint Surg* 64A(4):1008-1017, 1986.
41. Moller E, Andersen NS, Niedermann B: Treatment of fractures of the shaft of the humerus with the Sarmiento bandage, *Ugeskr Laeger* 145(2): 94-95, 1983.
42. Moore TM et al: Results of compression-plating of closed Galeazzi fractures, *J Bone Joint Surg* 67-A(7):1015-1021, 1985.
43. Mueller ME et al: *Manual of internal fixation,* ed 3, New York, 1993, Springer-Verlag.
44. Müller ME et al: *Manual of internal fixation,* ed 2, New York, 1972, Springer-Verlag.
45. Naver L, Aalberg JR: Humeral shaft fractures treated with a ready-made fracture brace, *Arch Orthop Trauma Surg* 106(1):20-22, 1986.
46. Peeters PM et al: Early functional treatment of humerus shaft fractures by the Sarmiento method, *Aktuel Traumatol* 17(4): 150-152, 1987.
47. Rhinelander FW: The normal circulation of bone and its response to surgical intervention, *J Biomed Mater Res* 8(1):87-90, 1974.
48. Rhinelander FW: The normal microcirculation of diaphyseal cortex and its response to fracture, *J Bone Joint Surg (Am)* 50(4):784-800, 1968.
49. Rhinelander FW et al: Microangiography in bone healing. II. Displaced closed fractures, *J Bone Joint Surg (Am)* 50(4):643-662, 1968.
50. Rogers JF, Bennett JB, Tullos HS: Management of concomitant ipsilateral fractures of the humerus and forearm, *J Bone Joint Surg* 66-A(4):552-556, 1984.
51. Rush J: Closed nailing of the humerus—from down under, *Aust NZ J Surg* 57(10):723-725, 1987.
52. Sarmiento A, Cooper JS, Sinclair WF: Forearm fractures, *J Bone Joint Surg* 57A:297-304, 1975.
53. Sarmiento A et al: Functional bracing of fractures of the shaft of the humerus, *J Bone Joint Surg (Am)* 59(5):596-601, 1977.

54. Schatzker J, Tile M: *The rationale of operative fracture care,* New York, 1987, Springer-Verlag.
55. Schemitsch EH, Richards RR: The effect of malunion on functional outcome after plate fixation of fractures of both bones of the forearm in adults, *J Bone Joint Surg* 74-A(7):1068-1078, 1992.
56. Schmeling GJ, Wright RR, Schwab JP: The necessity of acute bone grafting in diaphyseal forearm fractures, *Orthop Trauma* Association Abstracts, 1994.
57. Shang TY, Gu YW, Dong FH: Treatment of forearm bone fractures by an integrated method of traditional Chinese and Western medicine, *Clin Orthop* 215:56-64, 1987.
58. Sharma VK et al: Non-operative treatment of fractures of the humeral shaft: a comparative study, *J Indian Med Assoc* 89(6):157-160, 1991.
59. Sim R, Liang TS, Tay BK: Autologous marrow injection in the treatment of delayed and non-union in long bones, *Singapore Med J* 34(5):412-417, 1993.
60. Smith CR, Binder AI, Paice EW: Lesions of the mid-shaft of the humerus presenting as shoulder capsulitis, *Br J Rheumatol* 29(5): 386-388, 1990.
61. Sonneveld GJ et al: Treatment of fractures of the shaft of the humerus accompanied by paralysis of the radial nerve, *Injury* 18(6):404-406, 1987.
62. Stern PJ, Drury WJ: Complications of plate fixation of forearm fractures, *Clin Orthop* 175:25-29, 1983.
63. Tarr RR, Garfinkel AI, Sarmiento A: The effects of angular and rotational deformities of both bones of the forearm: an in vitro study, *J Bone Joint Surg* 66-A(1):65-70, 1984.
64. Teipner WA, Mast JW: Internal fixation of forearm diaphyseal fractures: double plating versus single compression (tension band) plating—a comparative study, *Orthop Clin North Am* 11(3):381-391, 1980.
65. Trousdale RT et al: Radioulnar dissociation: a review of twenty cases, *J Bone Joint Surg* 74-A(10):1486-1497, 1992.
66. Van der Werken C et al: Sarmiento's treatment method for humeral shaft fractures, *Ned Tijdschr Geneeskd* 129(13): 583-586, 1985.
67. Victor J, Mulier T, Fabry G: Refracture of radius and ulna in a female gymnast: a case report, *Am J Sports Med* 21(5):753-754, 1993.
68. Viegas SF, Gogan W, Riley S: Floating dislocated elbow: case report and review of the literature, *J Trauma* 29(6):886-888, 1989.
69. Vince KG, Miller JE: Cross-union complicating fracture of the forearm. Part I: adults, *J Bone Joint Surg (Am)* 69(5):640-653, 1987.
70. Weber BG, Cech O: *Pseudarthrosis,* Bern, 1976, Hans Huber.
71. Weller S, Hierholzer G, Hermichen HG: *Late results after osteosynthesis,* Tübingen, 1984, H-J Köhler.
72. Wild JJ, Hbason GW, Bennett JB: External fixation use in the management of massive upper extremity trauma, *Clin Orthop* 164:172-176, 1982.
73. Wu CC, Shih CH: Treatment for nonunion of the shaft of the humerus: comparison of plates and Seidel interlocking nails, *Can J Surg* 35(6):661-665, 1992.

CHAPTER 21

Bony Disorders: Clinical Assessment and Treatment

STEPHEN M. GRYZLO

The elbow is susceptible to overuse injuries in skeletally immature individuals as well as in adults. In the young athlete, repetitive microtrauma associated with various sport-related activities is a major etiologic factor in producing not only soft-tissue injury, but also various bony disorders about the elbow. Prevention is the key to reducing the risk of injury. Proper conditioning, adequate warm-up, good body mechanics, and common sense can help produce and maintain a healthy state and minimize the chance of injury.

PANNER'S DISEASE

H.J. Panner, in 1929, is credited with the first written description of osteochondrosis of the capitellum. In his classic treatise,[20] Panner detailed the history and course of three peculiar elbow cases. In each instance, the individuals were male, were 10 years of age or younger, and had developed elbow pain and restricted range of motion after a history of trauma. Radiographs revealed changes confined entirely to the capitellum that included deformity and fragmentation of the whole ossific nucleus. Panner likened these changes to those seen in Legg-Calvé-Perthes disease.

The term *osteochondrosis* encompasses a large number of conditions characterized by disorderly endochondral ossification of the growth centers in children.[27] The events that induce the epiphyseal changes so characteristic of this disorder are not well understood. Some theorize that an initial avascular event occurs at or to the epiphyseal center, but there is disagreement on the exact mechanism.[26] The etiology of this entity remains unknown, but it is likely multifactoral. The radiographic stages of this pathologic condition have been well described; they begin with necrosis or degeneration of the growth center, followed by revascularization with concurrent new bone deposition and resorption. Finally, bone healing and sometimes residual deformity occur.

Clinical Features

Since Panner's original description, the clinical appearance of this condition has remained constant. The capitellum continues to be a rare site for osteochondrosis. Affected individuals typically are under the age of 10 years (range, 3 to 11 years). Males are more often affected than are females, and the right elbow is involved more often than the left. The history of an injury or accident may be obtained, but a direct correlation to trauma has yet to be proved. Elbow pain is the main complaint and is exacerbated by use. The physical examination may reveal an effusion, with tenderness to palpation over the lateral aspect of the elbow. These patients may demonstrate a decreased range of motion, with the primary loss being extension. Pronation and supination are rarely compromised except in extreme cases.

Radiographs usually reveal involvement of the entire ossific nucleus of the capitellum. The changes seen within this distal humeral growth center resemble those seen in the femoral epiphysis that are characteristic of Legg-Calvé-Perthes disease. The changes typically include fragmentation, rarefaction, and sclerosis of the entire capitellar epiphyseal center. The fragmentation is secondary to new bone deposition occurring in conjunction with bone resorption. This x-ray appearance typically is seen during revascularization and is associated with few or no symptoms. This process of revascularization may lead to an irregularity of the outline of the capitellum or the appearance of a "capitellum within a capitellum."[26] This represents new bone deposition at the periphery of the more dense central ossific nucleus. With time, the capitellum heals, and frequently the x-ray resumes a normal appearance. Although permanent radiographic deformities are rare, they can occur if the elbow is subjected to excessive stress during this period.

Treatment

Conservative management is the recommended treatment for osteochondrosis of the capitellum. Because the elbow is not considered a weight-bearing joint, the development of deformity is unlikely as long as the capitellum is protected against unusual or excessive forces. During symptomatic periods, rest and sling immobilization are encouraged.

Largely because the etiology remains unknown for Panner's disease, prevention of this condition remains elusive. Rather, early detection and prevention of deformity are the primary goals. All osteochondroses heal; however, this may take several years. Protecting the elbow and avoiding abnormal forces at the elbow must be stressed, especially during the revascularization phase, when the new bone is at its weakest state. Periodic reexamination and radiographs should ensure a successful outcome. Over time, a return to all activities may be allowed if full, painless elbow range of motion is present and radiographs reveal reconstitution of the normal capitellum.

OSTEOCHONDRITIS DISSECANS OF THE CAPITELLUM

The term *osteochondritis dissecans* was coined by Franz Konig in 1887 to describe a condition that he observed in the knee.[16] He theorized that a dissecting inflammation in the subchondral bone led to the detachment and formation of an osteochondral loose body. Since that time, the term *osteochondritis dissecans* (OCD) has been applied to other areas besides the knee, including the elbow, ankle, and hip.

Etiology

In general, osteochondritis dissecans is a clinical condition in which an osteochondral fragment develops at the superficial surface of a diarthrodial joint. This osteochondral fragment may be in situ, partially detached, or free within the joint[21] (Fig. 21-1). Although the true etiology remains unknown, Konig's belief that this was due to an inflammatory condition largely has been discounted.

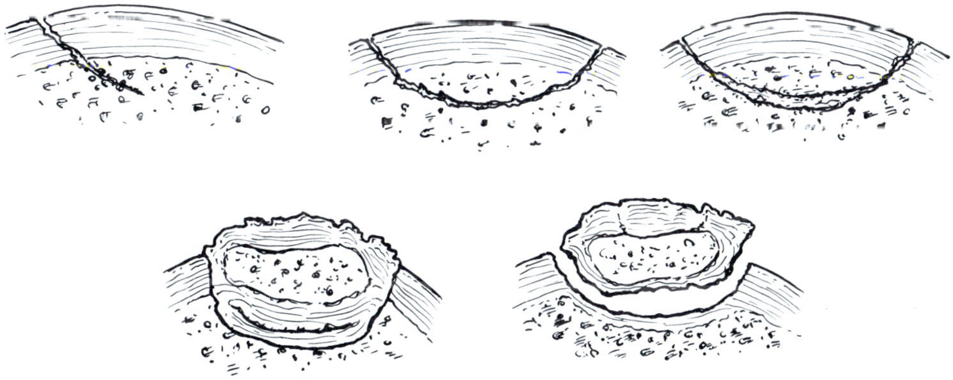

FIGURE 21-1 The development of an osteochondral fragment and potential loose body formation.

A better term for the condition now is *osteochondrosis dissecans.* Although less accurate, the term *osteocondritis* is difficult to abandon because of its historical connection.

In the elbow, osteochondritis dissecans is a lesion of bone and articular cartilage that often occurs on the anterolateral aspect of the capitellum. Anatomic vascular studies of the distal humerus, performed by Haraldsson,[13] revealed that the capitellum during skeletal growth had a predominantly posterior blood supply. Therefore it is the very anterolateral corner of the capitellum, which is relatively devoid of a rich vascular supply, that is at risk for development of osteochondritis dissecans if a vascular interruption should occur. Haraldsson further found no blood vessels that crossed the epiphyseal plate in a skeletally immature elbow, and after the growth plate had fused, many vascular channels connected the epiphyseal and metaphyseal region but the predominant blood supply remained posterior.

There is still confusion over whether osteochondritis dissecans (OCD) and the previous condition, Panner's disease, are separate entities or whether they are the same entity and represent different stages of the same progressive disorder of endochondral ossification.[23,25,28] However, there is no evidence to suggest that Panner's disease (osteochondrosis) is a precursor to osteochondritis dissecans.[6,7,26,35] Additionally, Panner's disease is a disease of young children, those less than 10 years old, but osteochondritis dissecans affects the adolescent and young adult. The onset of symptoms is relatively acute in patients with Panner's disease, but those with osteochondritis dissecans have a rather insidious onset of symptoms. Radiographically, the entire ossific nucleus of the capitellum is involved and fragmented in Panner's disease. In OCD, only the anterolateral corner of the capitellum is involved, with a subchondral bony island and surrounding lucency seen on x-ray. Panner's disease usually resolves without sequelae, but osteochondritis dissecans can progress with loose-body formation and late degenerative changes in the elbow.

The exact cause of osteochondritis dissecans has yet to be elucidated, and currently no pathogenetic theory is fully accepted. Strong etiologic factors to be considered include ischemia, trauma, hereditary factors, and a constitutional predisposition. The etiology is most likely multifactoral.

In the elbow, repetitive throwing has been implicated as the leading cause for osteochondritis dissecans.[21] The association of baseball pitching with OCD of the capitellum was first described by Bennett[5] in 1941, with many authors detailing its occurrence since.* As illustrated earlier in Chapter 15, during the late cocking and acceleration phases of pitching, the elbow experiences significant valgus stress (Fig. 21-2). This valgus stress produces compression and shear forces at the radiocapitellar joint (Fig. 21-3). In the adolescent thrower, these forces may injure the delicate underlying capitellar vascular channels and create an area of vascular insufficiency leading to an osteochondral lesion. This theory would account for the large preponderance of males seen with this entity versus females and also may explain why more right (dominant) elbows are seen afflicted than left (nondominant).

*References 1-4, 10-12, 14, 15, 17, 21, 22, 28-33, 35.

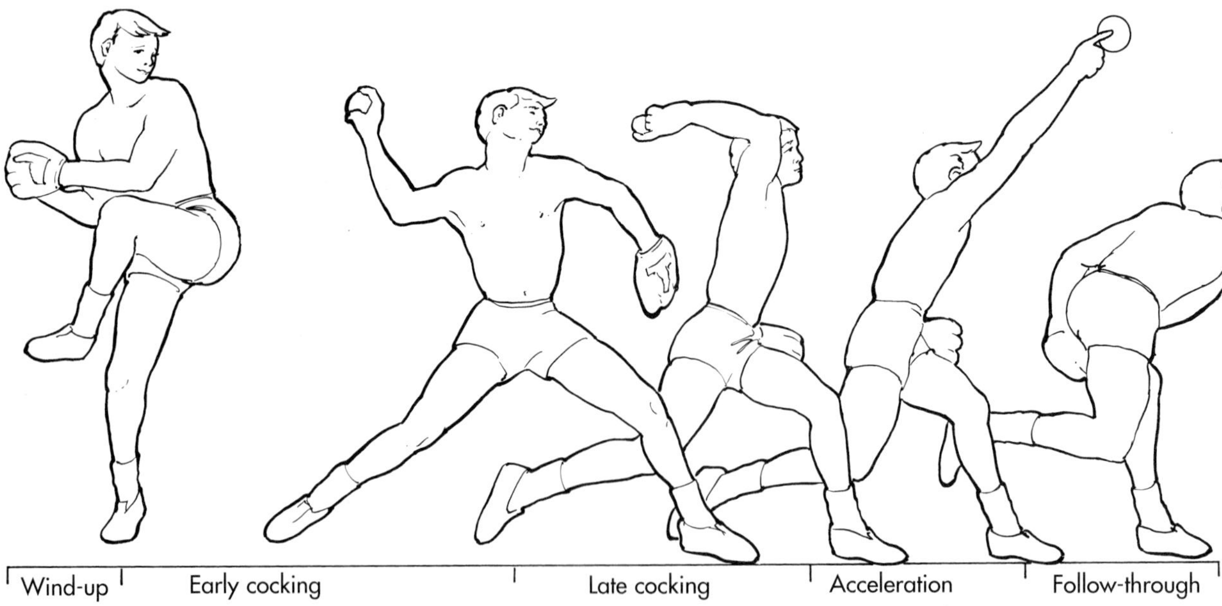

FIGURE 21-2 The five stages of pitching a baseball—wind-up, early cocking, late cocking, acceleration, and follow-through.

Medial-side tension and radiocapitellar compression forces also may explain the growing incidence and reports of OCD in the elbow in gymnasts. In these individuals, the arms must withstand additional weight-bearing stresses, and when these forces are combined with the previously mentioned abnormal forces (medial-side tension and lateral-side compression), osteochondritis dissecans may develop.[9,28] This theory of valgus stress, however, cannot explain all incidences of osteochondritis dissecans. Osteochondritis dissecans also may have a genetic factor. There are reports of osteochondritis dissecans in the nondominant elbow of individuals with no history of injury but with multiple family members having dissecans lesions in the capitellum.[18,24]

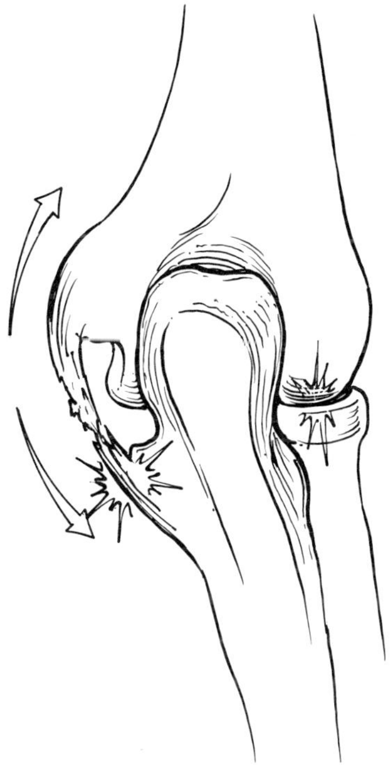

FIGURE 21-3 The valgus stress and compression laterally that occurs in the elbow when it is extended rapidly, such as during the acceleration phase of throwing.

Clinical Features

The typical patient is in the second decade of life (most commonly 10 to 15 years of age) and is more often male than female, with the right elbow affected more often than the left. Elbow pain, limitation of motion, sensations of "catching" or "locking" of the elbow, and swelling are common clinical symptoms.

Elbow pain is the most common complaint. Its onset, in most cases, is insidious, and often there is a delay of many months to years before the patient is seen by a physician. The pain is characterized as a diffuse dull ache and is worsened by activity and relieved by rest.

Loss of elbow motion is typical, and patients may develop a flexion contracture of 15° or more. There may be some loss of flexion, but pronation and supination are infrequently altered. Catching of the elbow may occur if the lesion is partially detached and subluxating in and out of its crater bed with elbow motion. Actual locking of the elbow usually is secondary to loose-body formation as the fragment becomes free within the joint. Additional findings may include localized tenderness over the lateral aspect of the elbow, an elbow effusion, and crepitus.

Radiographic Features

A wide variety of radiographic findings may be seen in osteochondritis dissecans. Early in this disease, the roentgenographic changes may be subtle, demonstrating only a patchy rarefaction with ill-defined borders and located near the anterolateral surface of the capitellum (Figs. 21-4 and 21-5). These changes typically are seen on the anteroposterior x-ray but are not clearly identified on the lateral view. With progression of the disease, the lesion can be easily identified in the routine anteroposterior and lateral x-rays. The characteristic appearance (so often described for osteochondritis dissecans) is an island of subchondral bone in the capitellum demarcated by a zone of lucency and surrounded by a bed of sclero-

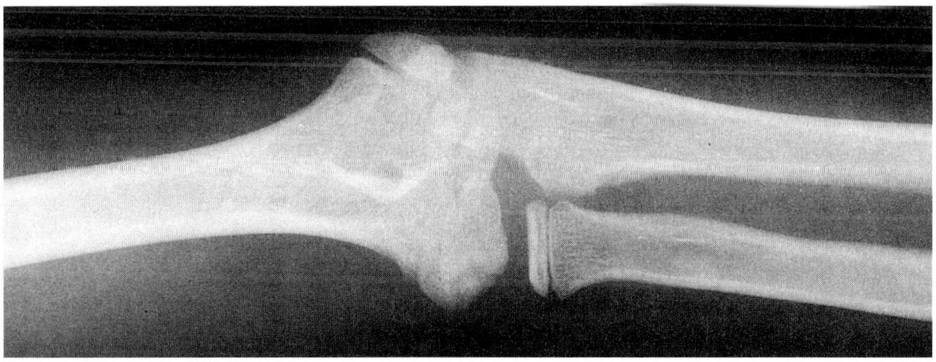

FIGURE 21-4 X-ray test of a 13-year-old's elbow with early typical OCD lesion at anterolateral corner of the capitellum.

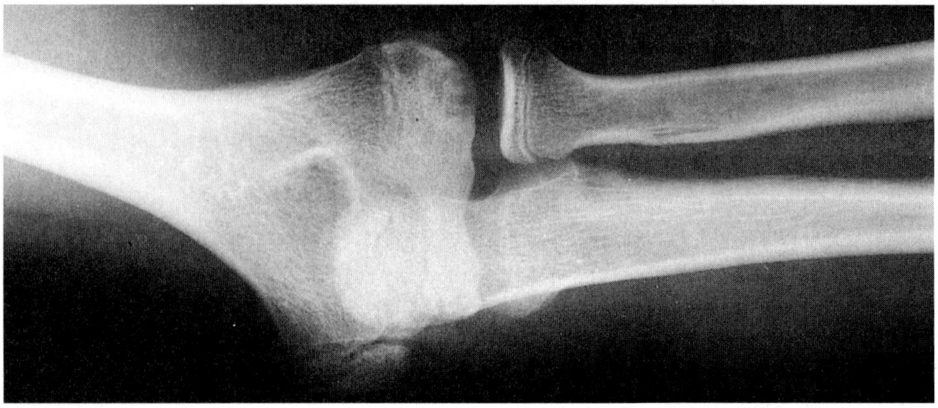

FIGURE 21-5 X-ray test of a 15-year-old's elbow with easily identified OCD lesion in the capitellum. Note the sclerotic border and patchy rarefaction.

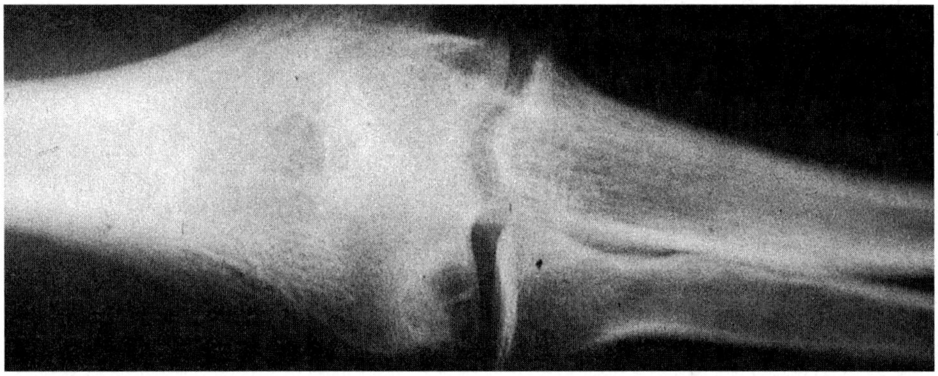

FIGURE 21-6 Cystic changes in the capitellum of a skeletally mature male elbow on plain x-ray test. (Courtesy Gordon Nuber, MD, Chicago.)

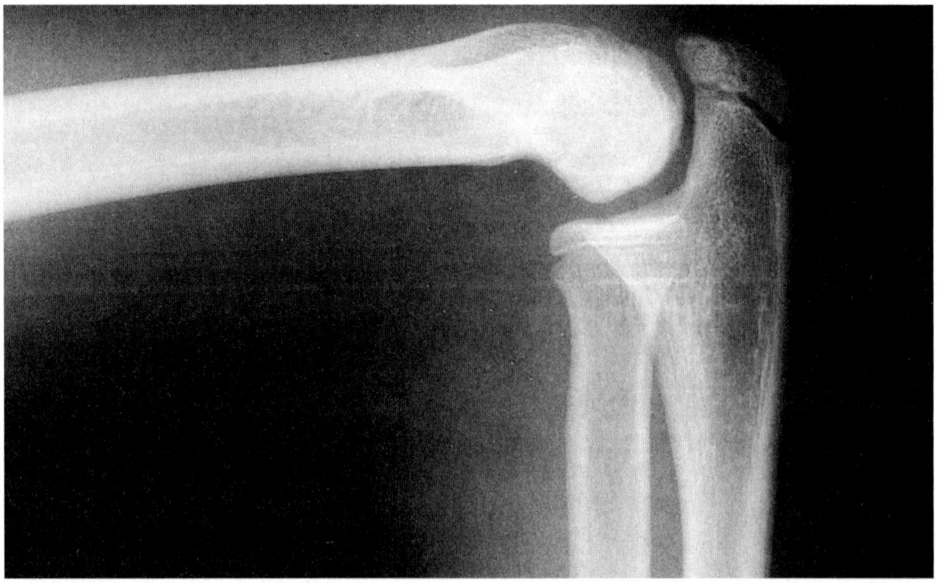

FIGURE 21-7 Lateral x-ray test of a 15-year-old with OCD. Note the irregular contour of the capitellum outline.

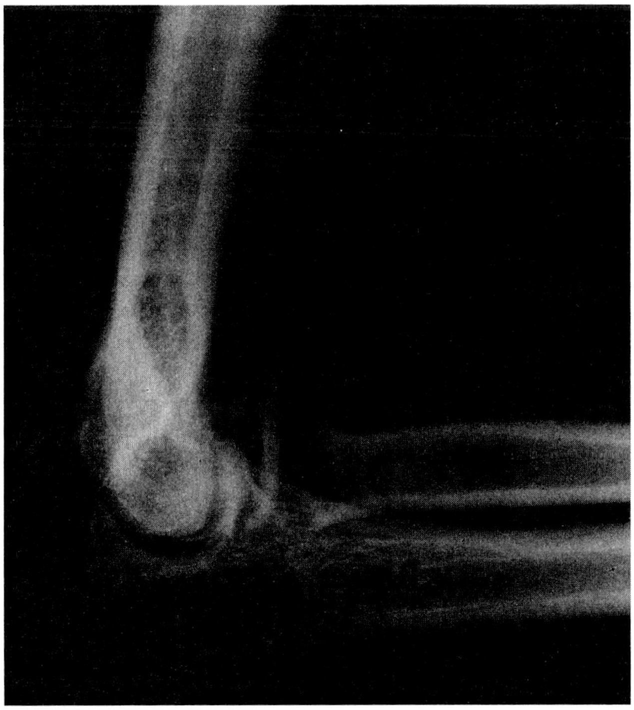

FIGURE 21-8 A skeletally mature 17-year-old with loose-body anterior elbow compartment secondary to OCD. (Courtesy John Sarwark, MD, Chicago.)

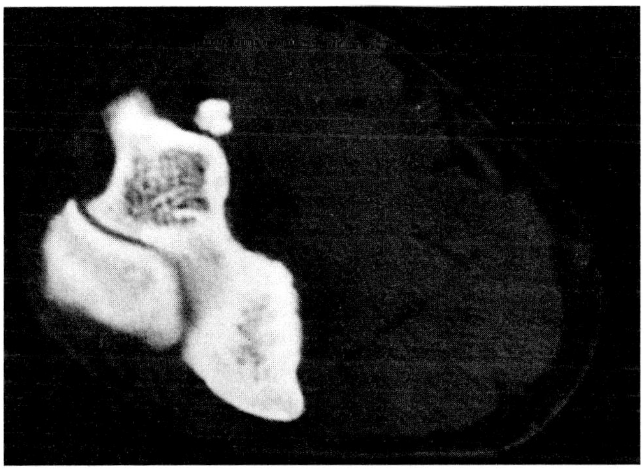

FIGURE 21-9 A CT scan of Figure 21-8 that demonstrates loose body in anterior elbow compartment. (Courtesy John Sarwark, MD, Chicago.)

sis. This lesion is sometimes better appreciated with tomography. The bony island may be multipartite and may show varying degrees of displacement into the joint. Cystic changes in the capitellum also may be present (Fig. 21-6).

In later stages, flattening and blunting of the capitellum may be seen on the lateral radiograph (Fig. 21-7). If the lesion separates from the underlying bone, one or more loose bodies may be seen on x-ray (Fig. 21-8). Further late changes include enlargement of the radial head when compared with the opposite elbow. Finally, the growth-plate can grow more rapidly and prematurely close, affecting the distal humerus and the proximal radius.

Additional studies frequently ordered when one is investigating this condition include arthrography, tomography, computerized tomography (CT), and magnetic resonance imaging (MRI). Historically, arthrography has been used to confirm loose-body formation. Care must be taken when interpreting these film results because reactive synovitis in the elbow may produce filling defects, which then can be misinterpreted as loose bodies. Tomography, with and without contrast, also has been used to evaluate the possibility of loose bodies and to determine articular changes. These studies, when performed early in the course of disease, may provide more accurate information about bony changes that are not readily seen on plain x-ray. Computerized tomography (CT) has been used to a lesser extent to confirm necrotic changes in the capitellum and the formation of loose bodies (Fig. 21-9). Recently, the use of MRI in evaluating elbow disorders has been expanding, and MRI appears to be a useful tool to investigate osteochondritis dissecans (Fig. 21-10). Magnetic resonance imaging may help in the early phases and in demonstrating abnormalities of bone or articular cartilage and even loose bodies displaced into the joint space. MRI is an attractive alternative because it is noninvasive and may reveal subtle bony and articular changes much earlier than all other available imaging techniques. Its use in this particular disorder should continue to increase.

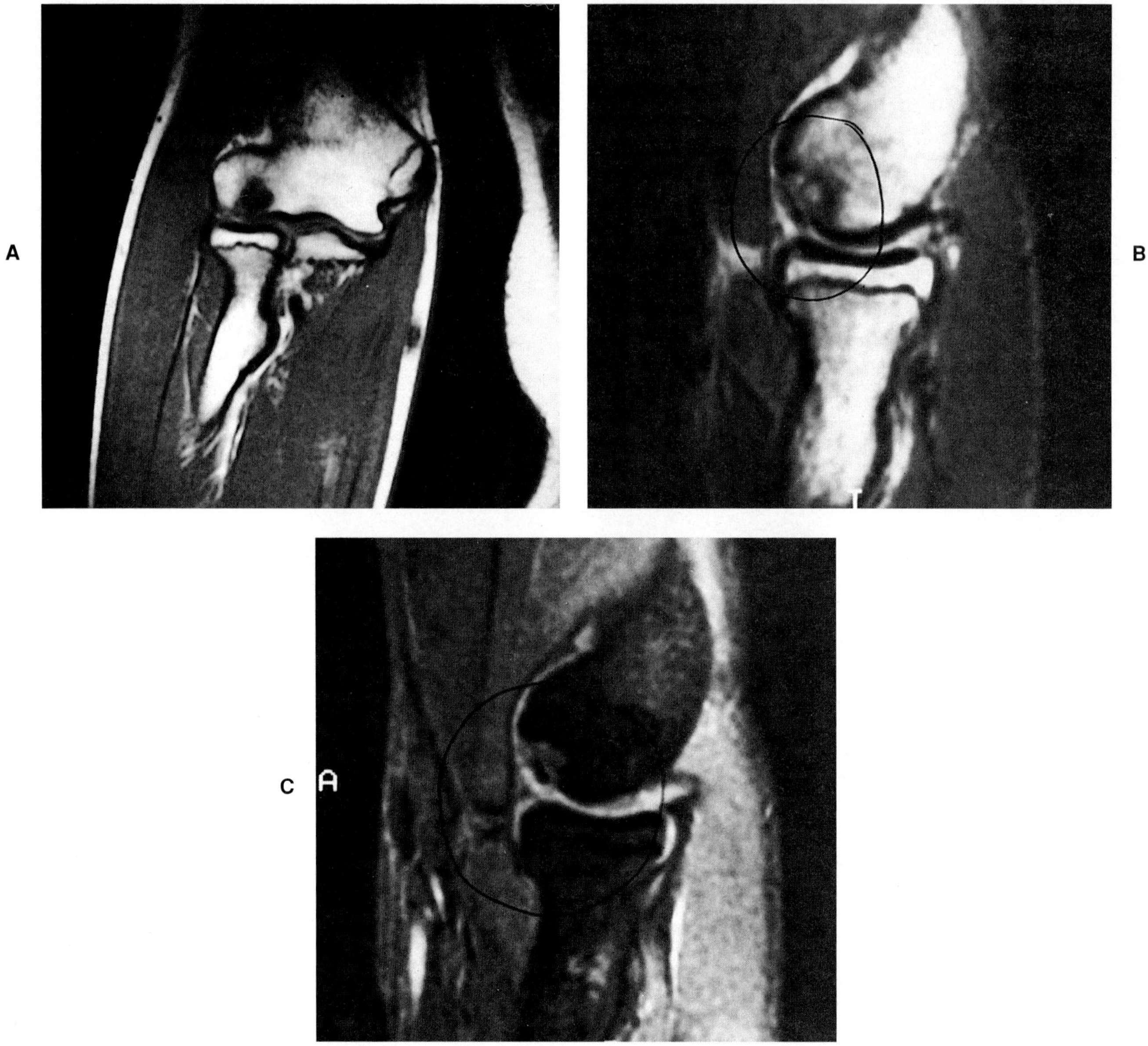

FIGURE 21-10 An MRI scan of a 15-year-old male's right elbow revealing OCD lesion in capitellum **(A)**. Sagittal T1 and T2 enlarged images of the same elbow demonstrating OCD lesion at anterolateral corner of capitellum **(B** and **C)**. During surgery, the fragment was found to be entirely cartilaginous and was removed. (Courtesy Gordon Nuber, MD, Chicago.)

Treatment

The essential theme in the treatment plan for osteochondritis dissecans of the elbow is to prevent the progression of the disorder, detachment of the osteochondral lesion, and/or degenerative changes of the articular cartilage. Thus the main focus is toward early recognition and prompt medical intervention. Unfortunately, this disease has an insidious onset, and in many cases the capitellar lesion is significantly progressed by the time of the initial evaluation and examination. If this is the case, one must determine whether the lesion has separated from its bed or is undergoing separation. Under these circumstances, the goal of preventing or reducing the likelihood of degenerative changes in the joint becomes paramount.

With these goals in mind, Pappas developed a classification scheme[21] for osteochondritis dissecans in 1981. These categories are based on the age of the patient and help guide the physician in treatment options and prognosis of the disease.

The category I lesion typically involves children who are in their early adolescence (13 years of age or less). Patients in this class exhibit subtle physical findings that normally include mild elbow pain and some restriction

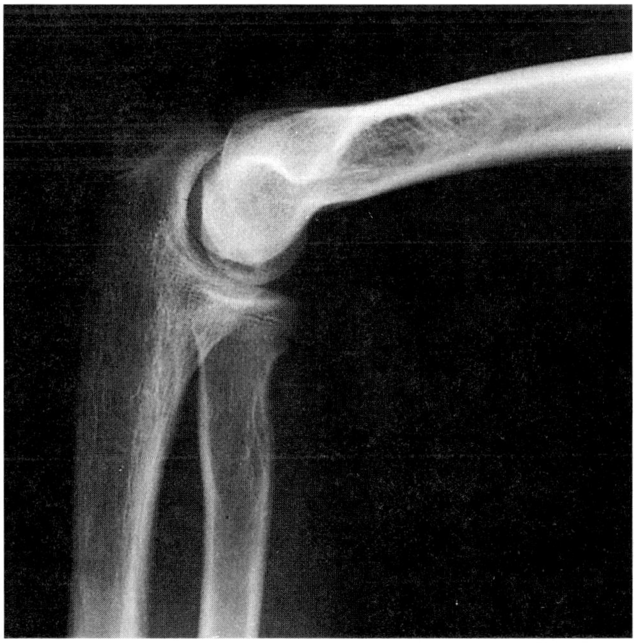

FIGURE 21-11 A lateral x-ray test of the elbow in an adolescent who is nearing skeletal maturity, revealing a subtle radiolucency in the capitellum with a sclerotic rim representing a stable lesion.

of motion secondary to synovitis. In some instances, these patients are identified when their lesions are discovered incidentally on a radiograph before any physical findings have evolved. The lesion on x-ray appears as a focal radiolucency in the capitellum (Fig. 21-11). This lesion is intact and seldom progresses to fragmentation or loose-body formation. The recommended treatment in this category obviously is nonoperative. This includes restriction of activities and cessation of sports, particularly if the individual is involved in an overhand sport (e.g., baseball, tennis, or gymnastics). For those who have had pain or limited range of motion, a temporary period of immobilization in a sling or long arm cast for 3 to 6 weeks may help to reduce the acute synovitis and localized tenderness. When the symptoms have resolved, therapy is begun to promote active range of motion and muscle strengthening. Some authors have recommended simply changing the position of the player (e.g., from pitcher to first base or right field) as an acceptable mode of treatment. In this age group, patient compliance may be difficult to obtain, and therefore the risk of continued injury to the elbow may be too great if the patient is allowed to play his sport, even with a change in position. The serious long-term sequelae of this disease, if treatment recommendations are not followed, must be explained to the patient, the parents, and the coaches. In most cases, these lesions will heal if not repetitively injured, and the prognosis for a favorable outcome is high with this group. Follow-up visits are essential because repeat x-rays are taken to document healing of the lesion. The elbow must be protected until radiographs reveal normal reconstitution of the capitellum before these patients are allowed to return to their sport.

The category II lesion involves individuals from adolescence to adulthood (13 to 20 years of age). This group usually has a history of repetitive, overuse activity (e.g., baseball pitching, gymnastics) and an insidious onset of pain, loss of motion, and swelling. The x-rays in this particular stage exhibit the classic subchondral bony island surrounded by a lucency and sclerotic crater rim. The concern at this stage is whether the lesion within the capitellum has separated or is undergoing separation from the underlying avascular bone. Initial treatment should include restriction of activity and immobilization of the extremity to allow resolution of the acute synovitis. If satisfactory pain relief occurs at 3 to 6 weeks after immobilization, only continued observation may be followed. If immobilization fails to control the symptoms or obvious separation of the lesion is discovered with imaging studies, however, operative intervention is warranted. Elbow arthroscopy provides an accurate evaluation of the cartilaginous surfaces of the radiocapitellar joint.

Arthroscopically, one may identify an intact appearance of the cartilage, partial detachment of a chondral or osteochondral lesion, or complete detachment of an osteochondral lesion. In lesions where intact cartilage overlies the bony defect, the demarcation between normal and abnormal cartilage may or may not be highlighted by fibrillated cartilage. Some authors have recommended drilling through the intact cartilage into the sclerotic subchondral bone in an effort to promote healing. However, the literature shows no advantage of drilling of an intact lesion versus simple rest and observation.

If a partially detached lesion is seen, the underlying osseous portion must be evaluated. If the flap is entirely cartilaginous without any underlying bone, arthroscopic débridement of the loose chondral lesion should be performed. This can be accomplished with standard arthroscopic equipment, removing all loose free cartilage and leaving a stable rim of cartilage behind. The exposed bone then can be curetted, burred, and even drilled. If the lesion is difficult to assess adequately via arthroscopy, the surgeon should employ an open anterolateral approach to the elbow to achieve thorough visualization.

If the partially detached lesion includes significant osseous involvement, reattachment is recommended. This should be performed open via an anterolateral approach. The osteochondral flap should be elevated, the underlying sclerotic bone is curetted and debrided of fibrous tissue, and then the flap is reattached. Retrograde pinning of the lesion with threaded or unthreaded Kirschner wires can be performed, with the wires exiting the lateral epicondyle for later removal. The ends of the pins should be positioned below the articular surface so that the wires do not penetrate the joint space. Newer bioabsorbable pins (e.g., Johnson & Johnson Orthosorb) and bioabsorbable screws have been developed as an alternative to K-wire fixation, but clinical studies supporting their use in the treatment of these lesions currently are lacking.

If the lesion is completely detached but not displaced within the joint, reattachment should be performed as stated previously. The use of bone graft in the treatment of these detached lesions of the lateral condyle has led to poor and unsatisfactory results[35] and therefore is discouraged.

If arthroscopy alone was performed, a short period of postoperative immobilization is recommended until the wounds are healed. Active range-of-motion exercises then are begun. Serial x-rays again are performed in the office, and activity may not be resumed until radiographs reveal complete healing of the osseous lesion. If pin fixation was performed, the pins are left in place for an average of 6 to 8 weeks while early active assisted range-of-motion exercises are instituted to prevent elbow contractures. Radiographic follow-up again is necessary to document healing of the bony lesion, and resumption of activities is delayed until adequate healing is seen on x-ray.

Category III lesions involve the adult patient usually over the age of 20 who has had intermittent symptoms for several years. In this stage, the lesion frequently has become fragmented, with more than one loose body commonly present within the joint. Joint incongruity and deterioration of the articular cartilage may include not only the radiocapitellar joint, but also the entire elbow. Arthroscopic removal of one or more loose bodies may help if there are symptoms of catching or locking.[19] Discomfort or symptoms secondary to degenerative changes unfortunately will not be changed dramatically by such treatment. Partial synovectomy and débridement of loose cartilaginous flabs of debris, however, may help in some individuals. On occasion, the loose body removed is much larger than the defect seen within the capitellum; therefore completely loose fragments generally should not be returned to their bed and pinned because of ensuing degenerative changes. If exposed bone is present on the capitellum, curettage and drilling of the crater bed may be beneficial. Overall, the prognosis in this group is generally poor because of the extent of the lesion at initial presentation and the inability to reconstruct a congruous articulation. If considerable degenerative changes are present within the radiocapitellar joint and pain is the primary complaint, radial head excision can be performed if these individuals have completed their growth.

In summary, early recognition is essential to optimal results. Although not all osteochondritis dissecans lesions require surgical intervention, diagnosis and operative elbow arthroscopy may be warranted in certain situations. These situations include persistent symptoms despite conservative care, a large osteochondral defect seen on plain x-rays or other imaging studies that is causing catching or grinding of the athlete's elbow, and mechanical symptoms caused by one or more loose bodies. Large osteochondral lesions may be fixed; however, the physician generally should not attempt to pin old detached loose bodies back in place, nor should the physician graft large defects within the capitellum.

OTHER BONY INJURIES TO THE SKELETALLY IMMATURE ELBOW

The elbow in an adolescent athlete participating in throwing sports is vulnerable to the same injuries and stresses as in an adult. Unique to the young are the open epiphyseal growth plates. These areas about the elbow are undergoing the fastest rate of growth and thus are the weakest link in the system and at greatest risk for injury.

Bennett,[5] in 1941, first drew attention to particular elbow ailments associated with professional baseball pitchers. Brogen[8] introduced the term "Little Leaguer's elbow" in 1960 as he described three cases of an avulsion injury to the medial epicondylar growth center in adolescent pitchers. Many authors also have chronicled the risks of Little League pitching for elbow injuries.* *Little Leaguer's elbow* now is a generic term for a whole host of elbow injuries. These include medial epicondylar fragmentation, avulsion, apophysitis, accelerated apophyseal growth with delayed closure of the medial epicondylar growth plate, osteochondritis dissecans capitellum, and changes within the radial head.

MEDIAL EPICONDYLE

The medial epicondyle of the elbow serves as the origin of the common flexor-pronator muscle group of the forearm. The medial epicondyle apophysis is the last growth plate in the elbow to fuse. This growth plate is at risk for injury in skeletally immature athletes who participate in overhead sports or activities that produce repetitive valgus stress at the elbow.

An injury to this area usually is the result of repetitive overhead use of the upper extremity, typically in pitching. The athlete may complain of elbow pain, loss of motion, and occasional swelling. The physical examination demonstrates point tenderness at the medial epicondyle, a flexion contracture, and accentuation of the discomfort with valgus strain of the elbow.

X-rays are essential and must include a comparison view of the opposite elbow. No demonstrable changes in the x-ray are seen early. In the subtle cases, where clinical suspicion is high, a bone scan is recommended to de-

*References 1, 12, 17, 29, 31, 32.

termine whether a growth-plate injury had occurred. Chronic, repetitive overuse may over time lead to radiographic changes of fragmentation of the medial epicondylar apophysis or simply widening of the growth plate. There may be accelerated growth of the growth plate and hypertrophy of the distal humerus. On occasion, a single traumatic event may avulse the medial epicondyle.

Treatment consists of immediate rest from all throwing or aggravating activities if no displacement of the medial epicondyle is seen. Four to 6 weeks of rest usually is sufficient time for the symptoms to resolve and for full motion to return. During this period, active range-of-motion exercises are begun, as are progressive resistive exercises for the entire upper extremity. Only when the elbow has regained full, pain-free range of motion and muscle strength has been restored should the athlete be allowed to resume his previous athletic activity.

If the medial epicondyle is avulsed and displaced more than 1 cm, open reduction and internal fixation is the treatment of choice. Woods and Tullos[34] recommended that any separation greater than 0.5 cm in the dominant elbow of an overhead athlete be operatively fixed.

SUMMARY

Micheli[36] identified risk factors in the young athlete that may lead to overuse injuries. In this group of skeletally immature individuals, training errors, muscle-tendon imbalance, anatomic malalignment, and growth may be risk factors for overuse injury. Safe training regimens and common sense are the keys to prevention. States have limited the number of innings a Little League pitcher may pitch per week to prevent injury. Prevention is the primary goal, because after significant chronic problems occur, the likelihood of successful treatment is poor.

References

1. Adams JE: Bone injuries in very young athletes, *Clin Orthop* 58:129-140, 1968.
2. Albright JA et al: Clinical study of baseball pitchers: correlation of injury to the throwing arm with method of delivery, *Am J Sports Med* 6:15-21, 1978.
3. Barnes DA, Tullos HS: An analysis of 100 symptomatic baseball elbows, *Am J Sports Med* 6:62-67, 1978.
4. Bennett GE: The elbow and shoulder lesions in baseball players, *Am J Surg* 98:484-492, 1959.
5. Bennett GE: Shoulder and elbow lesions in professional baseball pitchers, *JAMA* 117:510-514, 1941.
6. Bennett JB, Tullos HS: *The elbow and its disorders,* Philadelphia, 1985, WB Saunders.
7. Bianco AJ: *The elbow and its disorders,* Philadelphia, 1985, WB Saunders.
8. Brogdon BG, Crow NE: Little Leaguer's elbow, *Am J Roentgenol* 83:671-675, 1960.
9. Chan D et al: Chronic stress injuries to the elbow in young gymnasts, *Br J Radiol* 64:1113-1118, 1991.
10. Dehaven KE: Symposium: throwing injuries to the adolescent elbow, *Cont Surg* Sept 1976, p 9.
11. Grana WA, Rashkin A: Pitcher's elbow in adolescents, *Am J Sports Med* 8:333, 1980.
12. Gugenheim JJ et al: Little League survey: the Houston survey, *Am J Sports Med* 4:189-200, 1976.
13. Haraldsson S: Osteochondrosis deformans juvenilis capituli humeri including investigations of interosseous vasculature of the distal humerus, *Acta Orthop Scand Suppl* 33:1-232, 1959.
14. Indelicato PA et al: Correctable elbow lesions in professional baseball players: review of 25 cases, *Am J Sports Med* 7:72, 1979.
15. King JW, Brelsford HJ, Tullos HS: Analysis of the pitching arm of the professional baseball pitcher, *Clin Orthop* 67:116-123, 1969.
16. Konig F: *Lehrbuch der Allgemeinen Chirugie Fur Aerzte and Studirende,* Berlin, 1889, A Hirschwald, p 751.
17. Larson RL et al: Little League survey: the Eugene study, *Am J Sports Med* 4:201-209, 1976.
18. Nagura S: The so-called osteochondritis dissecans konig, *Clin Orthop* 18:110-119, 1960.
19. O'Driscoll SW, Morrey BF: Arthroscopy of the elbow, *J Bone Joint Surg* 74A:84-93, 1992.
20. Panner HJ: A peculiar affection of the capitellum humeri, resembling Calvé-Perthes disease of the hip, *Acta Radiol* 10:234, 1929.
21. Pappas AM: Osteochondrosis dissecans, *Clin Orthop* 158:59, 1981.
22. Pappas AM, Zawacki RM, Sullivan TJ: Biomechanics of baseball pitching, preliminary report, *Am J Sports Med* 13:216, 1985.
23. Pitt MJ, Speer DP: Imaging of the elbow with and emphasis on trauma, *Radiol Clin North Am* 28:293, 1990.
24. Roberts N, Hughes R: Osteochondritis dissecans of the elbow joint, a clinical study, *J Bone Joint Surg* 32B:348-355, 1950.
25. Ruch DS, Poehling GG: Arthroscopic treatment of Panner's disease, *Clin Sports Med* 10:629, 1991.
26. Salter RB: *Textbook of disorders and injuries of the musculoskeletal system,* ed 2, Baltimore, 1983, Williams & Wilkins.
27. Siffert RS: The osteochondroses, *Clin Orthop* 158:2, 1981.
28. Singer KM, Roy SP: Osteochondrosis of the human capitellum, *Am J Sports Med* 12:151-160, 1984.
29. Slager RF: From Little League to big league: the weak spot in the arm, *Am J Sports Med* 5:37-48, 1977.
30. Torg JS: Little League: the theft of a care-free youth, *Phys Sports Med* 1:72-78, 1973.
31. Torg JS, Pollick H, Sweterlitsch P: The effect of competitive pitching on the shoulder and elbow in pre-adolescent baseball pitchers, *Pediatrics* 49:267-272, 1972.
32. Tullos HS, King JW: Lesions of the pitching arm in adolescents, *JAMA* 220.264-271, 1972.
33. Tullos HS et al: Unusual lesions in the pitching arm, *Clin Orthop* 88:169-182, 1972.
34. Woods GW, Tullos HS: Elbow instability in medial epicondyle fractures, *Am J Sports Med* 5:23-30, 1977.
35. Woodward AH, Bianco AJ: Osteochondritis dissecans of the elbow, *Clin Orthop* 110:35-41, 1975.
36. Micheli LJ: Overuse injuries in children's sports: the growth factor, *Orthop Clinics of NA* 14:337, 1983.

CHAPTER 22

Biceps Rupture and Triceps Avulsion

DONALD F. D'ALESSANDRO
CLARENCE L. SHIELDS

In the context of athletic injuries about the elbow, isolated disruption of the distal biceps tendon from the radial tuberosity and avulsion of the triceps from the olecranon are relatively rare. Nonetheless, if not recognized and appropriately treated, these injuries can lead to significant disability not only affecting athletic performance but also interfering with activities of daily living and the workplace. Prompt anatomic repair usually results in full recovery of function and allows return to unrestricted athletic participation.

DISTAL BICEPS TENDON RUPTURE

Etiology and Pathology

Avulsion of the distal tendon of the biceps brachii represents 3% of all biceps ruptures, with proximal ruptures of the long head accounting for 96% and of the short head 1%.[29] Although this injury is uncommon, more than 200 cases have been reported in the world's literature, represented mostly by individual surgeons' accounts of two or three cases.* Dobbie[23] in 1941 collected 51 cases from 355 surgeons responding to a questionnaire. The surgeons performed conservative and surgical treatments, with all claiming essentially normal restoration of function. Only recently have series of at least 10 cases been published where treatment outcomes have been critically analyzed with isokinetic and functional testing.[1,7,22,54]

Distal biceps tendon ruptures usually occur in heavily muscled males[9,53,54,63] who often are laborers and average 40 to 50 years of age.[8,23,53,54] D'Alessandro et al have published the only series involving athletes, specifically weight lifters and bodybuilders who averaged only 40 years of age and seemed to be at risk for this injury be-

*References 8, 9, 20, 27, 35, 40, 56, 61, 68, 73, 74, 82.

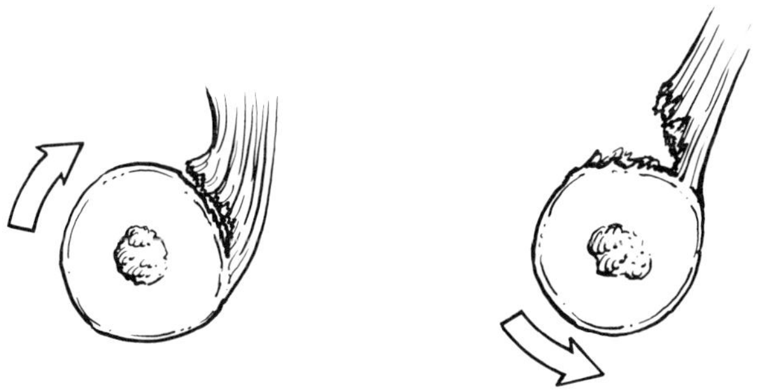

FIGURE 22-1 A proposed etiology of distal biceps tendon rupture is repetitive stress failure from pronation and supination in association with a local bony excrescence at the radial tuberosity. (Adapted from Davis WM, Yassine Z: An etiological factor in tear of the distal tendon of the biceps brachii, *J Bone Joint Surg* 38A[6]:1365-1368, 1956.)

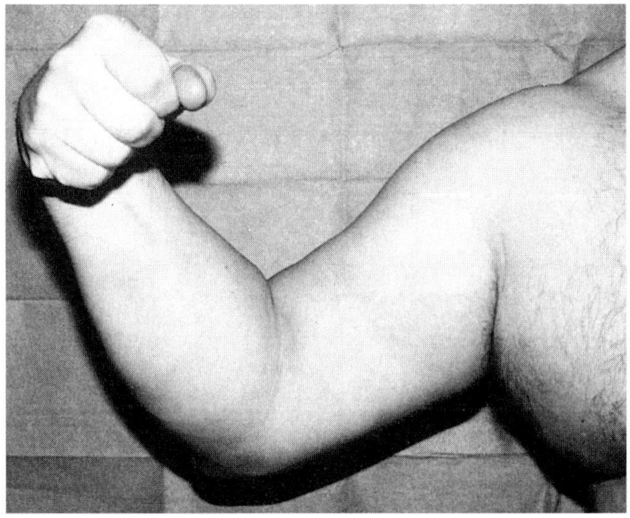

FIGURE 22-2 Clinical photograph of a patient 6 weeks after a distal biceps tendon rupture. With the swelling and ecchymosis resolved, the abnormal biceps contour with its proximal retraction can be appreciated.

cause of the large forces generated by their hypertrophied biceps muscles.[22] Morrey in 1991[12] recorded the only known case of this injury occurring in a female: a 38-year-old meat cutter who sustained a partial biceps tendon rupture.

The majority of ruptures involve the dominant extremity and usually result from a single traumatic event. The common mechanism of injury is an intense biceps contraction overwhelmed by an unanticipated extension force.[22,23,53] Most injuries occur when the person is lifting, pulling, or straining with heavy objects. Examples include catching a falling garage door, trying to lift the front end of an automobile, and jumping off a fire truck while holding the hose, which suddenly jammed.[22,23] Athletic activities that have led to injuries include spotting a falling gymnast, accidentally gripping a ring apparatus with a single arm, performing an unsuccessful biceps curl, striking the back of an opponent while playing handball, and not releasing a rein while being thrown while rodeo-riding.[7,22]

Complete avulsion of the distal tendon from the radial tuberosity is the rule,* with the exception of five case reports of attenuation and partial tearing of the tendon.[12,57] The fundamental cause of this injury has not been satisfactorily explained, although repetitive stress failure resulting from pronation and supination against a local bony excrescence has been suggested[21] (Fig. 22-1). Radiographic findings of slight irregularity and enlargement of the radial tuberosity support this concept.[12,21,53,54] Chronic degenerative changes of the tendon at the radial tuberosity insertion have been seen in cases of both partial and complete rupture.[12,17,21,23] Morrey recently postulated that chronic inflammation of the deep bicipital radial bursae at the radial tuberosity may contribute to degeneration of the biceps tendon.[52]

A direct relationship between anabolic steroid use and distal biceps tendon ruptures has not been identified. In a series of athletes with distal biceps tendon ruptures, 8 of the 10 were bodybuilders or weight lifters and denied using steroids before their injury.[22] However, recent experimental evidence does suggest that the use of anabolic steroids predisposes tendons to rupture. Miles et al[50] evaluated the histologic and biomechanical effects of anabolic steroids on rat tendon. The animals developed stiffer tendons that failed with less elongation and absorbed less energy before failing. The combination of increased muscle strength afforded by anabolic steroids and stiffer, weaker tendons may place an athlete at greater risk for tendon ruptures.[50]

Clinical Evaluation

The diagnosis often is determined by a history of a violent pull against a set forearm accompanied by an audible "pop." The patient experiences acute tearing-like pain and subsequent antecubital swelling and ecchymosis. The acute pain subsides within a few days and is followed by a dull ache that may last for several weeks. As the swelling diminishes, the asymmetric biceps contour with its proximal retraction can be appreciated (Fig. 22-2). Patients will experience weakness and fatigue pain with use of the arm. These symptoms are exacerbated by

*References 22, 23, 40, 53, 54, 61.

repetitive elbow flexion-and-supination activities, such as using a screwdriver and hammering. Flexion weakness may be present initially but decreases with time as the other elbow flexors, namely the brachialis and brachioradialis muscles, hypertrophy to adequately compensate for the loss of this biceps function.[16,40] A supination strength deficit will persist, however, and its clinical effect will depend on the individual's need to do supination activities. In addition, several patients have complained of loss of grip strength,[40,54] the biomechanical basis of which is unclear.

On physical examination, the deformity of the biceps may be disguised by antecubital swelling. Ecchymosis usually is present, but an intact lacertus fibrosus may contain the hematoma and limit the extent of ecchymosis. Similarly, an intact lacertus fibrosus may be misinterpreted as the biceps tendon. Palpation of the other arm will help define the normally substantial and discrete biceps tendon, helping to avoid this pitfall. An obvious defect in the antecubital fossa normally is present in the setting of the complete rupture. In the rare instance of attenuation and partial tearing, the tendon remains in continuity and is identifiable on examination.[12]

Strength testing of both elbow flexion and forearm supination is essential for diagnosis. Even on initial presentation, full range of motion should be possible with discomfort only at the extremes of flexion, extension, and supination. Decreased flexion strength usually is readily demonstrated on physical exam, with the exception of late-presenting cases where compensatory muscles have assumed this function. Weakness in supination always can be appreciated and particularly helps in revealing cases of biceps dysfunction resulting from a partial tear or a complete tear masked by an intact lacertus fibrosus.[12] If the diagnosis is still in question, formal isokinetic muscle testing can be used to objectively document strength deficits.[1,7,22,54]

As mentioned previously, the only radiographic finding associated with this injury is subtle hypertrophic changes at the radial tuberosity, and these changes frequently are not present. Magnetic resonance imaging, although usually not necessary for diagnosis of complete ruptures, can be useful in evaluating partial tears or in cases where the diagnosis is in question because of an intact lacertus fibrosus.

Treatment and Results

A review of the literature reveals considerable debate over the recommended treatment for acute distal biceps tendon ruptures. Carrol and Hamilton[16] are the only authors to unequivocally recommend conservative treatment. Their patients returned to work an average of only 4 weeks after the injury. No difference was found between the injured and uninjured sides when patients were tested in their ability to supinate and flex their elbows by lifting weights at 1 year after injury. Most investigators do not agree with this opinion, however. Although most patients treated nonoperatively will gain some improvement in arm strength with time,[33] they should expect diminished strength and endurance of elbow flexion and supination, because the biceps contributes substantially to these actions. Isokinetic muscle testing has documented elbow flexion strength deficits of 30% to 36% and supination strength deficits of 40% to 55% after conservative treatment.[7,54] Complaints of persistent weakness, fatigue pain with repetitive activities, and the permanent alteration of the shape and size of the arm argue against conservative treatment.[7,23,33,54,58]

The operative technique recommended for repair has varied in the literature, specifically in the site of reattachment of the tendon. Several reports claim good results with suturing the tendon to the brachialis muscle,* even though this shortens the muscle-tendon unit and sacrifices the contribution of the biceps to forearm supination. Dobbie, after analyzing the subjective results in 75 cases treated with a variety of surgical procedures, concluded that restoration of elbow flexion was the chief objective of biceps repair. He also stated that supination power was of secondary importance and could adequately be replaced by the muscles of the forearm, although no objective testing was conducted.[23] He and others advised repair to the brachialis because they thought acceptable clinical results were achieved without endangering the radial nerve, which would be at risk with anatomic repair to the radial tuberosity. However, recent isokinetic data on nonoperated patients[7,54] and on a patient whose tendon was repaired back to the brachialis[54] have shown permanent supination strength deficits.

An anatomic repair to the radial tuberosity has consistently yielded superior results in the literature†, and can safely be accomplished through the double-incision technique of Boyd and Anderson.[54] The recent literature offers compelling evidence that prompt anatomic repair of this injury is the treatment of choice. Five separate series, each including 10 patients or more, found that reattachment of the tendon to the radial tuberosity consistently yields excellent results with the restoration of essentially normal supination and flexion strength as documented by isokinetic muscle testing.[1,7,22,54,58]

Morrey et al[54] showed that immediate reattachment is preferable because the tract for the biceps tendon is easily identifiable in the acute setting and because delayed repair resulted in residual weakness in one of their patients.

A study by D'Alessandro et al is the only series consisting predominantly of weight lifters and bodybuilders with high functional demands that has evaluated their ability to return to their preinjury level of activity. These

*References 21, 23, 36, 39, 49, 63.

†References 1, 6-9, 13, 22, 27, 33, 40, 45, 53, 54, 58, 61, 78, 82.

patients elected to have surgery to maximize their potential for full recovery and to have the appearance of their biceps restored. All patients were satisfied with their functional and aesthetic results and returned to full unrestricted activity. Isokinetic muscle testing demonstrated that supination strength and endurance were normal in patients with a repaired dominant extremity. In flexion, they had normal strength but averaged 20% less endurance. Three patients had injured their nondominant extremity, and results in this group were less consistent. Although elbow flexion strength and endurance were essentially normal, one had complete recovery of supination strength, while the other two had only 56% and 58% recovery. The patient with a full recovery continues to weight train regularly, a bilateral activity. One patient with a marked supination deficit was an acrobat who had relied heavily on his dominant side when performing, while the other had elected to pursue racquetball and handball, sports that do not condition the nondominant extremity. In these athletes, flexion strength was restored, but significant supination deficits could reflect not only the lack of a formal rehabilitation program but also the relative disuse of the nondominant extremity with certain sports and activities of daily living. Agins et al[1] produced the only other study to consider repaired nondominant extremities. They had four patients whose repaired nondominant arms had 50% deficits in both strength and endurance of elbow flexion as compared with the noninjured dominant side. Supination function was not tested in their study. The compromised results also were attributed to the lack of a formal rehabilitation protocol for the nondominant arms.

In cases of delayed diagnosis, primary repair still can be accomplished within 4 to 6 weeks of the injury. Mobilization of the retracted tendon may be necessary, and delineation of the bicipital tunnel to the radial tuberosity is more difficult.

Morrey proposed a treatment rationale for late-presenting cases.[53] The specific patient complaints must be carefully assessed. The most likely scenario involves a patient whose occupation demands supination strength and endurance. Late reconstruction can be accomplished through either a ligament-augmentation device[53] or a fascia lata graft[33] to connect the retracted biceps to the radial tuberosity. No clinical results currently are available on these procedures. Surgical intervention for complaints of elbow-flexion weakness should be less likely because rehabilitation of the other elbow flexors should adequately compensate for the loss of this biceps function. If restoration of elbow-flexion strength is the purpose of surgery, direct repair to the brachialis muscle will give satisfactory results.

In conclusion, anatomic repair of distal biceps ruptures within the first week of injury should give consistently excellent subjective and objective results, allowing the athlete or laborer to return to the preinjury level of activity. Rehabilitation of the operative arm, particularly the nondominant repaired extremity, is essential for complete recovery.

Recommended Surgical Technique

The biceps tendon is reinserted into the radial tuberosity through a modification of the two-incision technique described by Boyd and Anderson.[13,78] The patient is placed in the supine position with the elbow extended and the forearm supinated on an arm board. An oblique curvilinear incision is made, beginning medially and proximal to the elbow crease and extending distally and laterally. We have found that this incision lies in the crease along the distal edge of the biceps muscle belly after repair and often is unnoticeable in the flexed posture (Fig. 22-3). The lacertus fibrosus may remain intact and should be released to unveil the underlying hematoma and biceps tendon. Care is taken to protect the lateral antebrachial cutaneous nerve, which lies just lateral to the biceps tendon and on top of the brachialis muscle. The end of the tendon is localized and débrided. Two nonabsorbable #1 sutures are placed in the tendon with a Bunnell stitch (Fig. 22-4). If the surgery is being performed within 7 days of injury, a tunnel vacated by the biceps tendon should lead directly to the radial tuberosity. The tendon invariably is cleanly avulsed from the tuberosity. When a delayed repair is being performed, this pathway may be obliterated by scar tissue, necessitating further dissection.

A curved clamp then is inserted between the radius and the ulna and directed posterolaterally, tenting the skin of the forearm (Fig. 22-5). The elbow is flexed, and a posterior longitudinal incision approximately 8 cm long is made paralleling the radial border of the ulna. Morrey's modification of the posterior approach is employed in an effort to decrease the chance of synostosis.[24,54] A limited

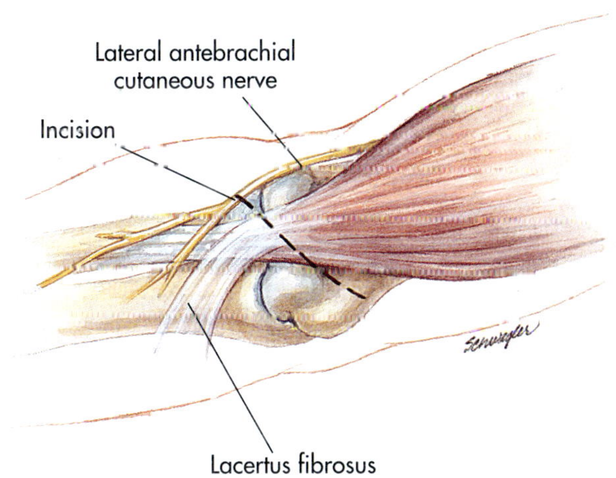

FIGURE 22-3 Anterior incision. An oblique curvilinear incision of approximately 5 to 7 cm in length provides adequate exposure and acceptable cosmetic result.

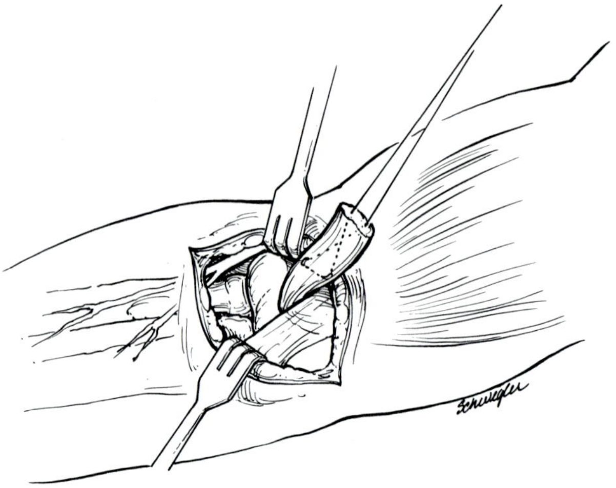

FIGURE 22-4 Biceps tendon identification and preparation. The end of the tendon is localized and débrided. Two nonabsorbable #1 sutures are placed in the tendon using a Bunnell stitch. (Adapted from Tibone JE: Repair of distal biceps tendon rupture. In Shields CF, editor: *Manual of sports surgery,* New York, 1987, Springer-Verlag.)

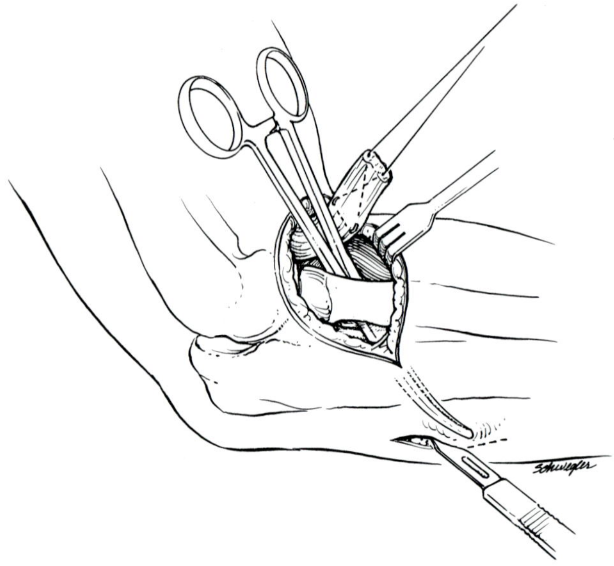

FIGURE 22-5 Posterior incision. A curved clamp is inserted between the radius and the ulna and directed posterolaterally. The tented skin localizes the center of the posterolateral incision of approximately 8 cm in length. (Adapted from Morrey BF: Tendon injuries about the elbow. In Morrey BF, editor: *The elbow and its disorders,* ed 2, Philadelphia, 1993, WB Saunders.)

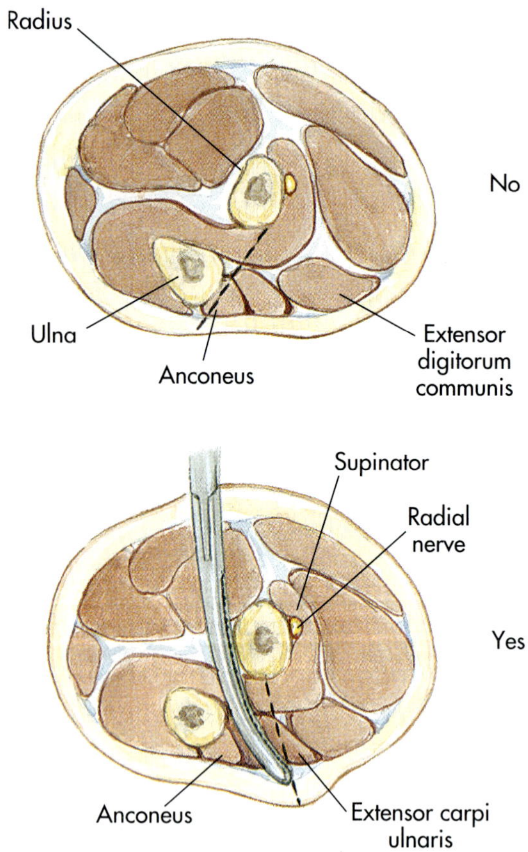

FIGURE 22-6 Posterior approach. Morrey has modified the posterior approach by recommending a limited muscle splitting approach through the extensor muscle mass in an effort to minimize the risk for synostosis. The periosteum over the ulna is not disturbed. See text for details. (Adapted from Morrey BF: Tendon injuries about the elbow. In Morrey BF, editor: *The elbow and its disorders,* ed 2, Philadelphia, 1993, WB Saunders.)

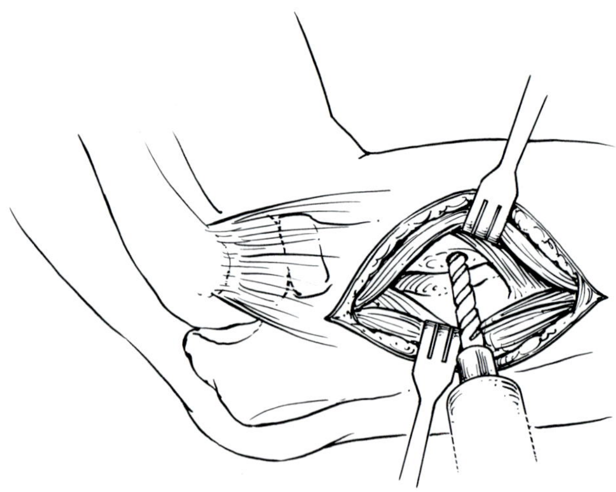

FIGURE 22-7 Radial tuberosity preparation. Radial tuberosity is cleared of soft tissue. A pilot hole in the radial tuberosity is made with a drill and then excavated using a high-speed burr. See text for details. (Adapted from Tibone JE: Repair of distal biceps tendon rupture. In Shields CF, editor: *Manual of sports surgery,* New York, 1987, Springer-Verlag.)

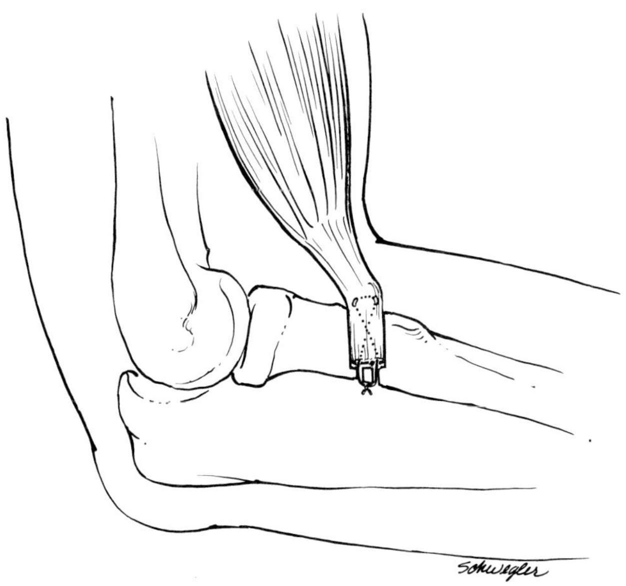

FIGURE 22-8 Securing the biceps tendon. Sutures are passed through the soft-tissue tunnel between the radius and the ulna and then through the cortex opposite the hole in the radial tuberosity. Before the sutures are tied, the forearm is supinated, and care is taken to be sure the tendon is well seated in the bone. (Adapted from Tibone JE: Repair of distal biceps tendon rupture. In Shields CF, editor: *Manual of sports surgery*, New York, 1987, Springer-Verlag.)

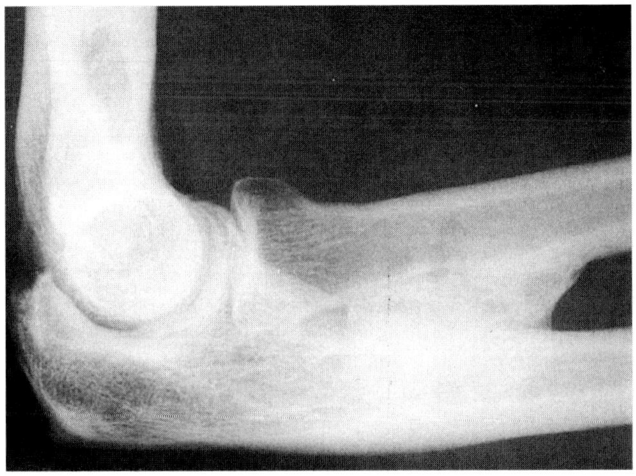

FIGURE 22-9 Proximal radial ulnar synostosis is an uncommon but severe complication of the two-incision technique for repair of distal biceps tendon ruptures. See text for details.

muscle-splitting approach through the extensor muscle mass while avoiding exposure of the ulna is performed to visualize the radial tuberosity (Fig. 22-6). The radial tuberosity then is cleared of soft tissue, and a $\frac{1}{8}$-inch drill is used to make a pilot hole in the tuberosity. The hole is enlarged with a $\frac{1}{4}$-inch drill, and the cavity is excavated with a high-speed burr if necessary (Fig. 22-7). Care is taken to remove bone dust with copious irrigation. Two smaller holes then are drilled across the tuberosity with a $\frac{5}{64}$-inch drill bit.

The tendon next is passed from anterior to posterior through the soft tissue tunnel between the radius and ulna. Nonabsorbable sutures are passed through the large drill hole into the radial tuberosity and out through the smaller holes using a 24-gauge wire as a suture passer. The sutures are pulled firmly with the arm supinated, making sure by direct palpation through the anterior incision that the tendon can be well-seated in bone (Fig. 22-8). Before tying the sutures, the surgeon deflates the tourniquet, obtains hemostasis, and closes the anterior incision over a drain. The elbow is then flexed 90°, and the forearm is supinated as the sutures are tied securely. The posterior wound then is closed over a drain.

Postoperative Management

The forearm is held in supination with the elbow in 90° of flexion for 3 weeks in a long arm splint. Gentle active range of motion in both the flexion-extension and pronation-supination planes is then begun. A gentle, progressive resisted strengthening program is started 6 weeks after surgery with a weight program that includes isometric and isotonic exercises instituted at 12 weeks. The patient is not permitted to return to unrestricted activities until 6 months after surgery. Continued rehabilitation is encouraged to restore full strength and endurance.

Complications

Before the development of the two-incision technique, the principal reason not to reattach the tendon to the radial tuberosity was the vulnerability of the radial nerve to injury through the extended anterior Henry approach.[31] Most radial nerve palsies proved to be transient, yet the potential for severe disability remained.[11,23,28,49] The two-incision technique has been successful at minimizing this risk, as we could find only one case of a transient radial neuropraxia, which resolved entirely by 3 months after surgery.[6]

As is often the case in medicine, the solution to one problem has led to another. Recently, Failla et al collected four cases of proximal radial ulnar synostosis with the use of the two-incision technique[24] (Fig. 22-9). The posterolateral approach involving subperiosteal elevation of the anconeus and extensor muscles and perforation of the proximal portion of the interosseous membrane may be responsible for synostosis formation with this procedure. The presence of a hematoma communicating with the radius and ulna also may contribute to the risk of synostosis. Resection of the synostosis with interposition of a Silastic sheath was successful in only half of the patients. The authors suggested that the posterior exposure be made with a small muscle-splitting approach through the extensor mass, avoiding periosteal elevation of the

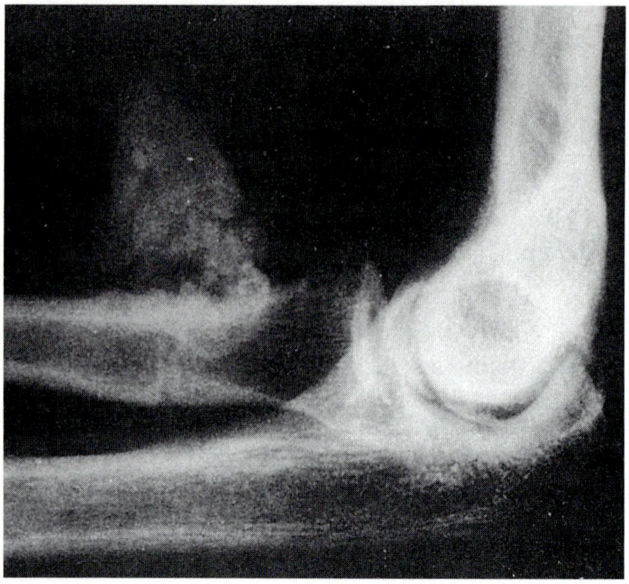

FIGURE 22-10 Calcification of the biceps tendon at the radial tuberosity after reattachment occurs rarely. Surprisingly, its presence has not been shown to compromise clinical results. See text for details. (From D'Alessandro DF et al: Repair of distal biceps tendon ruptures in athletes, *Am J Sports Med* 21[1]: 114-119, 1993.)

proximal ulna to decrease the chances of synostosis. Although this complication is relatively rare, adopting this modification probably is prudent.[24,53,54]

Calcification of the tendon at the site of its attachment to the radial tuberosity was seen in 20% of the patients in a recent series[22] (Fig. 22-10). This calcification did not affect the range of motion or clinical results. Norman et al[58] reported a loss of 10° to 20° in the pronation-supination arc in one third of their patients after operative repair. These patients were immobilized in a cast for 6 weeks after surgery, perhaps predisposing them to stiffness. Limitations of range of motion have not been a problem with splinting of the arm for only 3 to 4 weeks after surgery.[7,22,53]

Fortunately, complications with this procedure are relatively uncommon. We could not find a single case report of a recurrent rupture after operative repair.

TRICEPS TENDON AVULSION

Etiology and Pathology

Avulsion, or rupture, of the triceps tendon has been described as the least common of all tendon injuries.[83] Anzel et al reviewed a series of 1014 tendon injuries from the Mayo Clinic and identified only 8 cases of triceps tendon injury, and 4 of these were due to laceration.[3,53] Since Partridge documented the first case of a triceps tendon avulsion in 1868, approximately 50 cases have been recorded in the American and European literature.[15] The three largest series include Levy (16 cases), Pantazopoulos (7 cases), and Tarsney (7 cases). The remaining cases are from a number of individuals who provided only two or three case reports each.

Bach et al[5] reviewed the case reports and series available in the English literature up to 1987 and produced important epidemiologic data on triceps tendon injuries. The mean age at the time of injury was 26 years, ranging from 7 to 72. Seventy-one percent (29 of 41) of the patients were male. The right and left extremities were equally involved, and the side of rupture could not be correlated to the dominant or nondominant side.[5]

There are relatively few cases in the literature of triceps tendon injuries occurring in athletes. Before 1984, there are only two case reports of triceps avulsion injuries sustained while participating in athletics: One was a football player who was kicked on the posterior aspect of his outstretched arm, and the other was a skier whose ski struck his arm while he was falling. Since 1984, however, four triceps tendon injuries have occurred in body-builders and power lifters during the act of weight lifting.[5,15,32,66]

The mechanism of injury for triceps tendon avulsion is a fall on an outstretched arm in the majority of cases. The biomechanics of this injury have been described as "a deceleration stress superimposed upon a contracting triceps muscle, with or without a concomitant blow to the posterior aspect of the elbow."[25] Most commonly, the abrupt forceful eccentric contraction of the triceps is solely responsible for the avulsion injury. Less frequently, a concomitant direct blow to the posterior aspect of the triceps at its insertion may play a role in the mechanism of injury.* During athletic participation, the usual mechanism of injury also is a sudden forceful contraction, possibly associated with a direct blow to the posterior arm. The weight lifter, however, can incur this injury during a workout with a sustained extreme concentric contraction, as illustrated by four recent case reports.[5,15,32,36]

This injury has occurred in many systemically compromised patients in whom the tendon has ruptured spontaneously or as a result of trivial trauma. Tendon ruptures have been reported in association with renal osteodystrophy and secondary hyperparathyroidism,† chronic acidosis,[55] Marfan's syndrome,[69] and steroid treatment for lupus erythematosus.[79,84] The underlying pathophysiology is not well understood, but calcification resulting from the chronic hypercalcemia of secondary hyperparathyroidism has been implicated.[65] In addition, dialysis patients with renal osteodystrophy have had increased amounts of elastic fibers in their tendons, perhaps predisposing them to injury.[55]

*References 2, 10, 25, 60, 71, 76.

†References 18, 26, 44, 46, 47, 55, 64, 65, 70, 79.

The recent reports of triceps tendon injuries occurring in bodybuilders and weight lifters raises the question of the role of anabolic steroids.[5,32] The same reasons put forth to explain this group's predisposition to distal biceps ruptures are applicable to this injury. The detrimental effects of either local steroid injections on tendon[37,80] or systemic anabolic steroid use[34,38,50] on the strength of tendons and ligaments have been documented. In fact, a recent case report illustrates this risk. A bodybuilder who had received a series of six steroid injections for olecranon bursitis sustained an intrasubstance rupture of his triceps tendon while bench pressing.[75] He had a 5-year history of systemic anabolic steroid use as well. Athletes who use anabolic steroids are at risk for tendon ruptures because their excessive muscular strength is exerted on tendons that become stiffer and absorb less energy to failure.[50]

In 1933, McMaster demonstrated experimentally and clinically that musculotendinous ruptures occur in three locations, namely the muscle belly, the musculotendinous junction, and the osseous tendon insertion.[48] With regard to the triceps mechanism, the majority of authors have described tendoosseous avulsions, usually associated with a small fleck of bone.[25,53,76] Ruptures at the musculotendinous junction[29,32,51] and muscle belly tears of the triceps itself[4,51,60] both are extremely rare, having been seen in only a few cases.

Although complete disruption is the rule, incomplete or partial tears do occur.[15,25,76] A partial tear must be differentiated from a complete rupture because the former can be successfully treated nonoperatively; surgical repair is recommended for the complete lesion.

Associated injuries incurred as a result of falling on an outstretched arm must be considered. Levi et al[42,43] documented the association of radial head fractures with triceps ruptures in 16 patients. Lee[41] described the only case of a triceps rupture associated with a wrist fracture.

Triceps avulsion in the adolescent involves separation of the olecranon epiphysis, and it is an extremely rare injury.[62,67] The secondary ossification center of the olecranon appears in the area of the triceps insertion at about 9 years of age. The physis fuses in an anterior-to-posterior direction; this occurs at about 14 years of age.[14,77]

The epiphysis is enveloped by the triceps expansion, which extends distally, attaching to the metaphysis.[67] Consequently, an injury sustained when the physis is incompletely fused usually creates a Salter-Harris type II fracture.[30]

The avulsed fragment is larger than the typical fleck of bone seen in adults, but a small ossified metaphyseal fragment may be the only radiographic evidence that this injury has occurred. For significantly displaced fractures, open reduction and internal fixation is recommended. Depending on the size of the fragment, either a tension band wire technique[30,62,67] or fixation with a screw and washer[81] can be used with anticipated good results.

Clinical Evaluation

In the vast majority of cases, the patient will relate a history of falling on an outstretched arm accompanied by acute pain, a tearing sensation, and subsequent swelling and ecchymosis of the arm. As opposed to distal biceps tendon ruptures, a pop usually is not heard at the time of this injury.

The patient's complaints and physical findings will depend on whether the triceps is partially or completely torn. With a complete disruption, an indentation in the posterior contour of the arm often can be seen, particularly as swelling subsides. A defect in the triceps mechanism usually is palpable. If a partial injury has occurred, tenderness usually is localized to the musculotendinous junction, and a specific defect may not be felt. Complete loss of extension strength against gravity is experienced with a complete tear. An incomplete lesion is manifested by weakness but an ability to actively extend the elbow.

Extension strength can be difficult to evaluate because of the pain associated with an acute injury. In 1990, Viegas described a modification of the Thompson test[77] (traditionally used to identify complete ruptures of the Achilles tendon) for the assessment of a triceps injury.[81]

The modified test is performed with the patient seated and the arm draped over the back of the chair or with the patient in the prone position and letting the forearm hang over the table. In the normal extremity, squeezing the triceps muscle belly produces slight elbow extension, but no motion will occur if a complete rupture is present.[81] The results of this test may help the physician distinguish between partial and complete triceps tears.

The physician must look for associated injuries, especially if the injury was sustained while falling on an outstretched hand. Radial head fractures are most frequently associated,[42,43,76] but distal wrist injuries[41] also must be considered.

If a specific traumatic event is not elicited in the history, the differential diagnosis of isolated triceps weakness includes a C7-nerve-root lesion. As noted previously, spontaneous ruptures or injuries resulting from trivial forces may be the result of chronic medical conditions, including renal osteodystrophy with secondary hyperparathyroidism and long-term steroid use, as seen with systemic lupus erythematosus.

A lateral radiograph of the elbow can be very useful in confirming the diagnosis. A small avulsion fracture of the olecranon or "flake sign"[25,76] will be present in two thirds of the cases[32] and implies a complete rupture (Fig. 22-11). Ancillary studies such as MRI or ultrasound[15] may be useful in assessing partial lesions but usually are not necessary for the physician to make the diagnosis or determine an appropriate treatment plan in cases of complete rupture.

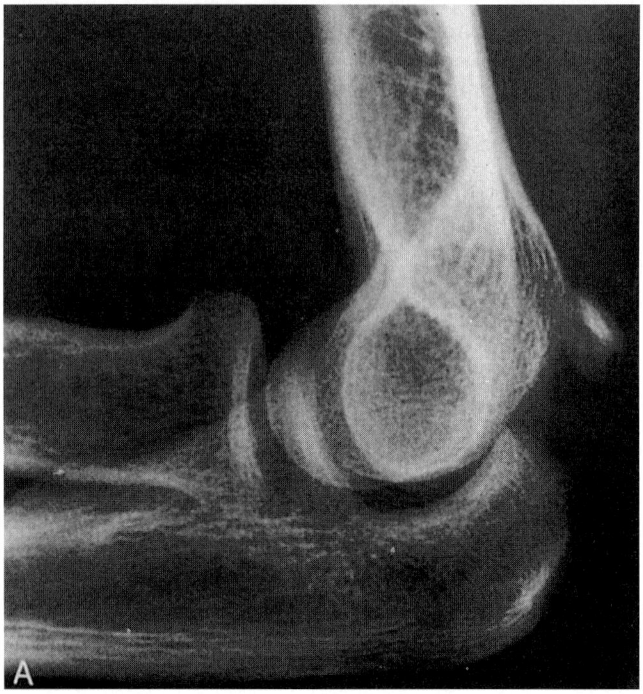

FIGURE 22-11 "Flake sign." A lateral radiograph of the elbow may reveal a small avulsion fracture of the olecranon signifying a complete triceps avulsion. (From Morrey BF: Tendon injuries about the elbow. In Morrey BF, editor: *The elbow and its disorders,* ed 2, Philadelphia, 1993, WB Saunders.)

Treatment and Results

Surgical repair is the treatment of choice for complete avulsions. Unlike in biceps tendon ruptures, other muscles cannot substitute for triceps function. Significant disability results from incontinuity of the triceps mechanism in the active population. Ritchie and Rocke reported on a 47-year-old bodybuilder treated nonoperatively with a complete rupture of the triceps in the presence of a patella cubiti.[66] At 3 years after injury, he declined operative repair even though his triceps strength was thought to be two thirds that of the other arm. In the chronically ill patients who sustain this injury, triceps function is essential for the use of ambulatory aids and transfers. Therefore operative repair is suggested in this group as well.

The surgical technique recommended for acute complete ruptures is basically the same throughout the literature. Anatomic reattachment of the triceps tendon is accomplished through drill holes in the olecranon using nonabsorbable suture most commonly. Surprisingly, in several cases where the diagnosis and treatment have been delayed for several months, as illustrated in case reports of 3-, 4½-, and 6-month delays in surgical treatment, primary repair has been accomplished with subsequent excellent results.[5,71,76] Others have suggested augmentation of the repair in the delayed setting or if poor-quality tissue is encountered at surgery.[19,25,53] Bennett described reinforcing the repair by reflecting a proximally based flap of posterior forearm fascia and suturing it to the triceps.[10] Clayton and Thirupathi used an inverted tongue of triceps fascia to supplement the repair in an elderly patient with chronic bursitis.[19] Carpentier et al suggested Z-plasty lengthening of the triceps to avoid undue tension when repairing a chronic rupture.[15]

The results of operative management are consistently excellent throughout the literature. In the majority of cases, however, the results are based on the patients' and physicians' subjective assessment of the restoration of function. Range of motion almost universally is reported as normal. Occasionally a loss of approximately 5° of terminal extension has been seen, which is thought to be of no functional significance.[14,47,72,73] Cybex evaluation provides an objective and accurate quantification of strength recovery but has been used by only two authors.[5,71]

An unusual combination of triceps injury and ulnar neuritis symptoms has been seen in two cases. In both instances, a delay in surgical intervention resulted in the formation of scar tissue encompassing the ulnar nerve.[2,32] Combined triceps repair and anterior transposition of the nerve has yielded satisfactory results.

Nonoperative treatment is appropriate for a partial injury. The extremity is splinted for 3 weeks as described previously, followed by progressive range-of-motion and strengthening exercises. With an adequate rehabilitation program, full restoration of strength and function can be anticipated after a partial tear.[4,15,25]

Recommended Surgical Technique

Early anatomic repair through bone holes in the proximal ulna is recommended for virtually all patients with acute complete avulsions.

The posterior approach to the arm and elbow can be employed with the patient in either a supine lateral or prone position. A tourniquet may be used for most of the procedure but must be deflated at the termination of the procedure to allow for a complete advancement of the triceps mechanism when the surgeon is tying the sutures. A posterior curvilinear incision is used passing lateral to the olecranon and parallel to the lateral border of the ulna (Fig. 22-12). The ulnar nerve should be identified and protected during the course of the dissection, but formal mobilization or transposition is not necessary. The small bone fleck often accompanying triceps avulsion is excised. If a large fragment has been avulsed, most probably in an adolescent patient, repair is amenable to tension-band technique or screw-and-washer fixation.

A nonabsorbable #5 suture is weaved through the freshened tendon in Bunnell fashion. Creating crisscrossed bone tunnels in the olecranon, as described by Morrey, is an excellent method to secure the sutures[53] (Fig. 22-13, *A* and *B*). Care should be taken not to tether the fascia encompassing the ulnar nerve to the repair. The suture is tied with the tourniquet deflated and the arm extended. Placing the knot on the lateral side will avoid sensitivity and ulnar irritation while the arm is resting on a hard surface (Fig. 22-13, *C*). After routine closure, the arm is splinted at 30° to 45° of elbow flexion, depending on the tension of the repair.

Postoperative Management

Postoperatively, the arm is immobilized in a posterior splint or cast at 30° to 45° of elbow flexion for 3 weeks. The duration of postoperative immobilization in the literature ranges from 10 days to 6 weeks, averaging about 3 weeks.[5] Gentle active range of motion is begun at 3 weeks after surgery, followed by progressive resisted exercises initiated at 6 weeks. Unrestricted activity can be resumed at 4 to 6 months after surgery, depending on the quality of the tissue repaired.

Complications

No significant complications, specifically rerupture or ulnar nerve injury, have been reported with operative repair of triceps avulsions. Wire sutures caused a bursa over the olecranon in one case and probably should be avoided.[59] The authors could not identify a single case of a failed repair in the literature.

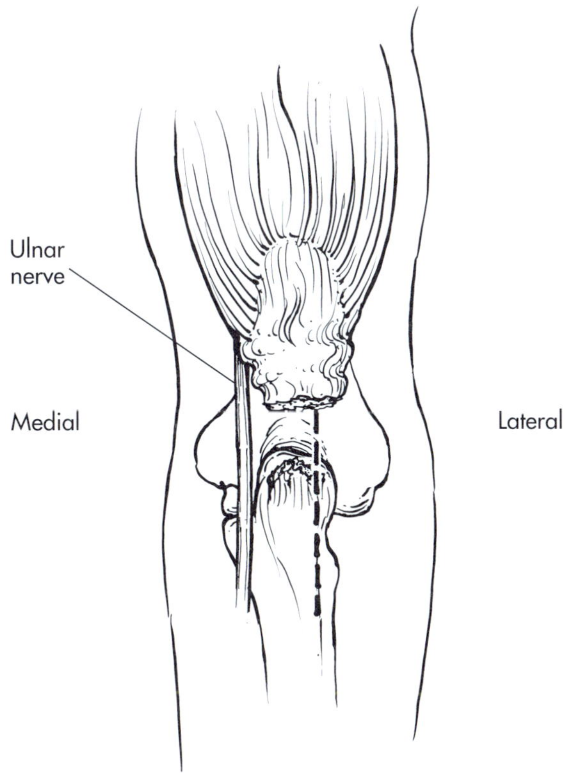

FIGURE 22-12 Posterior incision for triceps avulsion repair.

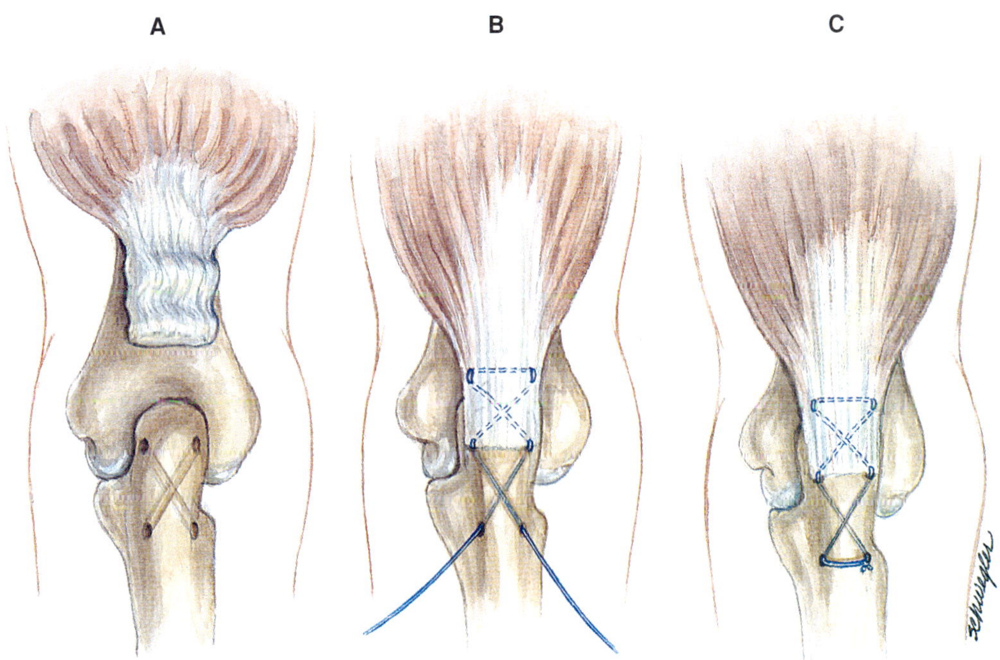

FIGURE 22-13 Surgical technique (Morrey) for repair of triceps tendon avulsion. See text for details. (Adapted from Morrey BF: Tendon injuries about the elbow. In Morrey BF, editor: *The elbow and its disorders,* ed 2, Philadelphia, 1993, WB Saunders.)

SUMMARY

Although distal biceps rupture and triceps avulsion are uncommon injuries, the physician treating an active athletic population or heavy laborers undoubtedly will encounter these injuries. In cases of complete disruption, prompt recognition and surgical repair are essential for obtaining optimal functional recovery, which should allow the laborer or athlete to return to full unrestricted activity.

Acknowledgment

The authors wish to thank Shirl Collier for her expert assistance and endless patience in the preparation of this manuscript.

References

1. Agins HJ et al: Rupture of the distal insertion of the biceps brachii tendon, *Clin Orthop* 234:34-38, 1988.
2. Anderson KJ, LeCocq JF: Rupture of the triceps tendon, *J Bone Joint Surg* 39A:444-446, 1957.
3. Anzel SH et al: Disruption of muscles and tendons: an analysis of 1,014 cases, *Surgery* 45:406, 1959.
4. Aso K, Torisu T: Muscle belly tear of the triceps, *Am J Sports Med* 12:485-487, 1984.
5. Bach BR, Warren RF, Wickiewica TL: Triceps rupture: a case report and literature review, *Am J Sports Med* 15:285-289, 1987.
6. Bak K, Haugegaard LM, Petersen OC: (Complete restoration of supination and flexion strength after surgical treatment of distal biceps tendon rupture by the Boyd-Andersson method), *Ugeskr Laeger* 154(10):629-631, 1992.
7. Baker BD, Bierwagen D: Rupture of the distal tendon of the biceps brachii: operative versus non-operative treatment, *J Bone Joint Surg* 67A(3):414-417, 1985.
8. Baker BE: Operative vs non-operative treatment of disruption of the distal tendon of biceps (abstract), *Orthop Rev* 11:71, 1982.
9. Bauman GI: Rupture of the biceps tendon, *J Bone Joint Surg* 16:966-967, 1934.
10. Bennett BS: Triceps tendon ruptures, *J Bone Joint Surg* 44A:741, 1962.
11. Boucher PR, Morton KS: Rupture of the distal biceps brachii tendon, *J Trauma* 7:626, 1967.
12. Bourne MH, Morrey BF: Partial rupture of the distal biceps tendon, *Clin Orthop* 271:143-148, 1991.
13. Boyd JB, Anderson LD: A method for reinsertion of the distal biceps brachii tendon, *J Bone Joint Surg* 43A(7):1041-1043, 1961.
14. Brodeur AE, Silberstein MJ, Graviss ER: *Radiology of the pediatric elbow*, Boston, 1981, GK Hall.
15. Carpentier E, Tourne Y, Vernay A: Les traumatismes fermes du tendon du triceps brachial, *J Chir* 129(2):99-102, 1992.
16. Carrol RE, Hamilton LR: Rupture of biceps brachii—a conservative method of treatment, *J Bone Joint Surg* 49A(4):1016, 1967.
17. Chevallier CH: Sur un cas de desinsertion du tendon bicipital inferieur, *Mem Acad Chir* 79:137, 1953.
18. Cirincione RJ, Baker BE: Tendon ruptures with secondary hyperparathyroidism: a case report, *J Bone Joint Surg* 57A:852, 1975.
19. Clayton ML, Thirupathi R: Rupture of the triceps tendon with olecranon bursitis, *Clin Orthop* 184:183-185, 1984.
20. Conwell HE, Alldredge RH: Ruptures and tears of muscles and tendons, *Am J Surg* 35(1):22, 1937.
21. Davis WM, Yassine Z: An etiological factor in tear of the distal tendon of the biceps brachii, *J Bone Joint Surg* 38A(6):1365-1368, 1956.
22. D'Alessandro DF et al: Repair of distal biceps tendon ruptures in athletes, *Am J Sports Med* 21(1):114-119, 1993.
23. Dobbie RP: Avulsion of the lower biceps brachii tendon: analysis of fifty-one previously unreported cases, *Am J Surg* 51:662-683, 1941.
24. Failla JM et al: Proximal radioulnar synostosis after repair of distal biceps brachii rupture by the two-incision technique: report of four cases, *Clin Orthop* 253:133-136, 1990.
25. Farrar EL, Lippert FG: Avulsion of the triceps tendon, *Clin Orthop* 161:242-246, 1981.
26. Fery A et al: Avulsion bilaterale simultanee des tendons quadricipital et rotulien et rupture du tendon tricipital chez un hemodialyse hyperparathyroidien, *Rev Chir Orthop* 64:175, 1978.
27. Fischer WR, Shepanek LA: Avulsion of the insertion of the biceps brachii, *J Bone Joint Surg* 38A(1):158-159, 1956.
28. Friedmann E: Rupture of the distal biceps brachii tendon: report on 13 cases, *JAMA* 184:60, 1963.
29. Gilcreest EL: Rupture of muscle and tendons, particularly subcutaneous rupture of the biceps flexor cubiti, *JAMA* 84(24):1819-1822, 1933.
30. Grantham SA, Kiernan HA: Displaced olecranon fractures in children, *J Trauma* 15:197-204, 1975.
31. Henry AK: *Extensile exposure,* ed 2, Baltimore, 1970, Williams & Wilkins.
32. Herrick RT, Herrick S: Ruptured triceps in a powerlifter presenting as cubital tunnel syndrome, *Am J Sports Med* 15:514-516, 1987.
33. Hovelius L, Josefsson G: Rupture of the distal biceps tendon: report of five cases, *Acta Orthop Scand* 48:280-282, 1977.
34. Hunter MB, Shybut GT, Nuber G: The effect of anabolic steroid hormones on the mechanical properties of tendons and ligaments, *Trans Orthop Res Soc* 11:240, 1986.
35. Johnson AB: Avulsion of biceps tendon from the radius [abstract], *NY Med J* 66:261-262, 1897.
36. Jorgensen U, Hinge K, Rye B: Rupture of the distal biceps brachii tendon, *J Trauma* 26(11):1061-1062, 1986.
37. Kennedy JC, Willis RB: The effects of local steroid injections on tendons: a biomechanical and microscopic correlative study, *Am J Sports Med* 4:11-21, 1976.
38. Kramhoft M, Solgaurd S: Spontaneous rupture of the extensor pollicis longus tendon after anabolic steroids, *J Hand Surg* 11B:87, 1986.
39. Kron SD, Satinsky VP: Avulsion of the distal biceps brachii tendon, *Am J Surg* 88:657, 1954.
40. Lee HG: Traumatic avulsion of tendon of insertion of biceps brachii, *Am J Surg* 82:290-292, 1951.
41. Lee MHL: Rupture of the triceps tendon, *Br Med J* 2:197, 1960.
42. Levy M, Fishel RE, Stern GM: Triceps tendon avulsion with or without fracture of the radial head: a rare injury? *J Trauma* 18:677-679, 1978.
43. Levy M, Goldberg I, Meir I: Fracture of the head of the radius with tear or avulsion of the triceps tendon, *J Bone Joint Surg* 64B:70-72, 1982.
44. Lotem M, Bernheim J, Conforty B: Spontaneous ruptures of tendons—a complication of hemodialyzed patients treated for renal failure, *Nephron* 21:201-208, 1978.
45. Louis DS et al: Distal biceps brachii tendon avulsion: a simplified method of operative repair, *Am J Sports Med* 14(3):234-236, 1986.
46. Mankin HJ: Rickets, osteomalacia, and renal osteodystrophy. Part I and II, *J Bone Joint Surg* 56A:101-128, 352-386, 1974.
47. Martin JR, Wilson CL, Mathews WH: Bilateral rupture of ligamenta patellae in case of disseminated lupus erythematosus, *Arthritis Rheum* 6:548-552, 1958.
48. McMaster PE: Tendon and muscle ruptures: clinical and experimental studies on causes and locations of subcutaneous ruptures, *J Bone Joint Surg* 15:705, 1933.
49. Meherin JM, Kilgore ES: The treatment of ruptures of the distal biceps brachii tendon, *Am J Surg* 99:636-640, 1960.
50. Miles JW et al: The effect of anabolic steroids on the biomechanical and histological properties of rat tendon, *J Bone Joint Surg* 74A:411-422, 1992.

51. Montgomery AH: Two cases of muscle injury, *Surg Clin Chic* 4: 871, 1920.
52. Morrey BF: Bursitis. In Morrey BF, editor: *The elbow and its disorders,* ed 2, Philadelphia, 1993, WB Saunders.
53. Morrey BF: Tendon injuries about the elbow. In Morrey BF, editor: *The elbow and its disorders,* ed 2, Philadelphia, 1993, WB Saunders.
54. Morrey BF et al. Rupture of distal tendon of the biceps brachii: a biomechanical study, *J Bone Joint Surg* 67A(3):418-421, 1985.
55. Murphy KJ, McPhee I: Tears of major tendons in chronic acidosis with elastosis, *J Bone Joint Surg* 47A:1253, 1965.
56. NCube BA, Singhal K: Rupture of the distal end of the biceps brachii tendon: an unusual occurrence in a horse rider, *Injury* 22(2):150-151, 1991.
57. Nielson K: Partial rupture of the distal biceps brachii tendon: a case report, *Acta Orthop Scand* 58:287-288, 1987.
58. Norman WH: Repair of avulsion of insertion of biceps brachii tendon, *Clin Orthop* 193:189-194, 1985.
59. Pantazopoulos T et al: Avulsion of the triceps tendon, *J Trauma* 15:827, 1975.
60. Penhallow DP: Report of a case of ruptured triceps due to direct violence, *NY Med J* 91:76, 1910.
61. Platt H: Observations of some tendon ruptures, *Br Med J* 1:611-615, 1931.
62. Poland J: *A practical treatise on traumatic separation of the epiphyses,* London, 1898, Smith, Elder & Company.
63. Postacchini F, Puddu G: Subcutaneous rupture of the distal biceps brachii tendon: a report on seven cases, *J Sports Med* 15(2):81-90, 1975.
64. Preston FT: Avulsion of both quadriceps tendons in hyperparathyroidism, *JAMA* 221:406-407, 1972.
65. Preston FS, Adicoff A: Hyperparathyroidism with avulsion at three major tendons, *N Engl J Med* 266:968, 1961.
66. Ritchie AJ, Rocke LG: Spontaneous rupture of the triceps in the presence of a patella cubiti, *Arch Emerg Med* 7:114-117, 1990.
67. Rockwood CA, Wilkins KE, King RE: *Fractures involving the proximal physis of the olecranon: fractures in children,* Philadelphia, 1991, JB Lippincott.
68. Rogers SP: Avulsion of tendon of attachment of biceps brachii: a case report, *J Bone Joint Surg* 21:197, 1939.
69. Schutt RC, Powell RL, Winter WG: *Spontaneous ruptures of large tendons,* American Academy of Orthopedic Surgeons Annual Meeting, New Orleans, January 25, 1982.
70. Searfoss R, Tripi J, Bowers W: Triceps brachii rupture: a case report, *J Trauma* 16:244-246, 1976.
71. Sherman OH, Snyder SJ, Fox JM: Triceps tendon avulsion in a professional body builder, *Am J Sports Med* 12:328-329, 1984.
72. Silberstein MJ et al: Some vagarities of the olecranon, *J Bone Joint Surg* 63:722-725, 1981.
73. Sleeboom C, Regoort M: Rupture of the distal tendon of the biceps brachii muscle, *Neth J Surg* 43(5):195-197, 1991.
74. Sonnenschein HD: Rupture of the biceps tendon, *J Bone Joint Surg* 14:416, 1932.
75. Stannard JP, Bucknell AL: Rupture of the triceps tendon associated with steroid injections, *Am J Sports Med* 21:482-485, 1993.
76. Tarsney FF: Rupture and avulsion of the triceps, *Clin Orthop* 83:177-183, 1972.
77. Thompson TC: A test for rupture of the tendo achilles, *Acta Orthop Scand* 32:461-465, 1962.
78. Tibone JE: Repair of distal biceps tendon rupture. In Shields CL, editor: *Manual of sports surgery,* New York, 1987, Springer-Verlag.
79. Twinning RH, Marcus WY, Garey JL: Tendon ruptures in systemic lupus erythematosus, *JAMA* 187:120-124, 1964.
80. Unverferth JL, Olix ML: The effects of local steroid injections on tendon, *J Sports Med* 1:31-37, 1973.
81. Viegas S: Avulsion of the triceps tendon, *Orthop Rev* 19(6):533-536, 1990.
82. Ware HE, Nairn DS: Repair of the ruptured distal tendon of the biceps brachii, *J Hand Surg* 17B(1):99-101, 1992.
83. Waugh RL, Hathcock TA, Elliott JL: Ruptures of muscle and tendons, *Surgery* 25:370, 1949.
84. Wener JA, Shein AJ: Simultaneous bilateral rupture of the patello tendon and quadriceps expansions in systemic lupus erythematosus: a case report, *J Bone Joint Surg* 56A:823, 1974.

CHAPTER 23

Nerve Entrapment Syndromes at the Elbow

JAMES R. BOATRIGHT
DONALD F. D'ALESSANDRO

The more common athletic injuries of the elbow, such as lateral or medial epicondylitis, medial collateral ligament laxity, and bony impingement of the olecranon, usually are encountered before the less common nerve entrapment syndromes. Compressive neuropathies of the ulnar, median, radial, and musculocutaneous nerves all occur in the athletic population. These lesions often present with vague pain, intermittent sensory symptoms, and occasionally weakness. Neurocompressive lesions can be a diagnostic dilemma for the physician evaluating elbow problems in the athlete because sparse objective findings can be difficult to demonstrate in the office setting; these lesions often require a specific athletic activity to provoke symptoms.

The anatomy of the elbow has several unique aspects that make the nerves particularly susceptible to either direct trauma or repeated traction and compression, ultimately resulting in recognized entrapment syndromes. The combination of generous joint mobility, longitudinal stresses, and unyielding fascial restraints makes nerve compressions about the elbow more likely. The lack of bulky muscle and adipose tissue about the elbow makes the nerves vulnerable to direct trauma. The nerves must pass into and around the numerous muscles that originate or insert at the elbow. The ulnar nerve enters the flexor carpi ulnaris, the median nerve enters between the ulnar and humeral heads of the pronator teres, and the dorsal interosseous nerve pierces the supinator. These points are notorious for their propensity to create nerve entrapments. The aforementioned sites of compression all are possibilities in individuals with normal anatomy. Individuals with anatomic anomalies have the threat of additional nerve insults. Anomalies such as vascular aberrations, abnormal fascial bands, a supracondylar process of the humerus, and the presence of an anconeus epitrochlearis muscle are well-documented causes of nerve impingement.

The athletic population is uniquely at risk for nerve entrapment lesions because the elbow is subjected to intense repetitive muscle actions and large joint forces during sports activities. For example, biomechanical studies of the throwing motion have shown that the elbow extends rapidly from 90° of flexion in the cocking phase to terminal extension on follow-through. Simultaneously, the medial elbow structures are placed under considerable valgus stress. The ulnar nerve therefore is under tension not only when the elbow is flexed, but also as a result of the valgus strain associated with the acceleration phase of throwing. Repetitive pronation and supination combined with firm gripping of a ball or racquet can cause median, radial, or musculocutaneous nerve irritation as the proximal forearm muscles with their associated fascial bands are repeatedly tightened across these nerves. Thus knowledge of the biomechanical aspects of specific athletic activities can help explain the etiology of nerve injury. Sicuranza and McCue provide an excellent discussion of various sports and the compressive neuropathies they produce in the upper extremity.[131]

The majority of nerve entrapment lesions in athletes could be categorized as neurapraxias,[14] defined as a conduction block in which all the nerve elements remain in continuity. Prognosis for complete nerve recovery is excellent provided that appropriate treatment is rendered before irreversible end-organ damage has occurred. Direct trauma to a nerve may result in a more severe injury termed *axonotmesis* in which axon degeneration occurs but the supporting connective tissue sleeve remains intact.[127] Although the prognosis is good, the time to recovery depends on the distance from the nerve lesion to the site of innervation. Complete nerve disruption, classified as neurotmesis, usually is associated with high-energy fractures, dislocations, or deep lacerations and fortunately occurs rarely in the athlete.[14,62]

The challenge to the physician is to elucidate the cause of symptoms and treat them appropriately, avoiding the morbidity of delayed diagnosis. The purpose of this chapter is to review the anatomy of the major nerves and their associated structures about the elbow, describe the clinical presentation of the common entrapment syndromes, and discuss the treatment alternatives.

THE ULNAR NERVE

The ulnar nerve is the major nerve about the elbow most susceptible to injury during sports activities. Compression, traction, and repeated irritation are the factors responsible for nerve injury, and all three are demonstrable in neurop-athies about the elbow. The superficial course of the ulnar nerve about the posterior-medial and convex aspect of the elbow contributes to its frequent direct trauma. The wide range of motion of the elbow and the valgus stresses applied here create traction stresses on the nerve, further traumatizing it. In throwing activities, the repetitive valgus stresses can lead to increased laxity of the medial collateral ligament. Not only does this add more traction to the nerve, but concomitant stretching of the arcuate ligament also can allow recurrent subluxation of the ulnar nerve anteriorly onto or over the medial epicondyle,[14] producing fibrosis about the nerve.

Racquet sports may produce effects on the elbow similar to throwing.[68] Nordic skiing has been implicated in ulnar neuropathy because of repetitive forceful pronation and extension elbow movements.[50] Medial epicondylitis is said to have an associated ulnar compressive neuropathy in 60% of cases.[105] Underlying conditions may precipitate compressive neuropathies of the ulnar nerve in the athlete, as illustrated by reports of ganglia,[44] lipoma,[42] osteochondromas,[42] osteophytes,[25] and inflamed olecranon bursae causing this problem. Old constrictive scar, as from a previous burn,[126] and secondary factors such as heterotopic bone formation[143] may contribute to a compressive effect on the nerve. Rheumatoid proliferative synovial reactions have produced not only nerve compression but also nerve ruptures.[102] Factors that increase the carrying angle of the elbow, either congenital or posttraumatic, can precipitate a tardy ulnar nerve palsy.[103,109]

In the contemporary literature, however, 30% of ulnar nerve entrapments at the elbow are occupation-related.[13] The recreational athlete's occupational demands should be strongly considered as the potential underlying cause of the compressive neuropathy.

Pathoanatomy

The ulnar nerve passes from the anterior to the posterior compartment at the midpoint of the arm by traversing the medial intermuscular septum (Fig. 23-1). It then continues distally, lying on the anterior border of the medial head of the triceps. The arcade of Struthers, which is present in 70%[133] of the population, is located about 8 cm above the medial epicondyle. These wispy fascial fibers course anterior and medial to the ulnar nerve from the medial head of the triceps to the medial intermuscular septum. Compression of the ulnar nerve occurs as it is taken anteriorly in transpositions. Enlargement of a more distal insertion of the medial head of the triceps can force the ulnar nerve upward against the intermuscular septum, causing nerve compression.[118] As the ulnar

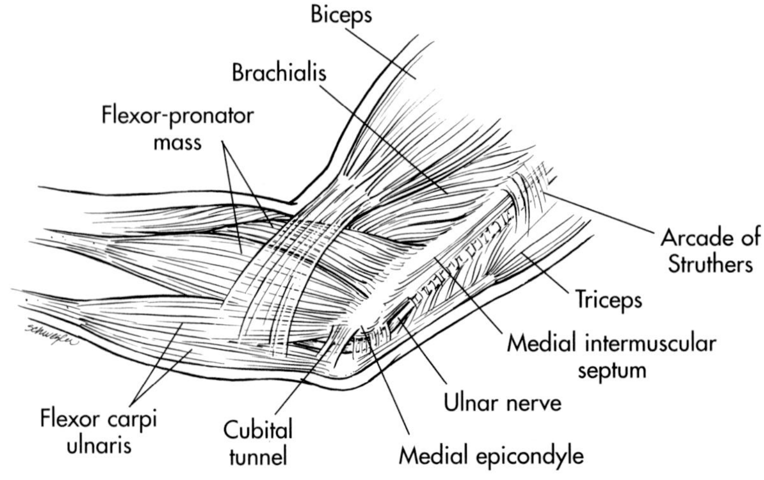

FIGURE 23-1 Anatomy pertinent to the course of the ulnar nerve around the elbow.

nerve enters the cubital tunnel, it is bounded posteriorly by the medial head of the triceps, posteromedially by the overlying arcuate ligament, anteriorly by the medial epicondyle, and laterally by the trochlea and olecranon. The passage for the nerve narrows by 54% and changes in configuration from oval to triangular as the elbow goes from full extension to full flexion.[5] As the elbow flexes, the arcuate ligament stretches approximately 5 mm for each 45° of flexion.[142] That tension on the arcuate ligament and the bulge of the medial collateral ligament with flexion[25] create increased tunnel pressure.[142] Combining wide shoulder abduction with elbow flexion and wrist extension can increase the tunnel pressure to as much as six times the pressures found in the anatomic position.[93,113] The "Osborne lesion" is a thickening of the arcuate ligament whose presence is highly correlated with compression of the ulnar nerve.[110] Certainly any congenital, acquired, or developmental anomalies can significantly increase the physiologic compressive or traction forces. Although the nerve is known to elongate by 4 to 7 mm with full elbow flexion,[5] tethering by scar in or about the nerve can double these intraneural pressures.[113] Old supracondylar fractures that have healed with exuberant callus, calcifications of the medial collateral ligament,[68] secondary genu valgus, and anomalies such as an anconeus epitrochlearis[62] can add further stress to or compression of the nerve.

The ulnar nerve then enters the forearm by passing between and underneath the humeral and ulnar heads of the flexor carpi ulnaris, ultimately resting on the surface of the flexor digitorum profundus muscle. The deep aponeurosis connecting the ulnar and humeral heads of the flexor carpi ulnaris also has been shown to be a source of ulnar nerve entrapment.[4] Rupture of the biceps tendon at the elbow has been said to contribute to ulnar nerve compression. The direct trauma causing the biceps rupture, the subsequent hematoma formation, and the flexed position of the elbow as it is immobilized for 6 to 12 weeks in protecting the biceps tendon repair are said actually to produce the neuropathy.[31]

The orientation of the nerve fascicles can partially explain the finding that sensory and hand intrinsic motor changes occur early and that motor changes in the flexor digitorum profundus (FDP) and flexor carpi ulnaris (FCU) occur very late. The nerve's sensory fascicles are located peripherally and anteromedially in the cubital tunnel, whereas the bundles of the proximal motors lie centrally and dorsally.[142,145] Sensory fibers within the ulnar nerve are more susceptible to compression[53]; therefore sensory symptoms usually are the first noted by the patient. This is also consonant with the finding that large fascicles in general,[92] and myelinated fascicles specifically, are more prone to damage from compressive forces.[24]

Awareness that anomalous innervation in the upper extremity is not uncommon will help prevent misdiagnoses. The Martin-Gruber anastomosis in 15% of the population[73] (median to ulnar nerve crossovers in the forearm), Riche-Cannieu anastomoses (ulnar to median motor fibers in the palm), and the anomalous radial nerve's innervation of the dorsum of the hand can present perplexing clinical pictures.[83] Differential nerve blocks can clarify these innervation variants.

Pathomechanics of the Throwing Athlete

The medial aspect of the dominant elbow in the overhead athlete, particularly in throwers, is subjected to repetitive large tensile forces. As a result of these forces, a number of associated pathologic conditions may occur. These factors may be a cause of the ulnar neuropathy or may simply coexist but must be addressed regardless. The throwing motion accentuates the normal anatomic and biomechanical factors that tend to create both compressive and traction forces on the ulnar nerve. Although

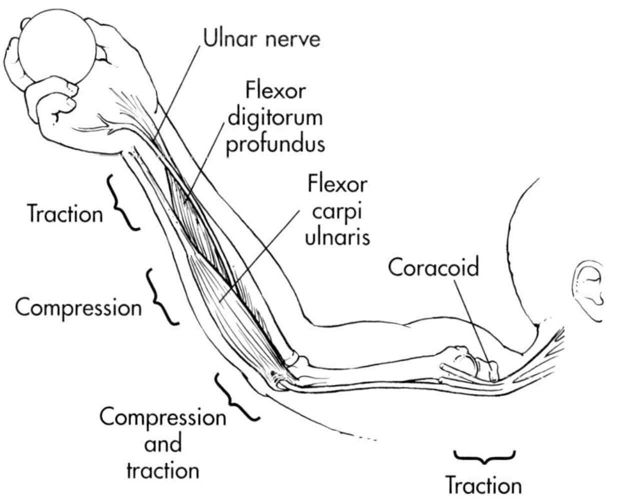

FIGURE 23-2 Effects on the ulnar nerve in the throwing arm. Traction and compression forces are produced on the nerve in the acceleration phase of throwing. The throwing arm in the acceleration phase produces valgus stress at the elbow.

the ulnar nerve normally can stretch and elongate 7 mm during flexion,[5] any tethering of the nerve from scar formation, traction spurs, calcific deposits about the medial collateral ligament, or degenerative changes in the ulnar groove can lead to traction neuropathy.[33,68,149] Continued throwing will produce further inflammation, adhesions, and fibrosis, leading to a progressive compressive neuropathy.

During the acceleration phase of the throwing motion, the elbow is flexed and the ulnar collateral ligament provides the restraint to valgus stress (Fig. 23-2). Chronic overuse, seen especially in the high-level thrower, can result in attenuation and partial rupture of this ligament.[20,70] Ensuing valgus laxity clearly increases tension on the ulnar nerve as the medial joint space widens. This laxity also precipitates olecranon impingement on the posterior medial humerus. Secondary degenerative changes, including spur formation and loose bodies, also may irritate the nerve.

The dominant arms of professional baseball players and top-level tennis players undergo adaptive changes over time in response to chronic repetitive use. These changes include bony hypertrophy of the humerus, olecranon, and olecranon fossa, frequently resulting in fixed flexion contractures of the elbow.[78] Muscle hypertrophy of the medial head of the triceps and flexor carpi ulnaris, often a result of weight-lifting, has been reported to cause ulnar nerve compression at this level.[25,54,93]

Finally, a friction neuritis may result from recurrent dislocation of the nerve from the ulnar groove. Childers reported that 16% of the population experiences recurrent dislocation of the ulnar nerve during elbow flexion. Hypermobility of the nerve usually is secondary to congenital or developmental laxity of the soft-tissue constraints that normally maintain the nerve within the groove. Those nerves that only sublux from the ulnar groove are particularly susceptible to direct trauma, but those that can completely dislocate anterior to the epicondyle are prone to develop friction neuritis as a result of repetitive flexion and extension.

Knowledge of ulnar nerve and cubital tunnel anatomy, the elbow biomechanics involved with the throwing motion, and the pathologic sequelae associated with chronic overuse is necessary for the physician to understand the propensity of the overhead athlete to develop ulnar nerve lesions.

Clinical Evaluation

Early symptoms may be wholly or partly paresthesias in the ring and little fingers. Aching in the medial elbow with radiation proximally or distally also may occur[39] and may extend into the ulnar side of the hand as the lesion progresses. The onset may be acute and may be the result of an injury. More frequently, however, the initial symptoms have an insidious beginning and are intermittent. Therefore a high index of suspicion for a compressive neuropathy is key to making an early diagnosis in the athlete because symptoms may be precipitated only by vigorous use. At first, only strenuous use, such as throwing, may be associated with the occurrence of symptoms, but later the symptoms may be constant regardless of activity. The athlete may voice complaints of heaviness and clumsiness in the hand and fingers during throwing.[149] Frank weakness usually is not experienced by athletes and rarely can be demonstrated on physical exam. Cramping with spasms in the ring and little fingers may occur. The majority of patients are recreational athletes, however, and the physician should seek historical clues to causative and aggravating maneuvers, vocational and recreational activities, and history of injury or medical illnesses that may predispose an individual to an ulnar compressive neuropathy. Details of the progression of symptoms, functional impairment, and treatment to date are useful in both the diagnosis and choice of treatment.

With progression of the problems, the symptoms may become more constant, and more classic ulnar nerve symptoms may ensue. A recurring subluxation of the nerve may produce sudden sharp pain at the elbow with radiating pain and numbness into the ring and little fingers.

The physical examination should start at the neck and proceed distally, taking care to exclude pathologic entities in the differential diagnosis. The physician should carefully palpate along the course of the nerve, looking for the presence of a supracondylar process, a mass lesion, hypertrophy of the medial triceps, cubitus valgus, and cutaneous evidence of recent or past trauma. A specific location of ulnar nerve tenderness might give an important clue about the underlying etiology of the nerve lesion. A Tinel's sign is significant only if strongly positive. Gentle manipulation of the ulnar nerve behind the medial epicondyle with the elbow flexed to 90° may demonstrate subluxation of the nerve and reproduce symptoms.[118,125] The elbow flexion test, performed by having the patient completely flex the elbows while fully extending the wrists for 3 minutes, is positive when ulnar nerve symptoms are evoked.[12,144] Fine reported a high correlation between a positive elbow flexion test and positive electromyographic findings.[46] However, this test must be interpreted in the context of other clinical findings since 50% of normal people were found to have similar symptoms with this maneuver.[117]

Sensory changes in the cutaneous distribution of the ulnar nerve should be sought. The earliest changes are evident with the threshold tests[28,30,32] of vibrometry or monofilament evaluations. Nerve-ending density tests such as two-point discrimination and moving two-point discrimination are positive later in the progressive course of compression. The expectation of dorsal sensory changes over the little and ring fingers as a result of ulnar nerve impairment above the wrist level can be foiled by anomalous innervation, but such is not common. The finding of diminished sensation on the dorsum of the ulnar side of the hand as well as on the palmar aspect implicates nerve compression above the distal third of the forearm.

Motor changes are seen earliest in the ulnarly innervated hand intrinsics, as may be determined by the finger-crossing test. Loss of pinch strength and accompanying Froment and Jean signs signal adductor pollicis weakness. Loss of adduction ability by the little finger (Wartenburg sign) and abductor digiti quinti weakness likewise may be apparent on testing. More significant compression, however, also may produce flexor digitorum profundus asthenia in the little and ring fingers and possibly flexor carpi ulnaris weakness. Frank atrophy is a late finding with poor prognostic connotations. Clawing may be evident if intrinsic weakness precedes FDP involvement.

In the overhead athlete, the physician must be careful to distinguish ulnar nerve compression from the often-associated pathologies involving the flexor-pronator muscle mass and ulnar collateral ligament. Pain elicited along the medial epicondyle with resisted wrist and finger flexion or forearm pronation may suggest the diagnosis of flexor pronator tendinitis, usually labeled medial epicondylitis. The ulnar collateral ligament of the elbow must be carefully evaluated. Tenderness to palpation along the ligament exacerbated with valgus stressing of the elbow signifies ulnar collateral ligament inflammation and possible attenuation.[70] Subtle instability may be appreciated by comparing the involved and uninvolved elbows. Ulnar nerve irritation may be only a secondary manifestation of medial collateral ligament laxity, and addressing both problems is imperative for successful treatment.[20,70]

The differential diagnosis must consider lesions of the ulnar nerve more proximal and distal to the elbow region. Cervical root compression, particularly C8, by cervical osteophytes or a herniated nucleus pulposus must be considered. Absence of the triceps jerk and symptoms with neck movement are common findings. Less commonly, a Pancoast tumor may produce symptoms similar to those of ulnar nerve compression. Thoracic outlet syndrome, in which the medial components of the brachial plexus usually are compressed, can produce vague symptoms in the ulnar nerve distribution. Rarely are objective neurologic deficits present, however. Symptoms may be recreated by shoulder abduction with external rotation (Roos' sign) or by applying pressure over the anterior scalene muscles. Distal compression of the ulnar nerve in Guyon's canal at the wrist must be specifically excluded. The double-crush phenomenon,[140] in which a proximal nerve compression coexists with a more distal compression along the same axon, also can be a diagnostic dilemma. An example of such would be a patient who has elements of a C8 nerve root compression and an ulnar compressive neuropathy at the elbow. Myocardial in-

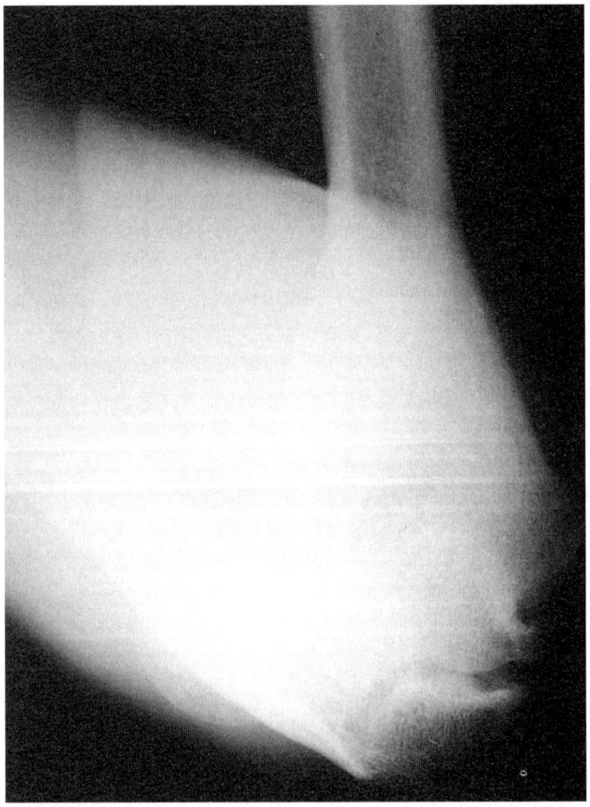

FIGURE 23-3 Cubital tunnel view showing groove impingement by osteophyte.

farction and diaphragmatic irritation lesions also must be considered in the differential diagnosis. Other medical causes of nerve dysfunction are vitamin B_{12} deficiency, folic acid deficiency, porphyria, diabetes mellitus, uremia, alcoholism, and prescription medications.[139] Diffuse intrinsic wasting with nerve sensory deficit could be caused by motor neuron disease.

Radiographic testing has limited value in the workup of compressive ulnar neuropathy. Exclusionary benefits are realized by evaluating the cervical spine and ruling out space-occupying lesions about the elbow, such as fracture callus, arthritic spurs, heterotopic bone, and a supracondylar process. A cubital tunnel view of the elbow particularly can demonstrate bony lesions within the cubital tunnel[144] (Fig. 23-3). Cystic lesions lend themselves to diagnosis by ultrasonography. Magnetic resonance imaging is helpful in evaluating soft-tissue mass lesions or the status of the medial collateral ligament.[7] Computed tomographic scans have limited use but can help in assessing degenerative changes or bony abnormalities.

Electrodiagnostic Testing

As mentioned previously, athletes tend to visit the physician early. Even mild compressive neuropathies that do not affect their activities of daily living can significantly compromise their sports performance. Electrodiagnostic studies, although confirmatory if positive, may be negative in mild ulnar nerve entrapment or ulnar neuritis.

A variety of nerve conduction parameters have been offered in the literature as diagnostic of nerve impairment. A decrease in motor nerve conduction velocity from above the elbow to the abductor digiti quinti of greater than 9 m per second is thought to be significant for early cubital tunnel syndrome.[37] Others consider conduction velocities of less than 41 m per second as significantly positive across the elbow.[67] Yet others report that a 10 m per second drop of conduction velocity across the elbow versus below the elbow is significant.[37] Comparison of right and left also is of some use in evaluating nerve function. Short segment stimulation techniques have proved to be useful in localizing a confined area of abnormal conduction.[74] Diffuse nerve conduction abnormalities should signal the possibility of a diffuse noncompressive neuropathy. A low-amplitude wave form seen on sensory conduction studies also suggests neuropathy.

Needle electromyography may indicate abnormalities of individual muscle innervation. The finding of fibrillation potentials and sharp positive waves in specific muscles, combined with the knowledge of the nerve or root that innervates those muscles, can help localize the site of the nerve lesion. Electromyography is particularly useful in differentiating cervical, elbow, and more distal nerve involvement.

Overall, the incidence of false negatives in electrodiagnostic testing is 10%.[96] The use of testing under conditions of stress is said to increase the detection of more subtle lesions.[96] This stress can be merely doing conduction studies with the arm and the elbow flexed, the wrist extended, and the shoulder abducted in position. The extreme stress may be testing after a standardized program of activities designed to provoke compression in a given area. Many clinicians think that normal electrodiagnostic studies alone should not preclude surgical treatment, nor should they be required of all patients if the remainder of the clinical assessment indicates ulnar nerve compression at the elbow.[30,54,149]

Thermography

Many have sought a diagnostic test that could verify specific pathology noninvasively, either qualitatively or with precision. Thermography has been investigated toward this end.[61,130,132] There is not yet conclusive evidence that thermography has a role in the diagnosis of ulnar compressive neuropathy.

Treatment

Conservative Treatment

The treatment of ulnar compressive neuropathy at the elbow depends on the degree of impairment in the nerve,[45] both motor and sensory. In an effort to standardize the expression of involvement, McGowen[98] published a classification system for this problem. He designated a grade I lesion as a "minimal lesion" with no motor weakness. A grade II was an "intermediate lesion," and a grade III or "severe lesion" involved paralysis of one or more ulnar intrinsics. No consideration was given to sensory impairment.

Dellon's grading system[30] is more specific in considering motor and sensory loss, defining each of his categories of mild, moderate, and severe. Although most athletes will present with chronic ulnar neuritis of a severity of McGowen grade I and should be treated with conservative measures initially, they usually require surgical intervention ultimately.[33,68,69,149] An exception may be when symptoms occur after an acute traumatic event in which conservative measures and the use of a padded elbow sleeve should be successful.[112] Conservative measures consist of rest, antiinflammatory medications, avoidance of throwing, and occasionally splint immobilization. Ice must be used cautiously because the subcutaneous location of the ulnar nerve makes it vulnerable to cold injury. When possible, biomechanical analysis of the patient's athletic activity may reveal factors that aggravate the condition. Local injection into the medial aspect of the elbow is not recommended.[33,149] In the general population, two series report success rates of 86% and 90% after conservative treatment emphasizing long arm splinting.[34,38] Unfortunately in most athletes, resumption of athletic activity prompts the return of symptoms, and surgical treatment is indicated. Before decompressing the ulnar nerve, the physician must rule out concomitant ulnar collateral ligament laxity and posteromedial olec-ranon impingement,[20,70] because medial elbow pain will recur if these problems are not addressed.

For patients whose classification falls into the McGowen grade II or III, or the Dellon category "moderate" or "severe," surgical intervention is the recommendation. Certainly, failure of conservative measures with grade I "mild" lesions also is an indication to proceed with surgery.

Surgical Treatment

When conservative management is unsuccessful or if the severity of the ulnar nerve lesion is deemed of a degree that warrants operative intervention, five choices are available. For most other nerves, treatment of the compressive disorder by surgical means is relatively straightforward with limited options. The following describes why we believe an anterior submuscular transposition is the best for treating the athlete with ulnar nerve problems.

The advantages of in situ decompression are its simplicity, low risk of impairing the blood supply of the nerve,[108] and lack of resulting scar.[13,143] Reports on this procedure show successful results in patients with a minimal compressive lesion characterized by mild pain and dysesthesias.[27,43,95,101] Simple decompression has proven not to be helpful with more advanced lesions[30] and should be avoided in cases of nerve subluxation, epicondylar tenderness, or osseous abnormality.[45] This procedure is not recommended in the overhead athlete because it does not eliminate the traction forces on the nerve associated with the throwing motion and does not address pathology within the cubital tunnel.

Removal of the medial epicondyle has many proponents in the literature,* but several aspects about the procedure make it undesirable for the athlete. The origin of the flexor pronator mass is altered in its repaired tension and could affect subsequent strength. The ulnar nerve is destabilized, allowing it to ride anteriorly and making it susceptible to direct trauma[95] and friction neuritis. Heterotopic bone formation also has been seen after medial epicondylectomy. Overall, the recurrence rate after medial epicondylectomy is the highest of all reported techniques.[30]

In the general population, subcutaneous anterior transposition is commonly employed.† The advantages of subcutaneous transposition include a relatively simple dissection; lack of risk of scar of the nerve within the muscle, of adjacent bone, or of a medial collateral ligament repair; and lack of requirement of immobilization. However, the detriments outweigh the benefits of this procedure. A less direct route of transposition increases the likelihood of kinking at entry and exit points.[11] Hypermobility of the nerve can result if it is not contained adequately by a fascial sling, and there is minimal protection from direct trauma in the subcutaneous position. In reality, the nerve can be sensitive along its subcutaneous course in thin individuals. There is only one report of anterior subcutaneous transposition being used successfully in baseball pitchers.[36]

Intramuscular anterior transposition has few proponents[17,18,52,79] because of its reputation for poor results secondary to neural scarring within the flexor-pronator mass.[85,141]

Anterior submuscular transposition is the best alternative in athletes for several reasons. The nerve's deep submuscular placement not only protects it from external trauma but also creates a nearly straight-line course from arm to forearm, avoiding the tension forces relevant to throwing. The extensile approach, removing the flexor-pronator muscles, allows for examination of the medial collateral ligament and its reconstruction if necessary. Overuse degenerative changes common in the overhead athlete, such as loose bodies or osteophytes in the posterior compartment of the elbow, also can be readily addressed during the procedure.[33] Many clinical series suggest that submuscular transposition gives the best results with the least recurrence.*

Authors' Preferred Operative Technique

The authors' preferred surgical technique in athletes is Learmonth's submuscular transposition of the ulnar nerve,[84] which also has been described in several articles

*References 21, 24, 45, 49, 60, 83, 93, 117, 143, 144, 147.

†References 1, 35, 47, 82, 91, 98, 104, 122.

*References 1, 30, 33, 66, 68, 69, 75, 85.

BOX 23-1

KEY STEPS IN ANTERIOR SUBMUSCULAR TRANSPOSITION OF THE ULNAR NERVE

1. Make posteromedial skin incision.
2. Ensure that the nerve is free to at least 8 cm above the medial epicondyle.
3. Excise a distal segment of the medial intermuscular septum.
4. Divide the arcuate ligament.
5. Divide the FDS-pronator aponeurotic band.
6. Elevate the entire flexor-pronator muscle origin off the medial epicondyle.
7. Inspect the medial collateral ligament of the elbow.
8. Place the ulnar nerve anteriorly adjacent to the median nerve in a fatty plane.
9. Ensure release of the ulnar head of the FCU.
10. Repair the flexor-pronator muscle origin without constricting the ulnar nerve.
11. Begin motion of the elbow within 2 weeks.

from the Kerlan-Jobe Orthopaedic Clinic.[54,149] Attention to details of the operative technique can prevent the creation of new entrapment sites along the nerve's transposed course[141] (Box 23-1). The medial curvilinear incision is centered just posterior to the medial epicondyle. Meticulous identification and mobilization of the branches of the medial antebrachial cutaneous nerve can minimize the risk of a painful postoperative neuroma in this area. The ulnar nerve can be identified first in the distal arm behind the medial intermuscular septum and freed proximally for 8 cm, taking care to release the arcade of Struthers (Fig. 23-5). The cubital tunnel is then released as the arcuate ligament is divided and the nerve is isolated with a Penrose drain. Continued mobilization is accomplished by sacrificing the articular branches, enlarging the interval between the flexor carpi ulnaris heads, and releasing the aponeurotic band of the flexor

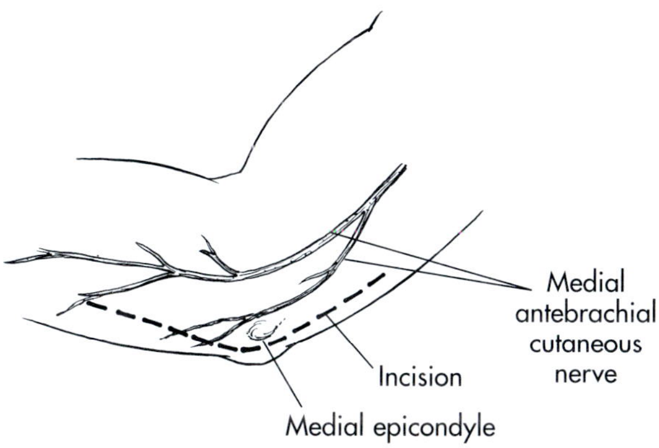

FIGURE 23-4 Posterior medial approach to the ulnar nerve. Note the course of the medial antebrachiocutaneous nerve and its branches, which are at risk.

digitorum sublimis origin. Care is taken to preserve the motor branches to these muscles. A nerve stimulator is helpful in this regard. If necessary, the first motor branch fascicle can be dissected proximally into the ulnar nerve to achieve mobilization anteriorly. A generous segment of the medial intermuscular septum, especially its distal insertion on the medial epicondyle, must be excised to prevent a transposed nerve from being kinked over its edge. The small collateral vessels posterior to the septum should be spared if possible.

The flexor-pronator muscle group is detached from the medial epicondyle, leaving 1 to 2 cm of the proximal tendon for reattachment. As the flexor-pronator muscle mass is reflected distally, the median nerve branches to the pronator and flexor digitorum sublimis are vulnerable to injury. The underlying ulnar collateral ligament of the elbow now can be examined. If its integrity is in question, an arthrotomy can be made via a longitudinal incision along the course of its fibers. A widened medial joint space resulting from attenuation of the ligament or granulation tissue within its substance suggests disruption and attempted healing of ligament fibers.[20,70] A posterior medial arthrotomy can be made to remove any osteophytes or loose bodies, often concomitant pathology in the athletic elbow.

The nerve is now transposed anteriorly, carefully inspecting for new entrapment sites proximally or distally. The transposed ulnar nerve now should lie adjacent to the median nerve in a fatty plane. The muscles are reattached with nonabsorbable suture to the proximal soft-tissue cuff or to drill holes made in the epicondyle, carefully placing them under direct vision to avoid injury to the nerve (Fig. 23-6). The elbow is then taken through a range of motion, testing the flexor-pronator muscle repair and confirming that there are no sites of ulnar nerve entrapment or tethering. The nerve should glide freely

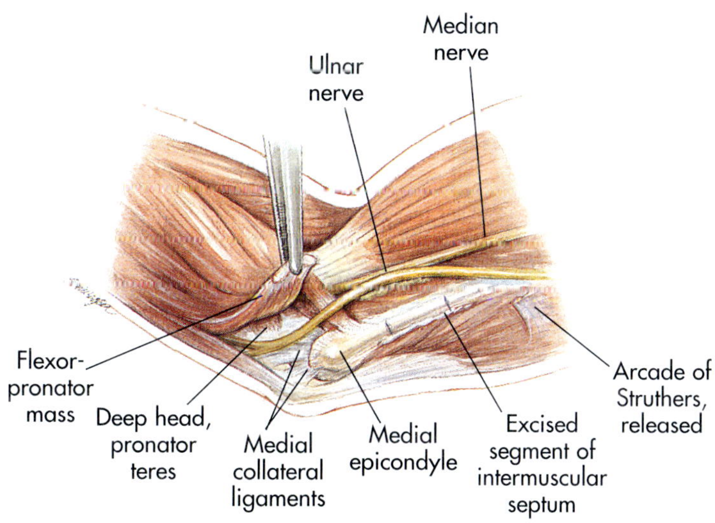

FIGURE 23-5 Anterior submuscular transposition of the ulnar nerve. (see Box 23-1).

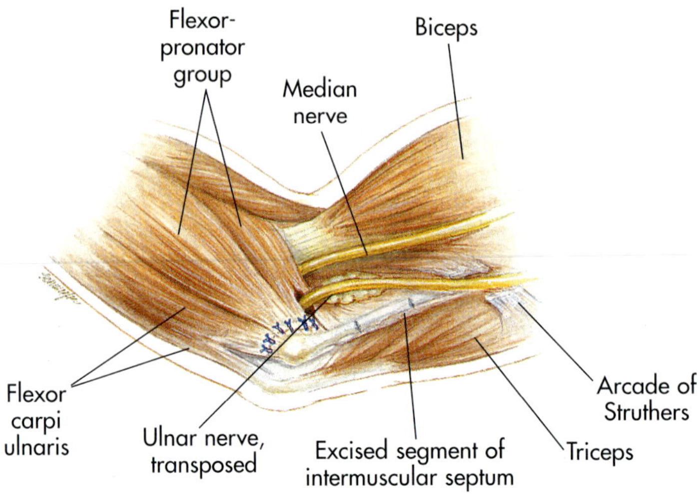

FIGURE 23-6 Completed anterior transposition of the ulnar nerve.

beneath the flexor muscle mass. The tourniquet is released, and hemostasis is obtained before skin closure. A well-padded posterior splint is applied with the elbow at 90° flexion for 10 days.

The postoperative rehabilitation protocol[149] begins 2 weeks after the operation with passive range-of-motion exercises. Active exercises are instituted at 3 to 4 weeks, followed by a strengthening program at 6 weeks after surgery. Two months after surgery, a well-supervised throwing program is started, beginning with ball tossing. Progressive increases in throwing duration and speed culminate in full activities at 4 months. This program has been applied to top-level athletes, and the flexor-pronator mass has not detached.[33,68] The results of this procedure depend on the degree of ulnar nerve involvement and the presence or absence of associated medial elbow pathology in the athlete. Patients with minimal sensory complaints and no motor weakness routinely recover completely,[30,33,85,86] but more advanced lesions involving muscle wasting have less consistent results. In athletes with the McGowen grade I (mild) lesion, the prognosis for return to their preoperative level of competition is excellent. Concomitant ulnar collateral ligament pathology or degenerative changes in the elbow joint often will play a larger role in militating against the athlete's return to competition.

Complications

The most common complication in surgery for ulnar compressive neuropathy at the elbow is involvement of the medial antebrachial cutaneous nerve with scar tissue or neuroma from contusion or laceration.[29,72] This problem is best prevented by identifying the cutaneous nerve and its branches that course across the region of the medial epicondyle.[97] The posterior branch and its subbranches are the most likely to be damaged by the medial surgical approaches. Race recommends making the longitudinal incision more posterior, approaching the midline to avoid this problem.[115]

The next most common complication is postsurgical bleeding. Attention to coagulation of small bleeding points, release of the tourniquet before closure of the wound, and drainage of the wound are advisable in this vascular region.

Persistence or recurrence of symptoms also is a complication and will be discussed next.

Failed Surgical Treatment

The average failure rate from all types of surgical treatment of ulnar nerve compression at the elbow is 20%; however, failure rates as high as 78% have been reported.[51] The causes of a failed procedure can be classified as those of failure to address the offending factors in the primary procedure, and those that were created by the procedure. Failure to diagnose accurately the primary neuropathic problem can be responsible for unsuccessful surgery. Examples include an unrecognized cervical root compression or compressive ulnar lesion in Guyon's canal. Compounding factors such as diabetes mellitus, alcoholism, and advanced age are associated with less-than-desired results from surgical intervention. Failure to release Struthers' arcade, to excise a segment of the intermuscular septum of the arm, to adequately release Osborne's band, or to release the flexor-pronator aponeurosis all can produce a poor result. Factors related to the actual procedure include (1) iatrogenic ulnar nerve injury, (2) development of elbow flexion contracture, (3) medial epicondylitis, (4) medial epicondyle nonunion if osteotomized, (5) cutaneous nerve injury or entrapment, (6) medial collateral ligament instability, (7) subsequent avulsion of the flexor-pronator mass, and (8) creation of a new entrapment by scar or by kinking of the nerve along its new path.

Postoperative persisting symptoms generally can be

treated conservatively; however, worsening pain or deterioration of nerve function after an improvement interval indicates a secondary problem and may warrant re-exploration. In Amadio's series, two thirds of the failures showed no postoperative improvement, signifying that the initial problem was not satisfactorily addressed.[51] The most common errors in the primary procedures were: (1) failure to resect a segment of the intermuscular septum, (2) failure to resect the arcade of Struthers, and (3) failure to incise the flexor-pronator aponeurosis distally.[11,51] Rogers found a high incidence of nerve scarring at the site of medial epicondylectomy.[123]

The decision to reoperate on a patient with a failed primary procedure should be made with great care. The statistical factors militating against a successful second procedure include: age greater than 50 years, more than one prior procedure, history of reflex sympathetic dystrophy, diabetes mellitus, alcoholism, electromyographic signs of denervation, and previous submuscular transposition.[51]

A failed primary procedure usually is best treated by anterior submuscular transposition.[51] Neurolysis alone has not met with success.[51] Intramuscular transposition has little in the literature to support it. Medial epicondylectomy failed in seven patients, as reported by Goldberg.[56] The results of anterior subcutaneous transposition as a salvage procedure are variously reported,[3,9,15,51,138] but Urbaniak prefers it in the failed submuscular transposition.[141]

According to Amadio,[51] the salient points of reoperation on the patient with failed ulnar nerve surgery at the elbow for entrapment are (1) explore the ulnar nerve proximal and distal to the previous dissection, (2) perform an external neurolysis if the nerve is encased in scar, (3) ensure that Struthers' arcade has been released, (4) excise a segment of the medial intermuscular septum in the arm if it persists, (5) explore sites of previously identified cutaneous neuromata (excise or transpose), (6) use intraoperative electrodiagnostic techniques to help determine the extent of neurolysis necessary,[16] (7) identify and incise the flexor-pronator aponeurosis distal to the joint, (8) identify and protect the medial collateral ligament, (9) perform intraneural dissection of the first branch to the flexor carpi ulnaris if anterior transposition is tethered by it.

For intractable pain, a transcutaneous electrical nerve stimulator (TENS) may be of value. In refractory cases, combining submuscular transposition with an implanted TENS has been of some benefit.[87]

THE MEDIAN NERVE

The median nerve is the least frequently entrapped of the major nerves about the elbow. There are two well-described syndromes of median nerve compression at the elbow that deserve consideration. Athletes are not immune to these conditions, and certain repetitive arm activities may induce them. Throwing involves repetitive forceful gripping, pronation, and ballistic extension at the elbow that can produce compression at the proximal margin in the pronator teres. Other sports, such as weight lifting, by their nature build muscle mass and can lead to nerve compressions that may not be manifest in the sedentary state.[71,114] The frequent repetitive arm motions in sports also can reveal underlying anomalous conditions, such as the supracondylar process and its attached Struthers' ligament with median nerve compression beneath it. Trauma to the upper limb, not uncommon in sports, can induce compressive neuropathies about the elbow as well.

Anatomy

The median nerve arises as a confluence of branches of the medial and lateral cords of the brachial plexus and has innervation from roots C6 thru T1.[63] As it courses down the medial aspect of the arm, the median nerve passes medial to the humerus, where the supracondylar process may lie. This is an atavistic bony tubercle off the medial aspect of the humerus in approximately 1% of humans, is located about 5 cm proximal to the medial epicondyle, and varies in size from insignificant to several centimeters in projection. A fibrous ligament extends from its tip to the medial epicondyle. This ligament of Struthers lies medial and anterior to the median nerve and brachial artery, which typically course through the foramen. The median nerve may be compressed in its passage through the forearm or tented over the supracondylar process itself. The median nerve exits the arm beneath the lacertus fibrosus and medial to the brachial artery. At the level of the elbow, the nerve enters into, between, or deep to the pronator teres muscle. The typical pattern is to pierce the interval between the superficial and deep heads of the pronator teres and then to give off the anterior interosseous branch posteriorly about 5 cm below the medial epicondyle. The anterior interosseous nerve then passes behind the median nerve and then proximal to the fibrous arcade between the two heads of the flexor digitorum sublimis muscle. Before exiting the pronator canal, the median nerve is crossed by branches of the radial artery and vein.

Pronator Syndrome

Compression of the median nerve in its course about the elbow can be produced by components of the foramen of Struthers, the lacertus fibrosus, the pronator muscle and its fibrous components, and the fibrous proximal margin of the flexor digitorum sublimis (Box 23-2). Although compression of the median nerve in the pronator canal is far less common than carpal tunnel syndrome, it must be considered with any median nerve impairment.

The pronator syndrome typically produces symptoms

BOX 23-2

COMMON SITES OF ENTRAPMENT OF THE MEDIAN NERVE AND ITS BRANCHES AT THE ELBOW

- Struthers' ligament or the supracondylar process
- Lacertus fibrosus
- Pronator teres or a fibrous band thereof
- Crossing branches of the radial artery and vein
- The fibrous arch between the two heads of the FDS muscle

of aching in the volar proximal forearm and distal arm and often is aggravated by forceful use of the extremity, especially involving pronation. Complaints of sensory loss in the median distribution and weakness or clumsiness are often noted.[59,81] Night pain is unusual.

The clinical examination may reveal tenderness of the pronator teres muscle or in the region of the lacertus fibrosus. Firmness of the pronator teres may be evident as well. A Tinel sign may be present but is often delayed in its appearance. A supracondylar process, if present, may be palpable. A Phalen sign usually is absent, but a concomitant carpal tunnel syndrome and pronator syndrome may be present, indicative of a double-crush phe-

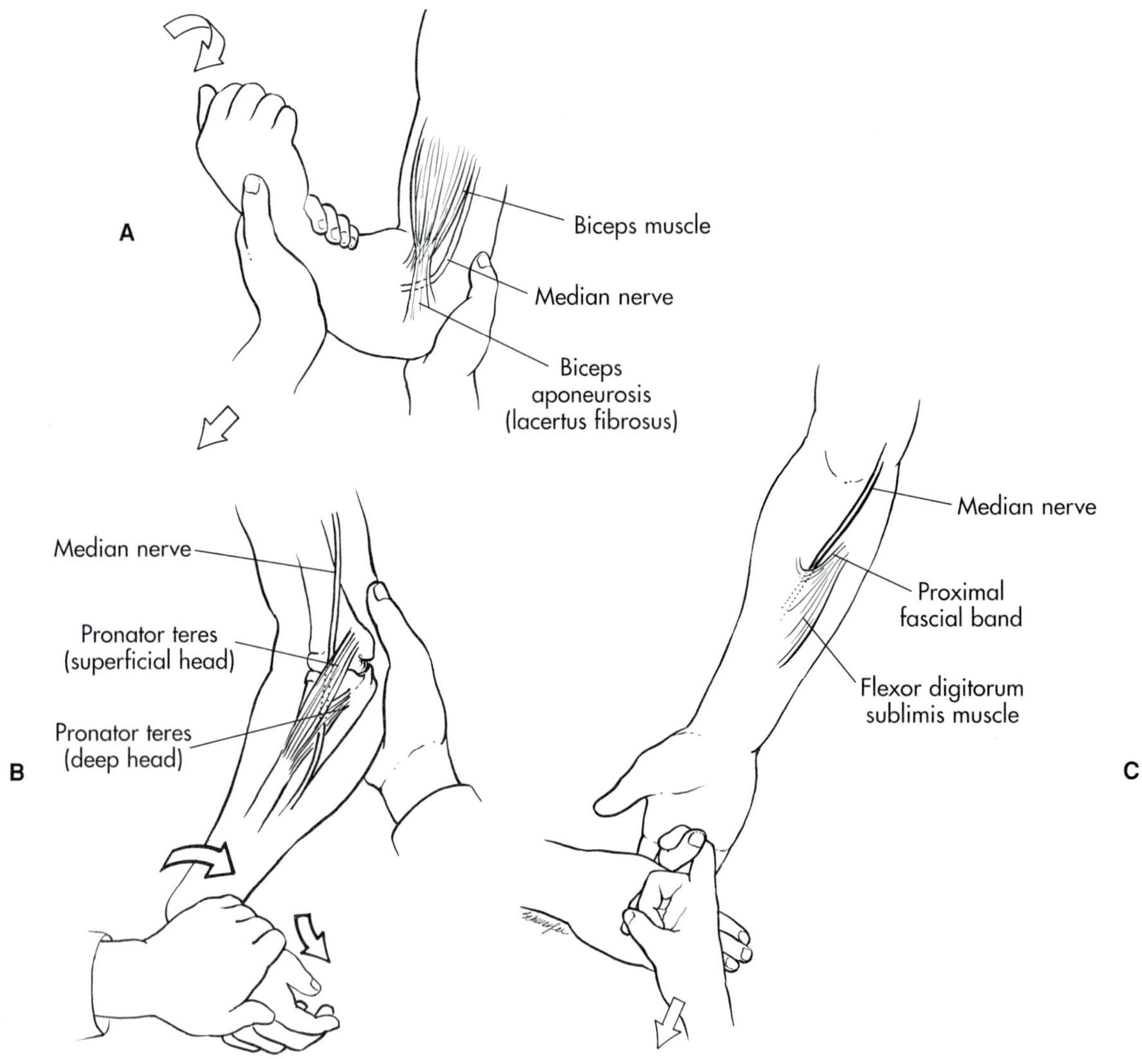

FIGURE 23-7 **A,** Provocative testing for median nerve entrapment by the lacertus fibrosus. Resistance given to patient's supination and flexion of the forearm causes proximal forearm pain. **B,** Provocative testing for median nerve entrapment by the pronator teres. Resistance to forearm pronation and passive wrist flexion may incite symptoms in the median distribution and create proximal forearm pain. **C,** Provocation testing for median nerve compression by the fibrous arch at the proximal flexor digitorum sublimis. Stressing the flexor digitorum sublimis by resisting long finger flexor may produce median paresthesias and proximal forearm pain.

nomenon. Weakness, if evident, may involve the flexor pollicis longus, abductor pollicis brevis, and less often the opponens and flexor digitorum profundus of the index and long fingers. Loss or diminution of sensibility on the palmar side of the radial three and one-half digits can be due to median nerve compression at the carpal tunnel or more proximal, but loss of sensation in the palmar cutaneous distribution is indicative of compression proximal to the carpal canal. Provocative testing often is useful in eliciting signs of the pronator syndrome (Fig. 23-7). Because compression by the lacertus fibrosus is a possibility, hyperflexion of the elbow past 120° with resistant forearm supination may reproduce forearm symptoms suggesting the lacertus as the offending structure. Resisted forearm pronation with the elbow flexed followed by elbow extension that increases symptoms suggest the pronator teres as the site of median nerve compression. Resisted contraction of the long finger flexor digitorum sublimis may elicit symptoms if the flexor digitorum sublimis arcade is the entrapment site.

Electrodiagnostic studies rarely are diagnostic for the syndrome. However, nerve conduction studies and electromyograms can help exclude coexisting pathology and may implicate other sources.

The treatment of the pronator syndrome will be discussed with that of the anterior interosseous nerve syndrome.

Anterior Interosseous Nerve Syndrome

The distinct clinical entity in which the anterior interosseous nerve function is impaired is termed the *anterior interosseous nerve syndrome.*[77] Thus its presentation is absence or diminished function of the flexor pollicis longus, pronator quadratus, and flexor digitorum profundus of the index finger. Because the anterior interosseous nerve has no cutaneous sensory component, numbness is not associated. Although the typical cause of this syndrome is a discrete compression of the anterior interosseous nerve after it diverges from the median nerve trunk, the cause may be differential compression of the fascicles destined to become the anterior interosseous nerve while they are still components of the median nerve up to 2.5 cm proximally. Variations in anatomy may yield somewhat atypical symptoms and findings. Examples include the intact flexor digitorum profundus to the index finger and, more rarely, the intact flexor pollicis longus. The differential diagnosis for the syndrome of motor weaknesses must include disruption of the musculotendinous units of the flexor digitorum profundus of the index or flexor pollicis longus. An intact tenodesis effect with passive wrist movement and interphalangeal flexion with pressure applied over the musculotendinous junction suggest a neurologic etiology. Electromyographic studies of the anterior interosseous nerve syndrome are more useful in making the diagnosis than in the pronator syndrome. The more common causes of anterior interosseous nerve compression are fibrous bands originating from the deep head of the pronator teres, thrombosed ulnar collateral vessels, other fibrous bands, and Gantzer's muscle (accessory head of the FPL from the medial epicondyle).

Treatment

The treatment of these median nerve impairments at the elbow initially is conservative because the appropriate time to intervene surgically is controversial. Certainly the degree of neurologic deficit, the progression of symptoms and findings, the time since onset of symptoms, and the failure to respond to conservative management play a role in determining the time for nonoperative treatment. Splinting the elbow at 90° with the forearm in neutral position is appropriate. Eight to 12 weeks of such treatment generally is sufficient before operative intervention is considered. Miller-Breslow presented evidence, however, that anterior interosseous nerve syndrome is a neuritis that can be treated successfully by watchful waiting in all cases of partial nerve involvement.[100]

Surgical treatment is exploration and decompression of the median nerve and anterior interosseous nerve, including inspection of all sites of potential entrapment that are mentioned in Box 23-2. The surgeon should note that all of the muscle branches off of the median nerve arise medially; thus dissection down the lateral side of the nerve is preferable (Figs. 23-8 and 23-9). Although the nerve must be freed of any compression by a pronator teres component, rarely must the deeper superficial head of the pronator teres be detached radially for visualization of the nerve. Fibrous bands should be excised, crossing vessels ligated and divided, the flexor digitorum sublimis arch split, and anomalous muscles sought.

Postoperative care includes splinting the elbow at 90° of flexion and the forearm in either neutral or slight supination with the wrist at neutral. At about 1 week, flexion and extension exercises may be started and slowly progressed. If the pronator teres has been detached and repaired, immobilization for about 3 weeks is required.

The prognosis for full recovery is generally very good, provided there is no long-standing muscle atrophy before surgery. If such atrophy is present, tendon transfers may be considered as the initial procedure.

THE RADIAL NERVE

One of the more difficult differential diagnoses in the upper extremity is distinguishing between radial tunnel syndrome and lateral epicondylitis. Both entities occur in those involved in sports activities, and not infrequently both are responsible for symptoms in the same patient. As with other compressive neuropathies, the underlying

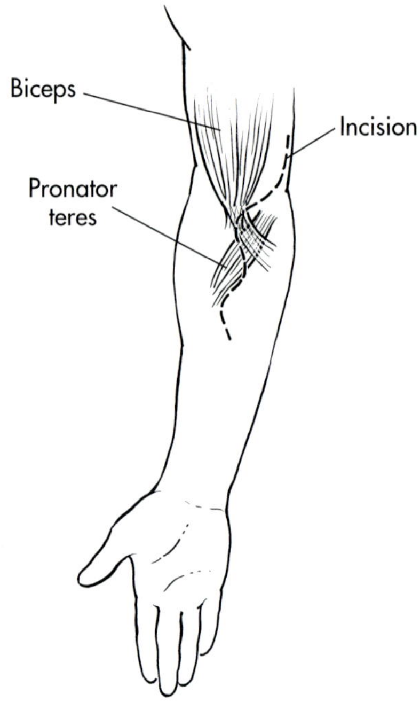

FIGURE 23-8 Anterior approach to median nerve at the elbow and proximal forearm. Dotted line—skin incision—median nerve traced from distal arm under lacertus fibrosus into head of pronator teres and under the flexor digitorum sublimis origin.

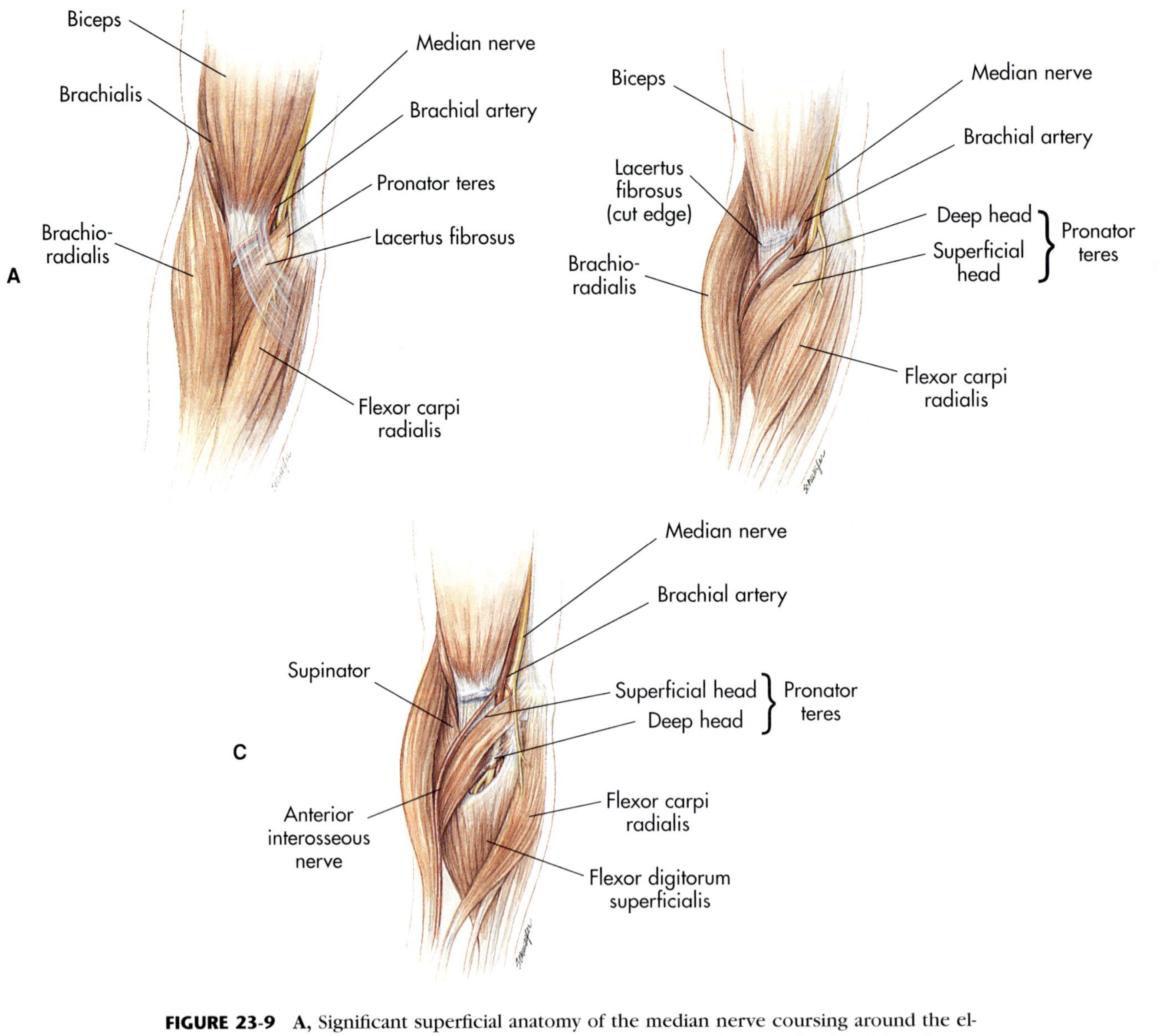

FIGURE 23-9 **A,** Significant superficial anatomy of the median nerve coursing around the elbow. **B,** Typical position of the median nerve coursing between the superficial and deep heads of the pronator teres. **C,** Deep anatomy of the course of the median nerve illustrating the fibrous arch of the flexor digitorum sublimis origin and fibrous bands from the pronator teres (see Box 23-2).

anatomic abnormality often is potentiated and the clinical problem made manifest by repetitive and strenuous use of the limb. The demands athletes place on their extremities easily replicate these conditions.

The forearm pronates during the acceleration and follow-through phases of the throwing motion, with the pronation occurring sooner for a fast ball than a curve ball.[76] Electromyographic analysis of the elbow in pitchers has shown peak activities of the pronator teres during these phases, which is consistent with the above concept.[55] The supinator acts to supinate the forearm during wind-up and early cocking, but more important, controls forearm rotation during the late cocking and acceleration phases. Interestingly, the magnitude of supinator activity is comparable for both the fast-ball and curved-ball deliveries. The primary function of the supinator is to decelerate forearm pronation that occurs during follow-through for all types of pitches.[55] The repetitive firing of the supinator against a pronating forearm may predispose the thrower to radial tunnel syndrome. The fibrous arcade at the lateral head of the triceps also can entrap the radial nerve with throwing activities. Frisbee throwing in particular has been associated with a posterior interosseous nerve compression.[48] Tennis-elbow-like symptoms often are present with lateral forearm pain caused by the radial tunnel syndrome. This syndrome also has been reported in a swimmer.[131] Problems in weight lifters have been described secondary to high radial nerve entrapment by a fibrous arch over the lateral head of the triceps in relation to repetitive elbow extension against resistance.[94] Distal entrapment with radial tunnel and posterior interosseous nerve symptoms also have been reported in weight lifters,[85] and injuries to the radial nerve have been reported in wrestlers. Obviously, trauma directly to the radial nerve or indirectly by fracture fragments can damage the nerve as well.

Anatomy

The radial nerve attains the lateral position on the arm as it winds around the middle third of the arm just below the radial groove on the upper border of the medial head of the triceps. At the junction of the middle and distal thirds of the humerus, the nerve lies between the brachioradialis laterally, the brachialis medially, and the lateral head of the triceps posteriorly. At this point it lies adjacent to the humeral shaft, where it is in jeopardy of being trapped by a spiral or oblique fracture of the humeral shaft. Sensory branches usually separate from the posterior interosseous nerve at this level, with the sensory component lying on the medial surface of the brachioradialis and following in this position to the midforearm. The posterior interosseous nerve passes deep to the origin of the extensor carpi radialis brevis (ECRB), which often has an accessory deep fibrous origin spanning anteriorly to the nerve, creating a potential compression site (Fig. 23-10). Wrist dorsiflexion and elbow extension further increase compression to this site. The posterior interosseous nerve proceeds distally and laterally. Just distal to the elbow, it is crossed by the radial recurrent artery and its concomitant veins. When the vessels are engorged, as with exercise or when thrombosed, the posterior interosseous nerve can be compressed. The posterior interosseous nerve continues laterally to the superior border of the supinator muscle on the neck of the radius. This fibrous, free margin of the supinator is known as the arcade of Frohse and is a site of potential posterior interosseous nerve compression.[111] As the nerve crosses the posterolateral aspect of the radial neck, it lies directly on bone in 25% of the population[26] and is in jeopardy of injury by fracture or by plate application. The nerve continues a longitudinal course distally between the two muscle layers of the supinator and exits at its inferior border as two major components. The superficial branch

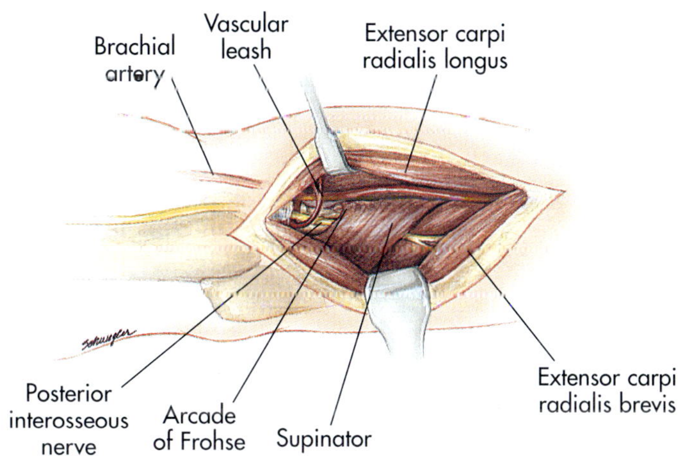

FIGURE 23-10 Posterior approach to the posterior interosseous nerve showing potential sites of entrapment over the posterior interosseous nerve. These sites include the following: (1) fibrous bands, (2) vascular leash, (3) proximal edge of ECRB, (4) arcade of Frohse, (5) distal fibrous edge of supinator.

turns proximally after emerging from the supinator to innervate the extensor digitorum communis, extensor digiti minimi, and extensor carpi ulnaris. This branch is in jeopardy of surgical trauma here, and care must be given to protect it. Some have suggested that the posterior interosseous nerve may be compressed as it exits from the inferior border of the supinator muscle.[136]

Radial Tunnel Syndrome

The radial tunnel syndrome, as described by Roles and Maudsley,[124] is a constellation of symptoms and findings resulting from dynamic compression of the posterior interosseous nerve in its course from the anterior capsule of the elbow joint proximally to the arcade of Frohse distally. The symptoms include deep, dull proximal dorsal forearm ache, often with distal radiation. Aggravation is created by resisted supination and extension, resisted extension in the metacarpophalangeal (MP) joint of the long finger with wrist extended,[88] and repetitive forearm pronation with a flexed wrist. The pain often is described as a cramp, and night pain is a common complaint.[58] In 5% of cases of tennis elbow, this syndrome is a major contributor to the symptoms, according to Werner[146] and as later corroborated by Jalovaara.[65] Sensory loss over the dorsoradial aspect of the second metacarpal suggests radial sensory branch involvement. Motor findings usually are absent. Electrodiagnostic studies rarely are useful in making a conclusive diagnosis but may be useful in identifying coexisting pathology.[116] Differentiating radial tunnel syndrome from lateral epicondylitis is a formidable responsibility for most clinicians. Injections into the lateral epicondyle and into the site of entry of the posterior interosseous nerve into the arcade of Frohse offer some distinction.[40]

Treatment

Conservative management in most cases is warranted. Simple rest from strenuous and repetitive use may be effective but frequently requires external elbow splinting for reinforcement of the recommendation. This should be applied with the elbow flexed, the forearm supinated, and the wrist extended. Treating suspected associated lateral epicondylitis with steroid injections, stretching, tennis-elbow exercises, massage, and ultrasound may successfully reduce some or all findings. Surgical treatment will be discussed with that of posterior interosseous nerve syndrome.

Posterior Interosseous Nerve Syndrome

Posterior interosseous nerve syndrome is a compression neuropathy that presents with weakness or loss of function of the finger and thumb extensors. Conversely, the radial tunnel syndrome is manifested by pain with little, if any, weakness. The symptoms may occur after an episode of strenuous arm and/or wrist use involving pronation and supination. Pain in the elbow and forearm may precede the weakness, which usually is rapid in progression and may be sequential. Posterior interosseous nerve syndrome is characterized by space-occupying lesions, such as ganglia[10] and lipomata[121] of the elbow, resulting in inability to extend the finger MP joints or abduct the thumb with the wrist at neutral. Other possible causes are synovitis of the radiocapitellar joint, entrapment by the fibrous edge of the ECRB, and compression by the leash of the radial recurrent artery. "Pseudo" clawing may be demonstrated. Although the wrist can be actively extended, it usually deviates radially because of the absence of the extensor carpi ulnaris to balance the extensor carpi radialis longus (ECRL) and the ECRB. Radial sensory changes are absent. In the differential diagnosis are metabolic or toxic neuropathies, most notably lead intoxication.[148] If the onset is secondary to a space-occupy-ing lesion and is gradual, the motor loss may proceed along the expected course of muscle innervation. Although the ECRL and ECRB may anomalously be innervated by the posterior interosseous nerve, the brachioradialis is not, and sensory involvement is absent. Computed tomographic scans, ultrasound, and magnetic resonance imaging can be effective in identifying space-occupying lesions responsible for this syndrome. Electromyography usually demonstrates denervation potentials in the involved muscle after 3 weeks.

Treatment

Unless space-occupying lesions are identified, open injuries are present, or chronic radial head dislocation is present, conservative management is indicated. Failure to respond in 12 weeks is an appropriate indication for surgical exploration.

Surgical Treatment

There are five well-recognized sites of posterior interosseous nerve compression in the radial tunnel: proximally by fibrous bands, the fibrous margin of the ECRB, the constricting leash of recurrent vessels, the arcade of Frohse, and fibrous bands at the distal end of the supinator muscle (Fig. 23-11). The operative approach depends on the suspected findings. If lateral epicondylitis is thought to coexist with radial tunnel syndrome, the common extensor origin should be released, and the posterior interosseous nerve decompressed as well. The extensive anterior approach is needed for complete nerve exploration from the arm through the entire supinator muscle. This is accomplished through the brachialis-brachioradialis interval, extending distally between the extensor carpi radialis brevis and the pronator teres. Care is taken to identify and protect the lateral antebrachial cutaneous nerve as it emerges lateral to the biceps tendon. The posterior interosseous nerve is freed from overlying fibrous tissue over the radiocapitellar joint (Fig. 23-12). Recurrent radial collateral vessels coursing over the nerve are ligated and divided. The leading edge of the ex-

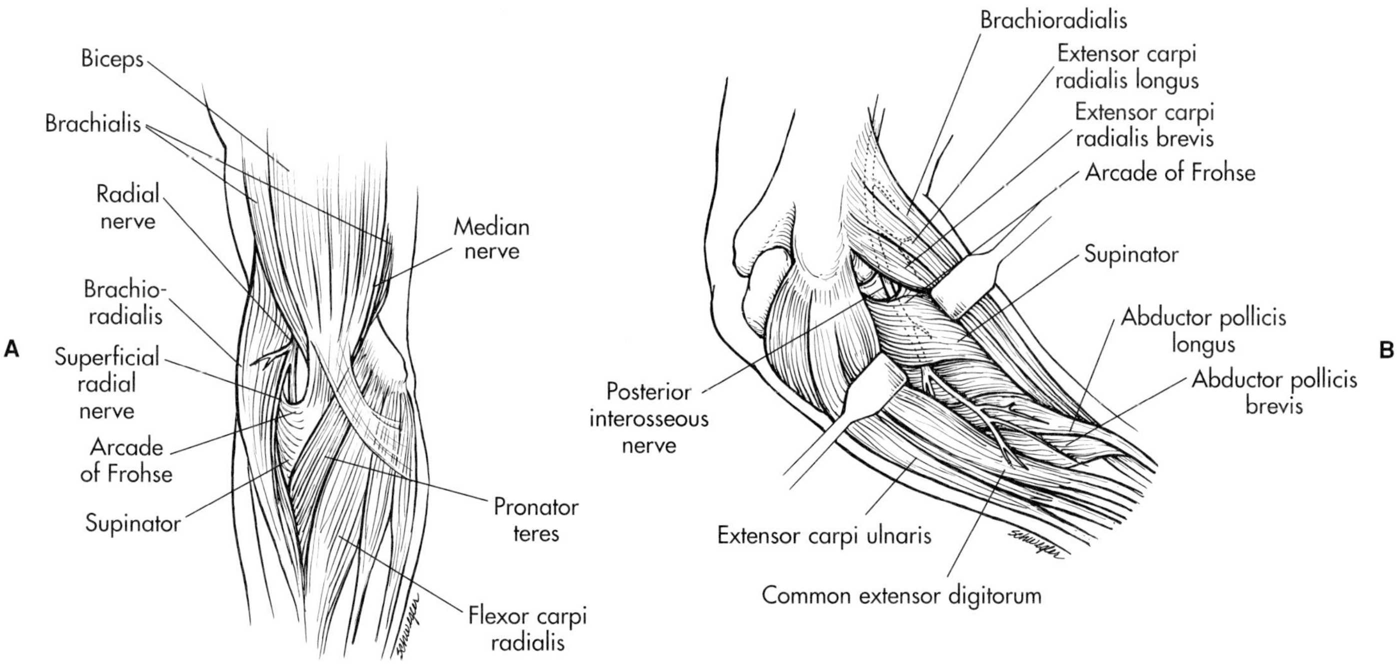

FIGURE 23-11 **A,** Anterior lateral approach to the radial nerve, posterior interosseous nerve, arcade of Frohse. **B,** The posterior approach is useful to explore the entire course of the posterior interosseous nerve from the radial tunnel through the supinator muscle.

tensor carpi radialis brevis is inspected. If any compression of the posterior interosseous nerve is seen, or if a pseudoneuromatous enlargement is present at that point, the fibrous edge is incised. The nerve is then followed into the arcade of Frohse, and the effect of pronation and wrist palmar flexion is studied. The fibrous arcade is divided, and the nerve is carefully identified into the supinator muscle. Some have identified offending fibrous bands within the supinator and thus recommend following the nerve entirely through the muscle. Dellon advocates releasing all potentially compressive sites. Elbow joint procedures can be carried out through this extensive approach, as can dissection of space-occupying masses. The scar is long and obviously placed, however.

The posterior approach of Thompson[137] is useful in exploring the entire supinator and branches of the posterior interosseous nerve distal to it. The incision is posterior from the lateral epicondyle to the midforearm between the extensor carpi radialis brevis and the extensor digitorum communis. The dissection must start distally and proceed proximally. Care is taken to protect the recurrent branch of the posterior interosseous nerve to the extensor digitorum communis, extensor digiti minimi, and extensor carpi ulnaris.

Authors' Preferred Surgical Approach

The brachioradialis splitting incision[19,89] is radially placed from the elbow flexion crease to 6 cm distal in a lazy "S"

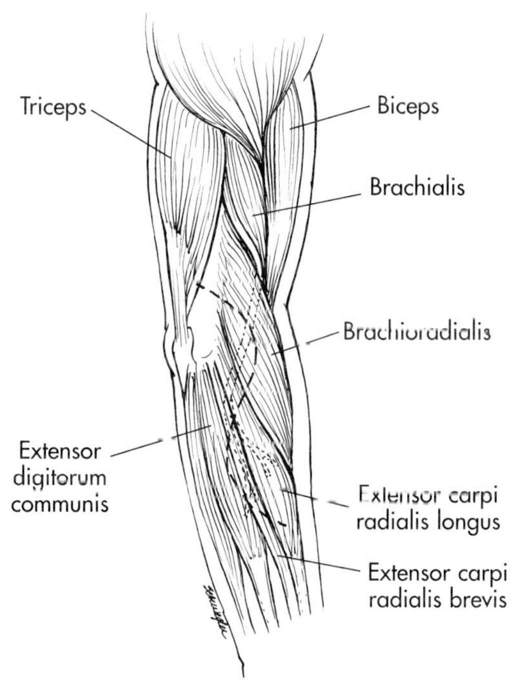

FIGURE 23-12 Posterior approach to the posterior interosseous nerve, skin incision, and underlying anatomy.

longitudinal orientation. The brachioradialis is dissected apart in the line of its fibers until the superficial radial nerve is exposed. One continues splitting the brachioradialis proximally and distally, aiming for the radial head to expose the posterior interosseous nerve and the proximal supinator; thus the radial tunnel is exposed from the radiocapitellar joint to the proximal supinator. The nerve is decompressed, as noted previously, although following it completely through the entire supinator is more difficult and in some cases may require distal extension dorsally. One should take care to release all potential sites of compression. Lister believes that the brachioradialis-splitting approach can easily be accomplished through a transverse incision at the level of the radial neck.[90]

Postoperative management includes prompt range-of-motion and progressive exercises at both the wrist and elbow. Early stretching exercises also are encouraged to promote nerve gliding. Progressive strengthening exercises will prepare the patient for the initiation of sport-specific activities at 6 to 8 weeks after surgery.

CUTANEOUS NEUROPATHIES

The superficial nature of the cutaneous nerves puts them at risk for direct trauma, but chronic compressive lesions are rare. The best-described lesion is compression of the musculocutaneous nerve at or proximal to the elbow. The nerve lies in the intermuscular plane between the brachioradialis muscle and the biceps brachii in the middle and distal thirds of the forearm (Fig. 23-13). Progressing distally as the biceps becomes tendinous, the nerve emerges lateral to the tendon 2 to 5 cm proximal to the elbow crease and here pierces the brachial fascia to lie subcutaneously. It then divides into posterior and anterior branches that supply sensation to the radial aspect of the forearm.

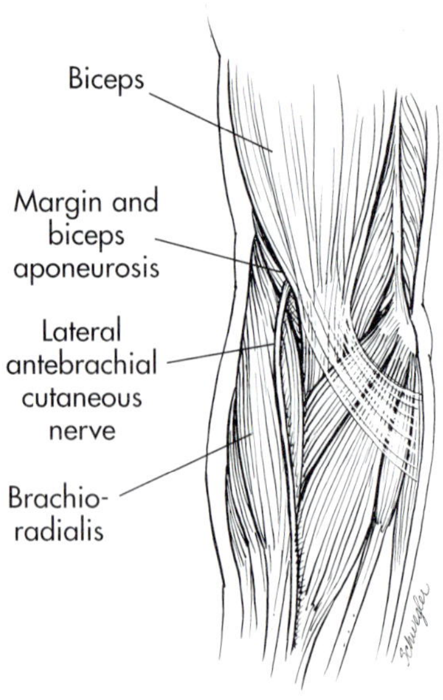

FIGURE 23-13 Course of the lateral antebrachial cutaneous nerve as it traverses the elbow.

Bassett described both chronic and acute types of compressive neuropathy.[8] Most had some history of hyperextension of the elbow with full pronation. One competitive backstroke swimmer and three tennis players with improper forearm strokes were included in his series of 11 patients. Pain in the anterolateral aspect of the forearm was uniformly present with occasional proximal radiation. Aggravation by forceful elbow extension and pronation was described, as was direct tenderness over the point of emergence of the musculocutaneous nerve from behind the biceps tendon. These patients previously were diagnosed erroneously with tennis elbow, carpal tunnel syndrome, and cervical radiculitis.

Treatment for the condition is antiinflammatories, rest, and often splinting with the elbow flexed and in a neutral position of rotation. The musculocutaneous tunnel is injected with steroids if unimproved at 6 to 12 weeks. Failure of conservative measures at 12 weeks is an indication for surgical decompression.[8]

The procedure is performed through a curvilinear incision in the antebrachial fossa. The musculocutaneous nerve is located just lateral to the biceps tendon and is followed proximally. At the point that it dives deep to the biceps tendon, a triangular section of biceps tendon is removed. Care is taken to observe the nerve with manipulation of the elbow in pronation and supination, to ensure that no entrapment persists.[8] Postoperative splinting for 2 to 3 weeks is followed by active motion as tolerated.

References

1. Adelaar RS, Foster RC, McDowell C: The treatment of cubital tunnel syndrome, *J Hand Surg [Am]* 9:90-95, 1984.
2. Adson AL: The surgical treatment of progressive ulnar paralysis, *Minn Med* 1:455-460, 1918.
3. Alissimi M, Pecorelli F, Pimpinelli G: Ulnar nerve compression at the elbow level, *Ital J Orthop* 12:395-399, 1986.
4. Amadio PC, Beckenbaugh RD: Entrapment of the ulnar nerve by the deep flexor-pronator aponeurosis, *J Hand Surg [Am]* 11:83, 1986.
5. Apfelberg DB, Larson SJ: Dynamic anatomy of the ulnar nerve at the elbow, *Plast Reconstr Surg* 51:76-81, 1973.
6. Aulicino PL: Neurovascular injuries in the hands of athletes, *Hand Clin* 6(3):455, 1990.
7. Barron JL et al: MRI of the elbow in baseball pitchers, unpublished data.
8. Bassett FH, Nunley JA: Compression of the musculocutaneous nerve at the elbow, *J Bone Joint Surg [Am]* 64:1050, 1982.
9. Bergfield TG, Schneider LH, Hunter JM: Ulnar neuritis at the elbow: results of surgical management, *Jefferson Orthop J* 16:41-43, 1987.
10. Bowen TL, Stone KH: Posterior interosseous nerve paralysis caused by a ganglion at the elbow, *J Bone Joint Surg [Br]* 48B:774-776, 1966.
11. Broudy AS, Leffert RD, Smith RJ: Technical problems with ulnar nerve transposition at the elbow: findings and results with reoperation, *J Hand Surg [Am]* 3:85-89, 1978.

12. Buehler MJ, Thayer DT: The elbow flexion test: a clinical test for the cubital tunnel syndrome, *Clin Orthop* 233:213-216, 1986.
13. Buzzard EF: Traumatic and toxic ulnar neuritis, *Lancet* 1:317-319, 1922.
14. Cabera JM, McCue FC: Nonosseous athletic injuries of the elbow, forearm and hand, *Clin Sports Med* 5(4):681, 1986.
15. Campbell JB, Post KD, Morantz RA: A technique for relief of motor and sensory deficits occurring after anterior transposition, *J Neurosurg* 10:405-409, 1974.
16. Campbell WW et al: Intraoperative electromyography: management of ulnar neuropathy at the elbow, *Muscle Nerve* 11:75-81, 1988.
17. Chan RC, Paine KWE, Varaghese G: Ulnar neuropathy at the elbow: comparison of simple decompression and anterior transposition, *Neurosurgery* 7:545-550, 1980.
18. Childress HM: Recurrent ulnar nerve dislocation at the elbow, *J Bone Joint Surg [Am]* 38:978-984, 1956.
19. Comtet JJ, Chambaud D: Paralysie "spontanée" du nerf inter-osseux posterieur par lesion inhabituelle, *Rev Clin Orthop* 61:533-541, 1975.
20. Conway JE et al: Medical instability of the elbow in throwing athletes, *J Bone Joint Surg [Am]* 74(1):67-83, 1992.
21. Craven RR, Green DP: Cubital tunnel syndrome: treatment by medical epicondylectomy, *J Bone Joint Surg [Am]* 62:986-990, 1980.
22. Cravens G, Kline DG: Posterior interosseous nerve palsies, *Neurosurgery* 27:397-402, 1990.
23. Curtis BF: Traumatic ulnar neuritis: transplantation of the nerve, *J Nerve Ment Dis* 25:480-481, 1898.
24. Dahlin LB et al: Effects of nerve compression or ischemia on conduction properties of myelinated and non-myelinated nerve fibers: an experimental study in the rabbit common peroneal nerve, *Act Physiol Scand* 136:97-105, 1989.
25. Dangles CJ, Bilos ZJ: Ulnar nerve neuritis in a world champion weight lifter, *Am J Sports Med* 8:443-445, 1980.
26. Davies F, Laird M: The supinator muscle in the deep radial (posterior interosseous) nerve, *Anat Rec* 101:243-250, 1948.
27. Davies MA et al: Results of ulnar neuropathy at the elbow treated by decompression or anterior transposition, *Aust NZ J Surg* 61:929-934, 1991.
28. Dellon AL: Clinical use of vibratory stimuli to evaluate peripheral nerve injury and compression neuropathy, *Plast Reconstr Surg* 65:466-476, 1980.
29. Dellon AL, McKinnon SE: Injury to the medial antebrachial cutaneous nerve during cubital tunnel surgery, *J Hand Surg [Br]* 19:33-36, 1985.
30. Dellon AL: Review of treatment results for ulnar nerve entrapments at the elbow, *J Hand Surg* 14:688-699, 1989.
31. Dellon AL: Think nerve in upper extremity reconstruction, *Clin Plast Surg* 16:617-627, 1989.
32. Dellon AL: Patient evaluation and management consideration in nerve compression, *Hand Clin* 8(2):230, 1992.
33. Del Pizzo W, Jobe FW, Norwood L: Ulnar nerve entrapment syndrome in baseball players, *Am J Sports Med* 5:182-185, 1977.
34. Dimond ML, Lister GD: Cubital tunnel syndrome treated by long-arm splintage (abstract), *J Hand Surg* 10:430, 1985.
35. Eaton RG, Crowe JF, Parkes JC III: Anterior transposition of the ulnar nerve with a non-compressing fasciodermal sling, *J Bone Joint Surg [Am]* 62:820-825, 1980.
36. Eaton RG: Anterior subcutaneous transposition. In Gelberman RH, editor: *Operative nerve repair and reconstruction,* Philadelphia, 1991, JB Lippincott.
37. Eisen A: Early diagnosis of ulnar nerve palsy: an electrophysiological study, *Neurology* 24:256, 1974.
38. Eisen A, Danon J: The mild cubital tunnel syndrome, *Neurology* 24:608-613, 1974.
39. Eversmann WW: Compression and entrapment neuropathies of the upper extremity, *J Hand Surg* 8:759-766, 1983.
40. Eversmann WW: Entrapment and compression neuropathies. In Green DP, editor: *Operative hand surgery,* ed 2, New York, 1988, Churchill Livingstone, p 1455.
41. Ewald FC et al: Capitello-condylar total elbow arthroplasty, *J Bone Joint Surg [Am]* 62:1259-1263, 1980.
42. Fahmy NR, Noble J: Ulnar nerve palsy as a complication of osteochondromatosis of the elbow, *Hand* 13:308-310, 1982.
43. Feindel W, Stratford J: The role of the cubital tunnel in tardy ulnar palsy, *Can J Surg* 1:278, 1958.
44. Ferlic DC, Ries MD: Epineural ganglion of the ulnar nerve at the elbow, *J Hand Surg* 15A:996-998, 1990.
45. Ferlic DC: Clinical assessment and conservative treatment of cubital tunnel syndrome. In Gelberman RH, editor: *Operative nerve repair and reconstruction,* Philadelphia, 1991, JB Lippincott.
46. Fine EJ, Wongjirad C: The ulnar flexion maneuver (Abstract), *Muscle Nerve* 8:612, 1985.
47. Foster RJ, Edshage S: Factors related to the outcome of surgically managed compressive neuropathy at the elbow level, *J Hand Surg* 6:181-192, 1981.
48. Fraim CJ, Peters BH: Unusual cause of nerve entrapment, *JAMA* 242:2557, 1979.
49. Froimson AI et al: Ulnar nerve decompression with medial epicondylectomy for neuropathy at the elbow, *Clin Orthop* 265:200-206, 1991.
50. Fulkerson JP: Transient ulnar neuropathy from Nordic skiing, *Clin Orthop* 174:230-231, 1980.
51. Gabel GT, Amadio PC: Reoperation for failed decompression of the ulnar nerve in the region of the elbow, *J Bone Joint Surg [Am]* 72:213-220, 1990.
52. Gay JR, Love JG: Diagnosis and treatment of tardy paralysis of the ulnar nerve: based on a study of 100 cases, *J Bone Joint Surg* 29:1087-1097, 1947.
53. Gelberman RH et al: The carpal tunnel syndrome, *J Bone Joint Surg [Am]* 63(3):380-383, 1981.
54. Glousman RE: Ulnar nerve problems in athlete's elbow, *Clin Sports Med* 9:365-377, 1990.
55. Glousman RE et al: An electromyographic analysis of the elbow in normal and injured pitchers with medial collateral ligament insufficiency, *Am J Sports Med* 20(3):311-317, 1992.
56. Goldberg BJ, Light TR, Blair SJ: Ulnar neuropathy at the elbow: results of medial epicondylectomy, *J Hand Surg* 14:182-188, 1989.
57. Goldberg V et al: Total elbow arthroplasty, *J Bone Joint Surg [Am]* 70:778-783, 1988.
58. Hagert CG, Lundberg G, Hansen T: Entrapment of the posterior interosseous nerve, *Scand J Plast Reconstr Surg* 11:205-212, 1977.
59. Hartz CR et al: The pronator syndrome: compressive neuropathy of the median nerve, *J Bone Joint Surg* 63A:885-890, 1981.
60. Heithoff SJ et al: Medial epicondylectomy for the treatment of ulnar nerve compression at the elbow, *J Hand Surg* 15A(1):22-29, 1990.
61. Herrick RT, Herrick SK: Thermography in the detection of carpal tunnel syndrome an other compressive neuropathies, *J Hand Surg* 12A:943-949, 1987.
62. Hirasawa Y, Sawamura H, Sakakida K: Entrapment neuropathy due to bilateral epitrochleoanconeus muscle: a case report, *J Hand Surg* 4:181-184, 1979.
63. Hollinshead WH: *Anatomy for surgeons. the back and limbs,* ed 3, Philadelphia, 1982, WB Saunders, pp 352-353.
64. Inglis AE, Pellicci PM. Total elbow replacement, *J Bone Joint Surg [Am]* 62:1252-1259, 1980.
65. Jalovaara P, Lindholm RV: Decompression of the posterior interosseous nerve for tennis elbow, *Arch Orthop Trauma Surg* 108:243-245, 1989.
66. Janes PC, Mann RJ, Farnworth TK: Submuscular transposition of the ulnar nerve, *Clin Orthop* 238:225-232, 1989.
67. Jebsen RH: Motor conduction velocities in the median and ulnar nerves, *Arch Phys Med Rehabil* 48:185-194, 1967.

68. Jobe FW, Fanton GS: Nerve injuries. In Morrey BF, editor: *The elbow and its disorders,* Philadelphia, 1985, WB Saunders, pp 497-501.
69. Jobe FW, Huber G: Throwing injuries of the elbow, *Clin Sports Med* 5:621-636, 1986.
70. Jobe FW, Stark H, Lombardo SJ: Reconstruction of the ulnar collateral ligament in athletes, *J Bone Joint Surg* 68A:1158-1163, 1986.
71. Johnson RK: Soft tissue injuries of the forearm and hand, *Clin Sports Med* 5(4):701, 1986.
72. Jones RE, Gauntt C: Medial epicondylectomy for ulnar nerve compression syndrome at the elbow, *Clin Orthop* 139:174-178, 1979.
73. Kaplan EB, Spinner M: Normal and anomalous innervation patterns in the upper extremity. In Omer GE, Spinner M, editors: *Management of peripheral nerve problems,* Philadelphia, 1980, WB Saunders, p 75.
74. Karakmedala RV et al: Ulnar nerve entrapment at the elbow localized by short segment stimulation, *Arch Phys Med Rehabil* 69:959-963, 1988.
75. Kelan RK et al: Throwing injuries of the shoulder and elbow in adults, *Curr Pract Orthop Surg* 6:41-58, 1975.
76. Ketlinski R: How is a curveball thrown? *Athle J* 51(5):54, 75-76, 1971.
77. Kiloh LG, Nevin S: Isolated neuritis of the anterior interosseous nerve, *Br Med J* 1:850-851, 1952.
78. King J, Brelsford HJ, Tullos HSJ: Analysis of the pitching arm of the professional baseball pitcher, *Clin Orthop* 67:116, 1969.
79. Kleinman WB, Bishop AT: Anterior intramuscular transposition of the ulnar nerve, *J Hand Surg [Am]* 14:972-979, 1989.
80. Kondo M et al: A new method of electrodiagnosis during operations on the brachial plexus and peripheral nerve injuries, *Int Orthop* 9:115-121, 1985.
81. Kopell HP, Thompson WAI: Pronator syndrome: a confirmed case and its diagnosis, *N Engl J Med* 259:712-715, 1958.
82. Laha RK, Panchal PD: Surgical management of ulnar neuropathy, *Surg Neurol* 11:393-398, 1979.
83. Learmonth JR: A variation of the radial branch of the musculospiral nerve, *J Anat* 53:371, 1919.
84. Learmonth JR: A technique for transplanting the ulnar nerve, *Surg Gynecol Obstet* 75:92-93, 1942.
85. Leffert RD: Anterior submuscular transposition of the ulnar nerve by the Learmonth technique, *J Hand Surg [Am]* 7:147-155, 1982.
86. Levy DM, Apfelberg DB: Results of anterior transposition for ulnar neuropathy at the elbow, *Am J Surg* 123:304-308, 1972.
87. Lewis RM et al: *Peripheral nerve stimulation for chronic pain,* presented at the third annual meeting, American Society for Reconstructive Surgery, Baltimore, Md, September 17, 1988.
88. Lister GD: *The hand: diagnosis and indications,* Edinburgh, 1977, Churchill-Livingstone.
89. Lister GD, Belsole RB, Kleinert HE: The radial tunnel syndrome, *J Hand Surg* 4:52-59, 1979.
90. Lister GD: Radial tunnel syndrome. In Gelberman RH, editor: *Operative nerve repair and reconstruction,* Philadelphia, 1991, JB Lippincott, pp 1023-1039.
91. Lugnegard H, Waldheim G, Wrenberg G: Operative treatment of ulnar neuropathy in the elbow region, *Acta Orthop Scand* 48:168-176, 1977.
92. Lundborg G: *Nerve injury and repair: a biological approach,* Edinburgh, 1988, Churchill-Livingstone, pp 1-222.
93. Macincol MF: Extraneural pressure affecting the ulnar nerve at the elbow, *Hand* 14:5-11, 1982.
94. Manske PR: Compression of the radial nerve by the triceps muscle, *J Bone Joint Surg* 59A(G):835, 1977.
95. Manske PR et al: Ulnar nerve decompression at the cubital tunnel, *Clin Orthop* 274:231-237, 1992.
96. Marin EL, Vernick S, Friedmann LW: Carpal tunnel syndrome: median nerve stress test, *Arch Phys Med Rehabil* 64:206, 1983.
97. Masear VR, Meyer RD, Pichora DR: Surgical anatomy of the medial antebrachial cutaneous nerve, *J Hand Surg [Am]* 14:267-271, 1989.
98. McGowan AJ: The results of transposition of the ulnar nerve for traumatic ulnar neuritis, *J Bone Joint Surg [Br]* 32:293-301, 1950.
99. Mendoza FX, Main K: Peripheral nerve injuries of the shoulder in the athlete, *Clin Sports Med* 9(2):331, 1990.
100. Miller-Breslow A, Terrona A, Millender LH: Nonoperative treatment of anterior interosseous nerve paralysis, *J Hand Surg* 15A:493-496, 1990.
101. Miller RG, Hummel EE: The cubital tunnel syndrome: treatment with simple decompression, *Ann Neurol* 7:567, 1980.
102. Moore JR, Weiland AJ: Bilateral attritional rupture of the ulnar nerve at the elbow, *J Hand Surg* 5(4):358-360, 1980.
103. Murakami Y, Uomiyama Y: Hypoplasia of the trochlea and the medial epicondyle of the humerus associated with ulnar neuropathy, *J Bone Joint Surg [Br]* 60:225, 1978.
104. Murphy JB: Transposition of the ulnar nerve, *Clin JB Murphy* 4:1101-1107, 1915.
105. Nirschl RP: Prevention and treatment of elbow and shoulder injuries in the tennis player, *Clin Sports Med* 7(2):289, 1988.
106. Norwood LA, Shook JA, Andrews JR: Acute medial elbow ruptures, *Am J Sports Med* 9:16-19, 1981.
107. O'Driscoll SW et al: Origin of the medial ulnar collateral ligament, *J Hand Surg* 17A(1):164-168, 1992.
108. Ogata K, Manske PR, Leaker PA: The effect of surgical dissection on regional block flow to the ulnar nerve in the cubital tunnel, *Clin Orthop* 193:195, 1985.
109. Ogino T, Minami A, Fukuda L: Tardy ulnar nerve palsy caused by cubitus varus deformity, *J Hand Surg* 11B:352-356, 1986.
110. Osborne GV: The surgical treatment of tardy ulnar neuritis. In: proceedings of the British Orthopaedic Association, *J Bone Joint Surg [Br]* 39:782, 1957.
111. Papadopoulos N, Paraschos A, Pelekis P: Anatomical observations on the arcade of Frohse and other structures related to the deep radial nerve: anatomical interpretation of deep radial nerve entrapment neuropathy, *Folia Morphologica* 37:319-327, 1989.
112. Payan J: Anterior transposition of the ulnar nerve: an electrophysiological study, *J Neurol Neurosurg Psych* 33:157-165, 1970.
113. Pechan J, Julius I: The pressure measurement in the ulnar nerve: a contribution to the pathophysiology of the cubital tunnel syndrome, *J Biomech* 8:75-79, 1975.
114. Posner MA: Compressive neuropathies of the median and radial nerves at the elbow, *Clin Sports Med* 9(2):343, 1990.
115. Race CM, Saldana MJ: Anatomic course of the medial cutaneous nerves of the arm, *J Hand Surg* 16A:48-52, 1991.
116. Raimberu G, Saint-Cast Y, Pelier-Cady MC: Radial tunnel syndrome. Study of a continuous and homogenous series of 35 cases, *Rev Clin Orthop* 76:177-184, 1990.
117. Rayan GM, Jensen C, Duke J: Elbow flexion test in the normal population, *J Hand Surg [Am]* 17:86-89, 1992.
118. Reis ND: Anomalous triceps tendon as the cause for snapping elbow in ulnar neuritis, *J Hand Surg* 5:361-362, 1980.
119. Rennels GD, Ochoa J: Neuralgia amyotrophy manifesting as anterior interosseous palsy, *Muscle Nerve* 3:160-164, 1980.
120. Rettig AC: Neurovascular injuries in the wrists and hands of athletes, *Clin Sports Med* 9(2):389, 1990.
121. Richmond DA: Lipoma causing a posterior interosseous nerve lesion, *J Bone Joint Surg [Br]* 35:83, 1953.
122. Richmond JC, Southmayd WW: Superficial anterior transposition of the ulnar nerve at the elbow for ulnar neuritis, *Clin Orthop* 164:42-44, 1982.
123. Rogers MR, Bergfield TG, Aulicino PL: The failed ulnar nerve transposition, *Clin Orthop* 269:193-200, 1991.
124. Roles NC, Maudsley RH: Radial tunnel syndrome: resistant tennis elbow as a nerve entrapment, *J Bone Joint Surg [Br]* 54:499-508, 1972.

125. Rolfsen L: Snapping triceps tendon with ulnar neuritis, *Acta Orthop Scand* 41:74-76, 1970.
126. Salisbury RE, Dingeldein GP: Peripheral nerve complications following burn injury, *Clin Orthop* 163:92-97, 1982.
127. Seddon HJ: Three types of nerve injury, *Brain* 66:237, 1943.
128. Seyffarth H: Primary mycoses in the m pronator teres as cause of lesion of the n medianus (the pronator syndrome), *Acta Psychiatr Scand [Suppl]* 74:251-254, 1951.
129. Shelty S: Surgical treatment of T and Y fractures of the distal humerus, *Injury* 14:345-348, 1938.
130. Shilo R et al: Thermography as a diagnostic aid in tennis elbow, *Hand Chirurgie* 8:101-103, 1976.
131. Sicuranza MJ, McCue FC III: Compressive neuropathies in the upper extremity of athletes, *Hand Clin* 8(2):263-273, 1992.
132. So YT, Olney RK, Aminoff MJ: Evaluation of thermography in the diagnosis of selected entrapment neuropathies, *Neurology* 39:1-5, 1989.
133. Spinner M, Kaplan EB: The relationship of the ulnar nerve to the medial intermuscular septum in the arm and its clinical significance, *Hand* 8:239-242, 1976.
134. Spinner M: Management of nerve compression lesions of the upper extremity. In Omer GE, Spinner M, editors: *Management of peripheral nerve problems,* Philadelphia, 1980, WB Saunders, pp 569-592.
135. Spinner RJ, Spinner M: Partial median nerve entrapment in the distal arm because of an accessory bicipital aponeurosis, *J Hand Surg* 16A:236-244, 1991.
136. Sponseller PD, Engber WD: Double-entrapment radial tunnel syndrome, *J Hand Surg [Am]* 8:420-423.
137. Thompson JE: Anatomical methods of approach in operations on the long bones of the extremities, *Ann Surg* 68:309, 1918.
138. Thomsen PB: Compression neuritis of the ulnar nerve treated with simple decompression, *Acta Orthop Scand* 48:164-167, 1977.
139. Tsairis P: Differential diagnosis of peripheral neuropathies. In Omer GE, Spinner M, editors: *Management of peripheral nerve problems,* Philadelphia, 1980, WB Saunders, pp 712-726.
140. Upton ARM, McComas AJ: The double crush in nerve entrapment syndromes, *Lancet* 2:359-362, 1973.
141. Urbaniak JR, Gabel GT: Perspective on the operative treatment for cubital tunnel syndrome. In Gelberman RH, editor: *Operative nerve repair and reconstruction,* Philadelphia, 1991, JB Lippincott.
142. Vanderpool DW et al: Peripheral compression lesions of the ulnar nerve, *J Bone Joint Surg [Br]* 50:792, 1948.
143. Vorenkamp SE, Nelson TL: Ulnar nerve entrapment due to heterotopic bone formation after a severe burn, *J Hand Surg [Br]* 50: 792-803, 1968.
144. Wadsworth TG: The external compression syndrome of the ulnar nerve at the cubital tunnel, *Clin Orthop* 124:189-204, 1977.
145. Wadsworth TG: *The elbow,* New York, 1982, Churchill-Livingstone, p 273.
146. Werner C: Lateral elbow pain and posterior interosseous nerve entrapment, *Acta Orthop Scand* [Suppl] 174:1-62, 1979.
147. Wilson FD et al: Valgus extension overload in the pitching elbow, *Am J Sports Med* 11(2):83, 1983.
148. Woltman HW, Kernohan JW: Disease of peripheral nerves. In Baker AB, editor: *Clinical neurology,* New York, 1955, Hoeber-Harper, p 1629.
149. Zemel NP, Jobe FW, Yocum LA: Submuscular transposition/ulnar nerve decompression in athletes. In Gelberman RH, editor: *Operative nerve repair and reconstruction,* Philadelphia, 1991, JB Lippincott, p 1100.

CHAPTER 24

Forearm Compartment Syndromes

DARRYL KAN

Compartment syndrome of the forearm, although much less commonly seen than that of the lower extremity, is an important diagnosis to consider in the athlete with forearm pain. This syndrome can have either an acute or chronic onset and may involve the dorsal compartment, volar compartment, or both. Most of the clinical data regarding this entity have come from case reports because large patient series are uncommon.

MECHANISM OF INJURY

Acute

The pathophysiology of acute compartment syndrome has been well described.* The initiating factor is an increase in interstitial fluid pressure occurring in a closed myofascial compartment. This pressure comes from capillary blood flow causing a tamponade effect and vascular occlusion. Over time, this may lead to a decrease in tissue perfusion with subsequent ischemia and possible permanent damage to the myoneural elements within that closed space. There is, however, some maintenance of peripheral blood flow as arterial pulses remain intact because the intracompartmental pressure is generally less than the arterial pressure.[24]

In addition to ischemia, certain metabolic changes also appear to occur, resulting in pain, dysfunction, and necrosis of local tissues. Heppenstall et al compared muscle changes induced by tourniquet ischemia with those resulting from increased interstitial pressure produced by infused plasma in dogs.[15] They found an accelerated breakdown of high-energy phosphate and more extensive cellular acidosis in muscle under pressure.

*References 4, 7, 12, 15, 18, 21, 23, 26, 29, 34-36.

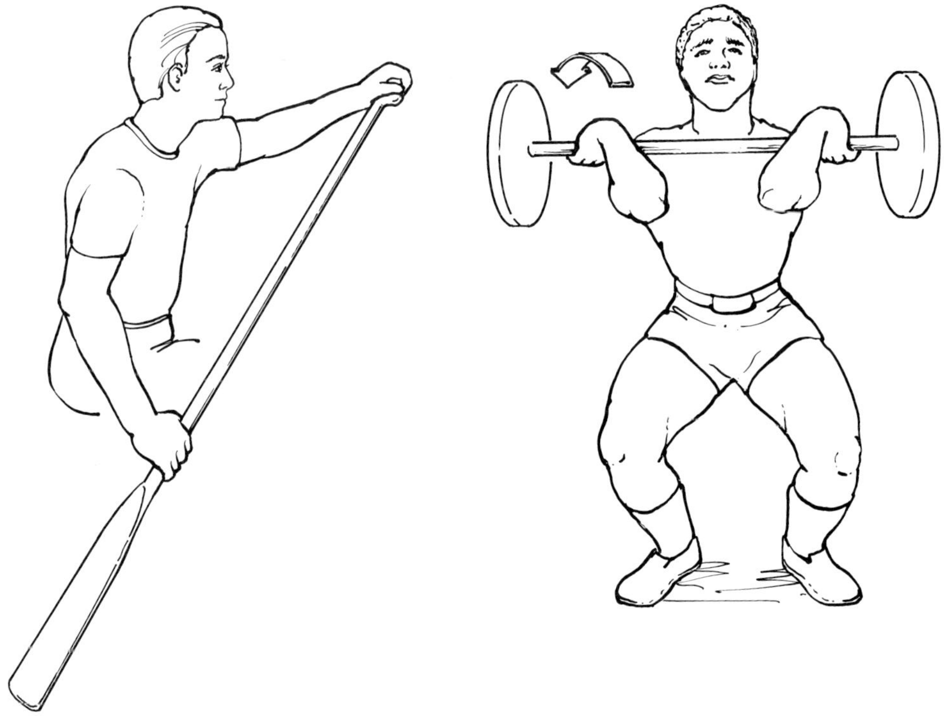

FIGURE 24-1 Although compartment syndrome has generally been associated with high-energy trauma, certain continuous repetitive activities, such as canoe paddling and weight lifting, have been implicated as etiologies.

They also theorized that elevated tissue pressure acts synergistically with ischemia to produce a more severe degree of cellular deterioration than produced by ischemia alone. The exact mechanism by which these metabolic changes occur, however, remains poorly understood.

In the acute form, this entire process often is irreversible without surgical intervention. There is usually an inciting event leading to intramuscular bleeding and swelling and subsequent increase in interstitial pressure. Traditionally, these etiologic events have included fractures, soft-tissue crush injuries, limb compression, severe contusion, burns, vascular trauma, injection injuries, and bleeding dyscrasias.[25,26] Recent case reports have described specific etiologies regarding sporting activities, including prolonged volar forearm contraction in a canoe paddler (Fig. 24-1), closed tendon avulsion in a car driver, and a Salter II fracture of the distal radius in an adolescent football player.[8,25,34] These reports demonstrate that acute compartment syndrome of the forearm can be seen in patients with trauma much less severe than traditionally has been expected. This is a particularly important point for those treating the athlete.

Chronic

As noted in the acute form, the basic pathophysiology process in chronic exertional compartment syndrome of the forearm is a rise in interstitial fluid pressure that impairs capillary circulation and compromises the delivery of metabolites to the tissues. In the chronic form, however, the rise in intracompartmental pressure is intermittent and reversible and usually is related to a muscular response to unaccustomed or overly strenuous exercise.

Exercise with either an isometric or isotonic contraction produces a rise in intramuscular blood volume and an increase in muscle weight of as much as 20%.[7] Compression of this increased interstitial fluid during contraction leads to pressure elevation within the closed myofascial compartment.[12] With chronic exercise, resultant muscle hypertrophy also can increase compartment volume and contribute to pressure changes. This increased pressure, if sustained, may lead to capillary occlusion and compartmental ischemia. As in the acute form, there also may be a local accumulation of lactic acid resulting from decreased blood flow.[15,34]

The most critical intracompartmental pressures are related to the postexercise state.[7,26,31] During this period, clinical manifestations of ischemia are directly correlated to how quickly the muscle is able to reduce the swelling to preexercise levels. Intensity of muscular effort also is related.[7] The level of intracompartmental pressure after exercise, as well as the levels during contraction, distinguishes the normal athlete from those with chronic exertional compartment syndrome.[7,26,30,31] Pressures that are considered pathologic remain high both during and after exercise.

Tompkins has described the histology of muscle in chronic compartment syndrome of the forearm, noting an increase in interstitial edema and a reduction and sometimes an absence of transverse striations.[34] These histologic findings were quite different from those of purely ischemic muscle. The latter is characterized by retention of its striations and nuclear structure and is nearly indistinguishable from normal cells. Tompkins theorized that the differences seen in muscle subjected to chronic exertional compartment syndrome were in the accumulation of excessive metabolites that ultimately contributed to tissue necrosis.

Case reports regarding chronic exertional compartment syndrome of the forearm describe many different etiologies, but all seem to involve activities requiring strenuous and continuous contraction of both volar and dorsal compartment muscles. These activities include power lifting (see Fig. 24-1), motocross riding, and tennis.[1,3,33] Athletes involved in other sports requiring repetitive forearm contraction, such as bowling, archery, sport fishing, and windsurfing, also may be at risk.

CLINICAL PRESENTATION

Acute

The patient with acute compartment syndrome of the forearm may present after a traumatic event, whether minor or severe, or after cessation of vigorous exercise. The onset of symptoms usually is immediate but can occur several hours later. The patient complains of severe pain over the affected compartment that is characteristically out of proportion to what normally would be expected. The pain often increases with movement of the fingers, and there is associated forearm swelling with numbness of the fingers.

The earliest physical findings, according to Mubarak, are swelling and palpable tenseness over the involved compartment.[26,28] The patient usually will demonstrate exquisite tenderness, and the skin may be hot and erythematous. Many authors have described an increase in pain with passive range of motion of the digits, but Mubarak suggests that this may be subjective and unreliable because the pain could stem from direct trauma rather than muscle ischemia.[4,10,20,22,26]

Mubarak and Gelberman agree that the most frequent physical finding is a sensory deficit involving the median nerve, ulnar nerve, or both.[10,26] This deficit is best measured by two-point sensibility that may increase to 10 mm (normal is up to 6 to 7 mm) in the patient with acute compartment syndrome. The vascular examination usually is normal, with palpable and symmetric pulses and brisk capillary refill. Rarely is the rise in intracompartmental pressure high enough to occlude a major artery. Thus the examiner should not rule out an acute compartment syndrome based on a normal vascular exam.

Laboratory examination is of little value, although some authors have reported a rise in CPK and LDH levels.[3] Hematocrit and erythrocyte sedimentation rate usually are normal. The most valuable diagnostic tool is the direct measurement of intracompartmental pressure.

Chronic

In the patient with chronic compartment syndrome, symptoms usually are related to exercise. Pain, muscle tightness, and a cramping sensation are the most common complaints and may occur during or after the cessation of activity.[2,4,6,17,20,29,33] The patient often is forced to terminate exercise or at least decrease the intensity secondary to pain. With rest, the symptoms usually subside and the patient returns to a normal, asymptomatic state. The time required for relief is variable, ranging from minutes to hours, and often is proportional to the intensity of effort involved. Neurovascular symptoms are uncommon, but they do occur, and they also resolve with rest.

Investigating the patient's exercise program is helpful because many patients will report that the activity that precipitated the symptoms was initiated after a prolonged period of rest or that the intensity of effort was significantly increased from normal.[4,20] These are important clues in the diagnosis of chronic compartment syndrome. They can be elicited with a thorough and detailed history. Unfortunately, the physical findings associated with chronic compartment syndrome may be sparse, especially if the patient is seen during a pain-free interval. The examiner might ask the patient to exercise before the examination to recreate the symptoms. Tenderness over the affected myofascial compartment and exquisite tenderness can be seen under these conditions. In addition, the incidence of fascial defects is increased in patients with recurrent compartment syndrome.[7] Sensory and motor deficits are variable, and vascular occlusion, as noted with acute compartment syndrome, is uncommon.[9,14] Again, tissue-pressure monitoring is the most useful diagnostic tool.

DIFFERENTIAL DIAGNOSIS AND CLASSIFICATION

The signs and symptoms of acute compartment syndrome are easily recognized. When suspected, it should be investigated with intracompartmental pressure monitoring. The diagnosis of chronic compartment syndrome, on the other hand, can be subtle, and other conditions should be considered in the differential diagnosis. These include nerve compression syndromes, vascular disorders, tumors, osteomyelitis, tenosynovitis, and epicondylitis.[3,20,33] A detailed history and physical examination, as well as tissue-pressure monitoring when indicated, should determine the diagnosis.

Compartment syndromes of the forearm generally are classified according to chronology of symptoms (acute or chronic [recurrent]) and location (dorsal, volar, or both) (Fig. 24-2). Traditionally, the dorsal and volar compartments of the forearm were believed to be separated by the interosseous membrane, fibrous septa between the antebrachial fascia, and bone (radius and ulna), thus creating independent compartments, as in the lower extremity.[4]

Gelberman, however, has shown through compartment pressure measurements in cadavers that no firm fascial divisions exist, at least from a functional standpoint.[11] He noted that when intracompartmental pressure was experimentally elevated in the volar and dorsal compartments with plasma infusion, volar fasciotomy alone could lower pressures in both compartments to an acceptable range. The same could not be accomplished with an isolated dorsal fasciotomy. Gelberman thought that this was related to the amount of muscle mass directly decompressed. Thus, although the compartments are not completely independent, they are somewhat different in their mass composition, and classification by location is still beneficial.

SPECIAL ASSESSMENTS

Intracompartmental Pressure Measurements

The most useful diagnostic tool used to confirm the diagnosis of compartment syndrome is intracompartmental pressure monitoring. Several techniques have been described.[19,27,32,35,36] For years, the standard technique was to insert a needle manometer directly into the intramuscular compartment to be measured. Injection of saline was required so that the free fluid was present at

A

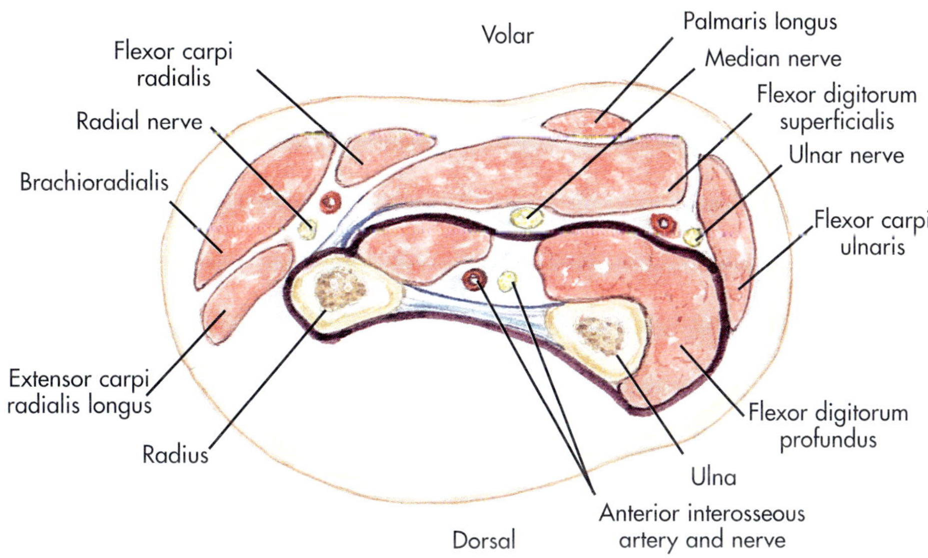

B

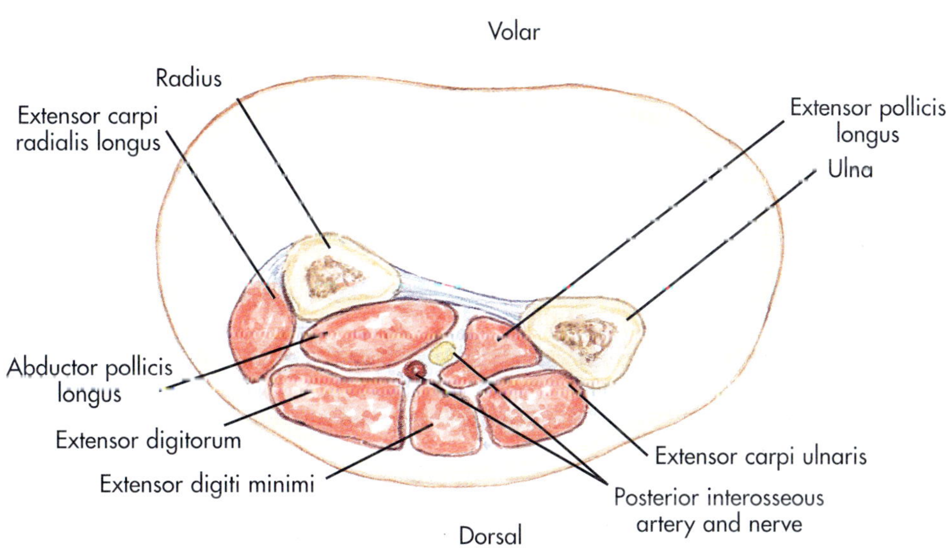

FIGURE 24-2 **A,** Volar compartment cross-sectional anatomy at midforearm. **B,** Dorsal compartment cross-sectional anatomy at midforearm.

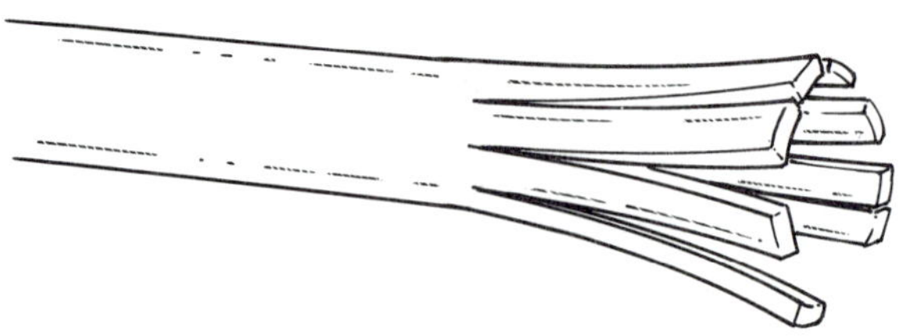

FIGURE 24-3 Slit catheter is composed of polyethylene tubing with 3 mm slits at the tip preventing occlusion of the bore.

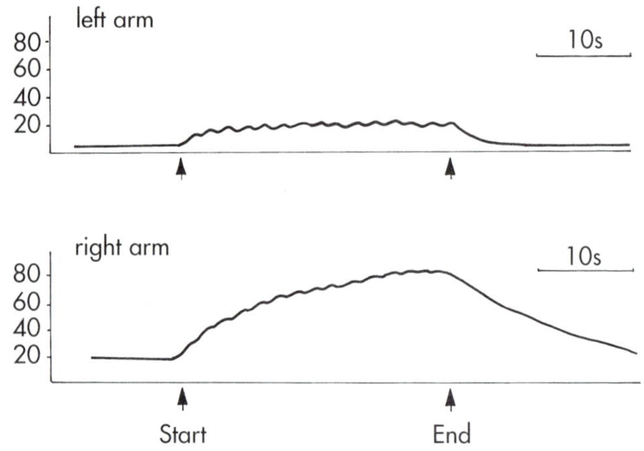

FIGURE 24-4 Intracompartmental pressure graph in symptomatic patient depicts increased levels at rest and before and after exercise.

the needle orifice. Some investigators, however, thought that this caused a disequilibrium, inflating the actual pressure measured.[27,32] In addition, the needle orifice could become obstructed with soft tissue, causing low reading at high pressures.

Mubarak described the use of the wick catheter in which fibrils made of the soluble braided Dexon suture protrude from the tip of the catheter assembly, providing an extensive contact area for fluid equilibrium and preventing obstruction.[27] This type of catheter was well suited to long-term continuous monitoring, which is required in the diagnosis of chronic compartment syndrome.

Recently, Rorabeck introduced the slit catheter[32] (Fig. 24-3). This device is made of polyethylene tubing with five symmetrical slits placed in the tip and extending 3 mm in length. The serrations and the small spaces between the serrations prevent total occlusion of the bore without the artifact of injected fluid, making this catheter ideal for continuous monitoring. Fronek, when comparing the wide and slit catheters, found that both catheters were equally accurate but that the slit catheter provided a higher-frequency response during exercise.[7]

As Martens noted, tissue pressure can be monitored through any of the above techniques.[20] Most important is that the examiner be experienced with the technique being used so that reliable data can be obtained.

In acute compartment syndrome, the clinical history and physical examination play the primary role in establishing the diagnosis. Tissue-pressure monitoring therefore should be used as an adjunct to confirm the diagnosis. Different parameters defining acute compartment syndrome have been described in the literature. In general, pressures reaching a threshold of 30 to 60 mm Hg below resting diastolic pressure should be considered as indications for fasciotomy.[23,35,36] In certain traumatic injuries, such as fractures and limb compression, the diagnosis may be evident based on symptoms and physical examination and delaying fasciotomy to measure intracompartmental pressures may not be warranted.

Parameters for Chronic Compartment Syndrome

In chronic compartment syndrome, measurement of intracompartmental pressures plays a larger role in diagnosis because the physical exam may be normal, especially if the patient is seen during an asymptomatic interval. Normal resting pressures in the forearm compartments range from 0 to 15 mm Hg and may rise to as high as 30 to 40 mm Hg during exercise[33] (Fig. 24-4). Pressures will return to resting values several minutes after the cessation of activity. There is some debate regarding which pressures are most important in the diagnosis. Some investigators believe that pressures obtained during exercise are of greatest value,[30,33] but others stress the importance of resting pressures and pressures obtained after exercise.[7,26,31] In general, the most consistent parameters identified for confirming the diagnosis of chronic exertional compartment syndrome are intracompartmental resting pressures greater than or equal to 15 mm Hg and/or 5 minutes after exercise greater than or equal to 25 mm Hg.[7,20,26,31] Patients usually will demonstrate higher-than-normal pressures during exercise, but it is more difficult to quantify an abnormal level at that time.

Ultrasound

Ultrasound has been used to quantify volume changes in myofascial compartments in normal subjects before and after exercise.[5,13] Gershuni et al reported a 10.1% increase in anterior leg compartment volume in asymptomatic joggers and an 8.6% increase in asymptomatic nonjoggers.[13] They believed that this difference was due to adaptive fascial compliance. They hypothesized that in joggers with low fascial compliance, swelling during exercise with concomitant muscle hypertrophy could produce prolonged muscle ischemia. Investigators have proposed that this test be used as an adjunct to intracompartmental measurements, but as yet no reports have described its use in compartment syndrome, so the diagnostic parameters are not known.

MRI

MRI scans generally are not helpful in the diagnosis of chronic compartment syndrome. They may show an increase in the circumference of the compartment and obscuration of previously well-defined fascial planes. However, these findings are nonspecific.[29] Certainly, in acute compartment syndrome, where timeliness in the diagnosis is of paramount importance, an MRI scan is not indicated.

NONSURGICAL TREATMENT

In acute compartment syndrome of the forearm, nonsurgical treatment is contraindicated. The treatment of choice is an expedient decompressive fasciotomy. In chronic compartment syndrome, conservative treatment also is of little value. In most cases, restriction of the offending activity will temporarily relieve symptoms. However, the majority of patients will have recurrence of symptoms on their return to those offending activities. Patients who refuse to modify their activities and have persistence of symptoms will require surgery.

PREFERRED SURGICAL TREATMENT

The preferred surgical treatment for both acute and chronic compartment syndrome of the forearm is decompressive fasciotomy. In the acute situation, surgery should be performed promptly because there is a very short time during which muscle ischemia is reversible. In chronic compartment syndrome, the symptoms themselves are reversible, allowing surgery to be performed on an elective basis.

The involved compartment, either volar or dorsal, should undergo an appropriate fasciotomy. If both are involved, then the volar compartment should be decompressed first and dorsal intracompartmental pressures measured. If these pressures are not greater than 20 to 30 mm Hg, then dorsal fasciotomy may not be required.[10,11] When clinical findings and pressures are equivocal, the safest choice is to decompress both compartments.

Surgical Technique—Volar Fasciotomy

Many techniques for volar fasciotomy have been described. We prefer the modified Henry approach, described by Gelberman,[10,11] with the skin incision beginning 1 cm proximal to the antecubital fossa and just medial to the biceps tendon (Fig. 24-5). The incision then is gently curved laterally across the fossa to the medial border of the brachioradialis. From here, it is brought back to the midline at the junction of the middle third and the distal third of the forearm, and then continued distally, ulnar to the palmaris longus and then across the carpal tunnel.

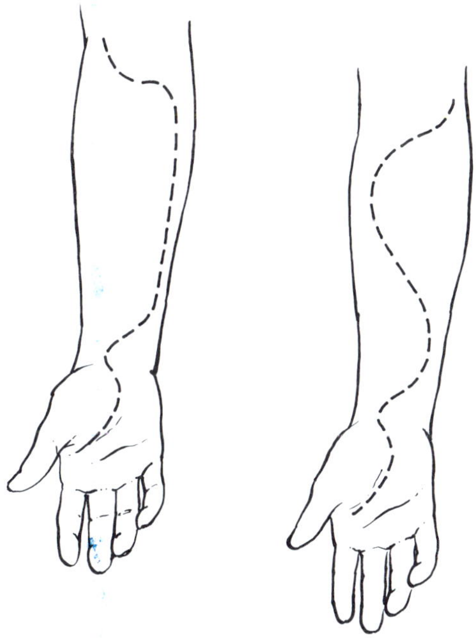

FIGURE 24-5 Curvilinear volar and volar-ulnar incisions described by Gelberman can be used for fasciotomy.

The lacertus fibrosus, encountered proximally, is divided, and a fasciotomy of the superficial compartment is performed starting 1 cm proximal to the elbow and ending at the wrist. The carpal tunnel then is decompressed. It is also important to release the deep volar compartment, which may have isolated involvement. The deep compartment is accessed through the interval between the brachioradialis and flexor carpi radialis, which is entered proximally (Fig. 24-6). The radial artery and superficial radial nerve are identified and retracted laterally with the brachioradialis. The fasciae over the flexor pollicis longus, flexor digitorum profundus, and pronator quadratus are incised individually to ensure an adequate decompression.

Gelberman notes that it is also important to inspect the potential sites of median nerve compression.[10] These include the lacertus fibrosus, which is always released, as well as the proximal edge of the pronator teres and the proximal edge of the flexor digitorum superficialis. Any constriction is carefully dissected free and removed. The skin and subcutaneous tissue usually are left open and are closed secondarily unless primary closure can be achieved without undue tension. The latter is more likely to be possible in chronic cases. Occasionally when the skin cannot be closed secondarily, a split-thickness skin graft is required.

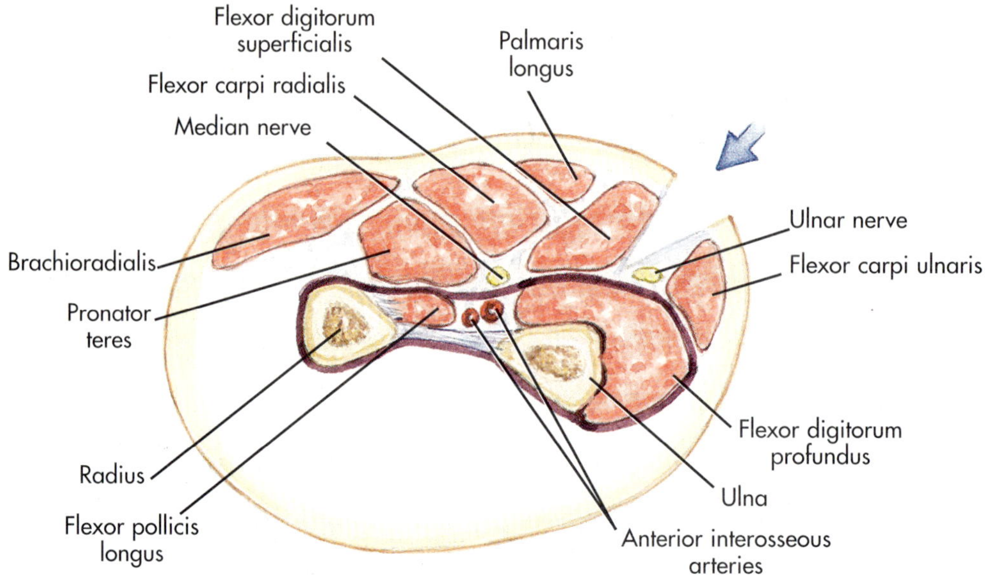

FIGURE 24-6 Deep volar compartment is entered through interval between flexor carpi radialis and brachioradialis. The superficial radial nerve and radial artery lie in this interval.

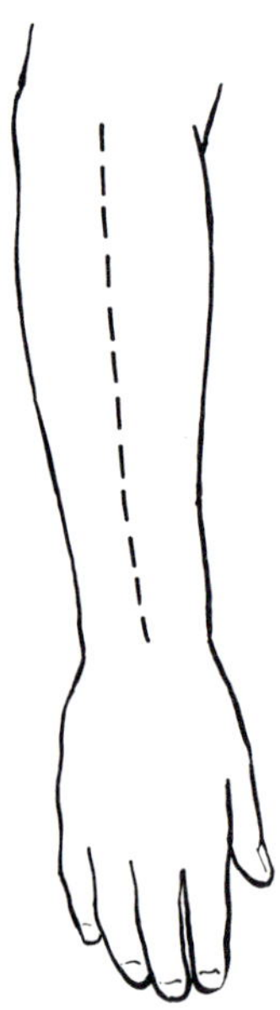

FIGURE 24-7 A straight midline incision is used for dorsal fasciotomy.

Surgical Technique—Dorsal Fasciotomy

Dorsal fasciotomy is achieved through a midline skin incision that begins 2 cm distal to the lateral epicondyle and ends just proximal to the wrist joint (Fig. 24-7). The dorsal fascia is incised directly in line with the skin incision. Some authors have recommended individual episiotomy of each muscle, but this is not thought to be necessary in most cases.* Fascial defects, if encountered, should not be closed. These are thought to be a manifestation of compartment syndrome, and recurrences have been associated with their closure.[7]

POSTOPERATIVE REHABILITATION

After the skin and subcutaneous tissue are closed, patients are immobilized in an above-elbow splint in 90° of flexion until the wounds have healed. The splint then can be discontinued, and active and passive range-of-motion exercises of the elbow, wrist, and hand are begun. Strengthening exercises are added when swelling is controlled and range of motion is improving. Recovery usually depends on the extent of involvement and, in acute cases, the time from onset of symptoms to surgery. In chronic cases, recovery is even more variable. This postoperative period can range from weeks to months.

SUMMARY

Compartment syndrome of the forearm can be seen in both the acute and chronic setting. When the diagnosis is suspected, intracompartmental pressure should be monitored. Treatment usually is surgical and involves a complete fasciotomy. Observation is contraindicated in the acute setting and usually is of little value in chronic cases. The key to treatment is making the diagnosis. The clinician should maintain a high index of suspicion in the athlete with acute or chronic forearm pain.

*References 3, 10, 11, 16, 23, 28.

References

1. Allen MJ, Barnes MR: Chronic compartment syndrome of the flexor muscles in the forearm: a case report, *J Hand Surg [Br]* 14:47, 1989.
2. Allen MJ, Barnes MR: Exercise pain in the lower leg: chronic compartment syndrome and medial tibial syndrome, *J Bone Joint Surg* 68B:818, 1986.
3. Bird CB, McCoy JW: Weight-lifting as a cause of compartment syndrome in the forearm: a case report, *J Bone Joint Surg [Am]* 65:406, 1983.
4. Black KP, Schultz TK, Cheung NL: Compartment syndrome in athletes, *Clin Sports Med* 9:471, 1990.
5. Brahim F, Zaccardelli W: Ultrasound measurement of the anterior leg compartment, *Am J Sports Med* 14:300, 1986.
6. Detmer DE et al: Chronic compartment syndrome: diagnosis, management and outcomes, *Am J Sports Med* 13:162, 1985.
7. Fronek MD et al: Management of chronic exertional anterior compartment syndrome of the lower extremity, *Clin Orthop* 220:217, 1987.
8. Gainor BJ: Closed avulsion of the flexor digitorum superficialis origin compartment syndrome: a case report, *J Bone Joint Surg [Am]* 66:467, 1984.
9. Garfin S, Mubarak SJ, Owen CA: Exertional anterolateral compartment syndrome: case report with fascial defect, muscle herniation, and superficial peroneal nerve entrapment, *J Bone Joint Surg [Am]* 59:404, 1977.
10. Gelberman RH et al: Compartment syndromes of the forearm: diagnosis and treatment, *Clin Orthop* 161:252, 1981.
11. Gelberman RH et al: Decompression of forearm compartment syndromes, *Clin Orthop* 134:225, 1978.
12. Imbriglia JE, Boland DM: An exercise induced compartment syndrome of the dorsal forearm: a case report, *J Hand Surg [Am]* 9:142, 1984.
13. Gershuni DG, Gosink BB, Hargens AR: Ultrasound evaluation of the anterior musculofascial compartment of the leg following exercise, *Clin Orthop* 167:185, 1982.
14. Hargens AR et al: Peripheral nerve-conduction block by high muscle-compartment pressure, *J Bone Joint Surg [Am]* 61:192, 1979.
15. Heppenstall RB et al: A comparative study of the tolerance of skeletal muscle to ischemia: tourniquet application compared with acute compartment syndrome, *J Bone Joint Surg [Am]* 68:820, 1986.
16. Imbriglia JE, Boland DM: An exercise induced compartment syndrome of the dorsal forearm: a case report, *J Hand Surg [Am]* 9:142, 1984.
17. Kutz JE, Singer R, Lindsay M: Chronic exertional compartment syndrome of the forearm: a case report, *J Hand Surg [Am]* 10:302, 1985.
18. Leach RE, Hammand G, Stryker WS: Anterior tibial compartment syndrome: acute and chronic, *J Bone Joint Surg [Am]* 49:451, 1967.
19. Logan JG, Rorabeck CH, Castle GSP: The measurement of dynamic compartment pressure during exercise, *Am J Sports Med* 11:220, 1983.
20. Martens MA, Moeyersoons JP: Acute and recurrent effort-related compartment syndrome in sports, *Sports Med* 9:62, 1990.
21. Matsen FA III, Drugmire RB Jr, King RV: Increased tissue pressure and its effects on muscle oxygenation in level and elevated human limbs: Nicholas Andry award, *Clin Orthop* 144:311, 1979.
22. Matsen FA III, Winquist RA, Krugmire RB Jr: Diagnosis and management of compartment syndrome, *J Bone Joint Surg [Am]* 62:286, 1980.
23. Matsen FA III: *Compartment syndromes,* New York, 1981, Grune & Stratton.
24. Matsen FA III et al: The effects of limb elevation and dependency on local arteriovenous gradients in normal human limbs with particular reference to limbs with increased tissue pressure, *Clin Orthop* 150:187, 1980.
25. Matthews LS: Acute volar compartment syndrome secondary to distal radius fracture in an athlete: a case report, *Am J Sports Med* 11:6, 1983.
26. Mubarak SJ, Hargens AR: *Compartment syndromes and Volkmann's ischemic contracture,* Philadelphia, 1981, WB Saunders.
27. Mubarak SJ et al: The wick catheter technique for measurement of intramuscular pressure: a new research and clinical tool, *J Bone Joint Surg [Am]* 58:1016, 1976.
28. Mubarak SJ et al: Acute compartment syndromes: diagnosis and treatment with the aid of the wick catheter, *J Bone Joint Surg [Am]* 60:1091, 1978.
29. Pedowitz RA, Toutounghi FM: Chronic exertional compartment syndrome of the forearm flexor muscles, *J Hand Surg [Am]* 13:694, 1988.
30. Puranen J, Alavaikko A: Intracompartmental pressure increase on exertion in patients with chronic compartment syndrome in the leg, *J Bone Joint Surg [Am]* 63:1304, 1981.
31. Rorabeck CH, Bourne RB, Fowler PJ: The surgical treatment of exertional compartment syndrome in athletes, *J Bone Joint Surg [Am]* 65:1245, 1983.
32. Rorabeck CH et al: Compartment pressure measurements: an experimental investigation using the slit catheter, *J Trauma* 21:446, 1981.
33. Rydholm U, Werner C, Ohlin P: Intracompartmental forearm pressure during rest and exercise, *Clin Orthop* 175:213, 1983.
34. Tompkins DG: Exercise myopathy of the extensor carpi ulnaris muscle, *J Bone Joint Surg [Am]* 59:407, 1977.
35. Whitesides TE Jr, Harada H, Morimoto K: Compartment syndromes and the role of fasciotomy, its parameters and techniques. In: *Instructional Course Lecture, The American Academy of Orthopaedic Surgeons,* vol 26, St Louis, 1977, CV Mosby, pp 179-196.
36. Whitesides TE Jr et al: Tissue pressure measurements as a determinant for the need of fasciotomy, *Clin Orthop* 113:43, 1975.

PART FOUR

The Wrist and Hand

CHAPTER 25

Biomechanics

THOMAS D. CAHALAN
WILLIAM P. COONEY

Understanding the biomechanics of the hand and wrist is important for the scientific evaluation, confirmation of the diagnosis, and management of sports-related injuries. Perhaps no area of the body is more important than the hand and wrist, which serve to deliver thrust, produced by body mechanics at the shoulder and elbow, to objects being thrown, batted, served, hit, or resisted. As a result of the combined forces of body momentum and acceleration generated through the shoulder and elbow, the hand and wrist become susceptible to a number of injuries related to the transmission of force. The purpose of this chapter is to consider methods of assessing force transmission (kinetics) through the hand and wrist, measure motion (kinematics) of the hand and wrist, examine recent biomechanical studies and their relationship to sports-related injuries, and discuss from a biomechanical point of view specific sports-related injuries and determine the role that biomechanics must have in developing more effective treatment.

MECHANISMS OF INJURY

Sports-related injuries to the hand and wrist are the result of tensile, compressive, or torsional loads applied directly to the hand and wrist from a fall or from striking an object, or indirectly from striking an object, such as with a bat or racquet. Laboratory studies have demonstrated that the majority of wrist-related injuries result from a combination of tensile loads on the palmar side of the wrist in combination with compression loads on the central and dorsal aspects of the wrist.[53] Fractures and dislocations of the hand involving the fingers and thumb also are a combination of compression loads from axially transmitted forces and both tensile and torsional load.[9] Thumb ligament injury, for example, may result from torsion applied through a ski pole to the resisting thumb and finger grip.

Studies of the mechanism of injuries at the wrist consistently demonstrate that hyperextension of the wrist is associated with volar tensile load. As a result, fractures and fracture-dislocations of the wrist, such as scaphoid fractures or purely ligamentous injuries of the wrist, such as scapholunate dissociation, depend on the degree of wrist extension, position of radioulnar deviation, and amount of force applied. Studies by Mayfield et al of perilunate injuries of the wrist as well as studies by Weber and Chao of scaphoid fractures and fracture-dislocations of the wrist demonstrated that a force of 150 to 200 kg applied to the hyperextended wrist will produce these specific injuries.[32,53] Linscheid and Dobyns have suggested that there is a spectrum of perilunate instability related to the amount of force, point of application, and resultant force distribution.[27] Investigators have demonstrated clinically that one or more fractures with or without ligament injuries can result from the same injury mechanism. With the wrist in hyperextension and radial deviation, a fracture of the scaphoid will occur. However, with the wrist in hyperextension and ulnar deviation, scapholunate dissociation will result. Scaphoid dissociation that involves all of the ligaments attached to the lunate progresses from its initial stages to perilunate dislocations as the final-stage result. In the younger individual, a scaphoid fracture can be produced by an extension loading mechanism, but in older patients fractures of the distal radius would occur. Based on the application and redistribution of applied force, fractures involving the wrist have been associated with fractures of the forearm, radial head, and distal humerus in the same extremity.

Fractures and dislocations involving the fingers and thumb have been observed after compression loads producing a typical "baseball finger" or jammed finger. In particular, these forces produce dorsal dislocations of inter-

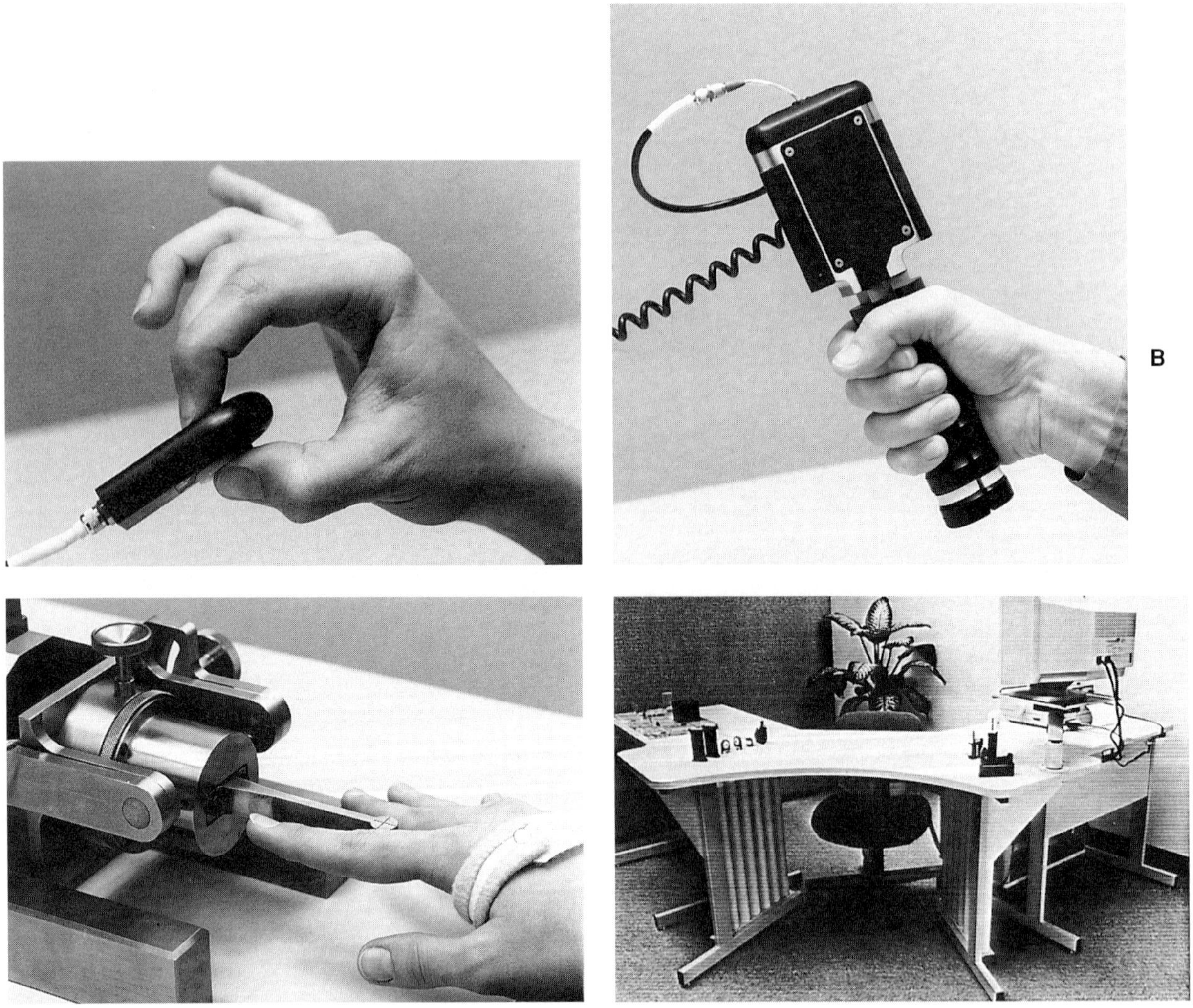

FIGURE 25-1 Strain-gauge instrumentation to assess **A,** pinch, **B,** grip, and **C,** intrinsic muscle abduction-adduction. **D,** These devices are now commercially available and can be computer integrated for a patient assessment program. (Courtesy NK Biotechnical Laboratories, Eden Prairie, MN.)

phalangeal joints. Torsional loads, such as those that produce skier's-thumb deformities, produce different effects on bones and joints, such as spiral fractures or joint-avulsion injuries. These require more specialized treatment modalities than would a fracture resulting from a direct blow, which might be inherently stable and require little or no reduction. Spiral fractures and avulsion injuries are associated with displacement, angulation, and rotational deformity.

Knowledge of the mechanism of injury therefore is very important in assessing the degree of bone and soft-tissue involvement in both the hand and wrist. The physician must evaluate associated bone and joint injuries both at the wrist and more proximally at the forearm, elbow, and shoulder. Treatment alternatives for specific injuries depend on the practitioner's knowledge of the injury mechanism. As part of understanding this mechanism of injury, it is important to perform a careful clinical examination of the patient to identify all areas of injury. The choice of radiographic tests and the plan for initial and subsequent treatment depend on a careful, complete initial examination.[10]

In addition to the clinical examination, the examiner now can employ a number of new measuring techniques and devices that will better evaluate the sports-related pathology.[1] These new assessment techniques include instrumented goniometers and dynamometers. Biplanar or triplanar goniometers can provide accurate measurements of loss of motion in the wrist or hand. The clinician can precisely determine strength with strain gauge instrumented pinch and grasp dynamometers, which provide comparative measurements of grip and pinch strength, rapid change-of-hand grip testing, and observations of weakness in grip and pinch in different wrist positions[37] (Fig. 25-1). The authors routinely use newer instruments for accurate isometric measurement of resisted wrist flexion and extension in our clinical assessment of patients (Fig. 25-2). Dynamic functional testing also is available, including measurement of maximum force output as well as endurance, work, and power, with the BTE and Lido upper-extremity assessment devices. To date, isokinetic measuring tools for the hand or for open versus closed chain exercise programs have not been developed. These would be valuable techniques, however, for measurement and testing of upper-extremity athletic injury. Although electromyographic studies have been applied to the shoulder and elbow,[14,50] no studies have examined the muscular contributions to strength and stability of the hand and wrist. Electromyographic techniques are being applied to sports-related injuries, and many areas of sports-related injuries to the hand and wrist structures remain to be clinically studied.

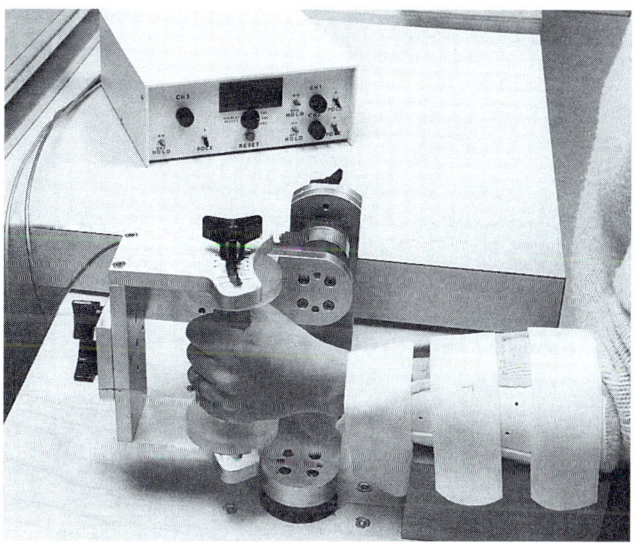

FIGURE 25-2 Isometric force measurement of wrist flexion using a strain gauge instrument, which is a hand-based dynamometer. The force peak and duration over time can be compared sequentially in the same person by using a patient-specific floppy disc or print recording. Fatigue-in-strength can be similarly assessed.

Wrist Kinematics

Wrist kinematics has been studied in a number of sports.[3,4,12,13,44] Using new techniques for motion analysis, three-dimensional motion of the wrist can be determined without interfering with the normal action and power of the hand or wrist in performing a specific sport. Biplanar electrogoniometers can be attached to the hand and distal forearm, and complex motions of the wrist, such as circumduction, can be measured while principal axes of planar motions of flexion-extension and radioulnar deviation are simultaneously determined[3,4] (Fig. 25-3). Magnetic field technology is another relatively new yet reliable study method, and uses magnetic position and orientation tracking systems to provide six degrees of freedom measurements of motion.[1] A "motion source" attached to the hand can be precisely plotted against a fixed "reference source" to record joint motion, changes in centers of joint rotation, and translation of carpal elements. For kinematic analysis, accelerometric methods can be used to measure the limb segment changes in velocity, giving a kinematic history of the joint of body part.[36] For example, accelerometers are used in analysis of throwing to determine maximum kinetic energy.

Most studies to date involving sports or daily activities have employed biplanar electrogoniometers. In golf, for example, studies demonstrate that wrist motion is integrated between two hands, with both hands assuming a certain amount of "cocking action" as the hands are preset to deliver force and direction to the golf swing[4] (Fig. 25-4). In both hands, wrist extension is associated with radial deviation and wrist flexion with ulnar deviation.

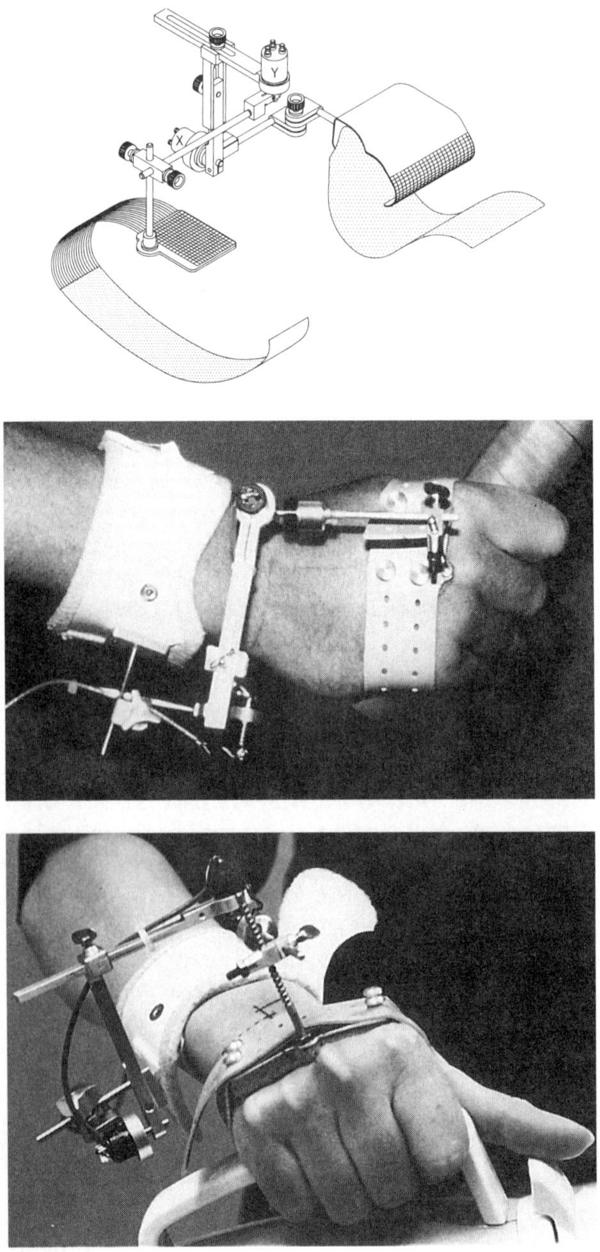

A

B

C

FIGURE 25-3 Biplanar wrist electogoniometer developed by E.Y.S. Chao, PhD. **A,** Potentiometers for wrist flexion-extension and, **B,** radioulnar deviation are with the base of the capitate, the instantaneous center of rotation. **B,** Dorsal alignment of the goniometer during the measurement of radioulnar deviation in tennis. **C,** Axial view of goniometer placement demonstration a "pouring grip" action. Note the alignment of dorsal potentiometer with the third metacarpal and the ulnar potentiometer with the midline of the distal ulna and the head of the capitate.

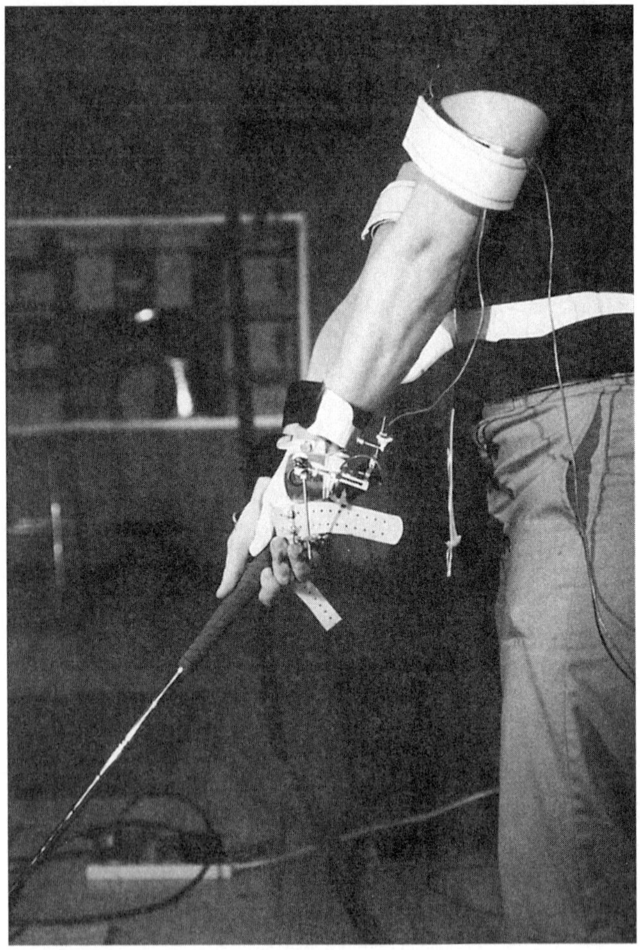

FIGURE 25-4 Analysis of the golf swing with biplanar electrogoniometers applied to both the left and right wrists. Elements of wrist "cocking phase" and position of the wrist at impact have been studied.

Radial deviation sets the hands for delivery, as does the hip turn and shoulder rotation, while ulnar deviation releases the power stored during the downswing to the impact phase to the golf stroke. The grip position of the left hand is a "power grip" position with the thumb on top of the club shaft, as with a hammer grip, while the right hand is positioned in prehensile or "precision grip," with the fingers and thumb, and not the palm, loosely gripping and controlling the club head in descent. Electrogoniometers made clear that the critical motion of the wrist was in a direction similar to that of "dart thrower's" wrist action, in which radial deviation and extension are linked in "cocking the wrist" and flexion and ulnar deviation deliver the thrust of power in "releasing the wrist."

Several authors have published data regarding maximum degrees of wrist motion (Table 25-1). Of the references noted, only Ryu et al[44] used an electrogoniometer in the assessment of motion, which we believe more accurately reflects total or global functional motion. Like

TABLE 25-1
Motion of the Wrist

Reference	Flexion (degrees)	Extension (degrees)	Radial Deviation (degrees)	Ulnar Deviation (degrees)
Hoppenfeld[19]	80	70	20	30
Cole[5]	90	70	20	30
Ryu et al[44]	79	59	21	38
Kapandji[21]	85	85	15	15
Engelberg[17]	60	60	20	30

Ryu et al, Palmar et al[39] assessed motion during various activities using a biaxial goniometer. Their studies found the normal useful range of flexion and extension to be a total of 133° (15° less than total motion) and the normal radial and ulnar deviation to be 40.5°. To complete most activities of daily living (excluding sports), Ryu et al found that 40° of wrist flexion and a combination of 40° of radial and ulnar deviation were needed.[44]

Flexion/extension motion (FEM) occurs through synchronous movement of the proximal and distal carpal rows. The center of rotation for the proximal row is located in the lunate, near the concavity, and the distal row locus is in the neck of the capitate. The overall wrist FEM locus is in the head of the capitate, midway between the individual raw loci.[28]

The total excursion of flexion and extension is equally distributed between the midcarpal and radiocarpal joints. Each carpal bone has a unique rotation and screw axis, which makes comparisons of relative motions somewhat complicated. The sum of relative motions is greater than the overall motion. For example, from full flexion to full extention, the capitate rotates 65.0° on the lunate, and the lunate rotates 58.6° on the radius. However, the capitate rotates 111.5° with respect to the radius. The apparent failure of the law of communication is explained by slightly out-of-plane rotations. In other words, the carpal bones not only flex and extend, they rotate as well.[22,43]

Radioulnar deviation (RUD) is more complex than FEM. The midcarpal joint contributes about 25% more motion than the radiocarpal joint contributes. The locus of RUD is in the head of the capitate, only a few millimeters from the sagittal plane locus. In the neutral position, the lunate and capitate are coaxially aligned. During radial deviation, laxity in the radiocapitate ligament allows palmar flexion of the proximal row. Conversely, ulnar deviation is accompanied by dorsiflexion of the proximal row. In addition, the distal row slightly supinates during radial deviation, and pronates during ulnar deviation.[28,43]

In the authors' biomechanics laboratory, differences in wrist motion among athletes were examined. The first study used biplanar electrogoniometers to assess the differences in wrist motion among the professional golfer, the amateur golfer, and patients (golfers) with disease involving the wrist. With different clubs and different strokes, clear differences in motion were seen. Professionals had a more repetitive, precise motion and delivery, but the "amateurs" of varying handicaps had considerable differences in the swing through the motion of the wrist and at the time of impact. In a previous study of normal wrist motion, most activities of daily living required only 40° of flexion-extension each and a total of 40° of radioulnar deviation. Golf was one functional activity, however, that required a maximum (above average) amount of radial deviation (25° to 30°) to set the wrist for power and club-head speed delivery (Fig. 25-5). Wrist flexion for golf was 65°, and wrist extension was 62°. With a golfer suffering from wrist disease, less flexion-extension motion (5° to 15°) and less accuracy than in age-matched normal wrists were observed. Ulnar deviation was the only wrist motion that was increased, and the increase appeared to result from a stronger effort to "pull-through" or force the club head farther through the swing phase. Wrist motion also was observed to vary during the different phases of the swing in the diseased wrist. With a change in the grip design to a "biocurved" handle, wrist motion and swing tempo improved, as did overall grip strength and tracking of the swing. With a large standard deviation between the normal and the involved wrists, however, statistical significance was observed only for ulnar deviation of the left wrist. Of interest, all other parameters of measurements of the golf swing (including club-head speed, club-head impact, and swing analysis) were unchanged with the biocurve grip compared with the normal grip. Further studies on the kinematics of the golf swing are needed not only to improve consistency but also to identify methods of limiting stress against the wrist in golfers with previous injury or disease affecting the wrist.[4]

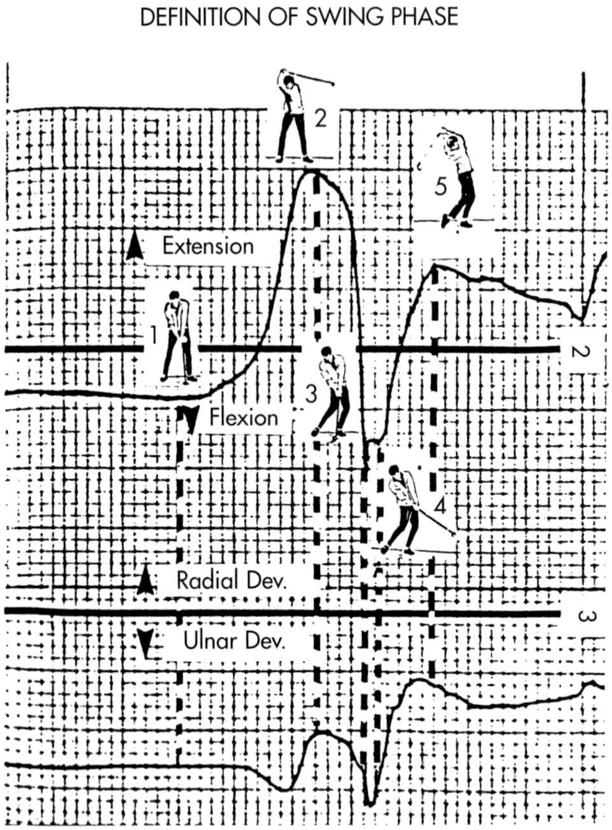

FIGURE 25-5 Tracing of wrist goniometric measurements during a golf swing. Position one represents the address, position two is the top of the back swing, position three is the hitting point (impact), position four is the wrist turn, and position five is the follow-through. Wrist flexion-extension is presented on the top tracing, and wrist radioulnar deviation is shown in the bottom tracing. Note the biphasic change in wrist motion during the five phases of the swing.

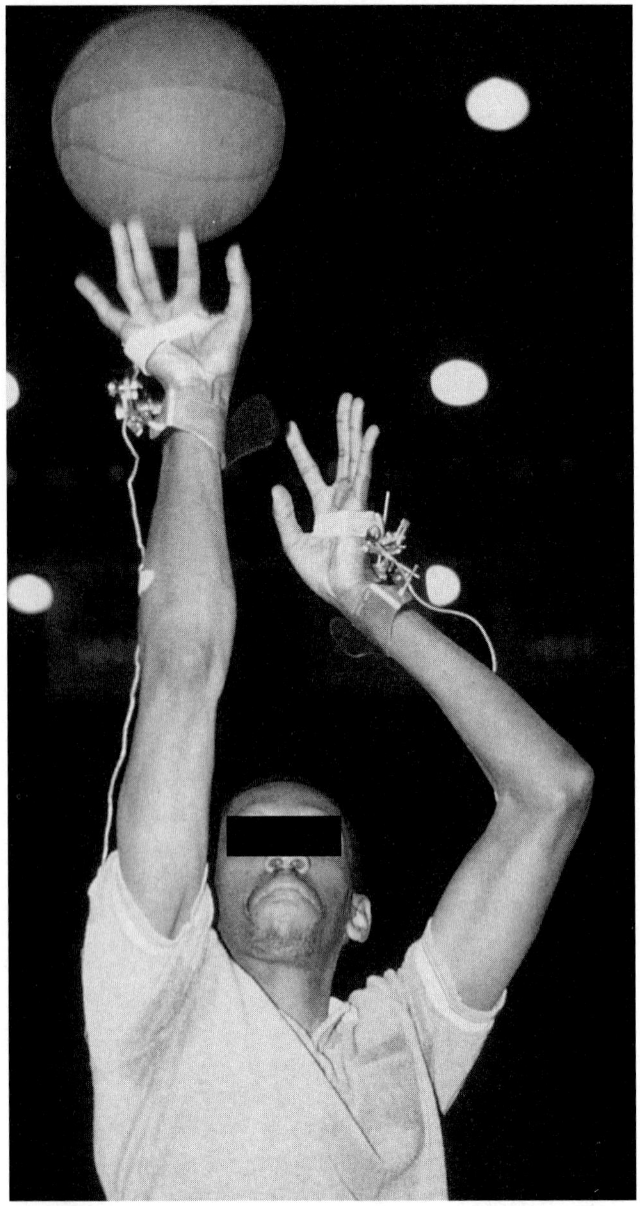

FIGURE 25-6 Analysis of shooting motion of the wrist in basketball. The "cocking phase" involved wrist extension–radial deviation; the "release phase" involved wrist flexion–ulnar deviation. These planes of motion are similar to other sports.

Motion of the wrist also has been studied in tennis, pitching, and basketball. Based on improved electrogoniometric technology, Ryu et al[44] studied wrist motion in six NCAA basketball players (Fig. 25-6). With the goniometer attached to the shooting hand (wrist), these authors determined that three phases of shooting were present: acceleration, velocity (constant), and deceleration. The wrist motion was (not surprisingly) similar to that in golf, with uniform flexion–ulnar deviation after the "cocking" position of extension–radial deviation. Some variation in acceleration-deceleration was noted, depending on the player, distance of the shot, and shot type (free throw versus jump shoot). Overall, wrist flexion-extension averaged 120° and radial deviation 23°. From a clinical perspective, Ryu et al suggested that a wrist ligament repair or partial fusion (STT fusion) preserved adequate motion for basketball shooting. However, when radial deviation of more than 20° is required, intercarpal fusions in particular may block this degree of motion. In fact, a study in the laboratory found that simulated STT fusion produced a wrist with 48° of extension and 68° of flexion, but radial deviation of 12° and ulnar deviation of 24°. Similar loss of radial deviation followed scaphocapitate fusion. The scaphoid after each fusion was observed to function as part of the distal carpal row. Therefore some loss of functional motion can be expected with operations on the wrist. These losses may affect the motion required to be effective in certain sports.[15]

In a study of wrist kinematics during the backhand

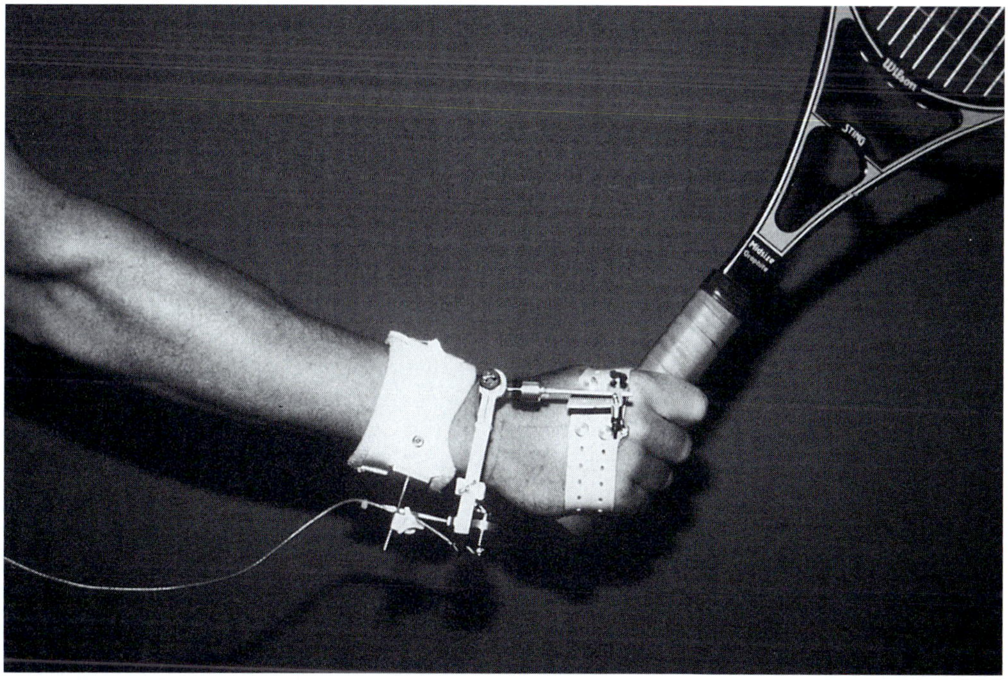

FIGURE 25-7 The backhand in tennis, novice vs. professional players, was studied with wrist goniometer. Changes in motion were observed in both the stroke and position of the wrist at the time of ball-racquet impact.

stroke in tennis (Fig. 25-7), novice players used a significantly different motion pattern than skilled players. At the moment of ball-racquet impact, novice players tend to have the wrist in a flexed position, but skilled players use an extended position. In addition, skilled players hit through the ball while using the wrist extensor muscles concentrically. Novice players attempt to hold the racquet stationary against the force of the ball, ending up with the extensor muscle working eccentrically. This phenomenon has been identified as the precipitating factor in lateral epicondylitis in novice tennis players.[3] Counterforce braces commonly used to lessen the symptoms of lateral epicondylitis have been reported to reduce EMG activity of the wrist extensors and reduce angular accelerations at the elbow. In the same study, a wrist brace was shown to reduce wrist angular acceleration; however, EMG recordings showed increased flexor and extensor activity.[16]

In a study of the loads exerted on a pommel horse, the wrists experienced very large forces. Peak forces averaged 1.12 to 1.52 BW (body weight units) and ranged as high as 2 BW. Mean support time ranged from 0.6 second to 1.18 seconds. The magnitude and duration of the forces depended on the maneuver being performed (e.g., hip circles, flares). In relationship to forces generated during other activities, the ground reaction forces during jogging are about 1.5 BW.[30]

WRIST AND HAND KINETICS

Forces across the wrist joint or hand have not been studied extensively in sports. In a review of recent texts that deal with athletic injuries of the upper extremity,[46] particularly the hand and wrist, there was little reference to the mechanism of injuries or the forces involved. However, researchers do have an active interest in wrist and hand force transmission, which could be applicable and the source for future studies. Force and pressure studies of the radiocarpal joint and distal radioulnar joint have increased our understanding of the basic mechanisms of these joints.[29,38] Static force analysis in the hand has been performed for both finger and thumb joints.[24] Studies show that with the application of one unit of force at the tip of the finger, there is a compression force of 6 kg at the proximal interphalangeal (PIP) joint and 10 to 12 kg at the metacarpophalangeal (MP) joint. Lateral stress or shear forces range from 1.5 to 3.5 times and torsional loads produce resistance to torque of 4 to 10 kg-cm. In the thumb, compression loads were measured at 2 kg for the IP joint, 7.5 kg for the MP joint, and 13 kg for the (TMC) joint. Torsion was calculated at 4 kg-cm.[6]

Combinations of bending and torsional loads appear responsible for most ligament injuries and sprains of the hand. Torsional loads appear responsible for finger and thumb collateral ligament injuries, spiral phalangeal and metacarpal fractures, and possibly Bennett's fractures of the thumb carpometacarpal (CMC) joint. Torque on the thumb can be considerable. For example, if a jar lid were 7.5 cm (3 inches) in diameter, the torque to turn the lid would be 7.5 cm times 4 kg-cm, or 30 kg-cm (132 lb-cm). In resisting the torque on the golf-club grip, the hands and wrist require 50 plus or minus 12 lb-in for a "biocurve" grip. Checking a swing in baseball could generate 16 to 20 kg-cm of force. A ball struck near the "hozzle" or handle of the bat would increase the inertial force such that if the bat did not break, the thumb or finger ligaments might rupture. Ligament forces have been calculated to resist dislocation forces at most of the finger and thumb joints. Moberg and Stenor[35] estimated that collateral ligaments resist 20 to 34 kg to bending. The amount of force for a PIP joint dislocation in a basketball or volleyball injury ranges from 125 to 150 kg, assuming the distance from the fingertip (point to applied load) to a PIP joint was 1.5 to 2.5 cm. An applied load of twice the player's body weight therefore would be needed to cause a dorsal PIP or lateral PIP joint dislocation. A protective splint or metal bar may provide protection from such injuries. A protective splint is applied after minor sprains to prevent more serious injury. In fact, newer designs of hockey gloves and ski gloves can protect the thumb or fingers by incorporating semirigid splints, which should reduce the risk of a primary injury as well as prevent recurrence of past injuries. Buddy-taping fingers together to protect a PIP joint injury or using a figure-eight wrap around the thumb to support the MP joint, however, undoubtedly is unsatisfactory protection, considering the potential forces that the fingers and thumb must resist.

In the wrist, forces resisted by the carpal ligaments were studied by Mayfield et al[31] and by Berger et al.[2] The palmar ligaments from the distal radius to and across the proximal carpal row are the strongest, often preventing hyperextension injuries where distal radius fractures or carpal fractures occur rather than ligament disruption. The dorsal ligaments are the next in strength, holding both the scaphoid across to the triquetrum and the distal radius to the lunate and triquetrum. The interosseous ligaments (scapholunate and lunotriquetral) are the weakest ligaments in the wrist. This fact accounts for the frequency of interosseous ligament injuries within the wrist. Even when high-energy injuries affect the wrist (as in gymnastics), perilunate dislocations or transscaphoid perilunate instabilities can result, with carpal bone fracture or rupture of the interosseous ligaments occurring more commonly than rupture of the extrinsic carpal ligaments. The high forces and significant displacement associated with carpal injuries in athletics explain the difficulty in treating these problems late. Only with early recognition, open reduction, and direct ligament repair can the physician be confident that a lasting, strong ligament support system can be reconstructed in the athlete. Delayed or late repairs have had only moderate success. Most surgeons favor intercarpal fusions for scapholunate dissociations with rotatory subluxation or midcarpal fusions for ulnar or midcarpal instabilities over ligament reconstruction.[9,25-27,34,41,48]

Although few bioengineering studies focus on sports-related injuries, data from recent basic biomechanics research may be applicable to the athlete. In biomechanics laboratories, researchers have studied compressive forces across the wrist with both Fuji film and implanted pressure transducers.[18,20,23,49,51] Using very pressure-sensitive film (super-low Fuji film) placed over the joint articular surfaces, bioengineers have measured the compressive forces across the scaphoid (60 N) and the lunate (47 N). Fuji film studies showed that the average pressure was 11.8 kg/cm^2 across the scaphoid fossa of the distal radius and 20.4 kg/cm^2 on the lunate fossa. The distal radius load-sharing proportions were 60% scaphoid and 40% lunate. With a ligament injury of the wrist producing a scapholunate dissociation with a gap of 6 mm, the contact pressure increased 40% between the radius and scaphoid and simultaneously decreased between the lunate and radius. With a positive ulnar variance, the load increased on the ulnocarpal complex and decreased in the radiocarpal joint. These changes correlate well with clinical observations of S-L advanced collapse (SLAC wrist) arthritis showing that compressive loads between the scaphoid and radial styloid occur first, followed by more generalized wrist-joint deterioration. Tencer and Viegas et al[49,51] have used pressure-sensitive film to confirm the changes in carpal force transmission that occur with changes in wrist position, ligament laxity, scaphoid fractures, and perilunate instability. Fuji film technology may help to explain further deformities of Kienböck disease, ulnocarpal abutment, and other ulnar-side wrist instabilities in the athlete.

Force-pressure-sensitive conductive rubber also has been used to measure contact (compression) force across the wrist[18] (Fig. 25-8). These studies demonstrate that dynamic wrist loading could be assessed using Fuji film in normal and pathologic conditions rather than in just static positions. Using a thin, uniformly compressible rubber mold with a pressure stabilizer, peak pressure under the scaphoid and lunate was measured while a 10-kg load was applied to the wrist. In this recent study, investigators found 2.4 Mpa pressure on the scaphoid, 1.5 Mpa on the lunate, and 1.1 Mpa pressure on the triangular fibro cartilage (TFC). These ratios of pressure were similar to those measured with Fuji film. However, a wrist position of ulnar deviation rather than radial deviation significantly influenced the peak pressure, with more pressure occurring on the scaphoid during ulnar deviation than radial deviation. In power grip (wrist extension and ulnar deviation) more force was present across the lunate fossa (Fig. 25-9), changing the scapholunate force ratio toward the lunate and suggesting that lunate force pressures are greater than anticipated during daily activities. Pressure-sensitive rubber, Fuji film, and rigid body spring models

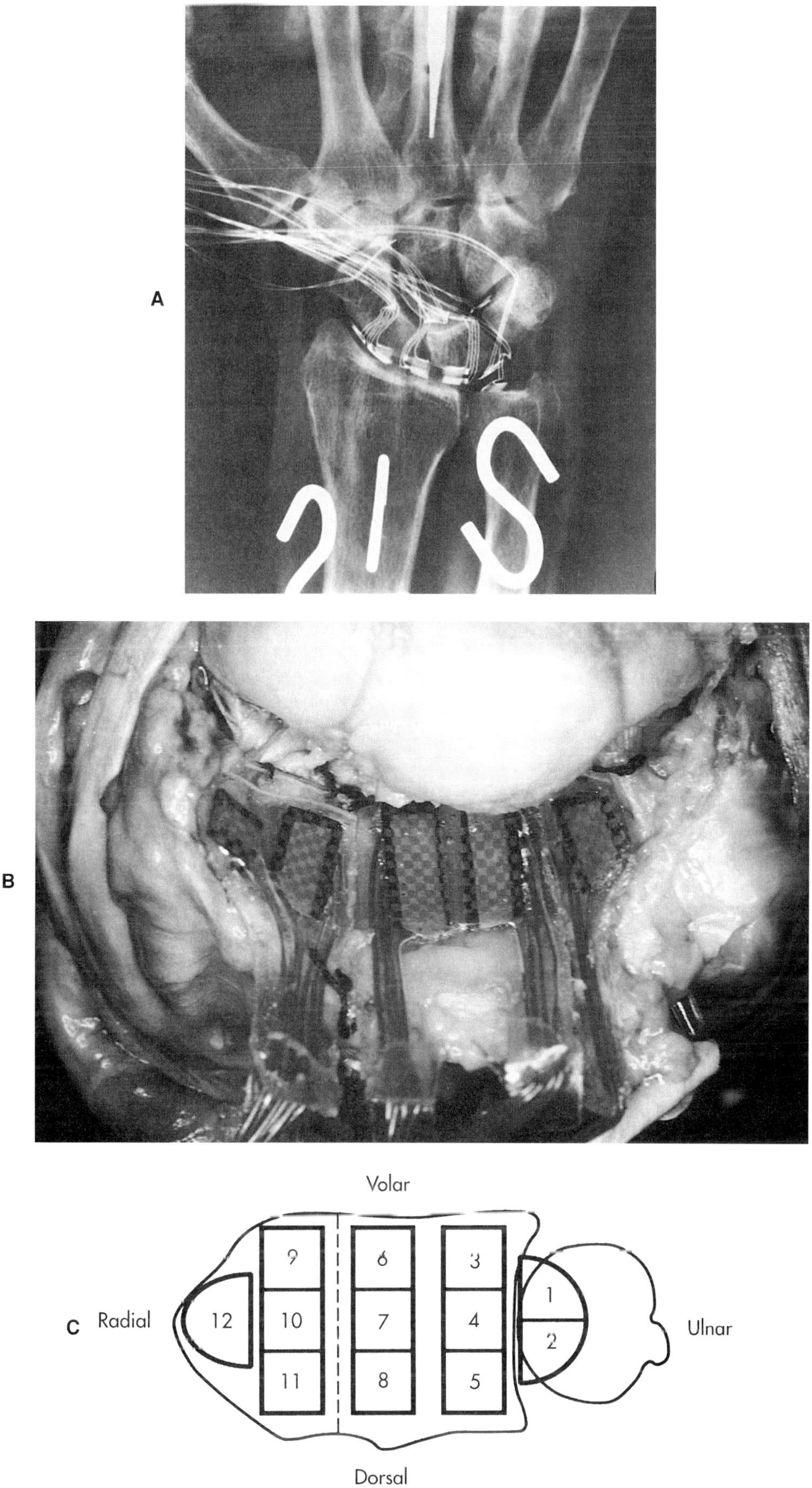

FIGURE 25-8 Pressure-sensitive conductive rubber sensors are placed in the radiocarpal joint. **A,** Radiographic appearance of sensors and connecting wires. **B,** Gross anatomic appearance of sensors covering the articular cartilage of the distal radius and triangular fibrocartilage. **C,** Graphic representation of location of 12 sensors in the radioulnocarpal joint.

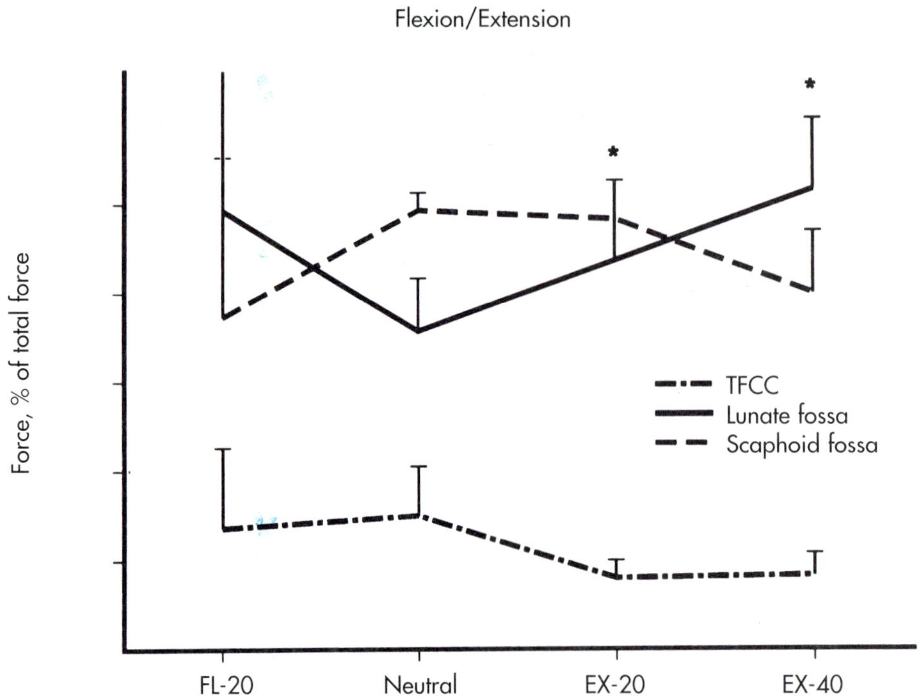

FIGURE 25-9 Proportional changes in force transmission during radioulnar deviation. Note the increase in lunate fossa force during ulnar deviation of 20°.[18]

(RBSMs) also have been used to examine the effect of malunited distal radius fractures,[40] Kienböck's disease,[20] distal radioulnar joint injuries,[38] and proximal scaphoid fractures.[52] The value of these studies in injuries such as gymnast wrist, radial styloid impingement, and ulnar impaction resulting from repetitive loading remains to be determined by laboratory assessment.

WRIST INJURIES

Scaphoid Fractures

Falls on the outstretched arm are everyday occurrences in many sporting events. As the athlete or anyone falls on the hand, the wrist may be forced into hyperextension and radial deviation. The styloid of the radius may impact against the waist of the scaphoid with sufficient force to fracture the carpal bone. More commonly, however, the scaphoid fails in tension when the palmar surface experiences an excessive bending moment.[52] This fracture, which may not become evident on plane radiographs for 2 weeks, often is misdiagnosed as a wrist sprain. If a fracture is suspected, even with negative radiographs, further diagnostic procedures such as technetium bone scans and trispiral tomograms may allow visualization of a fracture. If pain over the scaphoid is present, wrist immobilization with a thumb spica cast followed by reevaluation in 2 weeks is recommended.[7,34]

The scaphoid acts as a tie between the proximal and distal carpal rows. Fractures of the scaphoid therefore may alter the kinematics of the wrist. An unstable fracture can produce a "humpback" scaphoid, that is, a flexed stance of the distal fragment and an extended position of the proximal fragment (Fig. 25-10). The distal segment may become hypermobile, and the proximal fragment displays loss of motion. The resulting interfragmentary motion will compromise the healing potential, leading to delayed healing or nonunion.[45]

In cadaveric wrists, scaphoid fractures (simulated by osteotomy) produced increased wrist flexion, extension, and ulnar deviation. Increased motion resulted from loss of stability between the carpal rows. The distal carpal row displayed increased flexion, and the proximal row was allowed more extension.

Osteotomy site angulation occurs with as much as 36° of rotation between scaphoid segments.[45] Thus scaphoid fracture displacement apparently occurs at the time of injury rather than later, and the ideal time for primary fracture treatment appears to be early, before secondary changes of carpal instability occur. In the athlete, we recommend open reduction and screw fixation of the acute, displaced scaphoid fracture. If a compression screw is used, early motion and return to athletic competition may be possible for the athlete within 5 to 6 weeks.

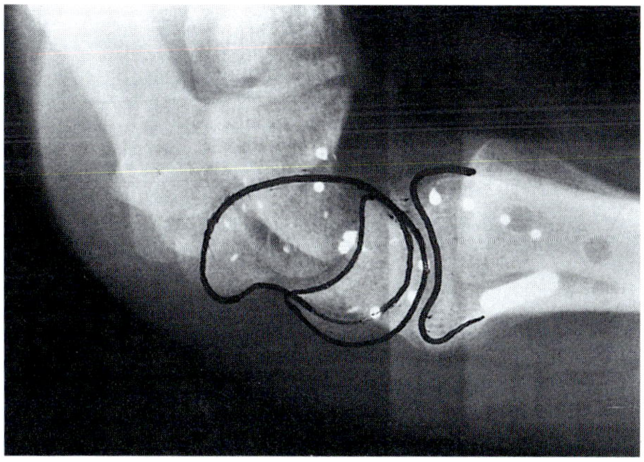

A

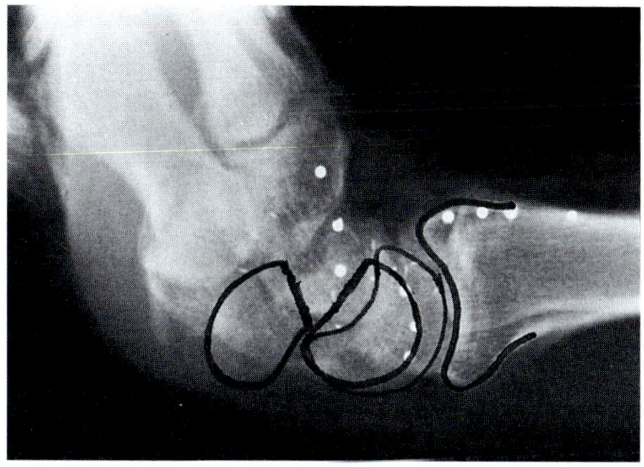

B

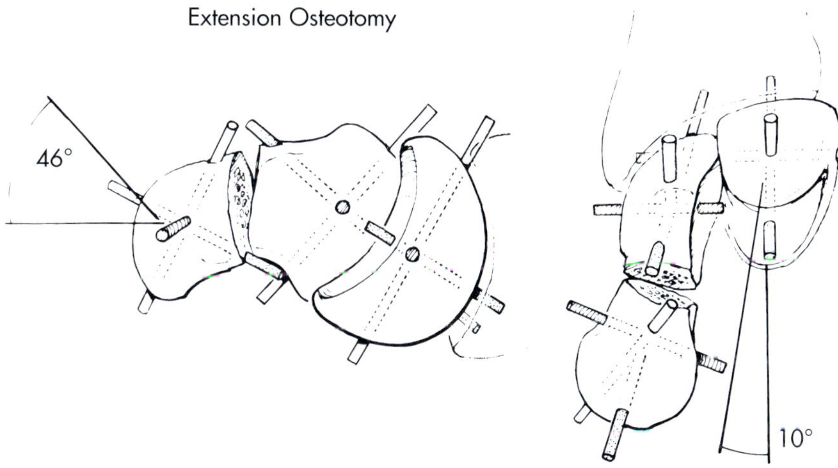

C

	Ext	Rd	Sup
Lunate	30	2	—
Prox scaph	49	2	—
Dist scaph	23	10	7

FIGURE 25-10 Scaphoid fractures involve an immediate angulation and displacement of proximal and distal fragments. **A,** Lateral radiograph, intact scaphoid. **B,** Lateral radiograph, fracture of scaphoid. **C,** Graphic representation of changes in scaphoid fracture components including scaphoid and lunate extension of 49° and 30°, respectively, and distal scaphoid 23°.[45]

SCAPHOLUNATE DISSOCIATION

The mechanism causing scaphoid fractures is very similar to the mechanism causing scapholunate dissociation, that is, extreme dorsiflexion. Instead of the bone fracturing, however, the scapholunate and deep radioscapholunate ligaments are ruptured. The subject complains of pain and weakness, may note a clicking of the wrist, or may report slipping of the bones with grasp or twisting maneuvers. The proximal pole of the scaphoid is allowed to subluxate as a result of the loss of ligamentous stability. Radiologically, the scaphoid will assume a palmar flexed position and the lunate becomes dorsiflexed[27,48] (Fig. 25-11).

Delayed diagnosis can lead to difficulty in obtaining satisfactory results. Therefore a high index of suspicion is needed with any dorsiflexion injury of the wrist. A variety of special radiographic views are available that attempt to emphasize the dissociation between the scaphoid and lunate.

Treatment consists of restoring the stability of the carpus. Early cast immobilization may be adequate, but pins may be necessary to obtain proper bony opposition. Documented scapholunate dissociation should be treated with direct sutures. In cases of subacute carpal instability (6 to 12 months after injury), ligamentous reconstruction may be necessary.

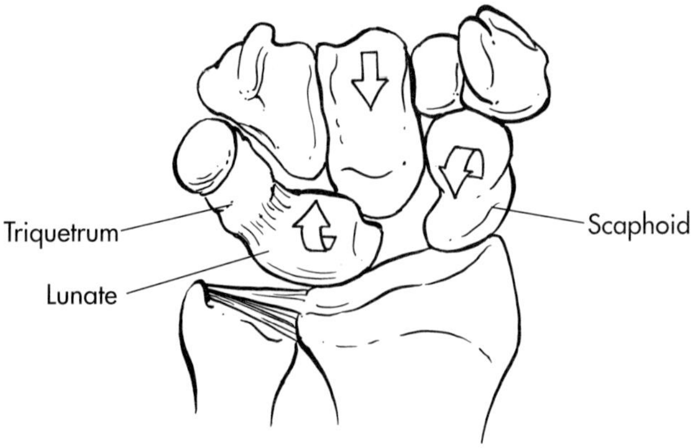

FIGURE 25-11 Graphic representation of scapholunate dissociation; (palmar view) scaphoid flexes (rotates) palmarly while lunate extends, resulting in a scapholunate diastasis and rotatory carpal instability. (Courtesy Surgical Rounds for Anatomy and Mechanics of Carpal Instability, Sept. 1989).

Arthrodesis is the surgical treatment preferred in cases of chronic carpal instability (of more than 12 to 18 months' duration). One of the most frequently performed limited intercarpal fusions involves the trapezium, trapezoid, and scaphoid, otherwise known as STT fusion. Fusion of the scaphocapitate (SC) joint has been advocated in cases of nonunions of the scaphoid as well as for carpal instability.

Global wrist motion is the result of composite rotation between bones of the two carpal rows. Fusion of two or more bones obviously will alter wrist kinematics.[8] Kinematic studies of cadaver wrist with STT fusions showed a loss of 12% of extension, 19% of flexion, 33% of radial deviation (RD), and 11% of ulnar deviation (UD). Wrists with SC fusions showed a 22% loss of extension, an 8% loss of flexion, and losses of 25% and 27% for RD and UD respectively.[15] Clinically measured losses were even greater. Patients who underwent STT fusions lost

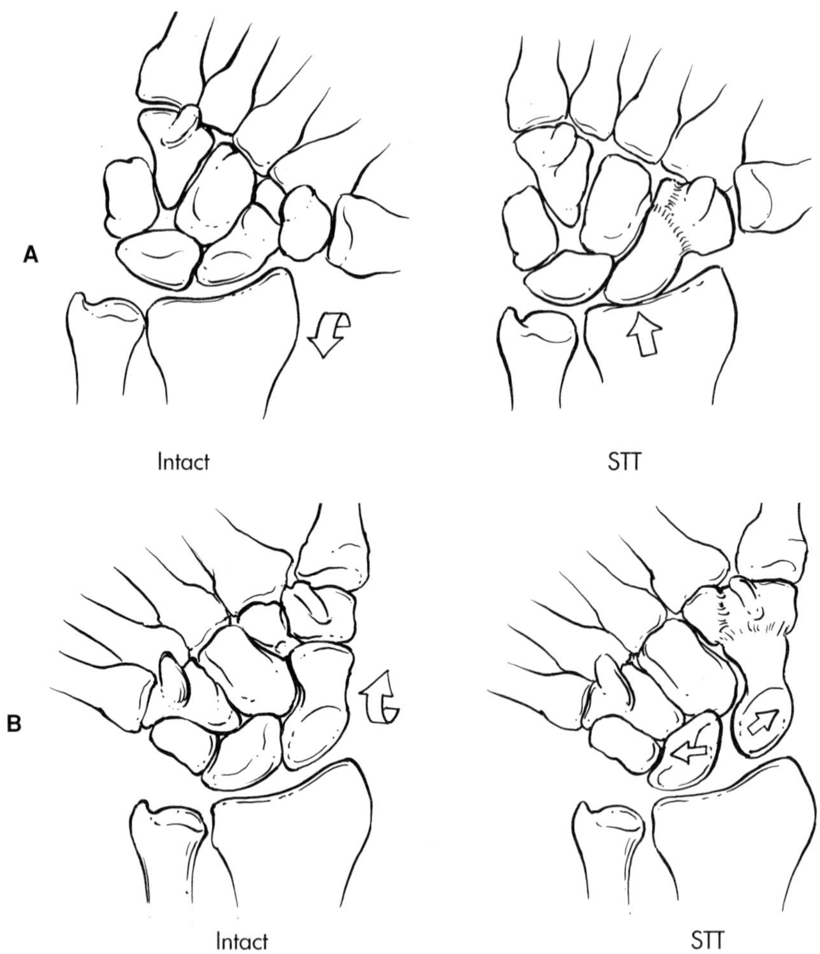

FIGURE 25-12 **A,** After STT fusion, compression forces increase between scaphoid and distal radius and radial deviation of the wrist is blocked, increasing the potential for arthritis in athletes. **B,** The scaphoid is locked to the distal carpal row so that it separates at the scapholunate area rather than rotates as in the intact wrist.

22% and 38% of their extension and flexion respectively, while patients with SC fusions lost 27% and 46%. Both STT and SC fusions lock the scaphoid to the distal carpal row (Fig. 25-12).

Such fusions alter force transmission as well as motion. In the loading model discussed previously, a 5% reduction in compressive load and a 3% decrease in peak pressure on the radiolunate joint were observed after STT fusion, while a 20% increase in pressure load was observed at the radioscaphoid joint. Fusions of scaphoid to the capitate resulted in similar results. On the other side of the wrist, fusions of the capitate and hamate resulted in decreased forces between the hamate and triquetral, and increased forces in the lunocapitate and scaphocapitate. However, no significant change was noted in the radioulnocarpal joint.[20]

OTHER FRACTURES OF THE WRIST

Fractures of the hook of the hamate have been reported in golfers.[33,34] The mechanism for this injury is a shearing force transmitted from the handle of the club to the hamate. This force often is the result of unexpectedly striking an object, such as a root or rock, and the club grip striking the hook as a result. Stress fractures of the hook also can result from tension exerted through ligamentous and muscular attachments. This type of injury has been noted in tennis, baseball, and softball, as well as golf.[26,34] Any activity where the handle of a club, stick, or tool rests in the palm of the hand may lead to fractures of the hook.

The hand and wrist also may be injured in baseball and softball. The hand is susceptible to blunt trauma in catching a baseball, leading to bruising and vascular occlusions.[47] "Jammed" fingers and wrist sprains are common in both baseball and softball. Impact injuries to any of the four finger joints or three thumb joints can occur when a batted or thrown ball hits the end of the unprotected digit. Such trauma can cause sprains, ligament disruptions, dislocation, intraarticular fractures, and avulsion injuries. The wrist may be injured through blunt trauma, such as being hit by a pitch, leading to fracture of the ulna, or by falling on an outstretched hand or using a poor sliding technique. Such a mechanism (i.e., hyperextension of the wrist) may result in scaphoid impaction, triquetrohamate impingement, and lunotriquetral tears.[26]

Many gymnastic activities require the wrist to be in full extension with some radial deviation while sustaining large loads.[10,11] This loading situation may lead to impaction of the radius on the scaphoid. The peak forces on the pommel horse are 1.12 to 1.52 times body weight. As noted previously, fracture or carpal instability may result. Another problem that may arise, especially in gymnasts or other athletes who repeatedly put the wrist under large loads with extension, is dorsal impaction. The individual suffering from this malady will complain of pain, weakness, and tenderness over the dorsoradial aspect of the wrist. Extension exacerbates the symptoms. With the wrist in slight flexion and ulnar deviation, the rim of the scaphoid may be palpated, eliciting point tenderness. Radiographs may exhibit a small ossicle on the scaphoid rim, or in chronic cases, a hypertrophic ridge may appear on the scaphoid.

Treatment consists of rest, avoidance of the causative mechanism, and possibly splinting and steroid injections. In cases of protracted disability, surgical excisions of osteophytes and loose bodies, synovial débridement, or other appropriate intervention may be warranted.[26,34]

ULNAR WRIST PAIN

In the athlete, ulnar wrist pain is secondary only to radial wrist pain, such as resulting from scaphoid fractures or carpal instability. On the ulnar side of the wrist, a continuum of injuries can occur that occasionally present with confusing signs and symptoms, making diagnosis difficult. With a fall or compression stress to the ulnar wrist, the physician can see tears of the extensor carpi ulnaris tendon sheath, triangular fibrocartilage tears or avulsion from the ulnar styloid, lunotriquetral ligament tears, or complete dissociation of the ulnar wrist from both the radial carpus and the distal radioulnar joint.[55] Carpal rotational subluxation has been recognized but is not well understood. In fact, the mechanism of injuries to the ulnar wrist is not well appreciated, and the amount and direction of force needed to produce these injuries remain speculative. A forceful hyperextension and ulnar deviation of the wrist with components of carpal rotation has been suggested as a cause by Mayfield et al[31] but never has been confirmed by laboratory study. A rotational stress seems reasonable because we see lunotriquetral ligament tears in association with TFC tears and subluxation instability of the distal radioulnar joint (DRUJ). Athletes, such as baseball players checking a hard swing or hockey players hitting a slap shot, have had combined DRUJ injury and ulnar wrist ligament tears. Hockey players in fact are notorious for recurrent ulnar wrist pain with repetitive injury to the ulnar wrist. Wrist arthroscopy more clearly presents these complex injuries and allows diagnoses that previously were only suspected.

Biomechanical studies by Viegas et al[51] and Horii et al[20] have shed new light on the motion and force-sharing of the ulnar wrist that clarifies the probable mechanism of injured structures. Both authors have analyzed carpal motion after division of the lunotriquetral ligaments. A palmar (or volar) rotation instability occurs only when both the intrinsic lunotriquetral (LT) ligament and one or more extrinsic ligaments have been injured. That is, LT ligament tears alone do not produce a VISI deformity, making x-ray diagnosis difficult. With division of the extrinsic ligaments, such as the dorsal radiotriquetral or

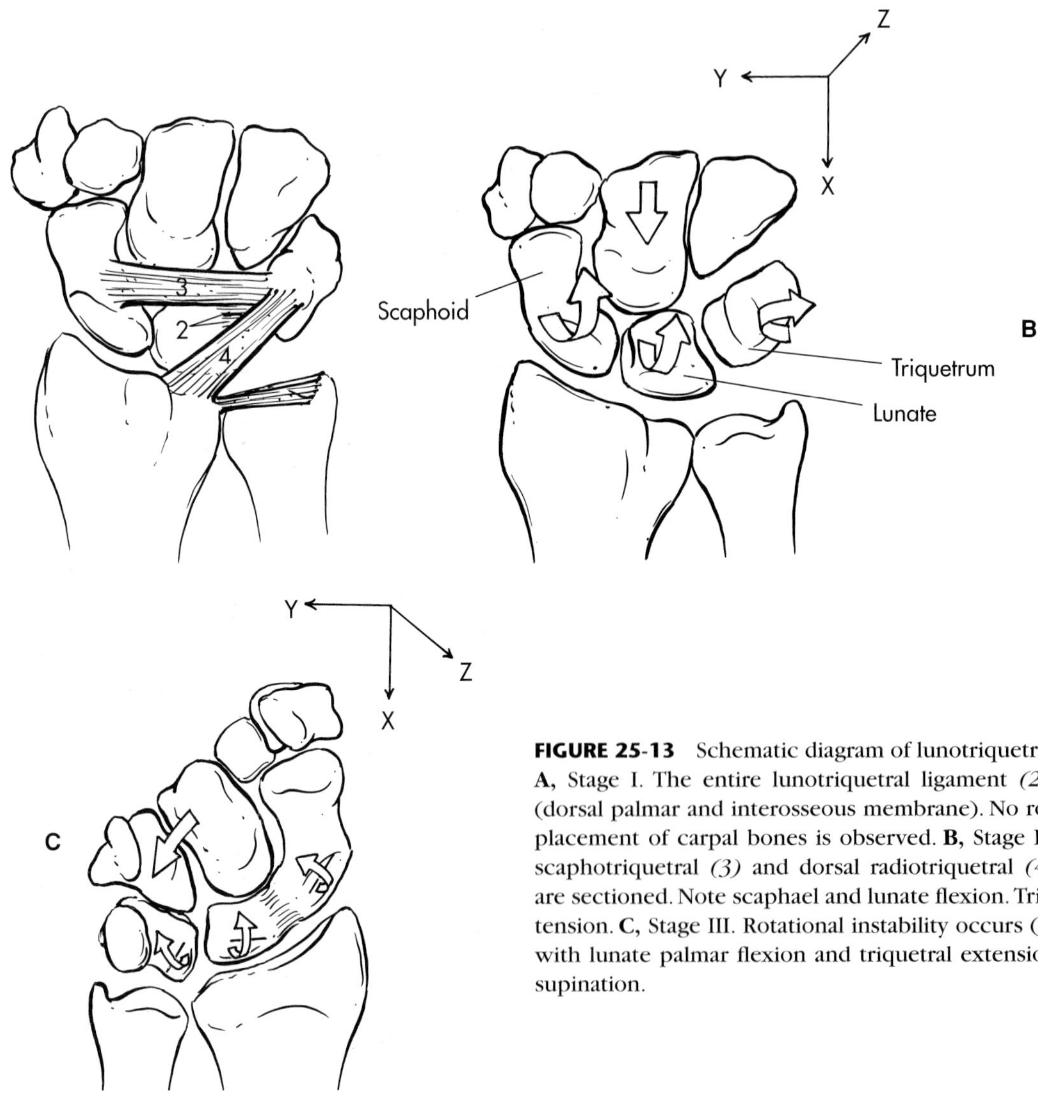

FIGURE 25-13 Schematic diagram of lunotriquetral ligaments. **A,** Stage I. The entire lunotriquetral ligament *(2)* is divided (dorsal palmar and interosseous membrane). No rotational displacement of carpal bones is observed. **B,** Stage II. the dorsal scaphotriquetral *(3)* and dorsal radiotriquetral *(4)* ligaments are sectioned. Note scaphael and lunate flexion. Triquetrum extension. **C,** Stage III. Rotational instability occurs (dorsal view) with lunate palmar flexion and triquetral extension and ulnar supination.

scaphotriquetral ligaments (or the palmar ulnotriquetral ligament) (Fig. 25-13), the LT tear will develop a separation of the lunate and triquetrum. The lunate stays tethered to the scaphoid while the triquetrum extends, rotates ulnarly, and supinates away from the remainder of the wrist. Unpublished laboratory studies at our institution suggest that dividing the dorsal and central parts of the LT ligament does not affect tensile load measurements and that the palmar third of the ligament and TFC attachments are the critical area of strength. When the palmar third gives way, the dorsal extrinsic ligaments alone cannot keep the lunate from separating from the triquetrum, and a VISI deformity results.

More studies are needed to determine the precise ligament strength (ultimate failure load), potential for ligament repair or reconstruction, and areas of interaction between the TFCC (triangular fibrocartilage complex) and ulnar carpal ligaments so that these injuries in athletes can be better understood and treated.

Sports Injuries of the Wrist—Distal Radioulnar Joint

Several studies have focused on ligament support, center of rotation, and mechanism of injury of the distal radioulnar joint (DRUJ).[29,38] The TFC clearly is the main stabilizer of the joint (Fig. 25-14). A TFC tear (or avulsion fracture) from the ulnar styloid insertion, from the lunate fossa of the distal radius (a radial-origin injury), or from the volar rim (ulnolunate and ulnotriquetral ligaments) can lead to instability. A complete tear of the TFC in association with disruption of the dorsal radioulnar ligament will lead to dislocation of the DRUJ. A supination

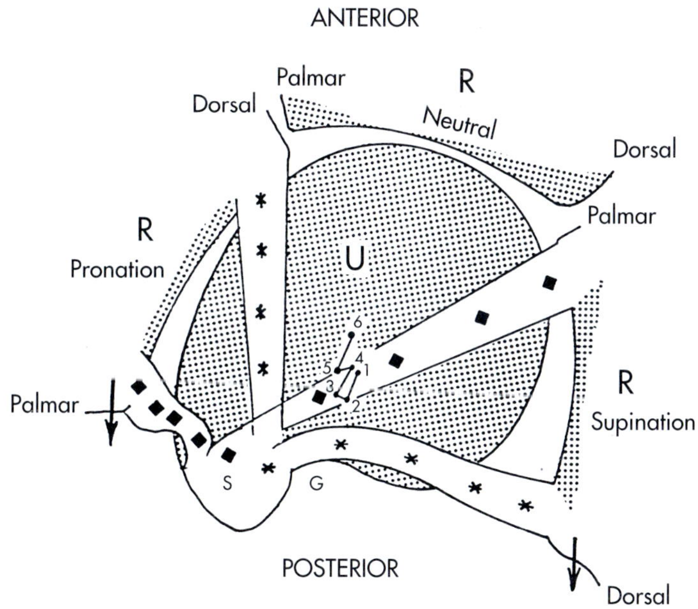

FIGURE 25-14 Axial view of the distal ulna relating changes in length of the distal radioulnar ligaments with forearm pronation-supination. *U,* Ulna; *R,* radius; *S,* ulnar styloid. The dorsal ligament *(asterisk)* is taut in pronation and neutral rotation; the palmar ligament *(blocks)* is taut in supination but lax in pronation. Athletic injuries of the DRUJ involve primarily tears of the dorsal radioulnar ligament or avulsion of the ulnar styloid.

injury results in a volar dislocation, and a pronation injury results in a dorsal dislocation. The associated structures that must be torn for these injuries to occur are not well delineated. This type of information is important so that reconstructive efforts can be improved. To date, we have had success with direct repair of the TFC (ulnarly and radially) alone or in association with ulnar recession osteotomy. At least two professional hockey players and one professional baseball player who led his team to a World Series had successful TFC repair and ulna recession. Still, a better understanding of the mechanics of such injuries is needed so that the ulnar risk-support ligaments can be repaired in an anatomically and biomechanically correct manner.

SPORTS INJURIES OF THE HAND

In the hand, sport injuries are frequent, usually the result of compression bending or torsion loads.[11] With the fingers and thumb relatively exposed and unprotected, joint injuries such as subluxations and dislocations, and tendon ruptures such as flexor tendon avulsions and mallet or boutonnière deformities are common. The mechanism of specific injuries often is unknown, but hyperextension of joints is certainly one of the most common. Dislocations result from hyperextension injuries, and hyperflexion injuries result in tendon ruptures. Torsional loads are evident with phalangeal or metacarpal fractures that have an oblique or spiral component. Axial compression generally results in intraarticular fractures or fracture-dislocations, such as the Bennett fracture of the thumb base or PIP joint dorsal fracture-dislocation.

Studies (see previous section on Wrist and Hand Kinetics) have demonstrated that a force must exceed 50 kg (110 lb) to produce a rupture of a ligament or an avulsion from bone in the hand.[42] Bending or torsional forces acting over a long lever arm, such as the thumb MP ligament, need 5 to 6 N-m (50 to 60 kg-cm) to produce rupture. That is, if the thumb length to the MP joint is 5 cm, an applied force at the thumb tip of 10 kg (22.5 lb) would potentially produce an ulnar collateral ligament tear. The amount of force, direction of application, and applied moment of inertia (mass and velocity) also will affect the injury pattern. For example, a baseball thrown at 100 mph (161 km/hr) striking the tip of a finger will produce an axial load and hyperextension moment resulting in a "baseball finger," that is, fracture-dislocation of the DIP or PIP joints. A volleyball or basketball of greater weight but less velocity also can cause a tendon rupture or a joint dislocation but rarely will lead to an actual fracture-dislocation of the joint.

Whatever the injury, joint reduction and fracture alignment are required to gain appropriate healing. For a pure ligament injury, a dorsal block splint is sufficient protection for 3 to 4 weeks, but a fracture-dislocation needs open surgical treatment to realign the joint and usually requires K-wires to prevent loss of alignment, especially if more than 30% of the joint articular surface is involved. In athletes in particular, anatomic reduction of joint surfaces and full joint reduction without subluxation are needed if the return to athletic performance is not to be compromised. With respect to the thumb, collateral ligament injuries of the MP joint are not infrequent and result from a number of different athletic activities. Although these ligament tears can result from any sport in which excessive stress is placed on the ulnar side of the thumb, the highest incidence follows stick-related or pole-related sports such as snow skiing. The frequency of ulnar collateral injuries with the latter, in fact, has lead to the name of skier's thumb for this injury. The ski pole has been identified as a causative factor in ulnar collateral ligament sprains or tears, because thumb injuries are not seen with snow boarders, who do not use a pole. A cantilever beam across the thumb MP joint results from the ski pole fixed in the hand against the thumb web space as the skier falls. A study on the mechanism of ulnar collateral ligament tears recently showed by mechanical testing that ligament rupture would occur at a failure torque of 5.77 N-m, which is equivalent to 50 kg-cm of load applied at the middle of thumb. A protective ski glove with a radial metal-reinforced angular joint within the glove required almost twice the torque (11 N-m) before a similar ulnar collateral injury would occur.[54] Maximum angular displacement also was improved from 44° to 30°. These authors concluded that the reinforced glove was beneficial in preventing "skier's thumb" when loads or displacement above the normal failure level are imposed in a fall when skiing. Athletic injuries such as this now are being studied by sophisticated mechanical testing techniques with the goal of preventing injury. The application of material technology to ice hockey, racquet sports, and other contact sports where finger joint injuries are frequent may help develop splints or wraps that protect both professional and amateur athletes.

References

1. An KN, Bejjani FJ: Analysis of UE performance in athletes and musicians, *Hand Clin* 6:393-403, 1990.
2. Berger RA, Kauer JMG, Landsmeer JMF: Radioscapholun ligament: a gross anatomical and histologic study of fetal and adult wrists, *J Hand Surg* 16A:350-355, 1991.
3. Blackwell JR, Cahalan TD: *Wrist positions in skilled and unskilled tennis players at ball racket impact: implications for the onset of lateral epicondylitis (tennis elbow),* abstracts of the First World Congress of Biomechanics, University of California at San Diego, 1990.
4. Cahalan TD et al: Biomechanics of the golf swing in players with pathologic conditions of the forearm, wrist, and hand, *Am J Sports Med* 19:288-292, 1991.
5. Cole TM: Goniometry: the measurement of joint motion. In Krusen FH, editor: *Handbook of physical medicine and rehabilitation,* ed 2, Philadelphia, 1971, WB Saunders Co.
6. Cooney WP, Chao EYS: Biomechanical analysis of static forces in the thumb during hand function, *J Bone Joint Surg* 59A:27-36, 1977.
7. Cooney WP: Sports injuries to the upper extremity, *Postgrad Med* 76:45-50, 1984.
8. Cooney WP, Horii E, Garcia-Elias M: *An in vivo and in vitro comparison of scaphocapitate and scaphotrapezial fusions of the wrist.* Proceedings of the 45th Annual meeting of the ASSH, Toronto, Ontario, Canada, Sept 1990.
9. Dobyns JH, Sim FH, Linscheid RL: Sports stress syndromes of the hand and wrist, *Am J Sports Med* 6:236-254, 1978.
10. Dobyns JH: Ligament injuries about the wrist. AAOS symposium on UE injuries in athletes. In Pettrone FA, editor: St Louis, 1986, Mosby, pp 134-141.
11. Dobyns JH: Short-shrift problems: a grab bag of athletic injuries. In AAOS Symposium on UE injuries in athletes. In Pettrone FA, editor: St Louis, 1986, Mosby, pp 170-173.
12. Elliot BC: Biomechanics of the serve in tennis, *Sports Med* 6:285-294, 1988.
13. Elliott BC, Marsh T: A biomechanical comparison of topspin and backspin forehand approach shots in tennis, *J Sports Sci* 7:215-227, 1989.
14. Funk DA et al: Electromyographic analysis of muscles across the elbow joint, *J Orthop Res* 5:529, 1987.
15. Garcia-Elias M et al: Wrist kinematics after limited intercarpal arthrodesis, *J Hand Surg* 14A:791-799, 1989.
16. Groppel JL, Nirschl RP: Mechanical and electromyographical analysis of the effect of various joint counterforce braces on the tennis player, *Am J Sports Med* 14:195-200, 1986.
17. Engelberg A, editor: *Guides to the evaluation of permanent impairment,* ed 3, Chicago, 1988, American Medical Association.
18. Hara T et al: Force distribution across the wrist joint: application of pressure-sensitive conductive rubber, *J Hand Surg* 17A:339-347, 1992.
19. Hoppenfeld S: *Physical examination of the spine and extremities,* Norwalk, Conn, 1976, Appleton-Century-Crofts.
20. Horii E et al: Effect on force transmission across the carpus in procedures used to treat Kienböck's disease, *J Hand Surg* 15A:393-400, 1990.
21. Kapandji IA: *The physiology of the joints,* vol 1, Edinburgh, 1982, Churchill Livingstone.
22. Kauer JMG: The interdependence of carpal articulation chains, *Acta Anat* 88:481-501, 1974.
23. Kazuki K, Kusunoki M, Shimazu A: Pressure distribution in the radiocarpal joint measured with a densitometer designed for pressure sensitive film, *J Hand Surg* 16A:401-408, 1991.
24. Kiefhaber TR, Stern PJ, Grood ES: Lateral stability of proximal interphalangeal joint, *J Hand Surg* 11A:661-669, 1986.
25. Linscheid RL, Dobyns JH: Carpal instability, *Curr Orthop* 34:106-114, 1989.
26. Linscheid RL, Dobyns JH: Athletic injuries of the wrist, *Clin Orthop* 198:141-151, 1985.
27. Linscheid RL, Dobyns JH: Wrist sprains. In Tubians R, editor: *The hand,* vol 2, Philadelphia 1985, WB Saunders.
28. Linscheid RL: Kinematic considerations of the wrist, *Clin Orthop* 202:27-39, 1986.
29. Linscheid RL: Biomechanics of the distal radioulnar joint, *Clin Orthop* 275:46-55, 1992.
30. Markolf KL et al: Wrist loading pattern during pommel horse exercise, *J Biomech* 23:1001-1011, 1990.
31. Mayfield JK, Johnson RP, Kilcoyne RK: Carpal dislocations: pathomechanics and progressive periulnar instability, *J Hand Surg* 5:226-241, 1980.
32. Mayfield JK, Johnson RP, Kilcoyne RK: Carpal dislocations: pathomechanics and progressive periulnar instability, *J Hand Surg* 5:226-241, 1980.
33. McCarroll JR: Golf: common injuries from a supposedly benign activity, *J Muskuloskel Med* 3:9-16, 1986.
34. McCue FC: The elbow wrist and hand. In Kulund D, editor: *The injured athlete,* ed 2, Philadelphia, 1988, JB Lippincott, pp 371-404.
35. Moberg E, Stener B: Injuries to the ligaments of the thumb and fingers: diagnosis, treatment and prognosis, *Acta Chir Scand* 106:166-186, 1953.

36. Morris JRW: Accelerometry—a technique for the measurement of human body elements, *J Biomech* 6:729-736, 1973.
37. O'Driscoll SW et al: Relationship between wrist position, grasp size, and grip strength, *J Hand Surg* 17:169-177, 1992.
38. Palmer AK, Wermer FW: Biomechanics of the distal radioulnar joint, *Clin Orthop* 187:26-35, 1984.
39. Palmer AK et al: Functional wrist motion: a biomechanical study, *J Hand Surg* 10A:39-46, 1985.
40. Pogue DJ et al: Effects of distal radius fracture malunion on wrist joint mechanics, *J Hand Surg* 15A:721-727, 1990.
41. Reagan DS, Linscheid RL, Dobyns JH: Lunotriquetral sprains, *J Hand Surg* 9A:502-514, 1984.
42. Rhee RY, Reading G, Wray RC: A biomechancial study of the collateral ligaments of the proximal interphalangeal joint, *J Hand Surg* 17A:157-163, 1992.
43. Ruby LK et al: Relative motion of selected carpal bones: a kinematic analysis of the normal wrist, *J Hand Surg* 13A:1-10, 1988.
44. Ryu J et al: Functional ranges of motion of the wrist joint, *J Hand Surg* 16:409-419, 1991.
45. Smith DK et al: The effects of simulated unstable scaphoid fractures on carpal motion, *J Hand Surg* 14A:283-291, 1989.
46. Strickland JW, Rettig AC: *Hand injuries in athletes,* Philadelphia, 1992, WB Saunders.
47. Sugawara M et al: Digital ischemia in baseball players, *Am J Sports Med* 14:329-334, 1986.
48. Taleisnik J: Carpal instability. In Tubians R, editor: *The hand,* vol 2, Philadelphia, WB Saunders, 1985.
49. Tencer AF, Viegas SF: Pressure distribution in the wrist joint, *J Orthop Res* 6:509-517, 1988.
50. Townsend H et al: Electromyographic analysis of the glenohumeral muscles during a baseball rehabilitation program, *Am J Sports Med* 19:264-272, 1991.
51. Viegas SF et al: Load transfer characteristics of the wrist—part I: the normal joint, *J Hand Surg* 12A:971-978, 1987.
52. Viegas SF et al: Simulated scaphoid proximal pole fracture, *J Hand Surg* 16A:485-500, 1991.
53. Weber ER, Chao EY: An experimental approach to the mechanism of scaphoid waist fractures, *J Hand Surg* 3:142-148, 1978.
54. Weiland AJ: Personal communication.
55. Wood MB, Dobyns JH: Sports related extra-articular wrist syndromes, *Clin Orthop* 202:93-102, 1986.

CHAPTER 26

Anatomy and Surgical Approaches: Hand, Wrist, and Forearm

NORMAN P. ZEMEL

ANATOMY

The outer covering of the forearm, wrist, and hand consists of skin, subcutaneous fat, and fascia. The fascia surrounds the individual muscles in the forearm and hand and forms various compartments to contain the muscles.

Skin overlying the extensor (dorsal) surface of the extremity is thinner and looser than on the flexor side. During contact sports, it is relatively more exposed and therefore is more vulnerable to injury. This dorsal skin is elastic and somewhat loose as it stretches with flexion of the wrist and fingers. Unlike the flexor side, it has few deep attachments. The subcutaneous layer contains various amounts of fat. This subcutaneous layer also contains the dorsal veins, lymphatics, and superficial nerves. Swelling on the dorsum of the hand and wrist, which is common after injury, drains proximally into the forearm through the venous and lymphatic systems.

Skin on the palmar side of the hand is thicker and less mobile, and contains the majority of fine nerve endings and sweat glands. This skin is less mobile than that on the dorsum of the hand, which allows for better grasping ability. Vertical fascial septa from the palm and lateral fascial septa from the periosteum of the fingers (Cleland and Grayson ligaments)[15] provide stability to the skin and prevent motion of the skin in the palm and fingers during grasp.

SKELETON

Forearm

The forearm skeleton is composed of the radius and ulna. Proximally, the radius articulates with the ulna (proximal radioulnar joint). This joint is minimally constrained and is stabilized by the annular ligament. The proximal radioulnar joint is part of the elbow joint complex and is contained within its synovial and fibrous capsule. Distally, the radius and ulna form a second minimally constrained joint (distal radioulnar joint) (Fig. 26-1). Stability at the distal radioulnar joint is provided primarily through the triangular fibrocartilage complex.[16]

Stability to the radius and ulna also is provided by the fibrous interosseous membrane. This broad fibrous sheet connects the two bones with fibers that extend between the lateral edge of the ulna and the medial edge of the radius. These fibers extend laterally and proximally from the ulna to the radius, which inhibits proximal migration of the radius.

The ligament and fibrous attachments between the radius and ulna are arranged to allow rotation of the radius relative to the ulna (forearm supination and pronation).

Wrist

The wrist is the connecting link between the hand and forearm. It is a complex structure consisting of the articular surface and distal end of the radius, the carpal bones and their articulations, the ulnocarpal space, and the carpometacarpal joints at the distal end.

At the proximal end of the wrist, the metaphysis of the distal radius flares into a large biconcave articular surface with facets to accommodate the scaphoid and lunate. At the ulnar edge of the radius is the attachment of the triangular fibrocartilage, which then inserts ulnarly into the styloid of the ulna with connection to the ulnocarpal ligaments (Fig. 26-2). In the sagittal plane, the distal radius has a palmar tilt of 10° to 12° (Fig. 26-3). Radial inclination in the coronal plane averages 22° to 23°, and the radial styloid height averages 11 to 12 mm.[10] The re-

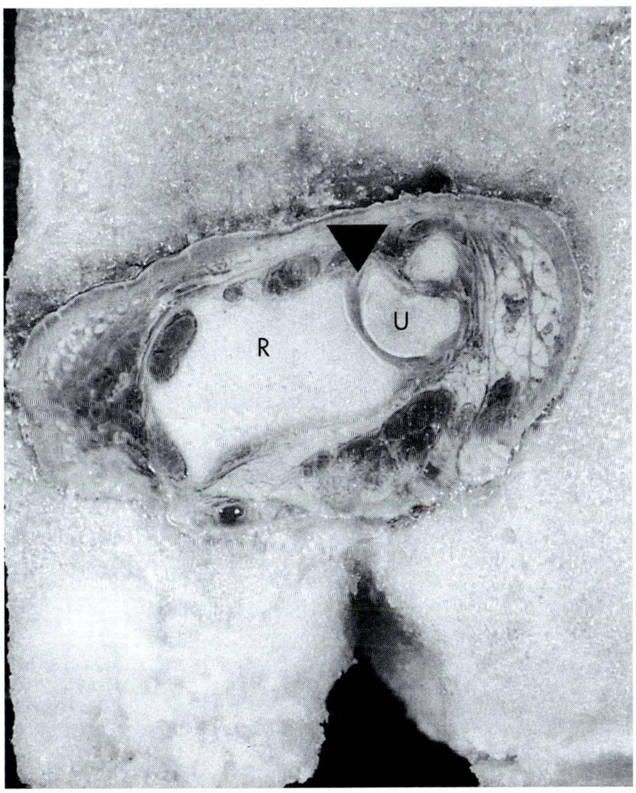

FIGURE 26-1 The minimally constrained distal radioulnar joint. *R,* Radius; *U,* ulna; *arrow,* distal radioulnar joint.

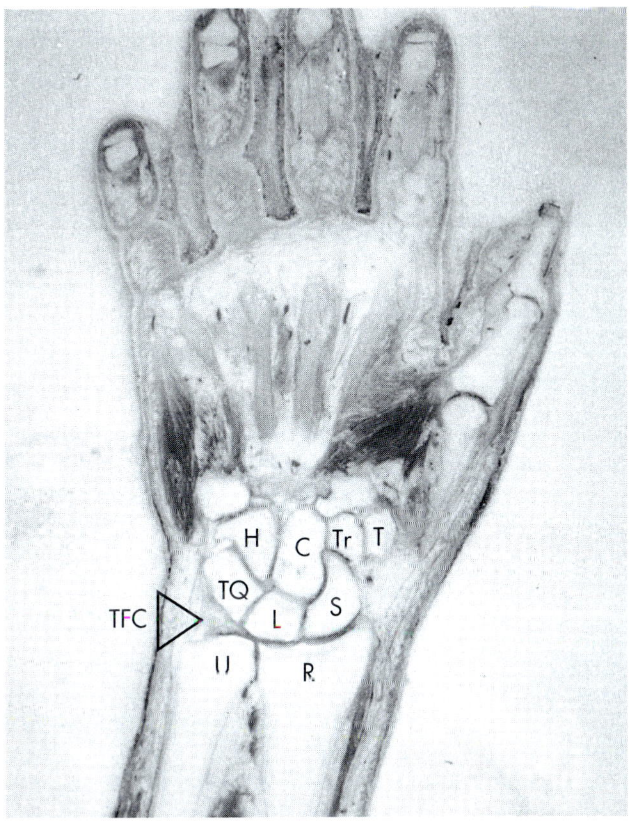

FIGURE 26-2 A coronal view of the carpus, distal radius, ulna, and triangular fibrocartilage. *R,* Radius; *U,* ulna; *T,* trapezium; *Tr,* trapezoid; *C,* capitate; *H,* hamate; *TQ,* triquetrum; *L,* lunate; *S,* scaphoid; *TFC,* triangular fibrocartilage.

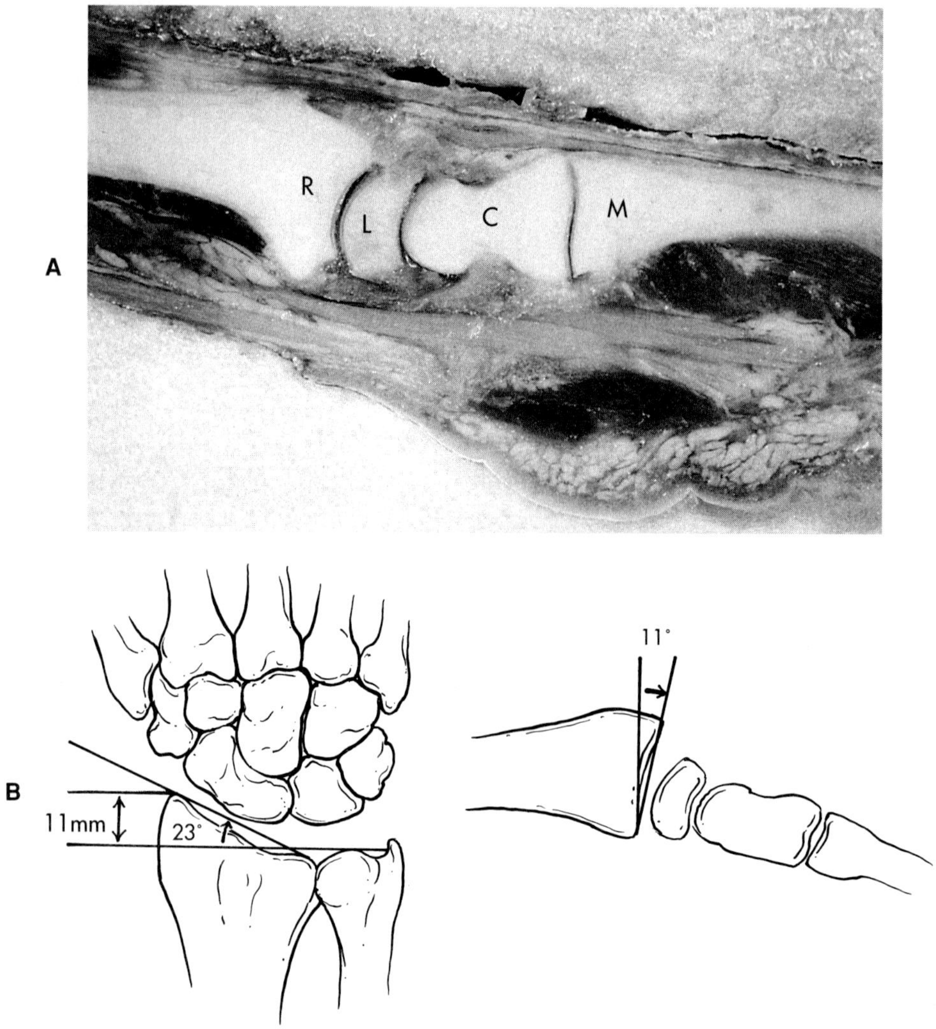

FIGURE 26-3 **A,** A sagittal view of the wrist showing the normal colinear relationship of the radius *(R),* lunate *(L),* capitate *(C),* and metacarpal *(M).* **B,** Diagram of the normal configuration of the distal radius.

lationship between the lengths of the distal radius and ulna is variable. The lengths of the distal articular surfaces of the radius and ulna are equal in 51% of individuals (zero variant), whereas 23% have a shorter ulna (minus variant), and 26% have a longer ulna (plus variant).[9]

There are eight irregularly shaped carpal bones in the wrist that are attached to each other (the radius, ulna, and metacarpals) through a complex ligamentous structure.[2,12-14,25,26] The bones, except for the pisiform, are arranged in two rows anatomically, although kinematically they have been described as having a columnar[22] or ring arrangement.[1] The scaphoid is the functional link between the proximal and distal carpal rows.

There are two major groups of ligaments in the wrist: extrinsic ligaments between the carpal bones and the radius, ulna, and metacarpals, and intrinsic ligaments that originate from and insert into a carpal bone.

The palmar extrinsic ligaments are the strongest and probably have a greater functional significance than the thinner dorsal ligaments. The palmar extrinsic ligaments are arranged in a proximal and distal inverted-V pattern with a weak area (space of Poirier) at the capitolunate joint. The more important palmar extrinsic ligaments, from radial to ulnar, are radiocapitate, radiolunate, radioscapholunate, ulnolunate, and lunotriquetral ligaments. The names of the ligaments are derived from their origin and insertion[26] (Fig. 26-4).

The intrinsic ligaments (interosseous ligaments, membranes) are short, thick ligaments connecting the carpal bones. Functionally the two important structures are the scapholunate and lunotriquetral ligaments. These ligaments extend from the dorsal to the volar surfaces of the bones and are important in maintaining carpal stability (Fig. 26-5).

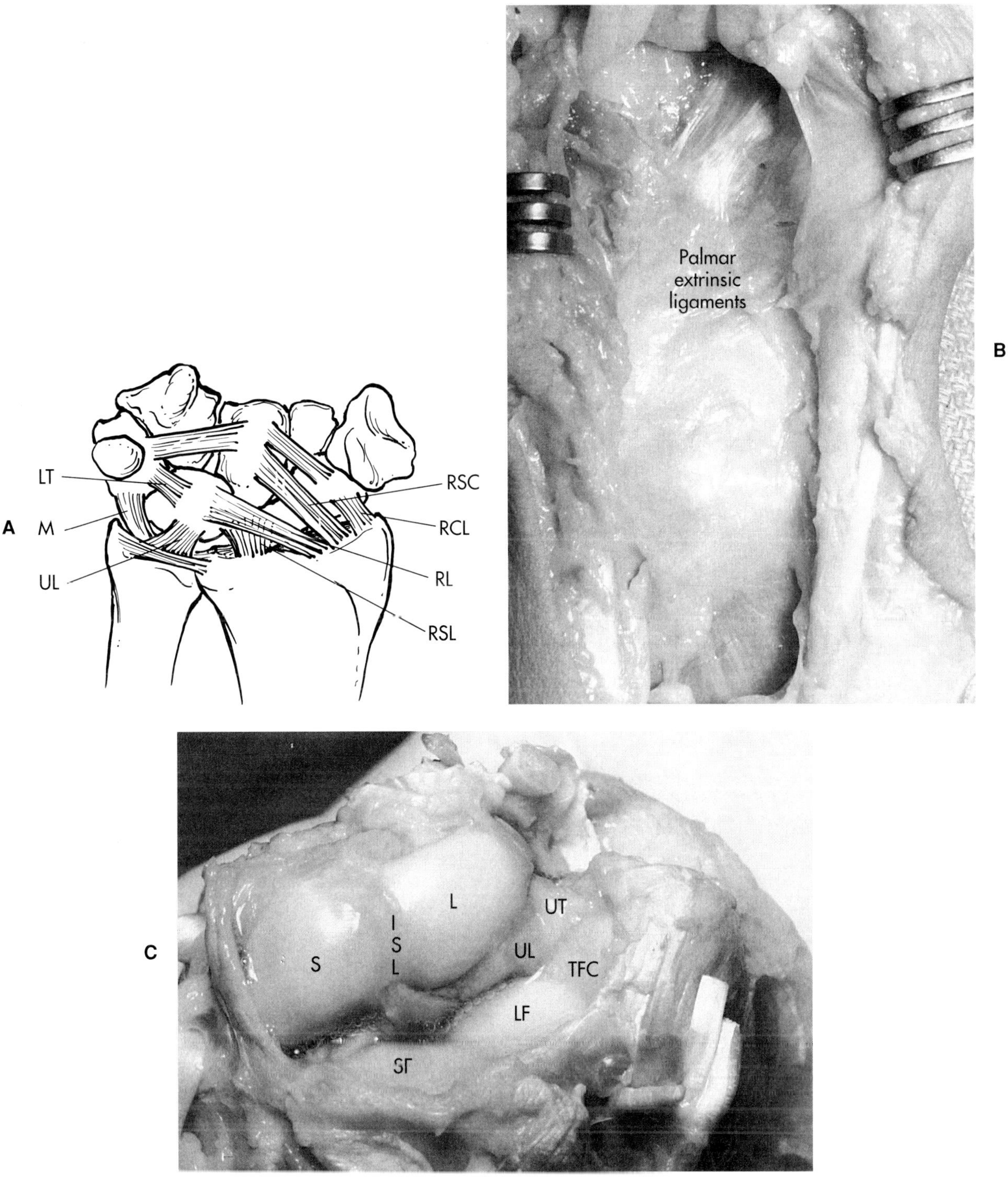

FIGURE 26-1 **A,** The palmar extrinsic ligaments of a right wrist. **B,** A palmar view of the palmar extrinsic ligaments of the wrist. The individual ligaments tend to blend into each other. **C,** A dorsal view of the palmar extrinsic ligaments, triangular fibrocartilage, and intrinsic ligament between the scaphoid and lunate. *S,* Scaphoid; *L,* lunate; *ISL,* interosseous scapholunate ligament; *UT,* ulnotriquetral ligament; *UL,* ulnolunate ligament; *TFC,* triangular fibrocartilage; *LF,* lunate facet of radius; *SF,* scaphoid facet of radius; *M,* meniscal homologue; *LT,* lunotriquetral ligament; *UL,* ulnolunate ligament; *RSL,* radioscapholunate ligament; *RL,* radiolunate ligament; *RCL,* radial collateral ligament; *RSC,* radioscaphocapitate ligament.

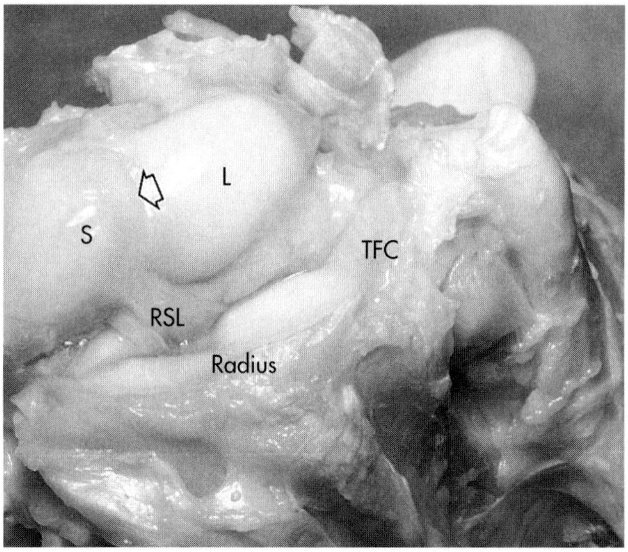

FIGURE 26-5 A dorsal view of the entire interosseous scapholunate ligament *(arrow)* as it extends volarward to join the extrinsic palmar ligaments. *S,* Scaphoid; *L,* lunate; *RSL,* radioscapholunate; *TFC,* triangular fibrocartilage.

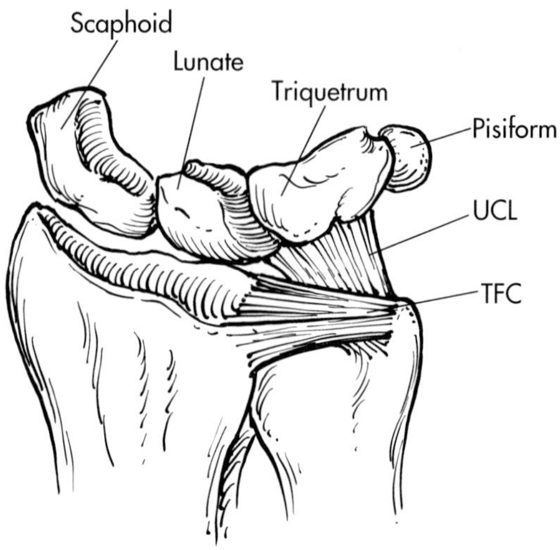

FIGURE 26-6 The triangular fibrocartilage complex showing the triangular fibrocartilage *(TFC)* and the ulnocarpal ligaments *(UCL).*

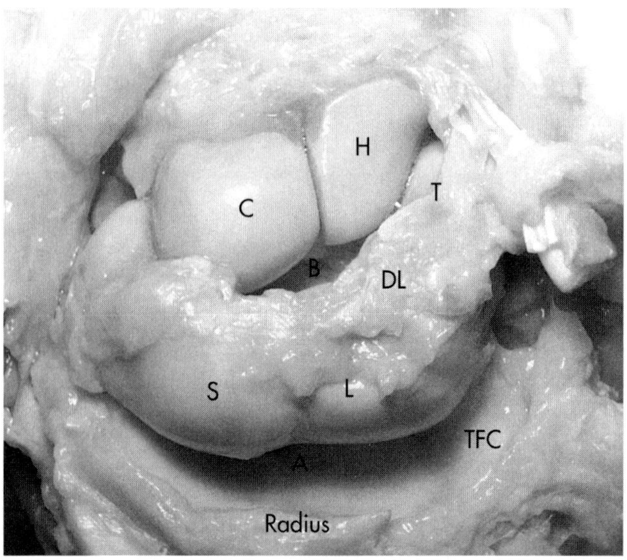

FIGURE 26-7 The radiocarpal and midcarpal joints as seen from the dorsum. The dorsal extrinsic ligaments are weaker than their counterparts on the palmar side. *A,* Radiocarpal joint; *TFC,* triangular fibrocartilage; *S,* scaphoid; *L,* lunate; *T,* triquetrum; *DL,* dorsal ligaments; *B,* midcarpal joint; *C,* capitate; *H,* hamate.

Stability on the ulnar side of the wrist is provided by the triangular fibrocartilage complex (Fig. 26-6). This is a homogeneous structure present between the distal radius, distal ulna, and ulnar carpus. This ligament complex arises from the distal aspect of the sigmoid notch of the radius and inserts into the base of the ulnar styloid, the ulnar carpus, and the base of the fifth metacarpal. The individual components of this ligament complex often are difficult to identify. The triangular fibrocartilage complex consists of a horizontal cartilaginous portion (the triangular fibrocartilage proper), the dorsal and palmar radioulnar ligaments, and the ulnolunate, ulnotriquetral, and ulnar collateral ligaments.[16,18] This ligament complex serves as the major stabilizer of the distal radioulnar joint and is a load-bearing column between the distal ulna and ulnar carpus. The thickness of the triangular fibrocartilage has an inverse relationship to a positive ulnar variance.[17]

This complex osseous ligamentous arrangement forms two essentially closed spaces; one is the radiocarpal with the ulnocarpal joints and the other is the midcarpal joint (Fig. 26-7). This is the basis for using wrist arthrography to evaluate wrist ligament injuries. In addition, this semiconstrained arrangement of the carpal bones allows significant wrist motion in several planes. The center of the axis of motion in flexion/extension and radial/ulnar deviation is through the head of the capitate.

There are no muscles or tendinous attachments to the wrist bones except for the insertion of the flexor carpi ulnaris into the pisiform.

Hand

The metacarpals and phalanges of the hand are arranged in longitudinal and transverse arches. The two transverse arches are located at the base and head of the metacarpals, respectively. The digital rays of the hand are the index, middle, ring, and little fingers (Fig. 26-8). The thumb forms the fifth digit of the hand.

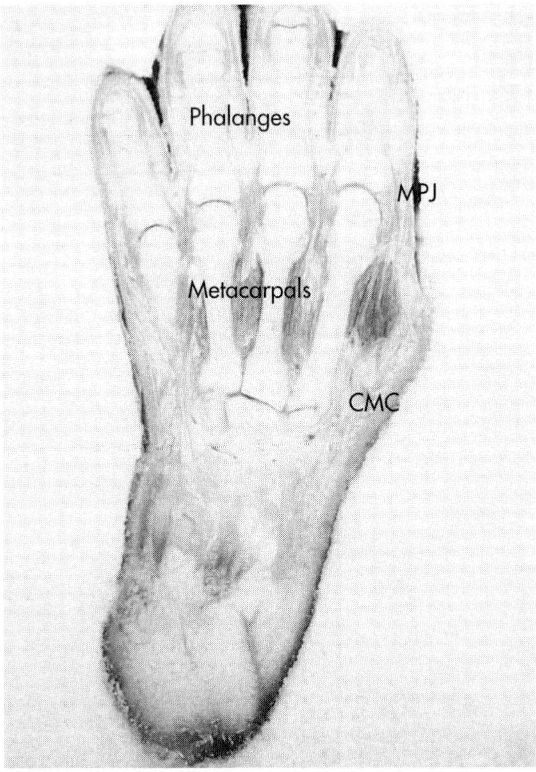

FIGURE 26-8 The metacarpals and phalanges form the arches of the hand. A coronal view of the bones, metacarpophalangeal joints *(MPJ)*, and carpometacarpal joints *(CMC)*.

At their bases, the thumb, ring finger, and little finger metacarpals are mobile, whereas the index and middle metacarpals are rigid in their attachments to the carpus. The proximal carpometacarpal joints, metacarpometacarpal joints, and metacarpal heads are stabilized by short interosseous ligaments.

Although the fingers usually seem straight in extension, in flexion their tips tend to point toward the tubercle of the scaphoid (Fig. 26-9).

Fingers

Metacarpophalangeal Joints

Each finger consists of a metacarpal and three phalanges. The most proximal articulation is between the convex metacarpal head and the shallow concavity of the base of the proximal phalanx. There is significant multiplanar motion at this joint, although its primary motion is flexion and extension. The head of the metacarpal is trapezoidal in shape (narrow dorsally and wider volarly). Depressions at the side of the head of the metacarpal serve as sites of origin of the collateral ligaments. Articular cartilage covers essentially the entire head of the metacarpal (Fig. 26-10).

Stability of the metacarpophalangeal joint is provided by its capsule, collateral and accessory collateral ligaments, volar plate, and musculotendinous units.

A

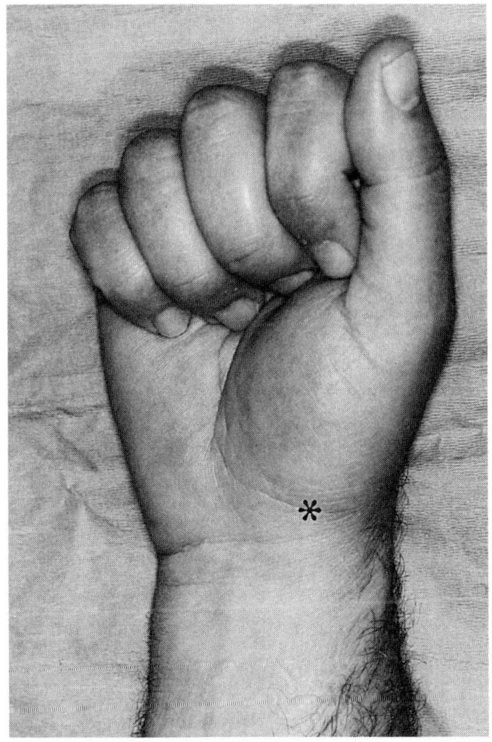

B

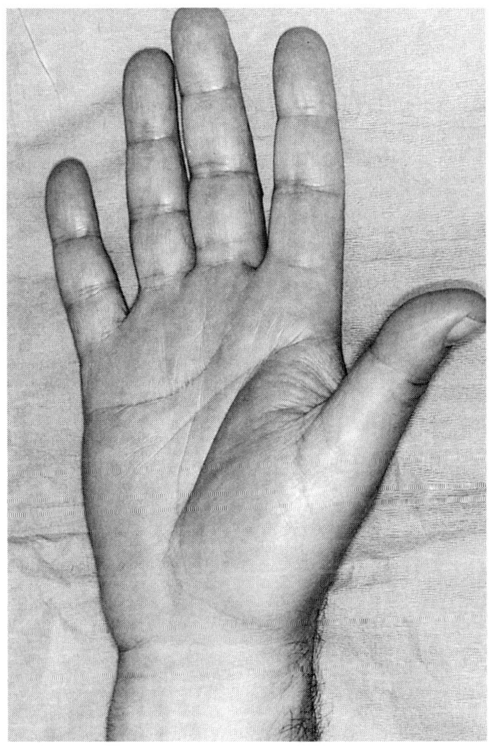

FIGURE 26-9 The fingers point toward the tubercle of the scaphoid *(star)* when flexed, but they are straight when extended.

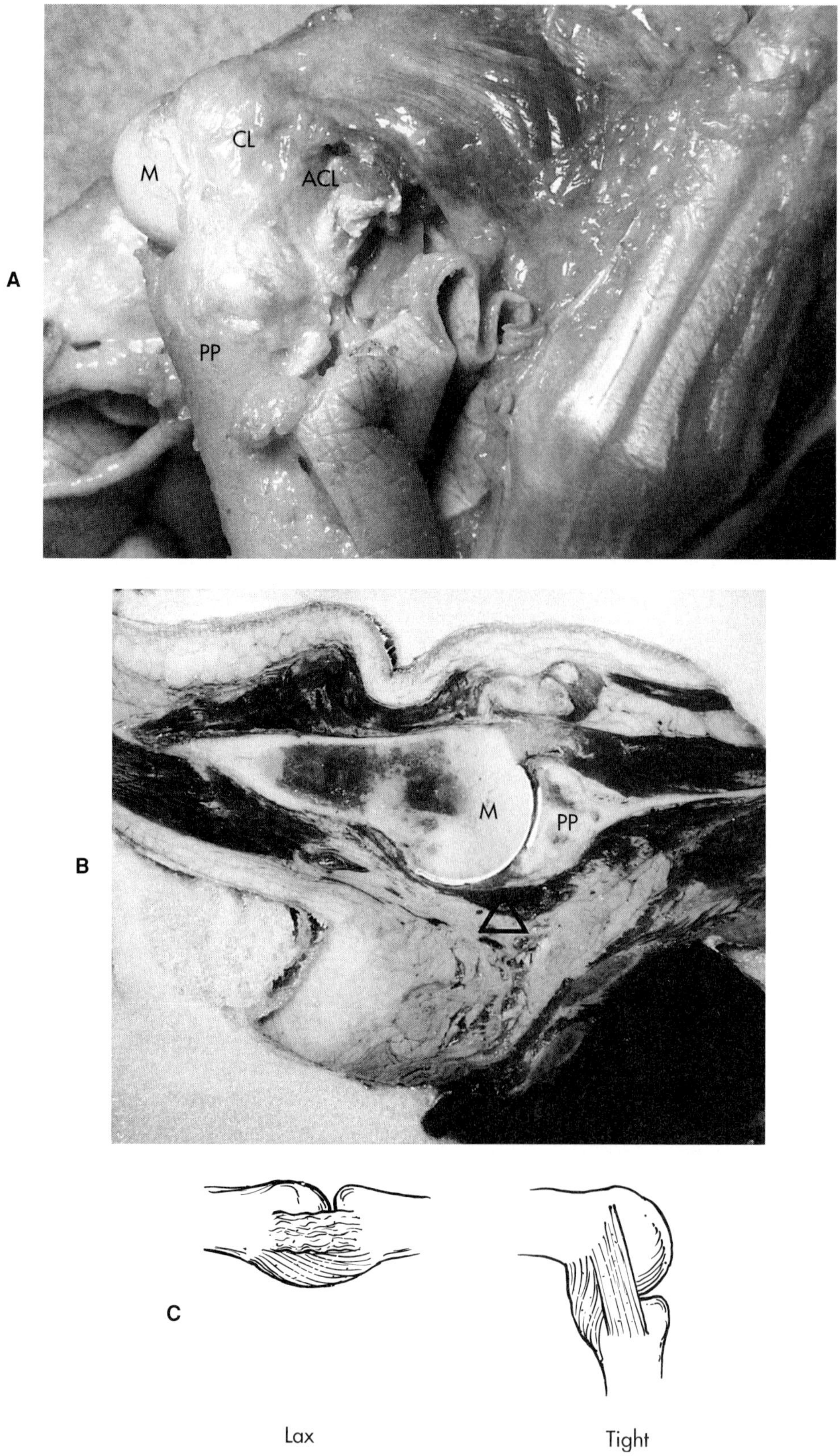

FIGURE 26-10 **A,** A lateral view of the metacarpophalangeal joint, which is stabilized by the collateral and accessory collateral ligaments. *M,* Metacarpal; *PP,* proximal phalanx; *CL,* collateral ligament; *ACL,* accessory collateral ligament. **B,** A sagittal view of the metacarpophalangeal joint. The articular cartilage on the metacarpal head essentially covers its entire surface. The volar plate *(arrow)* stabilizes the palmar side of the joint. *M,* Metacarpal; *PP,* proximal phalanx. **C,** The collateral ligaments of the proximal joint of a finger are lax in extension *(left)* and tight in flexion *(right).*

The laterally positioned collateral and accessory collateral ligaments stabilize the joint. The collateral ligament originates from the side of the metacarpal head and extends obliquely and distally to insert into a tubercle on the proximal phalanx. This is a thick, well-defined structure that originates dorsal to the flexion/extension axis of motion. In extension, the collateral ligament is lax, but with flexion of the fingers, the collateral ligaments tighten over the volar flare of the head of the metacarpal, and the ligaments are taut in complete flexion.[11] Volar to the origin of the collateral ligaments is the fan-shaped accessory collateral ligament, which extends distally to insert on each side of the volar plate. Because this ligament is volar to the flexion/extension axis of motion, it is lax in flexion and taut in extension. Lateral stability of the joint also is provided by the interosseous and lumbrical tendons and fibers of the extensor hood.

The fibrocartilaginous volar plate helps prevent hyperextension of the joint. The volar plate is loosely attached proximally to the metacarpal and firmly attached distally to the proximal phalanx. This loose, membranous attachment proximally creates a space (volar recess) that allows flexion of the proximal phalanx. The volar plate is continuous laterally with the deep transverse metacarpal (intervolar plate) ligament. This deep transverse metacarpal ligament separates the interosseous muscle-tendon (dorsal) from the lumbrical tendon (volar). In addition, the volar plate forms the dorsal wall of the flexor tendon sheath and A-1 pulley.

Interphalangeal Joints

The proximal and distal interphalangeal joints differ in their attachments between the ligaments and flexor/extensor tendons. However, the articular ends of the bones are similar. The heads of the proximal and middle phalanges are circular in the sagittal plane and are bicondylar. The corresponding joint surfaces of the middle and distal phalanges have two shallow concavities separated by a small ridge. Collateral and accessory collateral ligaments stabilize the joint on its lateral aspect. A strong volar ligament attaches distally at the lateral margin of the middle phalanx, where it is confluent with the fibers of the collateral ligament. In the central portion of the base of the middle phalanx, the volar plate is loosely attached to the periosteum. This arrangement permits the plate to retract from the base of the middle phalanx when the joint is flexed.[19] Proximally, the volar plate is anchored to bone just inside the walls of the second annular (A-2) pulley and is confluent with the origin of the proximal half of the first cruciate (C-1) pulley. This proximal bitailed origin of the volar plate allows branches of the digital arteries to reach the flexor sheath.[4]

Thumb

Carpometacarpal Joint

The metocarpotrapezial joint is minimally constrained and thus allows this joint a wide range of motion. The articular surface of the trapezium is both concave and convex (saddle shape), and the base of the thumb metacarpal has a ball-like surface. The trapezium is positioned so that the thumb metacarpal makes an angle of about 45° with the second metacarpal in the sagittal plane. A strong volar-ulnar ligament helps maintain stability of the thumb metacarpal in relation to the trapezium. The thumb rotates at the metacarpotrapezial joint to allow the thumb to touch the tips of the fingers and base of the little finger.

Metacarpophalangeal Joint

The head of the thumb metacarpal is larger than the finger metacarpals and is quadrilateral, with the dorsal side slightly wider than the volar side. The head articulates with both the proximal phalanx and the medial and lateral sesamoids, which are incorporated into the volar plate. The sesamoids act as part of the insertion of the adductor pollicis, flexor pollicis brevis, and abductor pollicis brevis tendons. Collateral and accessory collateral ligaments are present on each side of the joint. These ligaments are lax in extension and taut in flexion. The fibrous aponeurosis extending from the extensor tendon to the volar plate is much better developed on the ulnar side of the joint. It is an extension of the adductor pollicis tendon. On the radial side, the aponeurosis has an extension from the abductor pollicis brevis, but its fibers are less clearly separated from the radial collateral ligament. The proximal phalanx on the head of the thumb metacarpal has a slight radial inclination. On the volar aspect, the volar plate is part of the capsular supporting structure of the joint. This plate is tightly adherent to the base of the proximal phalanx and loosely attached to the neck of the metacarpal, thus allowing flexion and extension of the joint.

Interphalangeal Joint

This joint is primarily a hinge joint because of its anatomic configuration. It has sufficient ligamentous laxity to allow hyperextension of 10° to 40° and frequently has greater flexion than the metacarpophalangeal joint.

EXTENSOR MUSCLES AND TENDONS

On the dorsum of the forearm are superficial and deep groups of extensor muscles that move the wrist, fingers, and thumb. The exception is the brachioradialis muscle, whose primary function is to flex the elbow. The muscles on the dorsum of the forearm are innervated by the radial and posterior interosseous nerves (Box 26-1).

Superficial Muscles

Both the brachioradialis and extensor carpi radialis longus muscles arise from the lateral aspect of the supracondylar ridge of the humerus. The tendon of the brachioradialis muscle passes distally and inserts into the lateral side of the distal end of the radius. Arising as the

BOX 26-1
MUSCLE INNERVATIONS IN THE UPPER EXTREMITY

Musculocutaneous Nerve
Coracobrachialis
Biceps
Brachialis

Radial Nerve
Triceps
Anconeus
Brachioradialis
Extensor carpi radialis longus
Extensor carpi radialis brevis

Posterior Interosseous Nerve
Supinator
Extensor carpi ulnaris
Extensor digitorum communis
Extensor digiti minimi
Extensor pollicis longus
Extensor indicis propius
Abductor pollicis longus
Extensor pollicis brevis

Ulnar Nerve
Flexor carpi ulnaris
Flexor profundus (ring, little)
Hypothenar muscles
Adductor pollicis
Interosseous muscles
Lumbrical muscles (ring, little)
Flexor pollicis brevis

Median Nerve
Pronator teres
Flexor carpi radialis
Palmaris longus
Flexor superficialis (all fingers)
Abductor pollicis brevis
Opponens pollicis
Flexor pollicis brevis
Lumbrical muscles (index, middle)

Anterior Interosseous Nerve
Flexor pollicis longus
Flexor profundus (index, middle)
Pronator quadratus

most radial muscle from the common extensor tendon on the lateral epicondyle, the extensor carpi radialis brevis also arises from the radial collateral ligament and intermuscular septum. Crossing the wrist, the extensor carpi radialis longus and brevis tendons insert into the dorsoradial aspect of the base of the second and third metacarpals, respectively. They function to extend and radially deviate the wrist, although the extensor carpi radialis brevis is more of a pure extender of the wrist. Also arising as part of the common extensor tendon are the extensor digitorum communis tendons; the extensor digiti minimi, which shares a common muscle belly with the communis within the forearm; and the extensor carpi ulnaris, which is the most medial of the superficial group of extensor muscles (Figs. 26-11 and 26-12).

Deep Muscles

Deep to the superficial muscle group are the supinator, the abductor pollicis longus, extensor pollicis brevis, extensor pollicis longus, and extensor indicis proprius muscles. The supinator is a flat muscle in the upper forearm. It has two heads, between which the radial nerve passes from the flexor to the extensor surface of the forearm before it emerges as the posterior interosseous nerve. Except for the supinator, the remaining deep muscles have tendons that form in the middle and distal thirds of the forearm, continue through the extensor retinaculum on the dorsum of the wrist, and insert into the hand and fingers (Fig. 26-13).

The extensor retinaculum is a specialized structure of the forearm fascia that consists of supratendinous and infratendinous layers.[24] There are six synovial-lined compartments in the extensor retinaculum that are separated by vertical fibers that insert into the radius. The compartments are numbered one through six, with the first compartment being the most radial (Fig. 26-14).

Passing through the first extensor compartment are the abductor pollicis longus and extensor pollicis brevis tendons. There may be two to six tendons in this compartment because the abductor pollicis longus often has three to four tendons. The extensor pollicis brevis tendon inserts into the proximal phalanx of the thumb, and the abductor pollicis longus tendon inserts into the base of the thumb metacarpal. A septum may be present that divides the first compartment into two sections. The second extensor compartment contains the extensor carpi radialis longus and extensor carpi radialis brevis tendons. Ulnar to Lister's tubercle is the third compartment, which contains the extensor pollicis longus tendon. This tendon inserts into the distal phalanx of the thumb. Through the fourth compartment pass the extensor digitorum communis and the extensor indicis proprius tendons to the fingers. The fifth compartment contains the

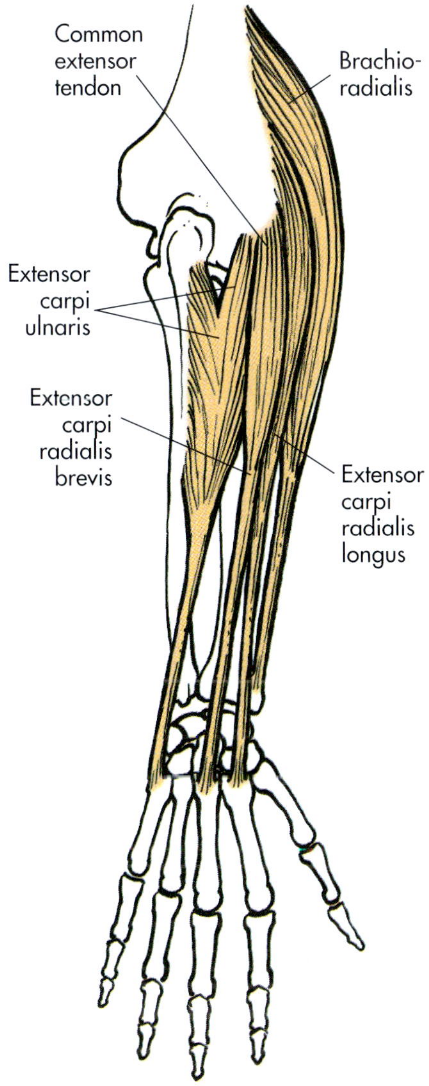

FIGURE 26-11 Superficial muscles on the extensor surface of the forearm.

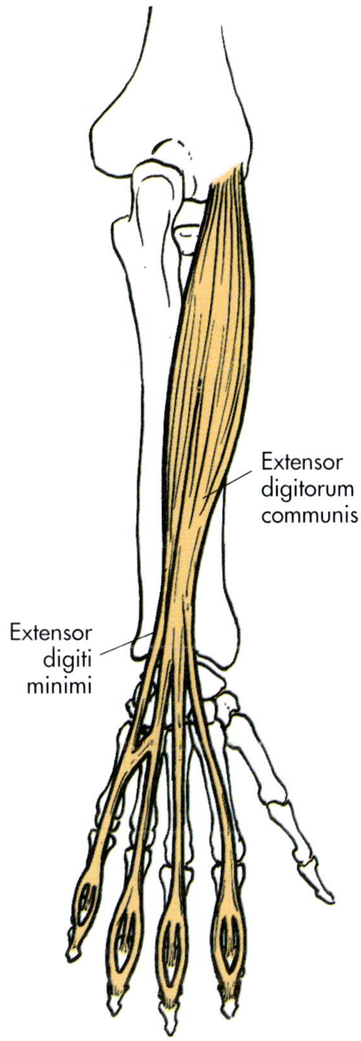

FIGURE 26-12 Extensor digitorum communis and extensor digiti minimi muscles.

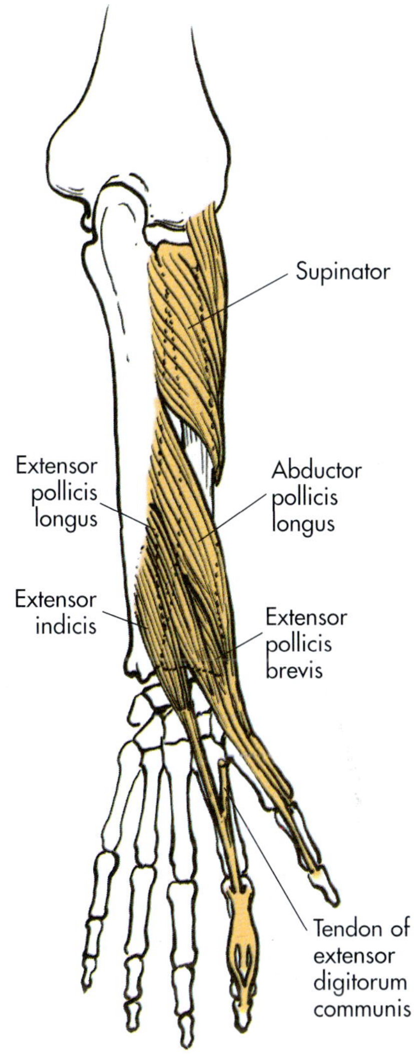

FIGURE 26-13 Deep muscles on the extensor surface of the forearm.

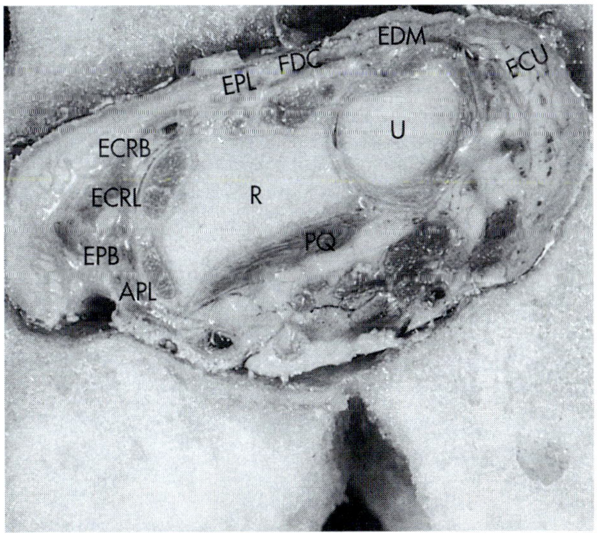

FIGURE 26-14 An axial view of the wrist showing the extensor tendons in their compartments. *R,* Radius; *U,* ulna; *APL,* abductor pollicis longus; *EPB,* extensor pollicis brevis; *ECRL,* extensor carpi radialis longus; *ECRB,* extensor carpi radialis brevis; *EPL,* extensor pollicis longus; *EDC,* extensor digitorum communis; *EDM,* extensor digiti minimi; *ECU,* extensor carpi ulnaris; *PQ,* pronator quadratus.

A

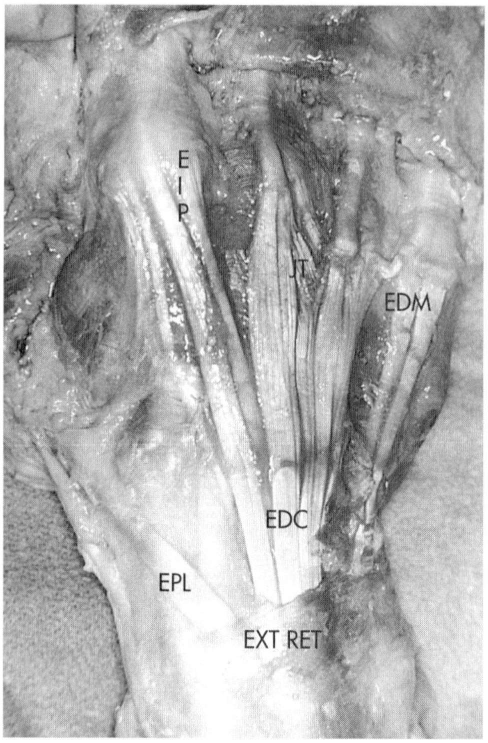

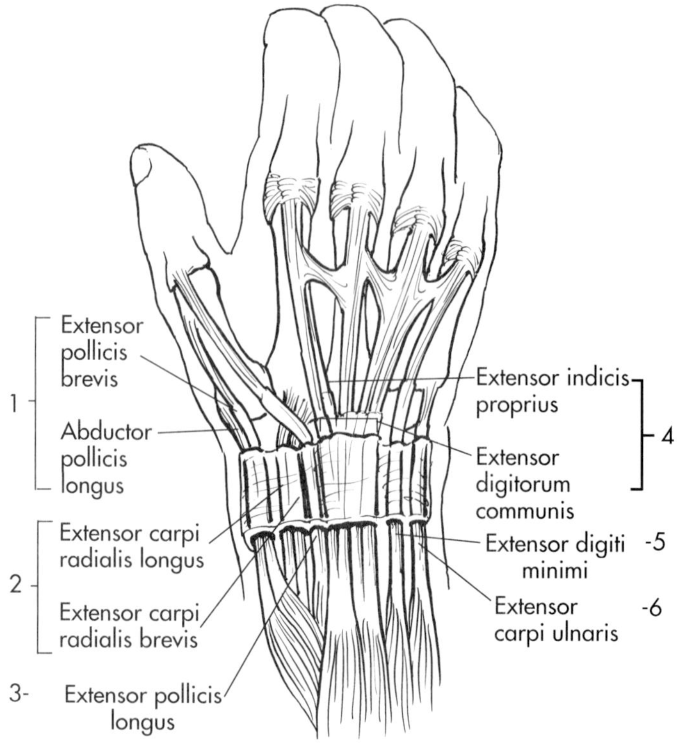

B

FIGURE 26-15 **A,** After the extensor tendons exit from the extensor retinaculum, they pass distally to the individual fingers. Juncturae tendinum connect and stabilize the extensor tendons on the dorsum of the hand. *EXT RET,* Extensor retinaculum; *EPL,* extensor pollicis longus; *EIP,* extensor indicis proprius; *EDC,* extensor digitorum communis; *EDM,* extensor digiti minimi; *JT,* juncturae tendinum. **B,** A schematic of the extensor retinaculum and the extensor tendons as they cross the wrist and pass distally to the fingers.

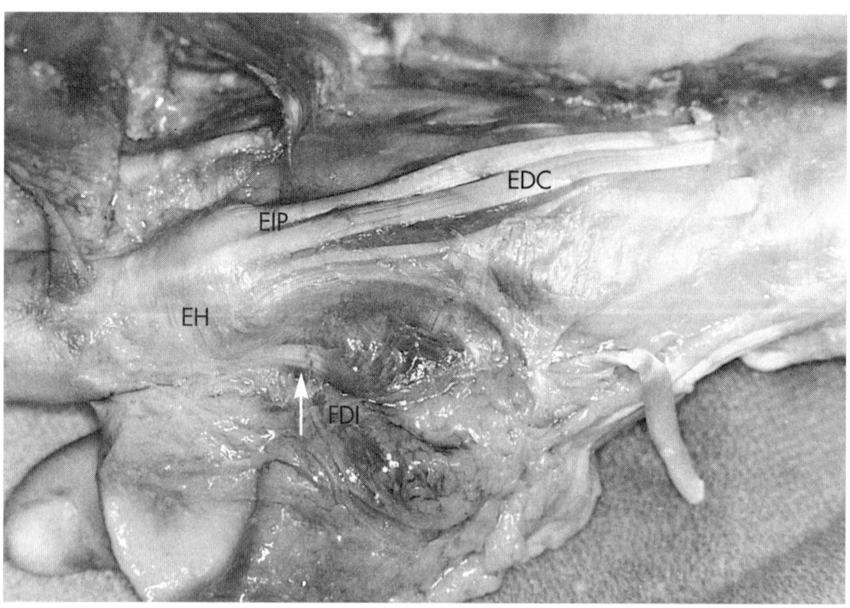

FIGURE 26-16 The extensor hood stabilizes the extensor tendon over the dorsum of the metacarpophalangeal joint of the finger. *EIP,* Extensor indicis proprius; *EDC,* extensor digitorum communis; *FDI,* first dorsal interosseous; *EH,* extensor hood.

extensor digiti minimi, which usually consists of two tendons. In the hand, the extensor indicis proprius and extensor digiti minimi tendons are on the ulnar side of their respective communis tendons. The sixth compartment, containing the extensor carpi ulnaris tendon, has a more complex structure. A fibrous tunnel surrounds the extensor carpi ulnaris tendon and extends from the base of the ulnar styloid to the triquetrum. The extensor carpi ulnaris tendon inserts into the base of the fifth metacarpal (Fig. 26-15).

This complex extensor retinaculum serves as a pulley system to prevent bow-stringing of the extensor tendons at the wrist. As the tendons pass across the dorsum of the hand, they are stabilized by interconnecting tendon bundles (juncturae tendinum) and sheets of fascia. Beneath the tendons are the metacarpals and fascia of the interosseous muscles, which provide a smooth surface over which the tendons can glide proximally and distally.

The extensor communis and proprius tendons cross the dorsum of the hand and pass distally to become part of the extensor mechanism of the fingers.

On the dorsum of the metacarpophalangeal joint of the finger, the extensor tendon is stabilized by a sling of fibers that extend from the lateral borders of the tendon volarward to insert into the proximal phalanx and volar plate. This structure is known as the sagittal band, extensor hood, or dorsal hood.[21] These fibers are superficial to the metacarpophalangeal joint capsule and phalangeal attachment of the interosseous tendon, but deep to the lateral band of the intrinsic muscles. The function of the extensor hood is to extend the proximal phalanx of the finger (Fig. 26-16).

The extensor tendon passes distally and divides into three slips; the central slip and two lateral slips. The central slip inserts into the dorsum of the middle phalanx. The two lateral tendinous slips cross the dorsal and lateral aspects of the proximal interphalangeal joint, receive fibers from the interosseous and lumbrical muscles, and form two lateral bands.[21,28] These structures converge over the distal half of the middle phalanx to form the terminal tendon, which inserts into the dorsal lip of the distal phalanx. The two lateral bands are maintained dorsally by the triangular ligament (Fig. 26-17).

At the proximal interphalangeal joint, the lateral bands are restrained by the transverse fibers of the transverse retinacular ligament. These fibers prevent excessive dorsal and volar shift of the lateral tendon bands.

The interdependence of motion of the proximal and distal interphalangeal joints of the fingers is due to the complex arrangement of the extensor tendons, intrinsic muscles of the hand, and oblique retinacular ligament. The latter extends obliquely and distally from the flexor pulley beneath the proximal phalanx to insert into the terminal extensor tendon. Its pathway is volar to the axis of motion of the proximal interphalangeal joint.

Extension of the thumb is caused by the abductor pollicis longus, extensor pollicis brevis, and extensor pollicis longus muscles. The abductor pollicis longus tendon inserts into the base of the thumb metacarpal after it exits from the first extensor fibroosseous compartment. This first compartment also contains the extensor pollicis brevis tendon, which is ulnar to the abductor tendon and inserts into the dorsal capsule of the metacarpophalangeal joint as well as the base of the proximal phalanx. Passing distally and ulnarly from the third extensor fibroosseous compartment is the extensor pollicis longus tendon, which inserts into the distal phalanx of the thumb. Fibers from the adductor pollicis on the ulnar side (adductor aponeurosis) and the abductor pollicis brevis on the radial side (abductor aponeurosis) insert into the extensor pollicis longus and assist in extending the distal interphalangeal joint of the thumb.

FLEXOR MUSCLES AND TENDONS

The muscles of the volar side of the forearm (flexor-pronator group) arise from the medial epicondyle, both directly and via a common flexor tendon, the ulna, the radius, and the interosseous membrane. These muscles are surrounded by a strong fascial covering both individually and as a group (antebrachial fascia). Significant injury to the muscles can result from prolonged swelling of the muscles within this rigid fascial structure.

These flexor forearm muscles are innervated by the median and ulnar nerves. The ulnar nerve innervates the flexor carpi ulnaris and the flexor digitorum profundus muscles to the ring and little finger, while the median nerve supplies the remaining forearm muscles (see Box 26-1). The musculotendinous juncture is found in the distal part of the forearm.

The flexor forearm muscles are grouped into three layers. The most superficial layer from the radial to the ulnar side consists of the pronator teres, flexor carpi radialis, palmaris longus, and flexor carpi ulnaris muscles. The flexor digitorum superficialis muscles are in the intermediate layer, and the flexor pollicis longus, the flexor digitorum profundus to the fingers, and the pronator quadratus are deep.

Superficial Group

The pronator teres arises from a humeral head (medial supracondylar ridge) and an ulnar head (coronoid process of the ulna) and extends obliquely and distally to insert through a short broad tendon into the lateral aspect of the middle third of the radius (Fig. 26-18). Passing between the two heads of the pronator teres, the median nerve leaves the antecubital fossa to enter the forearm.

Arising from the common flexor tendon, the flexor carpi radialis muscle passes distally and slightly radially. In the midforearm, it forms a flat tendon that enters a synovial-lined tunnel at the wrist. This tendon then lies in

A

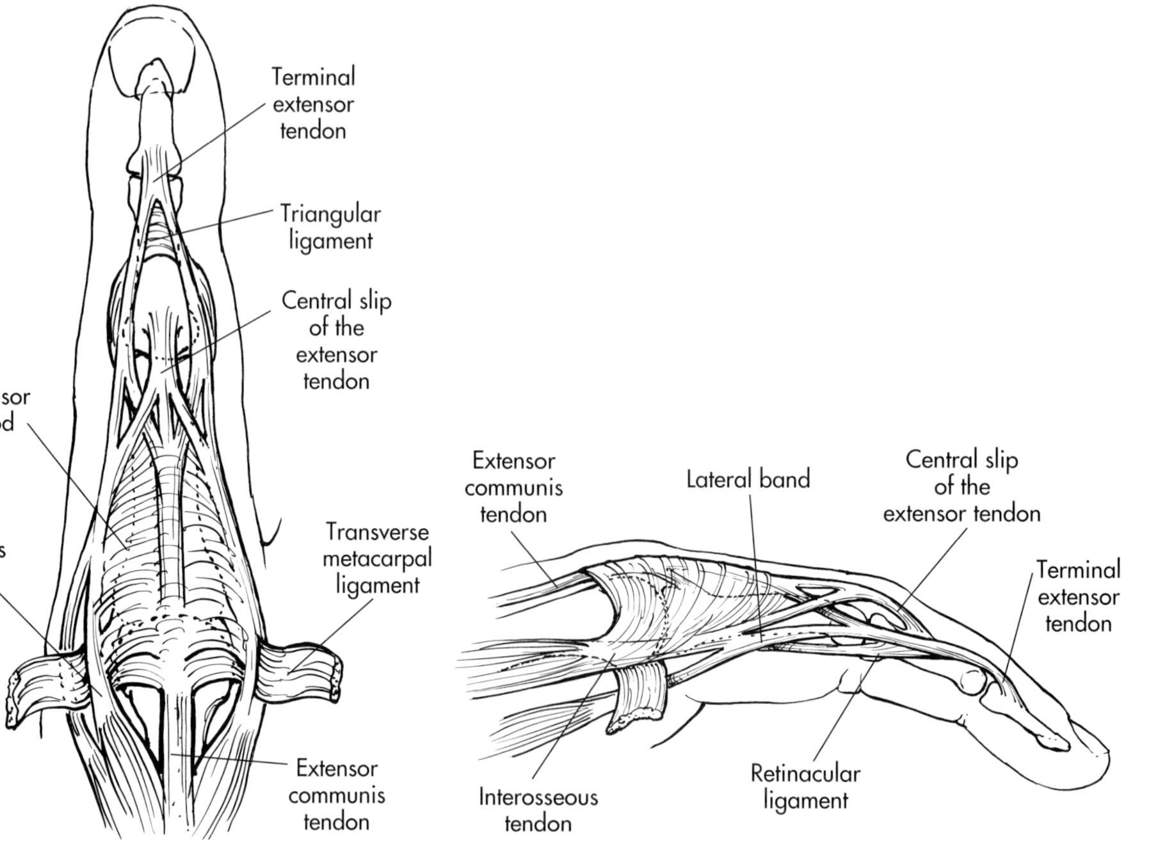

B

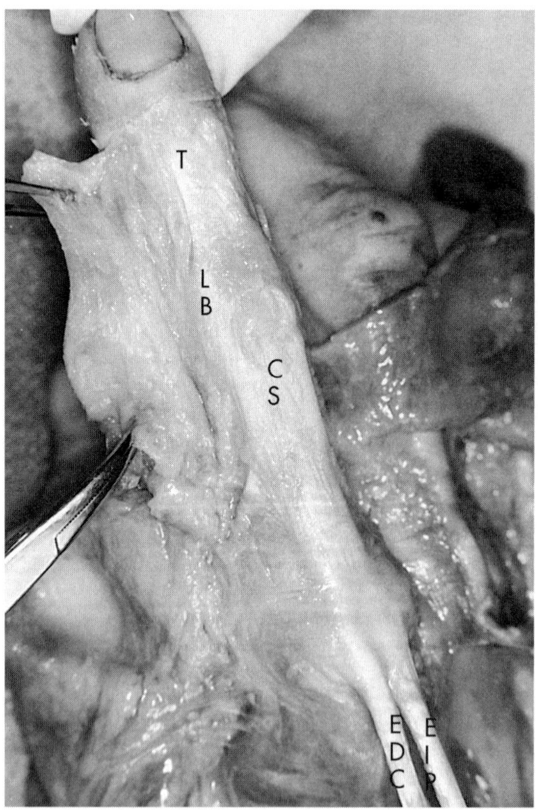

FIGURE 26-17 **A,** Coronal *(left)* and sagittal *(right)* views of the extensor mechanism of a finger. **B,** Extensor mechanism on the dorsum of the index finger. *EDC,* Extensor digitorum communis; *EIP,* extensor indicis proprius; *CS,* central slip; *LB,* lateral band; *T,* terminal tendon.

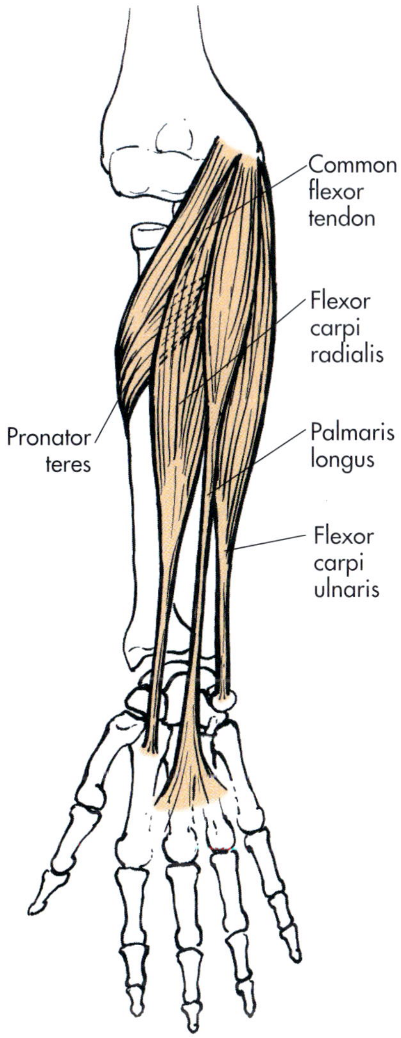

FIGURE 26-18 The superficial group of flexor muscles.

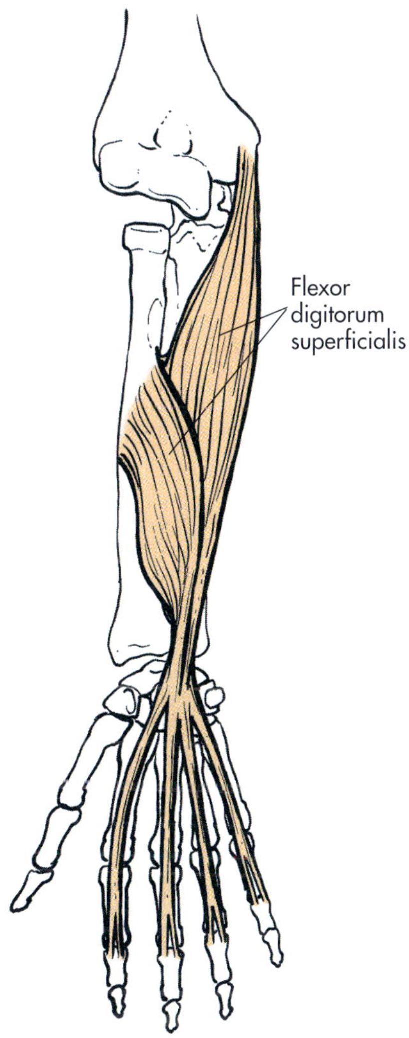

FIGURE 26-19 The intermediate group of flexor muscles.

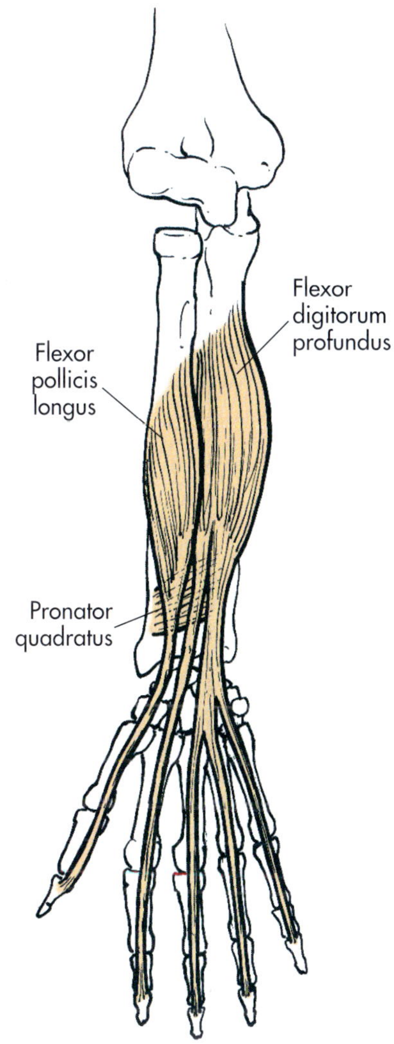

FIGURE 26-20 The deep group of flexor muscles.

a groove of the trapezium and inserts into the base of the second metacarpal and, not uncommonly, into the third metacarpal.

Also arising from the common flexor tendon is the palmaris longus. It is usually a short muscle ending in a long, thin tendon that passes superficial to the flexor retinaculum at the wrist and becomes continuous with the palmar aponeurosis. The palmaris longus is absent in 15% to 20% of individuals.

The two heads of the flexor carpi ulnaris muscle originate from the medial humeral epicondyle, the intermuscular septum, and the ulna. Just distal to the epicondyle, the two heads are covered by a fibrous arch. The ulnar nerve passes from the cubital tunnel beneath the fibrous arch and between the two heads of the flexor carpi ulnaris muscle and then lies superficial to the flexor digitorum profoundus muscles. The broad tendon of the flexor carpi ulnaris inserts into the pisiform. It covers and is medial to the ulnar artery and nerve at the wrist. After inserting into the pisiform, the tendon extends via the pisohamate and pisometacarpal ligaments to the hook of the hamate and to the base of the fifth metacarpal.

Intermediate Group

The origin of the flexor digitorum superficialis muscles extends from the medial epicondyle (common flexor tendon) and ulna to the proximal two thirds of the radius (Fig. 26-19). Its four tendons arise in the middle of the forearm and form two layers as they enter the carpal canal. The tendons to the middle and ring fingers are volar to the tendons of the index and little fingers.

Deep Group

The flexor digitorum profundus is a large muscle arising from the proximal two thirds of the ulna and the intermuscular septum (Fig. 26-20). The muscle divides into two parts. Laterally, an independent tendon passes to the index finger. Medially, a common tendon passes distally, and it does not separate into three tendons until it reaches the carpal tunnel.

The flexor pollicis longus muscle, on the same plane as the flexor digitorum profundus muscles, arises from the radius and the intermuscular septum and forms a large tendon that enters the radial side of the carpal tunnel.

The pronator quadratus is a flat muscle in the distal forearm, deep to the flexor tendons and muscles. It arises from the anterior surface of the ulna, and its transverse fibers pass laterally to the anterior surface of the radius.

WRIST AND HAND

There are two tunnels at the wrist that allow passage of tendons, nerves, and vessels from the forearm across the wrist into the hand. The carpal tunnel is formed by bone on its dorsal and lateral aspects, and it is completed on its volar side by the transverse carpal ligament. The tunnel extends about 5 cm from the transverse wrist crease to the midpalm. It is a synovial-lined tunnel and contains nine flexor tendons and the median nerve (Fig. 26-21). The wrist flexor tendons and the palmaris longus tendon do not pass through the carpal tunnel.

The ulnar tunnel (Guyon's canal) is 4 cm in length. Its

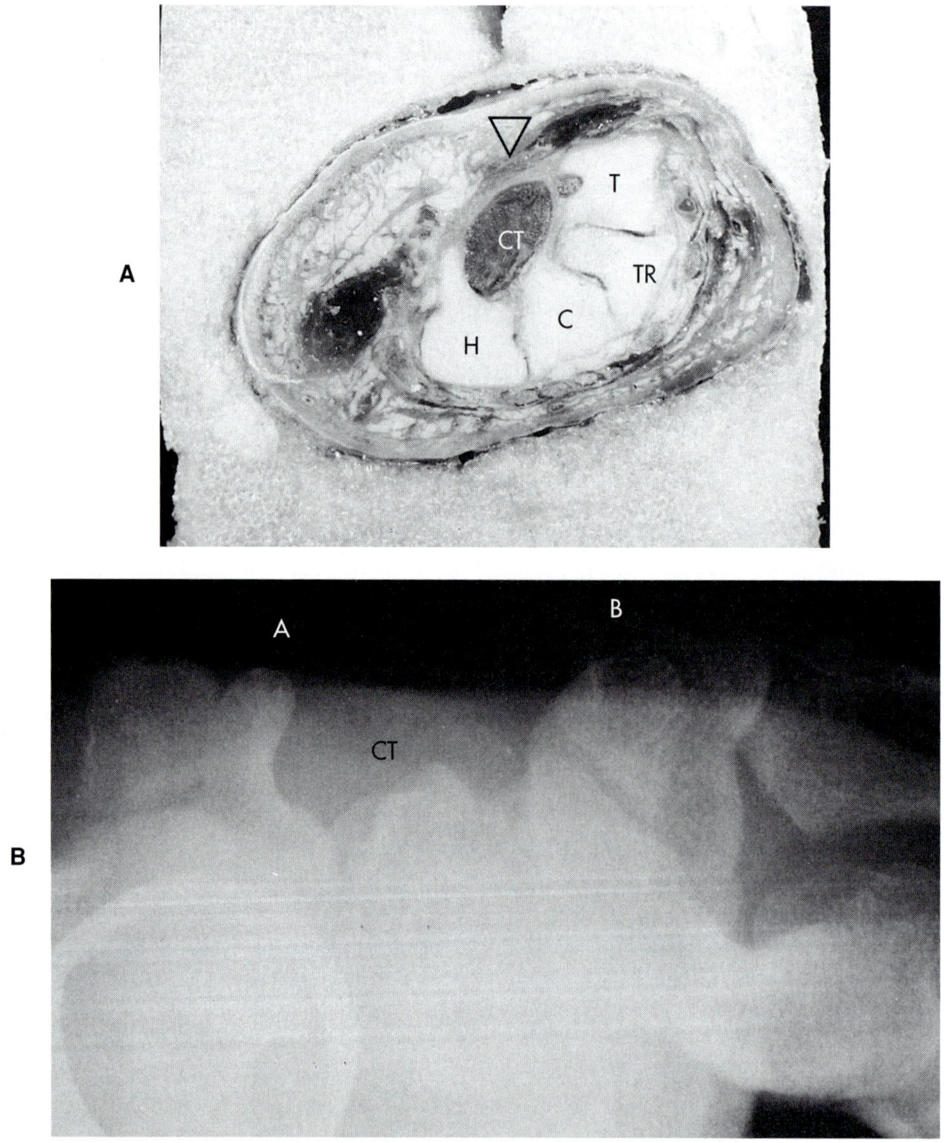

FIGURE 26-21 **A,** An axial section showing the carpal tunnel containing the median nerve and nine tendons. Carpal bones form the floor of the tunnel, and its roof is formed by the transverse carpal ligament. *CT,* Carpal tunnel; *T,* trapezium; *TR,* trapezoid; *C,* capitate; *H,* hamate; *arrow,* transverse carpal ligament. **B,** A radiographic view of the carpal tunnel. *A,* Hook of hamate; *B,* tubercle of trapezium; *CT,* carpal tunnel.

roof is formed by the volar carpal ligament, and its floor is formed by the pisohamate ligament and transverse carpal ligament. This tunnel contains the ulnar nerve, ulnar artery, and ulnar vein.

Beneath the skin in the palm is the palmar aponeurosis. This is a fascial covering over the nerves, arteries, and tendons. Beyond the carpal canal, the common flexor tendon sheath to the index, middle, and ring fingers ends in the midpalm. A continuous flexor sheath surrounds the tendons to the thumb and little finger and extends to the distal phalanx of these two digits.

The superficialis and profundus tendons to the fingers run in a fibroosseous tunnel. Doyle and Blythe[6] described the pulley system of the flexor sheath, which increases the mechanical efficiency of the flexor system. There are five annular pulleys and three cruciform pulleys. The description of this synovial-lined fibroosseous tunnel was updated by Doyle in 1989[7] (Fig. 26-22).

In the palm, the superficialis tendon to each digit is volar to the profundus tendon. In the proximal segment of the finger, the superficialis tendon splits into two slips. At the distal end of the proximal phalanx, the two slips converge and decussate with each other, inserting into the middle phalanx. This decussation (chiasm of Camper) occurs in such a manner as to not constrict the profundus tendon, which passes between the two superficialis slips and inserts into the distal phalanx. Within the flexor sheath, the tendons are nourished by synovial fluid and by blood vessels (vincula longa and breves). These vessels enter the flexor tendons and extend along the dorsal surface of the tendon (Fig. 26-23).

The thumb has only one flexor tendon, which inserts

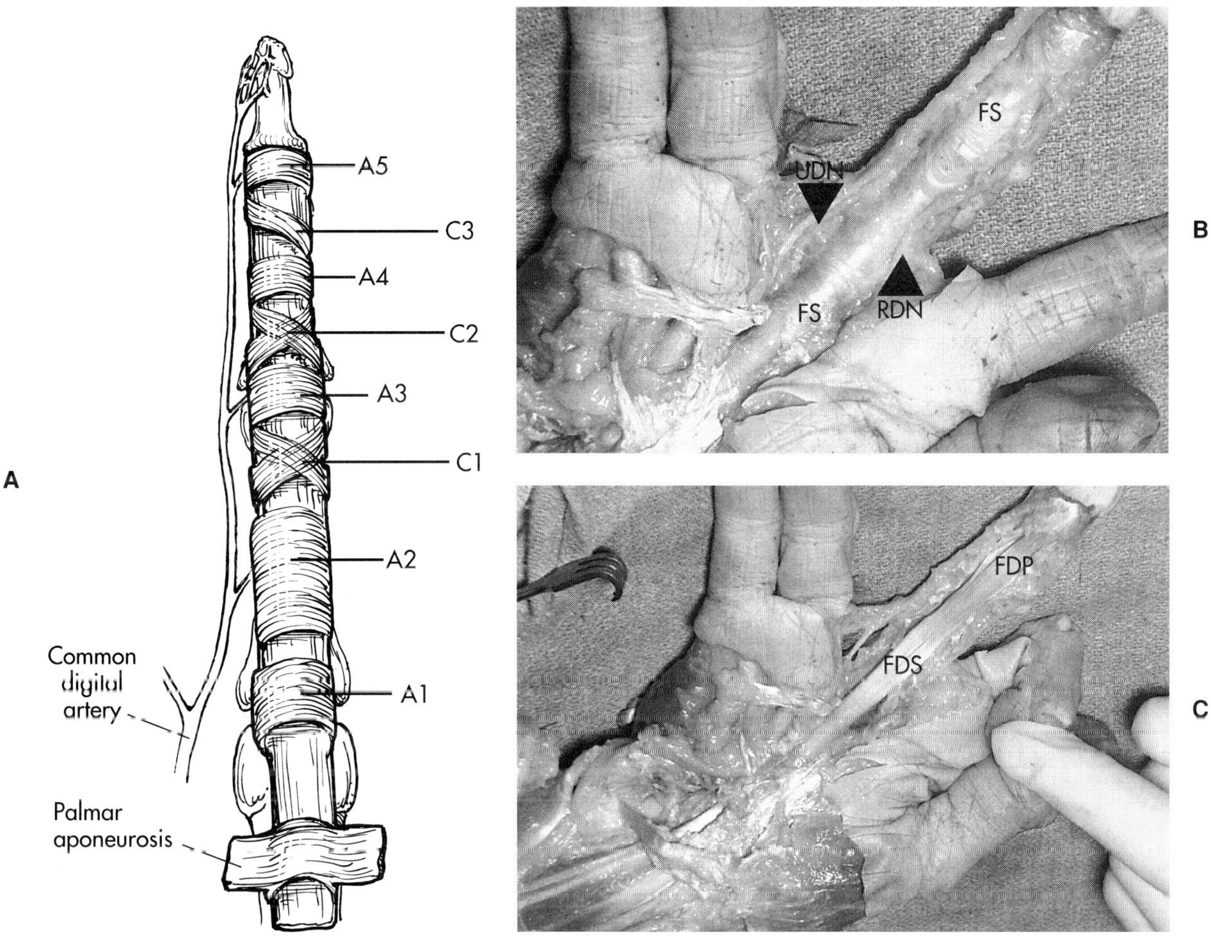

FIGURE 26-22 **A,** The flexor tendon sheath consists of a palmar aponeurosis pulley, five annular pulleys, and three cruciform pulleys. **B,** A volar view of the flexor tendon sheath in the middle finger. The digital nerves are on each side of the flexor sheath. *FS,* Flexor sheath; *UDN,* ulnar digital nerve; *RDN,* radial digital nerve. **C,** The flexor sheath has been removed. The flexor digitorum superficialis *(FDS)* and the flexor digitorum profundus *(FDP)* pass from the palm to insert into the middle and distal phalanges respectively. The flexor profundus tendon is dorsal in the palm and becomes volar in the finger.

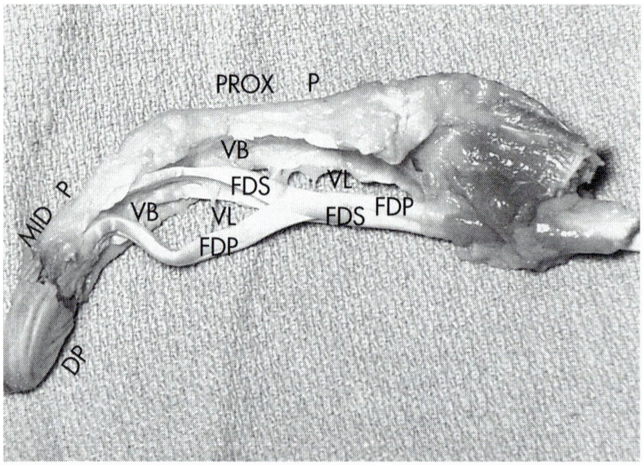

FIGURE 26-23 The decussation of the flexor superficialis tendon allows the flexor profundus tendon to pass distally and insert into the distal phalanx. Blood supply to the tendons, vinculum longum, and vinculum brevis enters the tendons from the dorsum. *FDP,* Flexor profundus; *FDS,* flexor superficialis; *VB,* vinculum brevis; *VL,* vinculum longus; *DP,* distal phalanx; *MID P,* middle phalanx; *PROX P,* proximal phalanx.

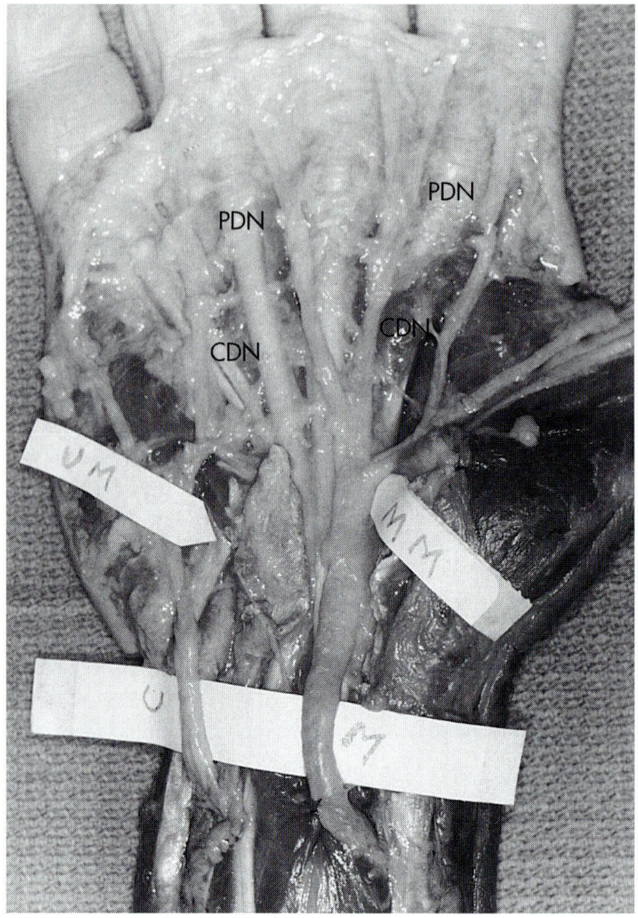

FIGURE 26-24 After median and ulnar nerves pass through their respective tunnels, they give off motor branches. The nerves then divide into common digital nerves, which in turn split into proper digital nerves to the fingers. *M,* Median nerve; *U,* ulnar nerve; *MM,* median motor nerve; *UM,* ulnar motor nerve; *CDN,* common digital nerve; *PDN,* proper digital nerve.

into the distal phalanx. There are three pulleys in the fibroosseous sheath of the thumb. These are the proximal transverse pulley at the metacarpophalangeal joint, an oblique pulley attaching to the proximal phalanx, and a small distal pulley at the distal interphalangeal joint.[8]

NERVES

The radial, median, and ulnar nerves provide motor and sensory function to the forearm, wrist, and hand.

Radial Nerve

After piercing the intermuscular septum at the lateral edge of the medial head of the triceps, the radial nerve continues in a spiral course between the bachialis and the brachioradialis muscles, and passes between the brachialis and extensor carpi radialis longus muscles into the anterior aspect of the forearm. At the level of the lateral epicondyle, the radial nerve divides into superficial and deep branches.

The superficial branch of the radial nerve passes deep to the brachioradialis muscle and emerges on the ulnar side of the brachioradialis tendon in the distal third of the forearm. It is a sensory nerve, and it supplies the radial and dorsoradial skin of the forearm and wrist, the dorsum of the thumb web, and the dorsum of the proximal segments of the thumb and index fingers.

The deep branch of the radial nerve (posterior interosseous nerve) passes beneath the thick fibrous edge of the supinator (arcade of Frohse). It emerges from the distal edge of the supinator, gives off branches to the extensor muscles, and continues on an interosseous membrane as a sensory nerve to innervate the dorsum of the wrist.

The muscles innervated by the radial and posterior interosseous nerves are listed in Box 26-1.

Median Nerve

The median nerve passes between the two heads of the pronator teres and beneath the flexor superficialis muscles; along with the ulnar artery, it continues to the wrist between the flexor superficialis and the flexor profundus muscles in the forearm. At the wrist it emerges radial to the tendon of the flexor superficialis to the middle finger and posterior and radial to the palmaris longus tendon. The nerve then passes through the carpal tunnel and continues to the palm, where it divides into motor and sensory branches (Fig. 26-24). The palmar cutaneous branch of the median nerve originates from the radial side of the main trunk of the median nerve in the distal forearm and innervates the skin at the base of the thenar

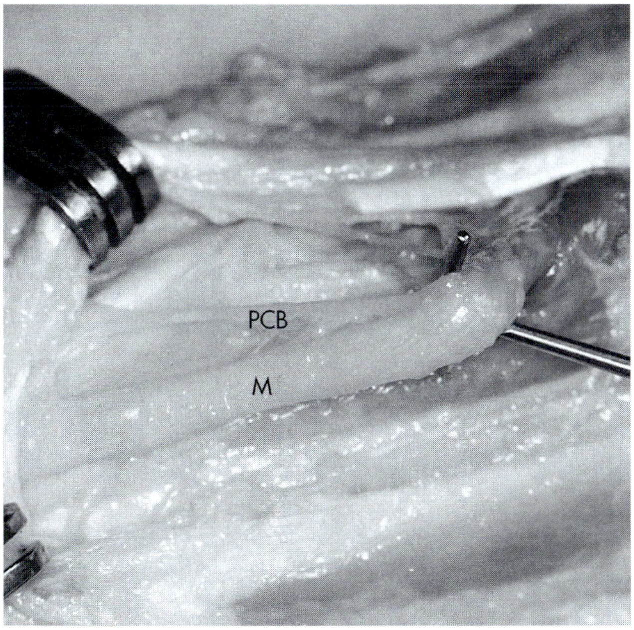

FIGURE 26-25 The palmar cutaneous branch arises from the radial side of the median nerve and innervates the skin over the base of the thenar eminence. *M,* Median nerve; *PCB,* palmar cutaneous branch.

eminence (Fig. 26-25). The median nerve provides sensibility to the palmar aspect of the thumb, the index and middle fingers, and the radial half of the ring finger. In addition, it innervates the dorsum of the distal segments of these digits. The muscles innervated by the median nerve are listed in Box 26-1.

Ulnar Nerve

The ulnar nerve courses posterior to the medial epicondyle in the cubital tunnel and continues between the two heads of the flexor carpi ulnaris muscle.

The ulnar nerve in the forearm lies on the flexor profundus muscles and courses along a stright line to the wrist, where it lies lateral to the pisiform, medial to the ulnar artery, and deep to the flexor carpi ulnaris tendon. The nerve passes through Guyon's canal and divides into motor and sensory branches (see Fig. 26-24). The terminal sensory branches in the hand provide sensibility to the palmar aspect of the little finger and ulnar half of the ring finger, as well as the dorsum of the distal segments of these digits. The dorsal sensory branch of the ulnar nerve, arising in the distal forearm, innervates the ulnar side of the hand and the dorsum of the proximal segments of the ring and little fingers. The muscles innervated by the ulnar nerve are listed in Box 26-1.

Function in the hand can vary after injury from a Martin-Gruber anastamosis (of the motor fibers from the median nerve to the ulnar nerve in the forearm).[22]

BLOOD VESSELS

Arteries

The brachial artery passes from the arm into the forearm with the biceps tendon on the radial side and the median nerve on its ulnar side. The artery then passes deep to the lacertus fibrosus and divides into the radial and ulnar arteries. These vessels continue to the wrist and palm, where they form the superficial and deep palmar arches.

The common interosseous artery arises from the ulnar artery in the forearm, and it branches to form the anterior and posterior interosseous arteries, which course along the interosseous membrane to the wrist.

Veins and Lymphatics

Many veins in the digits continue proximally into the extensive network on the dorsum of the hand. This subcutaneous venous system then extends proximally on both sides of the forearm. The ulnar side becomes part of the brachial vein, while the radial side becomes the antecubital vein and subsequently the cephalic vein.

The lymphatic system follows the veins on the dorsum of the hand and forearm.

SURGICAL APPROACHES

A great variety of incisions can be used to approach various areas on the dorsum and volar aspects of the fingers, hand, wrist, and forearm. The goals of the operation should be considered, and an intelligent surgical approach to an area should be chosen based on the regional anatomy.

Useful incisions on the dorsum of the fingers, hand, wrist, and forearm are outlined in Fig. 26-26.

The midlateral incision in the finger provides a useful approach for several procedures. This incision is made just dorsal to the flexor creases of the finger. The scar is then dorsal to the axis of finger motion and will not cause a flexion contracture of the digit (Fig. 26-27).

Incisions of the volar aspect of the fingers, hand, wrist, and forearm are outlined in Fig. 26-28.

Incisions on the radial side of the wrist and forearm and the lateral aspect of the thumb are shown in Fig. 26-29.

ARTHROSCOPIC ANATOMY OF THE WRIST

Arthroscopy of the wrist has developed into an excellent method for diagnosing and treating wrist lesions. The anatomic perspective of the radiocarpal, ulnocarpal, and midcarpal joints via the arthroscope is entirely different from that seen during an open operation. Using the arthroscope, one uses a series of small magnified views to evaluate a particular area.

The portals for wrist arthroscopy are located between the extensor tendon compartments on the dorsum of

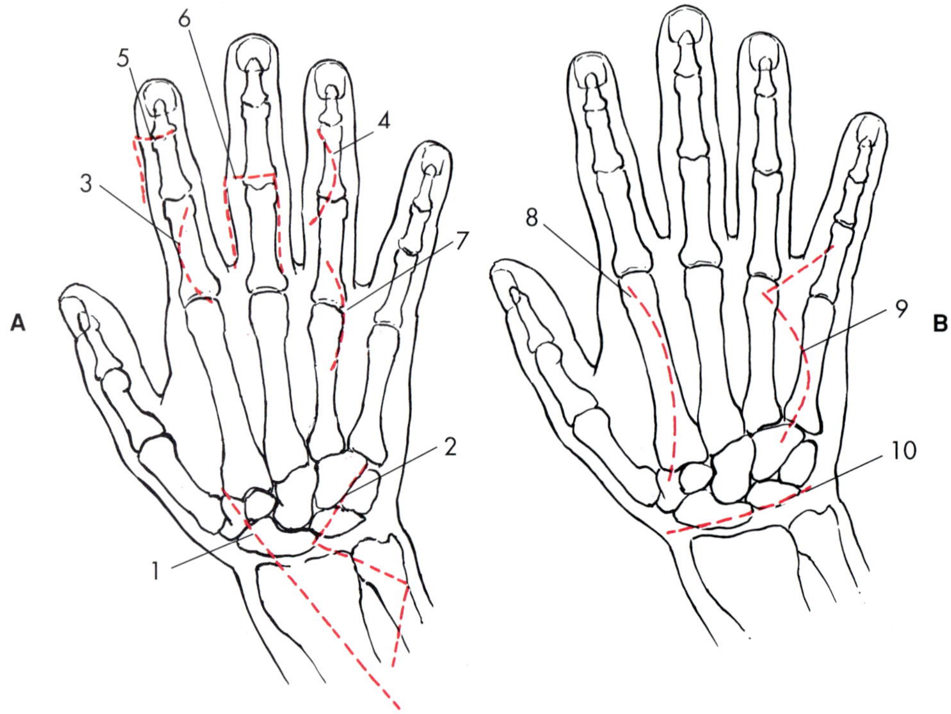

FIGURE 26-26 Incisions on the dorsum of the fingers, hand, wrist, and forearm:

1. Oblique incision on the dorsum of the hand, wrist, and forearm
   a. Open reduction and internal fixation of fractures of the radius, including the articular surface
   b. Open reduction and internal fixation of a scapholunate dissociation
   c. Midcarpal abnormality
   d. Limited or complete wrist function
   e. Extensor tendon repair or reconstruction
2. Zig-zag incision on the dorsoulnar aspect of the hand, wrist, and forearm
   a. Repair triangular fibrocartilage
   b. Open reduction and internal fixation of a fracture of the head of the ulna or the ulnar styloid
   c. Open reduction and internal fixation for a lunotriquetral instability
   d. Reconstruct the pulley for the extensor carpi ulnaris tendon
   e. The distal part of the incision can be used to approach the fifth metacarpohamate joint
3. Curved incision on the dorsum of the proximal phalanx
   a. Open reduction and internal fixation of a fracture of the proximal phalanx
   b. Osteotomy of the proximal phalanx
4. Curved incision on the dorsum of the middle phalanx
   a. Open reduction and internal fixation of a fracture of the middle phalanx
   b. Osteotomy of the middle phalanx
5. Transverse dorsal incision over the distal joint of the finger with a proximal midlateral extension
   a. Open reduction and internal fixation of an intraarticular fracture of the middle phalanx
   b. Open reduction and internal fixation of a fracture-dislocation of the distal phalanx
6. A transverse dorsal incision distal to the middle joint of the finger with a proximal midlateral extension on one or both sides
   a. Open reduction and internal fixation of an intraarticular fracture of the proximal phalanx
   b. Release of a contracture of the collateral ligaments
7. A curved incision on the dorsum of the proximal joint of the finger
   a. Exploration of the proximal joint of the finger
   b. Open reduction and internal fixation of an intraarticuar fracture of the proximal joint
   c. Reconstruction of the collateral ligaments
   d. Reconstruction of the extensor hood
8. A curved incision on the dorsum of the metacarpal
   a. Open reduction and internal fixation of a fracture of the metacarpal
   b. Osteotomy of the metacarpal
9. A zig-zag incision on the dorsum of two metacarpals
   a. Open reduction and internal fixation of a fracture of the metacarpals
10. A transverse incision over the dorsum of the radiocarpal joint
   a. Open reduction and internal fixation of a scapholunate dissociation (acute or chronic)
   b. Open reduction and internal fixation of a lunotriquetral instability
   c. Excision of the lunate

   With oblique extensions, this incision can be advanced proximally and distally.

FIGURE 26-27 Midlateral incisions of the finger, if placed properly, also can be used on the radial side of the index finger and on the ulnar side of the little finger.

1. a. Extensor and flexor tendolysis
   b. Flexor pulley reconstruction
   c. Repair of flexor tendons and digital nerves
   d. Open reduction and internal fixation of a fracture-dislocation of the middle phalanx
   e. An osteotomy for a malunited intraarticular fracture of the middle phalanx
   f. Flexor tendon graft (one-stage or two-stage)

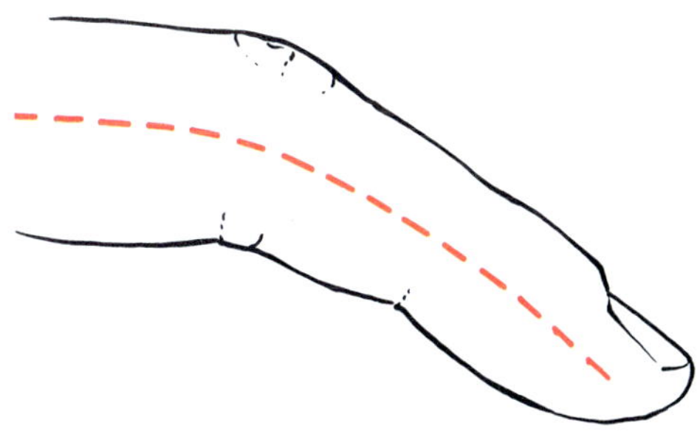

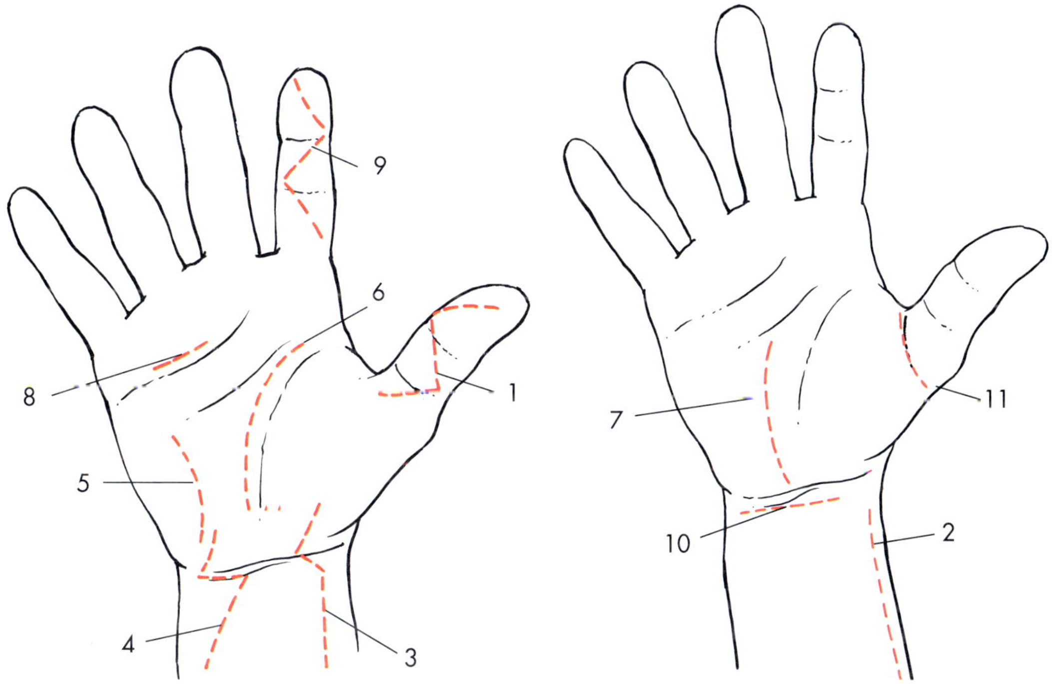

FIGURE 26-28 Incision on the volar aspect of the fingers, hand, wrist, and forearm.

1. Zig-zag incision of the thumb
   a. Flexor tendon and digital nerve repair
   b. Flexor tendolysis
   c. Reconstruction of the volar plate at the proximal joint
   d. Excision of a sesamoid bone
2. Longitudinal incisions on the volar radial aspect of the forearm: anterior approach of Henry, in which the dissection is radial to the radial artery
   a. Open reduction and internal fixation of fractures of the distal radius, including Barton's fracture
   b. Osteotomy of a malunited volar fracture of the distal radius by extension of this incision obliquely and ulnarward, allowing part or all of the carpal canal to be released
3. A longitudinal incision on the volar radial aspect of the forearm and wrist between the flexor carpi radialis tendon and the radial artery
   a. Open reduction and internal fixation of a fracture of the scaphoid
   b. Open reduction and internal fixation and bone graft of a nonunion of the scaphoid
   c. A decompression of the sheath of the flexor carpi radialis tendon
4. Zig-zag incision on the volar ulnar aspect of the wrist and forearm
   a. Decompression of Guyon's canal
   b. Excision of the pisiform
5. A curved incision on the dorsoulnar aspect of the base of the hand
   a. Excision of the hook of the hamate
6. A curved incision in the palm
   a. Flexor tendon reconstruction
   b. Nerve repair in the palm
7. A curved incision on the ulnar side of the palm
   a. Open release of the carpal tunnel
8. A short transverse incision in the distal palm just distal to the proximal joint
   a. Release of a trigger finger
9. A zig-zag incision on the volar aspect of the finger
   a. Flexor tendon and digital nerve repair
   b. Flexor tendon graft (one-stage or two-stage)
   c. Reconstruction of the volar plate of the middle joint of the finger
10. A transverse incision on the ulnar side of the wrist.
    a. Endoscopic carpal tunnel release
11. A transverse incision just distal to the proximal flexion crease of the thumb
    a. Release of a trigger thumb

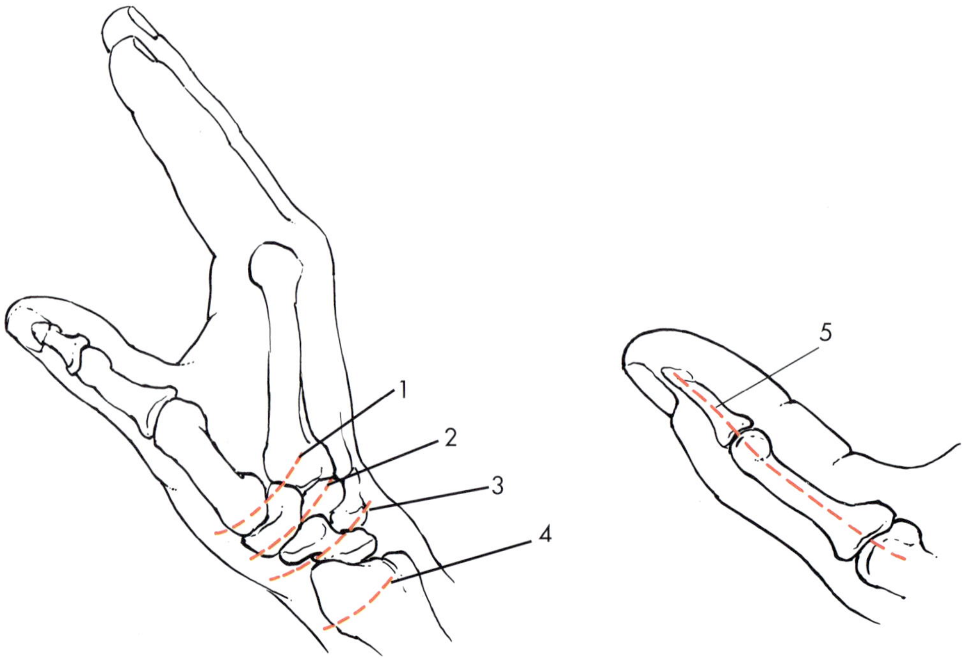

FIGURE 26-29 Incisions on the radial aspect of the wrist and lateral aspect of the thumb.

1. A transverse incision centered over the metacarpotrapezial joint
   a. Open reduction and internal fixation of a Bennett's fracture
   b. Open reduction and internal fixation of a recurrent dislocation at the metacarpotrapezial joint
   c. Reconstructive procedures for metacarpotrapezial arthritis
2. A transverse incision, centered over the scaphotrapezial joint, that can be extended proximally and distally
   a. Open reduction and internal fixation of fractures of the scaphotrapezial joint
   b. Reconstructive procedures for scaphotrapezial arthritis
3. A transverse incision over the radial carpal joint
   a. Open reduction and internal fixation of a fracture of the proximal pole of the scaphoid
   b. A radial styloidectomy
4. A short oblique incision over the pulley of the first extensor fibroosseous compartment
   a. Release of de Quervain's tenosynovitis
5. A midlateral incision of the thumb
   a. Flexor tendon and digital nerve repair
   b. Flexor tendon graft (one-stage or two-stage)
   c. Ulnar side: repair or reconstruction of the ulnar collateral ligament at the proximal joint; radial side: repair or reconstruction of the radial collateral ligament at the proximal joint

the wrist and are numbered accordingly. The 3-4 portal is between the third extensor compartment (extensor pollicis longus) and the fourth extensor compartment (extensor digitorum communis and extensor indicis proprius). The 6-R portal is located to the radial side of the sixth extensor compartment (extensor carpi ulnaris), and the 6-U portal is located on the ulnar side (Fig. 26-30).

The arthroscopic anatomy at the radiocarpal, ulnocarpal, and midcarpal joints has been described by several authors.[3,5,20,27,29]

Radiocarpal and Ulnocarpal Joints

In the radiocarpal joint, the scaphoid and lunate fossa of the radius, radial styloid, and radial recess can be seen. Distally, the proximal articular surfaces of the lunate, scaphoid, and scapholunate ligament are seen. Flexion and extension of the wrist will allow a better view of the dorsal and volar aspects of the bones and of the scapholunate ligament. Deeper within the joint, the palmar radiocarpal ligaments can be seen. From the radial to the ulnar side, they are the radioscaphocapitate, the radiolunotriquetral, and the radioscapholunate ligaments. The radioscapholunate ligament tends to be Y-shaped, with an identifying vascular tuft usually present. Sweeping to the ulnar side, the ulnocarpal ligaments (ulnolunate, ulnotriquetral) and the triangular fibrocartilage are seen. The proximal articular surfaces of the lunate and triquetrum as well as the lunotriquetral ligament can be identified and evaluated (Fig. 26-31).

Midcarpal Joints

Different portals are used for the midcarpal joints.[5,27] The midcarpal radial portal is in a soft spot proximal to the capitate, in line with the radial border of the third metacarpal, and is approximately 1 cm distal to the 3-4

A

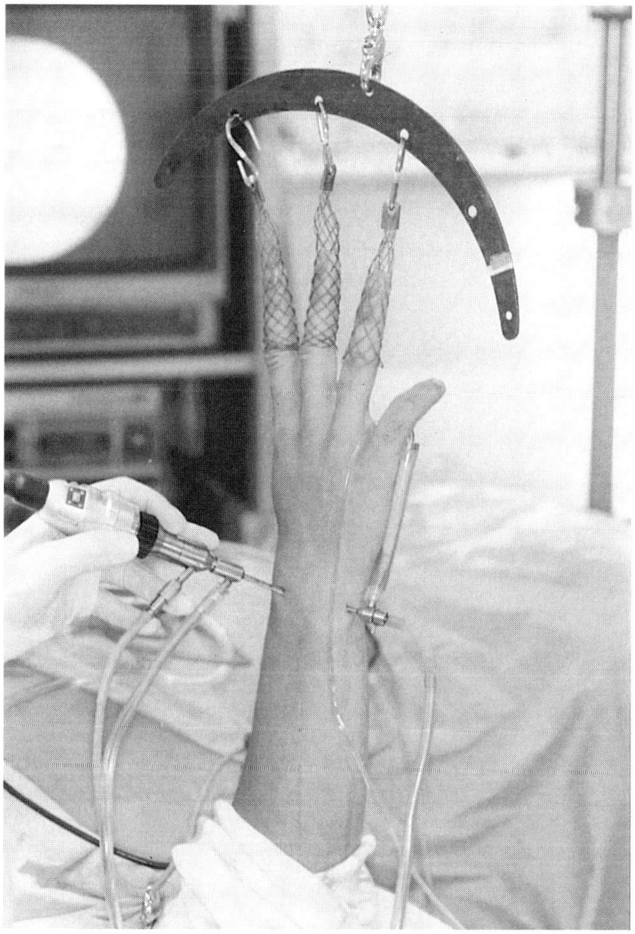

B

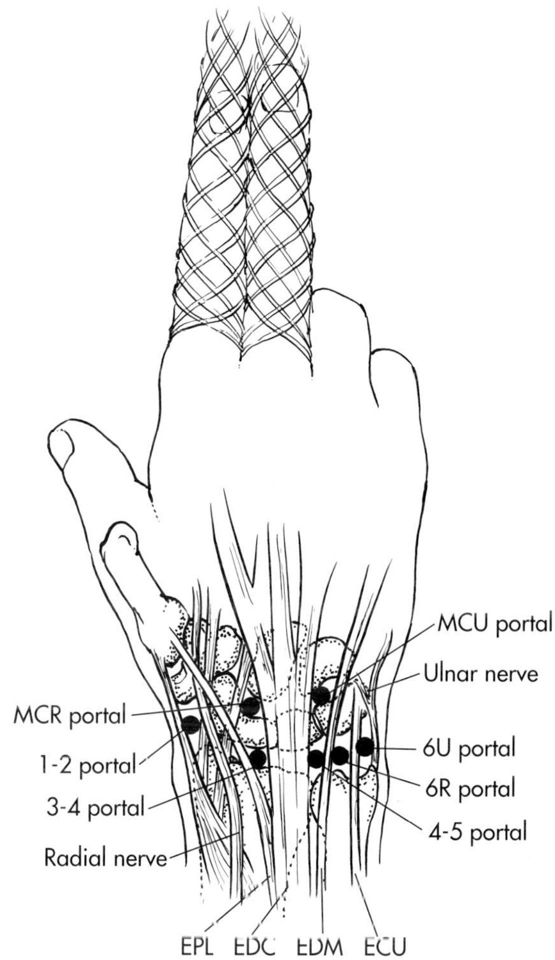

FIGURE 26-30 A right hand. **A,** The arthroscope is in the 3-4 portal, and the outflow is in the 6-B portal. **B,** The commonly used portals for wrist arthroscopy.

portal. This radial midcarpal portal is ulnar to the extensor carpi radialis brevis tendon and radial to the extensor digitorum communis tendons. Using this portal, the articular surfaces of the scaphotrapezium trapezoid joints, scaphocapitate joint, scapholunate joint, capitolunate joint, lunotriquetral joint, capitohamate joint, and triquetrohamate joint.

The midcarpal ulnar portal is in line with the center of the fourth metacarpal at the same level as the midcarpal radial portal. Ulnar structures are more easily seen through this portal, or this portal can be used as an accessory portal for instruments.

Structures that can be seen and evaluated through the various portals are noted in Table 26-1.[29]

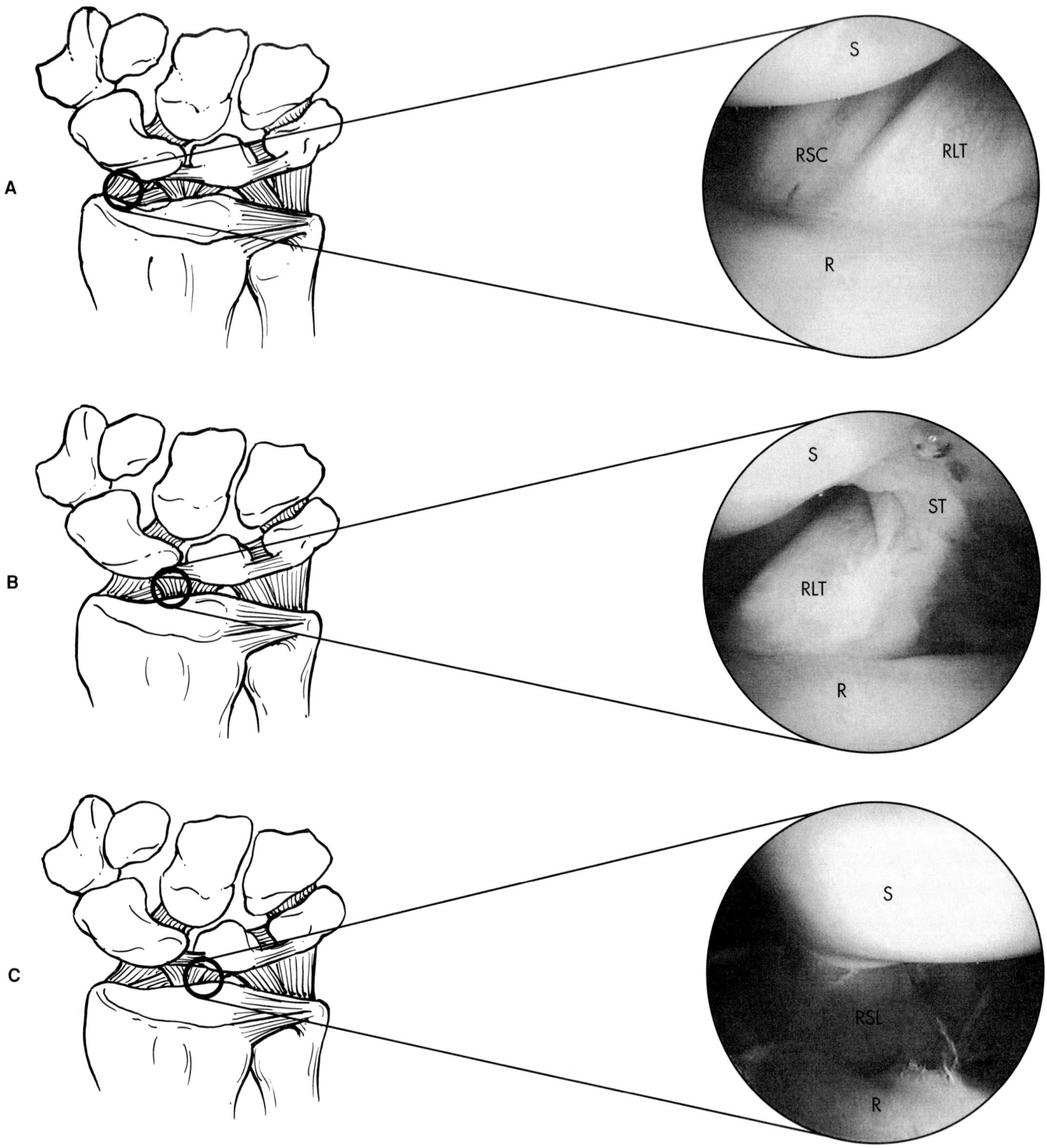

FIGURE 26-31 Drawing of ligaments with inset photos, a right wrist. **A,** The radioscaphocapitate *(RSC)* and radiolunotriquetral *(RLT)* ligaments. **B,** Radiolunotriquetral ligament *(RLT)* and the synovial tuft *(ST)* indicating the scapholunate joint. **C,** Radioscapholunate ligaments *(RSL)*.

D

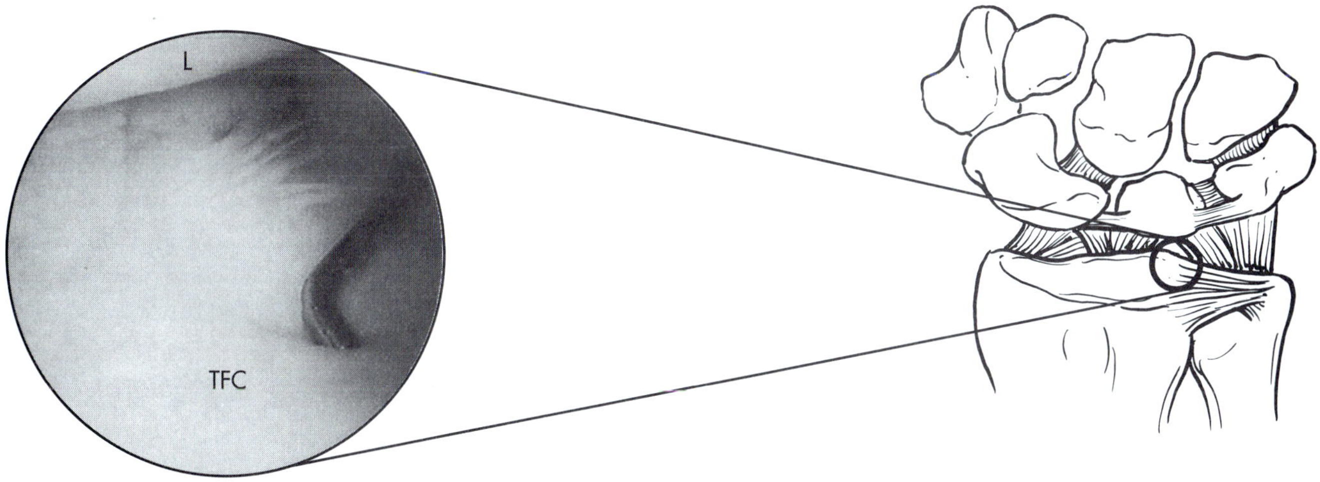

E

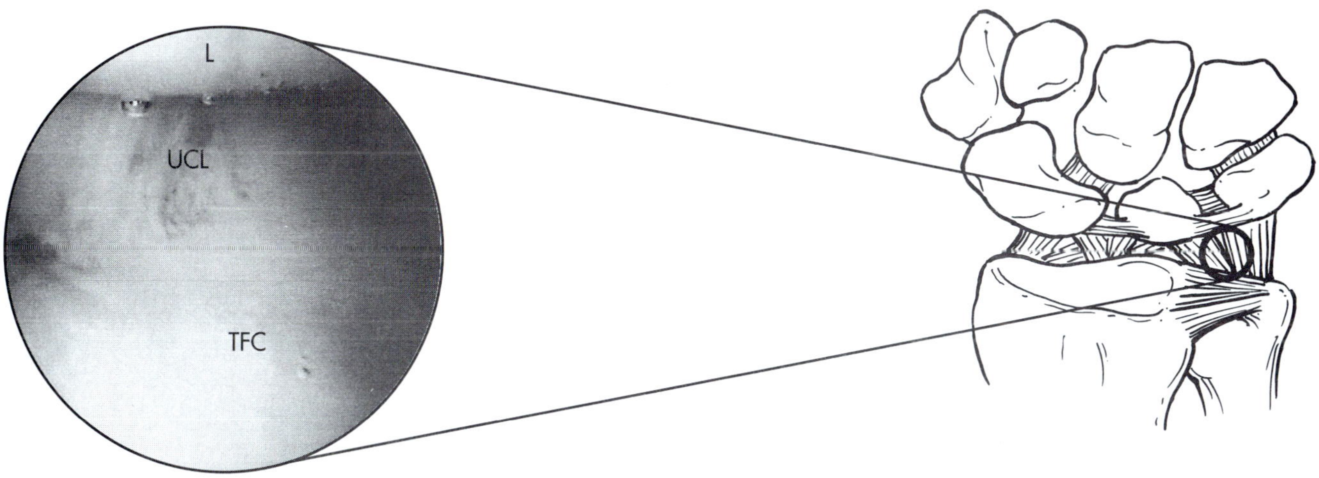

FIGURE 26-31—cont'd **D,** Triangular fibrocartilage *(TFC)*. **E,** Triangular fibrocartilage *(TFC)* and the ulnocarpal ligaments *(UCL)*. *R,* Radius; *S,* scaphoid; *L,* lunate.

TABLE 26-1
Structures Usually Seen Through the Various Arthroscopic Portals

Portals	Structures	Portals	Structures
Portal 1-2	Scaphoid facet	MC portal	Distal scaphoid
	Radial aspect of scaphoid		STT joint
Portal 3-4	Scaphoid and lunate facet of radius		Proximal capitate
	Radiocarpal and ulnocarpal volar ligaments		Distal lunate
	Triangular fibrocartilage		Proximal hamate
	Proximal carpal row		Distal triquetrum
Portal 4-5	Triangular fibrocartilage	DRUJ portal	Proximal triangular fibrocartilage
	Ulnocarpal ligaments		Ulnar head
Portal 6R-6U	Triquetrum		Sigmoid notch
	Ulnocarpal ligaments		
	Triangular fibrocartilage		

References

1. Alexander CE, Lichtman DM: Ulnar carpal instabilities, *Orthop Clin North Am* 15:307-320, 1984.
2. Bogumill GP: Anatomy of the wrist. In Lichtman DM, editor: *The wrist and its disorders,* Philadelphia, 1988, WB Saunders.
3. Botte MJ, Cooney WP, Linscheid RL: Arthroscopy of the wrist: anatomy and technique, *J Hand Surg* 14A:313-316, 1989.
4. Bowers WH et al: The proximal interphalangeal joint volar plate. I. An anatomical and biomechanical study, *J Hand Surg* 5:79-88, 1980.
5. Cooney WP, Dobyns JH, Linscheid RL: Arthroscopy of the wrist: anatomy and classification of carpal instability, *Arthroscopy* 6:133-140, 1990.
6. Doyle JR, Blythe WF: The finger flexor tendon sheath and pulleys: anatomy and reconstruction. In: *AAOS symposium and tendon surgery in the hand,* St Louis, 1975, CV Mosby, pp 81-87.
7. Doyle JR: Anatomy of the flexor tendon sheath and pulley system: a current review, *J Hand Surg* 14A:349-351, 1989.
8. Doyle JR, Blythe WF: Anatomy of the flexor tendon sheath and pulleys of the thumb, *J Hand Surg* 2:149-151, 1977.
9. Hulten O: Uber anatomische variationen der hand and gelen knochen, *Acta Radial* 9:155-169, 1928.
10. Jupiter JB: Current concepts review—fractures of the distal end of the radius, *J Bone Joint Surg* 73-A:461-469, 1991.
11. Kaplan EM: *Joints and ligaments in functional and surgical anatomy of the hand,* Philadelphia, 1965, JB Lippincott.
12. Kauer JMG: Functional anatomy of the wrist, *Clin Orthop* 149:9-20, 1980.
13. Mayfield JK, Johnson RP, Kilcoyne RF: The ligaments of the human wrist and their functional significance, *Anat Rec* 186:417-428, 1976.
14. Mayfield JK: Mechanism of carpal injuries, *Clin Orthop* 149:45-54, 1980.
15. Milford L: *Retaining ligaments of the digits of the hand,* Philadelphia, 1968, WB Saunders.
16. Palmar AK, Werner FW: The triangular fibrocartilage complex of the wrist: anatomy and function, *J Hand Surg* 6:153-162, 1981.
17. Palmar AK, Glisson RR, Werner FW: Relationship between ulnar variance and triangular fibrocartilage complex thickness, *J Hand Surg* 9A:681-683, 1984.
18. Palmar AK: Triangular fibrocartilage complex lesions: a classification, *J Hand Surg* 14A:594-606, 1989.
19. Posner MA, Kaplan EB: Osseous and ligamentous structures. In Spinner M, editor: *Kaplan's functional and surgical anatomy of the hand,* ed 3, Philadelphia, 1984, JB Lippincott.
20. Roth JH, Poehling GG, Whipple TL: Arthroscopic surgery of the wrist. In Bassett FH, editor: AAOS Instructional Course Lectures Park Ridge, Ill, American Academy of Orthopaedic Surgeons *ICL XXXVII,* 1988,
21. Smith RJ: Balance and kinetics of the fingers under normal and pathological conditions, *Clin Orthop* 104:92-111, October, 1974.
22. Spinner M: *Injuries to the major branches of peripheral nerves of the forearm,* ed 2, Philadelphia, 1978, WB Saunders.
23. Taleisnik J: The ligaments of the wrist, *J Hand Surg* 1:110-118, 1976.
24. Taleisnik J et al: The extensor retinaculum of the wrist, *J Hand Surg* 9A:495-501, 1984.
25. Taleisnik J: *The wrist,* New York, 1985, Churchill Livingstone, pp 1-38.
26. Taleisnik J: Current concepts review—carpal instability, *J Bone Joint Surg* 70-A:1262-1268, 1988.
27. Toby EB, Poehling GG, Koman AL: Midcarpal arthroscopy, *Surg Rounds Orthop* 23-27, Feb, 1989.
28. Tubiana R, Valentin P: The anatomy of the extensor apparatus of the fingers, *Surg Clin North Am* 44:897-906, 1964.
29. Whipple TL, Marotta JJ, Powell JH: Techniques of wrist arthroscopy,

CHAPTER 27

Fractures and Dislocations of the Fingers and Hand

NORMAN P. ZEMEL

Injuries to the hand and wrist occur in sports related activities either from a fall or direct blow or indirectly from a combination of forces directed against the hand and fingers. These forces usually are transmitted axially in combination with twisting or laterally directed loads. Injuries result from both one-time excessive and controlled stress and persistent repetitive controlled stress.[27] A survey of several sports centers indicated that hand, finger, and wrist injuries make up 3% to 9% of sports-related injuries.[89]

Although a few reports discuss hand injuries as they occur in a particular sport (professional football,[36] skiing,[108] wrestling[106]), most reports in the literature discuss the specific fracture or ligament injury. Any type of fracture, fracture-dislocation, or ligament injury can result from a sports-related injury; however, only those injuries commonly seen in athletes will be discussed here, with emphasis on the problem fractures and dislocations. Stress fractures of the fingers and hand are very uncommon.[25]

Most fractures and dislocations of the hand and fingers can be treated closed. Some are best managed by open reduction and internal fixation.

Certain principles for treating fractures of the hand are worth emphasizing. If these principles are followed, the end result of treatment is usually satisfactory. These are:

1. Fractures of the hand should be properly reduced and immobilized until they have healed sufficiently not to displace.

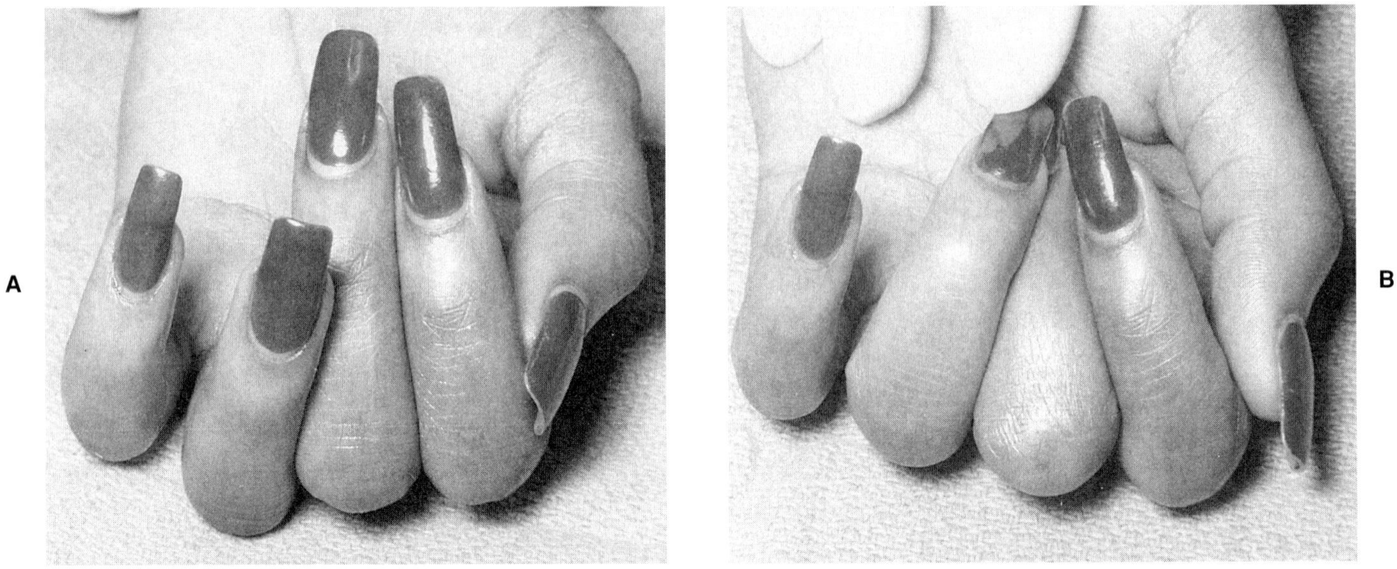

FIGURE 27-1 **A,** A displaced fracture of the ring finger causes it to rotate radially. **B,** The ring finger overlaps the middle finger with flexion.

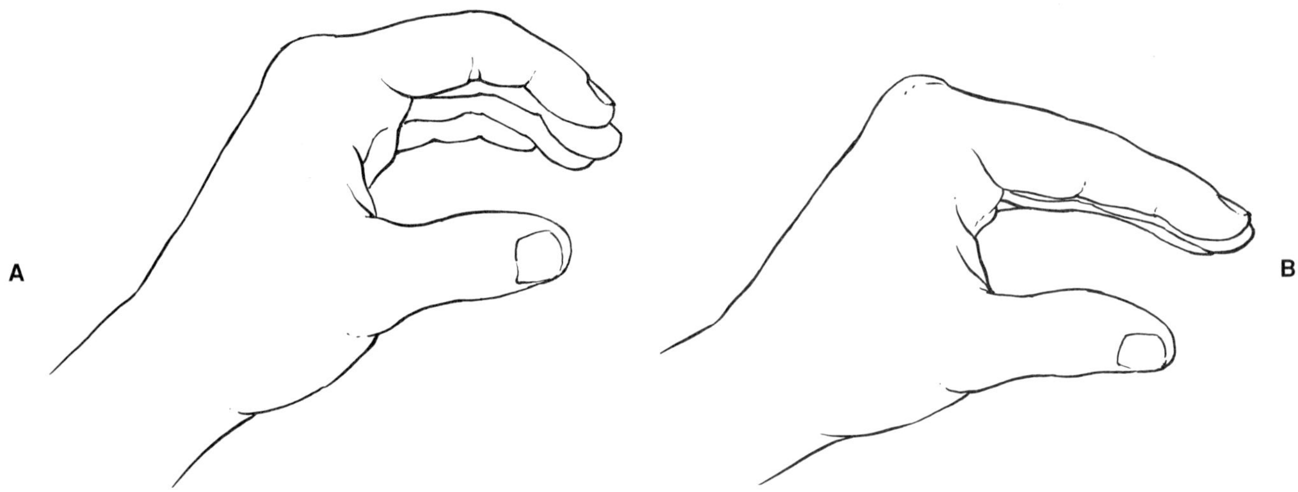

FIGURE 27-2 **A,** The authors prefer to immobilize the fingers in semiflexion. **B,** The other recommended position is with the fingers in the intrinsic-plus position (James).

2. Proper reduction includes aligning the fracture and correcting any malrotation. If fractures of the metacarpals and phalanges are not properly aligned and rotated, the fingers may deviate or overlap when flexed (Fig. 27-1). Although some dorsal or volar angulation of a finger can be tolerated, if a fracture heals in malrotation, there will be permanent deformity, regardless of the patient's age, and this will compromise finger and hand function.
3. Displaced intraarticular fractures must be reduced to restore a smooth gliding surface to the joint. If this is not done, the irregular joint surface will abrade the articular cartilage, eventually causing degenerative arthritis and a painful joint.
4. Most closed fractures of phalanges and metacarpals in adults, if treated conservatively, are sufficiently stable by 3 weeks to allow protected motion of the joints. Joints completely immobilized for more than 3 weeks have a tendency to stiffen.
5. Metacarpophalangeal and interphalangeal joints should be immobilized in semiflexion after the fracture is reduced (Fig. 27-2). The two collateral ligaments stabilize these joints. If these ligaments are splinted in extension, they tend to contract and become bound by scar tissue, and a fixed extension contracture often occurs. This complication usually can be avoided by maintaining the finger in a semiflexed position during the period of immobilization.

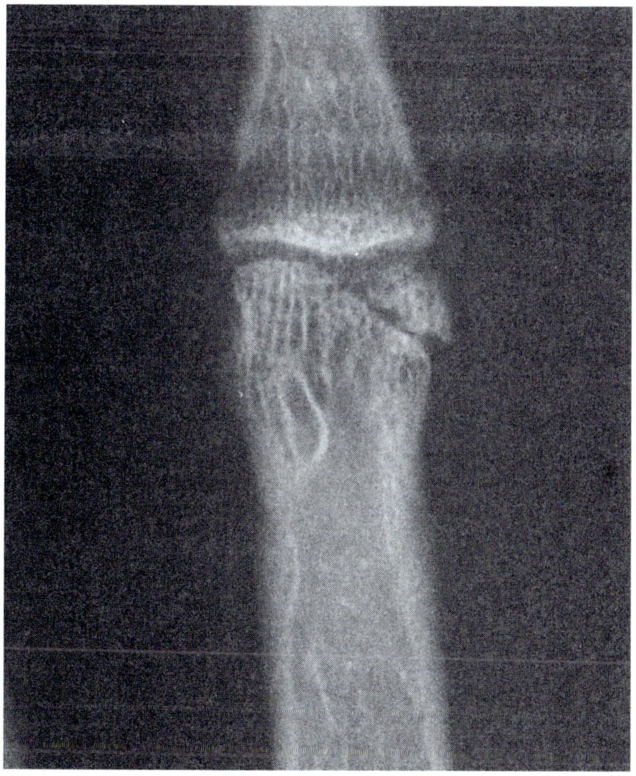

FIGURE 27-3 This intraarticular fracture has displaced laterally and volarly. The joint surface must be reduced through open reduction and internal fixation.

6. Because some of the muscles that move the fingers have tendons that cross the wrist, the physician must immobilize the wrist to maintain reduction of metacar-pal and proximal phalangeal fractures. Wrist immobilization is easily accomplished with a short arm cast, and the injured finger or fingers are immobilized in a splint. The uninjured fingers are allowed to move freely .
7. Posterior anterior, lateral, and oblique radiographs of all injured parts must be obtained both before and after fracture manipulation and immobilization. Special radiographic views also may be necessary for particular injuries.
8. Certain fractures of the phalanges and the metacarpals cannot be adequately reduced by closed methods (Fig. 27-3). These require open reduction and internal fixation to restore maximal function to the digits and hand. A variety of internal fixation devices are available.[115]

FINGERS

Distal Phalanx

Fractures of the tuft and body of the distal phalanx are usually a result of a crush injury. The fractures usually are undisplaced or minimally displaced and are associated with soft-tissue injury.[18] Significant pain may be associated with a subungual hematoma. This hematoma should be drained under sterile conditions. These injuries can be treated by splinting because the fracture usually heals with either a bony or fibrous union. The individual usually can return to sports within several days to 2 weeks, as soon as the pain has resolved.

A more significant problem is an intraarticular fracture of the distal phalanx.[99] This injury usually is a result of an axially loaded force (jam injury) and is the most serious injury in that spectrum.

Undisplaced intraarticular fractures of the distal phalanx should be treated by splinting the distal joint in extension. The joint should be splinted for 4 to 5 weeks because the pull of the flexor profundus tendon is stronger than that of the extensor tendon. A variety of splints are available and can be used on either the palmar or dorsal aspect of the joint. The joint should be splinted in 0° extension and not in hyperextension. Hyperextending the distal joint of the finger can result in necrosis of the skin over the dorsum of the joint.

Intraarticular fractures involving up to 50% of the joint surface that are displaced dorsally 1 to 2 mm, that are not rotated or tilted, and that maintain the articular contour of the joint surface also should be treated with a splint (Fig. 27-4). Wehbe and Schneider[111] and Schneider[95] in a subsequent report recommended that essentially all intraarticular fractures of the distal phalanx be treated by splinting. They reported that bony remodeling and restoration of the articular surface occurred in all their cases. All but one patient had a near-normal range of painless motion.

Fractures of the distal phalanx that involve more than one third of the joint surface, that are rotated or tilted, that have an incongruous joint surface, and that are associated with a palmar subluxation of the distal phalanx should be treated by an open reduction and internal fixation (Fig. 27-5). The operation is difficult because the fragments are small. The dorsum of the joint is opened by a curved incision without violating the nail matrix or the extensor tendon. One collateral ligament is divided, permitting a clear view of the joint (Fig. 27-6). If the phalanx is subluxated, it is reduced and immobilized with a transarticular Kirschner wire. The displaced dorsal lip fragment then is replaced into the defect, thereby restoring a nearly anatomic joint surface. The fracture is immobilized with two 0.028 Kirschner wires inserted parallel to the joint. The two parallel Kirschner wires are cut off beneath the skin. After the collateral ligament is repaired and the skin is closed, the finger is immobilized in a splint with the proximal interphalangeal joint in 30° of flexion. The transarticular Kirschner wire is removed in 3 to 4 weeks, and gentle joint motion is started. When the fracture has healed on radiographic examination, usually by 8 weeks, the remaining Kirschner wires are removed. An alternative approach is to divide the extensor tendon to reveal the fracture (Fig. 27-7).

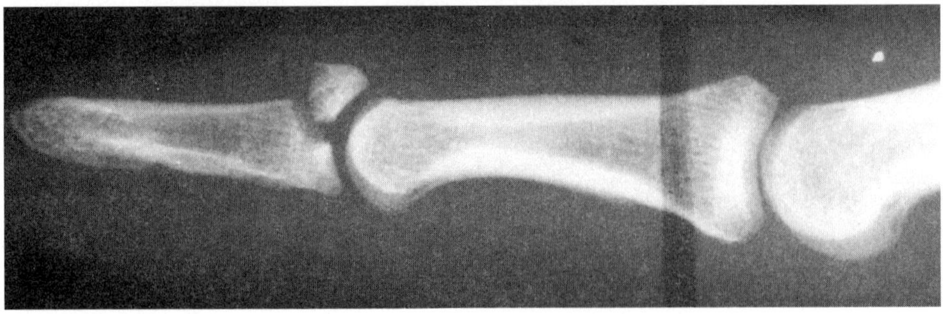

FIGURE 27-4 Although the distal phalanx is slightly displaced dorsally, the articular outline of the distal phalanx remains congruent.

A

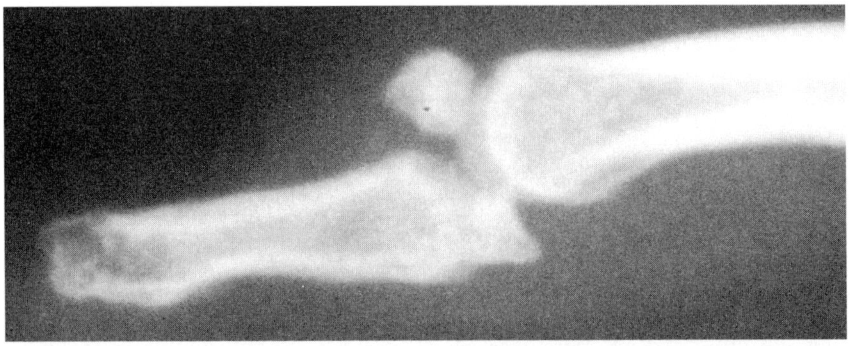

B

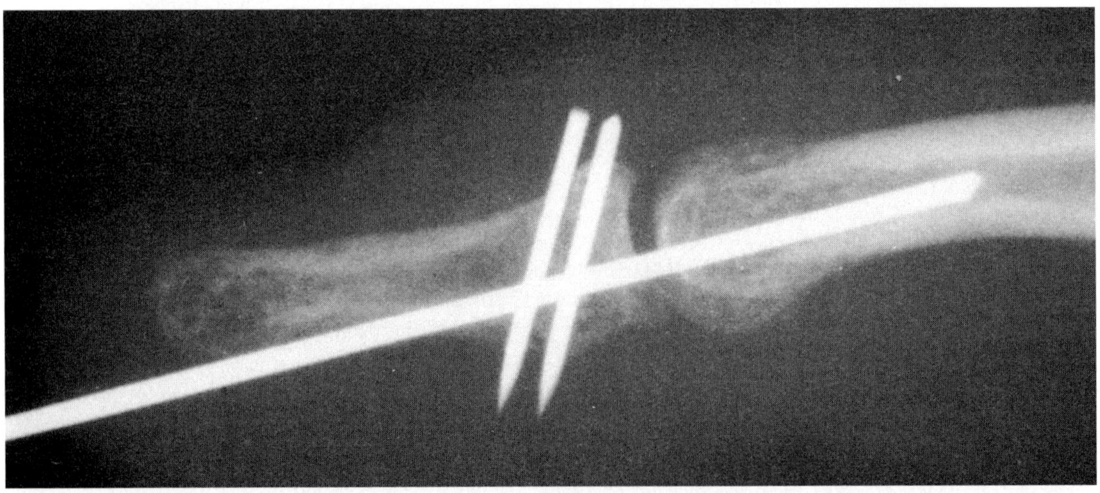

C

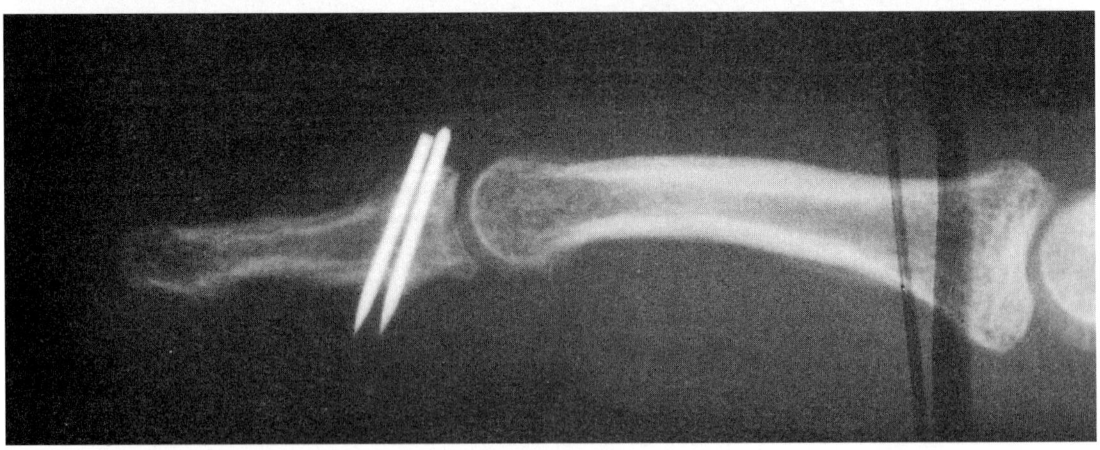

FIGURE 27-5 **A,** Fracture-dislocation of the distal joint of a finger. **B,** First the dislocation is reduced, and is stabilized with a transarticular Kirschner wire, and then the intraarticular fracture is immobilized. **C,** Three months after surgery the fracture has healed, and there is a good joint space.

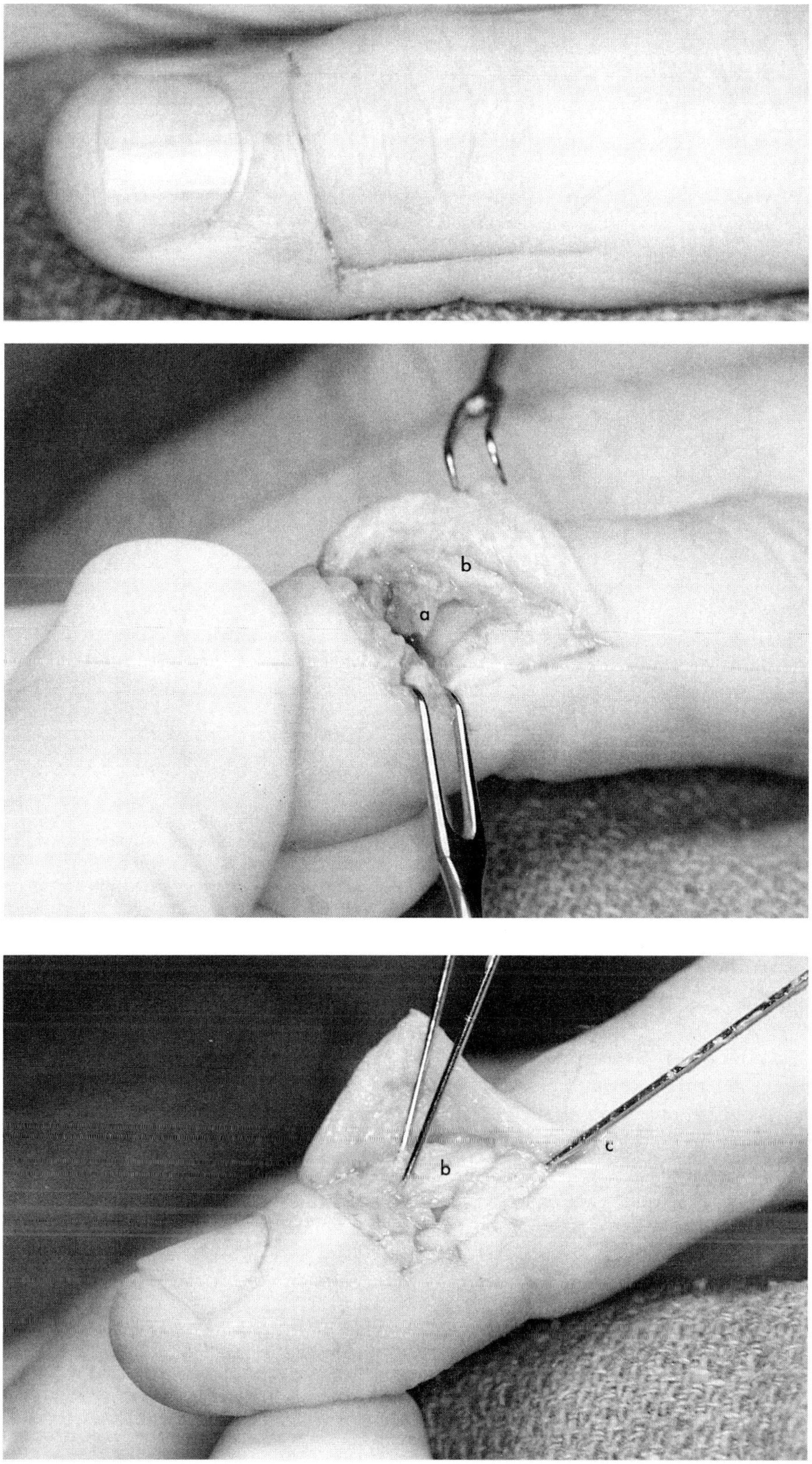

FIGURE 27-6 **A,** A curved incision is used to open the distal joint of the finger. **B,** After the collateral ligament is divided, the fracture fragment is identified *(a)* and attached to the extensor tendon *(b)*. **C,** After reduction, two Kirschner wires cross the fracture site and one Kirschner wire crosses the joint *(c)*. *b,* Extensor tendon.

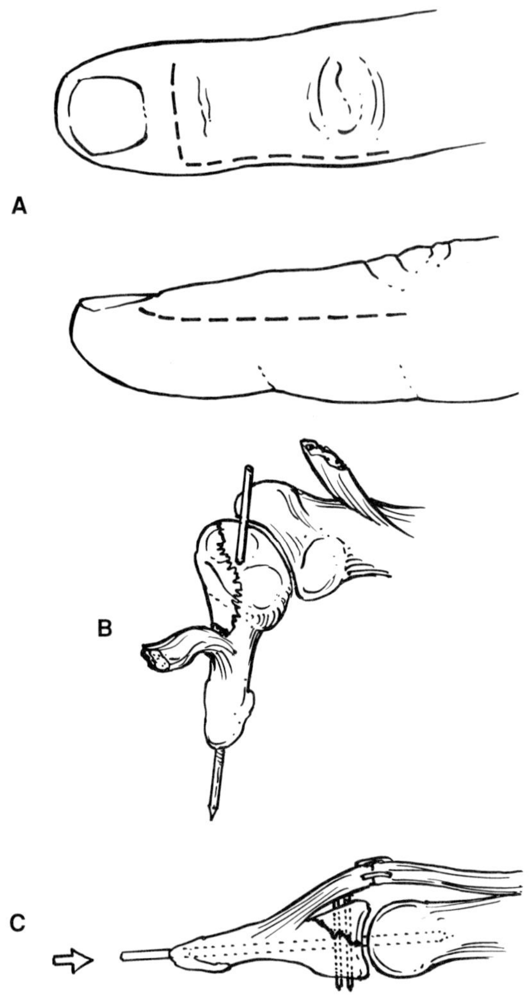

FIGURE 27-7 **A,** With a dorsal incision, **B,** the extensor tendon is divided and, **C,** the fracture and distal joint are stabilized.

Stark et al[101] reported on 36 fractures treated by open reduction and internal fixation. These patients maintained a good joint space and congruous joint surfaces an average of 46 months after the operation. Restoration of motion was excellent. The author prefers to treat these displaced fractures by open reduction and internal fixation.

Sprains and dislocations of the distal interphalangeal joint are uncommon. They are easily treated with splint immobilization, and they readily heal.

Middle Phalanx

An intracondylar (a fracture through a condyle) or an intercondylar (fracture between the condyles) fracture of the head of the middle phalanx disturbs the congruency of the joint surface.[71,115] These fractures are fairly common as a result of a sports injury. Although there may be ecchymosis and swelling, joint motion often is present, and the injury may be neglected by the patient and completely missed if proper radiographs are not obtained.

An intercondylar fracture is usually a short oblique fracture that is unstable because of shear forces at the fracture site (Fig. 27-8). The unstable condyle slides proximally, often rotates, and may tilt in a dorsal or volar direction. Both oblique radiographic views of the joint often are essential. The offset occurs at the joint surface, and, because of this, there may be an angular deformity through the joint. Because the fractured condyle is still attached to the collateral and accessory collateral ligaments, it is usually impossible to reduce the fracture by manipulation.

Accurate restoration of the joint surface is best attained through an operation. The joint is exposed through a dorsal skin incision (Fig. 27-9). At the distal interphalangeal joint, the extensor tendon usually can be elevated to expose the joint. The attachment of the collateral ligament to the fractured condyle is preserved. After anatomic reduction, the fracture is immobilized with either two Kirschner wires or a small lag screw. These are inserted parallel to the articular surface of the joint. Joint motion can be started in 3 weeks, or sooner if adequate stability of the fracture is obtained with the internal fixation. If this fracture is neglected or allowed to heal in a malunited position, improved motion can be restored to the joint by an osteotomy through the malunion site, providing that satisfactory articular cartilage is still present. If the joint cartilage has been sufficiently damaged and the joint is painful, a fusion is needed to improve function of the digit.

An intracondylar fracture results from an impaction, hyperextension, or crush injury of the joint. This produces osteochondral fragments of varying size and disrupts the gliding surface of the condyle. If the fragment is small, a CT scan may be necessary to identify the lesion. This fracture can be stabilized by small Kirschner wires passed in a retrograde fashion through the fragment and buried beneath the cartilage surface of the condyle. Joint motion can be started in 3 weeks, with a Kirschner wire functioning as an internal splint.

Fractures of the shaft of the middle phalanx can result from direct blows or twisting and torsional injuries. This discussion will deal with closed fractures. Any open fracture must be treated according to the demands of the wound and the accompanying soft-tissue injury.

Transverse fractures of the middle phalanx tend to be inherently stable, although the fracture can angulate. If the fracture is in the proximal one third of the bone, the angulation is usually apex dorsalward. When the fracture occurs distal to the insertion of the flexor digitorum superficialis tendon, the angulation is apex palmarward (Fig. 27-10).

If the transverse fracture is undisplaced or minimally displaced, the finger is splinted for 2 weeks. The finger is then buddy-splinted to allow range-of-motion exercises to increase joint mobility and decrease soft-tissue adhesions.[5,88] This regimen also can be used if the fracture is

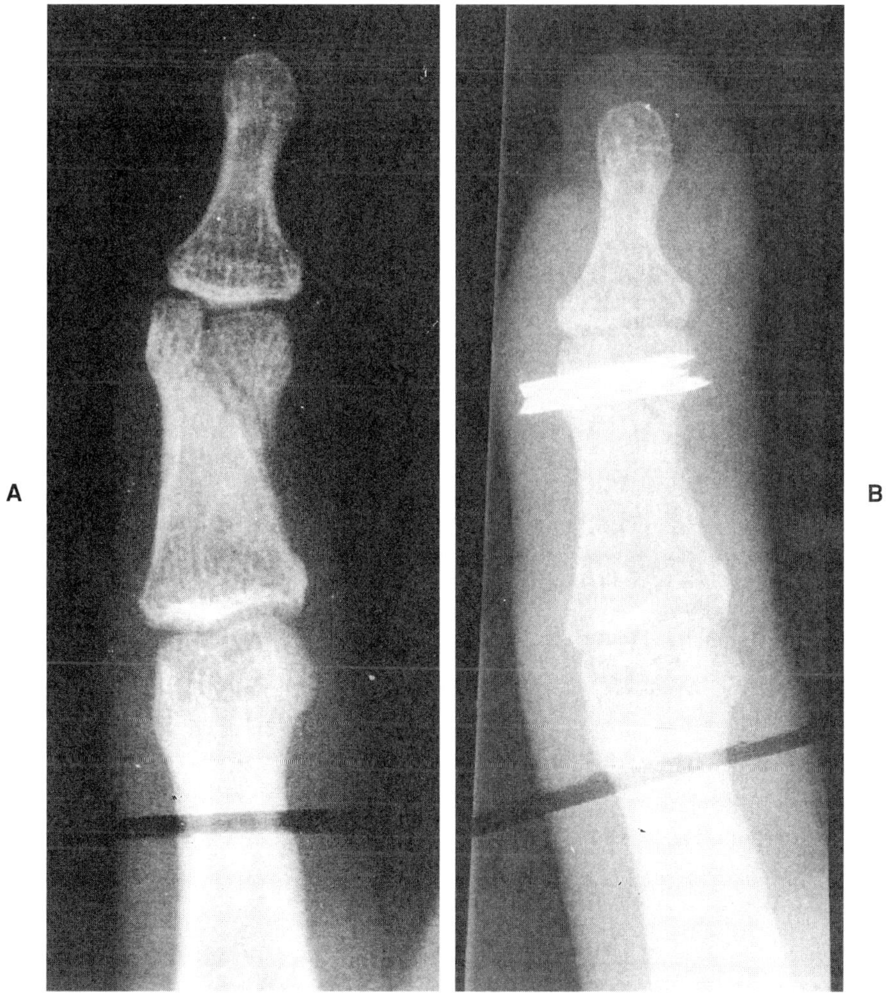

FIGURE 27-8 **A,** An intercondylar fracture of the middle phalanx that has displaced proximally and rotated volarly. **B,** The fracture is reduced and stabilized with three Kirschner wires.

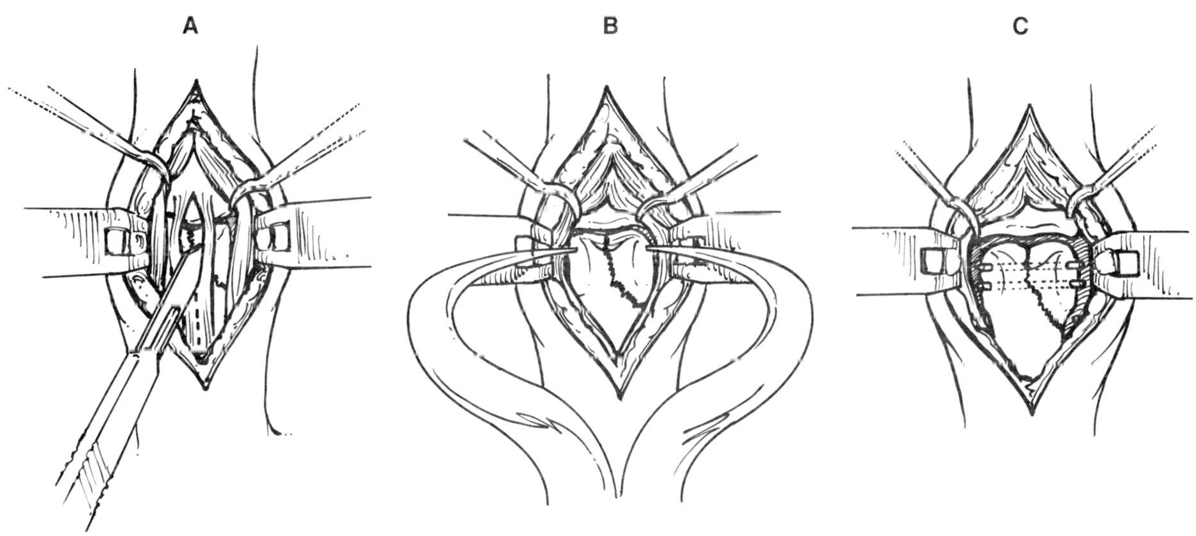

FIGURE 27-9 Approach to an intercondylar fracture of the middle phalanx. **A,** With an extensor tendon-splitting incision, **B,** the fracture is reduced and, **C,** immobilized with Kirschner wires or a screw.

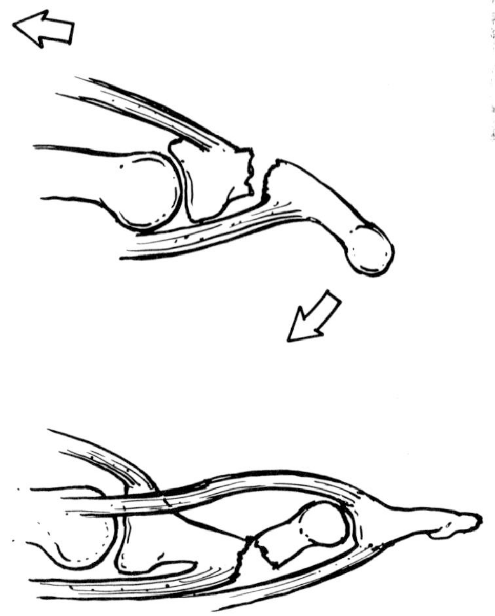

FIGURE 27-10 The angulation deformity of a fracture of the middle phalanx depends on the site of the fracture relative to the insertion of the flexor superficialis tendon.

stable after closed reduction. However, if for some reason a transverse fracture cannot be accurately reduced or maintained after a closed reduction, then either percutaneous Kirschner wires are inserted across the fracture site or an open reduction and internal fixation is needed. If an operation is needed, the best time to treat these fractures is early rather than late.

Spiral and long oblique fractures are inherently unstable. They tend to shorten and rotate along the long axis of the fracture (Fig. 27-11). This can cause the injured finger to overlap the adjacent finger when the individual is making a fist. A careful examination should be done to check alignment of the injured finger with the hand at rest. Comparing the alignment of the nail plate of the injured finger with the adjacent fingers or checking the opposite hand will allow the examiner to detect malrotation of the finger. Short oblique fractures tend to angulate. These unstable fractures should be treated with open reduction and internal fixation,[115] although some authors prefer percutaneous Kirschner wire fixation.[7,45] These authors apply the percutaneous technique to both proximal and middle phalangeal fractures.

An open reduction and internal fixation of the unstable fracture of the middle phalanx is performed either through an incision that splits the dorsal extensor tendon or through a mid-line incision with elevation of the intact extensor tendon. After the fracture is identified and reduced, it can be immobilized with either Kirschner wires[115] and interfragmentary lag screw[51] or a variety of other methods.[56] Because of the bulk of even the smallest plates, the author prefers not to use these in stabilizing fractures of the middle phalanx.

A

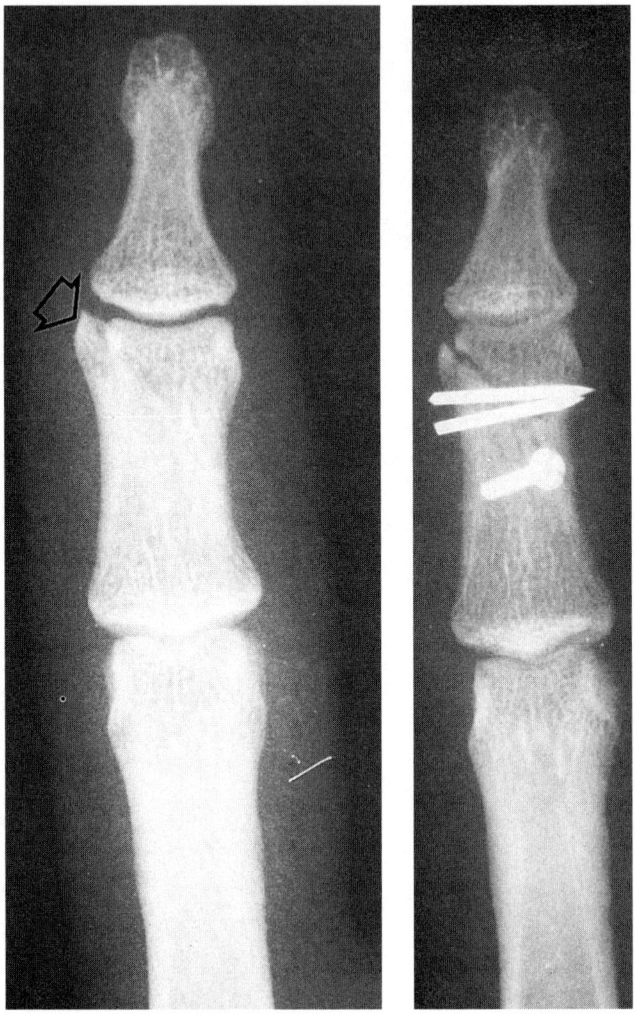

B

FIGURE 27-11 **A,** An oblique fracture in which the entire articular surface has shifted proximally. The bony spike *(arrow)* can impinge on the collateral ligament and restrict joint motion. **B,** The reduction was stabilized with Kirschner wires and a screw.

Comminuted fractures of the middle phalanx are unusual in sports-related injuries and should be treated by some type of open reduction and internal fixation.

If good internal fixation of the fracture is obtained, range-of-motion exercises can be started within 1 week after the operation. The athlete should undergo a supervised rehabilitation program for optimal return of finger function. Table 27-1 summarizes the treatment methods for shaft fractures of the middle phalanx. These methods also can be used for shaft fractures of the proximal phalanx.

Intraarticular fractures of the base of the middle phalanx usually are a result of the axial load associated with an extensor force and/or a laterally deviated force.[30,59] This results in a fracture of the volar lip of the middle phalanx, which can be associated with a dorsal dislocation of the shaft of the middle phalanx (Fig. 27-12). In ad-

A

B

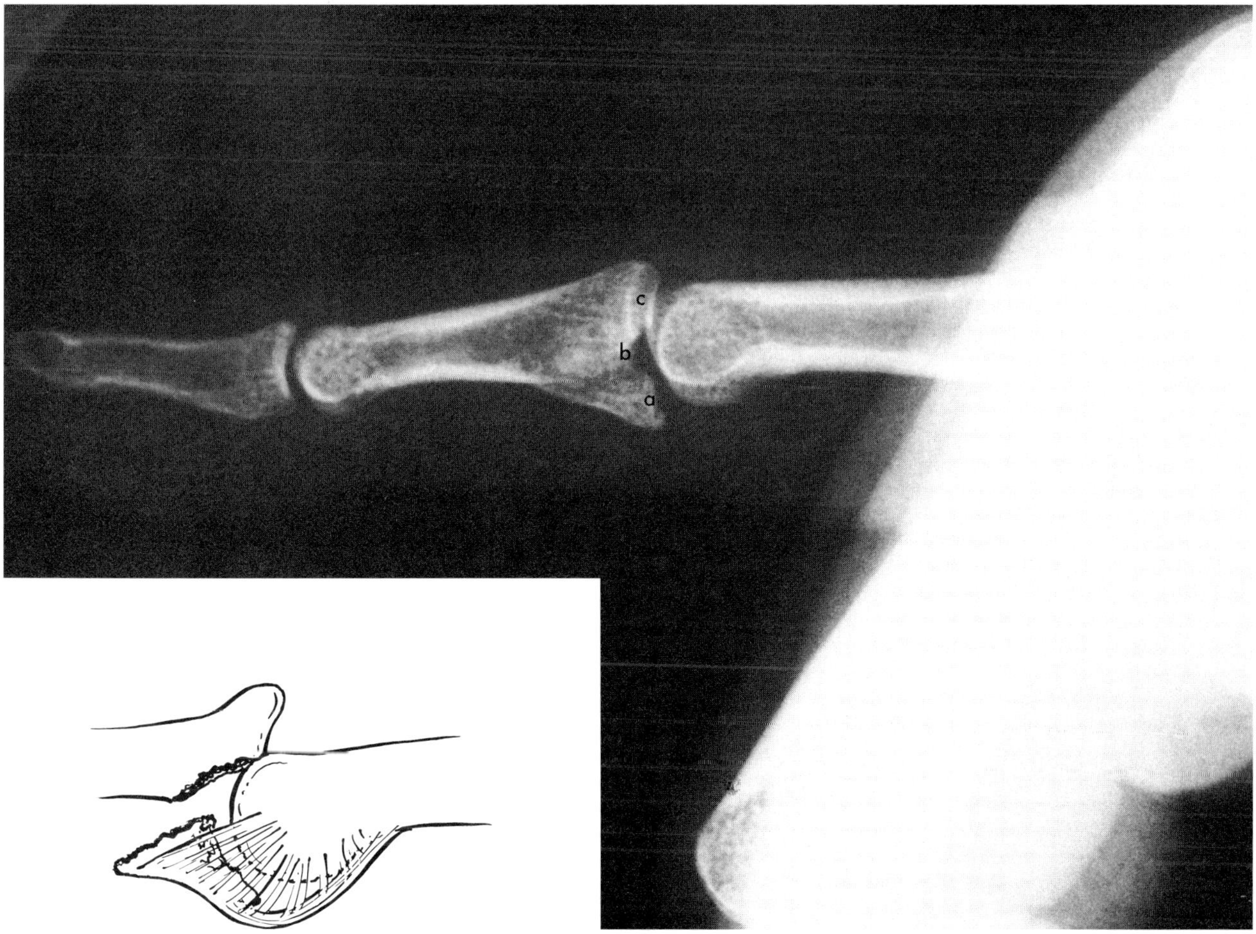

FIGURE 27-12 **A,** A fracture-dislocation of the middle joint of a finger with a large volar lip fragment *(a)*, a depressed joint surface *(b)*, and a dorsally subluxed middle phalanx *(c)*. **B,** Schematic of a fracture-dislocation of the middle phalanx.

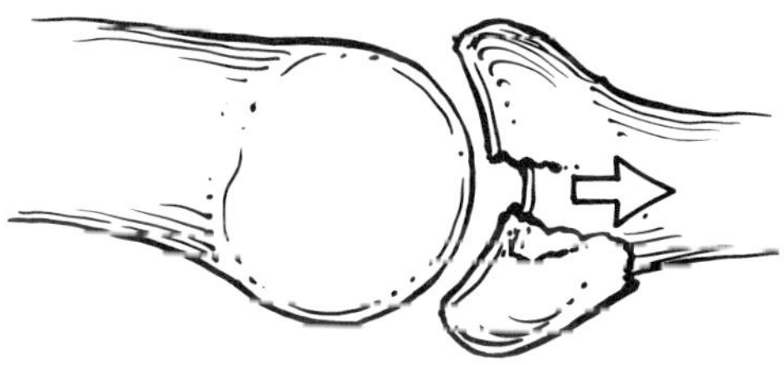

FIGURE 27-13 This fracture is primarily an impaction injury with depression of the midportion of the joint surface.

dition, there may be a depressed fracture involving the central one third of the articular surface of the middle phalanx (Fig. 27-13).

These injuries usually limit motion at the proximal interphalangeal joint, although the athlete frequently considers the injury a "sprain." It is imperative to obtain a good lateral radiograph of the proximal interphalangeal joint to accurately determine the extent of the injury.

If the injury causes a volar lip fracture involving less than one third of the articular surface of the middle phalanx, the fracture is undisplaced or minimally displaced, and there is no dislocation of the shaft of the middle phalanx, the fracture can be treated by splinting. Either splinting the finger in flexion or using an extension block splint is appropriate (Fig. 27-14).

A fracture-dislocation of the proximal interphalangeal joint that involves 30% to 40% of the joint surface but is stable after a closed reduction of the dislocation can be treated by extension block splinting. It is important to have reasonable congruity of the articular surface of the middle phalanx. The extension block splint technique of McElfresh et al[73] is preferred. A dorsal alumifoam splint is applied to the finger with the proximal interphalangeal joint in the degree of flexion needed to reduce the fracture. Active flexion of the finger is started when pain allows, but extension of the proximal interphalangeal joint is restricted. Extension is gradually increased over 3 to 4 weeks. Periodic radiographs should be taken to ensure that the reduction of the fracture is maintained during the exercise period.

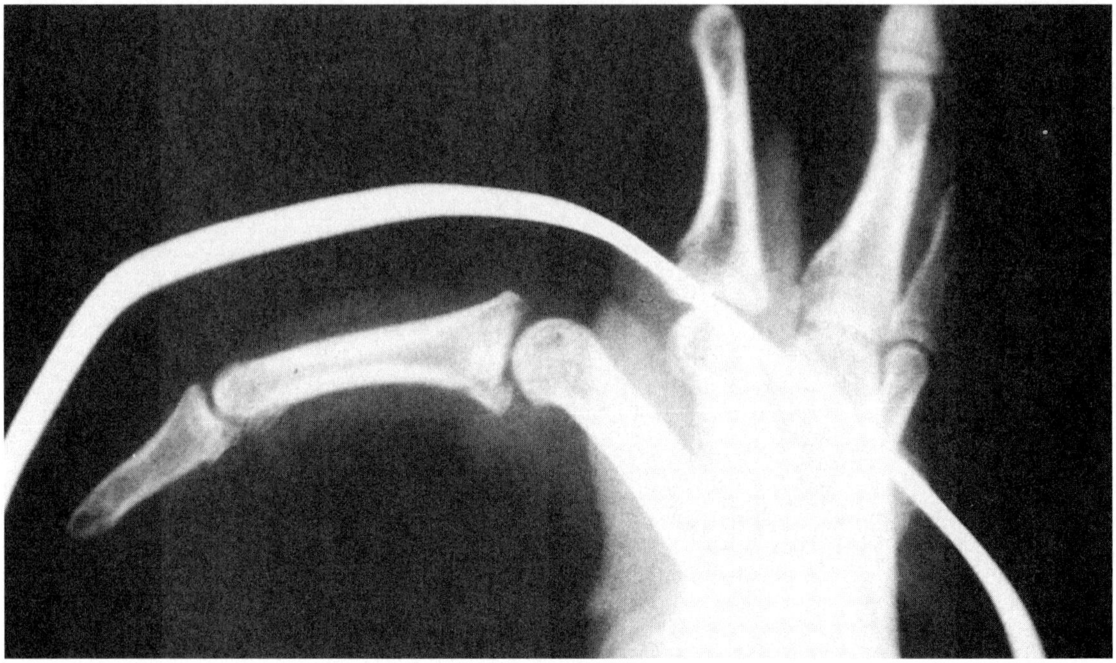

FIGURE 27-14 After reduction, the finger is immobilized in an extension block splint because the volar lip fragment is small.

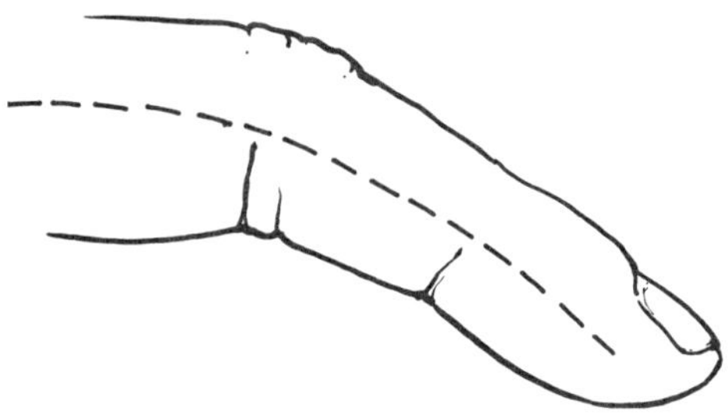

FIGURE 27-15 A midlateral incision in the finger is made just dorsal to the flexion creases of the finger.

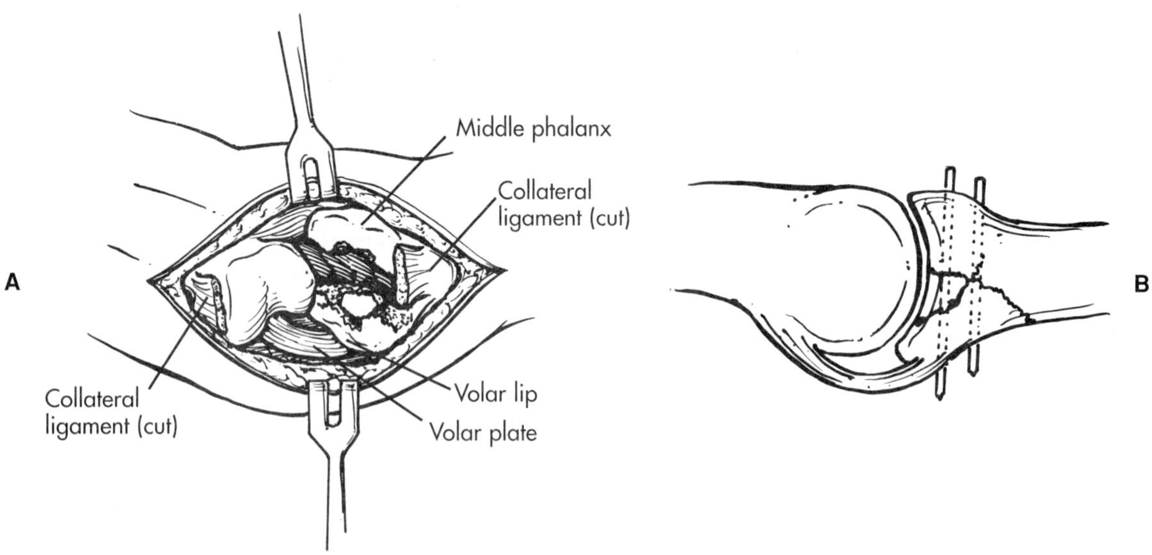

FIGURE 27-16 **A,** After the joint is opened and the fracture is identified, **B,** the fracture is reduced and stabilized with Kirschner wires placed parallel to the joint surface.

If the fracture-dislocation is unstable and the fracture involves 30% to 50% of the joint surface, an open reduction and internal fixation should be performed.[49,70,115]

The author prefers an open reduction and internal fixation using Kirschner wires to stabilize the dislocation and restore congruity to the articular surface of the middle phalanx. The joint is opened through a midlateral incision (Fig. 27-15). The transverse retinacular ligament and the collateral ligament are divided, the joint is opened, and the nature of the fracture is determined. If there is no central-third depression of the articular surface, the dislocation is reduced and immobilized in 45° of flexion with a transarticular Kirschner wire. The fracture fragment then is reduced and immobilized with two Kirschner wires placed parallel to the joint surface (Fig. 27-16). The Kirschner wires are cut off beneath the skin and do not interfere with joint motion. The transarticular Kirschner wire is removed 3 to 4 weeks after surgery, and joint motion is started.

Occasionally, the central third of the articular surface of the middle phalanx is depressed into the subchondral bone. The depressed segment should be elevated to its proper alignment, and a small bone graft from the radius should be inserted as a prop distal to the articular surface (Fig. 27-17). The fracture is then stabilized with two parallel Kirschner wires as mentioned previously. The divided collateral ligament and transverse retinacular ligaments are repaired, and the skin is closed.

If the fracture-dislocation is unstable and the volar lip bony fragment involves less than 30% of the joint surface or it is comminuted, then the volar plate arthroplasty described by Eaton will provide stability to the joint.[30,34] The proximal interphalangeal joint is opened through a volar radially based V-flap incision. After retracting the

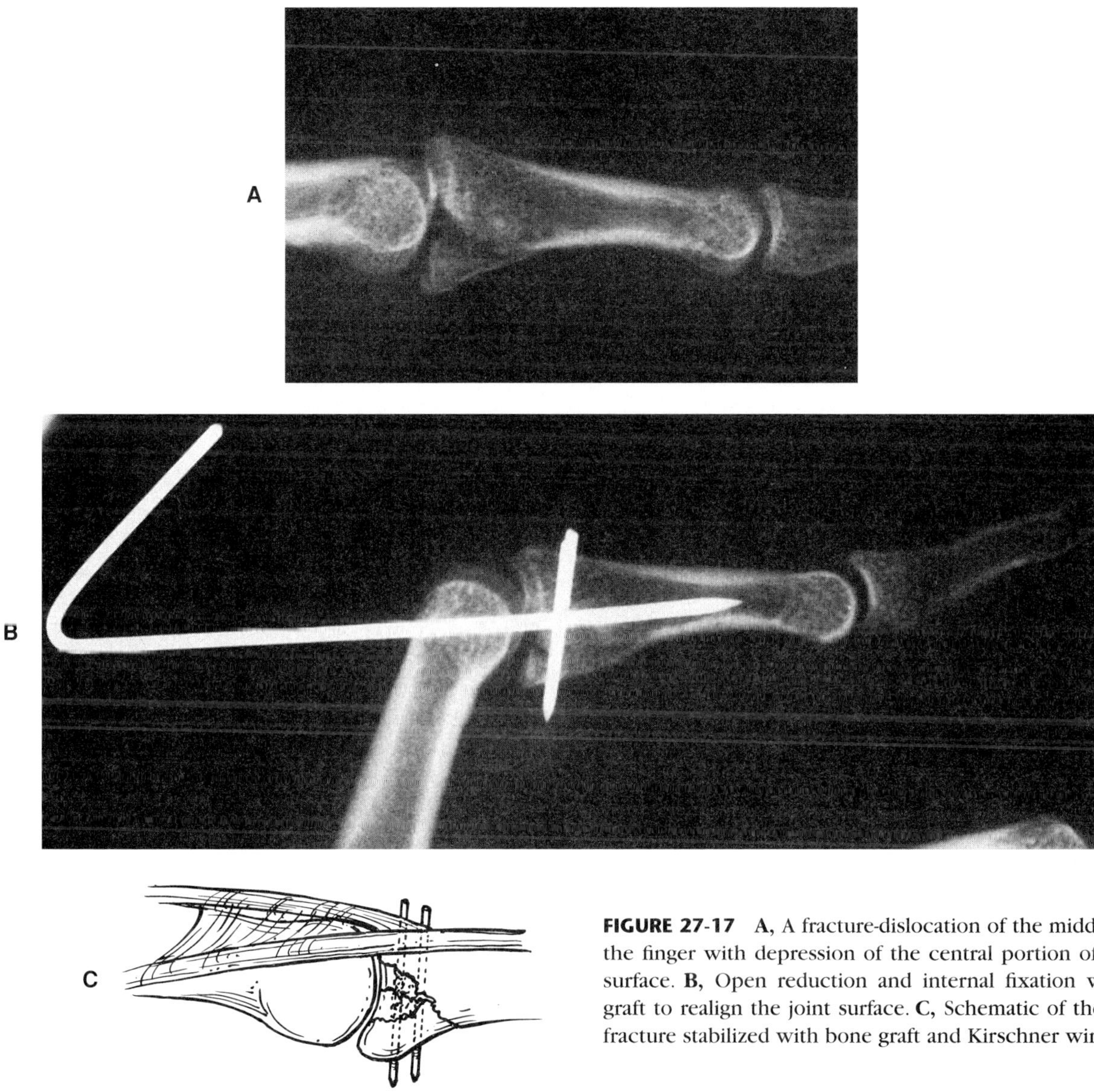

FIGURE 27-17 **A,** A fracture-dislocation of the middle joint of the finger with depression of the central portion of the joint surface. **B,** Open reduction and internal fixation with bone graft to realign the joint surface. **C,** Schematic of the reduced fracture stabilized with bone graft and Kirschner wires.

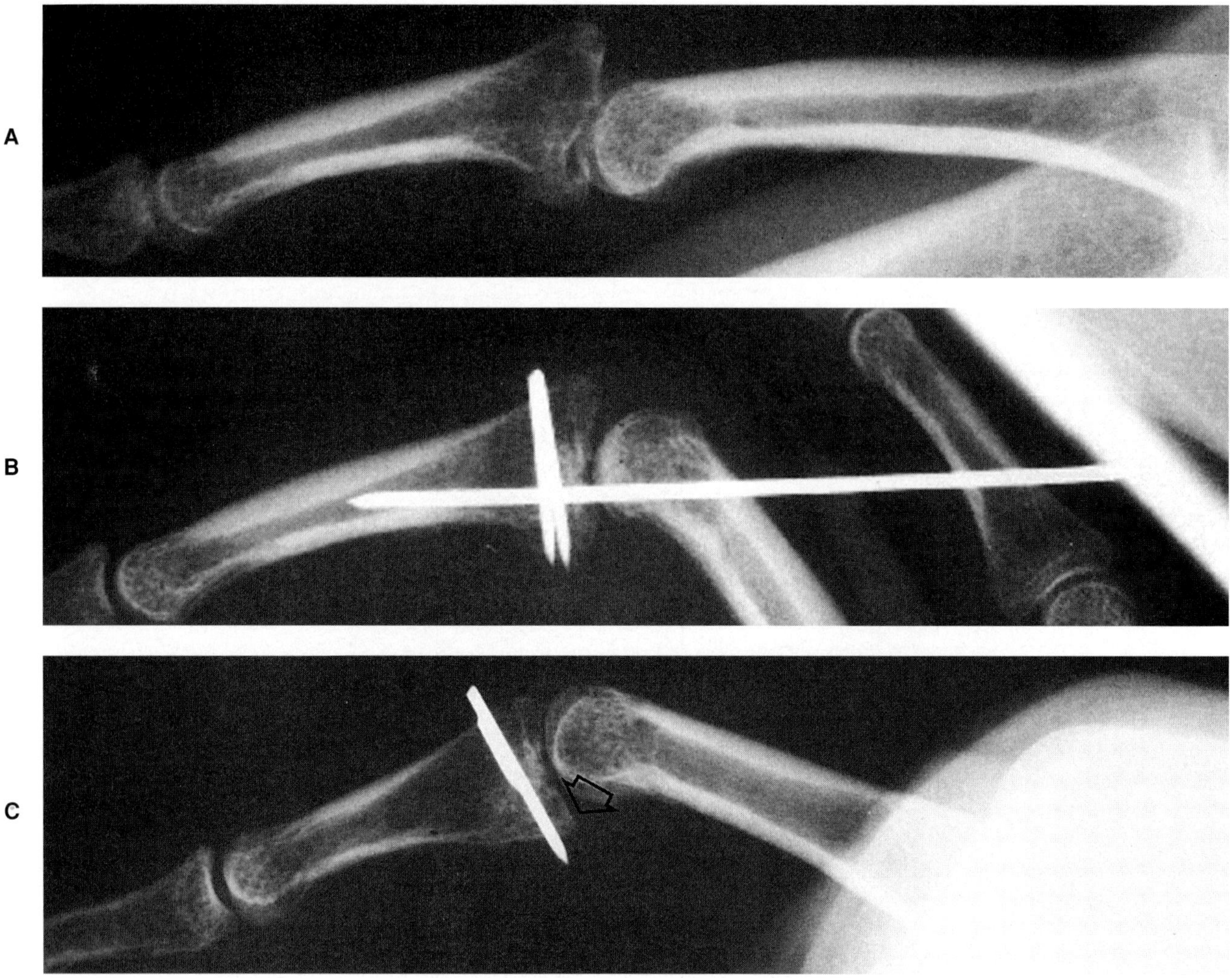

FIGURE 27-18 **A,** Two-month-old fracture-dislocation of the middle joint with a malunion of the volar lip of the middle phalanx. **B,** Osteotomy and bone graft of the malunited volar lip. **C,** Good restoration of the volar lip of the middle phalanx *(arrow)*.

flexor tendons, the surgeon can inspect the joint. The bony fragments are excised, and the defect in the middle phalanx is shaped into a transverse groove perpendicular to the long axis of the bone. Both collateral ligaments are detached, and the volar plate is advanced into the middle phalanx with a pull-out suture. A transarticular Kirschner wire is inserted to maintain the joint in 30° of flexion. The Kirschner wire is removed in 2 weeks, and range of motion is started with an extension block splint. Unrestricted exercises are started at 4 weeks. The patient may take up to 6 to 8 months to regain maximum range of motion.

In those cases where the fracture-dislocation has been neglected by the patient or the injury has been misdiagnosed and the volar lip fracture has healed in a malunited position, closed manipulation will not restore useful function to the proximal interphalangeal joint. Zemel et al[114] used an osteotomy of the volar lip fragment in conjunction with a small bone graft from the distal radius to restore congruity of the joint surface (Fig. 27-18). The operation is complex, but it will restore active flexion to these joints, even many months after injury, providing the articular cartilage is healthy. Motion of the proximal interphalangeal joint improved from an average of 30° before surgery to 68° after surgery. In 1966, Wilson[112] and Rowland used this technique in two patients and reported a successful result.

A volar fracture-dislocation in which the dorsal lip of the middle phalanx is fractured is uncommon. Often, the dislocation can be reduced, but the joint must be immobilized in extension for 3 to 4 weeks. The distal interphalangeal joint can be moved while the proximal interphalangeal joint is immobilized in a splint. An unstable volar fracture-dislocation of the proximal interphalangeal joint must be treated by an open reduction and internal fixation (Fig. 27-19).

A

B

C

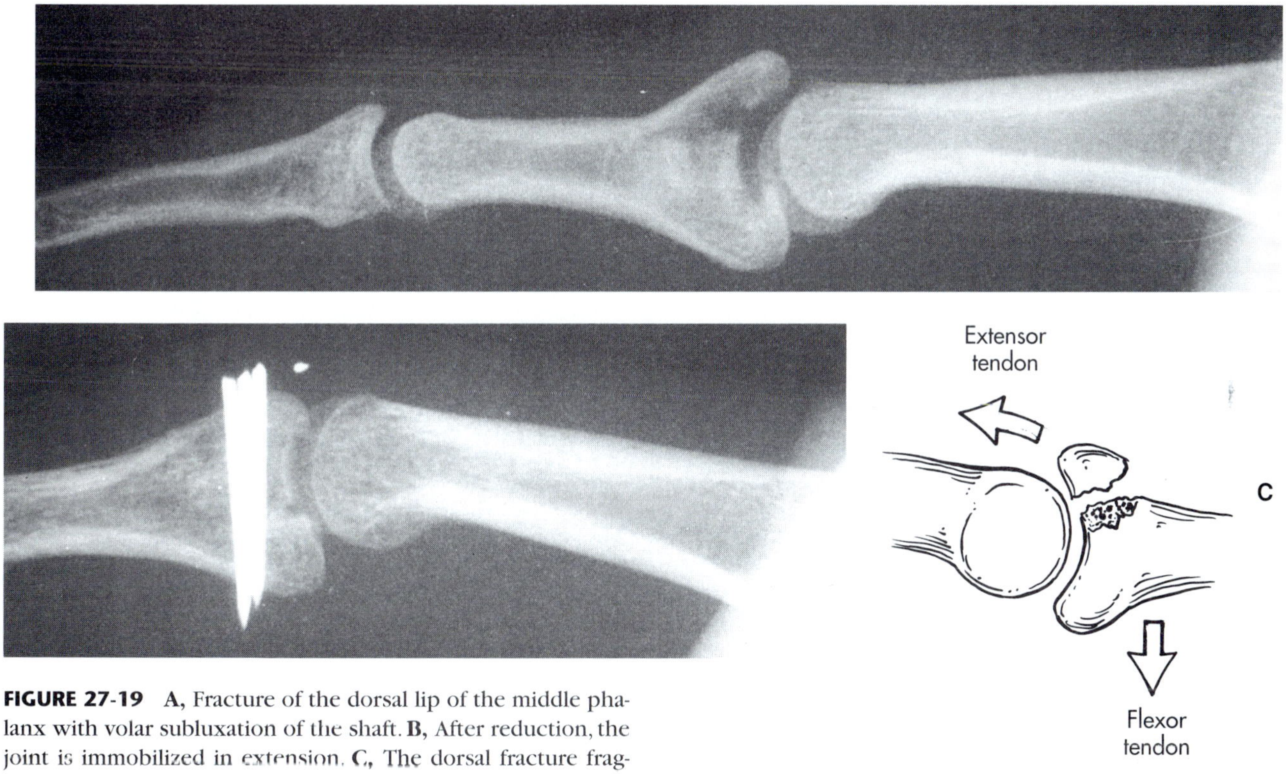

FIGURE 27-19 **A,** Fracture of the dorsal lip of the middle phalanx with volar subluxation of the shaft. **B,** After reduction, the joint is immobilized in extension. **C,** The dorsal fracture fragment is displaced by the extensor tendon, while the shaft of the bone is displaced by the flexor superficialis tendon.

PROXIMAL INTERPHALANGEAL JOINT—SPRAINS AND DISLOCATIONS

Although every joint in the fingers and thumb is susceptible to sprains (stretch injury to the ligament) or dislocations (tears of the supporting ligaments), the proximal interphalangeal joint of the finger seems especially vulnerable to this type of injury. The proximal interphalangeal joint is inherently stable throughout its arc of motion. Its stability is determined by the joint's articular contours, ligament structures, and secondary reinforcement of the tendons and retinacular system.[30] However, the principal stabilizing elements of the joints are the strong collateral ligaments and the accessory collateral ligaments joined to the thick palmar plate check ligament system[14,32,63] (Fig. 27-20).

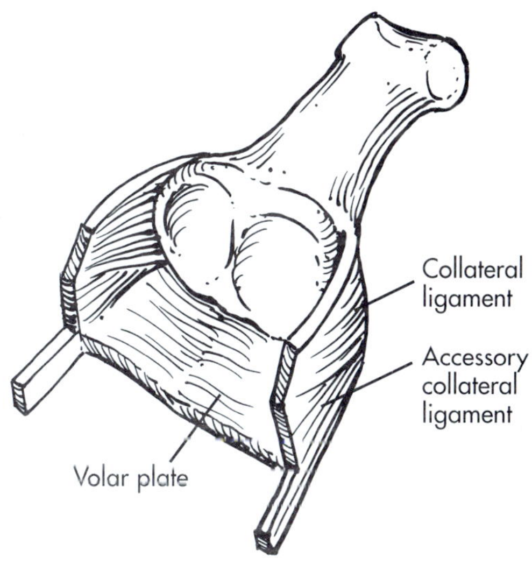

FIGURE 27-20 The ligament-box complex at the proximal interphalangeal joint, as described by Eaton.

Sprains or stretch injuries of the collateral ligaments are minor injuries. The injured finger may be taped or buddy-splinted to the adjacent digit, and the individual allowed to compete in sports.

Dislocation of the proximal interphalangeal joint can be dorsal, lateral, or volar (Fig. 27-21). These descriptions refer to the position of the middle phalanx in relation to the proximal phalanx.

Dorsal Dislocation

Dorsal dislocation of the proximal interphalangeal joint results from hyperextension stress associated with longitudinal compression of the joint. This results in disruption of the distal attachment of the ligament box complex.[32]

Dorsal displacement of the middle phalanx can be classified into three types[30]:

A

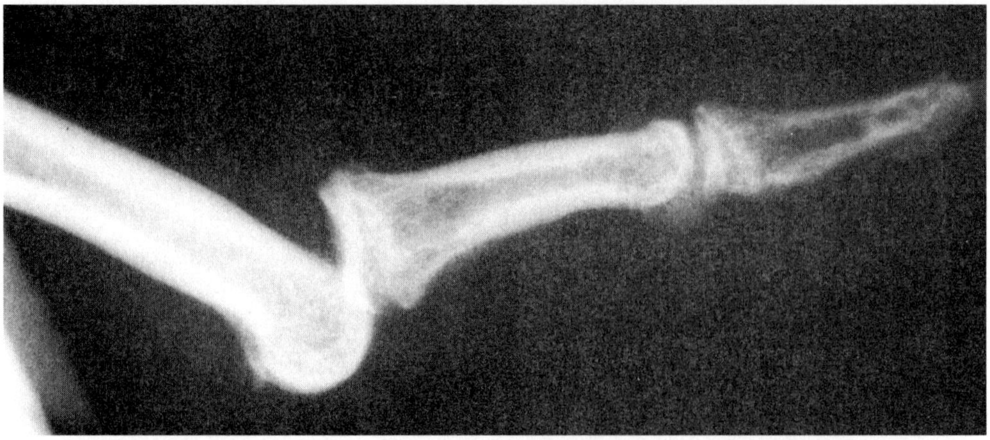

B

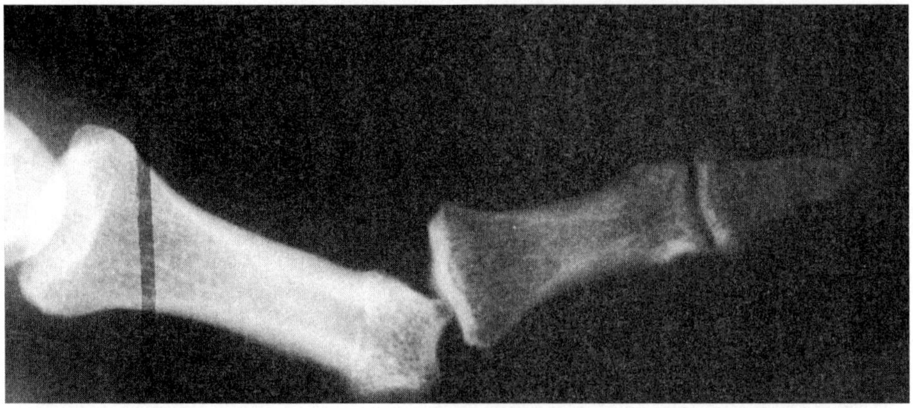

C

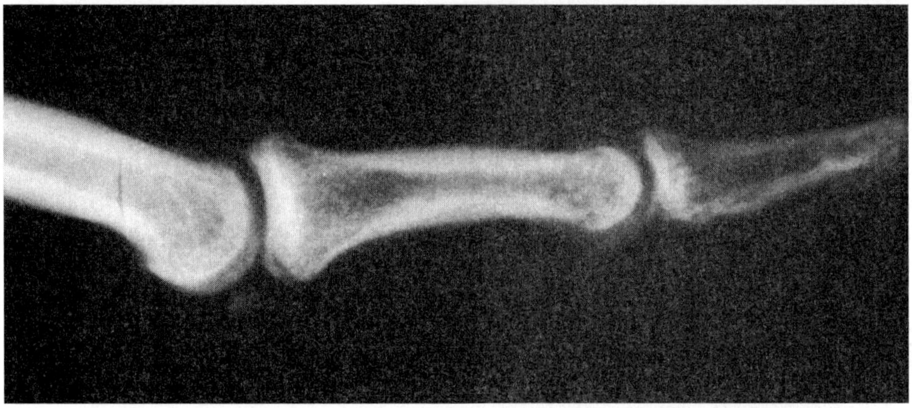

D

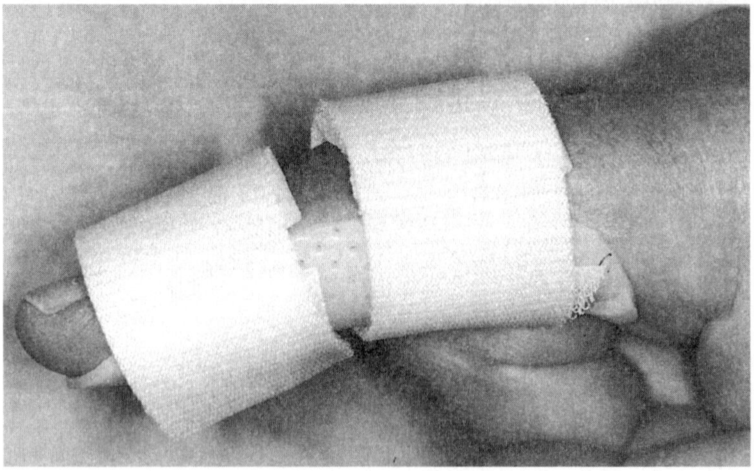

FIGURE 27-21 **A,** A dorsal and lateral, **B,** dislocation of the middle joint of the little finger. This injury involves the tearing of the volar plate and one collateral ligament. **C,** After the dislocation is reduced and determined to be stable, **D,** the finger is immobilized in a splint with the joint in about 20° of flexion.

Type I: hyperextension. The volar plate is avulsed from the base of the middle phalanx, and there is a minor longitudinal split in the collateral ligaments. The middle phalanx articulates with the dorsal third of the condyles of the proximal phalanx.

Type II: dorsal dislocation. The volar plate is avulsed from the middle phalanx and there are complete bilateral splits of the collateral ligaments with a complete dorsal displacement of the middle phalanx.

Type III: fracture-dislocation. This was previously discussed.

It is best to try and obtain a radiograph of the digit before attempting a closed reduction of the dislocation. A true lateral radiograph of the proximal interphalangeal joint is important to the assessment of the injury (Fig. 27-22). However, if pain is a factor or circulation is compromised, a closed reduction should be performed immediately and the patient definitively evaluated for further treatment.

Closed reduction of the dislocation usually suffices to restore joint congruity. The method of reduction includes exaggeration of the deformity, gentle longitudinal

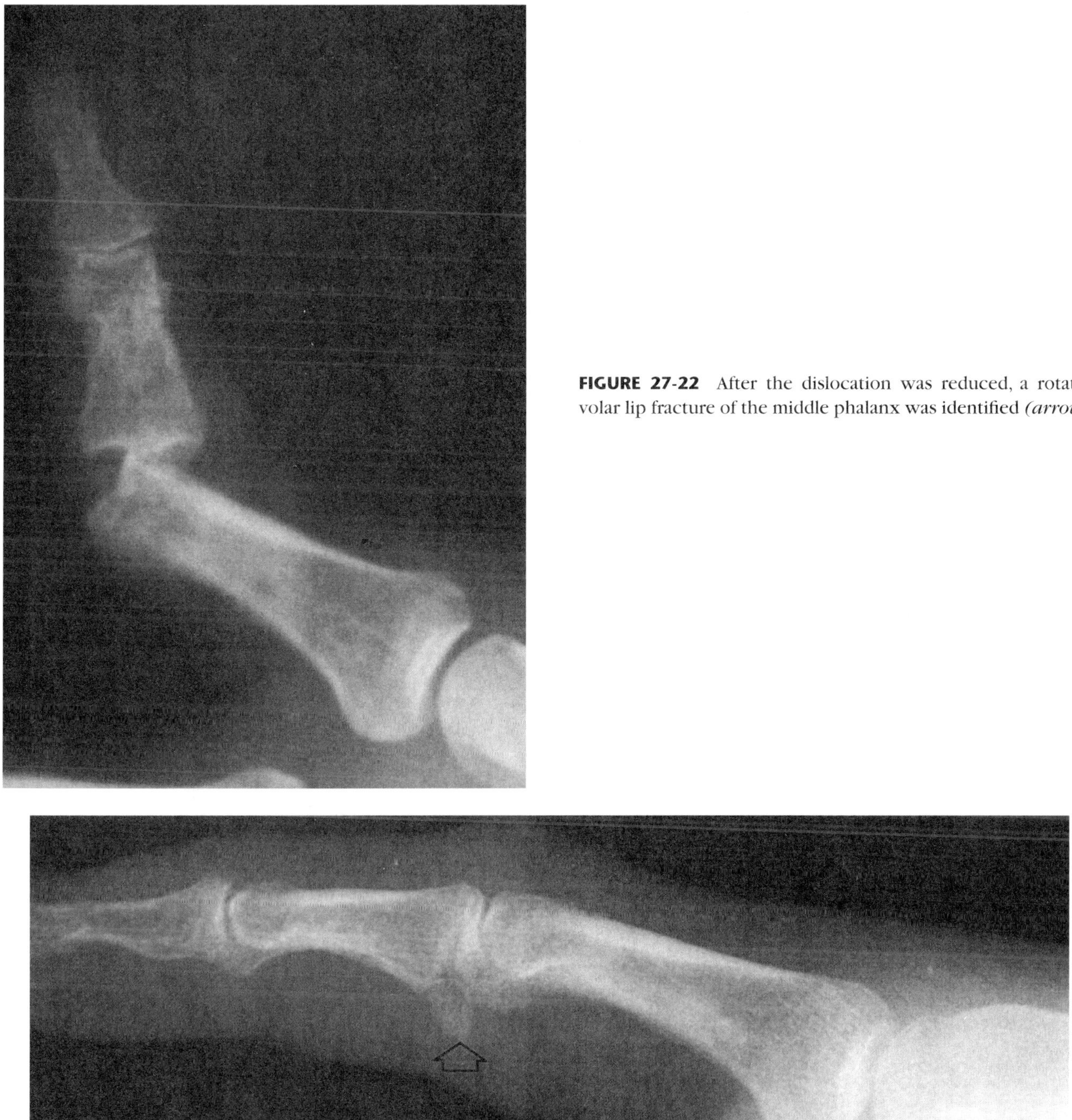

FIGURE 27-22 After the dislocation was reduced, a rotated volar lip fracture of the middle phalanx was identified *(arrow)*.

traction, and palmar flexion of the middle phalanx. When a congruent joint is obtained, postreduction radiographs should be taken to ensure that the joint is properly aligned. Eaton[33] recommended active and passive testing of the joint for postreduction stability. The patient actively moves the joint through an arc of motion to determine whether the dislocation will recur. The examiner also passively tests the joint laterally (collateral ligaments) and in the posterior-anterior plane (volar plate).

If the joint is stable, the digit is splinted in 15° to 20° of flexion for 2 to 3 weeks (see Fig. 27-21, *D*). When the patient is comfortable, the finger can be buddy-taped for 4 to 6 weeks, depending on the sporting activity and the degree of discomfort present. These joints tend to ache and remain enlarged and stiff for several months, and complete finger motion, especially proximal interphalangeal joint extension, often is not regained.

After attempted closed reduction of the dislocation, if

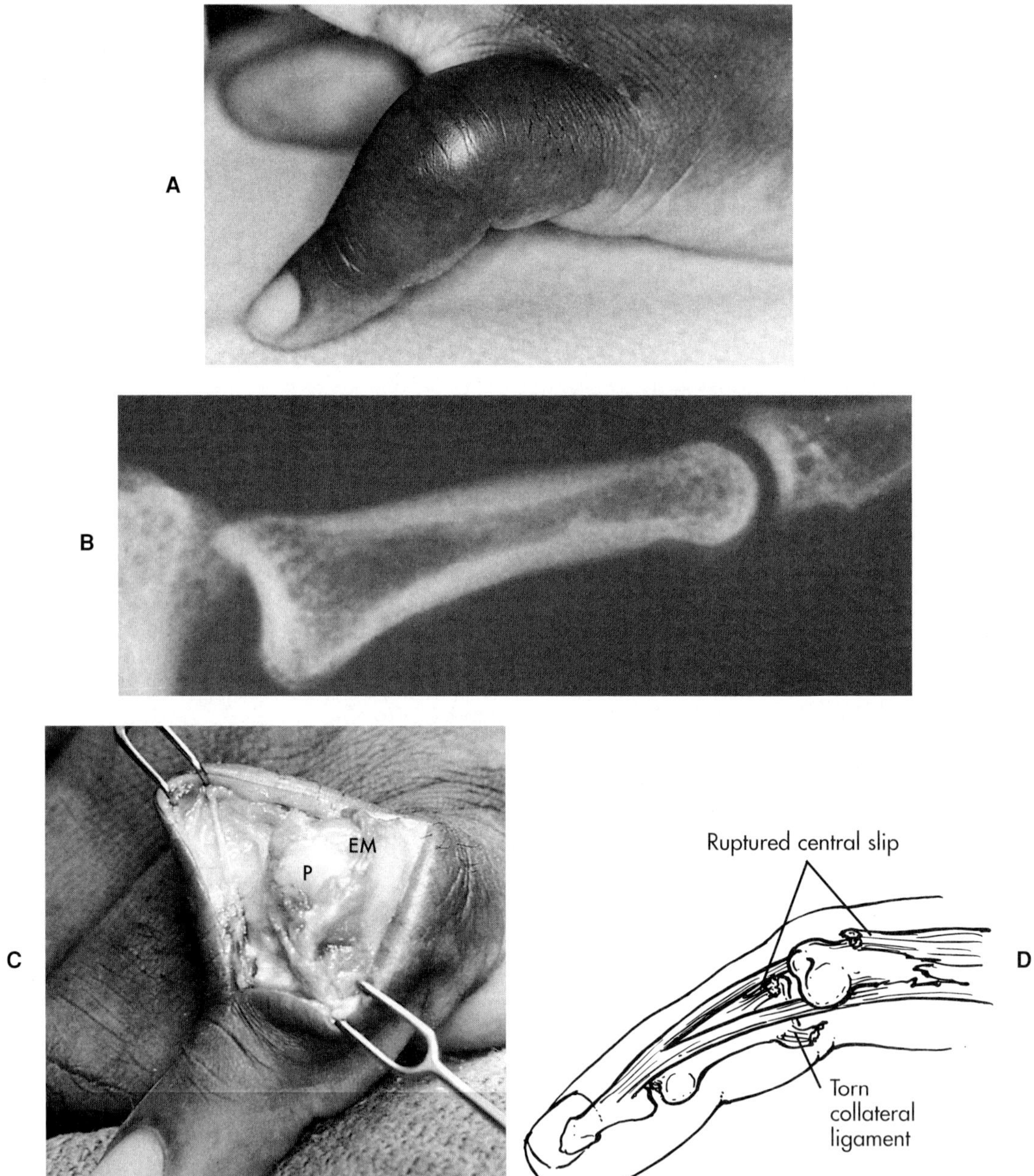

FIGURE 27-23 **A,** A fixed flexion deformity of the little finger, **B,** after a volar subluxation of the middle joint, **C,** associated with a tear of the central slip after the head of the proximal phalanx penetrated the extensor mechanism. **D,** Schematic of the condyle of the proximal phalanx through the extensor mechanism. *P,* Proximal phalanx; *EM,* extensor mechanism.

the reduction is unstable or it cannot be attained, an open reduction is indicated.[30,47] A volar or midlateral incision allows the clinician to determine the reason for failure of reduction and to remove any interposed soft-tissue, bony, or cartilaginous structures. The volar plate usually is the most common obstructing soft-tissue structure.

Lateral Dislocation

These injuries involve a tear of one collateral ligament as well as a tear (complete or partial) of the volar plate. After the joint is realigned, it usually is stable. Treatment consists of splinting the joint in 15° to 20° of flexion for 2 to 3 weeks, then buddy-taping the finger to an adjacent digit. Active range-of-motion exercises are started, and the buddy splints are continued for 4 to 6 weeks. Although some authors[1,71,91] have reported complete collateral ligament tears, operations rarely are indicated.

Volar Dislocation

Volar dislocation is rare and occurs when a rotatory longitudinal compression force is applied to a partially flexed middle phalanx. There is a tear of one collateral ligament and the volar plate, and the head of the proximal phalanx can rupture through the extensor mechanism (Fig. 27-23). The central slip can be torn, or the condyle can penetrate between the lateral band and the central slip of the extensor mechanism. If the joint cannot be reduced by gentle traction with the metacarpophalangeal and proximal interphalangeal joints flexed,[109] an open reduction is indicated.[30]

Chronic Subluxation

A chronic interphalangeal joint subluxation or hyperextension deformity can occur after a type I hyperextension injury (Fig. 27-24). This chronic instability results in a swan-neck deformity of the finger as the patient extends the digit. A painful snap of the lateral bands can occur when the individual flexes the finger, and flexion of the finger often must be assisted with the opposite hand. This interferes with the function of grasp. This most commonly occurs in the little finger and results from failure of healing of a torn volar plate. Operative treatment for this condition is necessary to restore joint stability. The author prefers to do a capsulodesis by advancing and reattaching the volar plate to the middle phalanx using a pull-out suture. This middle joint is stabilized in flexion with a transarticular Kirschner wire for 3 weeks,

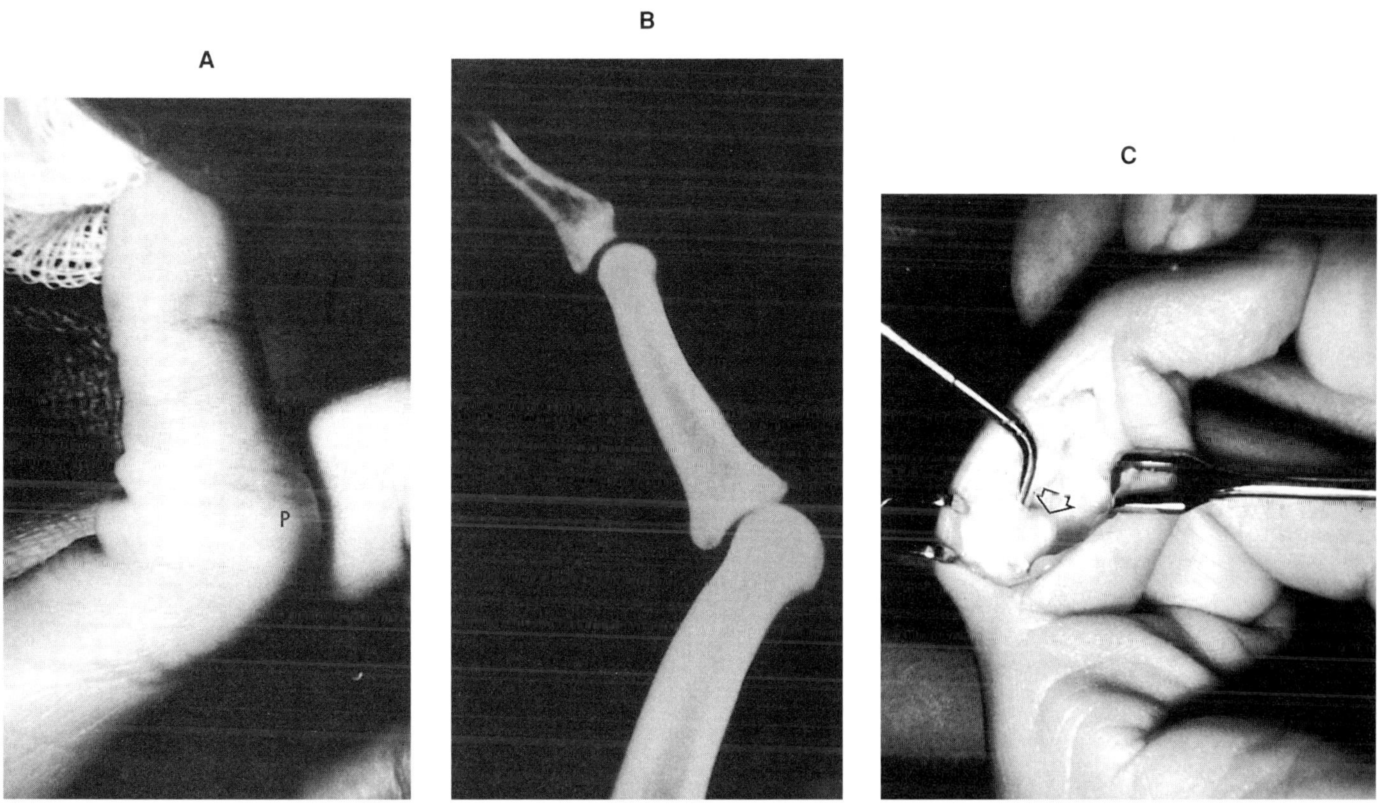

FIGURE 27-24 **A** and **B**, A tear of the volar plate that has not healed causes instability at the middle joint of the finger. **C**, The retracted volar plate *(arrow)* is identified at surgery. *P*, Palmar side of the joint.

then active range-of-motion exercises are started with splinting to restrict joint extension. Ideally, the athlete should have a 10° permanent flexion contracture at the proximal interphalangeal joint. Other authors use a flexor digitorum superficialis tenodesis to stabilize the joint.[24,30,71,84]

FRACTURES OF THE PROXIMAL PHALANX—FINGERS

Fractures of the proximal phalanx most commonly involve the condyles and shaft of the bone. Intraarticular fractures of the base of the proximal phalanx (metacarpophalangeal joint) are much less common but can be difficult to treat because they involve a joint surface (Table 27-1).

Fractures of the proximal phalanx, regardless of treatment, seem to have a worse prognosis for finger and hand function than injury to the other bones of the hand.[19,107] The proximal phalanx is covered dorsally and laterally by the extensor tendon mechanism and palmarly by the flexor tendons. These tendons are separated from the bone by only the periosteum and are vulnerable to injury from the fracture or from the tendons becoming stuck to callus during the healing process. Early motion is particularly important in treating fractures of the proximal phalanx, especially shaft fractures.

Undisplaced fractures of the proximal phalanx can be treated by splint immobilization for 3 weeks, then range-of-motion exercises and buddy-taping of the finger if needed. Although James[55] and others[113] emphasize splinting the hand in the intrinsic-plus position (70° of flexion at the metacarpophalangeal joints and extension of the interphalangeal joints), the author prefers to hold the hand and wrist in a position of function (wrist at 10° to 20° of dorsiflexion, metacarpophalangeal joints in 20° of flexion, and interphalangeal joints in 30° of flexion)

TABLE 27-1
Shaft Fractures of Middle and Proximal Phalanges

Fracture	Treatment
Transverse fracture	
Stable, undisplaced	Splint 2 weeks, buddy splint, and range-of-motion exercises
Closed reduction, stable	Same as above
Unstable postreduction	Open reduction and internal fixation, percutaneous K-wires
Short oblique	
Stable	Splint 2-3 weeks, buddy splint, range-of-motion exercises
Unstable	Open reduction and internal fixation, percutaneous K-wires
Long oblique or spiral—inherently unstable	Open reduction and internal fixation, percutaneous K-wires
Comminuted	Internal fixation (closed versus open)

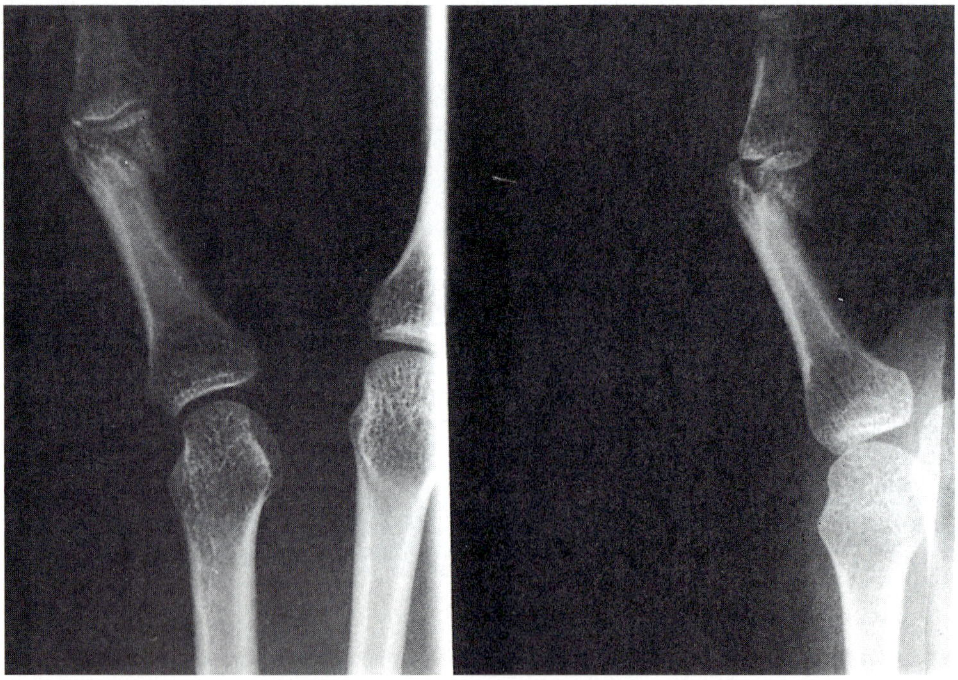

FIGURE 27-25 A displaced condylar fracture of the proximal phalanx.

(see Fig. 27-2). Even undisplaced fractures, if immobilized longer than 4 weeks, have worse results because of secondary stiffness caused by immobilization.[107]

Condylar fractures of the proximal phalanx rarely can be treated closed. Unicondylar fractures are especially troublesome because the fractured condyle tends to migrate proximally, frequently rotates, and also may tilt dorsally or palmarly (Fig. 27-25). It remains attached to its collateral ligament (similar to the fracture of the middle phalanx), and closed reduction usually is impossible. This fracture also is often missed because the individual can flex and extend the digit. An angular deformity also may be present at the proximal interphalangeal joint. Oblique radiographs may be necessary to identify the fracture and the malposition of the condyle.

Open reduction and internal fixation is performed through a dorsal skin incision. The interval between the lateral band and central slip of the extensor tendon is incised longitudinally, and the fracture is exposed. With the attachment of the collateral ligament to the condyle left intact, the bone is reduced and immobilized with Kirschner wires or small lag screws[80,83,105,115] (Fig. 27-26).

Unstable shaft fractures are treated the same as shaft fractures of the middle phalanx. Proximal-phalanx shaft fractures tend to angulate apex palmarward because of the pull of the interosseous muscles. Although some authors advocate closed reduction and percutaneous Kirschner wire fixation,[7,45,110] Barton[5] noted that it is often difficult to obtain complete reduction of the fracture and that Kirschner wires passing through the soft-tissue envelope may prevent or limit early mobilization of the digit. Others believe it usually is best to perform an open reduction and internal fixation of the fracture and to try to begin motion as soon as possible.[62,64]

The author prefers to use a dorsal incision and then incise the extensor tendon and periosteum longitudi-

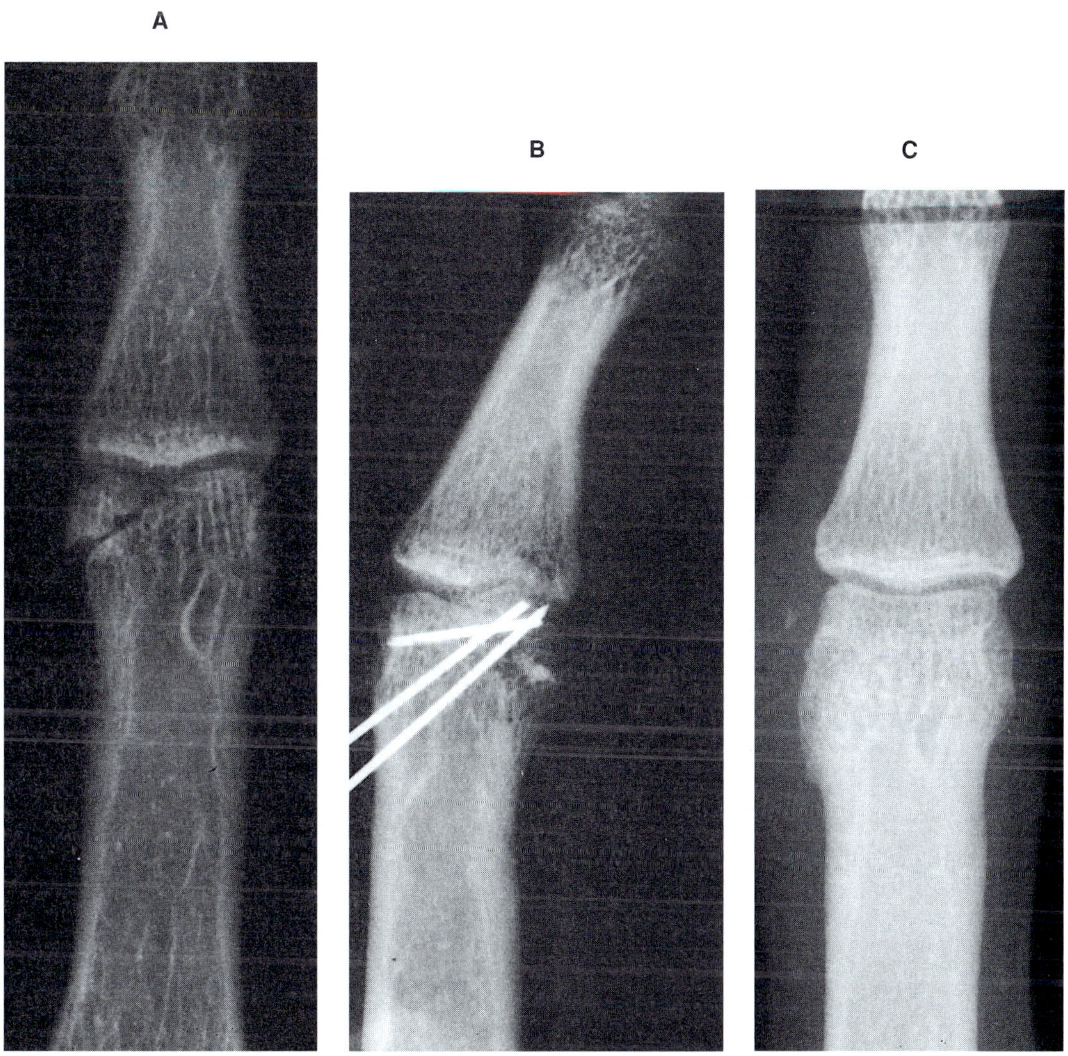

FIGURE 27-26 **A,** The displaced intercondylar fracture, **B,** was reduced and stablized with Kirschner wires. **C,** The joint surface 4 years later. The patient had good flexion but lacked 20° of complete extension of the joint.

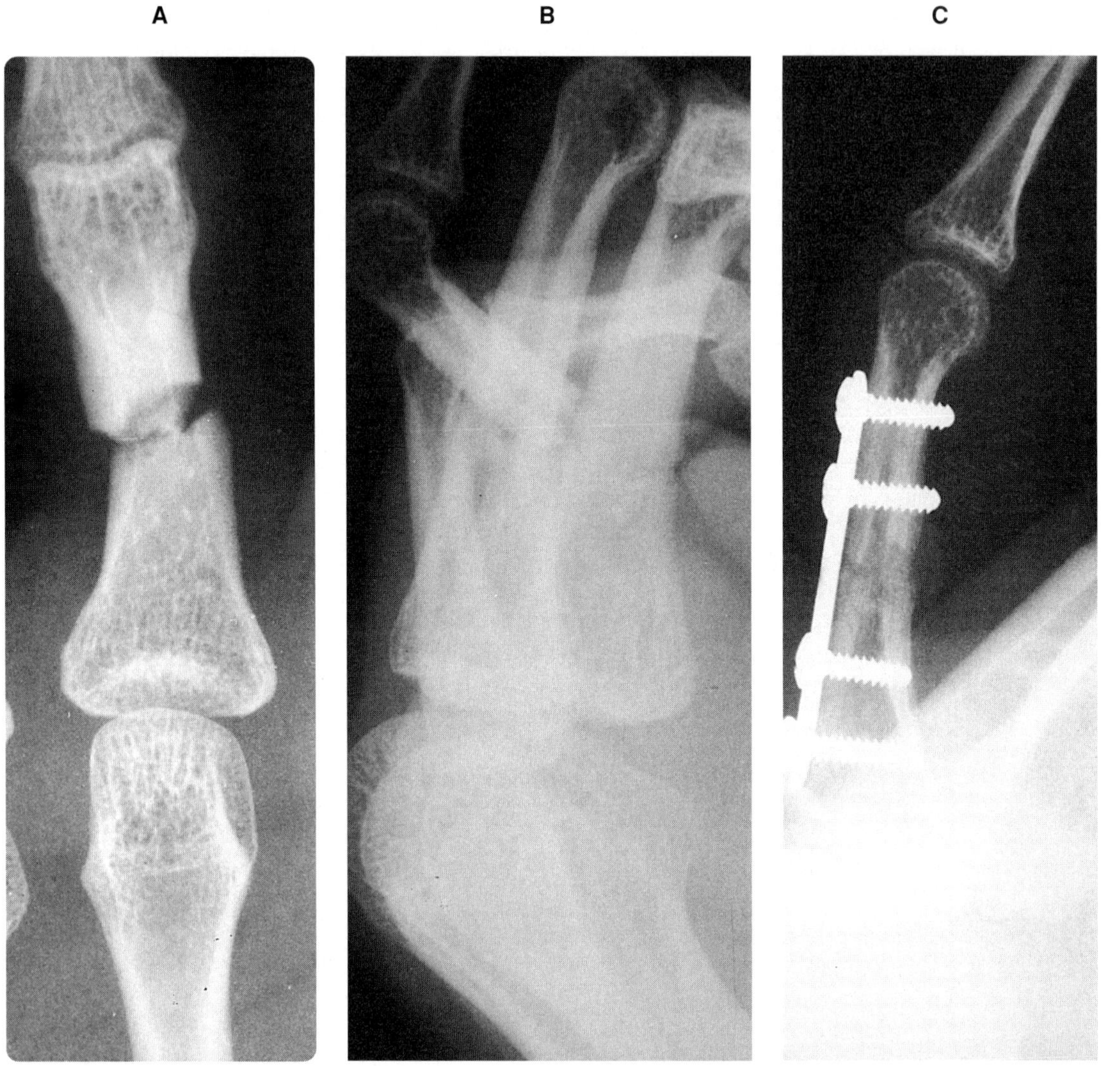

FIGURE 27-27 **A,** This displaced fracture of the proximal phalanx was comminuted, **B,** and severely angulated. **C,** Stable fixation was obtained with a plate and screws, and the finger motion after rehabilitation was excellent.

nally, elevating both structures as a single unit in an attempt to maintain a gliding surface between the tendon and bone. The fracture is reduced and stabilized with Kirschner wires cut beneath the skin, with small lag screws, or with a small plate as indicated by the fracture configuration (Fig. 27-27). Any rotational malalignment of the fracture must be corrected at the time of the open reduction and internal fixation. If this is not done, when the fracture heals, the injured finger will cross over when it is flexed. Small lag screws and plates provide more rigid fixation than Kirschner wires[8,23,50,102] and allow range-of-motion exercises to be started within 1 week of the operation. This seems to decrease the incidence of tendon adhesions and secondary joint contractures.

Intraarticular fractures of the base of the proximal phalanx occur as avulsion fractures attached to the collateral ligaments, as axially loaded compression fractures, or as vertical articular splitting fractures.[49,115]

If the fracture of the proximal articular surface of the proximal phalanx is a two-part fracture in which the spreading of the articular surface does not exceed 1 to 2 mm and the articular surface is not badly depressed, a fracture commonly seen in teenagers, these fractures can be treated with immobilization of the injured finger and wrist. If the fracture is displaced or malrotated, then open reduction and internal fixation is recommended (Fig. 27-28). Rotation of such a fracture fragment is more common in the proximal phalanx of the thumb than in a finger.

The preferred approach to this fracture is through a dorsal incision. The extensor tendon is incised longitudinally at its junction with the extensor hood. When the

A 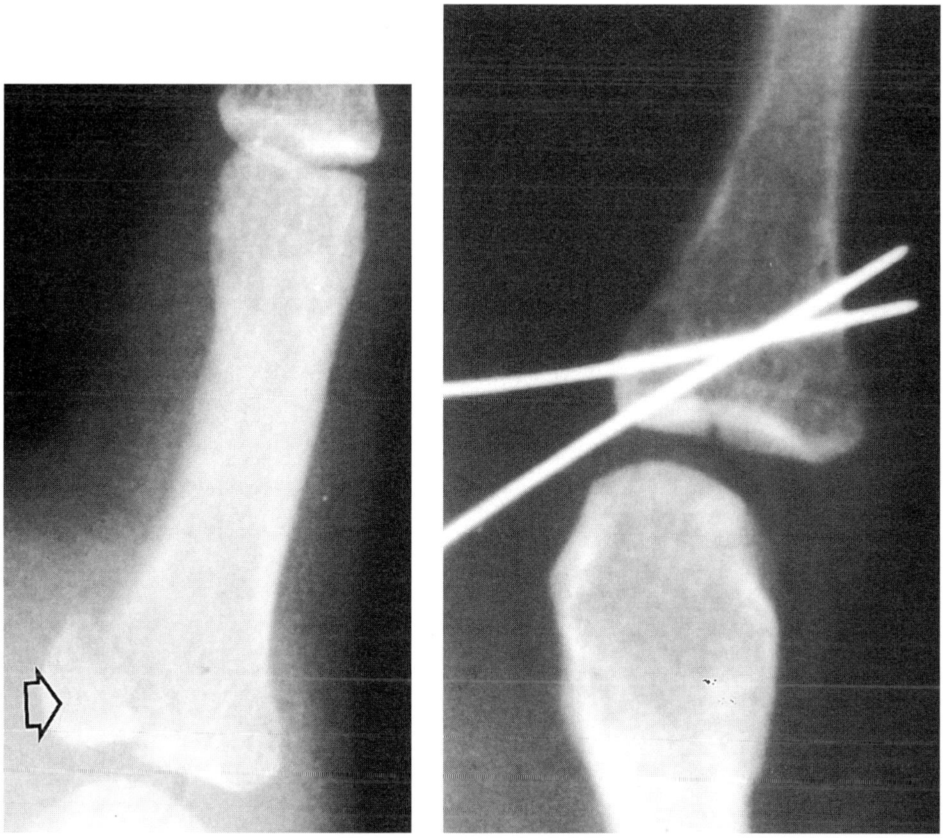 B

FIGURE 27-28 **A,** The radial fracture fragment *(arrow)* remains attached to the collateral ligament while the shaft of the proximal phalanx displaces ulnarward. **B,** Reduction of the fracture and fixation with Kirschner wires.

joint is flexed, the fracture can be identified, reduced, and immobilized with either Kirschner wires or a small lag screw. Depending on the stability of the fracture, motion can be started within 1 to 3 weeks.

A more complicated problem is a comminuted intraarticular fracture of the proximal end of the proximal phalanx. This fracture tends to have a greater crush component. Although the results after treatment of these fractures often are less than ideal, the only hope of achieving a painless, mobile joint is to restore the joint surface as best as possible. The multiple fracture fragments should be restored to their proper place and stabilized with small Kirschner wires. Because fixation of some of the fragments may be precarious, the joint should be immobilized for a full 3 weeks. Normal joint motion rarely is achieved after such an injury, but reasonable grip and useful motion can be expected. This injury often leads to painful degenerative arthritis of the metacarpophalangeal joint.

Complications after phalangeal fractures, particularly of the proximal and middle phalanges, are malunion (malrotation, volar angulation, lateral angulation, and shortening), nonunion, adhesions of flexor and/or extensor tendons, joint contraction, and infection (Fig. 27-29).

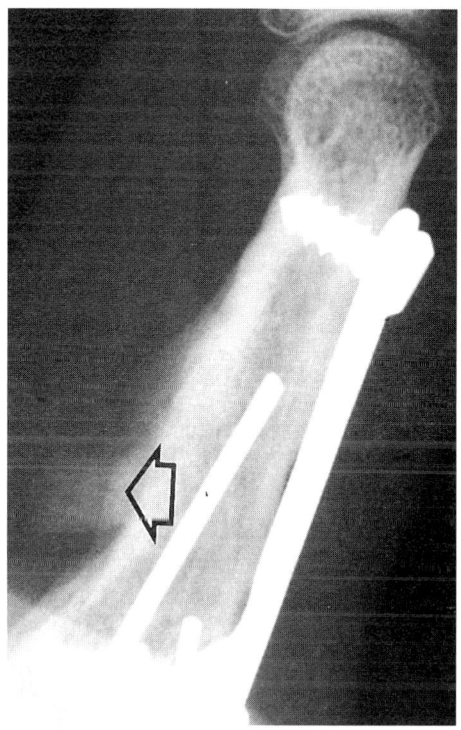

FIGURE 27-29 The large volar exostosis *(arrow)* can cause adhesions of the flexor tendons and a contracture of the middle joint of the finger.

METACARPOPHALANGEAL JOINT—SPRAINS AND DISLOCATIONS

Hyperextension injuries to the metacarpophalangeal joint of the finger often result in a tear of the proximal membranous attachment of the volar plate. The proximal phalanx hyperextends in its relation to the metacarpal, but some residual contact usually remains between the articular surfaces of both bones. These injuries are almost exclusively confined to the index and little fingers,[3,79] and provided that the volar plate remains palmar to the head of the metacarpal, they usually can be treated closed. One must take care to prevent the detached volar plate from sliding over the head of the metacarpal and becoming interposed between it and the base of the proximal phalanx. After reduction, the metacarpophalangeal joint is immobilized in approximately 30° of flexion for 2 to 3 weeks. A dorsal splint can be used that blocks joint extension but permits active flexion exercises.

A dorsal dislocation of the metacarpophalangeal joint is a much more severe injury, and the condition has been referred to as a complex or irreducible dislocation (Fig. 27-30). Unlike a hyperextension injury to the joint where some contact remains between the joint surfaces, there is no contact when the joint is dislocated. Closed reduction of these injuries usually is impossible.[52,79]

A

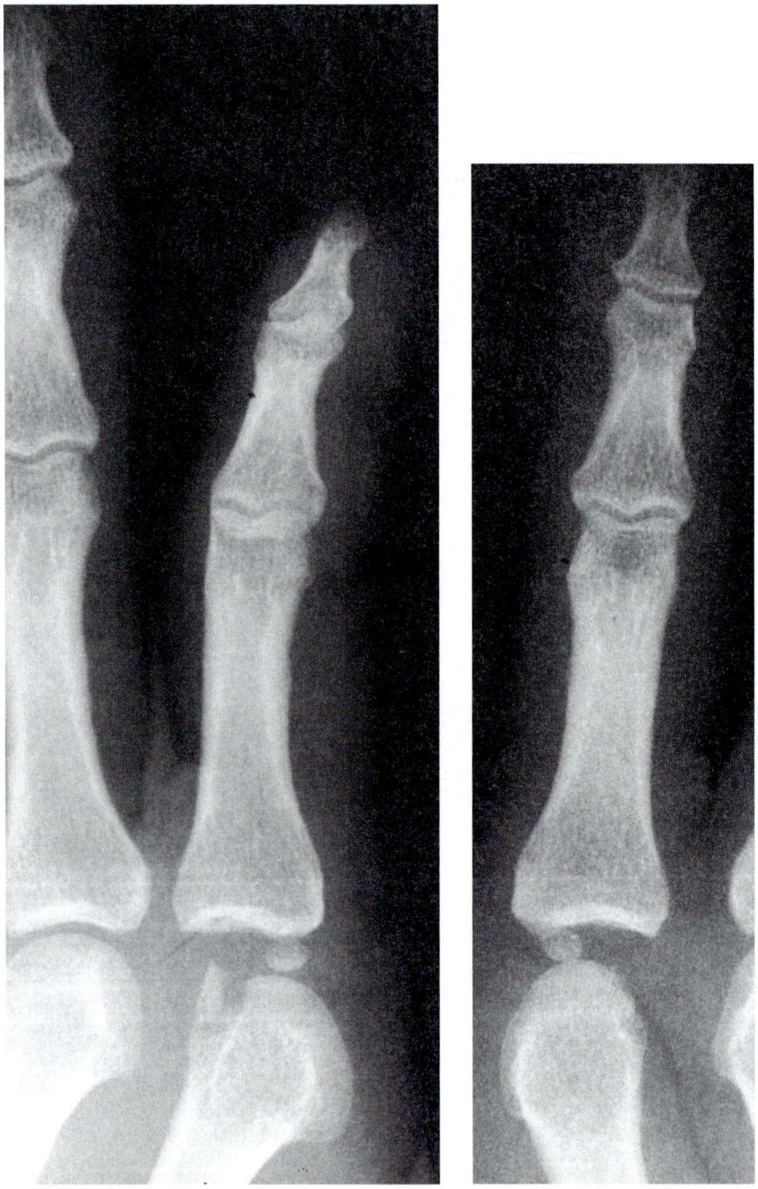

B

FIGURE 27-30 **A,** The proximal phalanx of the index finger is dislocated dorsally. A fracture of the head of the metacarpal also is present. **B,** The posteroanterior radiograph shows the sesamoid (attached to the volar plate) in the joint.

Kaplan,[60] in his classic article published in 1957, described the clinical and anatomic features of the injury that most commonly affects the index finger. The proximal phalanx is hyperextended, and both the interphalangeal joints are in slight flexion. The finger itself is deviated toward the middle finger and slightly overlaps it on its radial side. In the distal palm, there is a bony hard prominence that is the head of the second metacarpal, and on either side of this prominence the palmar skin may be puckered. The diagnosis of the dislocation is confirmed by radiographs of the hand, and three views always should be taken. Frequently, the dislocation is best seen on the oblique view. When sesamoid bones are present, they will displace with the phalanx and will be seen in the widened joint space. Occasionally, there may be a concomitant fracture of the metacarpal head or proximal phalanx.[37]

Investigators have clearly described the pathophysiologic features of the dislocation.[3,60] The lumbrical muscle is along the radial side of the neck of the second metacarpal, while the pretendinous band of the palmar fascia, the second cleft neurovascular bundle, and the flexor tendons, including the A-1 pulley, are around the ulnar side of the metacarpal. The volar plate, which is torn at its membranous portion, is displaced dorsal to the metacarpal head (Fig. 27-31). When the injury occurs to a little finger, both the lumbrical muscle and flexor tendons are radial to the head, while the hypothenar intrinsic muscles are on the head's ulnar side. Regardless of the finger that is injured, the metacarpal head is entrapped by the surrounding soft-tissue structures, and the entrapment has been likened to a Chinese finger trap. As with a finger trap, which tightens as greater traction is applied to it, when the physician attempts to reduce the dislocation by applying longitudinal traction, the soft tissues on both sides of the head, which already are tight, tighten even more and prevent reduction. Surgery is required for most of these injuries, and the standard operative approach is a volar one, as described by Kaplan.[60] A transverse incision is made between the proximal and distal volar creases, and it is extended to the radial side of the joint. Great care must be taken while making this skin incision because the radial nerve is tented over the head of the metacarpal and is immediately beneath the skin. An inadvertent laceration of the nerve can easily occur if the skin incision passes deeper than the dermal layer. After the nerve and its artery are identified and protected, the superficial palmar fascia and the proximal sheath of the flexor tendon are divided. Generally, the volar plate now can be freed from its entrapped position with the use of a probe. If this is not possible, the deep transverse metacarpal ligament is incised, which then frees the plate. After reduction, the joint is immobilized in approximately 30° of flexion with a dorsal extension block splint for 3 weeks. Active range-of-motion exercises can be started within 1 week. A dorsal operative approach also has been described to reduce these dislocations.[6,12] The advantages of this approach are that it permits a clearer view of the displaced volar plate, which is the prime structure blocking reduction, and the likelihood of damaging a neurovascular bundle is far less.

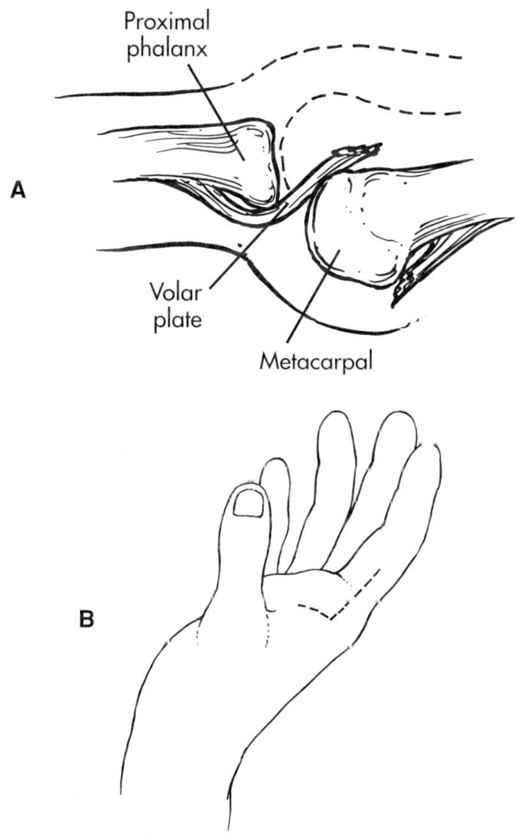

FIGURE 27-31 **A,** The volar plate interposed between the proximal phalanx and metacarpal head. **B,** The palmar incision used to approach the joint.

Occasionally, dorsal dislocations go untreated for weeks or even months. Satisfactory digital function still can be restored in these cases,[4,79] but the delay in treatment results in secondary contractures of the collateral ligaments that must be released in addition to release of the soft tissues entrapping the metacarpal head. Combined volar and dorsal operative approaches usually are necessary for chronic cases.

A volar dislocation of the metacarpophalangeal joint is a rare condition.

Injuries to the collateral and accessory collateral ligaments of the metacarpophalangeal joints of the finger are uncommon, particularly when compared with the same injuries in thumbs.[77] In the finger, the metacarpophalangeal joint is protected by its position close to the hand, by the adjacent fingers, and by the laxity of the collateral ligaments that permits the finger to absorb forces when it is in extension. Collateral ligament injuries result from sudden deviation of the finger, especially in an ulnar direction. This usually occurs when the joint is in flexion and the collateral ligament is already taut. Injuries also can result from forced twisting of the digit. The middle, ring, and little fingers are more commonly affected than the index finger.[29,30]

Collateral ligament injuries usually are either first-degree sprains (minimal injury with no damage to the integrity of the ligament) or second-degree sprains (partial tear of the ligament, causing slight laxity of the joint but no gross instability). Clinically, a second-degree sprain is characterized by tenderness over the injured ligament and slight laxity when the ligament is stressed. Ligament stability should always be tested with the joint in flexion because with the joint in extension the ligament normally is lax. Second-degree sprains are treated by immobilizing the joint in moderate flexion for 3 weeks and then buddy-taping the finger for an additional 3 to 4 weeks. Soreness and local tenderness over the injured ligament will persist for many months. Often the clinician can relieve patients' anxiety by telling them that 12 to 18 months often are required for injuries to reach a point of maximal improvement.

A third-degree sprain, which involves a complete tear of the ligament, is a serious injury causing joint instability (Fig. 27-32). These injuries sometimes are associated with a fracture, and a careful radiographic examination is important. The articular surfaces of the joint are best seen by either an oblique view or a Brewerton view. Collateral ligaments can tear at their metacarpal origin, their phalangeal insertion, or within their substance.[29] Surgery is recommended for clinical conditions in which there is gross instability of the joint in flexion, when the finger deviates away from its injured ligament in its resting position, and when there is a displaced bony fragment. Lateral deviation of the finger and a displaced fracture fragment, which represents the end of the avulsed ligament, require surgery even if weeks have elapsed from the time of the injury.[43]

The author's preferred treatment is to reattach the ligament to the bone. The extensor hood and joint capsule are opened to reveal the injured ligament and the articular surfaces of the joint. The avulsed ligament is reattached using a pull-out suture technique. Even in cases when treatment has been delayed and the ligament has undergone a mild contracture, the ligament usually can be gently stretched and reattached without the need to reconstruct it with a tendon graft. The ligament should not be repaired with the metacarpophalangeal joint in extension because this position likely will cause a residual extension contracture. After repair, the joint is often immobilized in flexion by using a transarticular Kirschner wire. The wire is removed after 3 weeks, and active range-of-motion exercises are started with the joint protected for an additional 3 to 4 weeks. In cases in which the ligament avulses with a large bone fragment from either the metacarpal or the phalanx, the fragment with its attached ligament is replaced and fixed, usually with Kirschner wires.

A

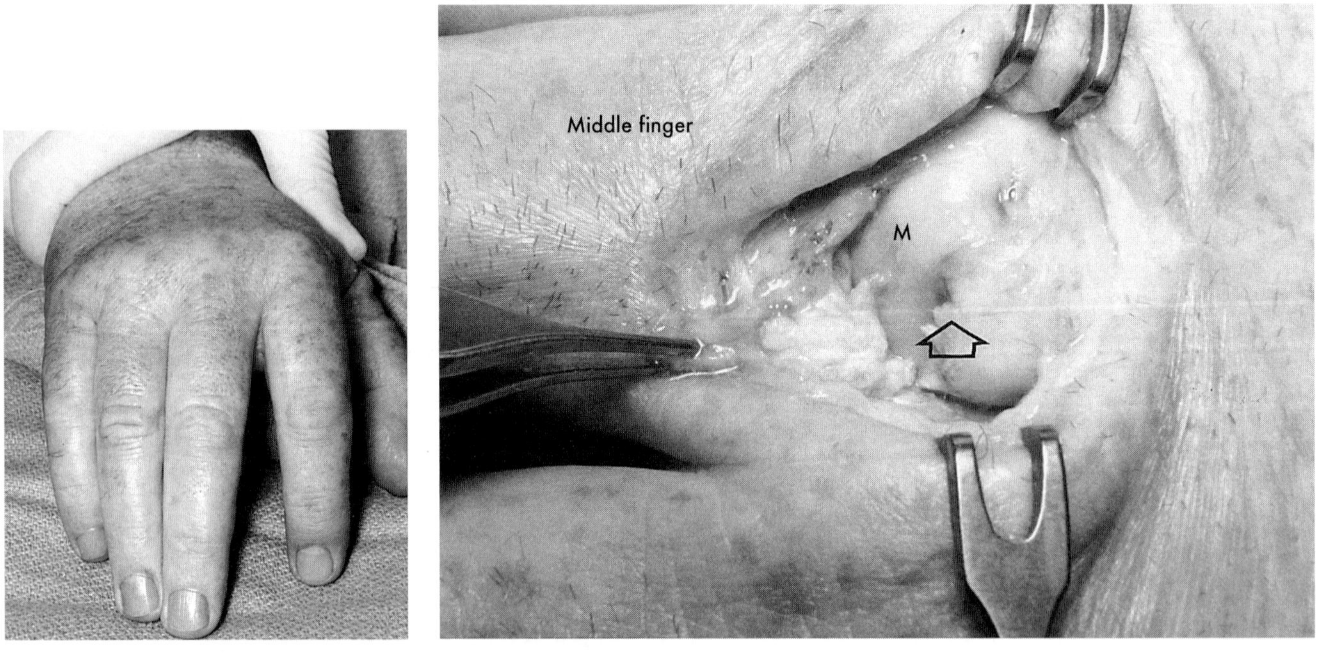

B

FIGURE 27-32 **A,** A tear of the radial collateral ligament of the proximal joint of the middle finger causes the finger to deviate ulnarward. **B,** The ligament *(arrow)* was torn near its insertion into the proximal phalanx. *M,* Metacarpal head.

METACARPAL FRACTURES

Fractures of the metacarpals that result most often from sports activities are intraarticular fractures of the head, shaft fractures (single or multiple), fractures of the neck of the fifth metacarpal (boxer's fracture), and fractures of the bases of the fourth and fifth metacarpals. These injuries are closed fractures, except possibly when they occur in motorcycle racing or auto racing.

Metacarpal Head Fractures

These fractures usually are the result of axial loading or direct trauma. The head of the metacarpal is entirely covered by articular cartilage, which permits the metacarpophalangeal joint to move in several planes. Even fractures that are not greatly displaced still will disrupt the contour of the head of the bone. A Brewerton radiographic view is useful to show the fracture (Fig. 27-33).[17,65] McElfresh and Dobyns[74] noted that injuries to the metacarpal head of the index finger were most common, followed in decreasing order of occurrence by the little, middle, ring, and thumb metacarpals. They described many fracture types in their report.

To restore joint congruity, an open reduction and internal fixation invariably is needed (Fig. 27-34).[49,74,75,115] The metacarpophalangeal joint is opened through a dorsal incision. The interval between the extensor tendon and extensor hood is incised, and the joint is opened. Depending on the fracture configuration, Kirschner wires or small lag screws can be used. A Herbert screw, which can be buried beneath the articular surface, may be particularly useful at this site.

Metacarpal Neck Fracture (Boxer's Fracture)

This injury occurs when a fist strikes a hard object, the head of the bone flexes palmarly, and the fracture angulates apex dorsally (Fig. 27-35). This is a result of the forces of the injury and the pull of the interosseous muscle. Although this fracture most commonly occurs in the ring and little fingers, the index and middle fingers occasionally may be injured in the same manner. Because of the mobility of the base of the fourth and fifth metacarpals, angulation of up to 50° to 60° usually can be tolerated without compromise of hand function.[35,53,68] Others believe an angulation of over 30° is not acceptable.[2,98]

A

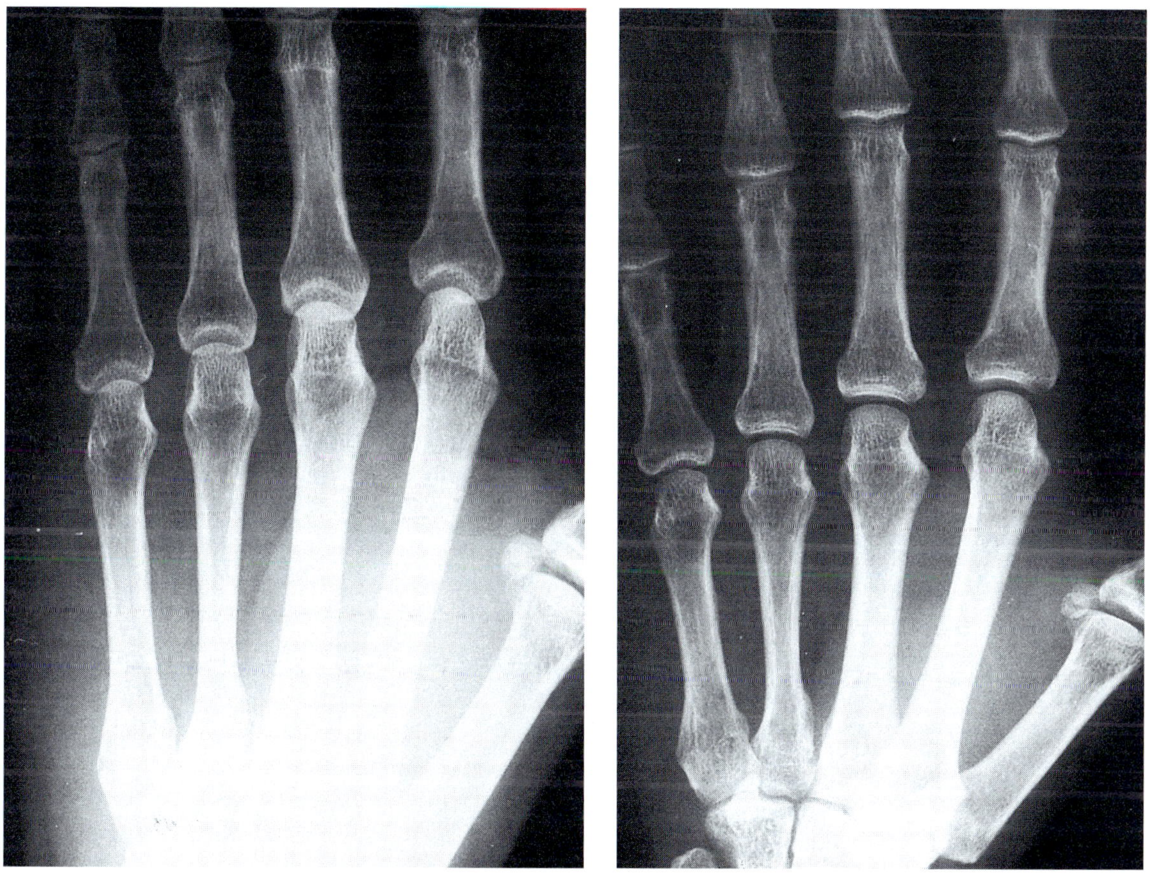

B

FIGURE 27-33 The metacarpal head can be better seen with the Brewerton view, **A,** than with a PA view, **B.**

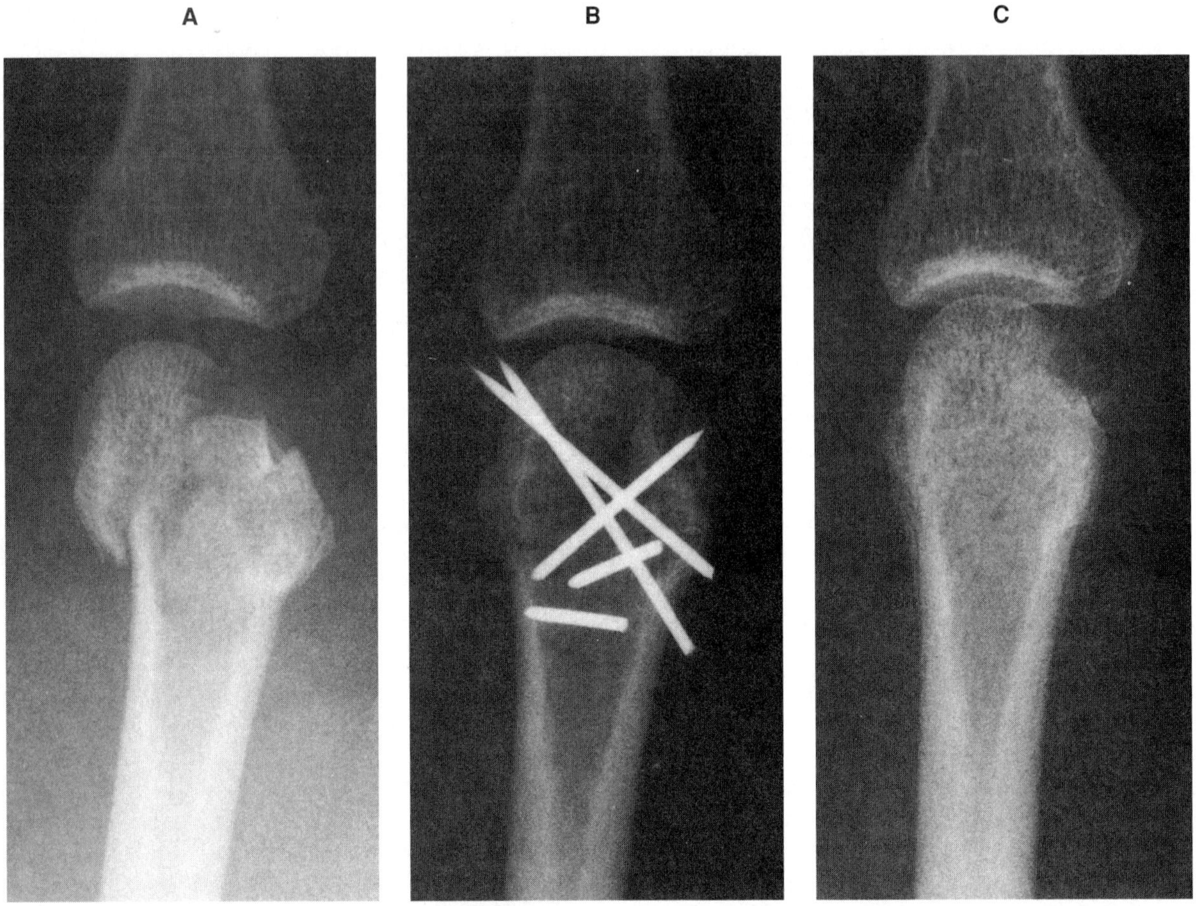

FIGURE 27-34 **A,** A comminuted displaced fracture of the metacarpal head, **B,** required multiple Kirschner wires to reduce the fracture. **C,** One year later the joint surface looked good but the patient had only fair flexion of the joint.

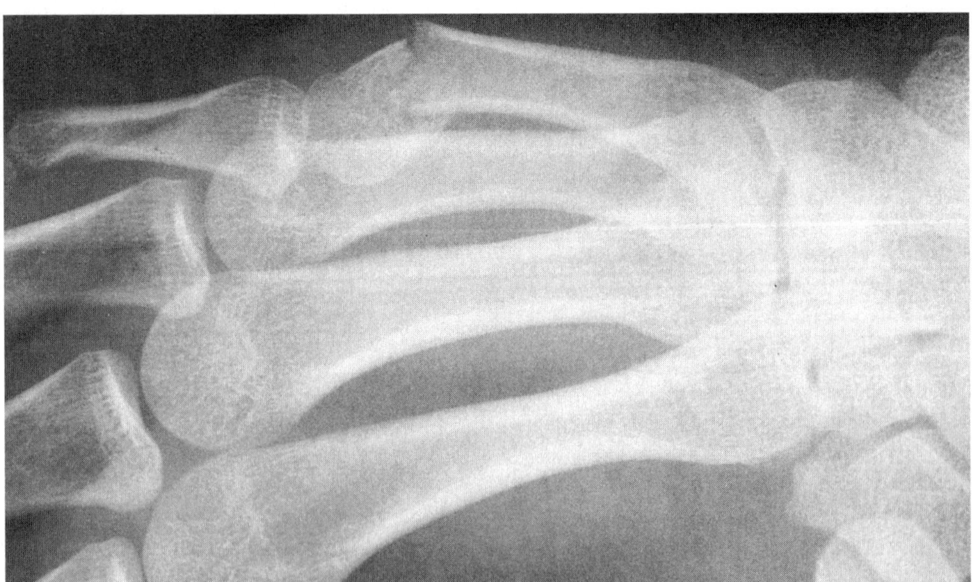

FIGURE 27-35 Boxer's fracture of the fifth metacarpal.

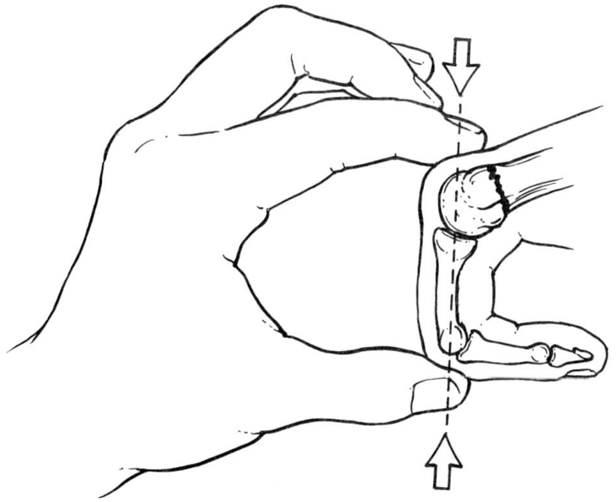

FIGURE 27-36 Jahss method of reducing Boxer's fracture.

The author prefers to attempt a closed reduction of the fracture, to decrease the 50° to 60° angulation to 20° to 30°, and to maintain this with a cast and splint to the injured digit. This is maintained for 3 weeks, and then range-of-motion exercises are started. The reduction method described by Jahss[54] is used (Fig. 27-36). The metacarpophalangeal and proximal interphalangeal joints are flexed 90°, and the proximal phalanx is pushed dorsally to decrease the angulation of the neck of the metacarpal. Although Jahss immobilized the hand in this position, this is not considered an acceptable method of immobilization of this fracture.

After the fracture heals, if the athlete has difficulty with grasp because of pressure from the metacarpal head in the palm, a corrective osteotomy can be done to realign the head of the metacarpal.

Because the constraints at the bases of the index and long metacarpals are fairly rigid, angulation of more than 10° to 15° at the neck of the index or long metacarpals is unacceptable.[2,86,98]

Metacarpal Shaft Fractures

Shaft fractures of the metacarpals, as with the phalanges, are transverse, oblique, or spiral.[57] Transverse fractures usually are produced by direct trauma to the hand. The fracture tends to angulate dorsally, and angulation of greater than 30° in the little finger, 20° in the ring finger, and 5° in the index and long fingers should be reduced. Angulation of a shaft fracture pushes the head of the metacarpal into the palm. Oblique and spiral fractures result from rotational forces, and these fractures can cause malrotation of the finger if not properly treated. Freeland et al[40] noted that 5° of malrotation in a metacarpal fracture can cause overlap of 1.5 cm in the finger. Opgrande and Westphal[82] stated that 1° of metacarpal shaft rotation causes 5° of rotation in the finger. Malrotation is best determined by examination of the hand.

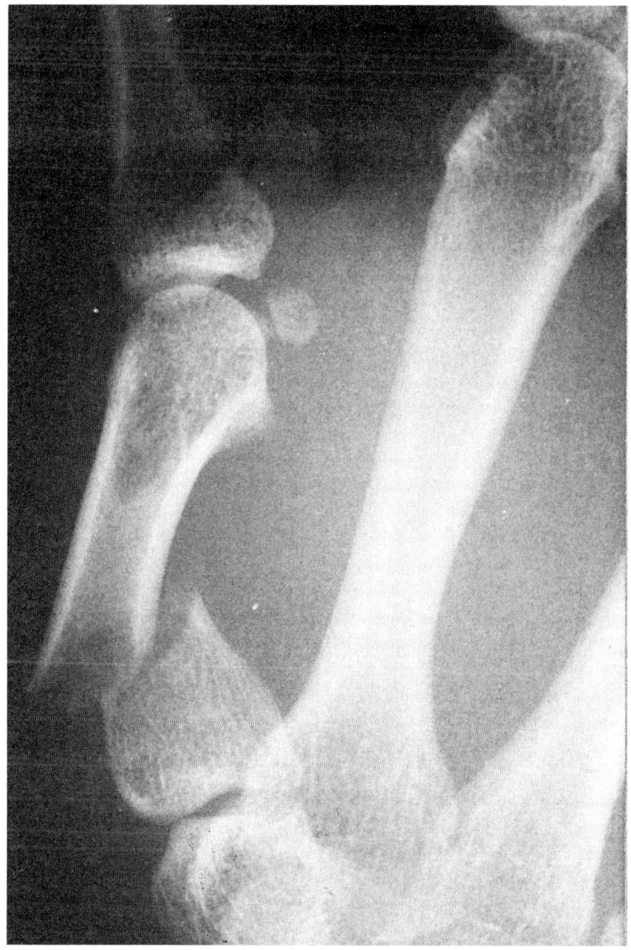

FIGURE 27-37 This slightly oblique thumb metacarpal fracture could not be reduced closed because the distal shaft had impaled the muscle.

Single Metacarpal Shaft Fractures

Single metacarpal fractures usually are transverse, minimally displaced, and stable. Even if there is some displacement, the fracture usually can be manipulated and reduced. If the fracture is stable, 3 to 4 weeks of immobilization will allow the fracture to heal. An ulnar or radial gutter splint will provide good support, and the athlete may participate in sports. Protective splints and buddy-taping can be used to protect the hand after adequate fracture healing. Occasionally a transverse completely displaced fracture is trapped in the interosseous muscle (Fig. 27-37) or an oblique or spiral fracture is so unstable that it cannot be controlled by splinting, and an open reduction and internal fixation is necessary (Fig. 27-38).[115] Small lag screws and small plates provide excellent fixation of a metacarpal fracture.[76] Range-of-motion exercises usually can begin within 1 week of fracture fixation.

Multiple Shaft Fractures

Multiple metacarpal shaft fractures are caused by significant trauma and often are associated with extensive soft-tissue injury. When displaced, these fractures are difficult

A B C

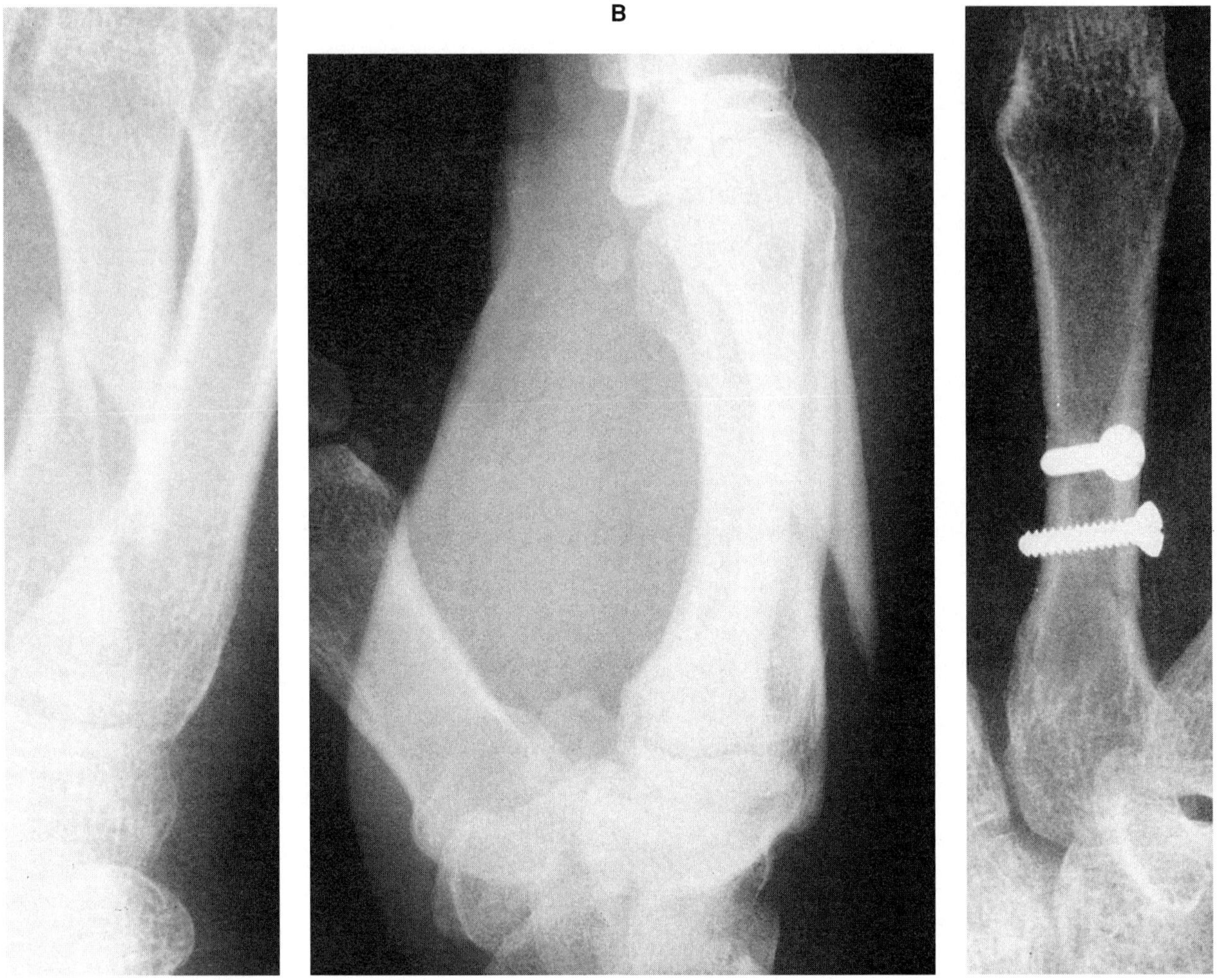

FIGURE 27-38 **A** and **B,** A long oblique fracture of the fourth metacarpal was extremely unstable and had to be stabilized with two screws, **C.**

A

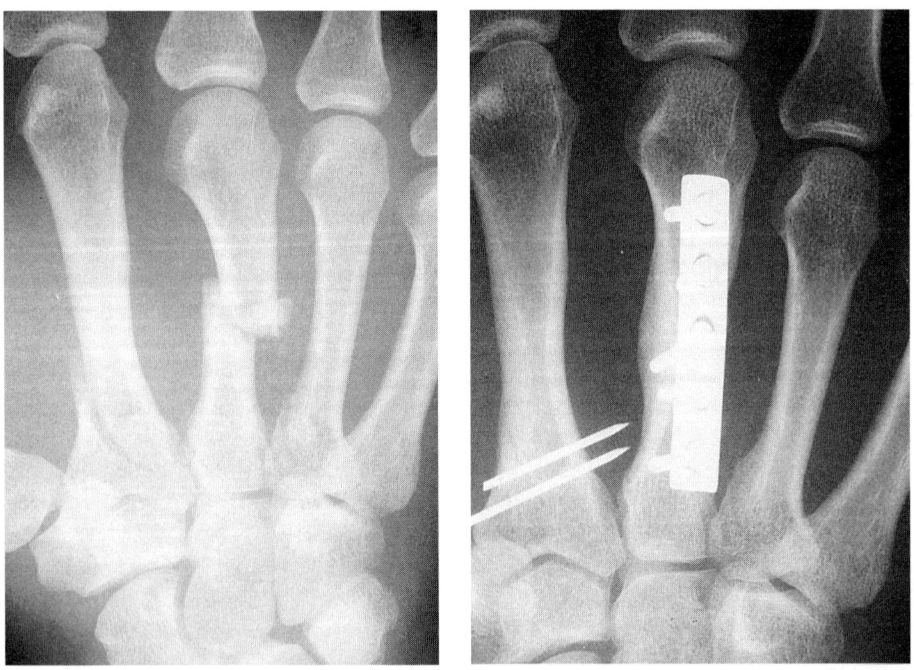

B

FIGURE 27-39 **A,** Multiple metacarpal fractures usually are unstable and, **B,** require open reduction and internal fixation.

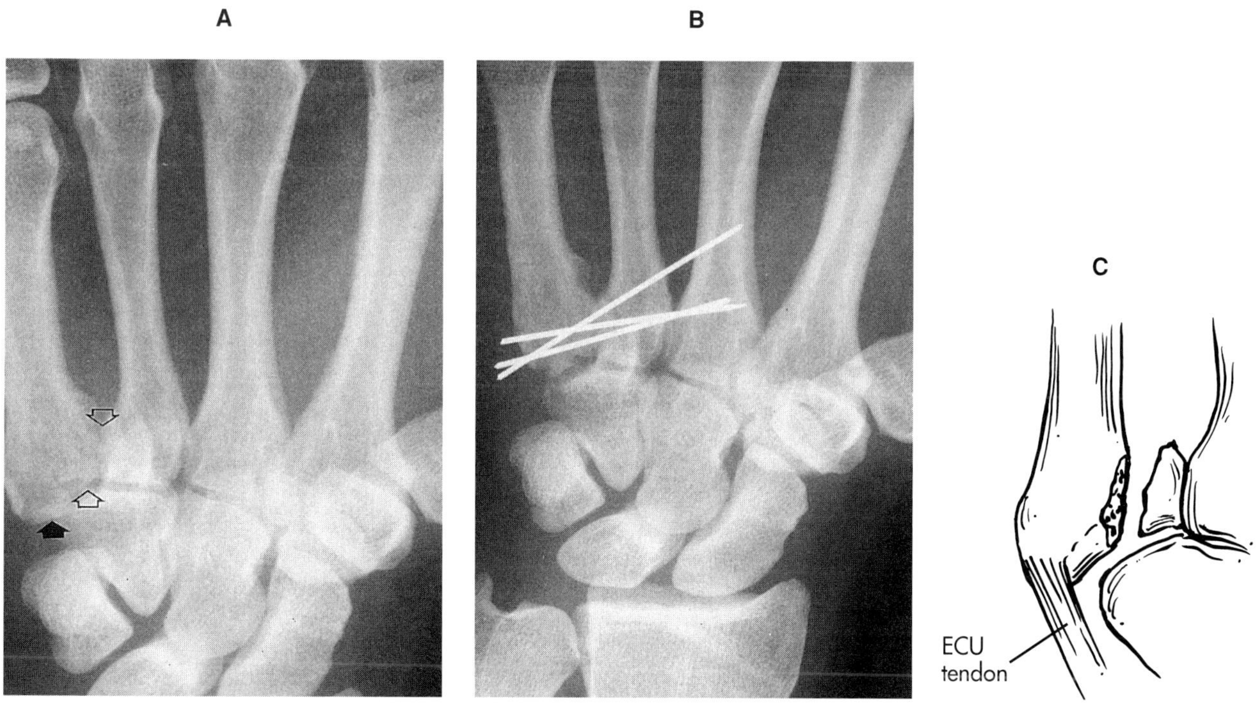

FIGURE 27-40 A, The shaft of the fifth metacarpal is displaced *(solid arrow)* while the radial fragment remains in place *(light arrows)*. **B,** Open reduction and internal fixation of the fracture-dislocation. The shaft of the fifth metacarpal is displaced by the pull of the extensor carpi ulnaris tendon **(C).**

to manipulate and reduce, and an open reduction and internal fixation is indicated (Fig. 27-39). Rigid internal fixation with screws[23,26,50] or plates[93,96] will allow rehabilitation to begin early and will prevent restricted finger motion because of tendon adhesions or joint contractures. Kirschner wires also will provide satisfactory internal fixation, but sometimes motion cannot be started for 3 weeks.

Fracture-Dislocation of the Base of the Fifth Metacarpal

This injury is a fracture-dislocation involving the fifth metacarpohamate joint. It is analogous to a Bennett's fracture.[61] After a force is directed longitudinally along the axis of the fifth metacarpal, the small radial fragment remains in place, while the rest of the metacarpal dislocates dorsally and ulnarly (Fig. 27-40). The dislocation results from the pull of the extensor carpi ulnaris tendon and the abductor digiti minimi tendon, as well as the slope of the hamate. This fracture is sometimes difficult to appreciate on radiographs. Bora and Didizian[13] recommended an anteroposterior view with the forearm pronated 30° (Fig. 27-41). A CT scan also may be useful. Occasionally the dorsal lip of the hamate also fractures, and this increases the instability at the joint. Although some authors advocate closed reduction and percutaneous Kirschner wire fixation of either the fracture or

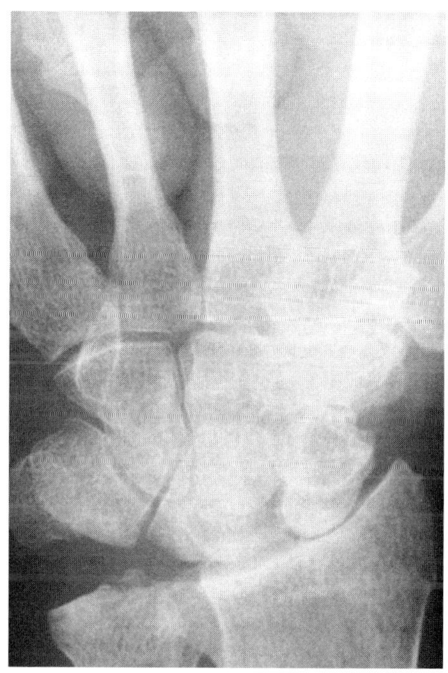

FIGURE 27-41 The pronated oblique view of the hand shows the base of the fifth metacarpal.

the fifth metacarpal to the fourth metacarpal,[13,28] the base of the metacarpal should be accurately reduced and a congruous joint surface restored by open reduction and internal fixation. If the joint surfaces remain offset, motion will be painful and the grip will be weak.[13] Secondary reconstructive procedures then will be necessary.

Multiple carpometacarpal dislocations are high-energy injuries, can occur in any configuration, and invariably require open reduction and internal fixation (Fig. 27-42).[67,81,90]

Complications of metacarpal fractures include malunion (with or without dorsal angulation), nonunion, tendon adhesions, and joint stiffness.

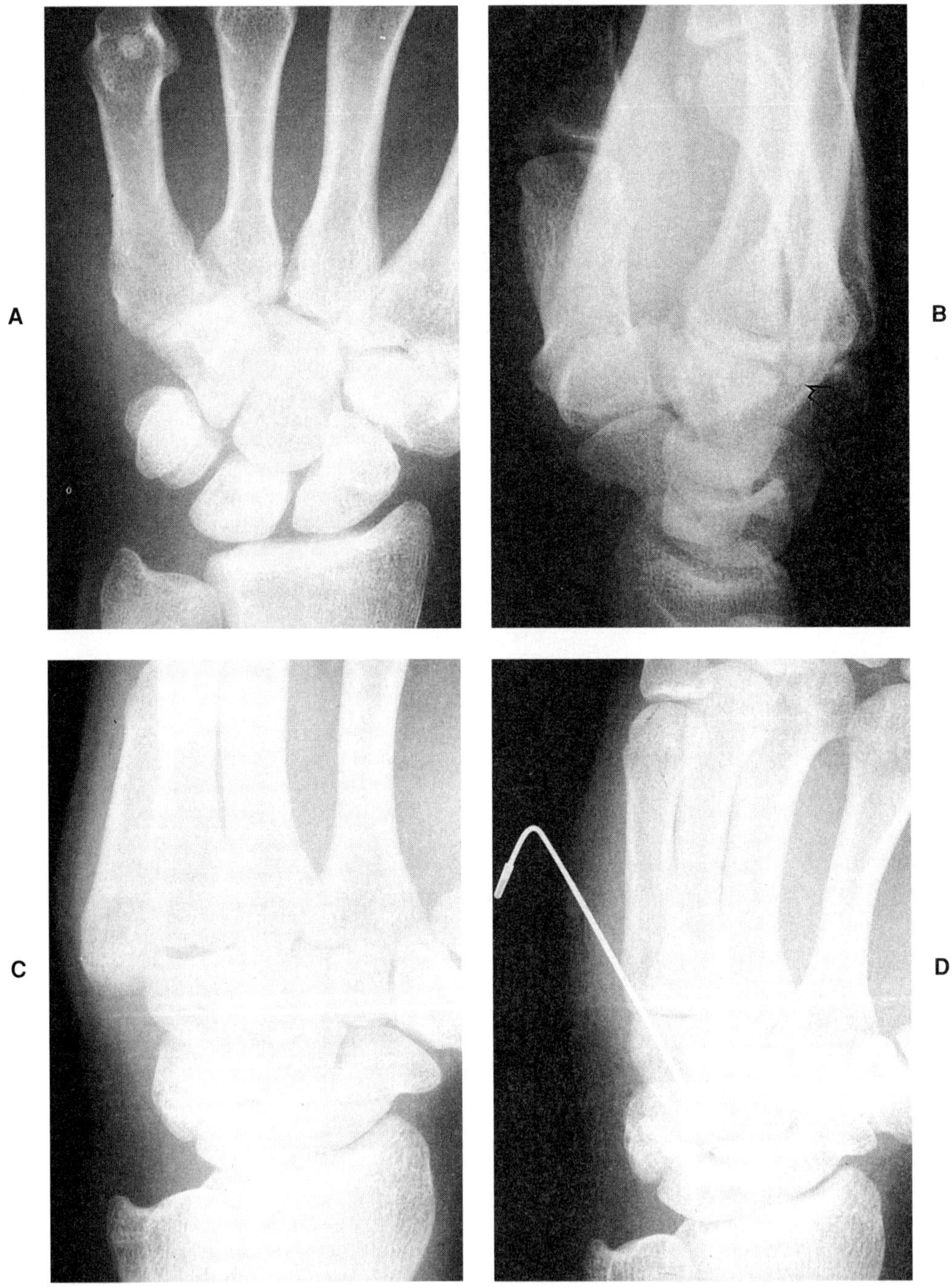

FIGURE 27-42 **A** and **B,** Anteroposterior and lateral radiographs showing a dislocation of the fourth and fifth metacarpals associated with a fracture of the hamate *(arrow)*. **C,** An isolated dislocation of the fifth metacarpal is unusual. **D,** It can be treated by closed reduction and percutaneous Kirschner wire fixation.

FRACTURES AND DISLOCATIONS OF THE THUMB

Fractures of the phalanges and metacarpals of the thumb are similar to those of the fingers and can be treated in the same way as previously described. Treatment depends on the configuration of the fracture.

Three entities commonly are found in sports-related injuries of the thumb: Bennett's fracture, closed rupture of the collateral ligaments of the metacarpophalangeal joint of the thumb, and the "irreducible" dislocation of the metacarpophalangeal joint of the thumb. These injuries will be discussed in greater detail.

Bennett's Fracture

In 1881 and 1886, Edward Hallaran Bennett[9,10] clearly described the mechanics and pathology of the fracture-dislocation at the metacarpotrapezial joint of the thumb that now bears his name. The fracture occurs through the volar-ulnar lip of the thumb metacarpal (Fig. 27-43). This fracture fragment, which can vary in size, stays in its anatomic position tethered by the anterior oblique ligament. This ligament extends from the volar lip of the metacarpal to the trapezium. The thumb metacarpal subluxes radially, dorsally, and proximally from the unopposed pull of the abductor pollicis longus tendon. This injury occurs when a thumb metacarpal is axially loaded and a flexion-adduction and supination force is applied to the base of the thumb.[85] Bennett's fracture is a common sports-related injury of the thumb.

It is important to suspect the injury when the thumb is swollen and the base of the thumb metacarpal is painful. Appropriate radiographs must be done to best visualize the fracture and evaluate the size of the volar-ulnar bony fragment. A true lateral radiograph, as described by Billing and Gedda,[11] and the hyperpronated (Robert's) view[66] will allow a good evaluation of the metacarpotrapezial joint (Fig. 27-44). The latter radiograph of the

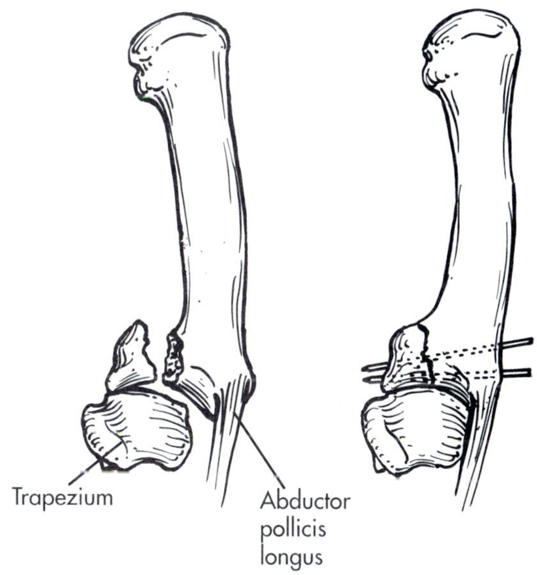

FIGURE 27-43 Bennett's fracture. The abductor pollicis longus tendon displaces the shaft of the thumb metacarpal.

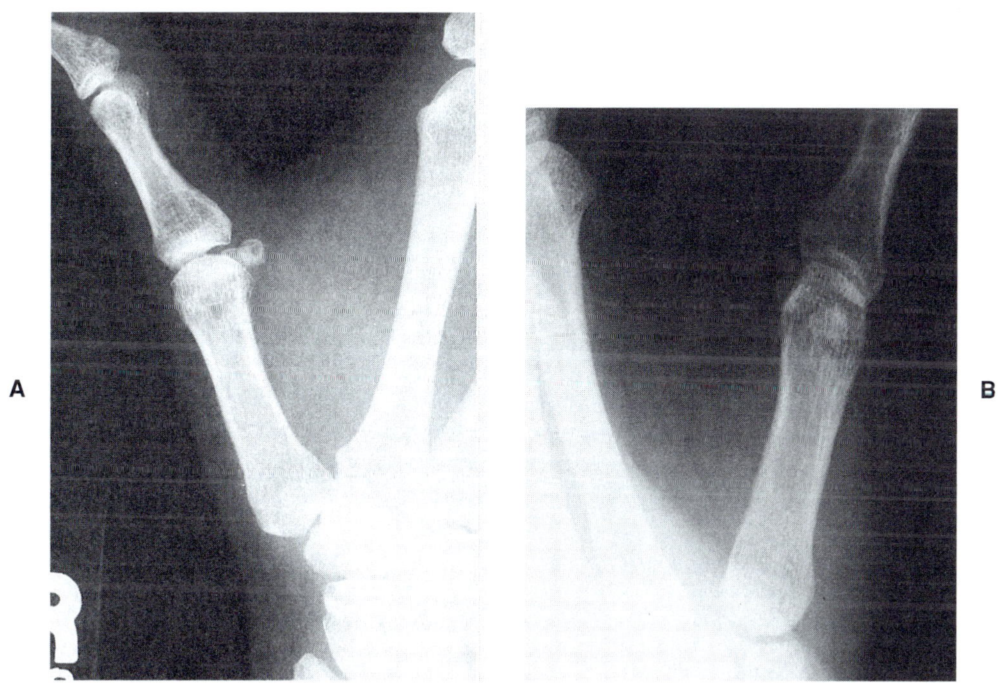

FIGURE 27-44 Radiographs showing **A,** lateral view of the base of the thumb metacarpal and, **B,** a hyperpronated (Robert's) view.

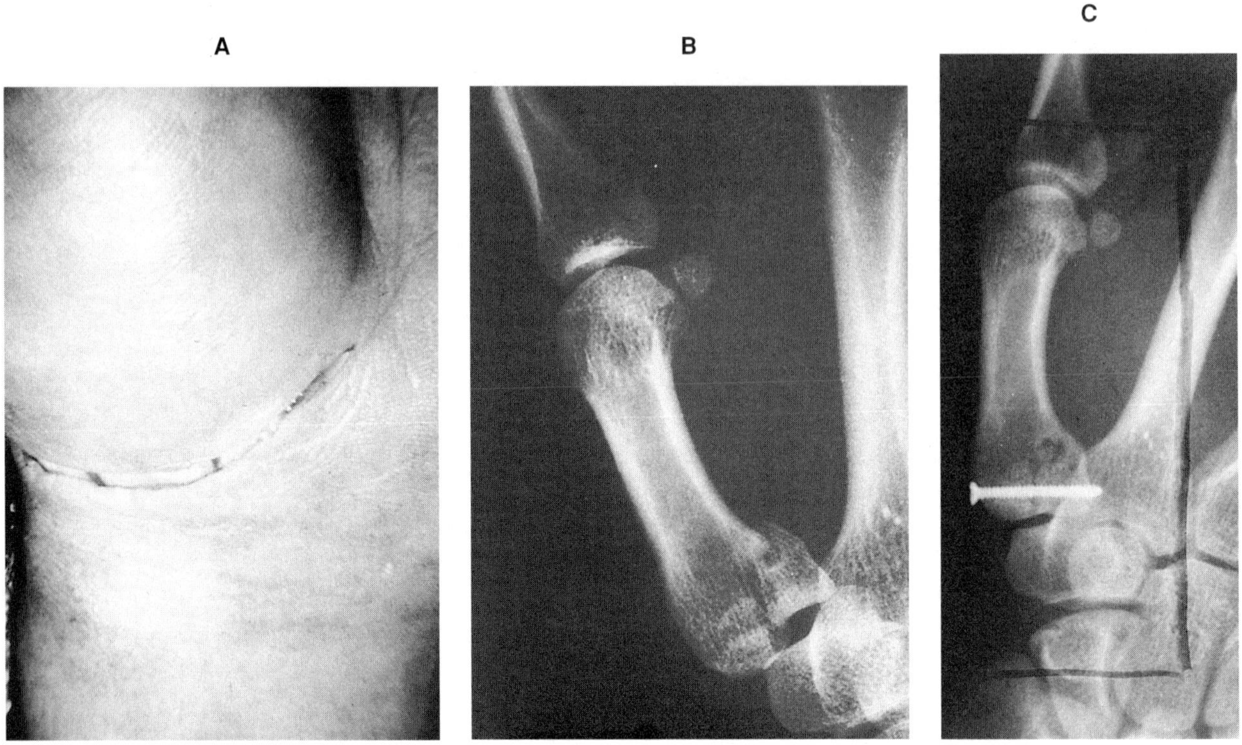

FIGURE 27-45 Bennett's fracture. **A,** The curved incision at the metacarpotrapezial joint of a left thumb. **B,** A significant offset is noted at the joint surface, and, **C,** the reduction is stabilized with a screw.

thumb is taken with the forearm on the table, the hand pronated 20°, and the thumb flat on the table. The x-ray tube is positioned 10° from the vertical in a distal-palmar direction.

The metacarpotrapezial joint of the thumb is very mobile, and joint stability is maintained by five ligaments. With thumb pinch and grasp, the compressive forces at the metacarpotrapezial joint increase 10 to 12 times.[22] Thus if there is loss of joint congruency resulting from an unreduced intraarticular fracture or loss of the soft-tissue stabilizing structures, degenerative arthritis can occur.[16,100]

There is no consensus as to the best method of managing a Bennett's fracture.[58,105] Two long-term reviews on the treatment of Bennett's fracture arrived at completely opposite conclusions. Livesley's[68] study, with an average follow-up of 26 years, noted poor long-term results with conservative treatment and recommended that these fractures be treated with an operation. The study of Cannon et al[20] had a mean follow-up of 9.6 years, and they concluded that conservative treatment was good.

As recommended by Gedda and Moberg,[42] accurate restoration of the joint surface is important to maintaining a healthy metacarpotrapezial joint. This is especially true if the incongruity of the joint is greater than 2 mm or there is an impaction component to the articular surface of the thumb metacarpal.[58]

The metacarpotrapezial joint of the thumb is exposed through a curved volar and radial incision (Fig. 27-45). By subperiosteal dissection, the thenar muscles are elevated from the proximal end of the metacarpal. The joint capsule is opened, and the hematoma is removed. Longitudinal traction on the thumb metacarpal and elevation of any depressed articular fracture fragments will reduce the articular surface of the thumb metacarpal in relation to the undisplaced volar lip fragment. The fracture is stabilized with Kirschner wires[7] or a lag screw.[38] A thumb spica cast is used for 4 weeks, and active thumb range-of-motion exercises are begun. The athlete usually can return to sports within 6 weeks of surgery with a splint to protect the thumb.

Rolando[92] described a three-part intraarticular fracture at the base of the thumb metacarpal. The fracture configuration is a Y or T with an extension into the joint (Fig. 27-46). Depending on the separation and displacement of the articular component of the fracture, and the degree of comminution of the smaller fracture fragments, the treatment will be a cast or an operation.[38]

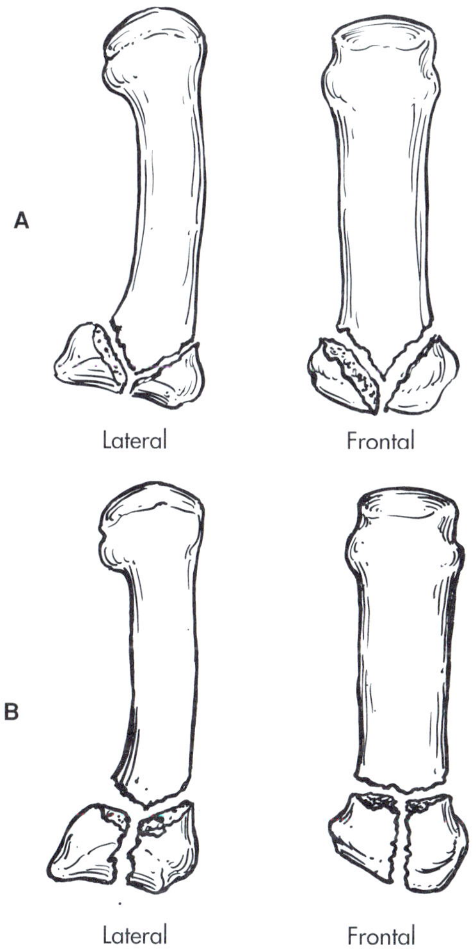

FIGURE 27-46 Rolando fracture. The fracture is intraarticular and can be in either a Y **(A)** or T **(B)** configuration.

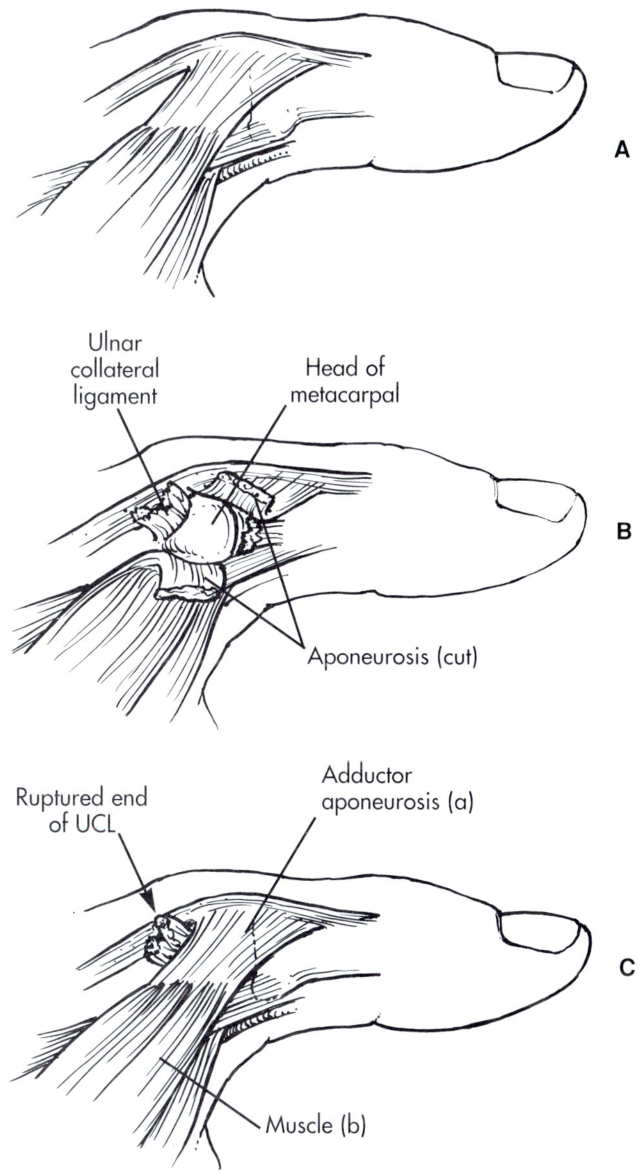

FIGURE 27-47 **A,** The adductor aponeurosis *(a)* and the adductor pollicis muscle *(b)*. **B,** After dividing the adductor aponeurosis, the surgeon can see the ulnar collateral ligament *(UCL)*. **C,** A Stener lesion in which the ulnar collateral ligament has retracted proximally *(arrow)*.

COLLATERAL LIGAMENT INJURIES

Metacarpophalangeal Joint of the Thumb

The metacarpophalangeal joint of the thumb, which functions primarily in flexion and extension, is stabilized by soft-tissue constraints consisting of capsule, ligaments, and musculotendinous units. Strong lateral support is provided by the ulnar and radial collateral ligaments.

Injuries of the ulnar collateral ligament are much more common than of the radial collateral ligament. Although originally referred to as a gamekeeper's thumb, these injuries most often result from a ski injury and now are called skier's thumb.[21,44,78] This condition also can result from an injury in football, hockey, and baseball.

The mechanism of injury of the ulnar collateral ligament is a radially directed force (abduction); the reverse is true for the radial collateral ligament. The ligament invariably is torn from its distal attachment to the proximal phalanx. Occasionally a fracture of the proximal phalanx accompanies the collateral ligament injury, and the fragment can vary from a bony flake to more than 10% to 15% of the joint surface.[39]

Stener,[104] in 1962, described a complete tear of the ulnar collateral ligament in which the ligament retracted proximally so that the adductor aponeurosis was interposed between the ligament and its insertion site at the proximal phalanx. This lesion does not heal without surgical intervention (Fig. 27-47).

A good examination of the thumb is extremely important in differentiating between a partial and complete rupture of the collateral ligament. The ligament stability should be tested with the metacarpophalangeal joint in both flexion and extension. If the injury is only a mild sprain, a small splint to protect the joint or taping of the joint will suffice. A moderate sprain, in which there is an end point to gentle lateral stress of the joint and the joint opens less than 30°, can be treated with a thumb spica cast for 3 to 4 weeks. The joint is protected when the athlete returns to sports.

However, if there is no apparent end point to lateral stress of the joint, the joint opens 30° or more, or a mass is palpable at the proximal end of the joint (possible Stener's lesion), an operation is indicated (Fig. 27-48). Radiographs should be taken to determine whether a fracture is present, and stress views also may be taken if they are felt to be necessary to evaluate the integrity of the ligament. Arthrography or an MRI of the joint usually is not necessary.

Although a variety of operative methods for treating the ligament have been described,[30] the author prefers a direct repair of the ligament to its insertion on the proximal phalanx using a pull-out suture.

The ulnar side of the metacarpophalangeal joint is opened through a midlateral incision. A branch of the dorsal sensory radial nerve, usually present in the wound, is identified and protected. The adductor aponeurosis is divided, and the ligament is identified. The joint is evaluated to determine whether there is any intraarticular injury. Often the dorsal capsule is partially torn. The ligament, which tends to shorten or fold as it retracts, is gently stretched and inserted into the proximal phalanx with a pull-out suture tied onto a button. A transarticular Kirschner wire fixes the metacarpophalangeal joint in 10° to 20° of flexion to protect the ligament repair. The adductor aponeurosis is repaired, and the skin is closed. A thumb spica cast is used to immobilize the joint for 4 to 5 weeks.

If a small bony fragment is attached to the ligament, it is excised (Fig. 27-49). If the fragment is sufficiently large, it is reduced and fixed to the proximal phalanx with Kirschner wires.

A chronic ulnar collateral ligament injury, with retraction and scarring of the ligament, presents a more diffi-

A
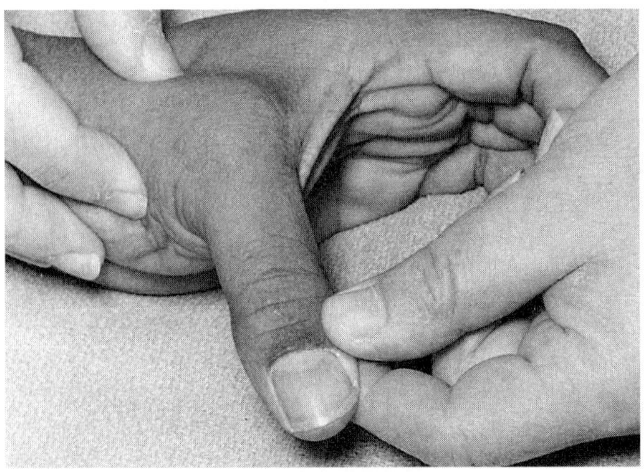
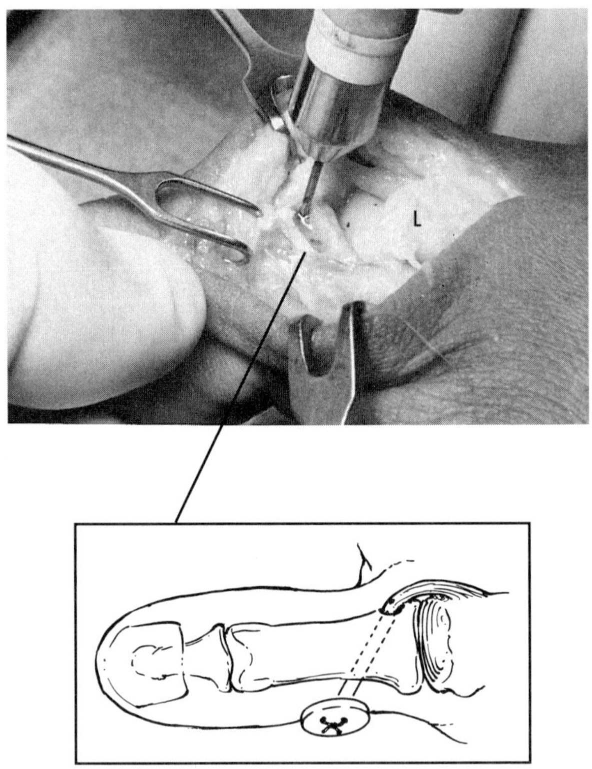

B
C
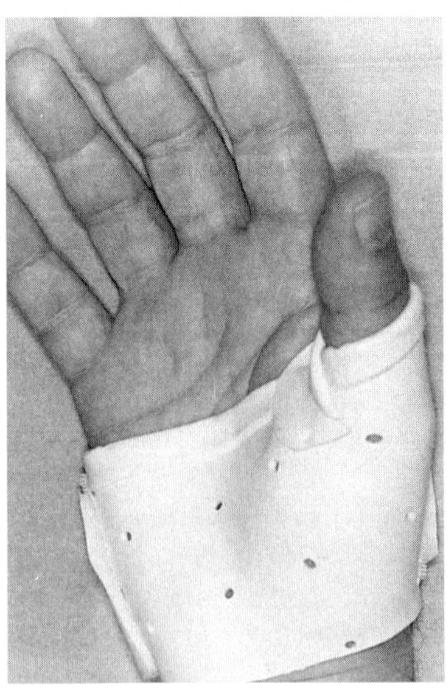

FIGURE 27-48 **A,** Examination of the ulnar collateral ligament shows significant laxity. **B,** At operation the ligament *(L)* was torn. Drill holes are made in the proximal phalanx to reattach the ligament to bone. **C,** After the cast is removed, the thumb is protected with a splint.

cult problem. A variety of reconstructive procedures[30] have been recommended, including reconstruction of the ligament with a piece of tendon to stabilize the joint. The author prefers to use the remnant of the ligament and its bridging scar tissue to provide stability of the joint. If no local material is available, then stabilization of the joint with a tendon graft is the recommended procedure.[15,30,41,97]

Despite design changes in the ski poles, pole grips, and gloves, skier's thumb remains a significant ski injury.[87]

Injuries to the radial collateral ligament of the metacarpophalangeal joint of the thumb, although much less common, are treated in a similar fashion (Fig. 27-50).[31] The anatomic relationship between the abductor pollicis brevis aponeurosis and the radial collateral ligament is less distinct than the corresponding anatomy on the ulnar side of the joint.

A hyperextension force on the metacarpophalangeal joint of the thumb can produce a dorsal dislocation of the proximal phalanx with an interposed volar plate and the accompanying sesamoid bones, which are part of the plate.[103] Although this dislocation has been described as "irreducible," it usually can be reduced by gentle manipulation under local or regional anesthesia. If a closed reduction is unsuccessful, an open reduction is indicated.[87]

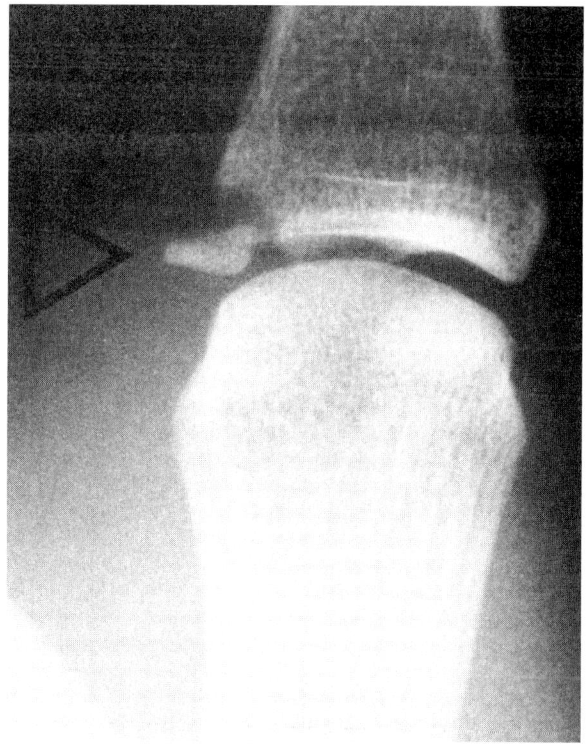

FIGURE 27-49 This bony fragment *(arrow)* is small and could be excised at the time of ligament repair.

A

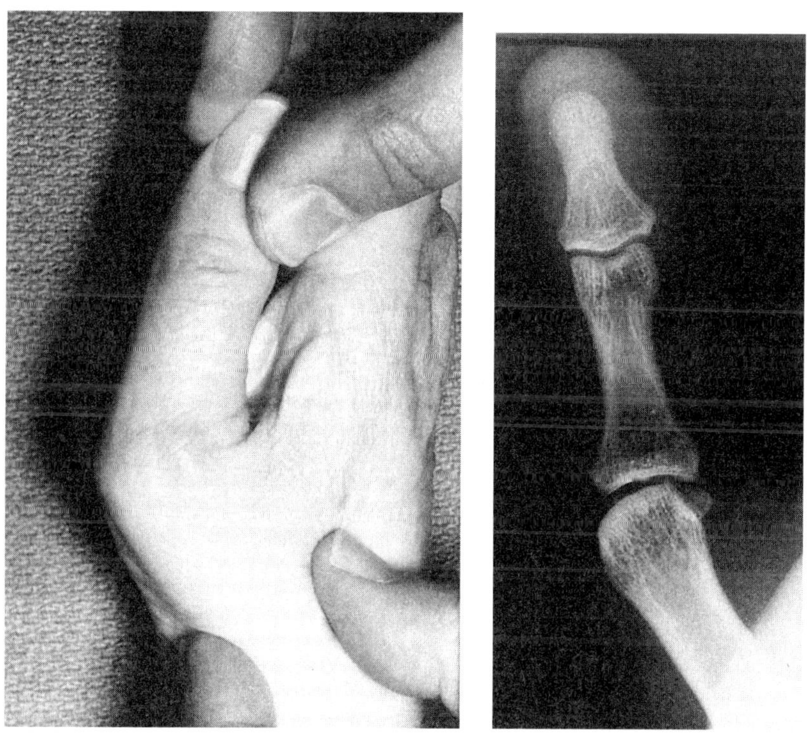

B

FIGURE 27-50 **A,** The radial collateral ligament is torn, as determined by examination and, **B,** by stress radiographs.

JUVENILE AND ADOLESCENT HAND INJURIES

In the juvenile and adolescent athlete, the tensile strength of the ligaments is greater than the strength of the open physeal plates. Fractures and dislocations occur in their physeal plates, and a variety of Salter-Harris fractures can occur.[94] These injuries frequently can be treated by closed manipulation and splinting. However, this carries the danger of growth-plate disturbance, and the parents should be advised of this potential complication. Although the potential for remodeling is best for fracture deformities in the anteroposterior plane, it decreases with the increasing age of the athlete. Remodeling *will not* correct rotational deformities or angulation in the medial-lateral plane.[48]

REHABILITATION

The triad of diagnosing the injury, treating the injury, and providing a comprehensive rehabilitation program is equally important in returning the athlete to sports. The goal is to return the individual to the sport as rapidly as possible as long as the management of the hand injury is not compromised.

Before the athlete is allowed to return to competition, several factors must be considered. The particular injury (fracture, dislocation), the treatment needed to stabilize the bone or joint (manipulation versus operation), the location of the injury, the particular sport, and the player's position in that sport (football lineman versus quarterback) must be considered.[48]

Hand injuries generally heal within 3 to 12 weeks. Stiffness after injury and immobilization must be treated with an aggressive therapy program, which may include intermittent use of protective splints, casts, or taping.

The rehabilitation program must consider the specific characteristics of the injury, age of the patient, sport played, and level of competition at which the individual plays. In general, the rehabilitation program should include restoration of motion, strength, power, and endurance.[72] Early active range of motion is preferred over passive motion. Active assisted range of motion is started when the soft-tissue healing allows it and when a reasonable passive range of motion is present. Dynamic splints are used when indicated to maintain joint motion and to relieve joint contractures. After pain-free motion has been restored, progressive resistive exercises are started and progressively increased. A weight program with low weights and high repetitions is used to increase endurance. Sport-specific exercises also are used.

SUMMARY

The fingers and hand can suffer a spectrum of soft-tissue and bony injuries as a result of athletic activities. These injuries must be properly diagnosed and appropriately treated, and the hand must be restored to good function with a comprehensive rehabilitation program. All this is done expeditiously to allow a rapid return to athletic competition and without compromising medical treatment of the injury or hand function.

References

1. Ali MS: Complete disruption of the collateral mechanism of proximal interphalangeal joints of fingers, *J Hand Surg* 9B:191-193, 1984.
2. Amadio PC et al: Fractures of the hand and wrist. In Jupiter JB, editor: *Flynn's hand surgery,* ed 4, Baltimore, 1991, Williams & Wilkins, pp 122-185.
3. Baldwin LW et al: Metacarpophalangeal joint dislocations of the fingers, *J Bone Joint Surg* 49A:1587-1590, 1967.
4. Barenfeld PA, Weseley MS: Dorsal dislocation of the metacarpophalangeal joint of the index finger treated by late open reduction, *J Bone Joint Surg* 54A:1311-1313, 1972.
5. Barton NJ: Fractures of the hand, *J Bone Joint Surg* 66-B:159-167, 1984.
6. Becton J, Christian JD, Jackson JC: A simplified technique for treating the complex dislocation of the index metacarpophalangeal joint, *J Bone Joint Surg* 57A:698-700, 1975.
7. Belsky MR, Eaton RG, Lane LB: Closed reduction and internal fixation of proximal phalangeal fractures, *J Hand Surg* 9A:725-729, 1984.
8. Belsole R: Physiological fixation of displaced and unstable fractures of the hand, *Orthop Clin North Am* 11:393-404, 1980.
9. Bennett EH: Fractures of the metacarpal bones, *Dublin J Med Sci* 73:72-75, 1882.
10. Bennett EH: On fractures of the metacarpal bone of the thumb, *Br Med J* 11:12-13, 1886.
11. Billing L, Gedda KO: Roentgen examination of Bennett's fracture, *Acta Radiol* 38:471-476, 1952.
12. Bohart PG et al: Complex dislocations of the metacarpo-phalangeal joint, *Clin Orthop* 164:208-210, 1982.
13. Bora FW Jr, Didizian NH: The treatment of injuries to the carpometacarpal joint of the little finger, *J Bone Joint Surg* 56A:1459-1463, 1974.
14. Bowers WH et al: The proximal interphalangeal joint volar plate. I. An anatomical and biomechanical study, *J Hand Surg* 5:79-88, 1980.
15. Breed JC et al: Free tendon grafting to repair the metacarpo-phalangeal joint of the thumb: surgical technique and a review of 70 patients, *J Bone Joint Surg* 71B:383-387, 1989.
16. Breeu TF, Gelberman RH, Jupiter JB: Intra-articular fractures of the basilar joint of the thumb, *Hand Clin* 4:491-501, 1988.
17. Brewerton DA: A tangential radiographic projection for demonstrating involvement of metacarpal heads in rheumatoid arthritis, *Br J Radiol* 40:233, 1967.
18. Brunet ME, Haddad RJ Jr: Fractures and dislocations of the metacarpals and phalanges, *Clin Sports Med* 5:773-781, 1986.
19. Burton RI, Eaton RG: Common hand injuries in the athlete, *Orthop Clin North Am* 4:809-838, 1973.
20. Cannon SR et al: A long-term study following Bennett's fracture, *J Hand Surg* 11B:426-431, 1986.
21. Carr D, Johnson RJ, Pope MH: Upper extremity injuries in skiing, *Am J Sports Med* 9:378-383, 1981.
22. Cooney WP et al: The kinesiology of the thumb metacarpotrapezial joint, *J Bone Joint Surg* 63A:1371-1381, 1981.
23. Crawford GP: Screw fixation for certain fractures of the phalanges and metacarpal, *J Bone Joint Surg* 58A:487-492, 1976.
24. Curtis RM: Treatment of injuries of the proximal interphalangeal joints of the fingers, *Curr Pract Orthop Surg* 2:125-135, 1964.
25. Daffner RH, Pavlov H: Stress fractures: current concepts, *Am J Radiol* 159:245, 1992.

26. Dewaker HN, Stothard J: The role of internal fixation in closed fractures of the proximal phalanges and metacarpals in adults, *J Hand Surg* 11B:103-108, 1986.
27. Dobyns JH, Sim FS, Linscheid RL: Sports stress syndrome of the hand and wrist, *Am J Sports Med* 6:236-254, 1978.
28. Dommisse IG, Lloyd GJ: Injuries of the fifth carpo-metacarpal region, *Can J Surg* 22:240-245, 1979.
29. Dray G, Millender LH, Nalebuff EA: Rupture of the radial collateral ligament of a metacarpo-phalangeal joint to one of the ulnar three fingers, *J Hand Surg* 4:346-350, 1979.
30. Dray GJ, Eaton RG: Dislocations and ligament injuries in the digits. In Green DP, editor: *Operative hand surgery,* ed 3, New York, 1993, Churchill Livingstone.
31. Duham JW, Khuri S, Kim MH: Acute and late radial collateral ligament injuries of the thumb metacarpo-phalangeal joint, *J Hand Surg* 18A:232-237, 1993.
32. Eaton RG: *Joint injuries of the hand,* Springfield, Ill, 1971, Charles C Thomas, pp 3-34.
33. Eaton RG, Littler JW: Joint injuries and their sequelae, *Clin Plast Surg* 3:85-98, 1976.
34. Eaton RG, Malerich MM: Volar plate arthroplasty of the proximal interphalangeal joint: a review of 10 years experience, *J Hand Surg* 5:260-268, 1980.
35. Eichenholtz SN, Rizzo PC: Fracture of the neck of the fifth metacarpal bone—is over-treatment justified? *JAMA* 178:151-152, 1961.
36. Ellsasser JC, Stein AH: Management of hand injuries in a professional football team, *Am J Sports Med* 7:178-182, 1979.
37. Flatt AE: Fracture-dislocation of an index metacarpo-phalangeal joint and an ulnar deviating force in the flexor tendons, *J Bone Joint Surg* 48A:100-104, 1966.
38. Foster RJ, Hastings H II: Treatment of Bennett, Rolando and vertical intra-articular trapezial fractures, *Clin Orthop* 214:121-129, 1987.
39. Frank WE, Dobyns JH: Surgical pathology of collateral ligament injuries of the thumb, *Clin Orthop* 83:102-114, 1972.
40. Freeland AE, Jabaley ME, Hughes JL: *Stable fixation of the hand and wrist,* New York, 1986, Springer-Verlag.
41. Frykman G, Johansson O: Surgical repair of rupture of the ulnar collateral ligament of the metacarpo-phalangeal joint of the thumb, *Acta Chir Scand* 112:58-64, 1956.
42. Gedda KO, Moberg E: Open reduction and osteosynthesis of the so-called Bennett's fracture in the carpo-metacarpal joint of the thumb, *Acta Orthop Scand* 22:249-257, 1953.
43. Gee TC, Pho RWH: Avulsion-fracture at the proximal attachment of the radial collateral ligament of the fifth metacarpo-phalangeal joint—a case report, *J Hand Surg* 7:526-527, 1982.
44. Gerber C, Senn Edgar, Matter P: Skier's thumb, *Am J Sports Med* 9:171-177, 1981.
45. Green DP, Anderson JR: Closed reduction and percutaneous pin fixation of fractured phalanges, *J Bone Joint Surg* 55-A:1651-1654, 1973.
46. Green DP: Complications of phalangeal and metacarpal fractures, *Hand Clin* 2:307-328, 1986.
47. Green SM, Posner MA: Irreducible dorsal dislocation of the proximal interphalangeal joint, *J Hand Surg* 10A:85-87, 1985.
48. Hankin FM, Peel SM: Sports-related fractures and dislocations in the hand, *Hand Clin* 6:429-453, 1990.
49. Hastings H II, Carroll C IV: Closed articular fractures of the metacarpo-phalangeal and proximal interphalangeal joints, *Hand Clin* 4:503-527, 1988.
50. Heim V, Pfeifer KM, Mueli HD: *Small fragment set manual. Technique recommended by ASIF Group (Swiss Association for Study of Internal Fixation),* New York, 1974, Springer-Verlag.
51. Heim V, Pfeifer KM: *Internal fixation of small fragments,* ed 3, New York, 1988, Springer-Verlag.
52. Hubbard LF: Metacarpo-phalangeal dislocations, *Hand Clin* 4:39-44, 1988.
53. Hunter JM, Cowen NJ: Fifth metacarpal fractures in a compensation clinic population: a report on one hundred and thirty three cases, *J Bone Joint Surg* 52A:1159-1165, 1970.
54. Jahss SA: Fractures of the metacarpals: a new method of reduction and immobilization, *J Bone Joint Surg* 20:178-186, 1938.
55. James JIP: Fractures of the proximal and middle phalanges of the fingers, *Acta Orthop Scand* 32:401-412, 1962.
56. Jones WW: Biomechanics of small bone fixation, *Clin Orthop* 214:11-18, 1987.
57. Jupiter JB, Silva MA: Fractures of the metacarpal and phalanges. In Chapman MW, editor: *Operative orthopaedics,* Philadelphia, 1988, JB Lippincott, pp 1235-1250.
58. Jupiter JB, Belsky MR: Fractures and dislocations of the hand in skeletal trauma. In Browner BD et al, editors: *Skeletal trauma*, Philadelphia, 1992, WB Saunders, pp 925-1024.
59. Kaplan EB: Extension deformities of the proximal interphalangeal joints of the fingers, *J Bone Joint Surg* 18A:781-783, 1939.
60. Kaplan EM: Dorsal dislocation of the metacarpo-phalangeal joint of the index finger, *J Bone Joint Surg* 39A:1081-1086, 1957.
61. Ker HR: Dislocation of the fifth carpo-metacarpal joint, *J Bone Joint Surg* 37B:254, 1955.
62. Kilbourne BC: Management of complicated hand fractures, *Surg Clin North Am* 48:201-213, 1968.
63. Kuczynski K: The proximal interphalangeal joint: anatomy and causes of stiffness of the fingers, *J Bone Joint Surg* 50B:656-663, 1968.
64. Lampier TA: Improper reduction of fractures of the proximal phalanges of fingers, *Am J Surg* 94:926-930, 1957.
65. Lane CS: Detecting occult fractures of the metacarpal head: the Brewerton view, *J Hand Surg* 2:131-133, 1977.
66. Lasserre C, Pauzat O, Dereunes R: Osteoarthritis of trapezio-metacarpal joint, *J Bone Joint Surg* 31B:534-536, 1949.
67. Lawless JF III, Gunther SF: Carpo-metacarpal dislocations, *J Bone Joint Surg* 73A:52-58, 1991.
68. Livesley PJ: The conservative management of Bennett's fracture-dislocation: a 26 year follow-up, *J Hand Surg* 15B:291-294, 1990.
69. Lowden IMR: Fracture of the metacarpal neck of the little finger, *Injury* 17:189-192, 1986.
70. Lubahn JD: Dorsal fracture dislocations of the proximal interphalangeal joint, *Hand Clin* 4:15-24, 1988.
71. McCue FC et al: Athletic injuries of the proximal interphalangeal joint requiring surgical treatment, *J Bone Joint Surg* 52A:937-956, 1970.
72. McCue FC III, Mayer V: Rehabilitation of common athletic injuries of the hand and wrist, *Clin Sports Med* 8:731-776, 1989.
73. McElfresh ED et al: Management of fracture dislocations of the proximal interphalangeal joint by extension block splinting, *J Bone Joint Surg* 54A:1705-1711, 1972.
74. McElfresh EC, Dobyns JH: Intra-articular metacarpal head fractures, *J Hand Surg* 8:383-393, 1983.
75. Margles SW: Intra-articular fractures of the metacarpo-phalangeal and proximal interphalangeal joints, *Hand Clin* 4:67-74, 1988.
76. Melone CP Jr: Rigid fixation of phalangeal and metacarpal fractures, *Orthop Clin North Am* 17:421-435, 1986.
77. Moberg E, Stener B: Injuries of the ligaments of the thumb and fingers: diagnosis, treatment and prognosis, *Acta Chir Scand* 106:166-186, 1953.
78. Morgan JV, Davis PH: Upper extremity injuries in skiing, *Clin Sports Med* 1:295-308, 1982.
79. Murphy AF, Stark HH: Closed dislocation of the metacarpo-phalangeal joint of the index finger, *J Bone Joint Surg* 49A:1579-1586, 1967.
80. O'Brien ET: Fractures of the metacarpals and phalanges. In Green DP, editor: *Operative hand surgery,* New York, 1988, Churchill Livingstone.
81. Oni OOA, Mackenny RP: Multiple dislocations of the carpo-metacarpal joints, *J Hand Surg* 11B:47-48, 1986.

82. Opgrande JD, Westphal SA: Fractures of the hand, *Orthop Clin North Am* 14:779-792, 1983.
83. O'Rourke SK, Gaur S, Barton NJ: Long-term outcome of articular fractures of the phalanges: an eleven year follow-up, *J Hand Surg* 14B:183-193, 1989.
84. Palmer AK, Linscheid RL: Chronic recurrent dislocation of the proximal interphalangeal joint of the finger, *J Hand Surg* 3:95-97, 1978.
85. Pellegrini VD Jr: Fractures at the base of the thumb, *Hand Clin* 4:87-102, 1988.
86. Posner MA: Injuries to the hand and wrist in athletes, *Orthop Clin North Am* 8:593-618, 1977.
87. Posner MA, Retaillaud JL: Metacarpo-phalangeal joint injuries of the thumb, *Hand Clin* 8:713-732, 1992.
88. Pun WK et al: A prospective study on 284 digital fractures of the hand, *J Hand Surg* 14A:474-481, 1989.
89. Rettig AC, Ryan RD, Stone JA: Epidemiology of hand injuries in sports. In Strickland JW, Rettig AC, editors: *Hand injuries in athletes,* Philadelphia, 1992, WB Saunders.
90. Rawles JG Jr: Dislocations and fracture-dislocations at the carpometacarpal joints of the fingers, *Hand Clin* 4:103-112, 1988.
91. Rodriquez AL: Injuries to the collateral ligaments of the proximal interphalangeal joints, *Hand* 5:55-57, 1973.
92. Rolando S: Fracture de la base du premier metacarpien, et principalement sur une variete non encore decrite, *Presse Med* 33:303, 1910.
93. Ruldi TP, Burri C, Pfeiffer KM: Stable internal fixation of fractures of the hand, *J Trauma* 11:381-389, 1971.
94. Salter RB, Harris WR: Injuries involving the epiphyseal plate, *J Bone Joint Surg* 45A:58B-622, 1963.
95. Schneider LH: Fractures of the distal phalanx, *Hand Clin* 4:537-547, 1988.
96. Simonetta C: The use of AO plates in the hand, *Hand* 2:243-245, 1970.
97. Smith RJ: Post-traumatic instability of the metacarpo-phalangeal joint of the thumb, *J Bone Joint Surg* 59A:14-21, 1977.
98. Smith RJ, Peimer CA: Injuries to the metacarpal bones and joints, *Adv Surg* 2:341-374, 1977.
99. Stark HH, Boyes JH, Wilson JN: Mallet finger, *J Bone Joint Surg* 44A:1061, 1962.
100. Stark H et al: Fusion of the first metacarpo-trapezial joint for degenerative arthritis, *J Bone Joint Surg* 59A:22-26, 1977.
101. Stark HH et al: Operative treatment of intra-articular fractures of the dorsal aspect of the distal phalanx of digits, *J Bone Joint Surg* 69:892-896, 1987.
102. Steel WM: The AO small fragment set in hand fractures, *Hand* 10:246-253, 1978.
103. Stener B: Hyperextension injuries to the metacarpo-phalangeal joint of the thumb—rupture of ligaments, fracture of the sesamoid bones, rupture of the flexor pollicis brevis: anatomical and clinical study, *Acta Chir Scand* 125:275-293, 1963.
104. Stener B: Displacement of the ruptured ulnar collateral ligament of the metacarpo-phalangeal joint of the thumb: a clinical and anatomical study, *J Bone Joint Surg* 44B:869-879, 1969.
105. Stern PJ: Fractures of the metacarpals and phalanges. In Green DP, editor: *Operative hand surgery,* New York, 1993, Churchill Livingstone.
106. Strauss RH, Lanese RR: Injuries among wrestlers in school and college tournaments, *JAMA* 248:2016-2019, 1982.
107. Strickland JW et al: Phalangeal factors: factors influencing digital performance, *Orthop Rev* 11:39-50, 1982.
108. Tapper EM: Ski injuries from 1939 to 1976: the Sun Valley experience, *Am J Sports Med* 6:114-121, 1978.
109. Thompson JS, Eaton RG: Volar dislocation of the proximal interphalangeal joint, *J Hand Surg* 2:232, 1977.
110. Von Saal FH: Intramedullary fixation in fractures of the hand and fingers, *J Bone Joint Surg* 35A:5-16, 1953.
111. Wehbe MA, Schneider LH: Mallet fractures, *J Bone Joint Surg* 66-A:658-669, 1984.
112. Wilson JN, Rowland SA: Fracture-dislocation of the proximal interphalangeal joint of the finger, *J Bone Joint Surg* 48A:493-502, 1966.
113. Wright TA: Early mobilization in fractures of the metacarpals and phalanges, *Can J Surg* 11:491-498, 1968.
114. Zemel NP et al: Chronic fracture dislocation of the proximal interphalangeal joint—treatment by osteotomy and bone graft, *J Hand Surg* 6:447-455, 1981.
115. Zemel NP, Stark HH: Problem fractures and dislocations of the hand. In: *AAOS instructional course lectures,* vol 37, Park Ridge, Ill, 1988, American Academy of Orthopaedic Surgeons.

CHAPTER 28

Neurovascular Disorders

NORMAN P. ZEMEL

During athletic competition, the cervical spine, spinal nerves, and brachial plexus can be injured, producing symptoms of burning, weakness, pain, and loss of function in the upper extremity. However, similar complaints can result from neurovascular or musculotendinous lesions originating in the extremity.

Neurovascular abnormalities in the upper extremity can occur anywhere along the pathway of the nerve or vessel. The peripheral nerves and vessels pass beneath muscles or fascial tunnels in their course from the neck to the tip of the digits. Certain sites are more prone to injury, usually by compression, and a knowledge of the anatomy is useful in localizing, evaluating, and diagnosing these injuries. A detailed examination of the extremity, including various diagnostic tests, will assist the physician in determining the exact diagnosis and thus provide the proper treatment.

Stress placed on the hand, wrist, and forearm of athletes as a result of repeated blunt trauma, sustained forceful gripping, and stretching during the various postures of the extremity while playing can lead to neurovascular abnormalities. However, neurovascular disorders in the upper extremity of athletes are uncommon when compared with musculoskeletal injuries. Injuries to the nerves and vessels of the upper extremity in an athlete are predominantly closed injuries.

NEUROLOGIC DISORDERS

Neurologic problems in the upper extremity of athletes are infrequent when compared with injuries of bone, muscles, tendons, and ligaments.[25] When these injuries occur, they are generally the result of blunt trauma, repetitive overuse, stretching, or repetitive forceful gripping. These neurovascular injuries rarely are due to open wounds.[34] Most nerve abnormalities in the upper extremity are compressive neuropathies or entrapment syndromes. Generally, the extent of the injury to the

TABLE 28-1
Nerve Injury

Seddon	Sunderland
Neurapraxia	First-degree nerve injury
Axonotmesis	Second-degree nerve injury
	Third-degree nerve injury
Neurotmesis	Fourth-degree nerve injury
	Fifth-degree nerve injury

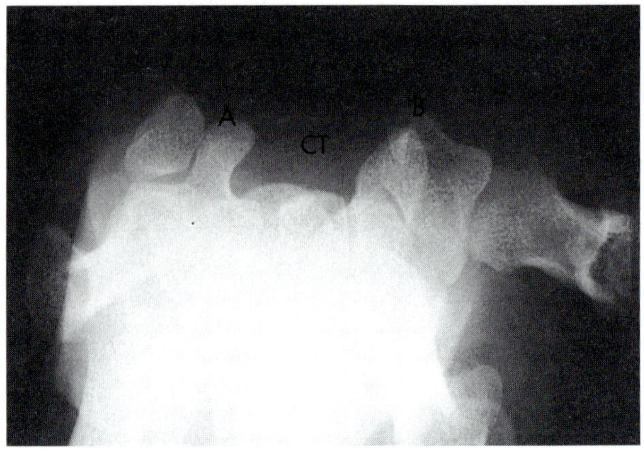

FIGURE 28-1 A radiograph showing the carpal tunnel. The bony borders of the tunnel are the hook of the hamate *(A)* and the tubercle of the trapezium *(B)*.

nerve is a neurapraxia (Seddon) or first-degree nerve injury (Sunderland).[38] Table 28-1 compares the Seddon and Sunderland classification of nerve injury. A neurapraxia, the least severe type of injury to the nerve, is characterized by transient loss of nerve function with no disruption of the integrity of the nerve fibers or sheath. Fortunately, these nerves usually recover, although the process can take weeks to months.

Axonotmesis is the next level of injury. This indicates a loss of axonal continuity at the lesion site; however, the endoneural tubes remain intact. This lesion usually is found in an advanced nerve compression injury or a crush or traction injury. Although these lesions also can resolve, the time for recovery depends on the time required for the axons to regenerate and pass through the endoneural tubes. Neurotmesis indicates complete severance of the nerve or destruction of the perineurium and endoneural tubes so that the internal anatomy of the nerve trunk is disorganized at the site of injury. Spontaneous regeneration usually does not occur, and surgery often is required.

The exact pathophysiologic changes associated with compressive neuropathies still are not clear. Theories of nerve compression include anoxia caused by venous obstruction within the nerve and a mechanical lesion that causes local structural changes to the myelin sheath.[41] These lesions, if left untreated, cause progressive damage to the nerve. The peripheral fibers tend to be involved initially while the central fibers are preserved. If the compression continues, the central fibers also become involved.[12,47] Depending on the forces and the extent of injury, the damage to the nerve can include a combination of neurapraxia, axonotmesis, and neurotmesis.

Evaluation

A detailed history and physical examination of the patient are critical in establishing whether the injury involves a peripheral nerve or vessel and where the lesion is located. In general, the clinician should perform both motor and sensory evaluations of the upper extremity and compare the results with the contralateral side when testing nerve function. Motor function is tested for both its presence and power. Sensibility can be tested by pinprick, Semmes-Weinstein nylon filaments, and two-point discrimination (static and moving).[3] In a study of controlled external compression of the median nerve, Semmes-Weinstein and vibration testing (threshold tests) reflected the decreases in nerve function, but innervation and density tests (two-point discrimination and moving two-point discrimination) remained normal until almost all sensory conduction of the nerve ceased.[19] Loss of sensibility usually precedes loss of motor function in a compressive neuropathy.

When evaluating peripheral nerve injuries or nerve compression, the clinician must include an electromyogram and a nerve conduction study in the diagnostic evaluation of the injured athlete. These studies are important in localizing the lesion and also help to objectively quantify the neuropathy. These studies evaluate the neurophysiologic integrity of the entire lower motor neuron.[42] Nerve conduction studies, both motor and sensory, measure the conduction time (latency) between any two points along the course of the nerve. Dividing the surface distance of these two points by the latency allows one to calculate the conduction velocity, or the speed at which a nerve impulse is traveling. A focal slowing of the conduction velocity (distal latency) identifies a localized nerve compression or injury.

Needle electromyography identifies denervation in muscles supplied by specific peripheral nerves. This test also differentiates a localized peripheral lesion from a more proximal lesion in either the brachial plexus or cervical nerve root. It is extremely important to always evaluate the paraspinal muscles when testing for a peripheral nerve disorder.

Imaging techniques can help determine whether a peripheral nerve is a cause of upper-extremity pain or numbness. Posterior-anterior, lateral, or oblique roentgenograms should be taken to evaluate the bony architecture and joints in the area being investigated. This is particularly useful in evaluating the cubital tunnel and carpal tunnel (Fig. 28-1). If an abnormality is noted, additional information often can be obtained with a CT scan. MRI often can provide useful information about the nerve itself.

Systemic diseases such as thyroid disorders and diabetes mellitus also should be considered in the overall evaluation of the athlete.[32]

PERIPHERAL NERVE INJURY

Lacerations

Nerves in the upper extremity rarely are lacerated during sporting activities. Nerves usually are injured by blunt trauma, repeated stretching, or compression.

COMPRESSION NEUROPATHIES

Superficial Radial Nerve

The superficial branch of the radial nerve passes deep to the brachioradialis muscle and emerges on the ulnar side of the brachioradialis tendon in the distal third of the forearm. It is a sensory nerve and supplies the radial and dorsoradial skin of the forearm and wrist, dorsum of the thumb web, and dorsum of the proximal segments of the thumb, index, and sometimes the middle fingers.

An isolated entrapment of the superficial radial nerve (cheiralgia paresthetica, Wartenberg's syndrome) can occur in the distal third of the forearm as the nerve emerges from beneath the brachioradialis tendon (Fig. 28-2). In athletes, this usually is caused by blunt trauma or repeated rotation of the forearm. With the forearm pronated, the extensor carpi radialis longus tendon crosses beneath the brachioradialis tendon and thus can repetitively pinch or compress the superficial branch of the radial nerve. Burning or pain usually is present in the distribution of the superficial radial nerve, and there is tenderness or tingling over the nerve in the distal third of the forearm.[13,18]

A diagnostic nerve block using local anesthesia can help verify the diagnosis.

If a trial of conservative treatment, including splinting, rest, therapy, and antiinflammatory medications, is unsuccessful, then surgical decompression of the nerve should be performed.

A longitudinal incision is made over the midportion of the forearm on the dorsal radial aspect, centered over the site of maximum tingling of the nerve. The superficial radial nerve is identified as it emerges between the tendons of the extensor carpi radialis longus and the brachioradialis. The fascia is released for 5 to 6 cm, competely releasing the nerve. Care must be taken not to injure the nerve as it branches distally.

This condition must be differentiated from a lesion of the more proximal radial nerve and from de Quervain's tenosynovitis.

A
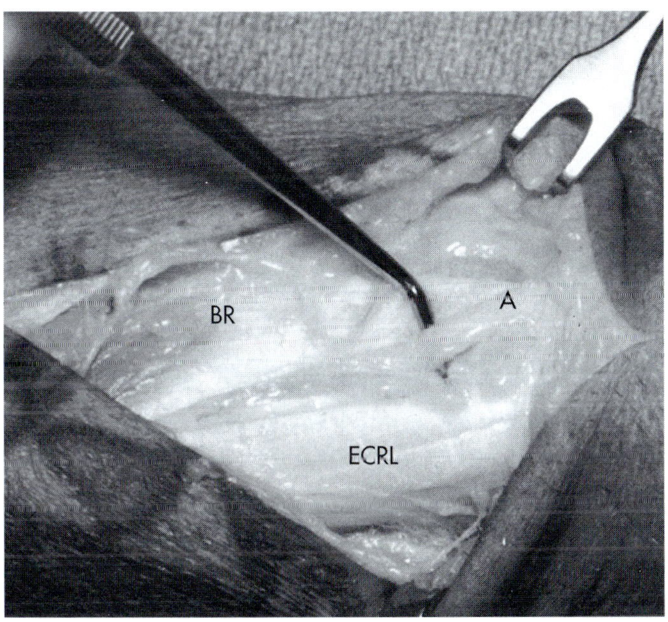

B
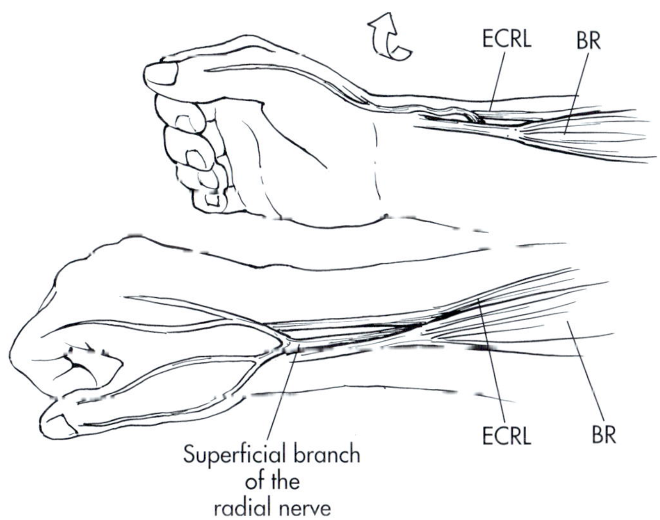

FIGURE 28-2 **A,** Compression of the superficial branch of the radial nerve in the forearm (Wartenberg's syndrome). *A,* Superficial radial nerve; *BR,* brachioradialis; *ECRL,* extensor carpi radialis longus. **B,** Schematic showing forearm rotation compressing the superficial radial nerve.

Distal Posterior Interosseous Nerve

The posterior interosseous nerve that innervates the deep extensor muscles has a lateral branch that continues along the posterior radial border of the radius to the wrist as the sensory branch of the posterior interosseous nerve. This nerve branch can be injured by repeated dorsiflexion motions of the wrist. The patients will present with pain over the dorsum of the wrist that is aggravated by forced wrist dorsiflexion. Tenderness also is noted over the dorsum of the wrist, and this tenderness is aggravated by wrist flexion. Xylocaine injected 3 cm proximal and 1 cm ulnar to Lister's tubercle usually will eliminate the patient's complaints and act as a diagnostic test.[8] If the complaints do not subside after extended conservative treatment, the terminal portion of the posterior interosseous nerve is transected, and a segment is removed. Operative findings have shown an enlarged nerve as it crosses the wrist, associated with perineural fibrosis. This entity has been called the *distal posterior interosseous nerve syndrome.*[8]

Median Nerve

Disorders of the median nerve in the athlete usually result from repetitive activity. This activity can cause compression of the nerve by hypertrophy of normal or abnormal muscles, by fascial thickening, or by flexor tenosynovitis. The two most common sites of compression of the median nerve are the proximal forearm and the wrist.

Carpal Tunnel Syndrome

Although compression of the median nerve at the wrist (carpal tunnel syndrome) is fairly common in the general population, it is relatively uncommon as a sports-related injury. In athletic activities, carpal tunnel syndrome results from forceful repetitive gripping, throwing, or any activity that involves repetitive flexion and extension of the wrist.[31,34]

The carpal canal is formed by the volar wrist capsule and carpal bones on the floor or dorsal aspect, and the roof is formed by the tranverse carpal ligament, which extends from the tubercle of the trapezium and the tuberosity of the scaphoid to the hook of the hamate and the pisiform. The median nerve passes through the carpal canal with the eight flexor profundus and superficialis tendons, as well as the flexor pollicis longus tendon.

The median nerve gives off a motor branch, usually from its radial side but occasionally from the ulnar side. The motor branch usually leaves the main trunk within the carpal canal or immediately after the nerve exits from the canal (Fig. 28-3). Beyond the distal edge of the transverse carpal ligament, the median nerve branches into common digital branches, which pass to the radial and ulnar side of the index finger, the radial and unlar side of the middle finger, and the radial side of the ring finger (Fig. 28-4).

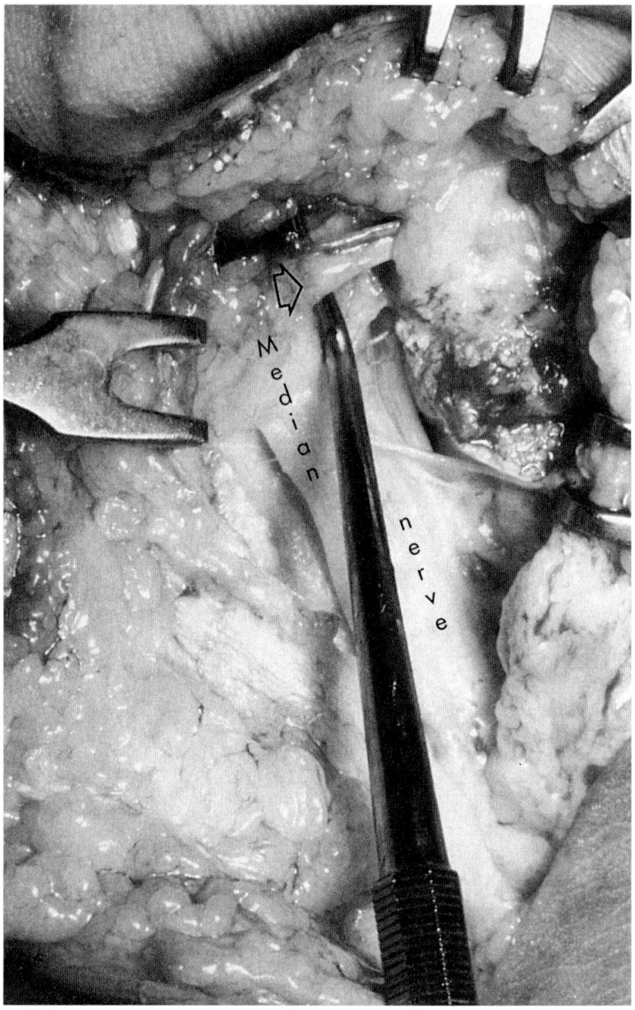

FIGURE 28-3 The motor nerve (thenar) *(arrow)* as it branches from the radial side of the median nerve.

Based on 246 hands in which the carpal tunnel was explored at surgery, Lanz described the anatomic variations of the median nerve in the carpal canal.[30] In about 50% of the cases, the motor branch of the median nerve was extraligamentous. Based on his study of the branching of the nerve, Lanz reiterated the importance of approaching the median nerve from the ulnar side when releasing it from the carpal tunnel.

Gelberman et al[20] showed that the pressure within the carpal canal in normal subjects rose tenfold with acute flexion and extension of the wrist. In patients with carpal tunnel syndrome, the pressure was three times greater than when the measurements were taken at neutral.

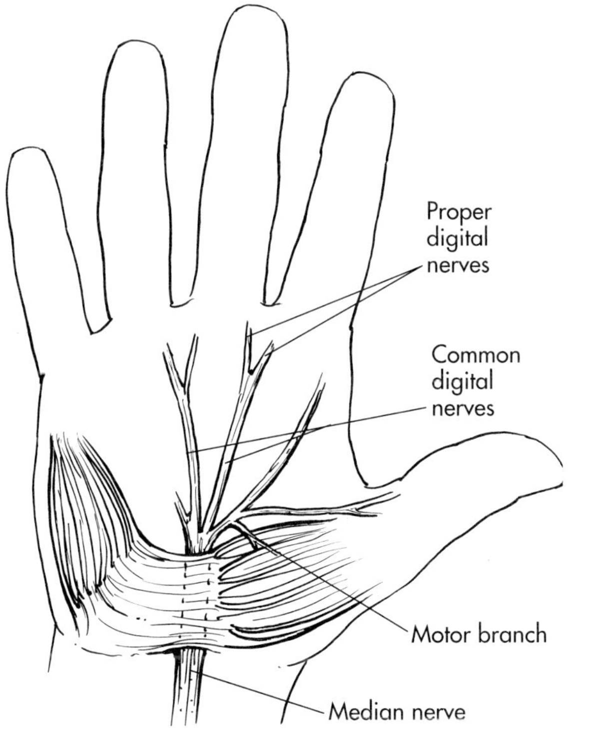

FIGURE 28-4 After it leaves the carpal tunnel, the median nerve branches into its motor and sensory components.

Typical complaints are numbness and tingling in the thumb, index finger, and middle and radial half of the ring finger, night pain or numbness in the wrist and fingers, and exertional activity either aggravating or initiating these complaints. Occasionally pain is referred proximally to the shoulder.[29]

Phalen's test (wrist flexion test) (Fig. 28-5) and percussion of the median nerve at the wrist (Tinel's sign) are important physical findings that help to localize the compression of the median nerve to the wrist.[39] Sensibility testing will show decreased sensation in the thumb, index finger, and middle finger when compared with the sensation in the small finger, which is innervated by the ulnar nerve. This allows the patient to appreciate the difference during the test. Thenar atrophy is a late finding (Fig. 28-6).

Routine roentgenograms should include three views of the wrist and a carpal tunnel view to rule out bony abnormality in the carpal canal. An MRI of the wrist also may provide useful information about the median nerve or flexor tendons within the canal, but this test should not be performed routinely.

Electromyography and nerve conduction studies are extremely valuable in confirming the diagnosis of carpal tunnel syndrome. These tests help to localize the lesion at the wrist as well as to determine the severity of nerve compression. Although these tests have a 10% incidence of false-negative findings, especially during the early stages of nerve compression,[53] one can overcome this by stressing the upper extremity to recreate the symptoms and then retesting the individual.

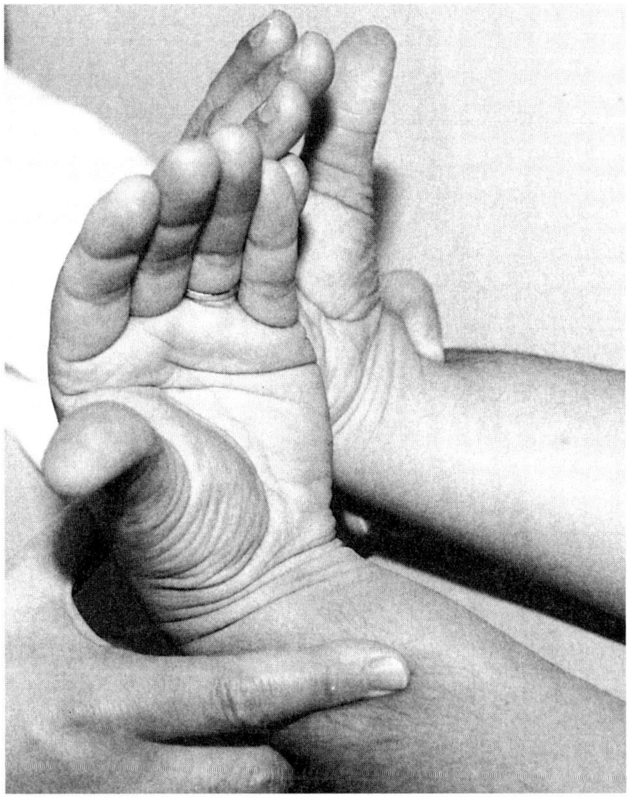

FIGURE 28-5 The wrist flexion test (Phalen test). Performing the test on both wrists simultanenously gives the patient a reference against which the abnormal extremity can be compared.

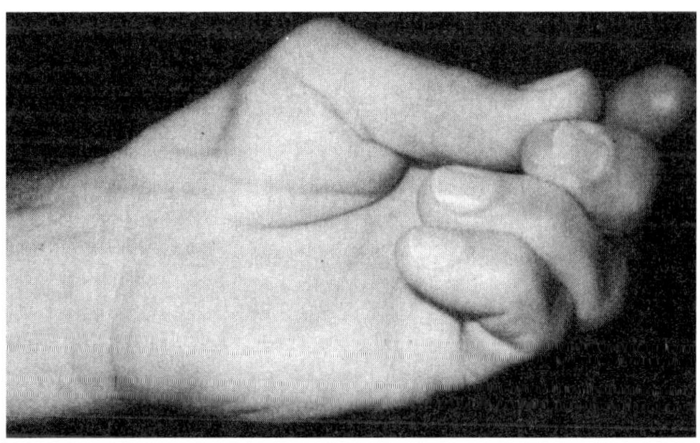

FIGURE 28-6 Thenar atrophy usually indicates a long-standing compression neuropathy of the median nerve.

The initial treatment of carpal tunnel syndrome in the athlete is conservative. A program of splinting both during the day and at night often is useful in relieving the patient's complaints. If there is significant synovial swelling, the application of ice also is useful. In addition,

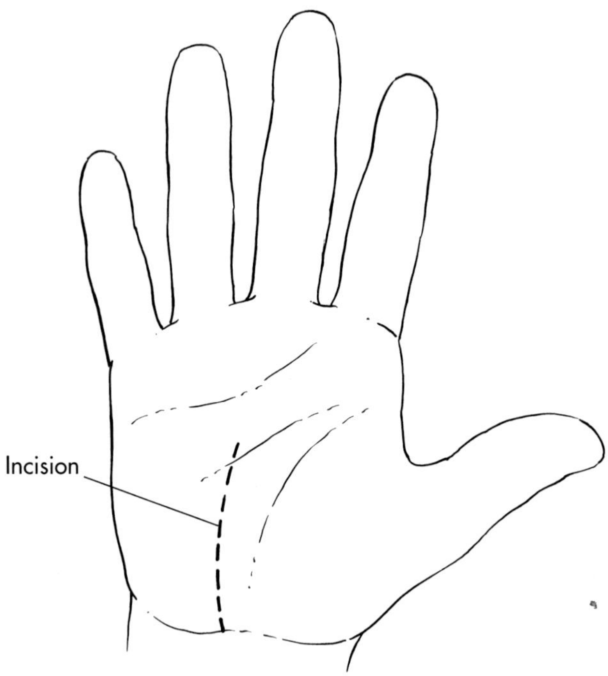

FIGURE 28-7 For an open carpal tunnel release, the incision is located toward the ulnar side of the palm in line with the fourth metacarpal. One usually need not cross the wrist crease.

antiinflammatory medication may be used to reduce the synovitis within the carpal canal. If these modalities do not provide significant and timely relief, one can inject the carpal tunnel with Xylocaine and a water-soluble steroid.[21]

In cases resistant to conservative treatment, surgical decompression of the median nerve at the wrist is indicated. During an open release, the palm is opened through a curved interthenar incision (Fig. 28-7). Skin flaps are elevated, and the hook of the hamate is identified, which locates the most ulnar aspect of the carpal canal. The transverse carpal ligament then is incised just radial to the hook of the hamate. By elevating the skin at the wrist flexion crease, the surgeon can release the transverse retinacular ligament and the distal edge of the antebrachial fascia without extending the skin incision across the wrist flexion crease. The entire ligament must release to ensure complete relief of the patient's symptoms (Fig. 28-8); however, the surgeon need not routinely perform a flexor tenosynovectomy or internal neurolysis of the median nerve.

An alternative approach is an endoscopic release of the median nerve at the wrist. A two-portal[9,43] and a single-portal technique have been described.[1] The one-portal technique is useful for the idiopathic carpal tunnel

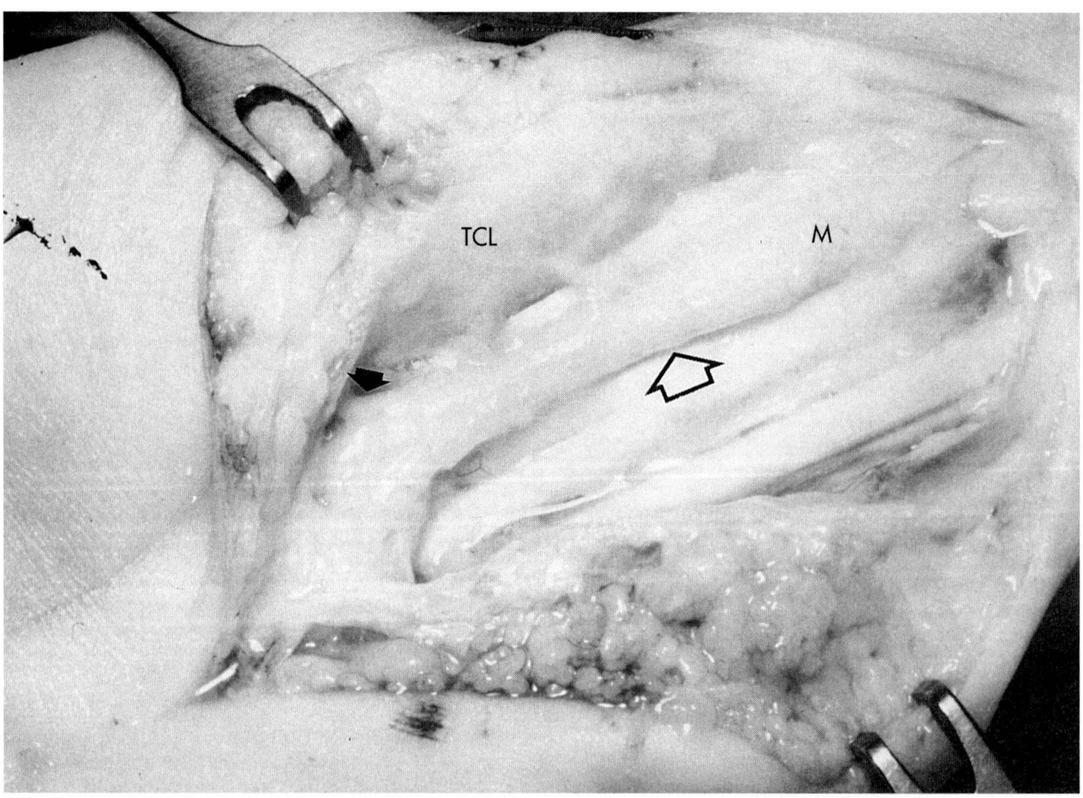

FIGURE 28-8 The median nerve can be constricted in a long-standing carpal tunnel syndrome. This is a right hand. *TCL,* Transverse carpal ligament; *dark arrow,* motor branch; *light arrow,* constriction in the median nerve; *M,* median nerve.

syndrome, but is not recommended when there is extensive flexor tenosynovitis, the patient has had a prior carpal tunnel release, or a mass or bony fragments are present within the carpal canal.

The wrist is opened through a transverse incision at the wrist flexion crease, extending from the palmaris longus tendon to the flexor carpi ulnaris tendon (Fig. 28-9). A U-shaped distally based fascial flap is elevated, and the distal edge of the proximal forearm fascia is incised. The median nerve is elevated from the volar aspect of

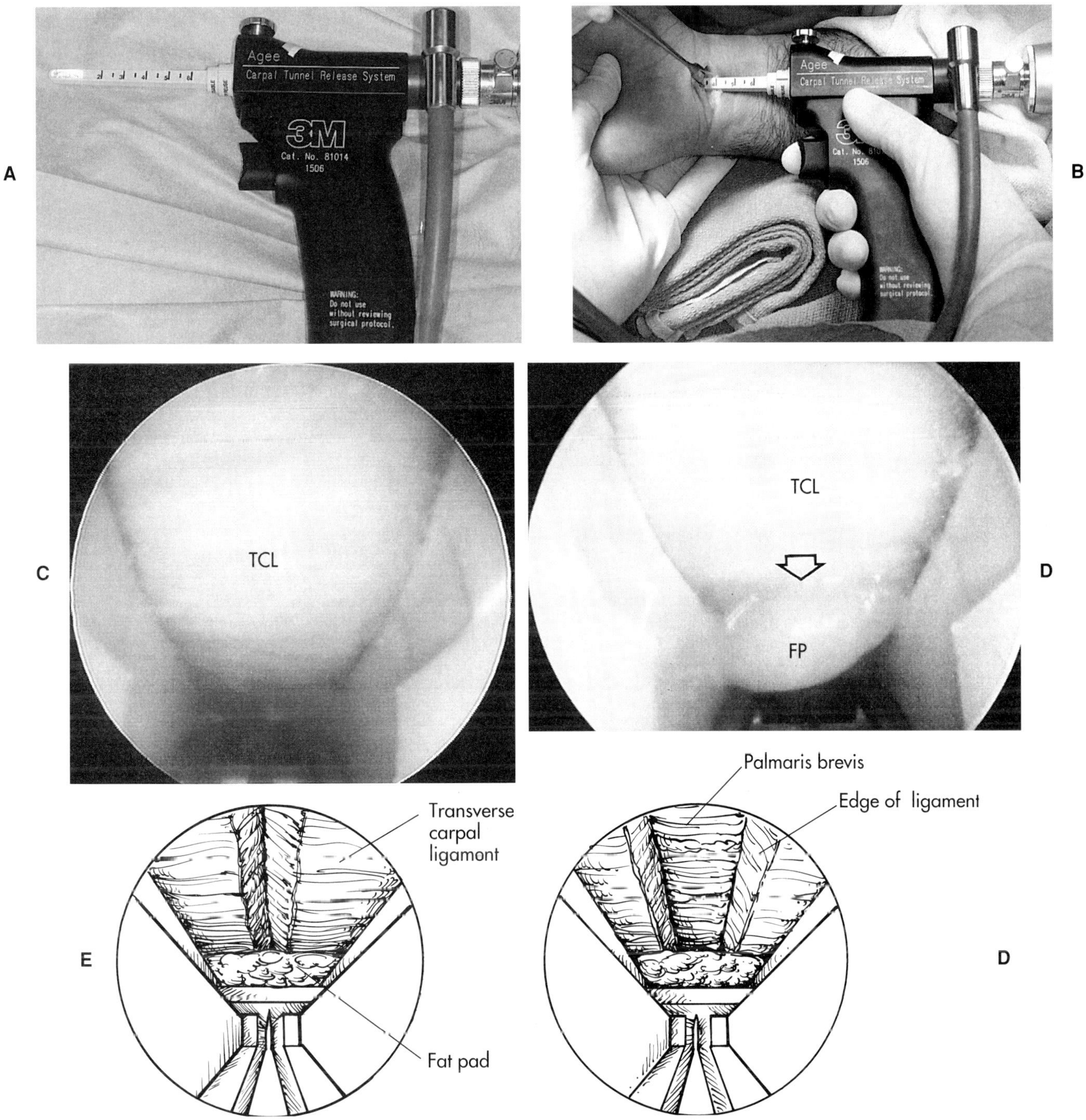

FIGURE 28-9 **A,** The Agee device used for the one-portal endoscopic carpal tunnel release. **B,** The endoscope is inserted into the carpal tunnel through a volar ulnar skin incision. **C,** The transverse carpal ligament (dorsal surface) as seen through the endoscope. **D,** The distal edge of the transverse carpal ligament *(arrow)* and beyond it the fat pad. *TCL,* Transverse carpal ligament; *FP,* fat pad. **E,** The completely divided ligament has a trapezoid shape.

the transverse carpal ligament with special dilators. The endoscope is then inserted into the carpal canal. The dorsal surface of the transverse carpal ligament is visualized, and the distal end of the ligament is identified by the presence of a fat pad. The blade of the endoscope should not extend beyond the distal edge of the transverse carpal ligament. Two passes usually are required to transect the ligament and decompress the nerve. The fibers of the palmar fascia usually are not divided, providing a residual pulley for the nerve and flexor tendons. When placing the nose piece of the endoscope into the carpal canal, the surgeon must hold the nosepiece against the radial side of the hook of the hamate and direct it in line with the ring finger. The surgeon stops dividing the transverse carpal ligament when a V-shaped defect in the transverse carpal ligament converts to a trapezoidal-shaped defect. Healing of the tissues and return to activities are faster with the endoscopic approach compared with the open release of the median nerve. However, at about 3 months, there does not seem to be a clinically significant difference between these two groups of patients.[5]

After surgical release, a progressive rehabilitation program is extremely important.[44] About 1 week after surgery, therapy is prescribed to decrease pain and edema in the operative area, increase range of motion, and desensitize the scar. Tendon gliding exercises also are performed.

Within 3 weeks, light weight lifting is initiated in conjunction with protective night splints as indicated. At 5 to 6 weeks, progressive resistive strengthening exercises are performed to improve grip and pinch strength. Between 6 and 8 weeks, sport-specific activities are begun. The throwing athlete gradually progresses from short tossing to full-speed throwing. The specific sports mechanics may need to be altered to prevent a recurrence of the athlete's symptoms.

The differential diagnosis of carpal tunnel syndrome should include compression of the median nerve in the proximal forearm, brachial plexus injury, and cervical radiculopathy. The coexistence of carpal tunnel syndrome and cervical radiculopathy, usually at the C6 or C7 level, or brachial plexus lesions also has been reported.[2,35] This double-crush syndrome[14,35,50] is thought to be due to impairment of axonal transport in the distal direction, which allows the distal portion of the nerve to be more susceptible to trauma.[12,35,50]

Palmar Cutaneous Branch of the Median Nerve

The palmar cutaneous branch of the median nerve originates from the radial side of the median nerve 2 to 3 inches above the wrist crease, passes distally, and crosses to the ulnar side of the flexor carpi radialis tendon at the wrist (Fig. 28-10). The nerve then passes into the short

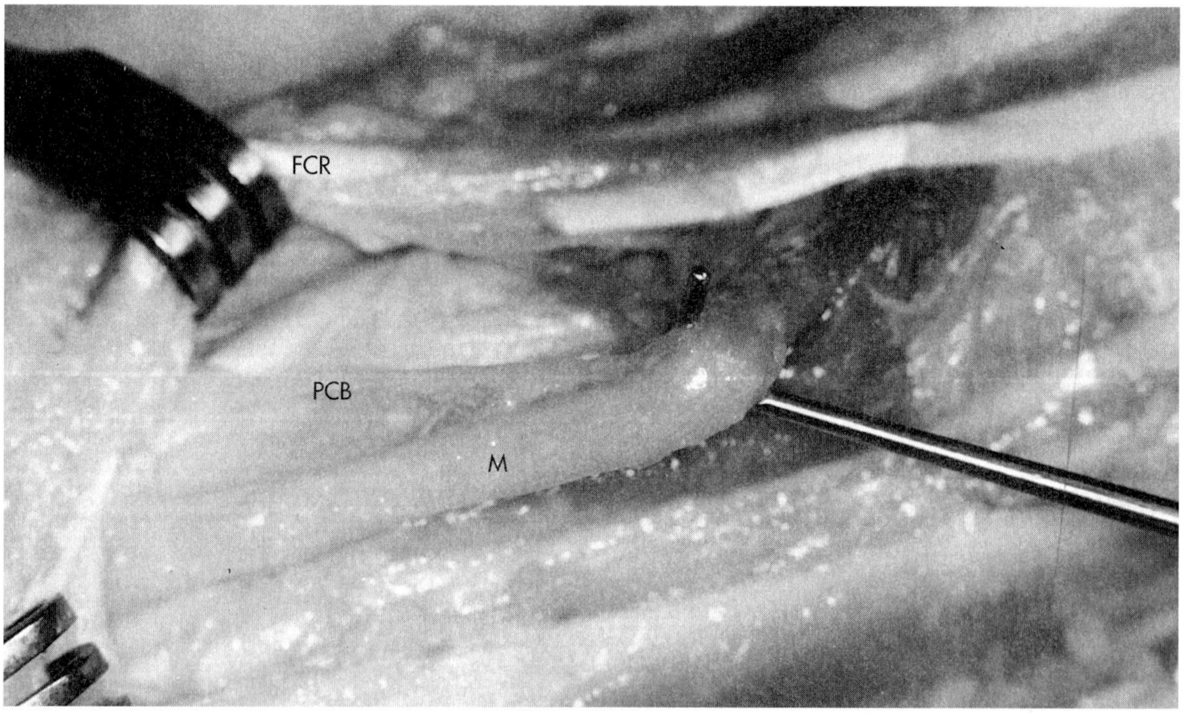

FIGURE 28-10 The palmar cutaneous branch *(PCB)* as it branches from the radial side of the median nerve *(M)*. *FCR,* Flexor carpi radialis.

tunnel within the transverse carpal ligament and divides into several branches. This nerve can be injured by blunt trauma. The patient may complain of pain or tingling at the wrist crease and base of the thenar eminence. This injury usually can be treated conservatively. Transient neurapraxia of the nerve usually resolves completely.

However, if there is sufficient perineural fibrosis and the patient has persistent symptoms, the palmar cutaneous branch of the nerve can be excised.

Digital Nerve Injuries

Isolated digital nerve injuries to the hand are unusual in athletes.

Bowler's thumb is a result of repeated friction or pressure on the ulnar digital nerve of the thumb.[14] This usually results from pressure on the thumb as it sits in the hole of the bowling ball. One case of bowler's thumb has been reported in a baseball player.[4]

Examination shows a thick tender area on the ulnar side of the base of the thumb. Tinel's sign may be positive. Sensibility to the thumb is usually normal.

Treatment generally is conservative, especially in the early stages of the condition. This usually consists of rest, splinting, a change in the grip on the ball, and a change in the thumb hole in the ball.

If this treatment is unsuccessful, surgery may be needed to allow the individual to continue in the sport.[4,14,16,36] The surgeon removes the perineural fibrosis, mobilizing and transposing the nerve to a more dorsal ulnar position in the thumb.

Handball players can sustain repetitive trauma to their digits with injury to the digital neurovascular bundles. These injuries usually resolve with conservative treatment.

Ulnar Nerve Disorders

The ulnar nerve is most commonly compromised at the elbow. However, the nerve also can be injured or compressed at the wrist. This compression occurs at or within Guyon's canal. Invariably this is a result of a single injury or repetitive trauma. Shea and McClean[45] described three types of ulnar nerve compression at the wrist. The symptoms vary depending on the site of compression. These three types of nerve compression injuries correspond to the anatomy of the nerve as it branches within the structure of Guyon's canal.[32]

Type I occurs proximal to or within the canal of Guyon and produces both sensory and motor symptoms. Type II is an isolated compression of the deep (motor) branch of the nerve at the hook of the hamate. Type III also can occur at the hook of the hamate but involves only the superficial (sensory) branch. Thus a type II lesion produces only motor abnormalities: weakness or atrophy of the ulnarly innervated intrinsic muscles of the hand, and type III produces only loss of sensibility in the ring and little fingers (Fig. 28-11). Lesions of the ulnar

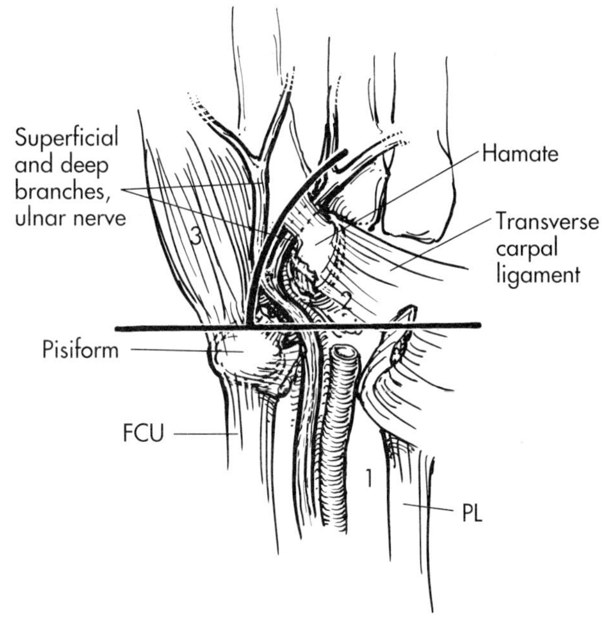

FIGURE 28-11 The ulnar nerve as it passes through Guyon's canal and separates into its motor and sensory branches. The three zones of injury are superimposed on the nerve.

nerve at the wrist spare the dorsal sensory branch of the ulnar nerve and do not affect the profundus tendons to the ring and little fingers.

Complaints include numbness and tingling of the ring and little fingers, and pain in the hypothenar eminence. The patient presents with decreased sensibility in the ring and little fingers, tingling with tapping over the ulnar nerve in Guyon's canal, and possible weakness or atrophy of the hypothenar or first dorsal interosseous muscles. If there is weakness of the ulnarly innervated intrinsic muscles of the hand, a claw deformity of the ring and little fingers may be present (Fig. 28-12). An Allen test should be done to ensure that the patient's complaints do not result from an injury to the ulnar artery.

The ulnar nerve at the wrist also may be injured by a single direct blow, a fracture of the hook of the hamate,[48] injuries to the pisiform,[24] or repeated power grip (Fig. 28-13). These injuries occur most commonly in baseball, tennis, golf, racquetball, and gymnastics.

Roentgenograms of the wrist should include a carpal tunnel view to evaluate the hook of the hamate and pisiform. If necessary, a CT scan of these areas should be done. Electrodiagnostic studies will help differentiate ulnar nerve lesions at the wrist and elbow from the more proximal lesions of the brachial plexus and cervical spine.

Initial treatment consists of rest, ice, splinting, and nonsteroidal antiinflammatory drugs. If the patient's symptoms persist, surgical decompression of the nerve

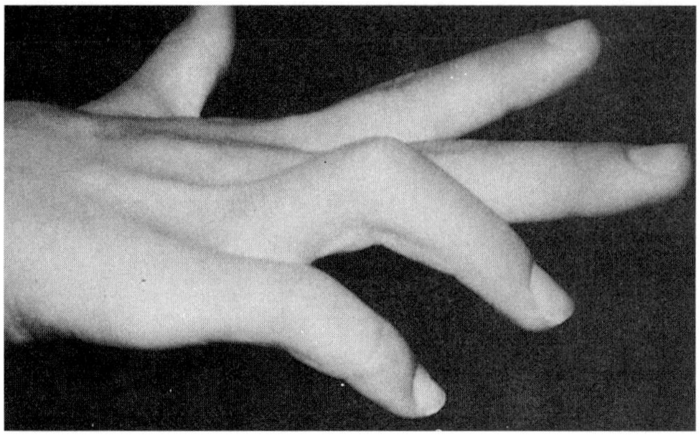

FIGURE 28-12 Claw deformity of the ring and little fingers.

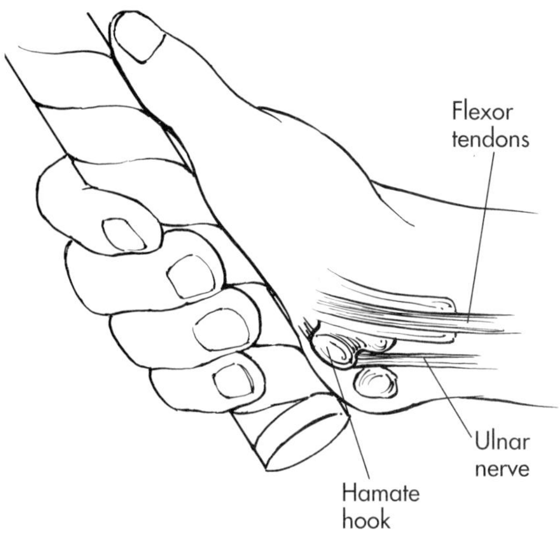

FIGURE 28-13 The ulnar nerve at the wrist can be injured secondarily from a fracture of the hook of the hamate. This fracture occurs most commonly in racquet sports, golf, and baseball.

may be necessary. However, if the nerve complaints are due to a bony injury, that is, a fracture of the hook of the hamate, treatment should be directed to the cause of the nerve irritation. In this example, the ununited hook of the hamate should be excised.

To decompress the ulnar nerve at Guyon's canal, the surgeon opens the ulnar side of the hand and wrist through a curved incision. After identifying the flexor carpi ulnaris tendon, the surgeon retracts it ulnarward and identifies the ulnar nerve and artery in the distal forearm. The ulnar nerve is deep and ulnar to the artery. Both structures are traced distally to Guyon's canal. The canal roof is incised, and the nerve is decompressed throughout the canal. Care must be taken to identify the motor and sensory branches of the nerve and ensure that each branch is not compressed by a fibrous band or some other structure.

Rehabilitation can be started in 10 to 14 days after surgery, and the sport may be gradually resumed after about 6 weeks.

Cyclist's Palsy

Bicycle riding has increased in popularity with the current fitness boom. Long-distance riding and prolonged riding trips have resulted in a compression neuropathy of the ulnar nerve at the wrist known as handlebar palsy or cyclist's palsy.[7,17,46] As a result of the riding position, a part of the rider's weight is supported by the handlebars. This causes direct, often prolonged pressure on the hypothenar eminence as the wrist is held in an extended position (Fig. 28-14). The pressure on the hand and the extended portion of the wrist tends to stretch and compress the ulnar nerve. This, in conjunction with poorly padded handlebars or gloves, may lead to the injury of the ulnar nerve.[23] The resulting neuropathy usually involves both motor and sensory components of the ulnar nerve. Wilmarth et al[52] noted that the distal sensory latencies of the ulnar nerve at the wrist in long-distance cyclists were significantly longer than in a group of controls. They concluded that there may be adaptive changes in the nerve in these cyclists resulting from the

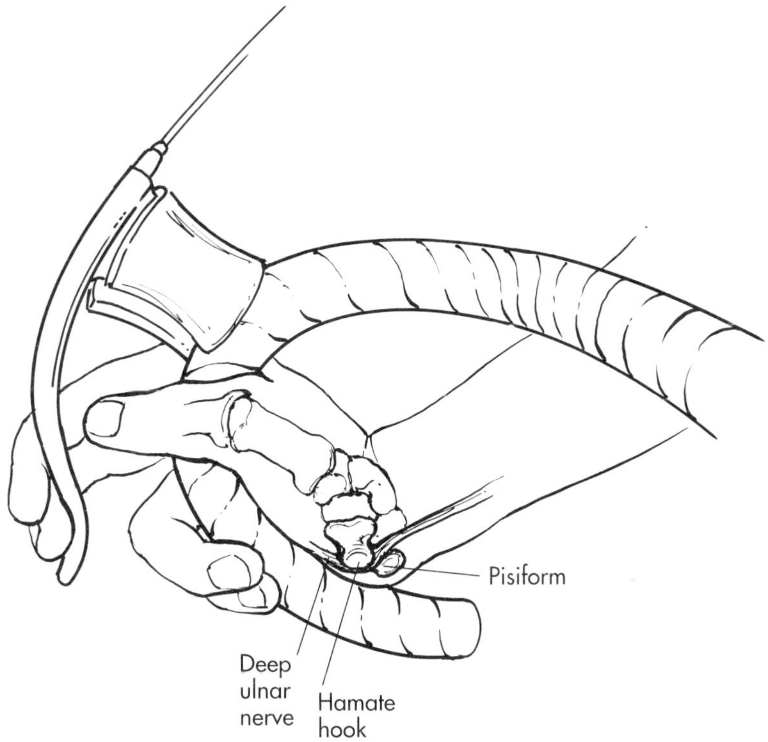

FIGURE 28-14 The ulnar nerve at the wrist can suffer compression after long-distance bicycle riding when the wrist is positioned in dorsiflexion for an extended time.

repeated compressive forces applied to the nerve at the wrist.

This neuropathy most commonly involves the dominant hand. Symptoms usually resolve spontaneously with a reduction in or temporary cessation of riding.

The athlete can prevent the injury through proper position of the handlebars, proper position of the rider on the bicycle, frequent hand position changes, padded gloves and handlebars, and, if necessary, interruption of a long or difficult ride with rest stops.

Vascular Disorders

Vascular disorders in the upper extremity of an athlete are uncommon. Open arterial injuries usually are associated with fractures. They are rarely found in finger, hand, and wrist injuries but are more likely at the elbow. This disorder can occur in conjunction with a fracture or dislocation of the elbow or a supracondylar fracture of the humerus. Acute angulated fractures of a finger can cause "circulatory embarrassment" of the finger distal to the injury. This disorder also may occur with a severely angulated dislocation of a finger joint. These injuries are best treated with immediate correction of the angular deformity of the digit. This may have to be performed as an emergency procedure in the field or in the locker room. If a persistent loss or decrease in circulation is apparent in spite of various conservative measures, then a revascularization procedure may be indicated.

Amputations or "avulsions" of a thumb resulting from rodeo roping contests[37] or of fingers resulting from water skiing[15] have been reported. These are treated the same way as any finger avulsion injury.[51] The clinician should evaluate the avulsed digit for possible replantation or revascularization.

In terms of frequency, blunt trauma to the vascular tree is much more common in association with sports-related injuries. These injuries tend to occur in athletes in whom there is a significant energy absorption in the wrist or hands from either a single traumatic event or repeated trauma. Injuries occur primarily to the ulnar artery at the wrist and to the digital arteries in the distal palm or the fingers.

Anatomy

The ulnar and radial arteries pass through the forearm to the wrist. They join the hand to form the superficial and deep palmar arches.

At the wrist, the ulnar artery along with the ulnar nerve passes through the canal of Guyon. As it exits Guyon's canal and until it passes beneath the palmar aponeurosis, the ulnar artery is susceptible to injury because it is poorly protected by soft tissue. The ulnar artery is the primary source of the superficial palmar arch. The arch is completed by the superficial palmar branch of the radial artery. The common volar digital arteries arise from the superficial palmar arch and are the primary arterial supply to the digits. The princeps pollicis artery comes from the deep branch of the radial artery and is the important arterial supply to the thumb. Coleman and Anson[10] noted that 80% of hands have a complete superficial arch, whereas 20% have incomplete arches (Fig. 28-15). Hands with incomplete arches may have vascular compromise of some of the digits after injury to the feeding artery of the incomplete arch. The deep palmar arch is complete in 97% of hands.

Blunt trauma to the ulnar artery at the wrist, from a single episode or from repeated trauma, can result in thrombosis of the artery if the intima is damaged or in a true aneurysm if the tunica media of the vessel wall is damaged (Fig. 28-16). A true aneurysm often is associated with fusiform swelling of the vessel. In addition, there may be spasm of the ulnar artery. Spasm of the artery is reversible if detected early. If it is prolonged or untreated, the vessel may occlude with secondary distal ischemic changes. These entities have been referred to as the hypothenar hammer syndrome.[11]

Ulnar artery thrombosis has been reported from baseball, karate, judo, hockey, and handball injuries.[40] The ath-

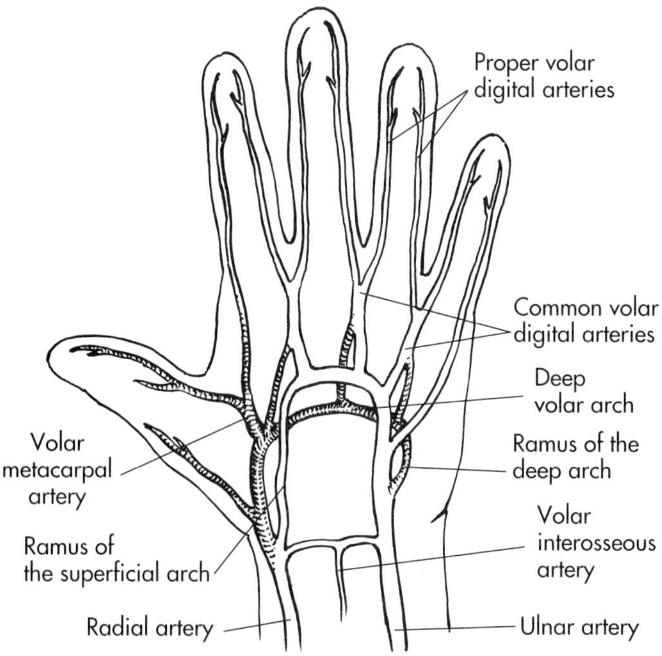

FIGURE 28-15 The radial and ulnar arteries form the superficial and deep palmar arches in the hand, which in turn send arterial branches to the fingers.

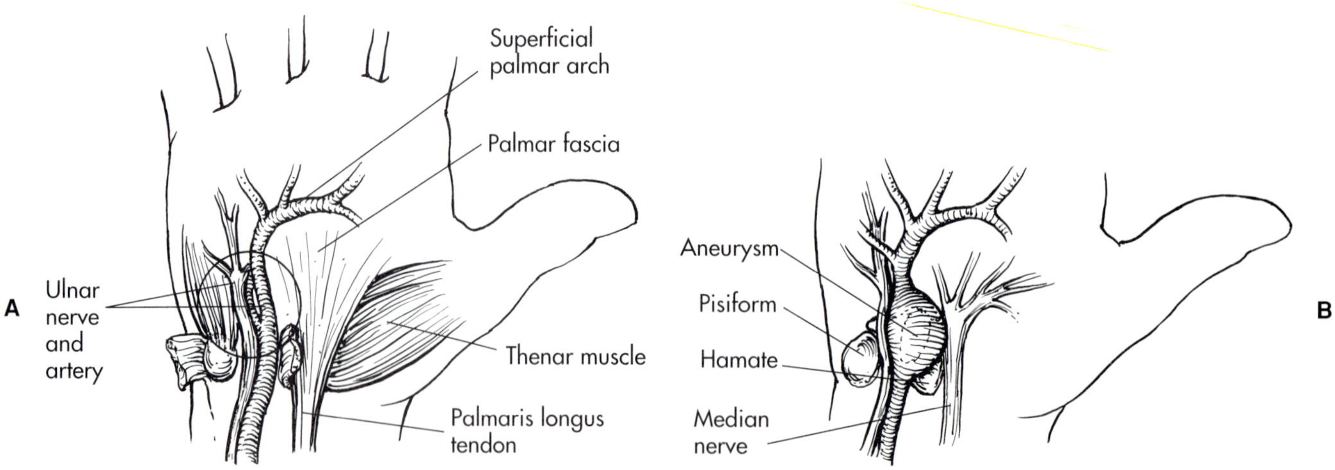

FIGURE 28-16 **A,** The ulnar artery is susceptible to injury after it leaves Guyon's canal *(circle)*. **B,** The site of aneurysm or thrombosis of the artery.

lete complains of pain, paresthesias, and Raynaud's phenomenon on the ulnar side of the hand. The ring and little fingers may be cool. There is usually no mass in the wrist or palm. The Allen test is abnormal (Fig. 28-17). Various noninvasive diagnostic examinations (Doppler digital plethysmography and radionuclide flow studies) are useful in establishing the diagnosis. Arteriography probably should not be used unless surgical reconstruction is planned. If conservative treatment is unsuccessful, excision of the thrombosed segment of artery with or without reconstruction is recommended. If backflow is good, ligation of the vessel alone should relieve the patient's complaints. However, if backflow is poor, reconstruction of the artery is indicated.[28,40]

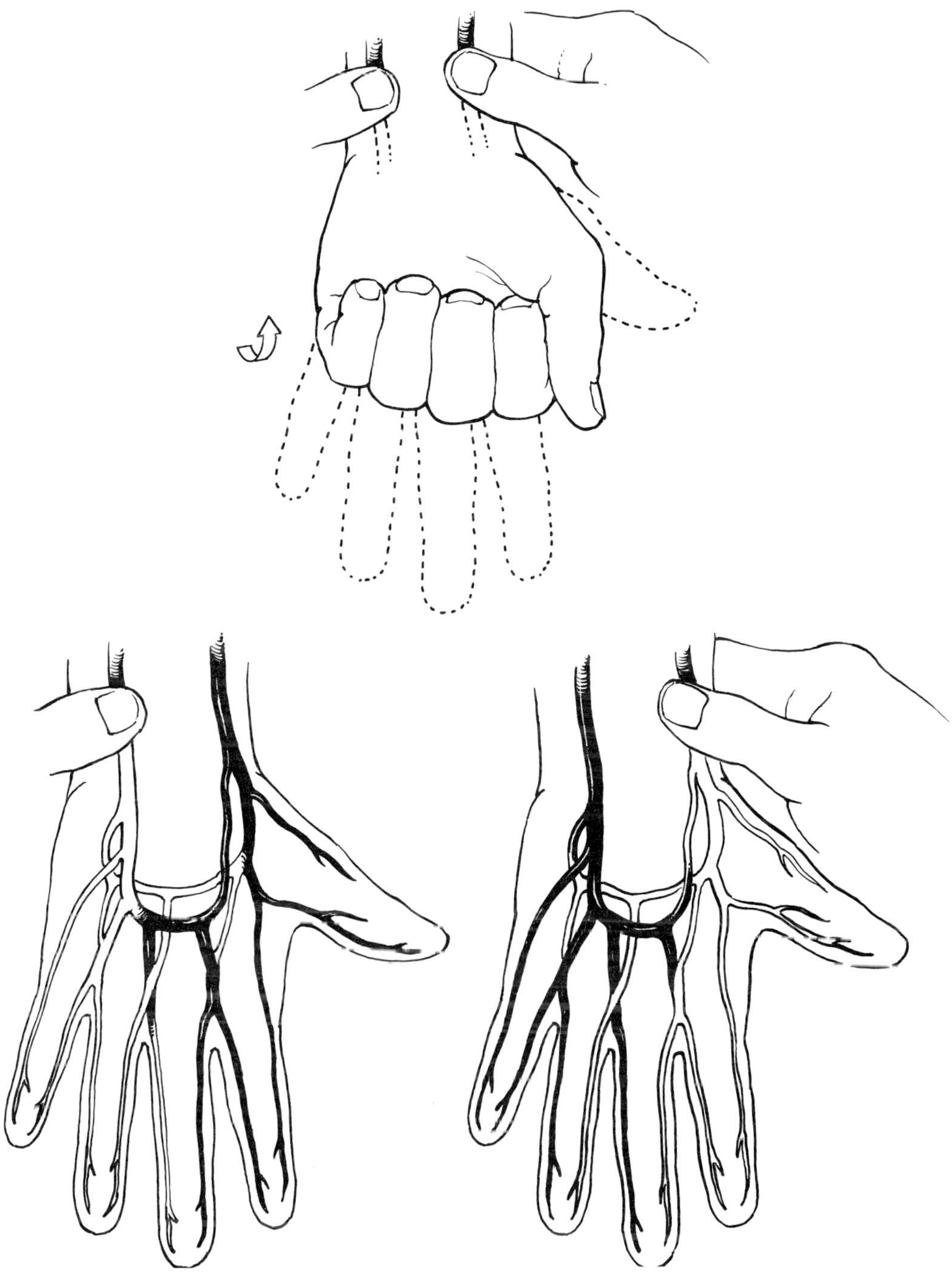

FIGURE 28-17 Allen test for patency of the radial and ulnar arteries. The Allen test is negative when there is good blood flow to the fingers and is positive when the blood flow is obstructed (e.g., in ulnar artery thrombosis).

A true aneurysm of the ulnar artery will present with similar symptoms. Examination will show a palpable mass at the wrist, and a bruit may be present. The Allen test probably will be normal. A positive Tinel`s sign at the wrist indicates ulnar nerve compression.

The treatment includes resection of the aneurysm with or without arterial reconstruction. If the superficial arch is incomplete, then arterial reconstruction will be needed. True aneurysms of the ulnar artery have been found in athletes playing football, basketball, lacrosse, and volleyball.[2,26]

A false aneurysm of an artery usually occurs after a penetrating injury and is extremely rare as a result of an athletic injury.

Digital Ischemia

Repeated blunt trauma has been blamed for ischemia in the hands of baseball, handball, karate, and volleyball players.[33,49] Baseball players[6] are at the greatest risk for injury. Lowrey and Chadwick[33] noted 13 of 22 baseball catchers had digital ischemia and hypertrophy of their left index fingers as a result of repeated injury from catching a baseball. The affected finger was cooler than the other digits. These injuries usually can be treated by padding the glove; however, some athletes object to this because it decreases ball control. Oral vasodilating agents and abstention from smoking also are useful treatment modalities. Sugawara et al[49] also noted a predilection for digital ischemia in the index finger in baseball players. They found that digital artery occlusion occurred distal to the proximal interphalangeal joint. Digital ischemia was more common in high school and college baseball players, apparently because of increased time in the sport.

Handball players were found to have more diffuse injury with multiple digits involved.[6] Using thermography, Buckhout and Warner noted multiple areas of decreased digital perfusion in 17 of 22 players. The risk of injury in handball players increased if the player had more than 2 years' experience or greater than 200 hours of accumulated playing time.

Vasospastic disorders of the index finger of baseball pitchers are thought to result from overstimulation of the local sympathetic nervous system secondary to repeated pressure of the ball on the finger. This disorder often responds to rest and oral vasodilation medication. However, Itoh et al[27] noted three cases where the neurovascular bundles to the finger were compromised by hypertrophy of the lumbrical muscles or by the proximal edge of Cleland's ligament. These three patients were relieved of their complaints after an operation to decompress the neurovascular bundles.

References

1. Agee J et al: Endoscopic release of the carpal tunnel: a randomized prospective multicenter study, *J Hand Surg* 17:987-995, 1992.
2. Aucilino PL: Neurovascular injuries in the hands of athletes, *Hand Clin* 6:455-466, 1990.
3. Bell-Krotoski J: Advances in sensibility evaluation, *Hand Clin* 7:527-546, 1991.
4. Belsky M, Millender LH: Bowler's thumb in a baseball player: a case report, *Orthopaedics* 3:122-123, 1980.
5. Brown RA et al: Carpal tunnel release: a prospective, randomized assessment of open and endoscopic methods, *J Bone Joint Surg* 75A:1265-1275, 1993.
6. Buckhout BC, Warner MA: Digital perfusion of handball players, *Am J Sports Med* 8:206-207, 1980.
7. Burke ER: Ulnar neuropathy in bicyclists, *Phys Sports Med* 9:53-56, 1981.
8. Carr D, Davis P: Distal posterior interosseous nerve syndrome, *J Hand Surg* 10A:873-878, 1985.
9. Chow JCY: Endoscopic release of the carpal ligament for carpal tunnel syndrome: 22 month clinical result, *J Arthroscopy* 6:288-296, 1990.
10. Coleman SS, Anson BJ: Arterial patterns in the hand based upon a study of 650 specimens, *Surg Gynecol Obstet* 113:408-424, 1961.
11. Conn J, Bergan JJ, Bell JJ: Hypothenar hammer syndrome: post-traumatic digital ischemia, *Surgery* 68:1122-1128, 1970.
12. Dahlin LB, Rydevik B: Pathophysiology of nerve compression. In Gelberman RH, editor: *Operative nerve repair and reconstruction*, Philadelphia, 1991, JB Lippincott, pp 847-866.
13. Dellon AL, Mackinnon SE: Radial sensory nerve entrapment in the forearm, *J Hand Surg* 11A:199-205, 1986.
14. Dobyns JH et al: Bowler's thumb, diagnosis and treatment: review of 17 cases, *J Bone Joint Surg* 54A:751-755, 1972.
15. Dobyns JH, Sim FH, Linscheid RL: Sports stress syndromes of the hand and wrist, *Am J Sports Med* 6:236-253, 1978.
16. Dunham W, Haines G, Spring J: Bowler's thumb (ulnovolar neuroma of the thumb), *Clin Orthop* 83:99-101, 1972.
17. Eckman PB, Perlstein G, Altrocchi PH: Ulnar neuropathy in bicycle riders, *Arch Neurol* 32:130-131, 1975.
18. Ehrlich W, Dellon AL, Mackinnon SE: Cheiralgia paraesthetica (entrapment of the radial sensory nerve), *J Hand Surg* 11A:196-199, 1986.
19. Gelberman RH et al: Sensibility testing in peripheral-nerve compression syndromes, *J Bone Joint Surg* 65-A:632-638, 1983.
20. Gelberman RH, Hergenroeder PT, Hargeus AR: The carpal tunnel syndrome: a study of carpal canal pressures, *J Bone Joint Surg* 65A:632-638, 1983.
21. Green DP: Diagnostic and therapeutic value of carpal tunnel injection, *J Hand Surg* 9A:850-854, 1984.
22. Gross MS, Gelberman RH: The anatomy of the distal ulnar tunnel, *Clin Orthop* 196:238-247, 1985.
23. Haloua JP, Collin JP, Couderre L: Paralysis of the ulnar nerve in cyclists, *Ann Chir Main* 6:282-287, 1987.
24. Helal B: Racquet player's pisiform, *Hand* 10:87-90, 1978.
25. Hirasawa Y, Sakakida K: Sports and peripheral nerve injury, *Am J Sports Med* 11:420-426, 1983.
26. Ho PK, Dellon AL, Wilgis EFS: True aneurysms of the hand resulting from athletic injury, *Am J Sports Med* 13:136-138, 1985.
27. Itoh Y et al: Circulatory disturbances in the throwing hand of baseball pitchers, *Am J Sports Med* 15:264-269, 1987.
28. Koman LA, Urbaniak JR: Ulnar artery insufficiency: a guide to treatment, *J Hand Surg* 6:16-24, 1981.
29. Kummel BM, Zazanis GA: Shoulder pain as the presenting complaint in carpal tunnel syndrome, *Clin Orthop* 92:227-230, 1973.

30. Lanz V: Anatomical variations of the median nerve in the carpal tunnel, *J Hand Surg* 2:44-53, 1977.
31. Layfer LF, Jones JV: Hand paraesthesias after racquetball, *Ill Med J* 190:191, 1977.
32. Leffert RD: Diabetes mellitus initially presenting peripheral neuropathy in the upper limb, *J Bone Joint Surg* 51A:1005-1010, 1969.
33. Lowrey CW, Chadwick RO, Waltman EN: Digital vessel trauma from repetitive impact in baseball catchers, *J Hand Surg* 1:236-238, 1976.
34. McCue FC et al: Hand and wrist injuries in the athlete, *Am J Sports Med* 7:275-286, 1979.
35. Massey EW, Riley T, Pleet AB: Coexistent carpal tunnel syndrome and cervical radiculopathy (double crush syndrome), *South Med J* 74:957-959, 1981.
36. Minkow FV, Bassett FH: Bowler's thumb, *Clin Orthop* 83:115-117, 1972.
37. Morgan RF et al: Rodeo roping thumb injuries, *J Hand Surg* 9A:178-180, 1984.
38. Omer GE, Spinner M: *Management of peripheral nerve problems,* Philadelphia, 1980, WB Saunders.
39. Phalen GS: The carpal tunnel syndrome: clinical evaluation of 598 hands, *Clin Orthop* 83:29-40, 1972.
40. Porubsky GL, Brown SI, Urbaniak JR: Ulnar artery thrombosis: a sports related injury, *Am J Sports Med* 14:170-175, 1986.
41. Posner MA: Compressive neuropathies of the median and radial nerves at the elbow, *Clin Sports Med* 9:343-361, 1990.
42. Read RL: Stress testing in nerve compression, *Hand Clin* 7:521-526, 1991.
43. Resnick C, Miller B: Endoscopic carpal tunnel release using the subligamentous two portal technique, *Contemp Orthop* 22:269-277, 1991.
44. Rettig AC: Neurovascular injuries in the wrists and hands of athletes, *Clin Sports Med* 9:389-417, 1990.
45. Shea JD, McClain EF: Ulnar nerve compression syndrome at and below the wrist, *J Bone Joint Surg* 51A:1095-1103, 1969.
46. Smail DF: Handlebar palsy, *N Engl J Med* 292:322, 1975.
47. Spinner M: *Injuries to the major branches of peripheral nerves of the forearm,* ed 2, Philadelphia, 1978, WB Saunders.
48. Stark HH et al: Fracture of the hook of the hamate, *J Bone Joint Surg* 71A:1202-1207, 1989.
49. Sugawara M et al: Digital ischemia in baseball players, *Am J Sports Med* 14:329-334, 1986.
50. Upton RM, McComas AJ: The double crush in nerve-entrapment syndromes, *Lancet* ii:359-362, 1973.
51. Urbaniak JR, Evan JP, Bright DS: Microvascular management of ring avulsion injuries, *J Hand Surg* 6:25-30, 1981.
52. Wilmarth MA, Nelson SG: Distal sensory latencies of the ulnar nerve in long distance bicyclists: pilot study, *J Orthop Sports Phys Ther* 9:370-374, 1988.
53. Wood MB, Dobyns JH: Sports related extra-articular wrist syndromes, *Clin Orthop* 202:93-102, 1986.

CHAPTER 29

Soft-Tissue Stress Injuries

NORMAN P. ZEMEL

Nonosseous injuries of the upper extremity can be as disabling as any bony injury. Soft-tissue injury may result from blunt trauma or repetitive use. In either instance, there can be direct or indirect injury to the muscles, tendons, tendon pulleys, tenosynovium, skin, or capsuloligamentous structures. Most of these injuries have an excellent prognosis if they are properly diagnosed and appropriately treated, if a good rehabilitation program is undertaken, and if the athlete is returned to the sport properly protected.[21]

Although these soft-tissue injuries are not always caused by sports-related activities, the injuries that tend to frequently result from athletic activities will be discussed.

MUSCLE STRAINS

Muscle strains are not nearly as common in the upper extremity as they are in the lower extremity. Most muscle injuries tend to result from direct trauma (e.g., the forearm is struck by a helmet during football). The resultant bruising usually will heal with conservative treatment. Hematoma within the muscle also can result from overuse or trauma. These are relatively minor injuries that rarely prevent an early return to competition.

Occasionally a large hematoma develops within the fascial sheath containing the muscles or in the subcutaneous tissue as a result of extreme muscle exertion during weight training. This can cause an acute or chronic compartment syndrome. In the acute phase, the diagnosis can be made clinically and can be verified by measuring forearm compartment pressures. In the chronic stage, the individual can present with an enlarged and painful forearm. An MRI usually will delineate the location of the hematoma. A complete discussion of the diagnosis and treatment of compartment syndrome of the forearm may be found in an earlier chapter.

TENDINITIS

Tendinitis refers to the symptomatic inflammation of the tendons and peritendinous structures. Tendons are the mechanical link between bone and muscle and as such are exposed to tensile, shear, and compressive stresses.

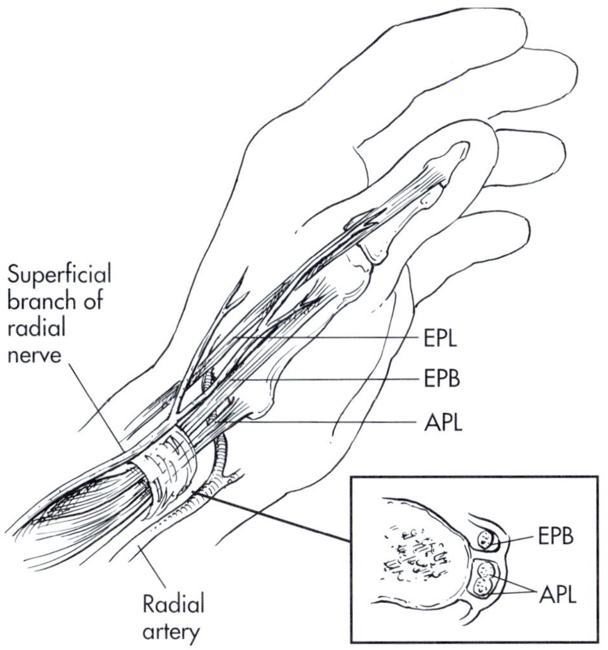

FIGURE 29-1 The first extensor fibroosseous compartment. The inset shows a septum creating two compartments. Both compartments must be released to relieve the patient's complaints.

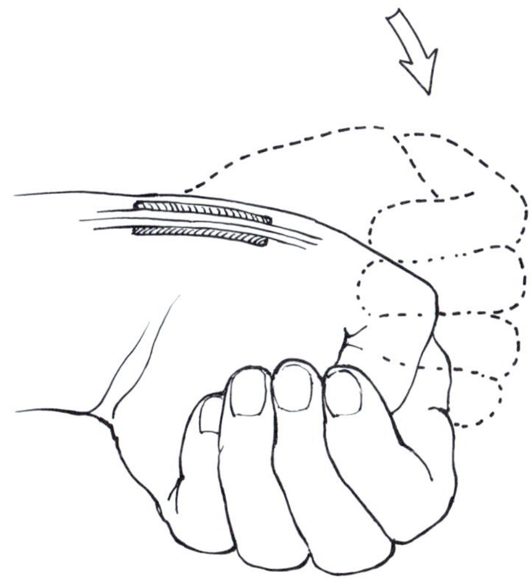

FIGURE 29-2 The practitioner performs a Finkelstein's test by clasping the thumb with the fingers and ulnarly deviating the wrist. This maneuver is painful when the patient has de Quervain's tendinitis.

As a result of these forces, the tendon becomes deformed. If the deformation of the tendon exceeds its elastic limits, cumulative microfailure of the molecular links between tendon fibrils can occur (fibrillar creep).[30] This cumulative microfailure may occur if (1) the load is too great or (2) the time between loads is too short to allow the tendon to recover to its resting length. These events have been considered analogous to a stress fracture in a bone.

As a result of this injury, swelling and thickening of the tendon sheath and occlusion of blood flow within the mesotendon can interfere with the tendon's ability for repair. The thick, swollen tendon and peritendinous tissue then may impinge on nearby nerves and lead to pain in the affected area.[22] Tendinitis from athletic activities is invariably the result of overuse.

EXTENSOR TENDINITIS

This can affect any of the tendons in the six extensor fibroosseous compartments. De Quervain's disease consists of inflammation of the abductor pollicis longus and extensor pollicis brevis tendons located within the first extensor fibroosseous compartment. Inflammation of these tendons is less common in the younger athlete but seems to occur in the individual over the age of 40 who is involved in sports.

Several authors have noted significant anatomic variability in the number of tendons within the first extensor fibroosseous sheath.[15,17] A thickened area of the sheath is located just proximal to the radial styloid and is the consistent area of tendon entrapment.[20] The incidence of a septum separating the extensor tendons in the first extensor compartment varies from 20% to 58%[12,15,17,18] (Fig. 29-1).

De Quervain's tendinitis usually presents with a history of pain and swelling on the radial side of the distal forearm. The pain may radiate proximally and/or distally and is aggravated by use of the thumb with associated ulnar deviation of the wrist.

Examination reveals tenderness to palpation over the first dorsal extensor compartment, occasional swelling, and an occasional firm mass over the first extensor sheath. The mass may represent a small ganglion. Occasionally a snap or trigger phenomenon is noted with thumb motion.[32] Finkelstein's test is pathognomonic[9] (Fig. 29-2). This test reproduces or aggravates the patient's pain. It is performed by ulnarly deviating the wrist with the thumb held in adduction. If the maneuver is repeated with the thumb in abduction, the pain is much less.

De Quervain's tendinitis must be differentiated from degenerative arthritis at the base of the thumb (metacarpotrapezial and scaphotrapezial joints), Wartenberg's syndrome (entrapment of the superficial branch of the radial sensory nerve), and the intersection syndrome (a more proximal tendinitis).

The usual initial treatment for de Quervain's tendinitis consists of immobilization with a thumb spica splint and nonsteroidal antiinflammatory medication (Fig. 29-3). If this is not immediately successful, cortisone can be injected into the first extensor compartment, followed by

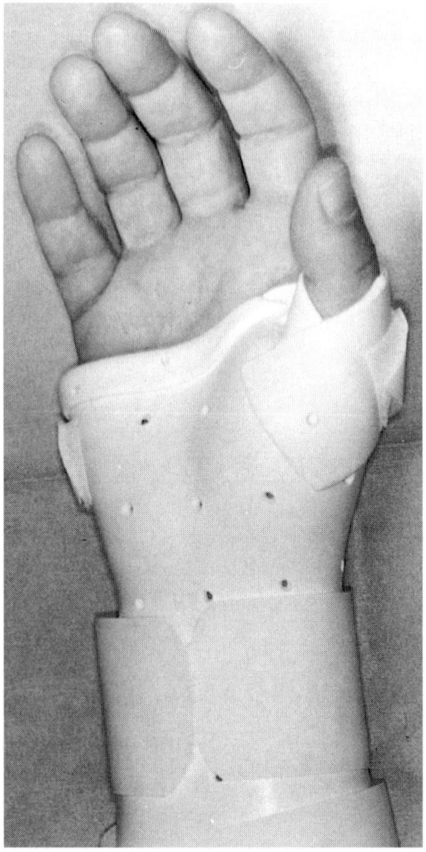

FIGURE 29-3 A thumb spica splint is useful as part of the conservative treatment for de Quervain's tendinitis.

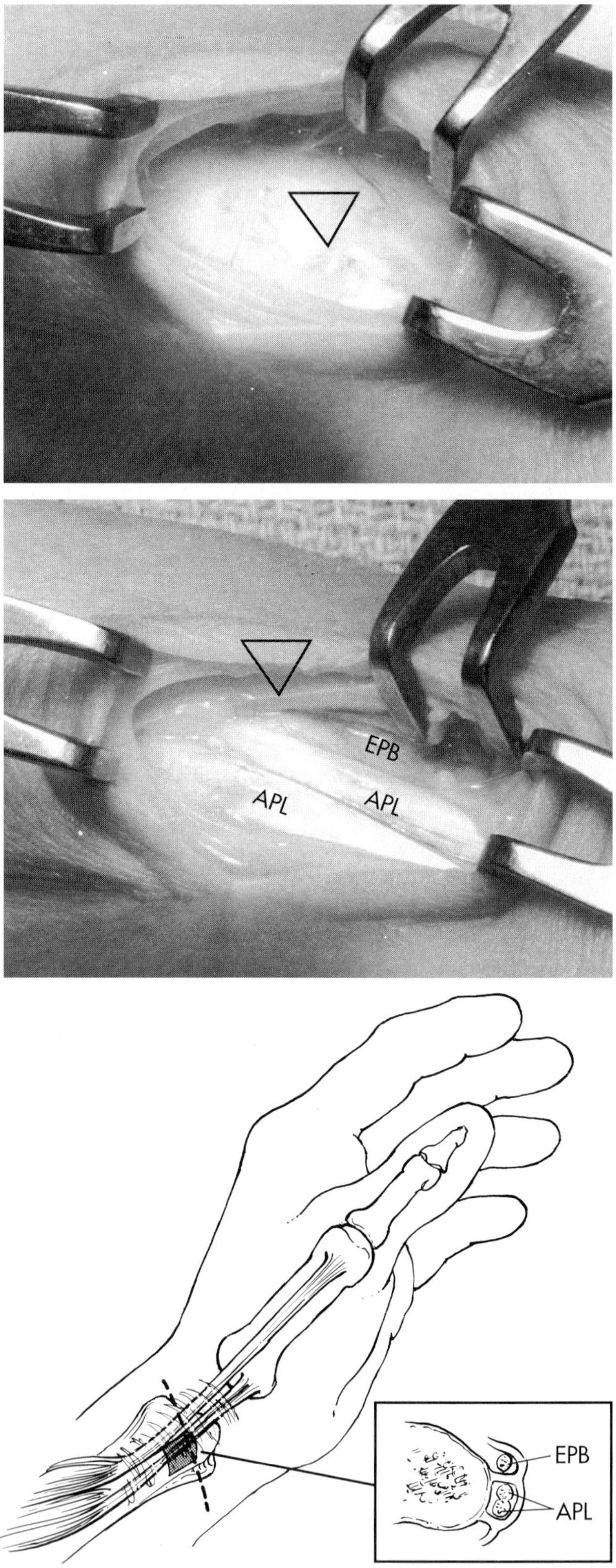

FIGURE 29-4 **A,** The thick extensor sheath is exposed, and cortisone deposits are noted *(arrow)*. **B,** After the sheath is excised *(arrow)*, the tendons all are within one compartment. *APL,* Abductor pollicis longus; *EPB,* extensor pollicis brevis. **C,** Diagram showing excision of the thick portion of the extensor sheath.

a splint for 10 days after the injection. This frequently results in an 80% cure of the symptoms.[12,18]

If conservative treatment fails, surgery may be necessary to release the first extensor fibroosseous compartment. This usually is performed under local anesthesia. An oblique short skin incision is made over the thick area in the first extensor sheath. The superficial branches of the radial sensory nerve are identified and gently retracted. The roof of the thick area in the extensor sheath is excised (Fig. 29-4). It is important to leave the sides of the pulley intact and leave the extensor sheath intact proximal and distal to the site of constriction. This will prevent radial subluxation of the tendons when the wrist is palmarly flexed. A careful examination is made for a separate compartment containing the extensor pollicis brevis tendon. If this is present, this compartment also must be released. The hand and wrist are immobilized for 2 weeks before range-of-motion exercises are started.

Although this is a common operation, complications can occur if it is not performed carefully. These complications usually include injuries to the branches of the radial sensory nerve or inadequate decompression of the extensor sheath, especially if a septum is present within the sheath.[1,2]

Intersection syndrome is a painful condition that occurs in the distal forearm 4 to 8 cm proximal to Lister's tubercle, where the abductor pollicis longus and extensor pollicis brevis muscles cross superiorly to the radial wrist extensor tendons[7,9,11] (Fig. 29-5). This condition presents as pain, swelling, redness, and occasional crepitus in the distal forearm. The basic pathology consists of tenosynovitis of the tendons of the second extensor compartment.[11] This condition frequently occurs in rowers, canoeists, weight lifters, and others whose sport involves repetitive wrist activity.[33] This condition also has been called "oarsman's wrist."[31]

The condition usually can be successfully treated with a combination of nonsteroidal antiinflammatory drugs, rest, splinting of the wrist in slight extension, and a cortisone injection. In recalcitrant cases, an operation to incise the fascia overlying the tendons and to remove the hypertrophied synovium or bursa generally is successful.[11]

Stretch injury and microtears of the insertion of the radial wrist extensors (i.e., the extensor carpi radialis longus and extensor carpi radialis brevis tendons) can be found in golfers, tennis players, and racquetball players where the wrist and hand are rapidly accelerated and decelerated.[16] These patients complain of vague pain along the radial side of the hand and wrist. This pain is aggravated by use of the involved extremity. Tenderness is noted over the insertion of the radial wrist extensor tendons at the base of the second and third metacarpals. A hard mass often is found at this site (carpometacarpal boss). This bony mass is best seen with a radiograph taken with the hand in 30° to 40° of supination and 20° to 30° of ulnar deviation[6] (Fig. 29-6). About 30% of these cases are associated with a small ganglion that usually contributes to the patient's pain.

Conservative management usually will relieve the pain and allow the patient to return to sports. If not, the surgeon can excise the osteophytes (boss), ganglion (if

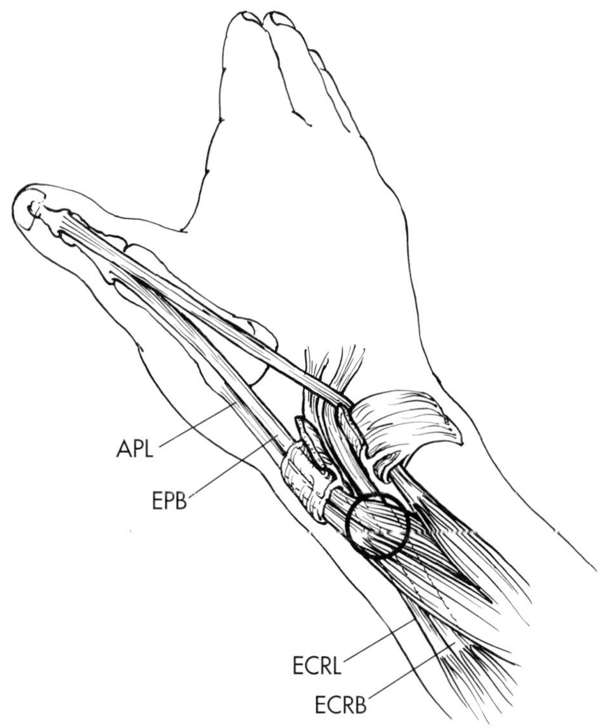

FIGURE 29-5 The arrow indicates the site of the pathology in an intersection syndrome.

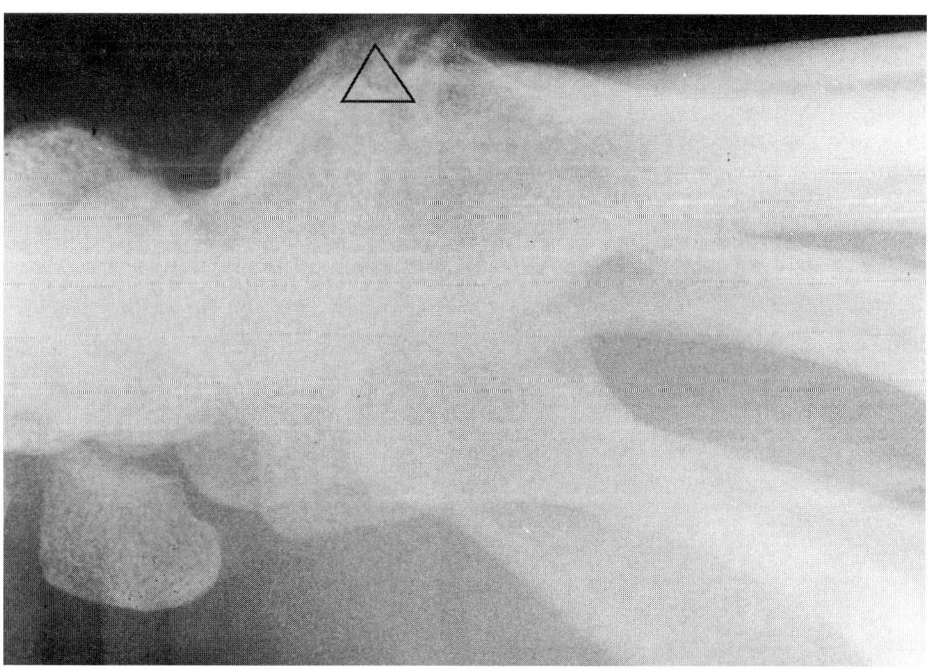

FIGURE 29-6 A carpometacarpal boss *(arrow)*.

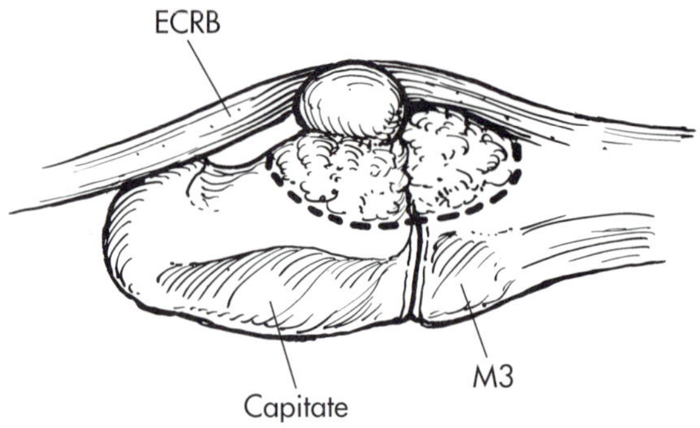

FIGURE 29-7 After the extensor tendons are elevated, all the reactive bone and a ganglion, if present, should be excised.

present), and any associated detritus about the tendon ends[6] (Fig. 29-7). Because the extensor tendons must be elevated from the bone during the operation, the hand and wrist are immobilized for about 3 to 4 weeks. A gradual return to sports can be started after 8 weeks.

Tendinitis or tenosynovitis of the other wrist extensor compartments can result from a variety of activities, frequently related to overuse. However, these conditions are uncommon as sports-related entities.[16,33]

In almost all instances, these conditions can be treated with rest, nonsteroidal antiinflammatory drugs, a cortisone injection into the affected extensor compartment, and a gradual return to athletic activity. If nonoperative treatment fails to relieve the patient's complaints, the clinician should suspect an anatomic variation. Occasionally, a muscle belly is more distal than usual and will intrude into an extensor compartment with finger motion. This often will lead to a painful inflammatory process.[28,29] Under these circumstances, surgical decompression usually is needed to alleviate the symptoms.

FLEXOR TENDINITIS

At the wrist, the flexor carpi ulnaris tendon, the flexor carpi radialis tendon, and the flexor tendons within the carpal canal can be affected by an inflammatory process. Involvement of the flexor tendons within the carpal canal will be discussed in the section on carpal tunnel syndrome. Trigger fingers can result from trauma to the distal palm or base of the thumb.

The flexor carpi ulnaris tendon is the wrist flexor tendon most often afflicted with tendinitis. Repetitive trauma, especially in racquet sports, is frequently the underlying cause.[13] Pain, swelling, and tenderness are present at the insertion of the flexor carpi ulnaris tendon into the pisiform. Passive wrist extension or resisted wrist flexion will be painful. Although radiographs usually are normal, occasionally calcific deposits are noted within the tendon (Fig. 29-8).

Conservative treatment invariably relieves the pain, and rest and immobilization also allow resorption of the calcified area within the tendon. Occasionally, surgery is needed to excise the pisiform.[5,13,24]

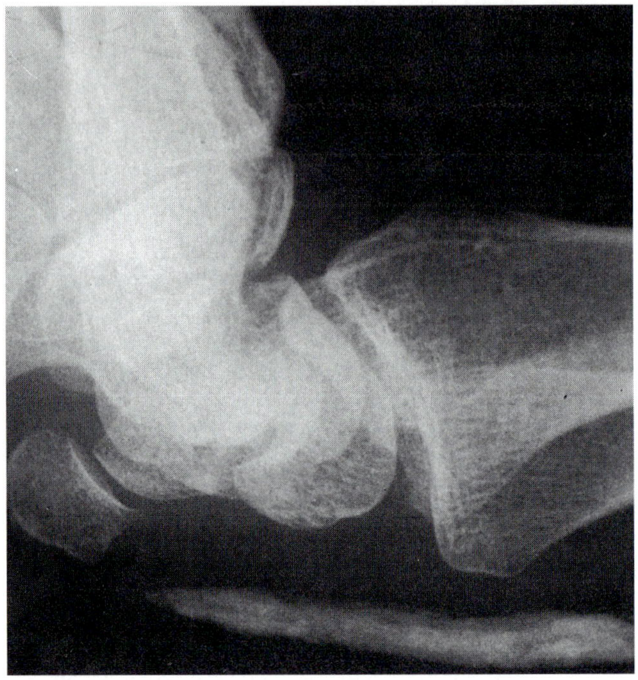

FIGURE 29-8 Calcification of the flexor carpi ulnaris tendon.

Flexor carpi ulnaris tendinitis should be differentiated from pisotriquetral joint pathology.

The flexor carpi radialis tendon passes through a synovial-lined tunnel at the wrist and inserts into the base of the second metacarpal[3] (Fig. 29-9). This tunnel is outside the carpal tunnel (Fig. 29-10). A tendinitis or tenosynovitis can result from a single direct blow to the tendon or from repetitive trauma or use. Pain, swelling, and local tenderness are the patient's primary complaints. Pain is aggravated by passive wrist extension or resisted wrist flexion.

If conservative treatment fails, then release of the synovial sheath and synovectomy of the flexor tendon usually will relieve the patient's symptoms. Occasionally, a partial tear of the tendon is found, and this can either be débrided if the tear is small or be repaired if the tear is large.[10]

In older patients, degenerative arthritis of the scaphotrapezial joint should be considered in evaluation of the patient's pain complaints. A radiograph usually will determine the presence of arthritis in the scaphotrapezial joint.

The flexor tendons at the A-1 pulley in the distal palm can be irritated by blunt trauma (Fig. 29-11). This more commonly occurs in handball players, baseball catchers, gymnasts, and weight lifters. Pain, swelling, and snapping or triggering of the involved finger(s) or thumb result from narrowing of the A-1 pulley at the metacarpal head.[8,14] Rarely, the patient also may have snapping at the

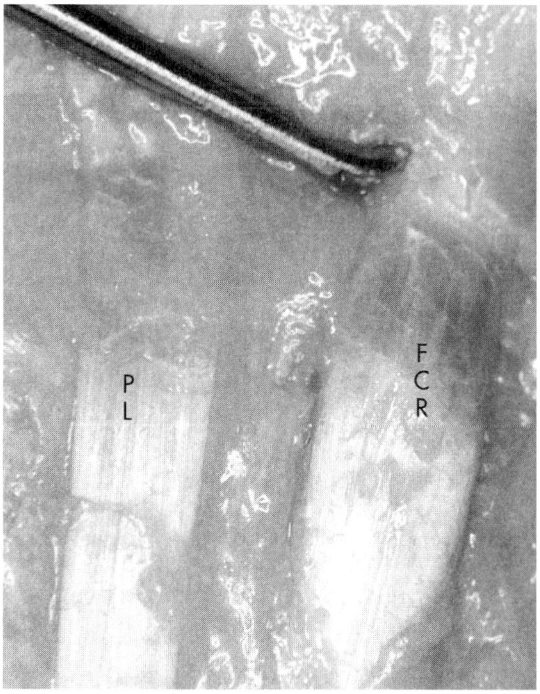

FIGURE 29-9 The pointer is at the entrance to the synovial-lined tunnel of the flexor carpi radialis tendon. *FCR,* Flexor carpi radialis; *PL,* palmaris longus.

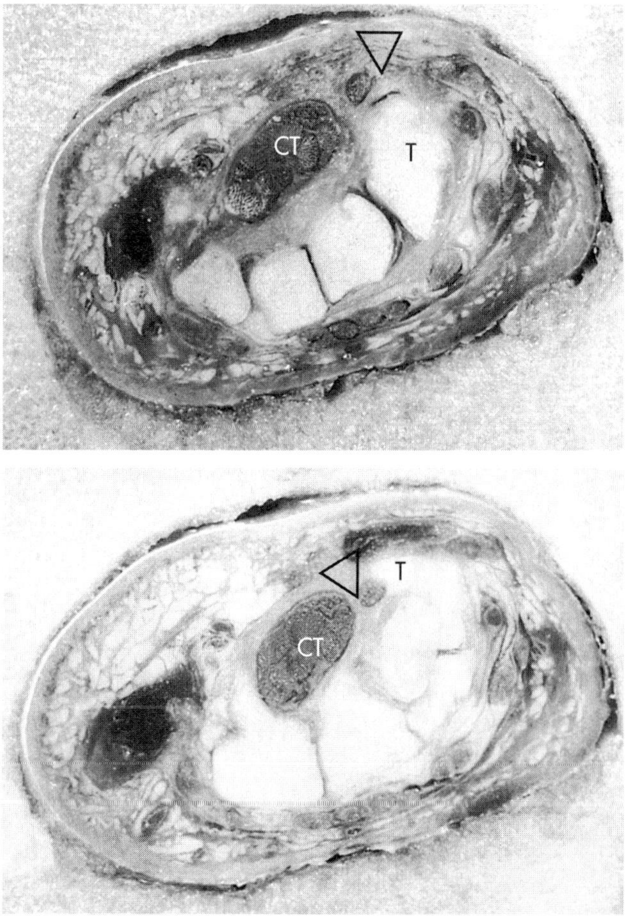

FIGURE 29-10 **A,** An axial view of the flexor carpi radialis tendon in its own sheath *(arrow)* and, **B,** in its groove *(arrow)* adjacent to the trapezium. *CT,* Carpal tunnel; *T,* trapezium.

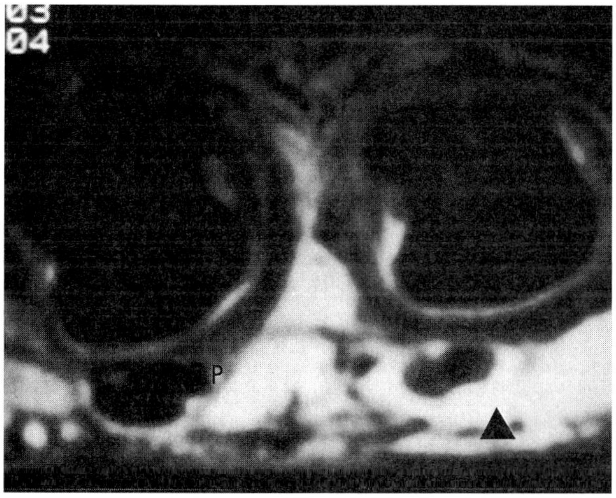

FIGURE 29-11 MRI showing edema around the flexor tendon within the flexor sheath *(arrow)*. *P,* Normal flexor tendons.

decussation of the flexor digitorum superficialis tendon in the finger.[26]

Successful treatment has been reported with splinting,[25] injection,[23] or a combination of both.[27] The author prefers to inject 1 ml of Celestone and 1 ml of Xylocaine into the flexor sheath without splinting the hand; this has an associated success rate of well over 80%.

Occasionally, surgery is needed to release the A-1 pulley in the distal palm (trigger finger) or at the proximal flexion crease of the thumb (trigger thumb) (Fig. 29-12). The operation is performed under local anesthesia. A short transverse incision is made over the A-1 pulley. The neurovascular bundles are retracted, and the roof of the pulley is excised. Traction should be placed on the flexor tendon(s) to ensure a complete release of the constricted area at the pulley and to check for a second distal site where snapping can occur. A soft dressing is applied to the hand for 7 to 10 days, and normal activity is then gradually resumed.

Linburg and Comstock reported on four patients with pain and tenderness over the volar radial aspect of the distal forearm. Surgical exploration revealed a tendinous connection between the flexor pollicis longus and the digital flexor profundus tendons, usually the index finger.[19] In their study of 194 individuals, they noted the anomaly was present in 31% unilaterally and in 14% bilaterally.

The characteristic physical finding is an inability to completely flex the thumb without flexing the index finger at the same time. When the patient is symptomatic, this motion of the thumb and index finger causes pain

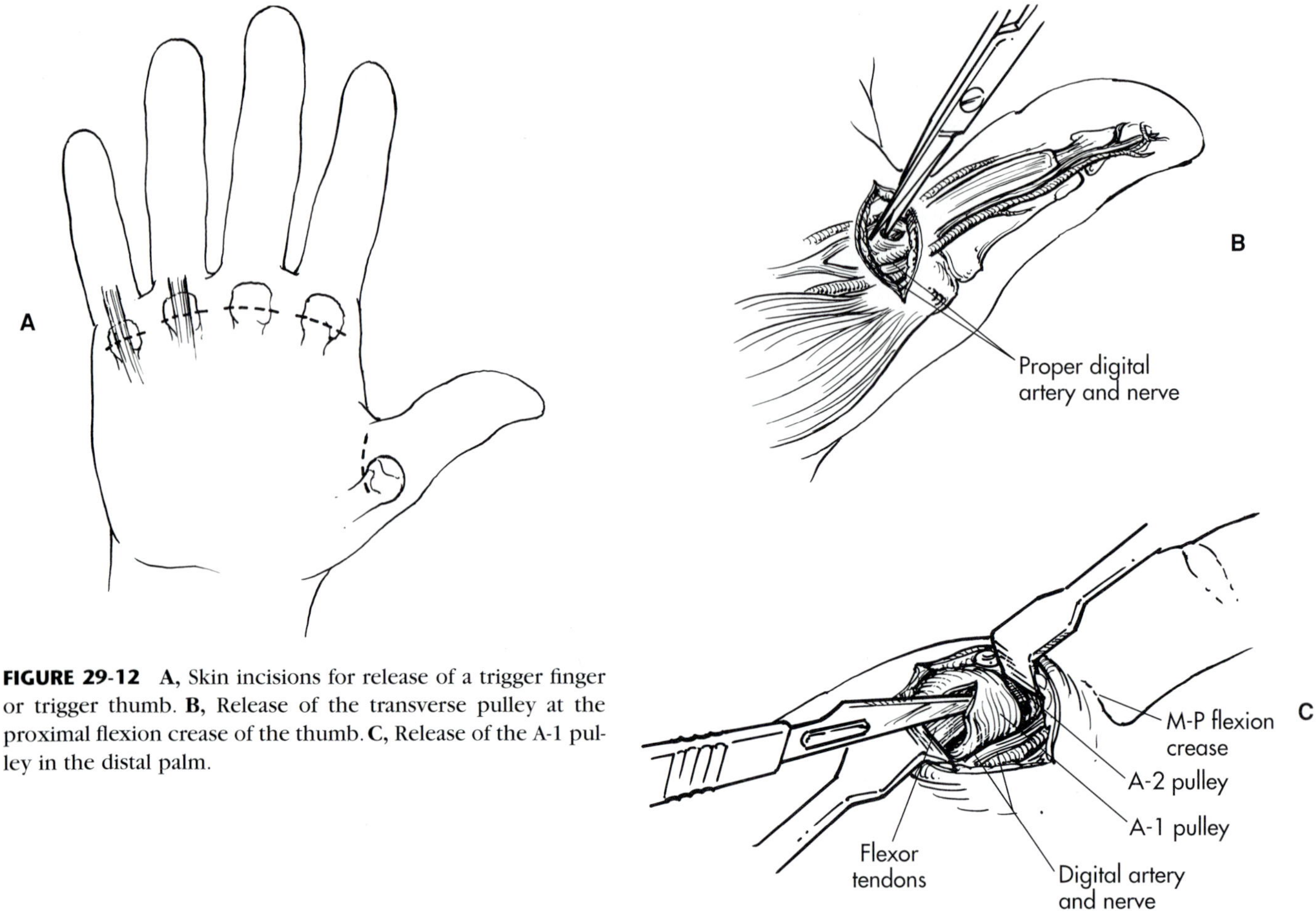

FIGURE 29-12 **A,** Skin incisions for release of a trigger finger or trigger thumb. **B,** Release of the transverse pulley at the proximal flexion crease of the thumb. **C,** Release of the A-1 pulley in the distal palm.

over the volar radial distal forearm. If index finger flexion is passively restricted, the pain is worsened.

If the condition is sufficiently symptomatic and correct conservative treatment fails, a surgical excision of the anomalous tendon slip will relieve the patient's symptoms.

SKIN CONDITIONS

Calluses and blisters are common in athletes such as gymnasts, weight lifters, and rowers who constantly exert frictional stress on their hands, primarily the palmar aspect of the hand and fingers.

Calluses can be controlled with appropriate taping and protective devices.[4] If they get too large, the calluses can be trimmed.

Blisters often are noted in the throwing hand of baseball pitchers. Appropriate conservative measures, such as ice, medication to toughen the skin, and aspiration of the blister to flatten it frequently resolve the problem. If the blister tears, the skin should be excised and the wound exposed.

Good hygiene to the skin of the hand and upper extremity will relieve many skin problems secondary to a variety of irritants, including excessive sweating.

References

1. Arons MS: De Quervain's release in working women: a report of failures, complications and associated diagnosis, *J Hand Surg* 12A:540-544, 1987.
2. Belsole RJ: De Quervain's tenosynovitis—diagnostic and operative complications, *Orthopaedics* 4:899-903, 1981.
3. Bishop AT, Gabel G, Carmichael SW: Flexor carpi radialis tendinitis. Part I. Operative anatomy, *J Bone Joint Surg* 76A:1009-1014, 1994.
4. Cabrera JM, McCue FC: Non-osseous athletic injuries of the elbow, forearm and hand, *Clin Sports Med* 5:681-700, 1986.
5. Carroll RE, Coyle MP: Dysfunction of the piso-triquetral joint: treatment by excision of the pisiform, *J Hand Surg* 10A:703-707, 1985.
6. Cuono CB, Watson HK: The carpal boss: surgical treatment and etiological considerations, *Plast Reconstr Surg* 63:88-93, 1979.
7. Dobyns JH, Sim FH, Linscheid RL: Sports stress syndromes of the hand and wrist, *Am J Sports Med* 6:236-253, 1978.
8. Fahey JJ, Bollinger JA: Trigger finger in adults and children, *J Bone Joint Surg* 36A:1200-1218, 1954.
9. Finkelstein H: Stenosing tendovaginitis at the radial styloid process, *J Bone Joint Surg* 12A:509-540, 1930.
10. Gabel G, Bishop AT, Wood MB: Flexor carpi radialis tendinitis. Part II. results of operative treatment, *J Bone Joint Surg* 76A:1015-1018, 1994.
11. Grundberg AB, Reagan DS: Pathologic anatomy of the forearm: intersection syndrome, *J Hand Surg* 10A:299-302, 1985.
12. Harvey FJ, Harvey PM, Horsley MW: De Quervain's disease: surgical or non-surgical treatment, *J Hand Surg* 15A:83-87, 1990.
13. Helal B: Racquet player's pisiform, *Hand* 10:87-89, 1978.
14. Hueston JT, Wilson WF: The aetiology of trigger finger, *Hand* 4:257-260, 1972.

15. Jackson WT et al: Anatomical variations in the first extensor compartment of the wrist, *J Bone Joint Surg* 68-A:923-926, 1986.
16. Johnson RK: Soft tissue injuries of the forearm and hand, *Clin Sports Med* 5:701-707, 1986.
17. Leao L: De Quervain's disease: a clinical and anatomic study, *J Bone Joint Surg* 40-A:1063-1070, 1958.
18. Leslie BM, Ericson WB, Morehead JR: Incidence of a septum within the first dorsal compartment of the wrist, *J Hand Surg* 15A:88-91, 1990.
19. Linburg RM, Comstock BE: Anomalous tendon slips from the flexor pollicis longus to the flexor digitorum profundus, *J Hand Surg* 4:79-83, 1979.
20. Lipscomb PR: Tenosynovitis of the hand and wrist: carpal tunnel syndrome, de Quervain's disease, trigger digit, *Clin Orthop* 13:164-181, 1959.
21. McCue FC, Cabrera JM: Common athletic digital joint injuries of the hand. In Strickland JW, Rettig AC, editors: *Hand injuries in athletes,* Philadelphia, 1992, WB Saunders, pp 49-94.
22. Manske PR, Ogata K, Lesker PA: Nutrient pathways to extensor tendons of primates, *J Hand Surg* 10B:8-10, 1985.
23. Newport ML, Lane LB, Stuchin SA: Treatment of trigger finger by steroid injection, *J Hand Surg* 15A:748-750, 1990.
24. Palmieri TJ: Pisiform area pain treatment by pisiform excision, *J Hand Surg* 7:477-480, 1982.
25. Patel MR, Bassini L: Trigger fingers and thumb: when to splint, inject or operate, *J Hand Surg* 17A:110-113.
26. Rayan GM: Distal stenosing tenosynovitis, *J Hand Surg* 15A:973-975, 1990.
27. Rhoades CE, Gelberman RH, Manjarris JF: Stenosing tenosynovitis of the fingers and thumb: results of a prospective trial of steroid injection and splinting, *Clin Orthop* 190:236-238, 1984.
28. Ritter MA, Ingles AE: The extensor indicis proprius syndrome, *J Bone Joint Surg* 51A:1645-1648, 1969.
29. Spinner M, Olshansky K: The extensor indicis proprius syndrome: a clinical test, *Plast Reconstr Surg* 51:134-138, 1973.
30. Thorson E, Szabo RM: Common tendinitis problems in the hand and forearm, *Orthop Clin North Am* 23:65-74, 1992.
31. Williams JGP: Surgical management of traumatic non-infective tenosynovitis of the wrist extensors, *J Bone Joint Surg* 59B:408-410, 1977.
32. Witczak JW, Masear VR, Meyer RD: Triggering of the thumb with de Quervain's stenosing tendovaginitis, *J Hand Surg* 15A:265-268, 1990.
33. Wood MB, Dobyns JH: Sports-related extra-articular wrist syndromes, *Clin Orthop* 202:93-102, 1986.

CHAPTER 30

Fractures and Ligament Injuries of the Wrist

NORMAN P. ZEMEL

The wrist is a complex structure consisting of multiple articulations involving eight carpal bones, the distal radius and ulna, and the bases of the five metacarpals. In addition to their bony configuration, the many joints within the wrist are stabilized by extrinsic and intrinsic ligaments. In a review of injuries at the Olympic training center in Colorado Springs, Colorado, from January 1977 to October 1986, hand and wrist injuries accounted for 9% of the injuries recorded. Fifteen sports accounted for 80% of these injuries, and about 50% of hand and wrist injuries were sprains.[123]

Most wrist injuries in athletes seem to result from a fall or injury to the dorsiflexed wrist. This places a tensile load on the palmar aspect of the wrist and a compression load on the dorsum of the wrist.[81] Hyperextension and radial deviation of the wrist result in a fracture of the scaphoid, whereas hyperextension and ulnar deviation of the wrist can produce a scapholunate dissociation. Mayfield and Johnson[91] described the stages of perilunate injuries that can occur with and without carpal fractures. These injuries result from a fall on the outstretched extremity with the wrist in dorsiflexion, ulnar deviation, and intercarpal supination.

Although any type of wrist injury can result from athletic activity, certain injuries seem to occur more often, and these will be discussed in this chapter.

Fortunately, most injuries about the wrist are minor sprains, strains, or contusions, and they readily heal with conservative treatment and intelligent rehabilitation. If seemingly minor injuries to the wrist do not improve with conservative treatment, and a nagging pain, weakness, or inability to actively participate in sports persists, additional evaluation is indicated. The clinician should not dismiss the individual's complaints. Misdiagnosing a serious injury, such as a scaphoid fracture or scapholunate injury as a minor sprain, can significantly increase the amount of time the athlete will lose from competition. In addition, a delay in treatment often can compromise the available treatment options.

FRACTURE OF THE CARPUS

Fractures of the scaphoid account for 8% of all fractures in organized sports[119] and for 70% of carpal bone fractures.[15,18,27] Although the other carpal bones are fractured infrequently, they must be considered in any acute wrist injury or an injury that does not readily respond to treatment. Although a fracture of the hamate is not common, the hook of the hamate can be fractured as a result of playing golf, tennis, baseball, racquetball, and squash.[165]

Any wrist injury must be accurately evaluated for a fracture of one of the carpal bones. The treating physician or trainer should have a high index of suspicion. Clinical findings often are minimal, and good radiographs of the wrist are extremely important because there is considerable overlap of the contours of the carpal bones. Special radiographic views may be needed to isolate the individual carpal bones.

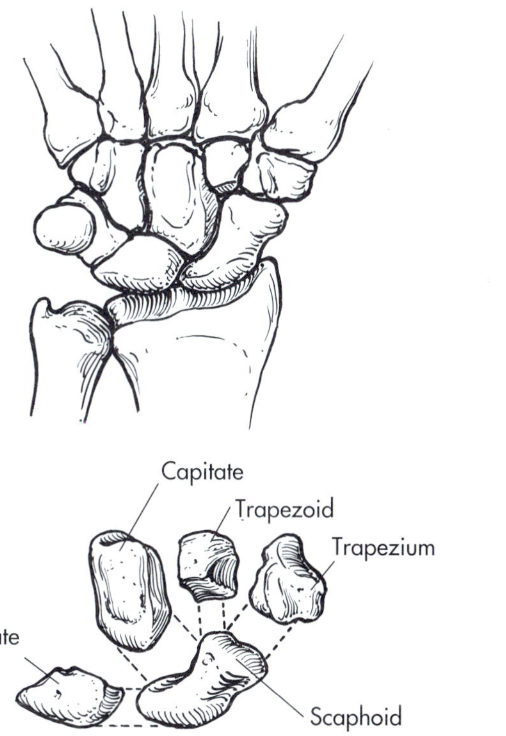

FIGURE 30-1 The scaphoid and its relationship to the carpal bones.

FRACTURE OF THE SCAPHOID

The scaphoid, which is almost completely covered by articular cartilage, articulates with the radius and lunate proximally and the capitate on its ulnar side, and it forms the scaphotrapeziotrapezoid joint distally (Fig. 30-1). It spans the proximal and distal carpal rows, and it acts as a mechanical link between these two rows of bones.[46] In normal wrists, a strong volar ligament (radioscaphocapitate) acts as a sling and maintains the bone in 30° to 60° of flexion in relation to the lunate.[80]

The scaphoid receives its blood supply through ligamentous attachments. Taleisnik and Kelly[141] described three main arterial groups that are the primary blood supply to the proximal two thirds of the scaphoid.

Gelberman et al studied the extraosseous and intraosseous vascularity of the human carpus.[54,111] The extraosseous blood supply comes from a network of dorsal and palmar arches from the radial and ulnar arteries. Additional anastomoses are supplied by the anterior interosseous artery. Between 70% and 80% of the intraosseous blood supply, including the proximal pole of the scaphoid, is from branches of the radial artery that enter the dorsal ridge of the bone near the waist. Gelberman and Menon[52] concluded that a volar operative approach to the scaphoid is the least harmful to the blood supply of the proximal pole of the scaphoid. The scaphoid is at risk for avascular necrosis after a fracture because it has large intraosseous areas that depend on one vessel.[111] Investigators estimate that 30% of middle-third fractures and almost 100% of proximal-fifth fractures of the scaphoid will develop avascular necrosis of the proximal pole of the bone.[102,129]

As a result of its position connecting the two carpal rows, the scaphoid is especially vulnerable to injury when the wrist is loaded in dorsiflexion. Weber and Chao[155] were able to produce fractures through the waist of cadaver scaphoids when the wrists were in 95° to 100° of dorsiflexion and the load was primarily on the radial side of the palm. The load forces between the articular surface of the scaphoid and radius were four times that on the palm. The proximal pole of the scaphoid was trapped between the radius and capitate, and the fracture occurred at the unsupported waist of the scaphoid. Experimentally, and probably clinically as well, the scaphoid waist fracture originates on the volar ulnar surface of the bone (tension side) and extends to the dorsal lateral surface (compression side).

In a study on fractures of the distal radius, Frykman was able to consistently produce fractures of the waist of the scaphoid when the waist was dorsiflexed more than 90° and also radially deviated.[48] If a lesser degree of dorsiflexion was present, the distal radius would fracture. Although the findings on physical examination may be

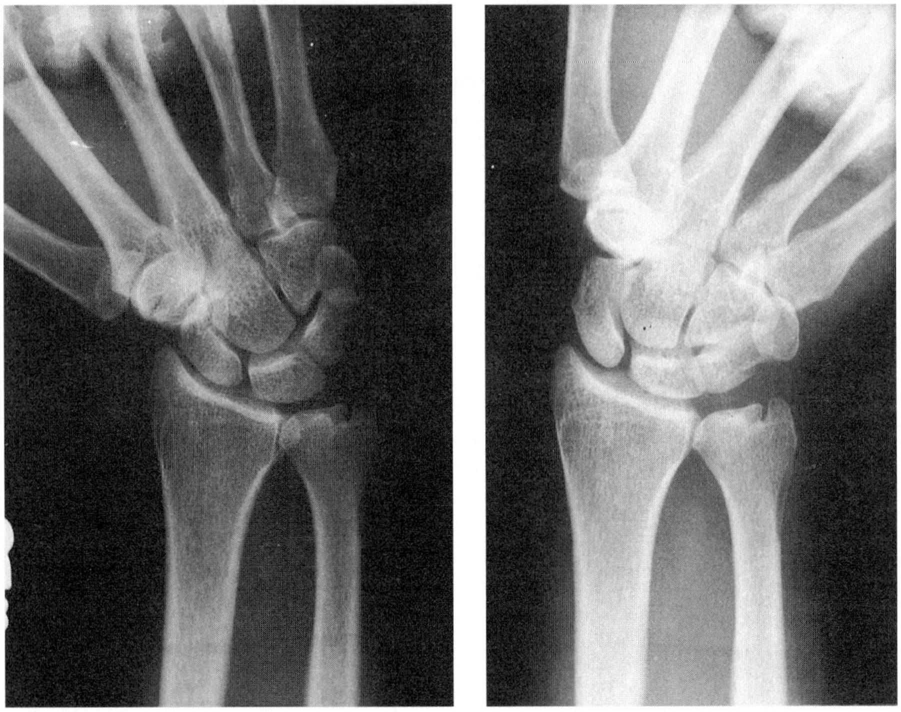

FIGURE 30-2 Stress views of the scaphoid allow the entire bone to be seen and can be used to show motion at a nonunion site of the bone.

only minimal, a history of a fall and injury to the wrist in an adult male between the ages of 17 and 30 should be considered a fracture of the scaphoid until proven otherwise. Swelling may be only slight, pain may be present with wrist motion, and wrist motion may not be significantly restricted. However, tenderness over the dorsoradial aspect of the wrist and in the anatomic snuff box should alert the physician to the possibility of a scaphoid fracture.

Radiographic examination of the wrist should include a six-view series (scaphoid series). This consists of a posterior-anterior (PA) view, lateral view, right and left oblique views, and stress views. The stress views are taken as a PA view of the wrist in radial deviation and ulnar deviation with the fingers curled into a fist (Fig. 30-2). By making a fist, the patient elevates the scaphoid into a more horizontal position, and ulnar deviation tends to profile the entire bone. If no fracture is seen, the wrist should be immobilized in a splint and the radiograph repeated in 2 weeks.[67,94,129] Resorption at the fracture site may allow the fracture to be seen on the subsequent radiographs. Other useful imaging modalities are bone scan, polytomography, and computerized tomography.[35,50,67] If the bone scan is negative, a fracture usually can be ruled out. However, if the bone scan is positive, more definitive studies, such as polytomograms or a CT scan, should be ordered. This author prefers the CT scan in the coronal and sagittal views as the best method of viewing the scaphoid.

Acute fractures of the scaphoid have been classified by various methods. Russe[129] classified scaphoid fractures into horizontal oblique (35%), transverse (60%), and vertical oblique (5%) based on the relationship of the fracture line to the longitudinal axis of the scaphoid. The first two types he considered stable because of compression forces at the fracture site, but the vertical oblique fracture was unstable and more at risk for delayed union or nonunion because of shear forces at the fracture site. Weber[156] and Cooney et al[27] distinguished between undisplaced and displaced fractures. Cooney et al[27] considered a fracture displaced and unstable if there was more than a 1-mm offset on the PA or oblique radiographic views. Other criteria used were a lunocapitate angle of more than 15° or a scapholunate angle of more than 45° on the lateral radiograph. The authors stressed the position of the lunate as an indicator of carpal instability secondary to fracture of the scaphoid. Dorsal angulation at the fracture site of the scaphoid causes the lunate to rotate dorsally and produces a dorsal intercalated segmental instability (DISI collapse deformity).[27,46,133] Herbert and Fisher[60] described a classification of scaphoid fractures that includes anatomy, stability, and time from injury. This classification is divided into four types (stable acute fractures, unstable acute fractures, delayed union, and established nonunion), and each major type is subdivided.

Investigators generally agree that approximately 70% of scaphoid fractures occur through the middle third

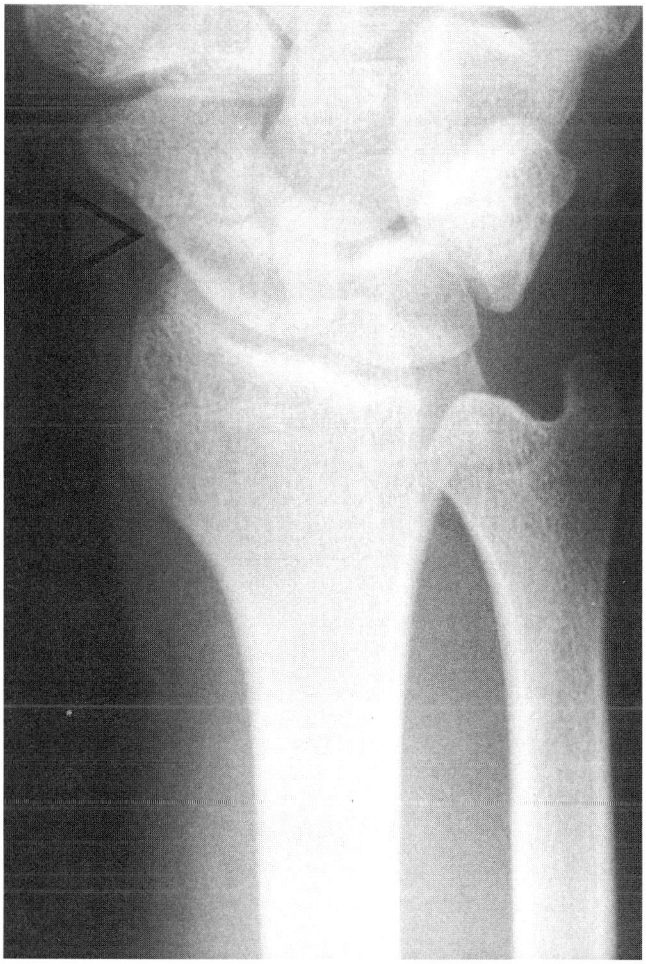

FIGURE 30-3 Undisplaced middle-third fracture of the scaphoid.

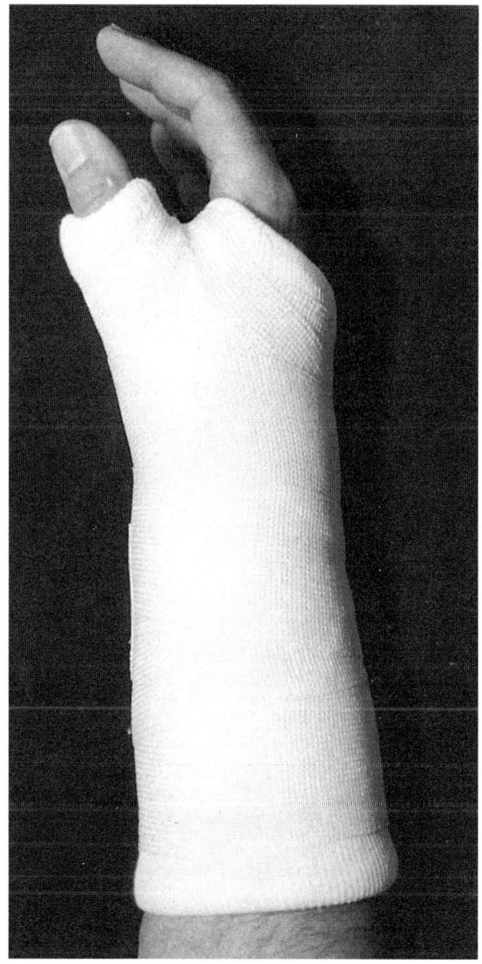

FIGURE 30-4 A below-elbow thumb spica cast for an acute undisplaced scaphoid fracture.

(waist), 20% through the proximal third, and 10% through the distal third of the bone.[129]

Middle-Third Fractures

These fractures account for 70% of scaphoid injuries. If diagnosed within a few days from injury and properly immobilized, 95% of undisplaced or minimally displaced fractures of the scaphoid will unite within 3 months[27,129,140,156] (Fig. 30-3).

A variety of cast types and wrist positions to treat this fracture have been described in the literature.[4,126] This author prefers to immobilize the wrist with a short arm thumb spica cast that holds the wrist in neutral (Fig. 30-4). The thumb is immobilized in abduction and opposition, and the cast can either include the tip of the thumb or stop ½ inch proximal to the distal flexion crease of the thumb. A snug, well-molded fiberglass cast is best because it does not tend to loosen as readily as plaster. The cast should be changed every 3 to 4 weeks. After the bone has healed, as verified by radiographic examination, the cast is discontinued and range of motion of the wrist is started. Athletes may return to competition using a rigid protective wrist splint. Strenuous use of the wrist without external protection should not be allowed for an additional 2 months. The specific rehabilitation program is determined by the sport and the athlete's level of competition.

Out of every 100 college-level U.S. football players, 1 athlete breaks the scaphoid each year. Riester et al[124] allowed 13 athletes with 14 scaphoid fractures to participate in contact sports while their fractures were being treated. Because NCAA and high-school rules do not allow the use of an unyielding material below the elbow, a custom-made Silastic short arm thumb spica cast was applied before and removed immediately after each game or practice. Plaster immobilization was used at all other times. All fractures were considered stable, and 10 of 11 middle-third fractures healed.

McCue et al[85] also used a silicone cast during athletic competition.

Some authors have advocated cast immobilization and electrical stimulation to treat scaphoid fractures.[49] This

A

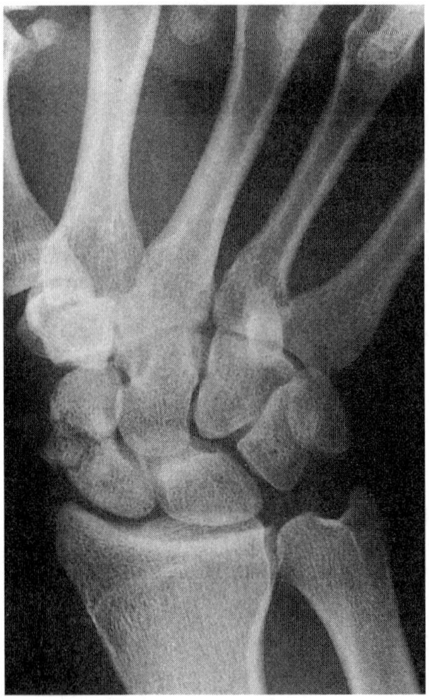

B

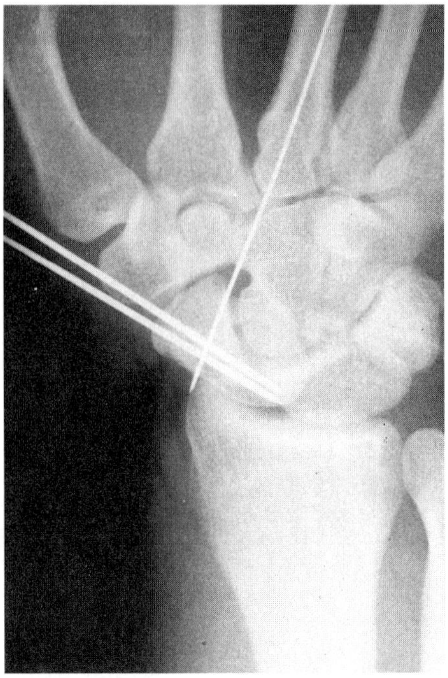

C

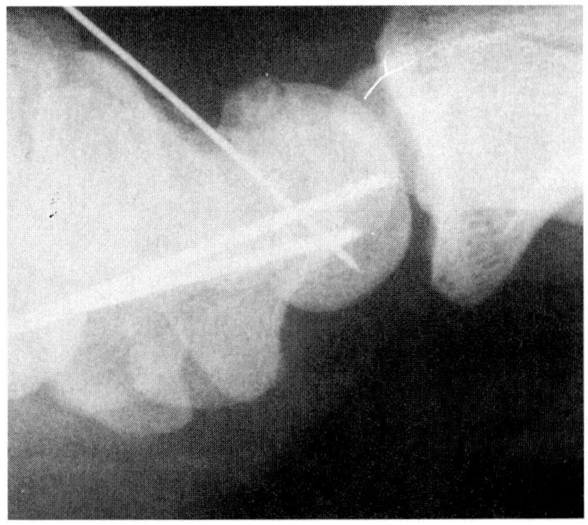

FIGURE 30-5 **A,** A comminuted middle-third fracture of the scaphoid. **B,** Good stability and reduction of the fracture was obtained on the AP view and, **C,** on the lateral view.

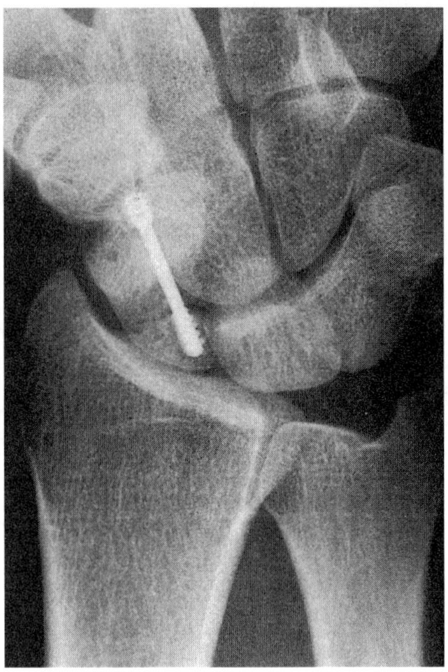

FIGURE 30-6 A proximal-third fracture of the scaphoid is stabilized with a Herbert screw.

method of treatment should be used only for undisplaced scaphoid fractures or stable nonunions.

If an acute scaphoid fracture is displaced, angulated, or associated with carpal instability or cannot be maintained by closed manipulation and cast immobilization, it should be treated with open reduction and internal fixation with either Kirschner wires or screws[46,60,61,90,165] (Fig. 30-5). This should be performed without delay. It is then easier to restore the articular surfaces of the bone, prevent malunion of the scaphoid, restore the lunate to proper alignment, and ideally prevent future arthritis of the wrist.

The volar radial aspect of the wrist is opened through the Russe approach[129] (see Fig. 30-10). A relatively avascular plane between the flexor carpi radialis tendon and the radial artery is used to approach the volar capsule of the radiocarpal joint. After the capsule is incised, the fracture usually is readily identified. By gently manipulating the bone fragments, the surgeon can reduce and immobilize the fracture. After the scaphoid fracture is reduced and stabilized, the malalignment of the lunate often is also corrected. Although the author generally prefers to use Kirschner wires cut off beneath the skin, the choice of internal fixation should depend on the surgeon's preference and personal experience[4,126] (Fig. 30-6). Whipple[161] recently described an arthroscopically assisted technique for scaphoid fracture fixation using a cannulated Herbert-Whipple screw. Intraoperative radiographs may be taken to determine whether the bony alignment has been corrected. Unless there is

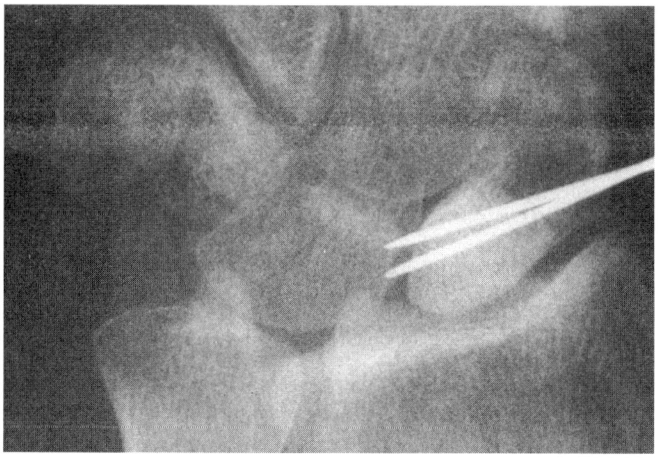

FIGURE 30-7 A healed scaphoid fracture in spite of avascular necrosis of the proximal pole.

significant comminution at the fracture site, a bone graft usually is not necessary in the treatment of acute scaphoid fractures.

The hand and wrist are immobilized in an above-elbow thumb spica cast for 6 to 8 weeks, followed by a below-elbow thumb spica cast until the fracture has united. Fracture union is determined by periodic radiographic evaluation of the scaphoid at the time of cast change. Avascular necrosis, which sometimes occurs in the proximal pole of the scaphoid, does not affect the rate of fracture healing, although it can prolong the time to fracture union (Fig. 30-7).

After fracture healing, an appropriate rehabilitation program is undertaken to allow the athlete to return to sports. The time to return to competition will depend on many variables, including the age of the individual, the sport, the level of competition, and the individual's degree of participation in the rehabilitation program.

If there is a persistent radiolucency at the fracture site after prescribed cast immobilization, the clinician must consider a delay in bony union (3 to 4 months) or a nonunion of the fracture (6 months). The scaphoid fails to heal in 5% to 10% of cases[74,129] (Fig. 30-8). Stress radiographs of the scaphoid can be taken to determine whether there is motion at the fracture site. Computed tomography is the most reliable method to determine the presence of bone across the fracture site[116] (Fig. 30-9). Even with a cast, multiplanar cuts of the fracture site can be obtained with a CT scan. If a delayed union is present, additional cast immobilization is indicated. If the scaphoid has not healed after 6 months of continuous immobilization, the surgeon should perform a bone-grafting procedure. Delayed union and nonunion of the scaphoid have been attributed to inadequate immobilization, fracture displacement, instability of the fracture fragments, carpal instability, and inadequate blood supply

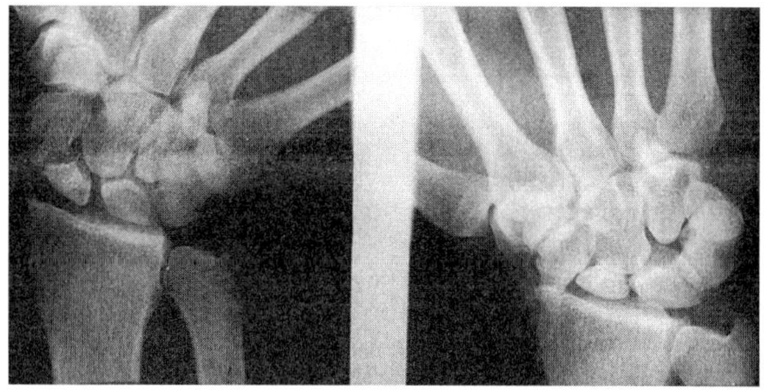

FIGURE 30-8 One year after an injury, radiographs show an ununited fracture of the scaphoid.

A

B

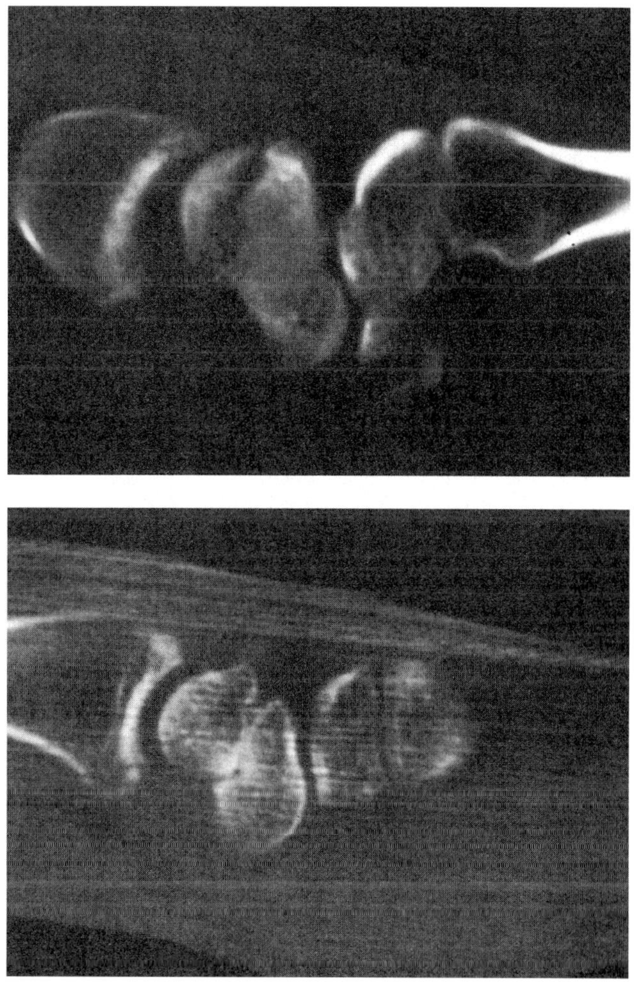

FIGURE 30-9 The CT scan in the sagittal plane shows **A**, minimal healing of the scaphoid fracture. **B**, This patient had partial healing of the bone, and treatment consisted of continued cast immobilization.

of the proximal fragment.[163] Bone grafting combined with some type of internal fixation of the scaphoid is the generally accepted method of treating a scaphoid nonunion.* Radiographic evidence of slight radiocarpal arthritis, cystic changes in the bone, and avascular necrosis of the proximal fragment is not considered a contraindication to bone grafting of a nonunited scaphoid. The iliac crest is the most popular source for the bone graft.

A variety of bone-grafting techniques and internal-fixation devices have been described.[4,126] The Matti-Russe bone-grafting method is the most widely used.[129] Green[57] reported on Russe's modification in which he inserted corticocancellous bone graft across the excavated nonunion site. He also reported a lower rate of successful union of the scaphoid if there is poor vascularity of the proximal fragment. If there is collapse and dorsal angulation at the nonunion site, the anterior wedge graft described by Fisk,[46] Fernandez,[43] and Cooney et al[31] is recommended. Herbert screw fixation, although difficult technically, is probably the most popular screw-fixation technique.[22,47,60,62,152] The results with this technique generally have been favorable.

This author prefers Kirschner wires for internal fixation of the scaphoid because they are easy to insert and later remove, they provide satisfactory stability to the scaphoid as well as stabilizing any associated carpal instability, they can be used in the presence of avascular necrosis, and they do not require extensive dissection of the scaphoid and adjacent joints.

The preferred technique for bone-grafting a scaphoid nonunion is as follows (Fig. 30-10): The radial side of the

*References 4, 27, 28, 56, 57, 60, 126, 137.

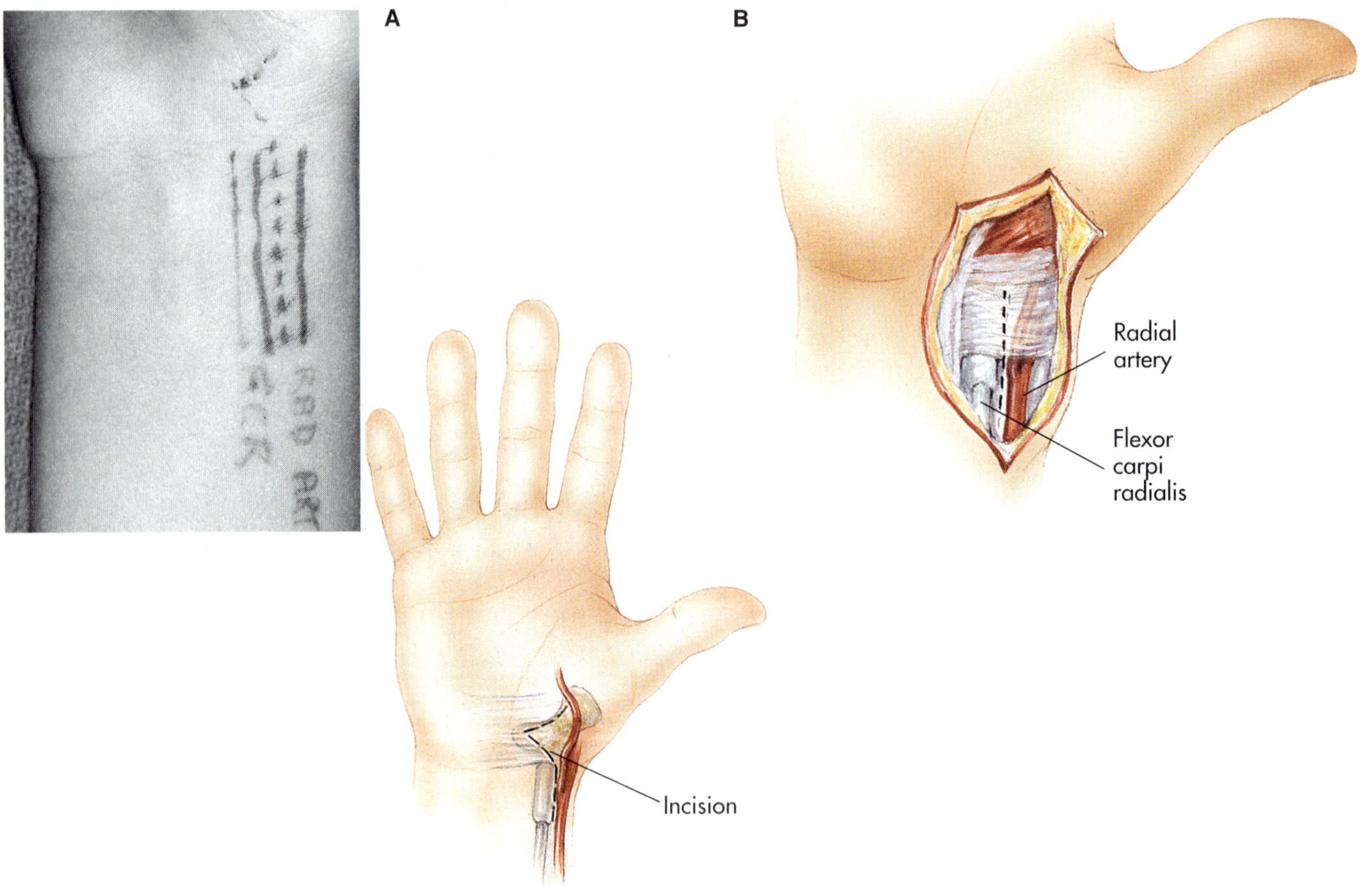

FIGURE 30-10 **A,** The Russe approach to the scaphoid between the radial artery and the flexor carpi radialis tendon. The hand is at the top. **B,** The radiocarpal joint is approached through this relatively avascular plane. **C,** Once the joint capsule is opened, the nonunion site is identified *(arrow)*. **D,** Detritus and scar are removed to create a cavity in which bleeding bone is seen on both sides of the nonunion site. **E,** Kirschner wires are inserted under direct vision and in order to accurately place them in the bone. **F,** After bone is packed into the scaphoid, the Kirschner wires are advanced into subchondral bone of the proximal scaphoid.

C

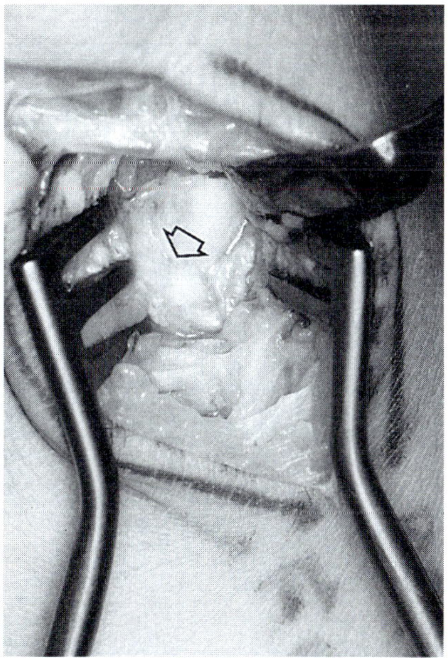

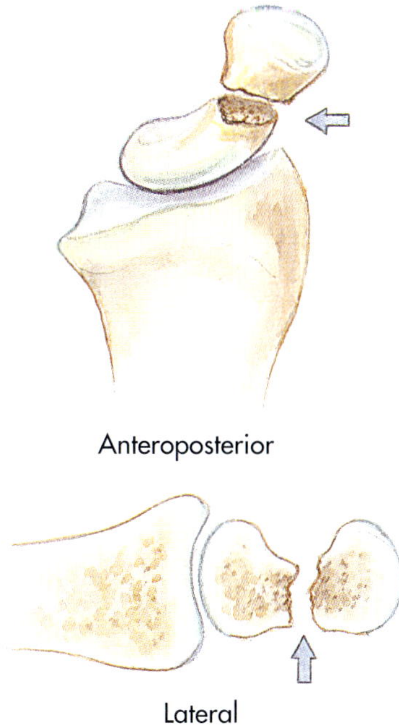
Anteroposterior
Lateral

D

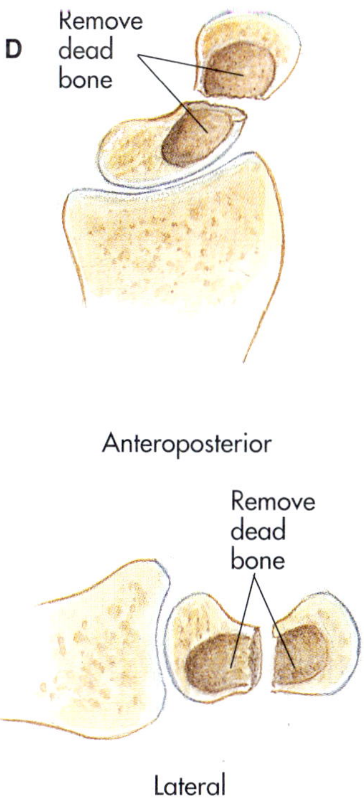
Remove
dead
bone
Anteroposterior
Remove
dead
bone
Lateral

E

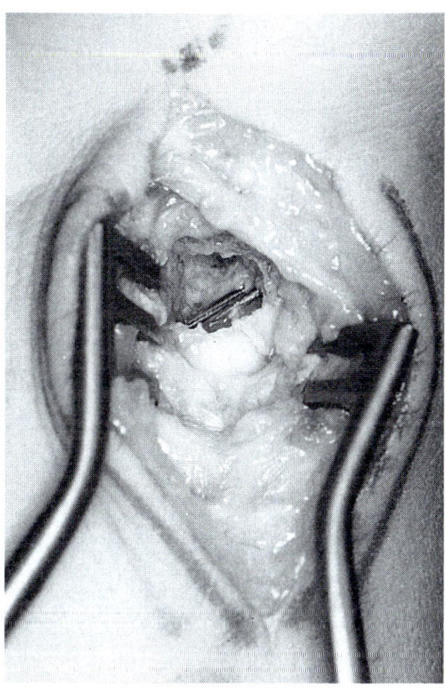

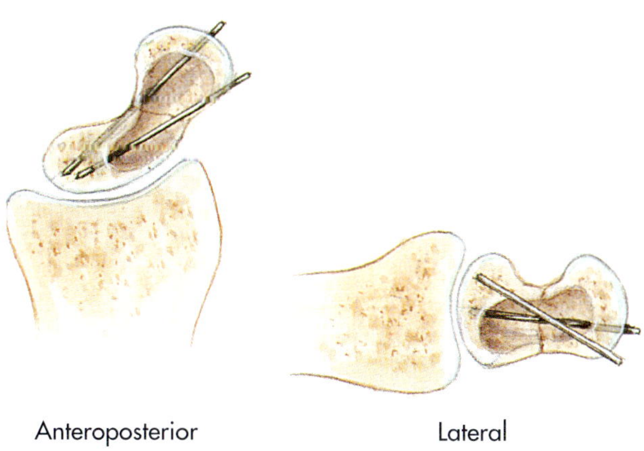
Anteroposterior
Lateral

F

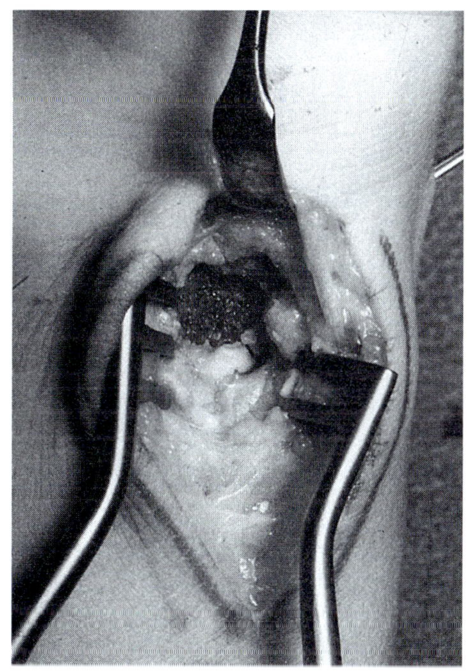

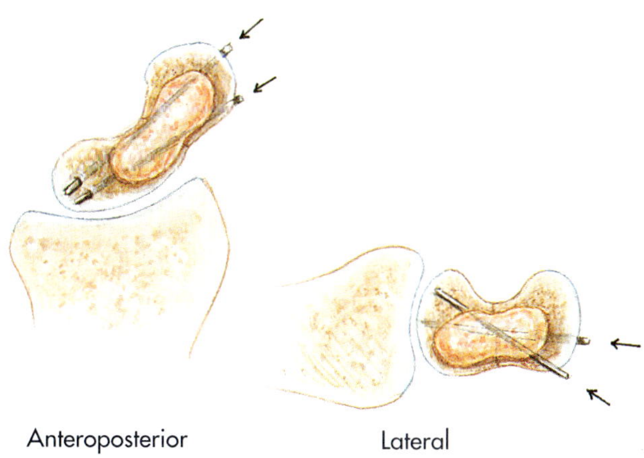
Anteroposterior
Lateral

wrist is opened through a longitudinal incision in the interval between the flexor carpi radialis tendon and the radial artery. The incision can be angulated across the wrist flexion crease if additional exposure is needed. An extension of the incision often is useful when a collapse deformity of the scaphoid is present and additional exposure is needed. The small branches of the radial artery are cauterized. This relatively avascular plane is used to proceed to the radiocarpal joint. The joint capsule and palmar radioscaphoid ligaments are incised. The nonunion site in the middle third of the scaphoid now is usually seen in the center of the field. Radial and ulnar deviation of the wrist will readily demonstrate motion at the nonunion site and also will improve visualization of the entire bone.

A small segment of cortical bone is removed from the palmar side of the proximal and distal halves of the scaphoid. This cortical window can be made with small osteotomes or a rongeur. This allows introduction of instruments to clean out the scar and sclerotic bone from the cavity of the scaphoid. The detritus is removed first with a low-speed burr, and then as bleeding bone is noted, a curette is used to excavate the cavity further and to prevent heat damage to the bone. The distal half of the scaphoid usually requires less débridement than the proximal side. In proximal-third nonunions, the débridement may have to extend to subchondral bone when the proximal fragment is being curetted. This part of the operation must be performed carefully to prevent perforation and injury to the articular cartilage.

After the débridement is completed, a Chandler retractor is used to reduce and approximate the cartilaginous edges of the dorsal and radial sides of the scaphoid. A smooth Kirschner wire (0.9 or 1.1 mm) is inserted percutaneously into the scaphoid with power equipment. The wires are inserted distal to the radial styloid in the direction of the proximal end of the scaphoid. Under direct vision, the position of the Kirschner wires can be adjusted as necessary. Usually two Kirschner wires are used. After the position is deemed to be satisfactory, both Kirschner wires are backed out until the tips are just out of the cavity but still within the bone of the distal half of the scaphoid.

Bone graft from the iliac crest is preferred over bone from other sites. Cancellous bone graft is packed into both sides of the cavity in the scaphoid. Further compressing the cancellous bone with a bone tamp provides additional stability across the nonunion site. A small cortical strut of bone can be inserted just beneath the edges of the window in the proximal and distal parts of the scaphoid if additional stability is needed. Both Kirschner wires then are advanced into the subchondral bone of the proximal scaphoid. The Kirschner wires should not be inserted into or across the radiocarpal joint. This is not always possible, however, especially in proximal-third nonunions. Kirschner wires then are trimmed so that the cut edges are beneath the skin (Fig. 30-11).

Severe resorption of the palmar side of the scaphoid produces increased flexion of the distal fragment with a secondary dorsal collapse deformity of the carpus. If there is a carpal instability associated with a collapse deformity of the scaphoid, an anterior wedge graft is used (Fig. 30-12). The edges of the scaphoid at the nonunion

A

B

C

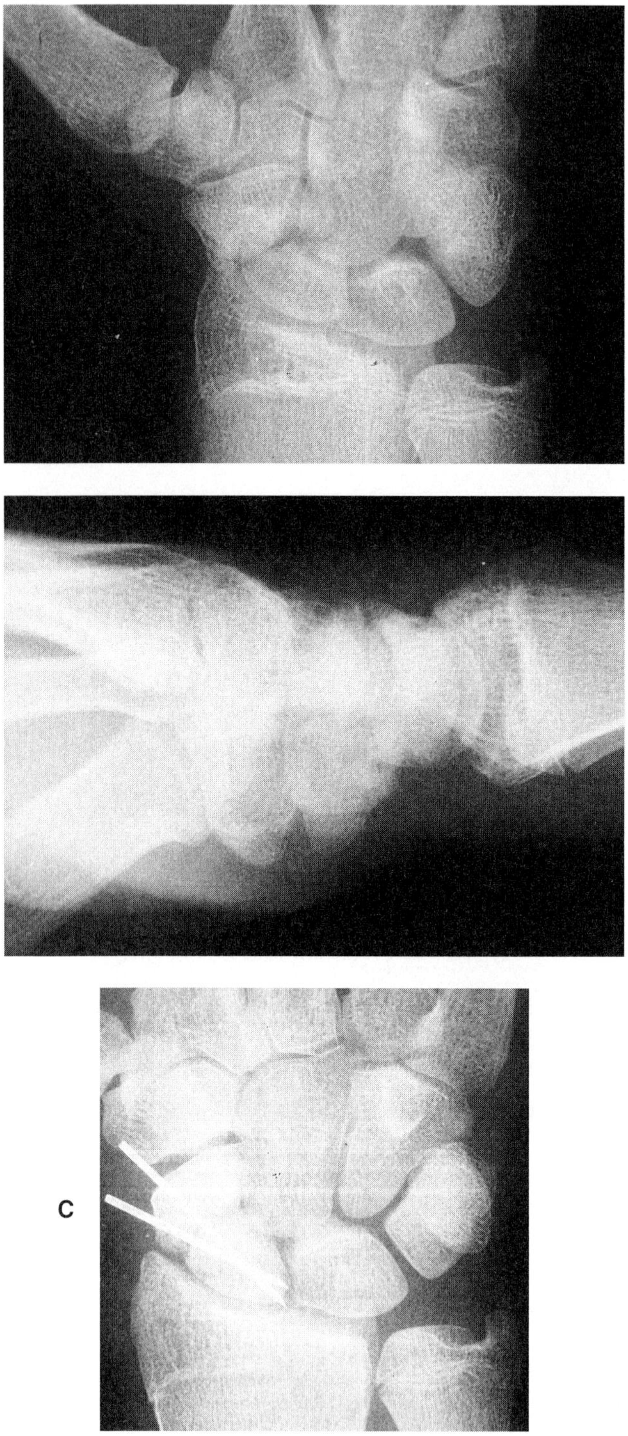

FIGURE 30-11 **A,** AP radiograph shows the middle third scaphoid nonunion while, **B,** the lateral view shows good carpal alignment. **C,** Open reduction, internal fixation, and bone graft of the scaphoid.

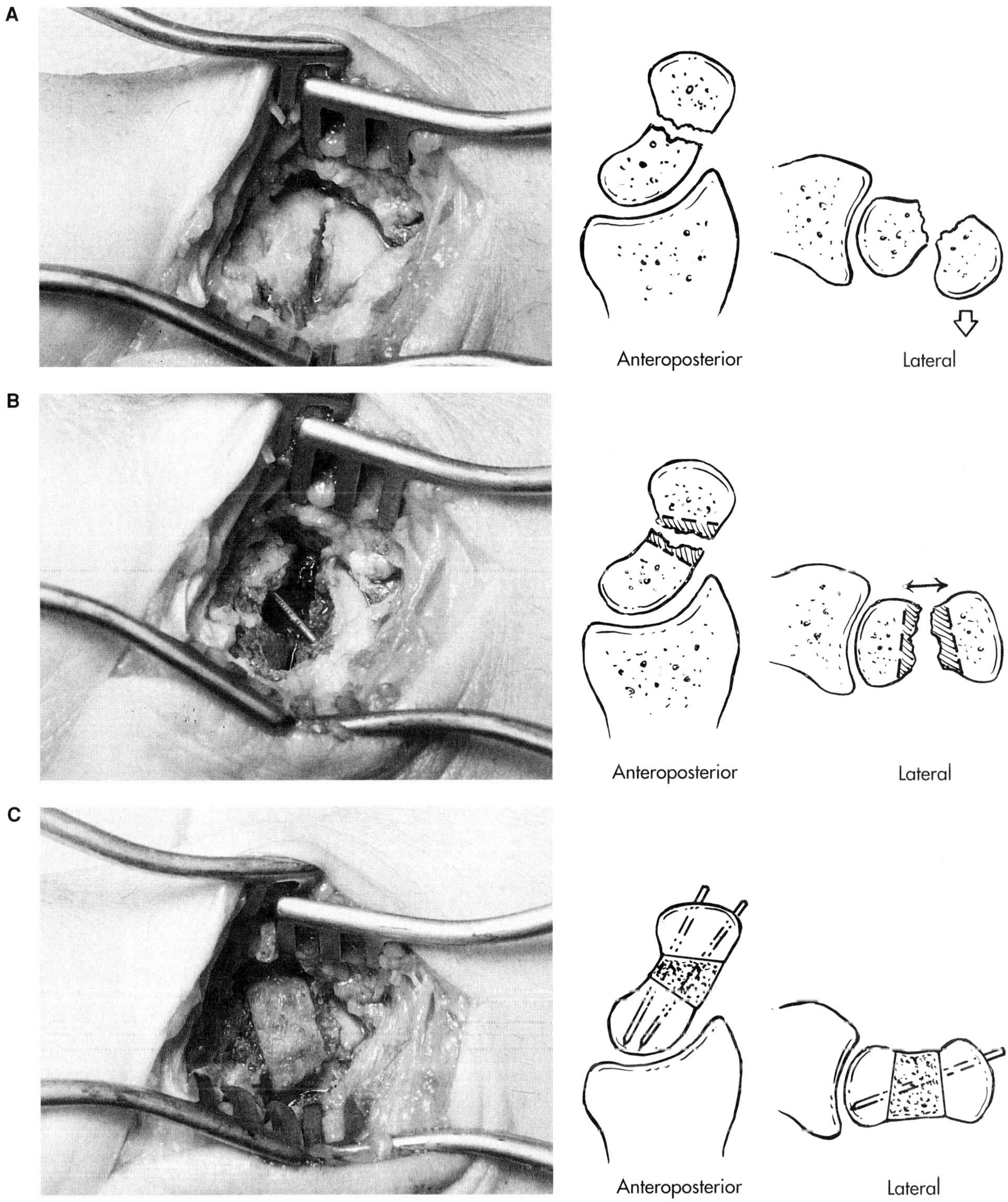

FIGURE 30-12 **A,** A collapse deformity of the scaphoid with dorsal angulation of the bone. The hand is to the left. **B,** Dead bone is removed and the angular deformity is corrected. This creates a trapezoidal-shaped defect in the bone. **C,** A trapezoidal-shaped bone graft is inserted into the defect in the scaphoid.

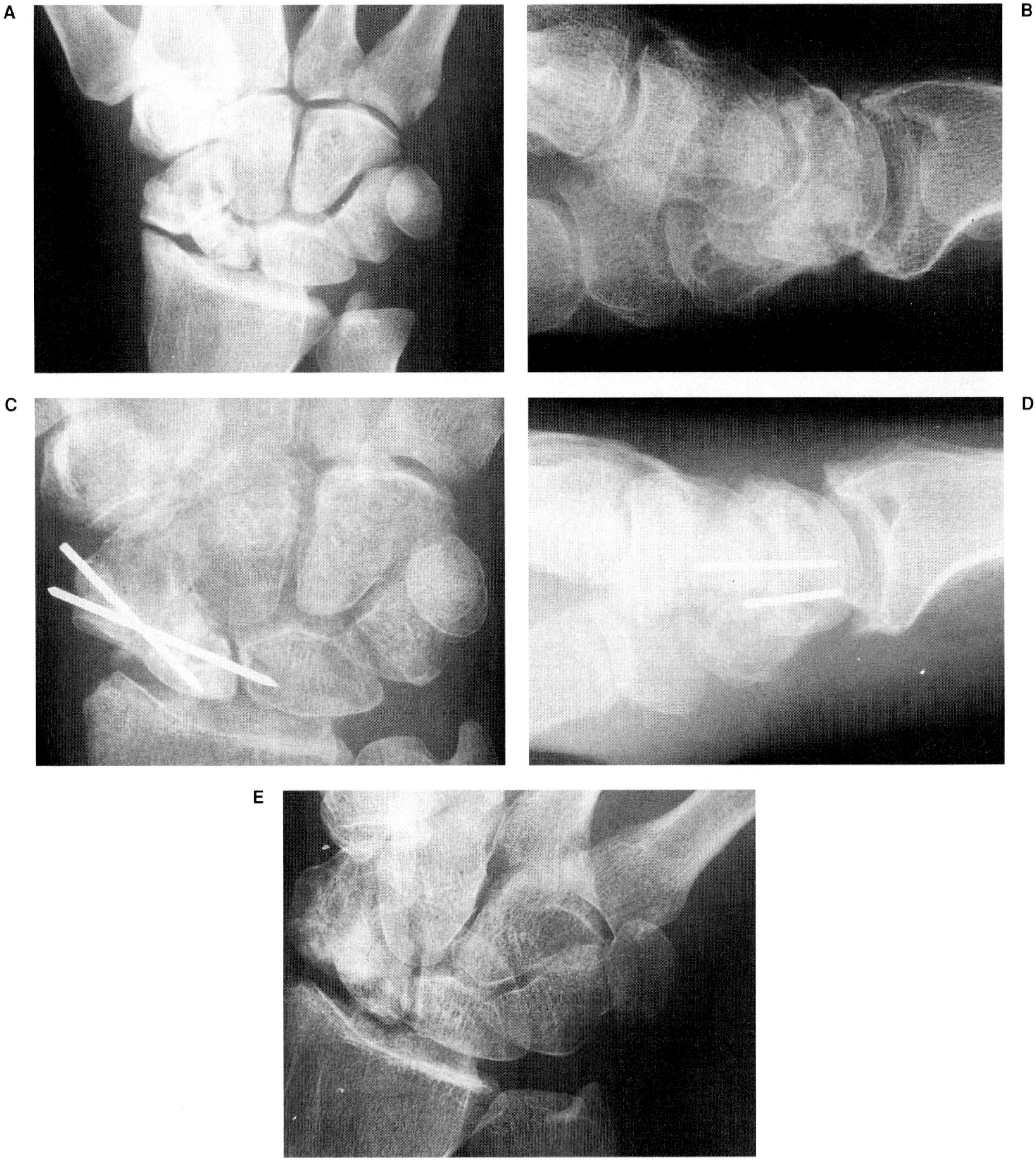

FIGURE 30-13 **A,** Long-standing scaphoid nonunion with early arthritic changes at the radial styloid-scaphoid articulation. **B,** The lateral view shows a DISI deformity. **C,** After open reduction and internal fixation, trapezoidal bone graft, and radial styloidectomy, **D,** the DISI was corrected and, **E,** the scaphoid healed $3\frac{1}{2}$ months after the operation.

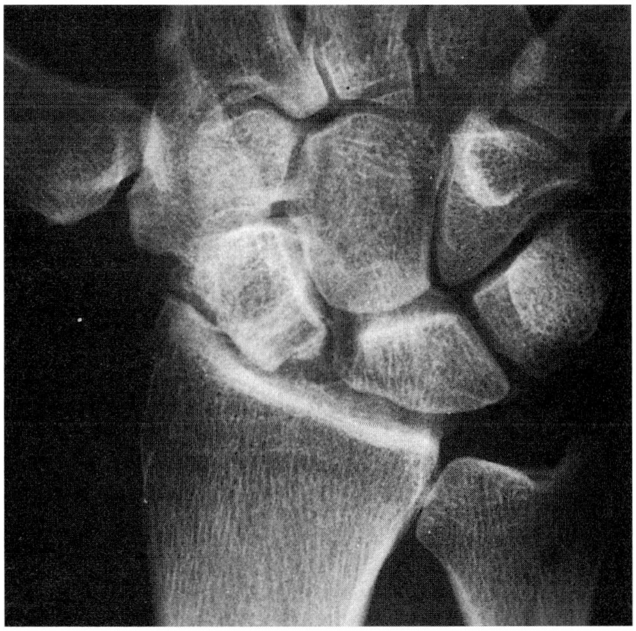

FIGURE 30-14 Degenerative arthritis at the radioscaphoid joint from an untreated fracture of the proximal scaphoid.

site are débrided, and a small spreader is used to reduce (straighten) the scaphoid, thus creating a large palmar defect. A Kirschner wire can be inserted into the lunate and used as a "joy stick" to aid in reducing the lunate, or reduction can be produced by manual pressure. It is not always possible or necessary to completely reduce the carpal instability. The longer the scaphoid nonunion has been present, the more difficult it is to correct the carpal malalignment. When the reduction has been obtained, Kirschner wires are inserted as previously described. A trapezoid-shaped corticocancellous bone graft is taken from the iliac crest and trimmed to fit the defect. The cortical side of the bone graft is palmar and also ulnar if it is necessary to maintain the reduction. The graft should be flush with the palmar surface of the scaphoid. After either procedure, the palmar radiocarpal ligaments are repaired.

Initially, the thumb, hand, and wrist are immobilized in a palmar plaster splint extended as an above-elbow cast. After 10 days, an above-elbow thumb spica cast is applied, and 6 weeks after the operation, a below-elbow thumb spica cast is used until the scaphoid heals as noted on radiographic examination (Fig. 30-13). Healing of a nonunion of the scaphoid usually takes 3 to 4 months. When the bone has healed, the Kirschner wires can be removed under local anesthesia.

Between 86% and 97% of scaphoid nonunions heal with bone-grafting procedures.[4,28,126,129,137] Jiranek et al[65] reported a significant relief of pain (92%), an ability to return to sports (88%), and an improvement in the quality of life enjoyed by the patients (92%). Other long-term follow-up studies[63,137] of scaphoid nonunion treated by bone grafting report long-term relief of pain and a return to a satisfactory lifestyle, including athletics. However, the treated wrists were rarely "normal."

Mack et al[88] and Ruby et al[125] have reported on the "natural history" of scaphoid nonunions. They noted the development of carpal malalignment and arthritis in the wrist if the nonunion is untreated for 5 to 10 years (Fig. 30-14). This degenerative progression of the wrist occurs even if the patient is asymptomatic.[79] The severity of the arthritis increased with time.

Various reconstructive procedures used to treat localized or generalized arthritis of the wrist after scaphoid nonunion can be found in hand-surgery textbooks.

Proximal-Third Fractures

Fractures through the proximal third of the bone account for 20% of scaphoid fractures (Fig. 30-15). Previously discussed vascular studies of the scaphoid[52,54,141] show that the proximal end of the bone is particularly at risk for avascular necrosis. Clinical studies also have shown that proximal-third scaphoid fractures take longer to heal.[27,129,137]

The treatment of proximal-third fractures of the scaphoid depends on the size, vascularity, and condition of the bone (fragmented) and the age of the fracture.

An acute undisplaced fracture of the proximal third of the scaphoid (or even a smaller proximal fragment) can be treated with cast immobilization. If the fracture is displaced, it should be treated with open reduction and internal fixation. The bone probably will unite in 3 to 4 months. When the proximal fragment is less than one third of the bone, a dorsal approach can be used to reduce and stabilize the fracture. De Maagd and Engber[36] used a Herbert screw, inserted freehand through a dorsal approach, to unite 11 of 12 scaphoid fractures.

If a nonunion develops, the treatment will depend on the size of the proximal fragment. If the proximal fragment is large enough and has sufficient bone, the surgeon should perform a bone graft in conjunction with internal fixation (Matti-Russe).[137] When the proximal fragment is very small, sclerotic, deformed, or fragmented, it can be excised and a hand-curved Silastic spacer inserted[162] (Fig. 30-16). Patients having this procedure, as reported by Zemel et al, were able to return to recreational sports such as golf, tennis, racquetball, baseball, and basketball. Silicone synovitis, a significant complication with complete scaphoid replacement,[69,134] has not proven to be a problem with replacement of small proximal pole fragments. A rolled-up tendon (palmaris longus) or fascia also can be used to replace an excised small proximal pole of the scaphoid.

Pulsed electromagnetic-field stimulation has been less effective in treating proximal-third nonunions (62.5%) than middle-third or distal-third injuries.[49]

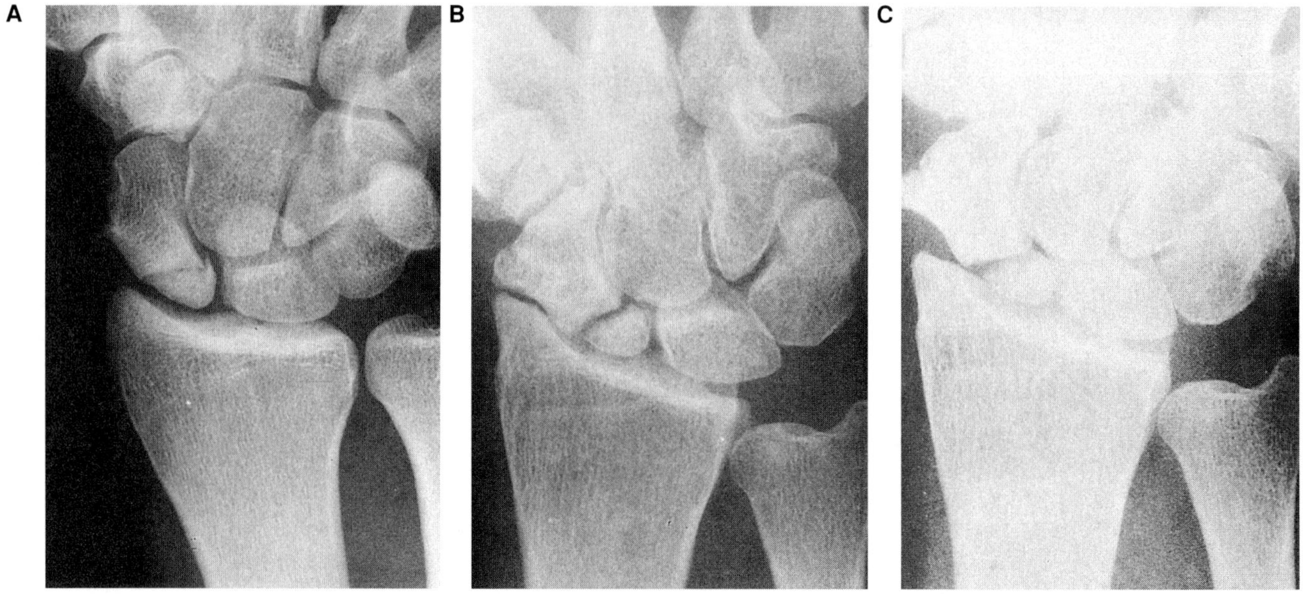

FIGURE 30-15 **A,** Fracture of the proximal third of the scaphoid. Stress view of the scaphoid shows a nonunion of a proximal third fracture. **B,** Radial deviation. **C,** Ulnar deviation.

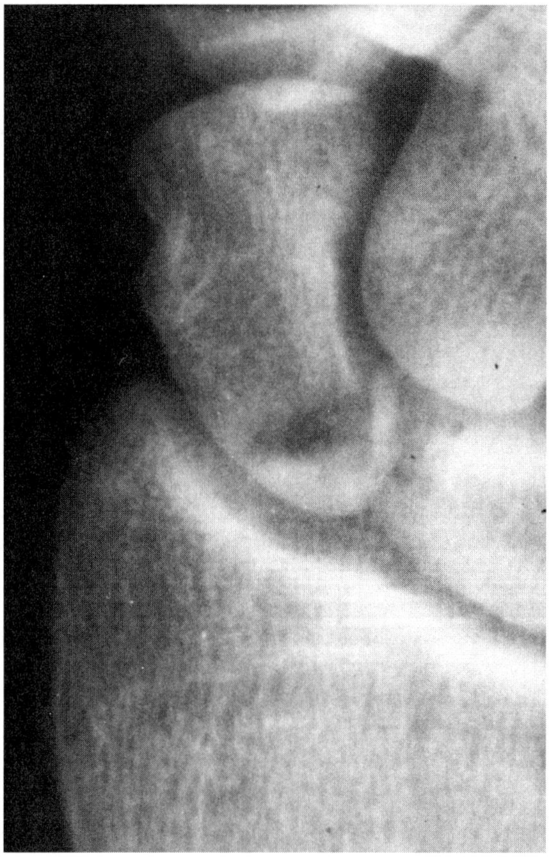

FIGURE 30-16 This very small proximal fragment should be excised.

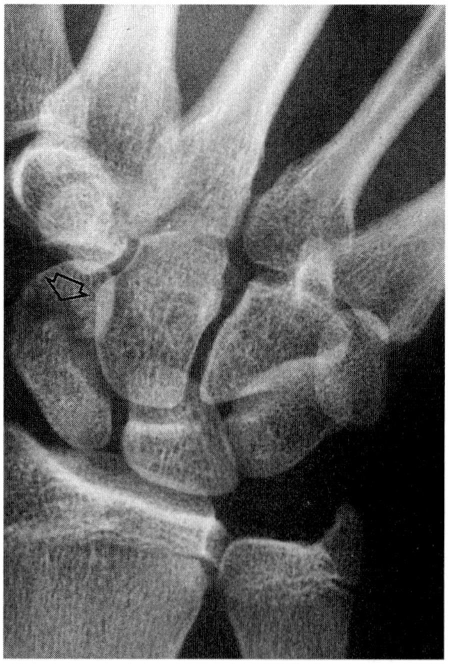

FIGURE 30-17 Fracture of the distal third of the scaphoid *(arrow)*. These generally occur in younger patients.

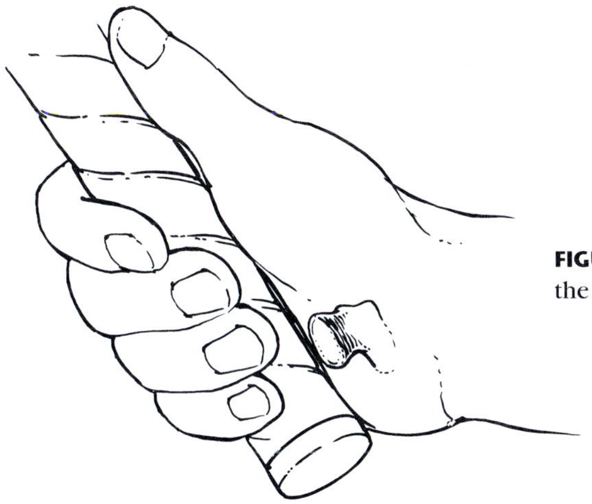

FIGURE 30-18 The hook of the hamate is usually fractured by the end of a racquet, golf club, or bat.

Distal-Third Fractures

Scaphoid fractures occur in the distal third at a rate of 10% or less (Fig. 30-17). Fractures involving the distal third of the bone or the scaphoid tuberosity are stable and readily heal within 6 to 8 weeks with cast immobilization.[129,137] If the tuberosity fails to unite and remains painful, it can be excised.

Prosser et al[120] classified distal scaphoid fractures into three types. Type II, a scaphotrapezial intraarticular fracture, must be treated with open reduction and internal fixation if the offset at the articular surface of the bone is unacceptable.

FRACTURE OF THE HAMATE

The body of the hamate is on the dorsoulnar aspect of the wrist, while the hook (hamulus) protrudes volarward into the base of the hypothenar eminence. The hook serves as an attachment for the pisohamate ligament, the short flexors and opponens muscles of the little finger, and the transverse carpal ligament. These structures afford stability to the hook, but when the hook is broken, they become deforming forces and interfere with bone healing by exerting intermittent tension on the bone fragment. This long bony prominence is found 1 to 2 cm radial and distal from the pisiform. The motor branch of the ulnar nerve passes on the ulnar side of the base of the hook of the hamate. Ulnar and adjacent to the apex of the hook is the sensory branch of the ulnar nerve and the ulnar artery. On the radial side of the base of the hook lie the flexor tendons to the ring and little fingers in the carpal tunnel.

The hook of the hamate most probably breaks as a result of direct trauma. In sports, fractures of the hook usually occur when an athlete is playing golf, tennis, baseball, squash, or racquetball.* Although the exact mechanism of injury is unknown, the most likely cause of the fracture is the handle of the bat, racquet, or club striking the hook of the hamate during a swing (Fig. 30-18). When the athlete grasps a cylindrical object, the end of the handle rests against the distal ulnar surface of the bone. Although the fracture can occur anywhere along the hook, it occurs most frequently in the proximal third of the bone near its base.[138] It invariably occurs in the hand near the end of the bat, club, or racquet. In baseball, the fracture occurs after a forceful or checked swing. In tennis, the fracture occurs when the athlete loses control of the racquet when trying to make a difficult shot. In golf, a fracture can occur at the end of a swing or when the club accidentally hits the ground or a hidden tree root.

This diagnosis must be considered in any athlete playing golf, tennis, baseball, squash, or racquetball or who has persistent pain on the ulnar side of the wrist and palm. This is especialy true if conservative treatment fails to resolve the athlete's complaints. This fracture is frequently misdiagnosed as a wrist sprain or tendinitis. Although activities of daily living will elicit few complaints, an attempt to play a sport that requires forceful gripping of a bat, club, or racquet will produce significant pain and cause the individual to play poorly or to cease playing. There is often tenderness with pressure directly over the tip of the hook in the hypothenar eminence, although occasionally pain can be elicited with pressure over the dorsoulnar aspect of the wrist. The latter occurs when the fracture is located at the base of the hook. Ulnar neuritis may be present, and ruptures of flexor ten-

*References 16, 23, 82, 112, 136, 138, 149.

dons have been reported in undiagnosed fractures of the hook of the hamate.[34,136,138]

Apparently the diagnosis is often missed because the fracture cannot be seen on routine radiographs. A carpal tunnel view described by Hart and Gaynor[59] frequently will show the fracture line in the bone (Fig. 30-19). A lateral profile of the hook can be seen on an oblique radiograph of the wrist with the forearm supinated and the wrist dorsiflexed[136] (Fig. 30-20).

If these special views do not show the fracture, a CT scan should be done.[40,163] Keeping the hands together in the prayer position and using axial cuts, the surgeon can see the hook of both hamate bones and can use the uninjured bone as a comparison (Fig. 30-21). Occasionally a partially healed fracture of the hook is identified on the CT scan. Sclerosis of a part of the hook is seen, and there may be a faint lucent line part of the way through the bone[138] (Fig. 30-22). At operation, this partially healed bony fragment usually is loose.

Although cast immobilization for acute fractures of the hook of the hamate[12,85] and bone grafting for nonunions of the hook[154] have been described, the best treatment for a fracture of the hook of the hamate is to excise the bony fragment[136,138] (Fig. 30-23).

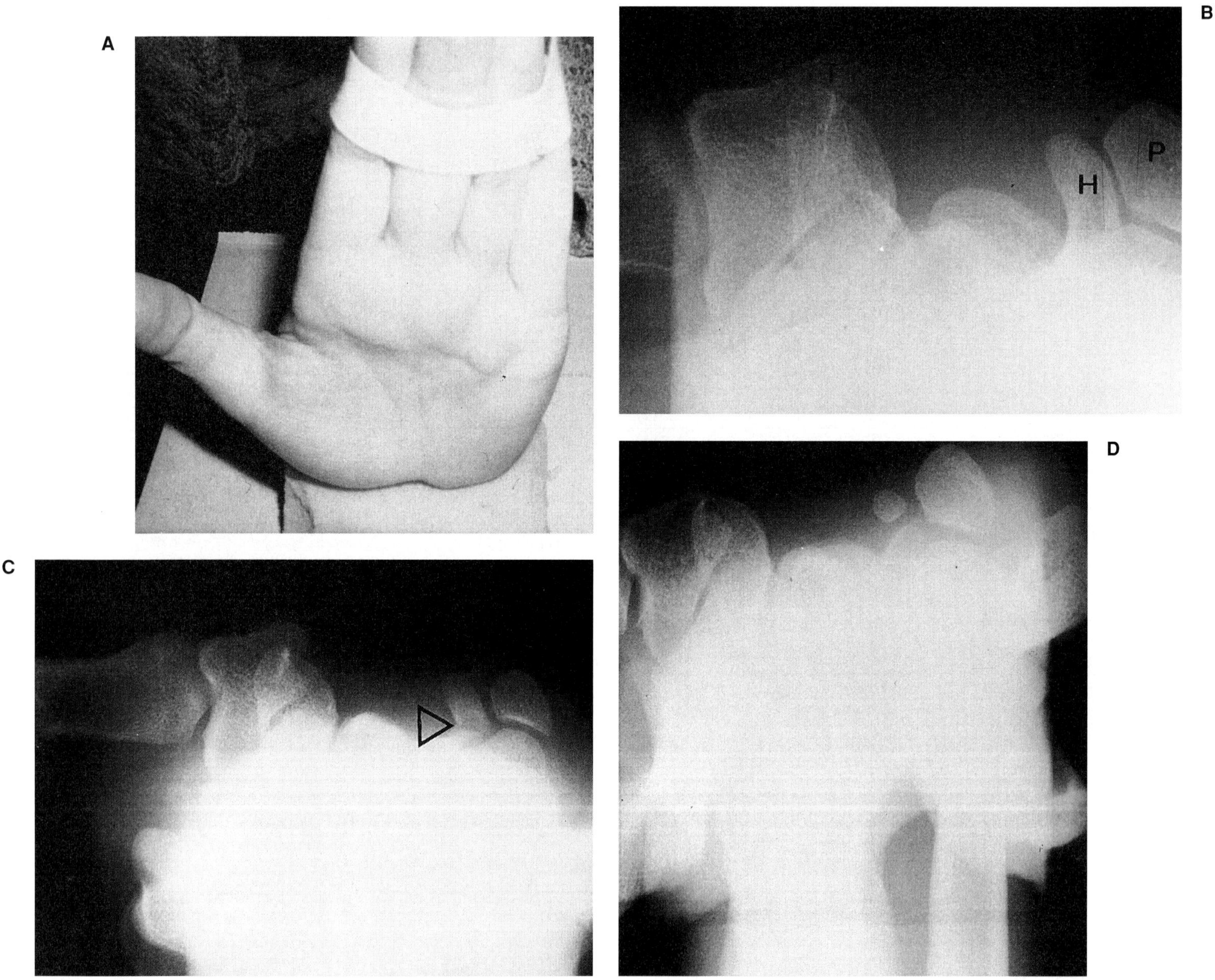

FIGURE 30-19 **A,** The Hart and Gaynor carpal tunnel view. The X-ray beam is directed 2.5 cm distal to the base of the fourth metacarpal and the tube is angled 25° toward the horizontal. **B,** A normal CT view showing the hook of the hamate *(H)*, pisiform *(P)*, and the tubercle of the trapezium *(T)*. **C,** A fracture of the hook of the hamate. **D,** Failure of union of the ossification center of the hook of the hamate.

A 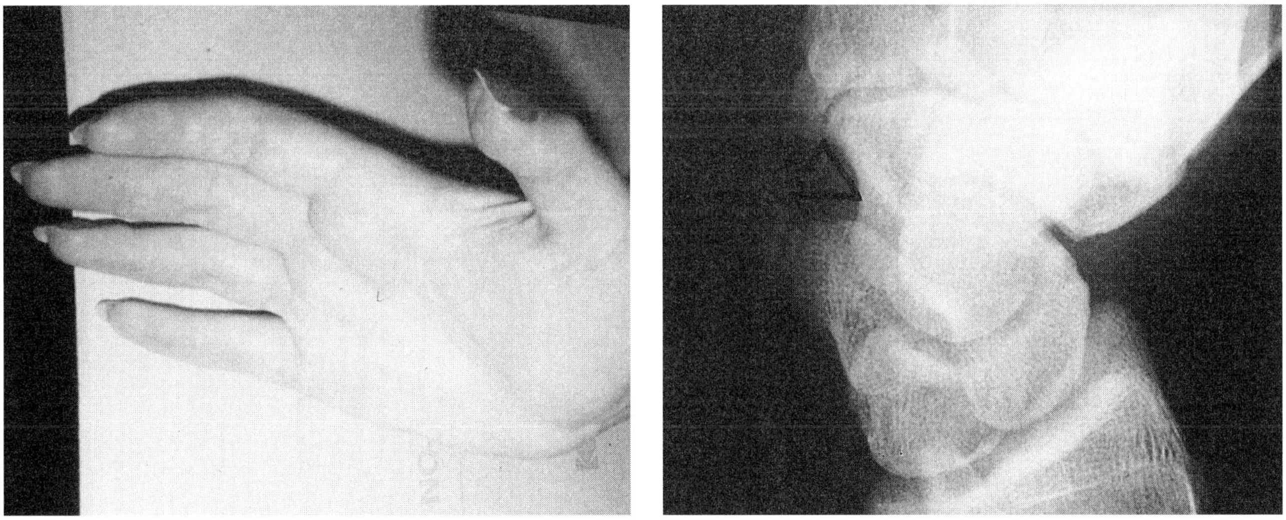 B

FIGURE 30-20 **A,** An oblique radiograph of the wrist is taken with the forearm supinated about 45° and the wrist dorsiflexed. **B,** A fracture of the hook of the hamate shown on a supinated oblique radiograph *(arrow).*

A 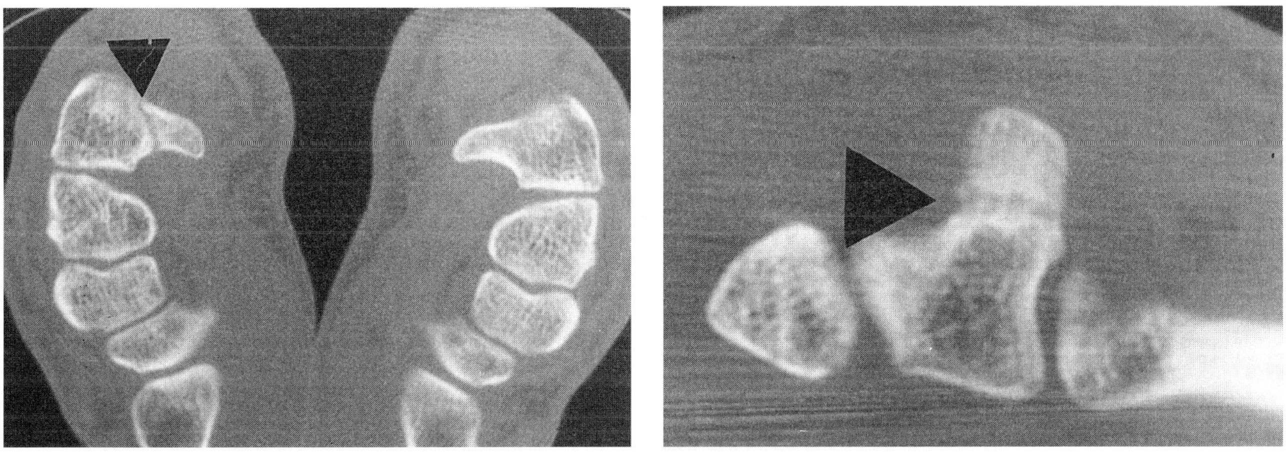 B

FIGURE 30-21 **A,** A fracture of the hook of the hamate can be seen on an axial view of both hands held in the prayer position and, **B,** on a sagittal view of the wrist.

A 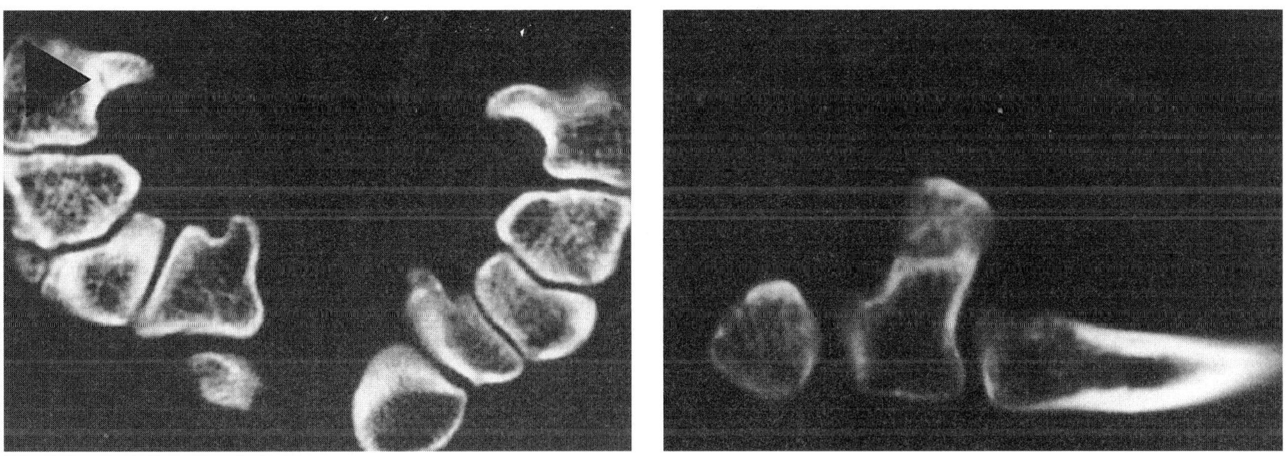 B

FIGURE 30-22 This golfer had a 2-year history of pain in his hand when playing golf. Routine radiographs including carpal tunnel views were negative. **A,** A CT scan of the wrist showed a partially healed fracture of the hook of the hamate *(arrow).* **B,** This can also be seen on the sagittal view.

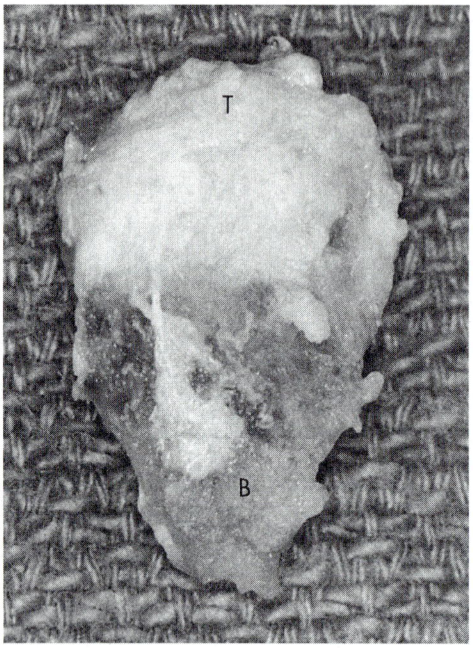

FIGURE 30-23 Hook of the hamate. *T,* Volar tip; *B,* fractured base.

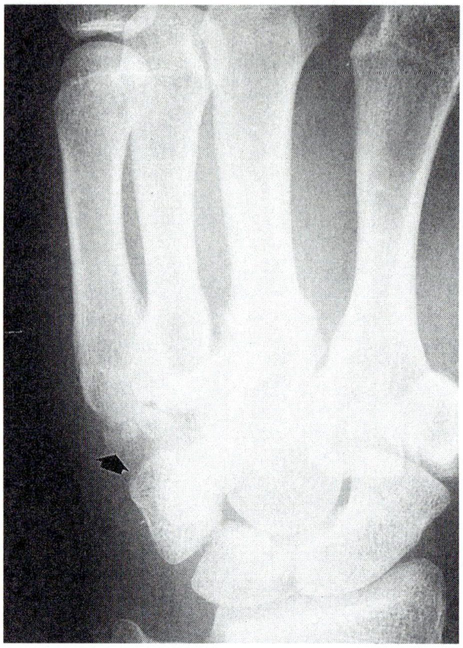

FIGURE 30-24 Fracture-dislocation of the bases of the fourth and fifth metacarpals associated with an intraarticular fracture of the hamate *(arrow).*

A curved palmar incision is centered over the tip of the hook in the hypothenar eminence. The ulnar nerve and artery are exposed and protected. After incising the periosteum over the tip, the surgeon exposes the bone by subperiosteal dissection down to its base. Care must be taken not to injure the motor branch of the ulnar nerve. The hook is removed, and the base of the bone is smoothed with a rongeur. The periosteum and adjacent fascial structures are repaired, and the hand and wrist are immobilized in a short arm cast for 3 weeks. Athletes can resume all activities as soon as scar tenderness has subsided, usually 6 to 8 weeks after the operation. Complete return of function is anticipated after the operation.[136,138]

Fractures of the body of the hamate are much less common in athletes and frequently occur in conjunction with fractures and dislocations at the base of the fourth and fifth metacarpals. An intraarticular fracture of the hamate at the carpometacarpal joint usually displaces proximally and dorsally. This injury frequently follows a direct blow on a hand, such as when striking a football helmet. The fracture is best seen on a radial or ulnar oblique view of the hand and wrist[14] (Fig. 30-24). If displaced, the fracture should be treated with open reduction and internal fixation. After operation, the hand and wrist are immobilized in a cast for 4 to 6 weeks, then rehabilitation is started.

Isolated fractures of the body of the hamate are rare. When the fracture is displaced, open reduction and internal fixation is recommended.[103]

The remaining six carpal bones are collectively injured much less frequently than the scaphoid and hook of the hamate, in both sports and daily activities. Nevertheless, they must be considered when the physician examines a painful wrist after a sports injury.

FRACTURE OF THE TRIQUETRUM

Although triquetral fractures are the second[8,15] or third[16,21] most common carpal fracture, they are not a significant problem to athletes (Fig. 30-25). They generally occur as a chip or avulsion fracture, and a fracture of the body of the bone is rare. These small avulsion fractures are best seen on oblique radiographs of the wrist. A fall on the outstretched hand with the wrist in dorsiflexion and ulnar deviation is the usual mechanism of injury. Either the hamate impinges on the triquetrum,[91] or the ulnar styloid impacts on the triquetrum to cause the fracture. These chip fractures often accompany a fracture of the scaphoid or distal radius. The usual finding is swelling and tenderness over the dorsal ulnar aspect of the wrist. After 4 weeks of immobilization, the pain subsides and the athlete can return to unrestricted activity.

FRACTURE OF THE CAPITATE

The capitate, the largest of the carpal bones, is well protected in its position in the wrist. Adler and Shaftan[2] described three types of injuries to the capitate: isolated fracture of the capitate, naviculocapitate syndrome, and capitate injuries combined with a variety of other carpal injuries (Fig. 30-26). Although a direct blow to the wrist can cause a fracture of the capitate, the most common

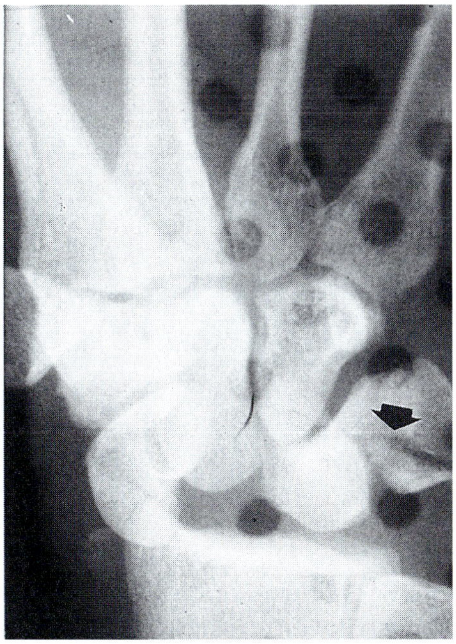

FIGURE 30-25 Although this fracture of the triquetrum *(arrow)* was associated with a perilunar dislocation of the wrist, the bone healed with cast immobilization.

mechanism of injury is a fall on the dorsiflexed wrist. While the wrist is in dorsiflexion and radial deviation, the waist of the scaphoid sometimes impinges against the radial styloid. With moderate force, only the scaphoid will fracture, but with greater force the capitate also can break. The proximal fragment of both broken bones may rotate, with the head of the capitate often rotating 180°.

Fenton[41] described this condition as the naviculocapitate syndrome. Using cadavers, Stein and Siegel[139] noted that the scaphoid fractures under tension when the wrist is dorsiflexed. Increased extension of the wrist forces the capitate under the dorsal lip of the radius, thereby fracturing the capitate. The proximal fragment of the capitate rotates as the wrist returns to the neutral position. Vance et al[150] reported that radiographs taken after injury show a scaphocapitate syndrome without the dislocation because the original dislocation often reduces spontaneously. They emphasized the importance of examining the relationship of the carpus and proximal pole of the capitate to the lunate and distal articular surface of the radius on lateral radiographs.

An acute fracture in which the head of the capitate is rotated 90° or 180° cannot be reduced by closed manipulation. If a scaphocapitate syndrome is present, both fractures must be treated with open reduction and internal fixation. The scaphoid can be exposed through a volar or dorsal approach, and the capitate is exposed through a dorsal approach. Both fractures can be stabilized by Kirschner wires or screws. The hand and wrist are immobilized until the fractures are healed. After a fracture, the head of the capitate is prone to avascular

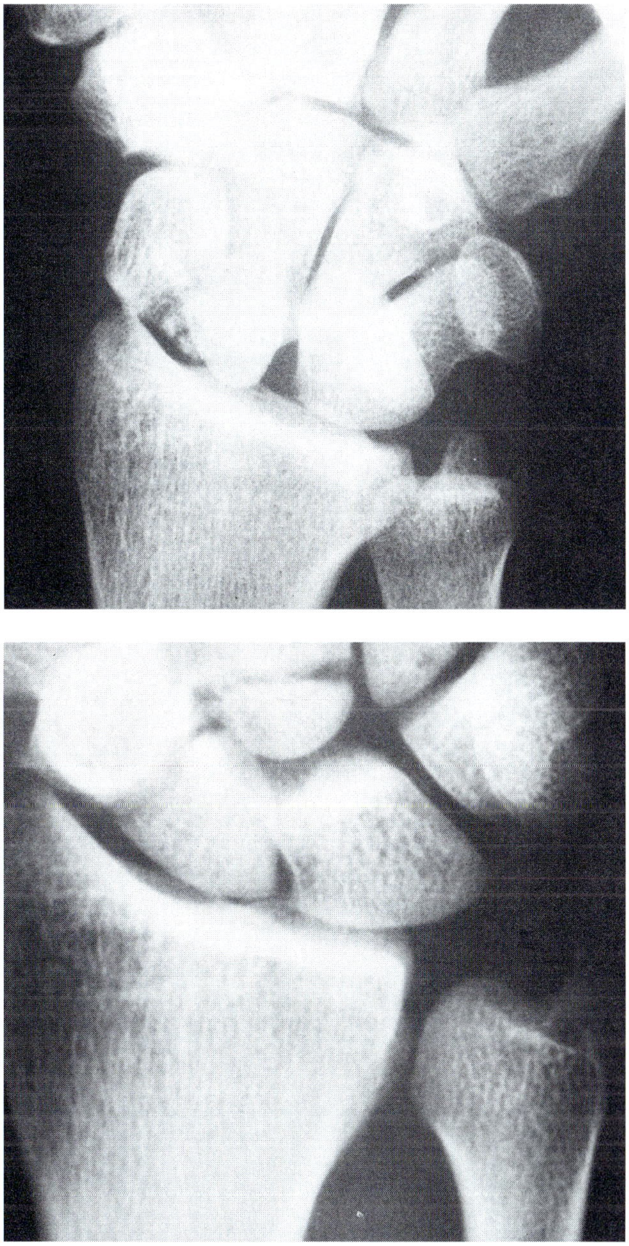

A

B

FIGURE 30-26 A transscaphoid transcapitate perilunar fracture-dislocation. **A**, Before reduction. **B**, After reduction.

necrosis because the proximal fragment is supplied by a single intraosseous artery.[111] If painful midcarpal arthritis develops, a midcarpal fusion is indicated.

FRACTURE OF THE LUNATE

Isolated fracture of the lunate accounts for 2% to 7% of carpal fractures.[16] Although a variety of fracture configurations can occur, the lunate is susceptible to compression between the radius and capitate when the wrist is in dorsiflexion and ulnar deviation. Initial radiographs may not show transverse or longitudinal fractures of the bone, and a CT scan or MRI may be needed. Undisplaced fractures can be treated with cast immobilization for 6 weeks, whereas displaced fractures should be treated with open reduction and internal fixation.[4] Tseisen and Hjarbaek[146] reviewed 17 cases of fresh lunate fractures and classified them into five groups. They followed 11 cases from 4 to 31 years, and none of the bones developed the progressive sclerosis and collapse typical of Kienböck's disease.

A relationship between an acute lunate fracture and the development of Kienböck's disease remains controversial (Fig. 30-27). Repeated stress or compression fractures leading to loss of blood supply and collapse and fragmentation of the bone may be the series of events leading to Kienböck's disease (lunatomalacia).[9,53,55] Individuals diagnosed with Kienböck's disease rarely recall a specific injury. This disease causes pain, stiffness, and swelling of the wrist.

A four-stage classification of Kienböck's disease, based on radiographic characteristics of the lunate, has been described by Lichtman.[77] Treatment generally is predicated on the stage of the disease.[4,126]

A detailed discussion of the treatment of Kienböck's disease is beyond the scope of this chapter. There are two basic principles of treatment. If the bone has not collapsed, a joint-leveling procedure to unload the lunate (radial shortening, ulnar lengthening, capitate shortening) or some procedure to augment the blood supply of the bone is recommended. If the bone has collapsed and fragmented, other reconstructive procedures may be performed.

Kienböck's disease has not been specifically related to sports injuries. Nakamura et al[101] reported on 10 patients who were identified as having Kienböck's disease while playing sports. Their clinical history and radiographic findings were similar to a group of 82 manual laborers with Kienböck's disease. The athletes had favorable results after treatment with radial shortening.

FRACTURE OF THE PISIFORM

The pisiform is a sesamoid bone located in the flexor carpi ulnaris tendon. It articulates with the triquetrum and forms the pisotriquetral joint. The pisiform is attached to the fifth metacarpal, triquetrum, and hamate by strong ligaments, although in some individuals the bone is mobile.

Fractures of the pisiform may be linear, comminuted, or of the avulsion type[151] (Fig. 30-28). About 50% of pisiform fractures are associated with fractures of other bones. These fractures are best seen on a 30° supinated oblique radiographic view of the wrist.

Isolated pisiform fractures usually are the result of direct trauma to the hypothenar eminence, such as when the heel of the hand is struck by a pitched ball. Undisplaced fractures can be treated by cast immobilization for about 4 to 6 weeks. If degenerative arthritis occurs at the pisotriquetral joint after injury to the pisiform or the joint, excision of the pisiform is curative and will permit the athlete to return to competition in about 8 weeks.

A

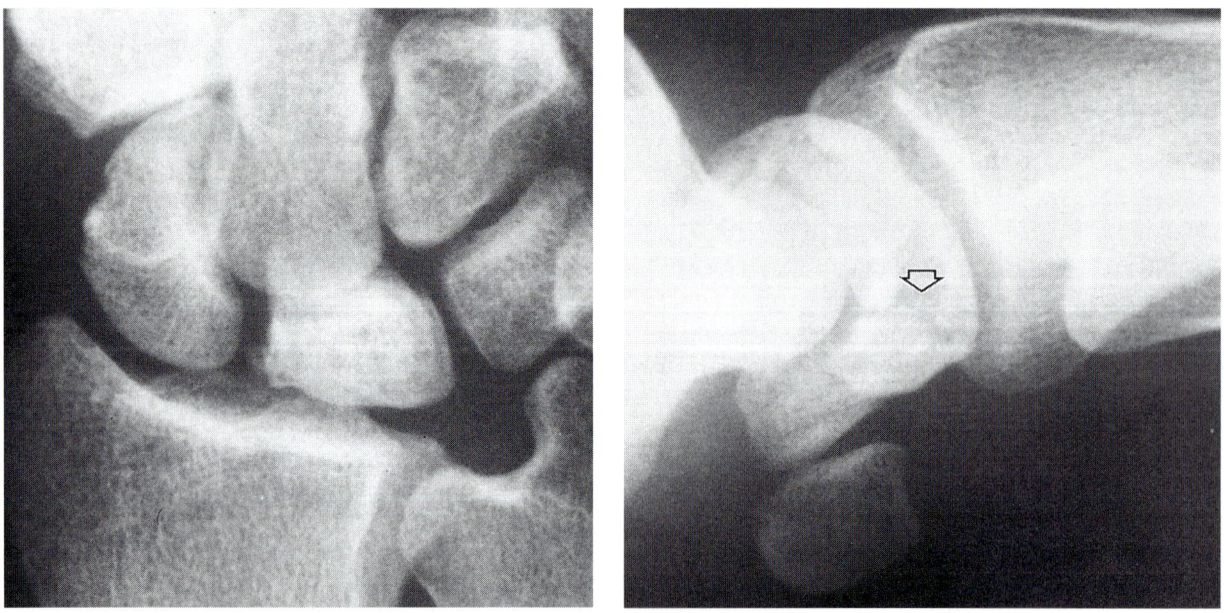

B

FIGURE 30-27 Kienbock's disease with collapse and fracture of the lunate *(arrow)* on the, **A,** PA view and the, **B,** lateral view.

FRACTURE OF THE TRAPEZIUM

Trapezial fractures make up less than 5% of carpal fractures. These fractures are either vertical fractures of the trapezium associated with a dislocation of the base of the thumb[33] or avulsion fractures of the ridge of the trapezium.[84,105] Ridge fractures often are missed because they cannot be seen on routine radiograph. A carpal tunnel view must be taken to make the diagnosis (Fig. 30-29).

Avulsion fractures of the trapezial ridge or undisplaced vertical body fractures of the trapezium are treated by immobilizing the wrist in a cast. Displaced small bony fragments can be excised, but larger fragments should be reduced and stabilized with Kirschner wires or screws.

FRACTURE OF THE TRAPEZOID

These fractures make up less than 1% of carpal injuries. Dorsal dislocation of the bone can occur after a significant hand and wrist injury.[16] This diagnosis must be considered in a patient with persistent pain over the base of the index finger. Closed or open reduction of the dislocation is indicated, but excision of the bone is not advised.

DISLOCATION OR FRACTURE-DISLOCATION OF THE CARPUS

A wide spectrum of bony and ligamentous injuries can occur to the wrist. These injuries can result in a variety of fractures and ligament disruptions that can present as single entities or in combination. Although these injuries are described according to their initial radiographic appearance (e.g., perilunate dislocation), in reality each wrist injury is a specific stage of a progressive disorder. The progressive disorder in a particular patient is determined by (1) the degree of force loading, (2) the duration and magnitude of the force, (3) the position of the hand at the time of impact, and (4) the biomechanical properties of the bones and ligaments of the individual.

The mechanism of carpal dislocation is ulnar deviation and supination of the wrist.[92] Mayfield et al.[91] described four stages of perilunar instability that varied from scapholunate diastasis (stage I) to volar dislocation of the wrist (stage IV) (Fig. 30-30). Fracture of the carpal bones about the lunate in conjunction with a lunate dislocation is called a greater arc injury, and dislocation of the perilunar carpal bones without a fracture is known as a lesser arc injury[66] (Fig. 30-31). Dorsal transscaphoid dislocations, dorsal perilunate dislocations, and palmar

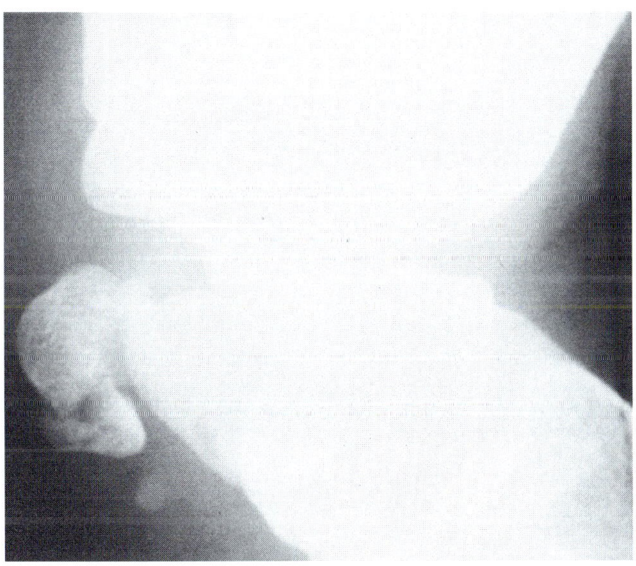

FIGURE 30-28 Fracture of the pisiform. This is a supinated oblique radiograph.

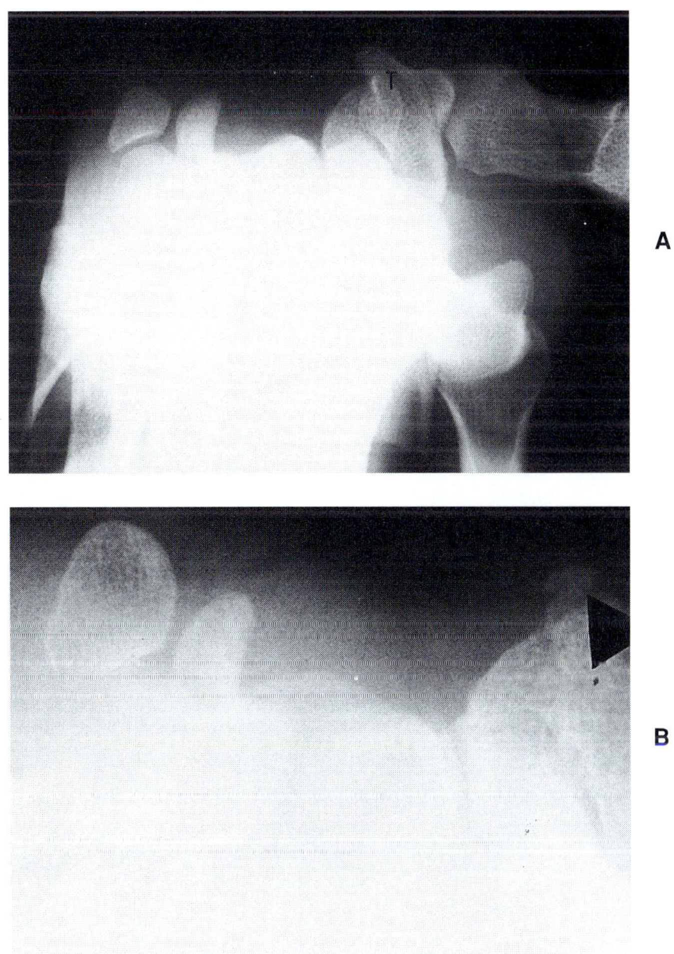

FIGURE 30-29 **A,** Carpal tunnel view to show the ridge or tubercle of the trapezium *(T)*. **B,** A fracture of the ridge (tubercle) of the trapezium *(arrow)*.

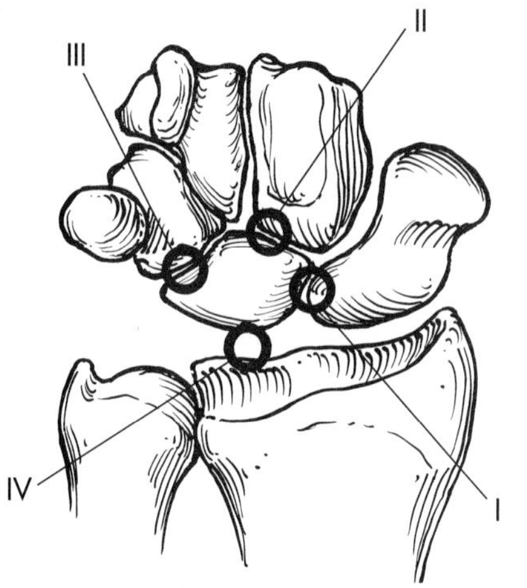

FIGURE 30-30 Progressive stages of perilunar instability: I (scapholunate separation), II (capitate dislocation), III (lunotriquetral separation), IV (lunate dislocation).

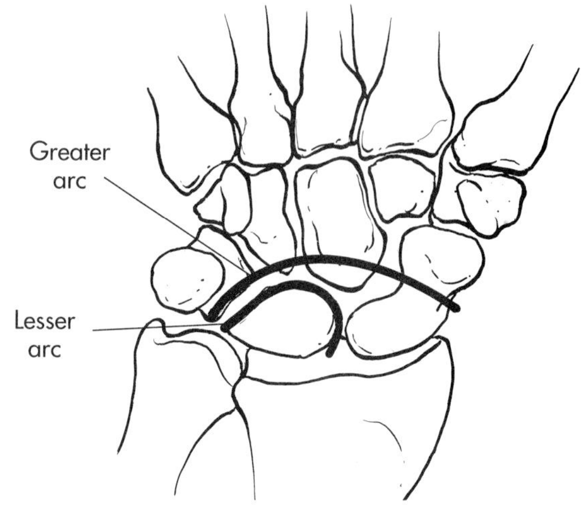

FIGURE 30-31 The arcs of injury to the bone and/or ligaments in the wrist. Greater arc injury is a fracture-dislocation. Lesser arc injury is a dislocation or ligament injury.

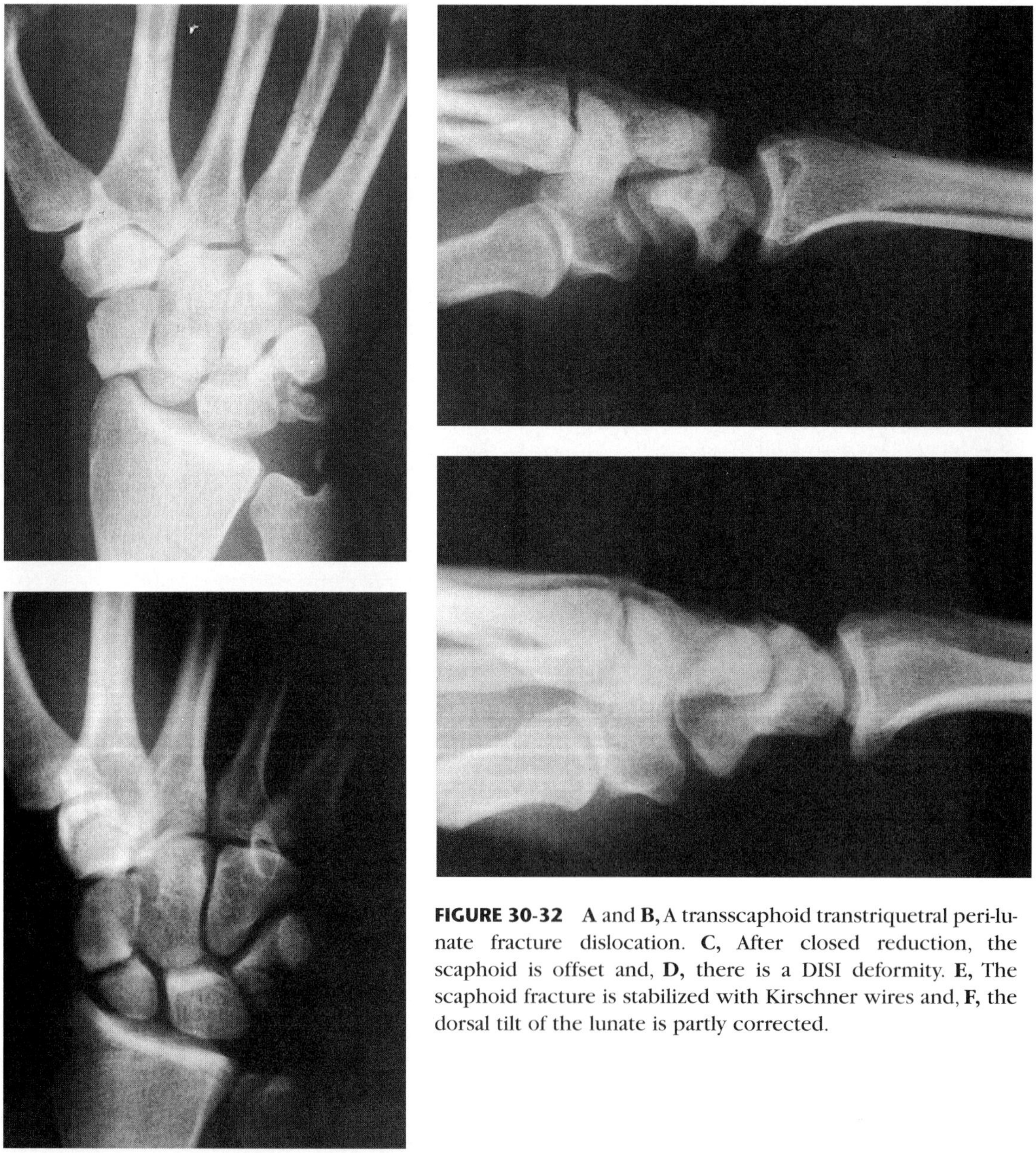

FIGURE 30-32 **A** and **B,** A transscaphoid transtriquetral peri-lunate fracture dislocation. **C,** After closed reduction, the scaphoid is offset and, **D,** there is a DISI deformity. **E,** The scaphoid fracture is stabilized with Kirschner wires and, **F,** the dorsal tilt of the lunate is partly corrected.

lunate dislocations sometimes are seen after athletic injuries (Fig. 30-32).

FRACTURE OF THE DISTAL RADIUS

The distal radius is the proximal end of the radiocarpal joint. Its articular surface has two concavities that contain the scaphoid and lunate. The sigmoid notch of the distal radius forms part of the distal radioulnar joint. In addition, the complex ligament structures of the carpus include attachments to the dorsal and volar surfaces of the radius. The types of injuries that occur to the distal radius depend on many factors: (1) the force exerted, (2) the energies absorbed, (3) the geometric configuration of the articular elements, (4) the strength of supporting ligaments and muscles, (5) the rigidity of the bony structures (age of the patient), (6) the position of the hand and wrist at the time of impact, and (7) the duration of exposure to the injury forces.

The distal articular surface of the radius has an average radial inclination (slope) of 23°, an average palmar tilt of 11°, and an average radial styloid height (in relation to the ulna) of 11 mm (Fig. 30-33). A fracture of the distal radius, either extraarticular or intraarticular, results in loss of the relationship of the distal end of the bone to the carpus (radiocarpal or midcarpal alignment) and to the ulna (distal radioulnar joint). If the fracture is intraarticular, it also disrupts the smooth cartilaginous surface of the joint and may predispose the joint to later degenerative changes. The goal of fracture treatment at the dis-

E

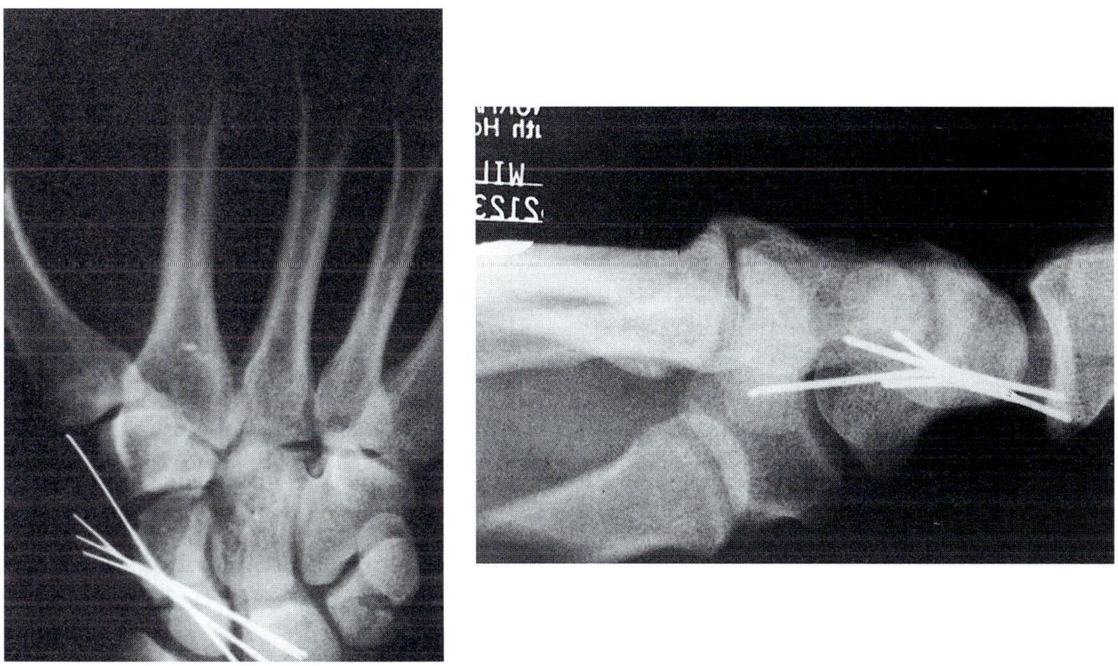

F

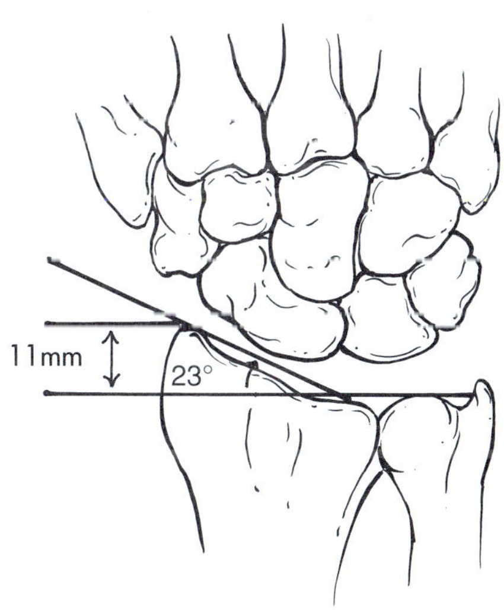

FIGURE 30-33 The normal configuration of the distal articular surface of the radius.

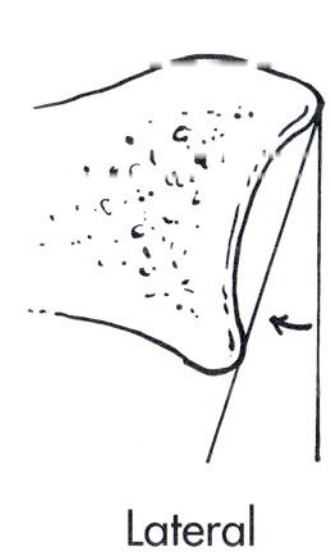

tal radius is to correct the basic deformities that occur: dorsal tilt of the distal radius fragment, dorsal displacement and radial deviation, and shortening of the radius. In addition, any disruption of the articular surface of the radius at the radiocarpal or distal radioulnar joints should be corrected.

Abraham Colles published his treatise on the fracture of the carpal extremity of the radius in the Edinburgh Medical Journal in 1814.[25] Since the publication of this essay on a fracture involving the distal 4 cm of the radius, knowledge of fractures of the distal radius has expanded significantly. However, the classification and treatment of the many varieties of distal radius fractures remain controversial even today.

A myriad of classifications of distal radius fractures have been published. Frykman's classification[48] is based on the extent of involvement of the articular surface of the radiocarpal and distal radioulnar joints. Older et al[104] classified metaphyseal Colles-type fractures into four groups. The classification is based on the extent of displacement, dorsal angulation, shortening of the distal radius fragment, and comminution of the dorsal metaphyseal cortex. Other studies[64,135] also concluded that the presence of dorsal comminution and the extent of the initial deformity are the best determinants of possible loss of reduction at a later time. In evaluating the use of external pin fixation in unstable Colles' fractures, Cooney et al[26] concluded that these displaced fractures tend to redisplace after reduction if there is significant comminution, severe dorsal angulation (20° or more), or extensive intraarticular involvement. Weber[157] noted that because the injury to the distal radius results from a fall on the outstretched hand, the dorsal cortex is compressed while the volar cortex of the radius has a tension load. He noted that if the depth of the dorsal cortex comminution extends volar to the midaxial plane of the radius, treatment in a cast will fail.

Several other classifications have been published, including those of Melone,[95] Fernandez,[44] Swiss association for the study of internal fixation,[100] the Mayo Clinic,[19] and Rayhack.[121] A universal classification also was published in a cooperative effort at a symposium on fractures of the distal radius.[29] A fracture classification using the anatomic type of fracture was described by McMurty and Jupiter.[86] Intraarticular fractures are described based on the number of parts: (1) two parts, including radial styloid, die-punch, and dorsal/palmar Barton's fractures; (2) three parts—the lunate and scaphoid facets separate from each other and the proximal portion of the radius; (3) four parts—the same as three parts except the lunate facet is further fractured at the dorsal and volar fragments; and (4) five parts or more, including a wide variety of comminuted fragments.

For a detailed discussion of the classifications, the reader is referred to the author's articles, standard texts, or monographs on distal radius fractures.[68,86,96,110] Although some authors decry the use of eponyms (e.g., Barton's, Colles', Smith's, Chauffer's, and die-punch) to describe fractures, this author finds them useful because most individuals are familiar with these terms. Until a universally accepted or understood classification is developed, these eponyms should not be discarded.

Radiographs of the distal radius in at least the PA, lateral, and oblique views are imperative in beginning the evaluation of the fracture. If the fracture is minimally displaced and easily seen, these views may be sufficient. A more complex fracture may require additional radiographs before or after traction or manipulation before the physician can accurately determine the nature of the fracture. Complex fractures (displaced, comminuted, intraarticular, involvement of the distal radioulnar joint) are best assessed with computed tomography.

Closed reduction and cast immobilization remains the standard treatment in 75% to 80% of fractures of the distal radius. This treatment is advocated for fractures that are extraarticular, minimally displaced, and inherently stable.[68,86,110,113] The results are worse after remanipulation of a fracture that has redisplaced.[24,87]

Fractures that are unstable (extraarticular or intraarticular) or that cannot be satisfactorily reduced for any reason should be stabilized by some type of fixation device, whether external, internal, or both.[86,110]

Fractures of the distal radius as a sports-related injury tend to occur in younger people and usually result from a high-energy injury. As a result, these fractures tend to be more comminuted and displaced and frequently involve the articular surfaces of the radius. They often are difficult to reduce and tend to redisplace in a cast. Congruency of the articular surfaces, both the radiocarpal and distal radioulnar joints, must be restored to maintain good function of these joints. Knirk and Jupiter[70] concluded that failure to reduce intraarticular fractures of the radius with more than 2 mm of displacement of articular congruity, especially in young adults, likely will lead to symptomatic posttraumatic arthritis. These high-energy injuries also can be associated with carpal instability and injury to the distal radioulnar joint.[11]

In a young athletic population, the following fractures should be treated aggressively to restore maximum function to the wrist. There is no single acceptable treatment procedure, and readers should use the technique with which they are most familiar, not necessarily the one currently in vogue. A closed technique that does not restore good alignment to the distal radius is unacceptable today.

1. Comminuted dorsal cortex extraarticular fractures of the radius, with a dorsal tilt of more than 20°, usually must be opened, reduced, bone-grafted, and internally or externally stabilized. This author usually opens these fractures through a dorsal approach and, if possible, uses a buttress T plate (Fig. 30-34). If the distal radius fragments are small,

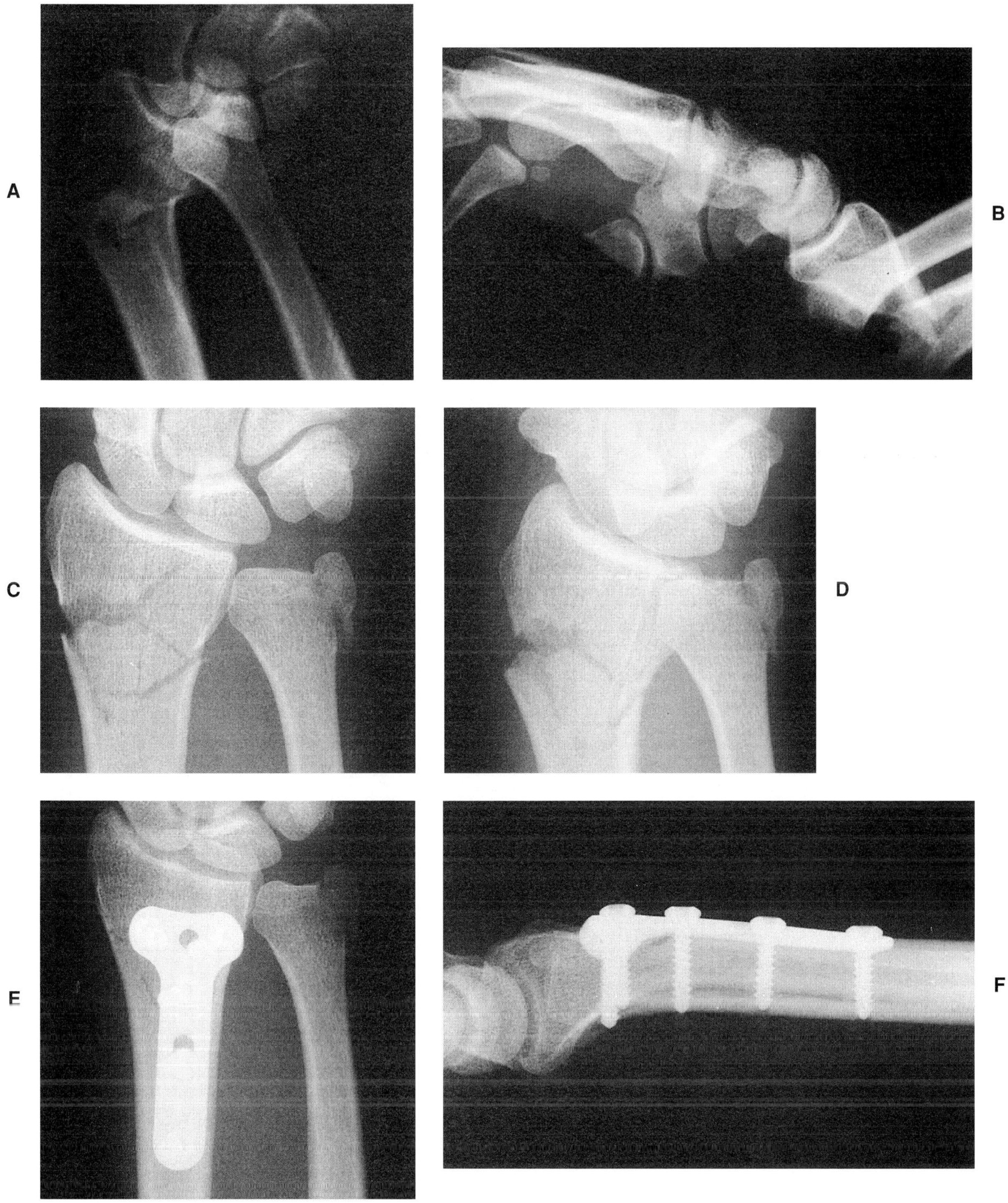

FIGURE 30-34 **A** and **B,** This high-energy displaced extraarticular fractures of the distal radius was, **C** and **D,** unstable following a closed reduction. **E** and **F,** Using a dorsal approach, the fracture was stabilized with a plate and screws. A bone graft was not needed.

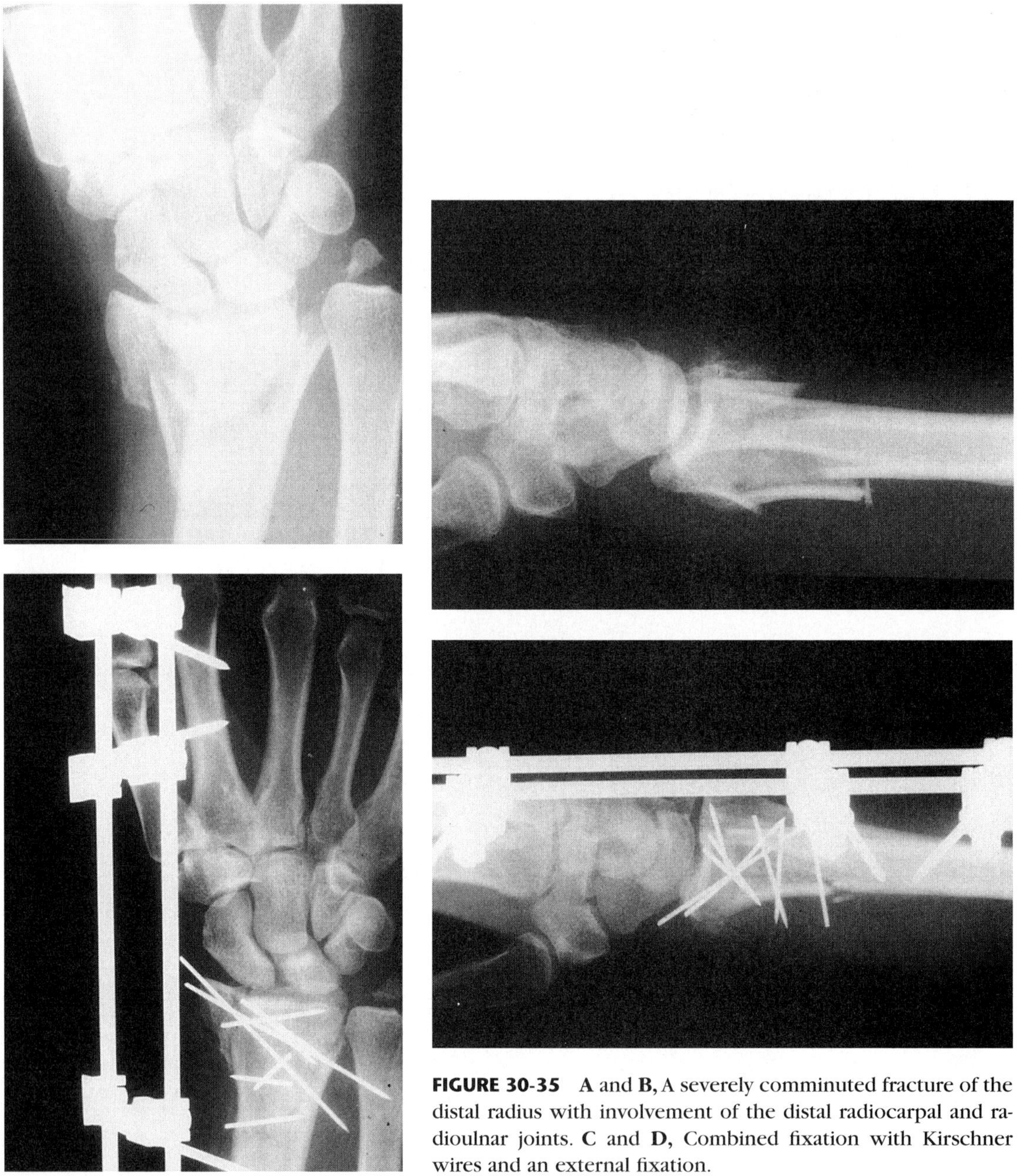

A B C D

FIGURE 30-35 **A** and **B,** A severely comminuted fracture of the distal radius with involvement of the distal radiocarpal and radioulnar joints. **C** and **D,** Combined fixation with Kirschner wires and an external fixation.

Kirschner wires can be used. When there is an intraarticular component, an external fixator can supplement the internal fixation devices (Fig. 30-35).

2. Dorsal and palmar Barton's fractures (two-part intraarticular fractures) are unstable and usually displaced, and require accurate open reduction and internal fixation. The dorsal or palmar wrist and forearm are opened, depending on the fracture site, and the fracture is stabilized with a buttress plate (Fig. 30-36).
3. Comminuted intraarticular fractures of the distal radius are the most difficult to treat. Accurate diagnosis often requires a CT scan (Fig. 30-37). Congruency of the joint surface must be restored. The use of limited open reduction techniques, as described by Seitz et al[130] and Axelrod et al,[6] arthroscopically assisted reduction of the fracture,[110,113] or a formal open reduction and internal fixation of the radius must be determined case by case. Although algorithms and protocols are useful, not all fractures will fit into the defined categories.[110]

Fractures of the ulnar styloid occur in association with 50% to 75% of fractures of the distal radius.[7,48] Most fractures of the ulnar styloid heal without complication. Careful evaluation of the ulnar side of the wrist should

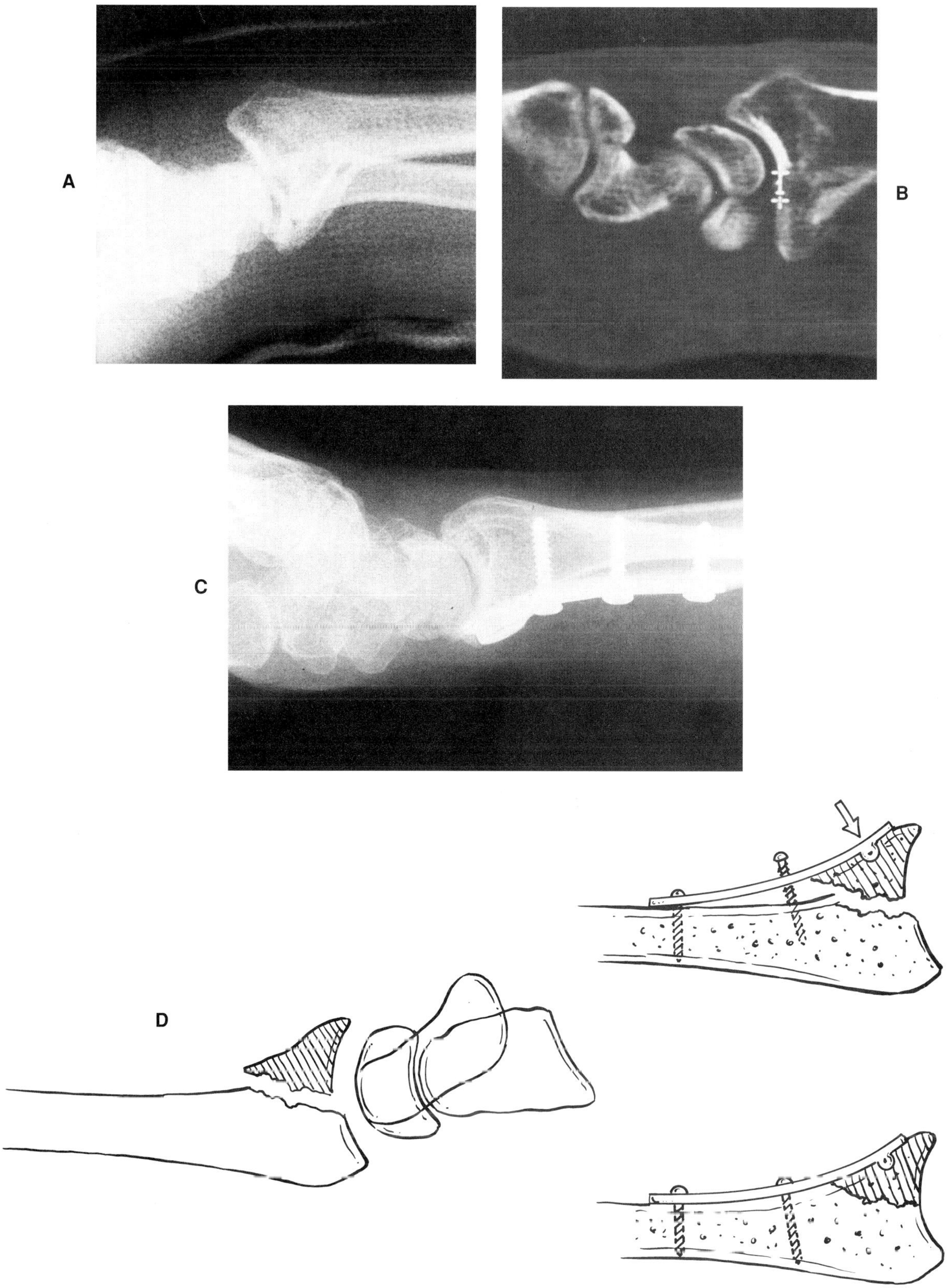

FIGURE 30-36 **A,** Volar Barton's fracture that was casted without being reduced. **B,** The volar lip fragment is comminuted. **C,** Reduction and stabilization of the fracture with a buttress plate. The carpus is relocated in the cup of the distal radius. **D,** A schematic of the reduction and plate fixation for a volar Barton's fracture.

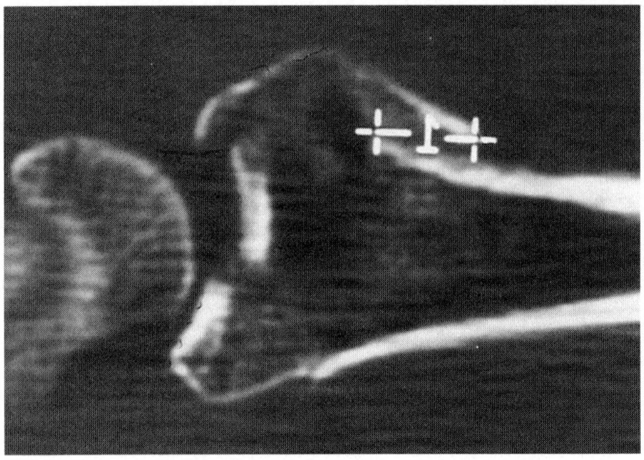

FIGURE 30-37 The sagittal view of the CT scan shows the depressed articular surface of the distal radius.

be done to ensure there is no injury to the triangular fibrocartilage, associated osteochondral injuries to the ulnar head, or ligamentous instability.

A displaced fracture of the ulnar head should be treated with open reduction and internal fixation to restore congruency to its relationship in the distal radioulnar joint.

Complications after fractures of the distal radius and ulna can involve both bone and soft-tissue structures.[72,164] Cooney et al[30] noted a complication rate of 30% to 35% after Colles' fracture. Several reports have documented a long-standing clinical impression that the greater the residual deformity of the fracture, the greater the tendency toward increased complications and functional limitations of the hand, wrist, and forearm.[7,39,51,132] Some of the complications that may follow fractures of

A

B

C

D

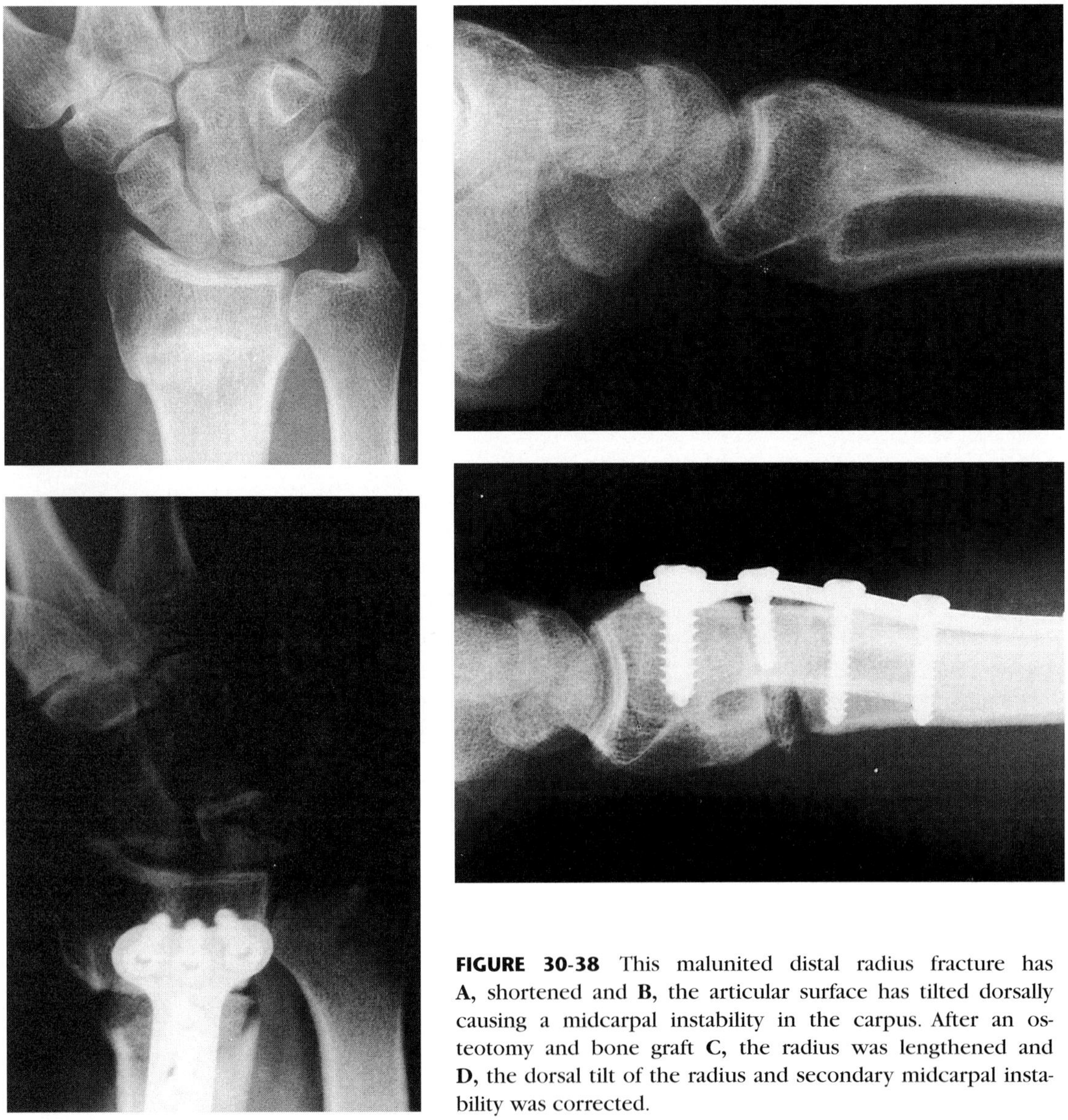

FIGURE 30-38 This malunited distal radius fracture has **A,** shortened and **B,** the articular surface has tilted dorsally causing a midcarpal instability in the carpus. After an osteotomy and bone graft **C,** the radius was lengthened and **D,** the dorsal tilt of the radius and secondary midcarpal instability was corrected.

the distal radius are (1) deformity of the distal radius, (2) carpal instability, (3) radiocarpal arthritis, (4) disturbance of the distal radioulnar joint, (5) ulnar styloid fracture, (6) injury to the triangular fibrocartilage complex, (7) compartment syndrome, (8) nonunion of the distal radius, (9) nerve compression, (10) tendon ruptures, (11) de Quervain's tenosynovitis, and (12) reflex sympathetic dystrophy.

A malunion of a distal radius fracture can occur despite our best attempts at treatment. Bone and joint alignment must be restored in patients under the age of 50 to 55, especially in the 20-to-40 age group, which is very active athletically. This should allow good long-term function of the extremity and a return to athletic activity.

Residual dorsal tilt of the distal radius that exceeds 10° can significantly interfere with wrist palmar flexion. Load transmission of the carpus is displaced dorsally and can create a prearthritic condition.[118,131] If the dorsal tilt exceeds 35°, dorsal subluxation of the carpus can occur, and the wrist is painful in palmar flexion.[80,143] Shortening of the radius of more than 6 mm can disrupt the distal radiocarpal joint. If there are no degenerative changes at the radiocarpal joint, an opening wedge osteotomy through the malunion site in the metaphysis of the radius in conjunction with a bone graft is an excellent method of restoring length to the radius, correcting the dorsal tilt of the joint surface, reducing the subluxation of the carpus, and improving the relationship of the distal radius to the distal ulna (Fig. 30-38). This author uses a dorsal appproach, corticocancellous bone graft from the iliac crest, and a buttress plate for fixation. This fixation can be supplemented with Kischner wires if necessary. The osteotomy is made just proximal to the sulcus of the distal radioulnar joint (Fig. 30-39). This technique has been described by Fernandez[42,45] and others.[86,110]

The distal radioulnar joint can be disturbed primarily or secondarily in association with a fracture of the distal radius. The joint is affected primarily if there is involvement of the sulcus on the ulnar side of the radius. An offset of the articular surface, bone spurs, or arthritic changes will cause pain and interfere with forearm rotation. Diastasis of the joint at the time of the radius fracture also can disrupt joint function.

Secondarily, the distal radioulnar joint is affected if there is radial shortening and/or dorsal tilt of the distal fragment of the radius, producing an ulnar-plus configuration, or if an injury involves the triangular fibrocartilage complex.

Shortening of the radius more than 6 mm alters the relationship of the radius and ulna. This can result in pain and loss of forearm rotation. Sometimes the altered relationship of the radius and ulna is restored by a corrective osteotomy of the radius. If not, and if a good articular surface is present, the author prefers to shorten the ulna. A variety of other reconstructive procedures have been de-

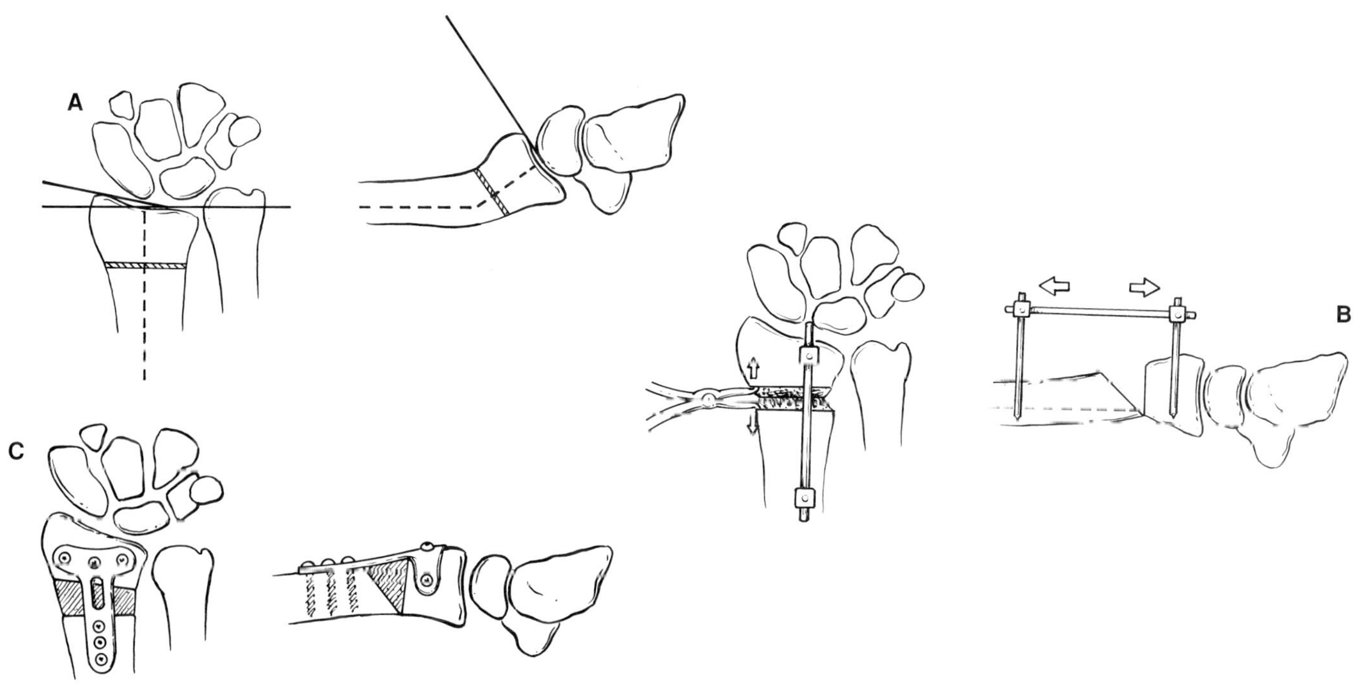

FIGURE 30-39 Using a dorsal approach, **A**, an osteotomy is made through the distal radius proximal to the distal radioulnar joint. **B,** A spreader or a distractor is used to restore appropriate length and tilt of the distal radius. **C,** A wedge-shaped graft from the iliac crest is inserted into the defect and a plate is used to rigidly stabilize the osteotomy of the radius.

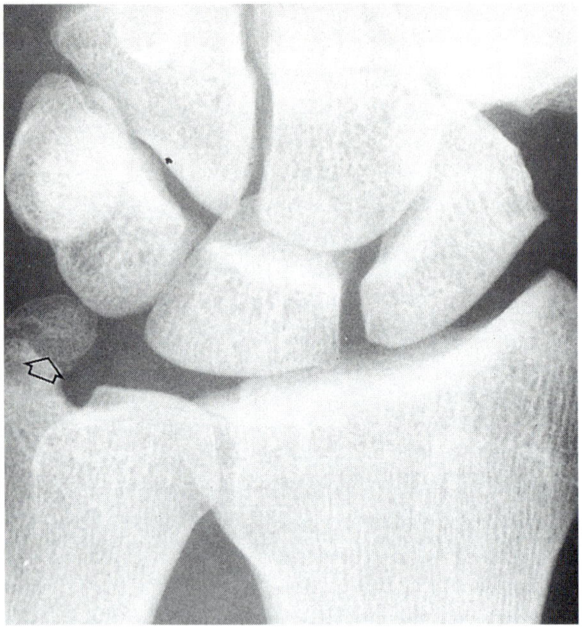

FIGURE 30-40 A painful fibrous union of the ulnar styloid. *(arrow).* The pain was relieved after the ununited styloid fragment was excised.

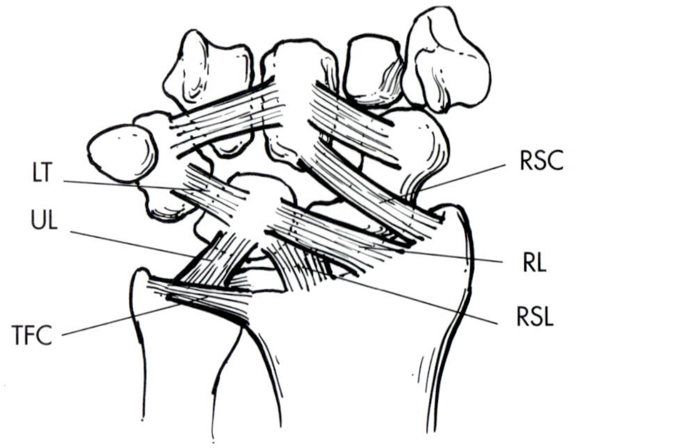

FIGURE 30-41 The volar wrist ligaments as described by Taleisnik. *RSC,* Radioscaphocapitate; *RL,* radiolunate; *RSL,* radioscapholunate; *UL,* ulnolunate; *LT,* lunotriquetral; *TFC,* triangular fibrocartilage.

scribed,[17] but their ability to restore an individual to a high level of athletic competition is doubtful. Excision of the distal ulna has been widely used, but in young patients the results are unpredictable and the procedure may produce weakness and instability on the ulnar side of the wrist.[10,17,42] A Darrach procedure is not recommended in a young athletic adult.

Although most ulnar styloid fractures heal without complication, up to 25% either heal by a fibrous union or fail to unite.[7] Pain on the ulnar side of the wrist after the fracture of the radius has healed can be due to a nonunion of the ulnar styloid. Palpation at the base of the styloid will reproduce the patient's pain. Radiographs will confirm the diagnosis. Radial and ulnar deviation views of the wrist may show movement of the ulnar styloid. If the nonunited ulnar styloid is sufficiently painful, subperiosteal excision of the bony fragment (styloid) usually provides good pain relief (Fig. 30-40). With this approach, the ligaments attached to the ulnar styloid are left intact.

The rehabilitation of an athlete who sustained a fracture of the distal radius is started within 24 hours of injury and treatment. The athlete should begin exercises to flex and extend the fingers and thumb, as well as range-of-motion exercises for the elbow and shoulder. When the wrist immobilization is discontinued or replaced with a removable device, the athlete should begin range-of-motion exercises to the wrist and elbow. Range-of-motion and strengthening exercises are gradually increased, and sport-specific exercises are added to restore strength, endurance, and joint motion.

LIGAMENT INJURIES OF THE WRIST

The two rows of carpal bones, the base of the four ulnar metacarpals, and the distal radius and ulna are supported and connected by the extrinsic wrist ligaments. These ligaments are thicker and stronger on the palmar side of the wrist (Fig. 30-41). The palmar ligaments are arranged in two arcades and in an inverted-V pattern. Radially, the more important ligaments are the radioscaphocapitate, radiolunotriquetral, and radioscapholunate, and on the ulnar side the significant ulnocarpal ligaments are the ulnolunate, the ulnotriquetral, and the triangular fibrocartilage complex.[142]

The intrinsic ligaments originate and insert onto the carpal bones and separate the intercarpal compartments (midcarpal and radiocarpal). The intrinsic ligaments are less stiff than the extrinsic ligaments and can be elongated to a greater degree before they will tear.[83] Injuries to the scapholunate and lunotriquetral ligaments are the most common.[93,122]

Linscheid et al[80] and Dobyns et al[37] published classic descriptions of posttraumatic carpal instability in 1972 and 1975, respectively. They defined traumatic instability of the wrist as "a carpal injury in which loss of normal alignment of the carpal bones develops early or late." Four types of carpal instability were described: dorsiflexion, palmar flexion, ulnar translocation, and dorsal subluxation. Dorsiflexion instability produces a zig-zag alignment of the radius, lunate, and capitate, which is called *dorsal intercalated segmental instability (DISI).* This condition is diagnosed on a lateral radiograph and is characterized by dorsal tilt of the lunate. This configuration is most commonly seen with scapholunate dissociation. Palmar flexion instability produces a volar intercalated segmental instability (VISI) characterized by palmar flexion of the lunate. Lunotriquetral injuries usually produce a VISI configuration (Fig. 30-42).

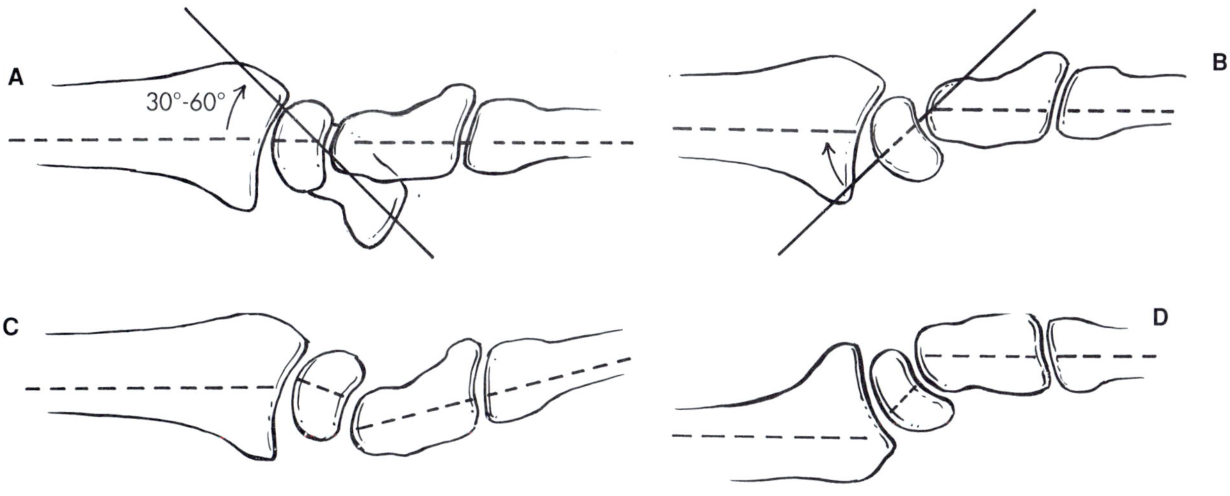

FIGURE 30-42 **A,** Normal carpal alignment; **B,** dorsal intercalated segmental instability (DISI), **C,** volar intercalated segmental instability (VISI); and, **D,** midcarpal instability.

Midcarpal instability[3,76,83] can occur primarily from extrinsic ligament injury or secondarily from a malunited fracture of the distal radius.[143]

Carpal instabilities have been further characterized as carpal instability dissociative (CID) and carpal instability nondissociative (CIND).[127] CID refers to loss of interosseous ligament support and dissociation of the bones of the proximal carpal row. CIND indicates loss of the extrinsic ligament support and a carpal instability with rotational deformity of an intact proximal carpal row.

Scapholunate, lunotriquetral, and midcarpal ligament injuries will be discussed further, but for a detailed discussion of carpal instability anatomy, biomechanics, pathomechanics, and treatment, the reader is referred to other studies.*

Injuries to the wrist ligaments occur after compressive load onto the wrist in some degree of dorsiflexion. Forearm rotation also is present as a component of the injury. Mayfield et al[91] loaded cadaver wrists into extension, ulnar deviation, and intercarpal supination, and this resulted in a progressive sequence of carpal ligament injury that they called "progressive perilunate instability." The progression occurred in four stages. As force was slowly applied to the radial side of the wrist, the proximal pole of the scaphoid migrated dorsally, creating a scapholunate instability (stage I). Further progressive loading of the wrist caused dorsal dislocation of the capitate from the lunate (stage II), dislocation of the triquetrum from the lunate, causing a lunotriquetral diastasis (stage III), and finally dislocation of the lunate (stage IV) (see Fig. 30-30). Loading the ulnar side of the wrist with the carpus pronated may cause lunotriquetral injury.[83]

*References 36, 37, 76, 78, 80, 83, 127, 144, 145.

In athletics, these injuries can result from a collision on the field, from a fall onto the outstretched hand, from injury to the wrist in a pile-up (football, rugby), or in a more subtle manner, such as when playing tennis or golf (hitting a bad shot). To make the diagnosis, the examiner must be aware of the different carpal instability injuries.

SCAPHOLUNATE INSTABILITY

This is the most common of the carpal instabilities. Symptoms are persistent wrist pain that has not resolved with conservative treatment. Occasionally the patient will complain of a click or snap in the wrist. This does not appear to occur very often. Examination usually shows swelling on the dorsum of the wrist and significant tenderness with pressure over the scapholunate joint. Passive wrist motion may produce a click. Sometimes pain can be elicited as the wrist is brought from ulnar to radial deviation with the examiner's thumb blocking flexion of the scaphoid by putting pressure over the scaphoid tubercle (Watson's test).

In a static deformity, radiographs will show a scapholunate angle greater than 70°, widening of the scapholunate joint of more than 3 mm, dorsiflexion of the lunate, and a cortical ring sign as the distal pole of the scaphoid in its palmarly flexed position is seen end on[127,145] (Fig. 30-43).

If the deformity is a dynamic instability, the routine radiographic changes may be more subtle, so stress views of the wrist are recommended. These stress views are PA views of the wrist taken in radial and ulnar deviation, with the fingers curled into a fist for compressive loading of the wrist and the forearm supinated. Comparison views should always be taken of the uninjured wrist (Fig. 30-44). When the diagnosis cannot be confirmed by routine and stress radiographs, the scapholunate ligament may be stretched or partially torn. An arthrogram of the

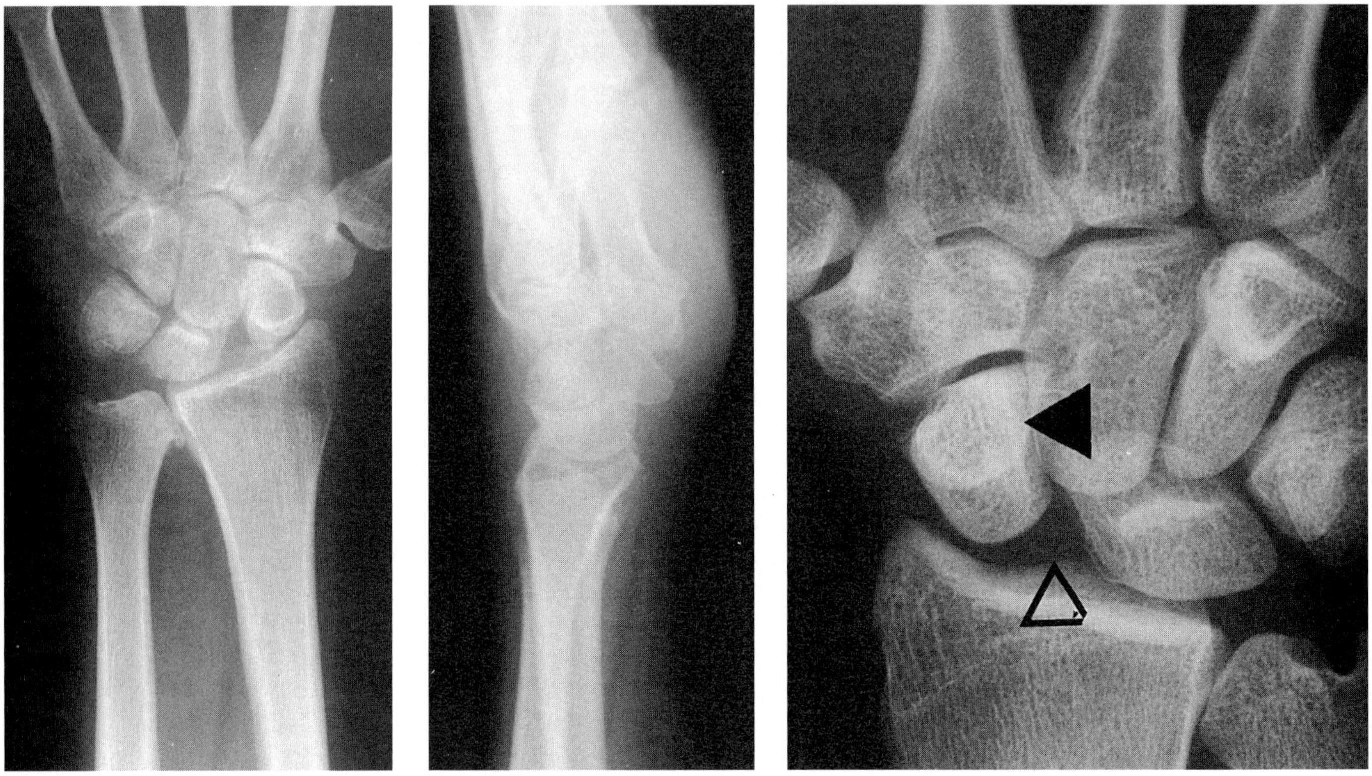

FIGURE 30-43 Static scapholunate instability. **A,** On the PA radiograph a significant separation is noted between the scaphoid and lunate and a ring sign is present. **B,** The lateral radiograph shows a DISI instability pattern. **C,** A close-up view of a ring sign *(solid arrow)* and the gap between the scaphoid and lunate *(arrow).*

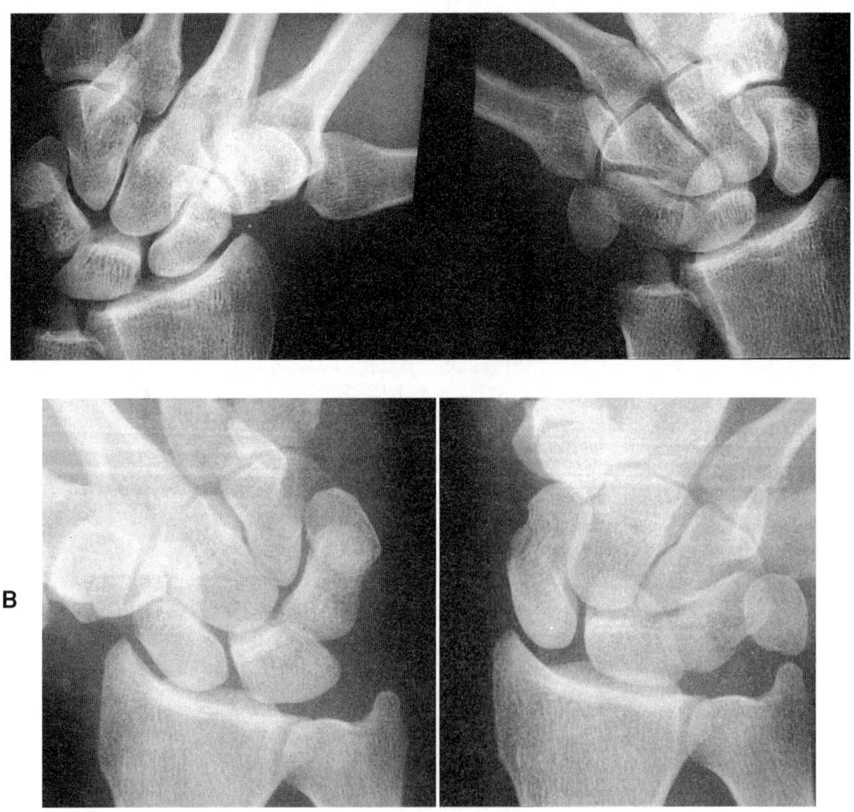

FIGURE 30-44 Dynamic scapholunate instability. **A,** The separation between the scaphoid and lunate is seen on the stress view. **B,** The opposite extremity is normal.

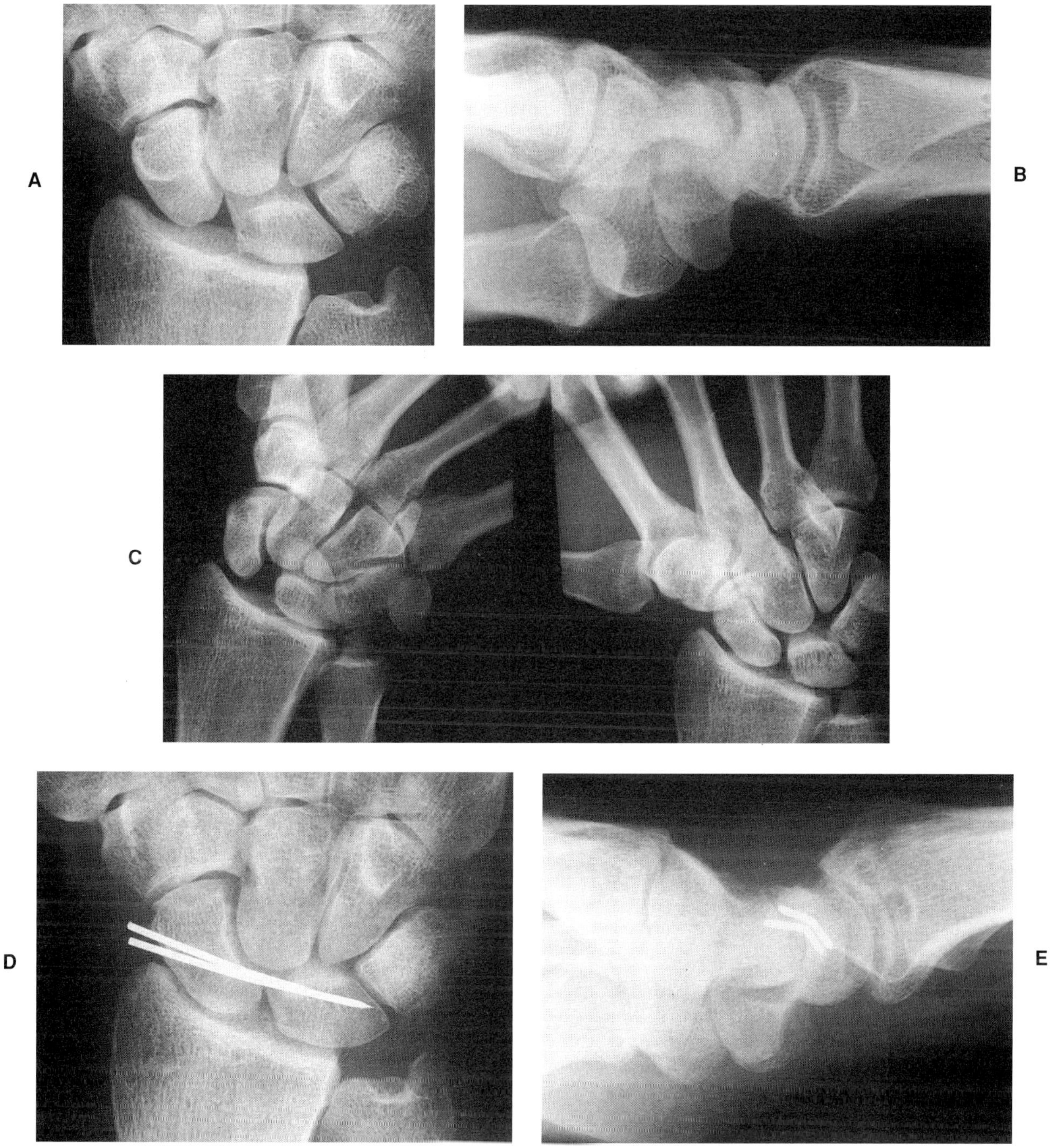

FIGURE 30-45 Four weeks after an injury to his wrist playing golf, the patient had persistent pain and swelling over the dorsum of the wrist. **A,** The PA radiograph showed a vertical tilt of the scaphoid and, **B,** the lateral view showed a dorsal tilt of the lunate. **C,** Stress radiographs confirmed the diagnosis of scapholunate instability. **D,** After ligament reconstruction and Kirschner wire fixation, **E,** carpal alignment is restored.

wrist may be useful in evaluating the integrity of the ligaments.

An acute scapholunate ligament tear with a DISI deformity and scapholunate joint widening of more than 3 mm on radiographs is best treated surgically. There is no place in the treatment of this disorder for cast immobilization of the wrist. When the scapholunate gap exceeds 4 to 5 mm, an open operation is best for reducing the scapholunate dissociation, repairing the torn ligaments, and immobilizing the reduced bones with Kirschner wires. This procedure produces excellent results and restores good function to the wrist[32,127,145] (Fig. 30-45).

This author prefers to approach the joint through a dorsal incision. The third and fourth extensor compartments are opened, the tendons are retracted, and the capsule of the radiocarpal joint is opened. This provides

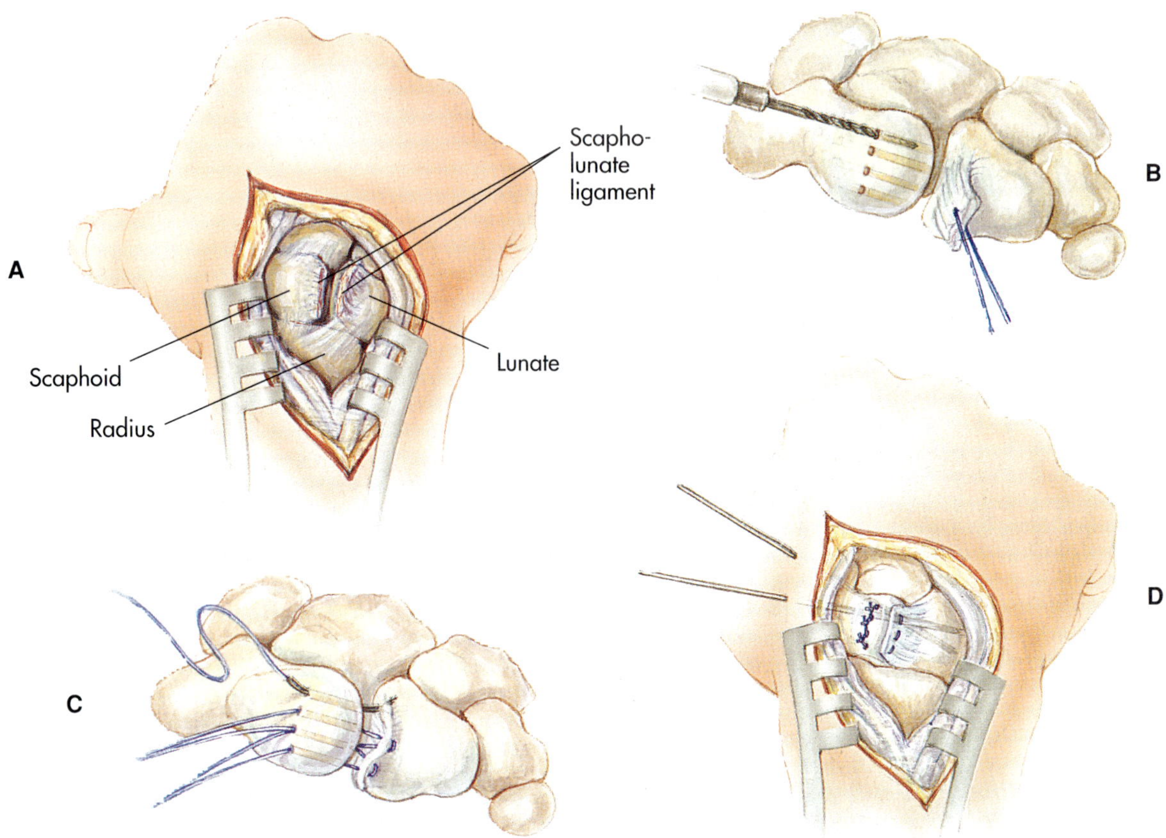

FIGURE 30-46 Schematic of reconstruction for scapholunate ligament tear. **A,** The wrist is opened through a dorsal incision and the torn scapholunate ligament identified. **B,** Drill holes are made in the proximal scaphoid. **C,** Sutures are passed through the ligament and the scaphoid. **D,** The scaphoid and lunate are reduced and immobilized with Kirschner wires. The sutures are tied against the scaphoid.

an excellent exposure of the proximal scaphoid and lunate. The ligament usually detaches from the scaphoid. A small cuff of tissue is left to allow a direct repair of the torn ligament. If not, drill holes can be made in the scaphoid and the ligament reattached[32,58,127] (Fig. 30-46). The hand and wrist then are immobilized for 8 weeks in a short arm cast, the Kirschner wires are removed, and rehabilitation is started. Loading of the wrist is not allowed for 3 months after the operation.

Arthroscopy has been advocated as a diagnostic and therapeutic tool in carpal instability injuries.[71,152] The physician can use the arthroscope both to identify extrinsic ligament injuries (using the 3-4 portal to examine the volar ligaments and the 1-2 portal for the dorsal ligaments) and to evaluate injuries of the intrinsic ligaments. Examination and palpation of the scapholunate ligament can be performed under direct visualization, and the extent of the tear can be accurately determined (Fig. 30-47). Débridement of partial ligament tears is reported to be successful in allowing athletes to return to complete activity in about 2 weeks.[71] Arthroscopic reduction and immobilization (ARIF) of acute scapholunate dissociations has been described by Whipple[152,159] and Ruch et al.[128] Whipple reports a 70% success rate in patients treated within 3 months of injury if the scapholunate interval measures less than 3 mm.

Treatment of the "chronic" scapholunate dissociation is more controversial. The definition of a chronic injury has been extended to 12 months or longer from the time of injury. At that time there are secondary structural changes in the carpal bones and ligaments caused by the unconstrained position of the bones. This makes reduction of the carpal bones more difficult.

If sufficient ligament is present and the bones can be reduced, ligament reconstruction is the preferred operation[32,58,73,127] (Fig. 30-48). This invariably requires drill holes placed into the proximal scaphoid to reattach the ligament and stabilization of the scaphoid and lunate by Kirschner wires in their reduced positions. This procedure can be augmented by the dorsal capsulodesis recommended by Blatt.[13] This involves using a flap of dorsal capsule based proximally to help stabilize the scaphoid.

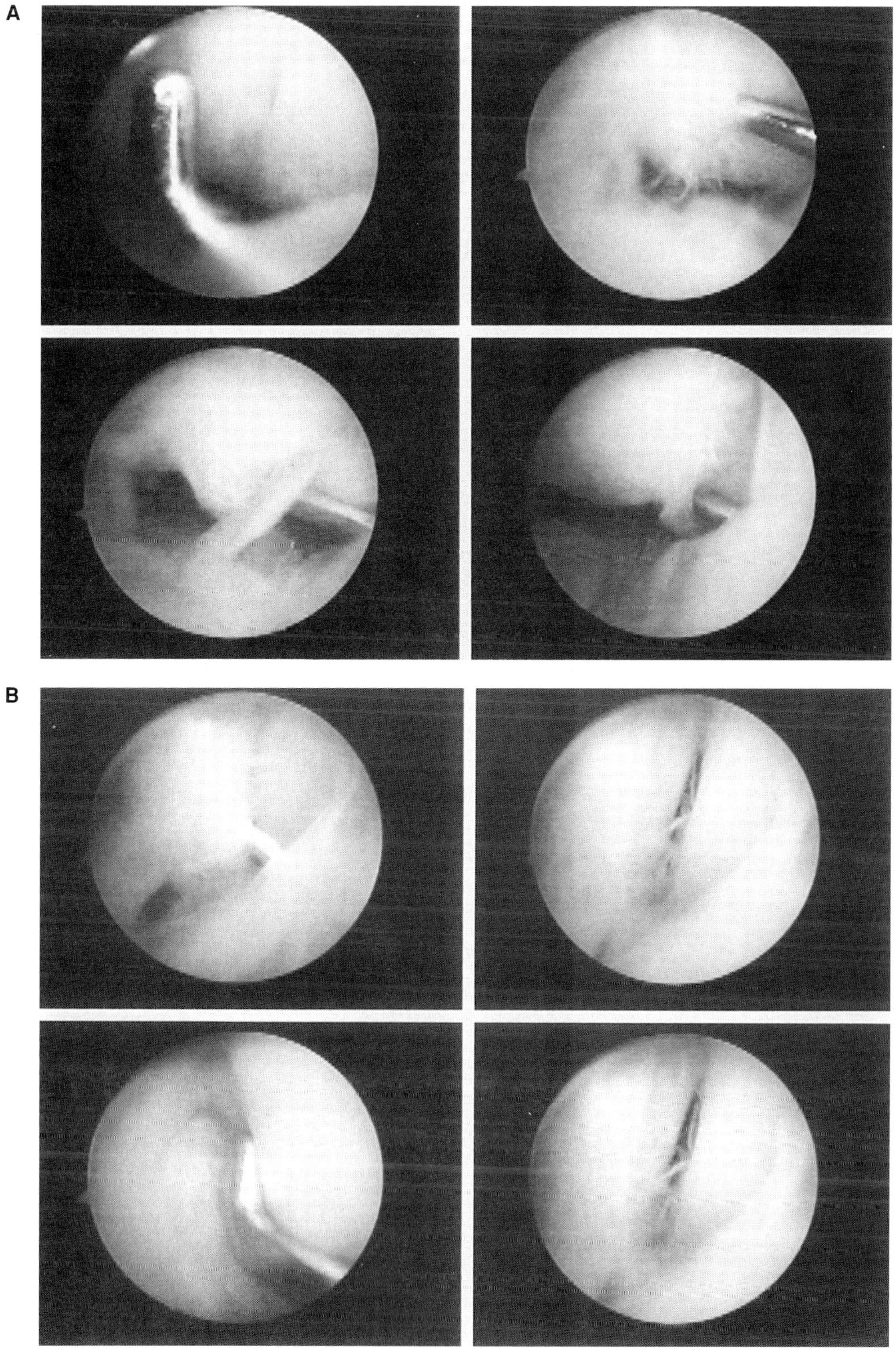

FIGURE 30-47 Right wrist arthroscope in the 3-4 portal. **A,** Partial tear of the interosseous scapholunate (probe). **B,** A complete tear of the interosseous scapholunate ligament with the probe in the scapholunate joint.

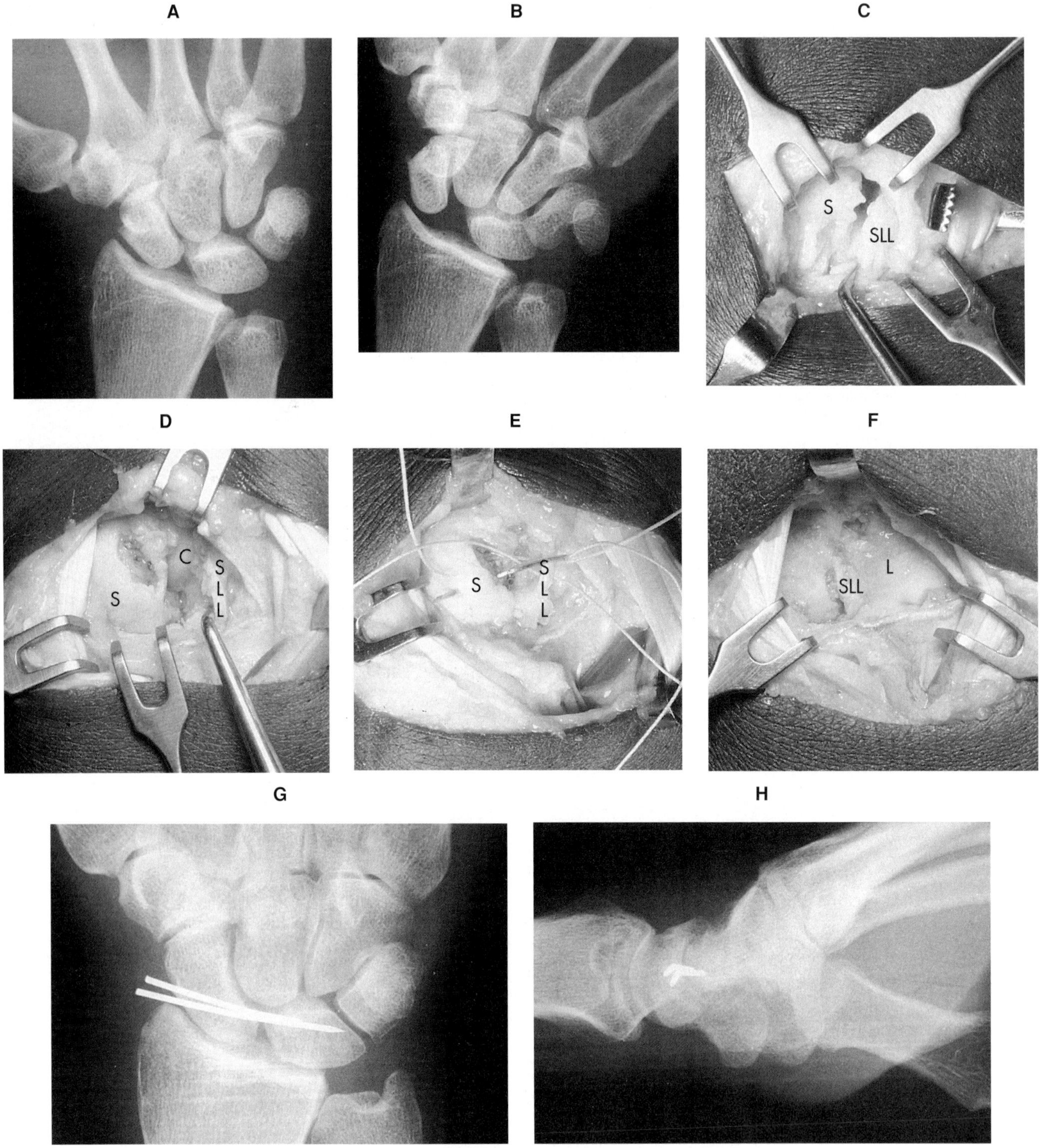

FIGURE 30-48 Right wrist. The injury occurred 9 months before treatment while playing basketball. **A** and **B**, Radiographs show a dynamic scapholunate instability. **C**, Using a dorsal approach, the wrist was opened. A complete tear of the scapholunate ligament was found (probe). The ligament had torn off the scaphoid. **D**, Drill holes are placed in the proximal scaphoid, **E**, sutures are passed through the scaphoid and the ligament, and, **F**, after the separation between the scaphoid and lunate is reduced and immobilized with Kirschner wires, the sutures are tied. **G** and **H**, Reduction of the scapholunate instability. *S*, Scaphoid; *SLL*, scapholunate ligament; *L*, lunate; *C*, capitate.

Occasionally the author has augmented the scapholunate ligament reconstruction with local tissue to enhance scar formation at the joint. This tissue is sutured directly to the bone. The wrist is then immobilized for 8 weeks in plaster, and rehabilitation is started after the Kirschner wires are removed. The rehabilitation procedure after reconstruction is much slower than for an acute injury, and the athlete is not allowed to return to unrestricted activity for 4 to 6 months. Individuals competing in sports requiring heavy lifting or repeated motion and compressive loads on the wrist are at risk for reinjury.

Ligament reconstruction using tendons placed through drill holes in the bone was unreliable and is no longer recommended.[127]

In cases where ligament reconstruction is not possible or when the scaphoid and lunate cannot be reduced, limited intercarpal fusion is recommended. Either the scaphotrapezial trapezoid fusion[153] (Fig. 30-49) or the scaphocapitate fusion[117] can be used. These fusions will cause some limitations of wrist motion, and residual weakness and pain may be present with forced loading of the wrist into dorsiflexion.

Untreated scapholunate dissociation will progress to degenerative arthritis of the wrist[127,145] (Fig. 30-50).

LUNOTRIQUETRAL INJURIES

These injuries are less common than scapholunate injuries. They also can result from a fall onto the outstretched hand. Symptoms include pain and swelling over the lunotriquetral joint on the ulnar side of the wrist and ulnocarpal joint pain. Examination indicates tenderness in the above areas, but usually there is no tenderness over the triangular fibrocartilage complex. Ballottement of the lunate and triquetrum in a dorsopalmar direction (Linscheid test) or ulnar to radial compression

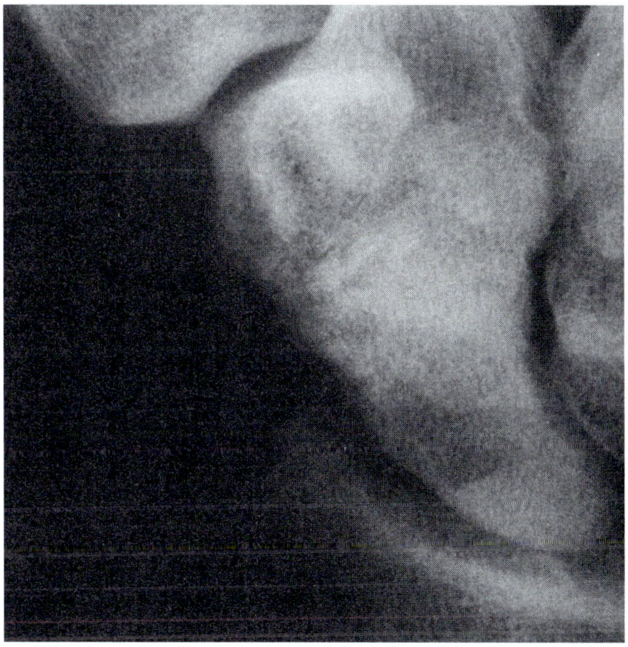

FIGURE 30-49 Scaphotrapezio-trapezoid fusion *(STT)* is one method of stabilizing a *chronic* scapholunate instability.

A

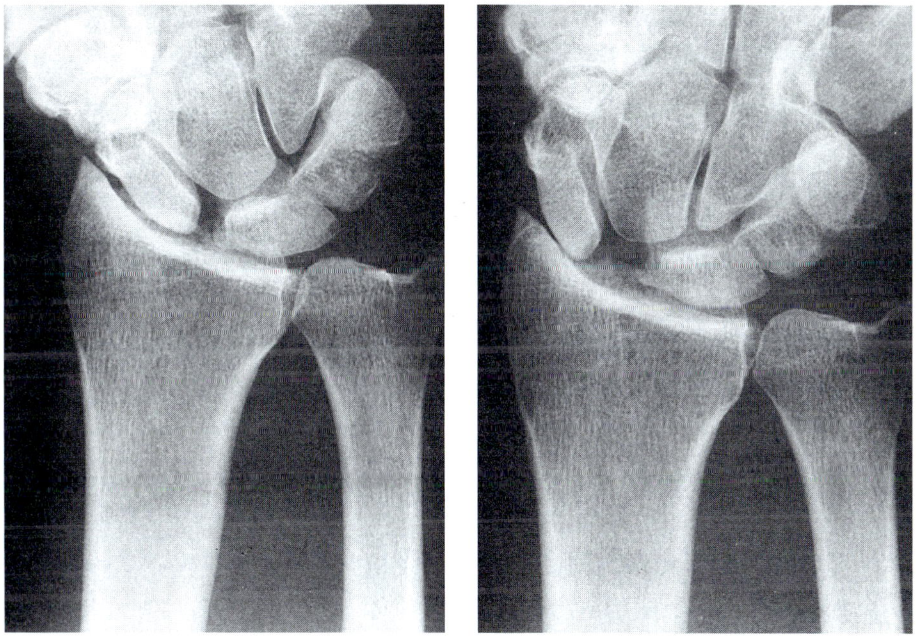

B

FIGURE 30-50 **A** and **B,** Significant degenerative arthritis at the radioscaphoid joint from an untreated scapholunate dissociation.

of the triquetrum against the lunate (Kleinman test) may elicit joint pain and is a useful diagnostic test.[32]

Radiographic changes in the wrist are not as dramatic as with a scapholunate dissociation. The lateral view may show a VISI configuration, and there may be a step-off between the lunate and triquetrum in the proximal convex articular line of the carpal bones on the PA view (Fig. 30-51). Stress views are rarely helpful. The best way to make a definitive diagnosis is by arthrography of the wrist. Both radiocarpal and midcarpal joints should be injected[75,107] (Fig. 30-52).

Acute injuries of the lunotriquetral joint usually can be treated with a cast and nonsteroidal antiinflammatory medication. These sprains usually resolve with conservative care.[71,145] Arthroscopic evaluation of the extent of the ligament tear often is useful in deciding the appro-

A

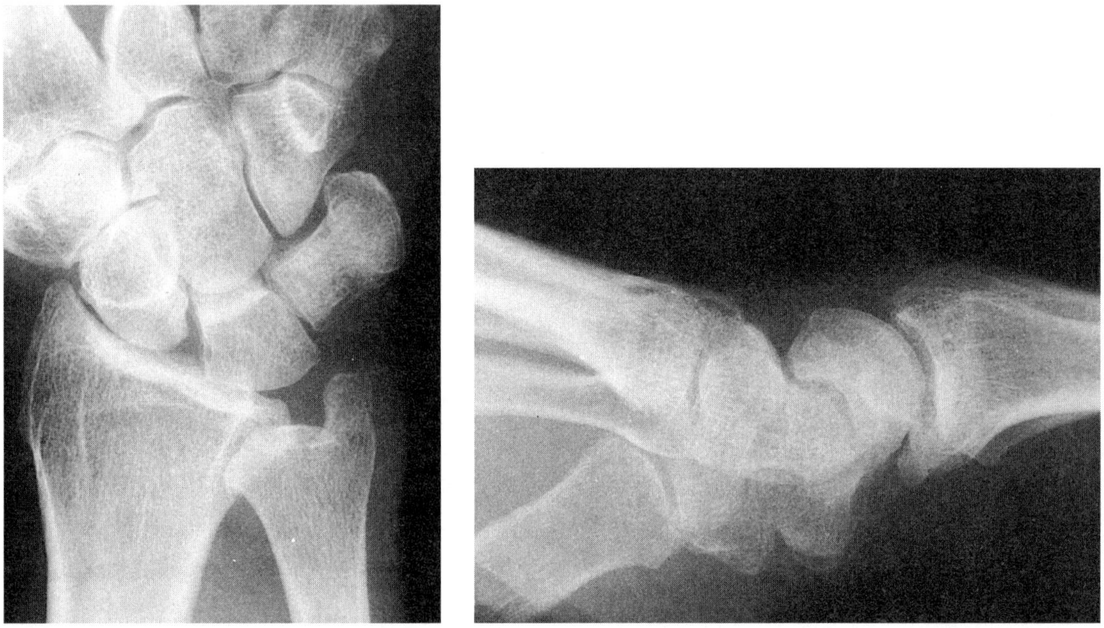

B

FIGURE 30-51 **A,** The PA radiograph shows a step-off at the lunotriquetral joint. **B,** A VISI instability pattern is seen on the lateral view.

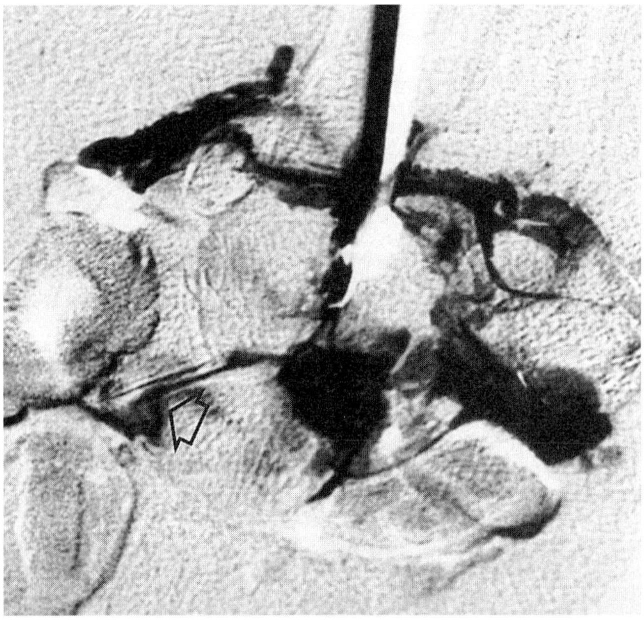

FIGURE 30-52 A midcarpal arthrogram of a left wrist shows dye leaking into the radiocarpal joint through a tear in the lunotriquetral ligament *(arrow)*.

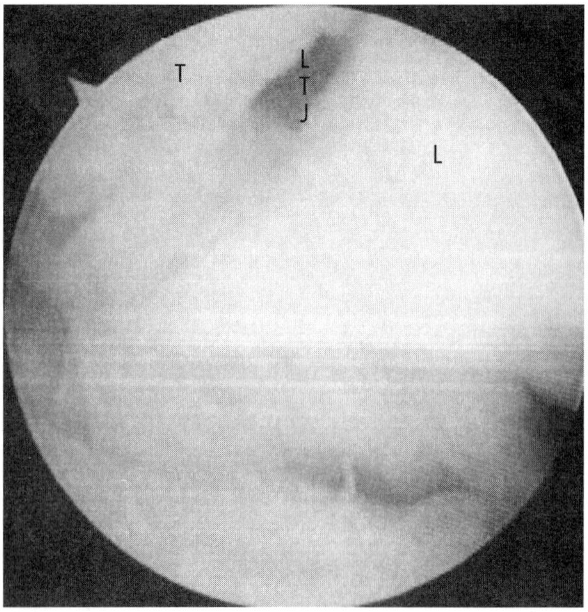

FIGURE 30-53 Left wrist with the arthroscope in the 6-A portal. A complete tear of the lunotriquetral ligament. *T,* Triquetrum; *L,* lunate; *LTJ,* lunotriquetral joint.

priate treatment (Fig. 30-53). If the ligament is discovered to be disrupted, arthroscopically assisted reduction and pinning of the joint has been employed.[71,99,152]

If the lunotriquetral instability becomes chronic and debilitating, either lunotriquetral ligament reconstruction with or without tendon augmentation or a lunotriquetral arthrodesis has been recommended[122] (Fig. 30-54).

Ulnar impingement syndrome (ulnar-plus configuration and tear of the triangular fibrocartilage complex) associated with a lunotriquetral injury is best treated with ulnar shortening.

MIDCARPAL INSTABILITY

Primary midcarpal instability that results from injury to the extrinsic ligaments of the wrist[3,76,83] presents with vague pain in the wrist and a loud clunk with wrist motion.[20,76] The diagnosis can be made with video radiography or arthroscopy. Attempts to reconstruct the extrinsic ligaments have not been particularly successful, especially in a high-demand individual such as an athlete.[71] Arthrodesis of the midcarpal joint will correct the instability, but wrist motion will be decreased by about 50%. This could be disabling for an athlete. If possible, symptomatic treatment with or without a wrist splint should be tried to allow the individual to try to continue in sports.

DISTAL RADIOULNAR JOINT INJURIES

Soft-tissue injuries at the distal radioulnar joint can be associated with radioulnar subluxation and cartilage and bony injury at the joint. The primary soft-tissue injury to this joint occurs through the triangular fibrocartilage and its associated ligaments.

The extrinsic ligaments on the ulnar side of the wrist include the ulnolunate, ulnotriquetral, and triangular fibrocartilage complex (see Fig. 30-41). A primary stabilizer of the distal radioulnar joint, the triangular fibrocartilage complex consists of the triangular fibrocartilage itself, meniscal homologue, radioulnar ligaments, the ulnar collateral ligament, and the sheath of the extensor carpi ulnaris tendon[106] (Fig. 30-55). Palmer et al[106] noted that the triangular fibrocartilage complex functions both as a cushion for the ulnar carpus and as a major stabilizer of the distal radioulnar joint.

Blood supply to the triangular fibrocartilage is restricted to the peripheral 15% to 20%, leaving the central articular disc relatively avascular. Triangular fibrocartilage thickness is related to ulnar variance.[108] A thicker disc is associated with an ulnar-minus variant, and a thin disc is present in an ulnar-plus individual (Fig. 30-56). Mikic showed that degenerative changes in the triangular fibrocartilage begin in the third decade and progress with age.[97] Palmer[109] has classified triangular fibrocartilage complex tears into traumatic (four subheadings describing location) and degenerative (with subheadings of increasing changes resulting from ulnocarpal abutment syndrome). However, younger athletes with an ulnar-plus variant who are involved in sports with significant loading of the ulnar side of the wrist can develop degenerative tears of the triangular fibrocartilage.

Injuries to the distal radioulnar joint often are associated with fractures of the radius and with Essex-Lopresti and Galeazzi fracture-dislocations. Isolated dislocations and subluxation of this joint occur, but they are less common. Injuries to the distal radioulnar joint result from a

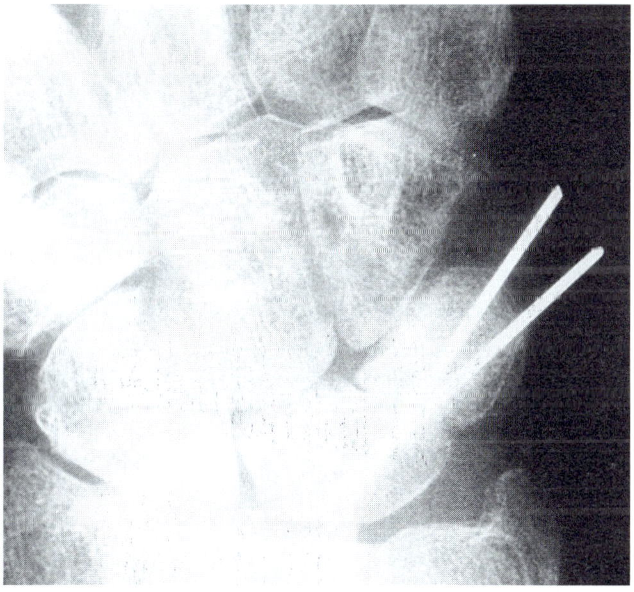

FIGURE 30-54 A lunotriquetral instability was stabilized by fusing the joint.

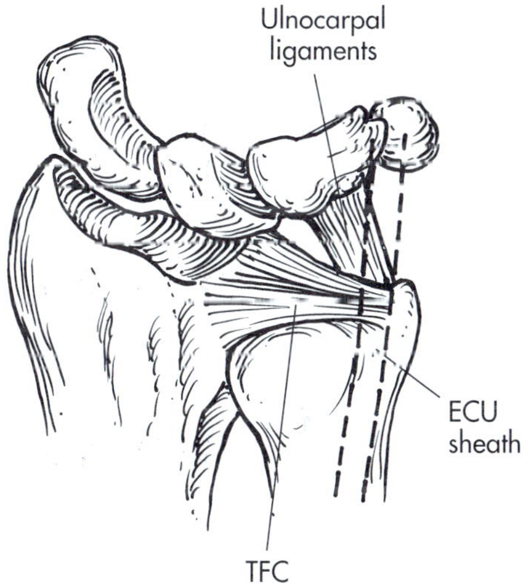

FIGURE 30-55 The schematic of TFC complex.

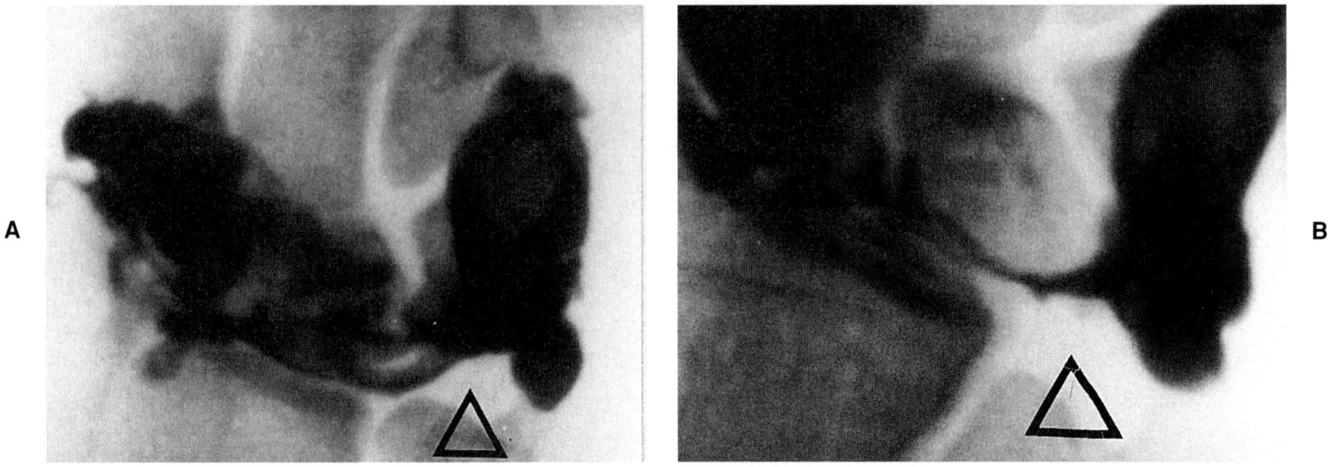

FIGURE 30-56 Arthrogram of right wrist showing, **A,** normal triangular fibrocartilage *(arrow)* and, **B,** a thicker than normal triangular fibrocartilage *(arrow)* associated with a shorter ulna.

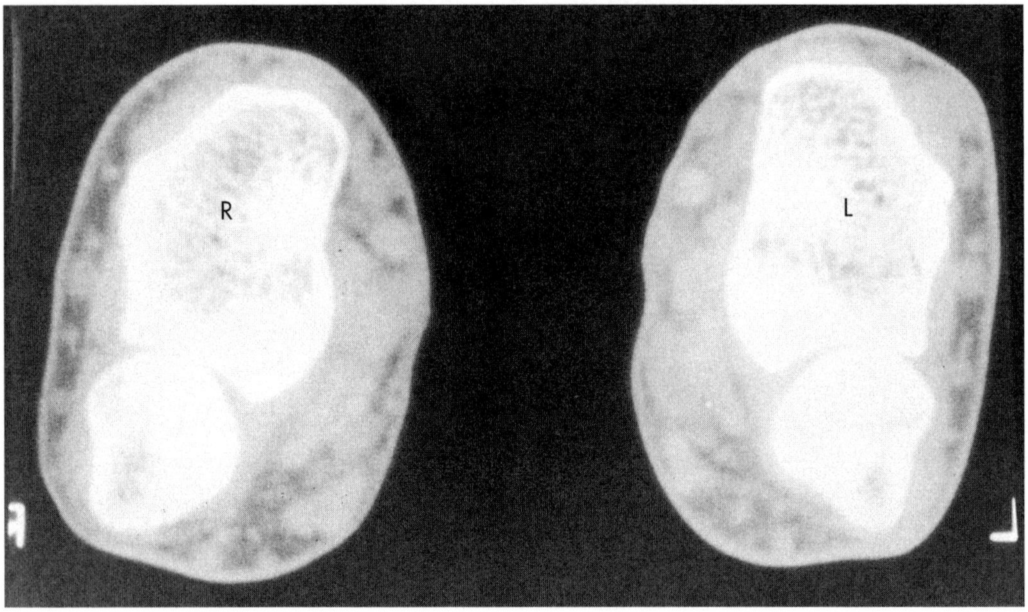

FIGURE 30-57 An axial view CT scan showing the normal relationship between the radius and ulna on the left *(L)*, while the head of the ulna is slightly dorsally subluxated on the right *(R)*.

fall or injury in which the dorsiflexed wrist is pronated and ulnarly deviated. Because the concavity on the ulnar side of the radius is shallow, stability of this joint depends on the ulnar-side ligaments and the distal portion of the interosseous membrane.

Symptoms will vary from mild pain on the ulnar side of the wrist to significant pain and swelling. Examination can show slight laxity of the joint, prominence of the head of the ulna either dorsally or palmarly, a clunk as the head of the ulna seats itself, or significant restriction of forearm rotation. A dislocation or subluxation of the head of the ulna is more common dorsally.

If radiographs are inconclusive, a CT scan of the joint in the axial view will be useful to show displacement of the head of the ulna[98] (Fig. 30-57). Arthrography of the wrist is useful in evaluating any associated injury to the triangular fibrocartilage complex, especially if there is an associated fracture of the base of the ulnar styloid (Fig. 30-58).

Acute injuries to the distal radioulnar joint are treated with cast immobilization of the forearm in supination for dorsal subluxations or dislocations of the ulna and in pronation for palmar displacement of the head of the ulna. Open treatment to repair the detached triangular fibrocartilage may be necessary.[123]

For chronic instability of the distal radioulnar joint, with persistent pain, weakness, and instability, a variety of reconstructive procedures have been described in the

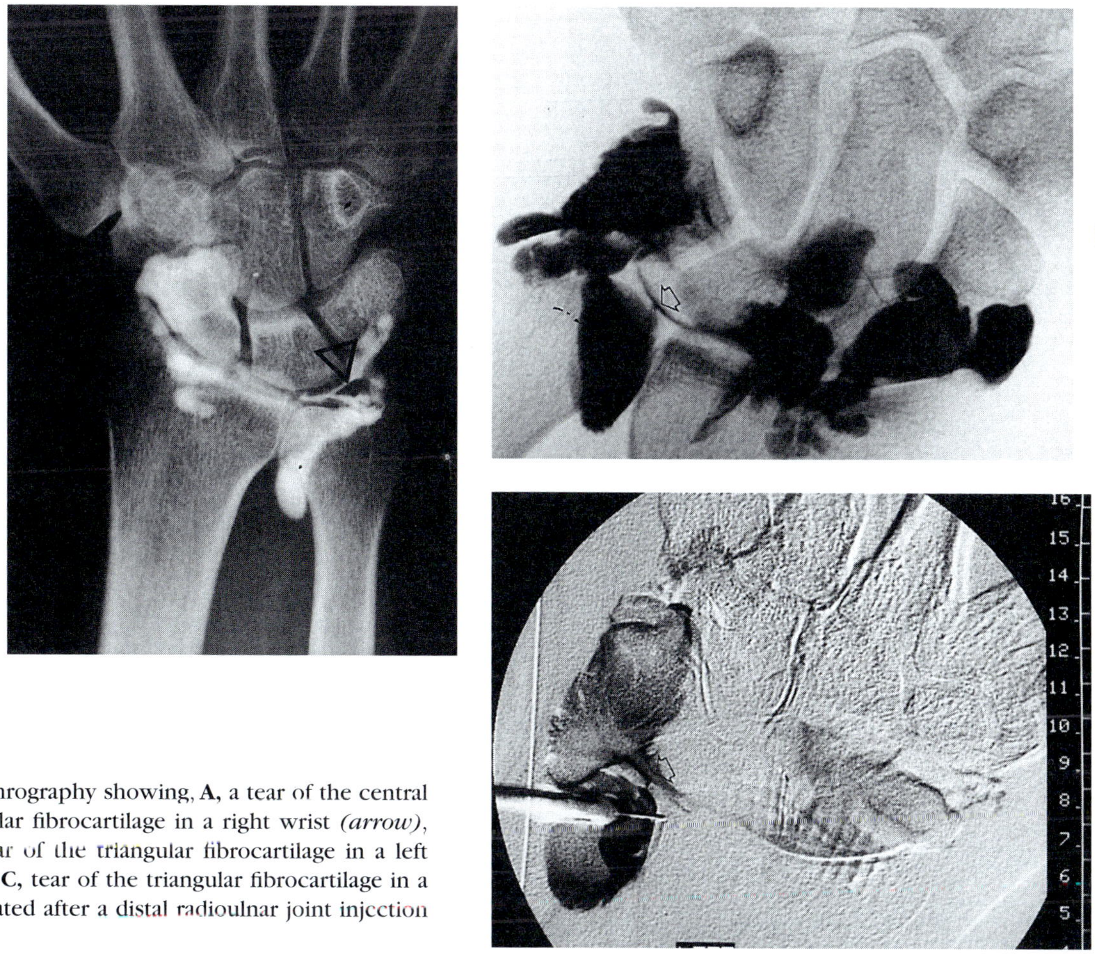

FIGURE 30-58 Arthrography showing, **A**, a tear of the central third of the triangular fibrocartilage in a right wrist *(arrow)*, **B**, a radial third tear of the triangular fibrocartilage in a left wrist *(arrow)*, and, **C**, tear of the triangular fibrocartilage in a left wrist demonstrated after a distal radioulnar joint injection *(arrow)*.

literature.[17] However, these procedures have not been uniformly successful.[114] This type of injury can significantly impair the performance of an athlete.

TRIANGULAR FIBROCARTILAGE INJURIES

Injuries to the triangular fibrocartilage complex can result in tears or perforations of this structure. These injuries include ulnotriquetral ligament disruptions, peripheral detachment of the triangular fibrocartilage from the ulna or radius, avulsion of the triangular fibrocartilage complex from the ulnar styloid, central tears, and complex injuries associated with subluxation of the head of the ulna.[71] The exact extent of the injury can be confirmed using arthrography and arthroscopy (Fig 30-59).

If an acute injury is not associated with a significant separation of the triangular fibrocartilage complex from the ulna or radius, it can be treated with cast immobilization. A peripheral tear of the radial or ulnar attachment of the triangular fibrocartilage should be repaired because the periphery of the structure has the potential to heal.[17,147]

A central linear or flap tear can be débrided arthroscopically with good results[152] (Fig. 30-60).

Ulnar-side wrist pain can be particularly disabling in golfers, tennis players, gymnasts, and throwing athletes. Chronic or degenerative tears of the triangular fibrocartilage complex often are associated with pain on forearm rotation and ulnar deviation of the wrist. These lesions are best diagnosed and treated arthroscopically. Synovitis, cartilage fibers, or central tears can be débrided arthroscopically.[1,71,152] If there are changes indicating an ulnar impingement syndrome, pain can be relieved with an ulnar shortening procedure. In a competitive athlete, an accurate diagnosis is imperative, and a specific treatment program for that individual must be developed. The more complex the ulnar-side wrist injury, the more difficult the return to high-level competitive sports.

GYMNAST'S WRIST

Over the past 10 to 20 years, participation in gymnastics has significantly increased in the United States. Athletes participate at the high-school, college, and club levels, and the sport has been especially popular with female athletes. The age of the participants ranges from 6 or 7

A

B

C

D

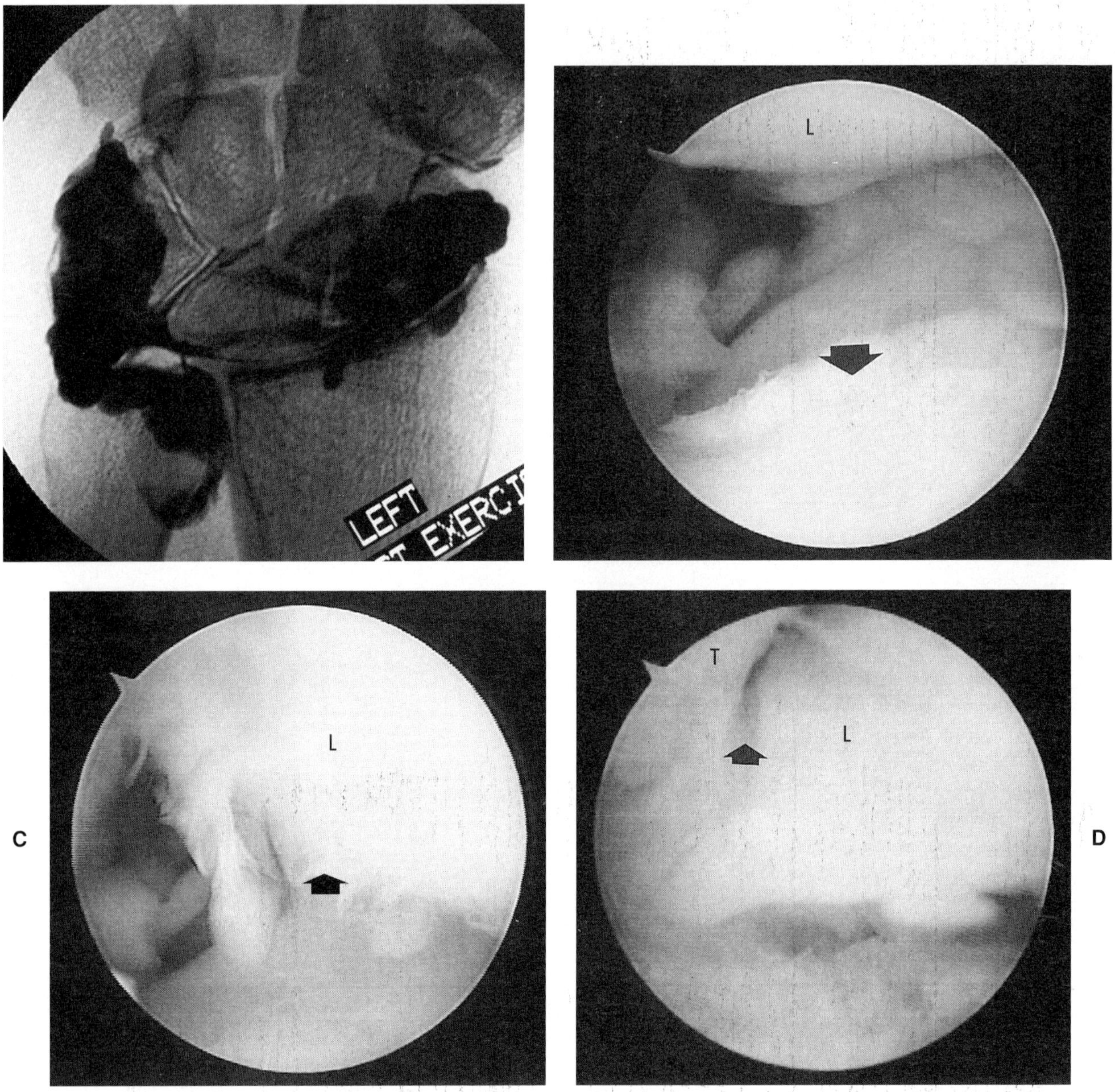

FIGURE 30-59 **A,** An arthrogram of this left wrist showed a tear of the triangular fibrocartilage and a tear of the lunotriquetral ligament. Arthroscopy showed, **B,** a tear of the triangular fibrocartilage *(arrow)*, **C,** chondromalacia of the lunate *(arrow)*, and, **D,** a tear of the lunotriquetral ligament *(arrow)*. *L,* Lunate; *T,* triquetrum.

years to 20 years. These individuals spend many hours each week practicing and competing.

The primary mechanism of loading of the wrist in gymnastics is compressive, and the most common position of the wrist is in dorsiflexion.[38] These repetitive compressive loads on the wrist, occurring with a significant frequency and intensity, superimposed on an immature skeleton, can cause a variety of wrist injuries. Chronic wrist injuries are significantly more common than acute injuries.[38,115] The incidence of chronic injuries in gymnastics ranges from 17% to 43%.[38] However, 80% to 90% of wrist complaints are related to chronic overuse of the wrist. Aronen[5] reported that "dorsal wrist pain is considered by gymnasts to be a direct consequence of the sport and not an injury."

Repetitive compressive loading and unloading of the wrist causes a spectrum of bony and soft-tissue injuries.[38,89,158] These injuries include stress reaction and injury to the physis of the distal radius and ulna, premature closure of the physis of the distal radius and ulna, scaphoid impaction syndrome, ulnar impaction syndrome, avascular necrosis of the capitate, acquired Madelung's deformity, carpal chondromalacia, chronic wrist capsulitis, wrist "splints," triangular fibrocomplex

A

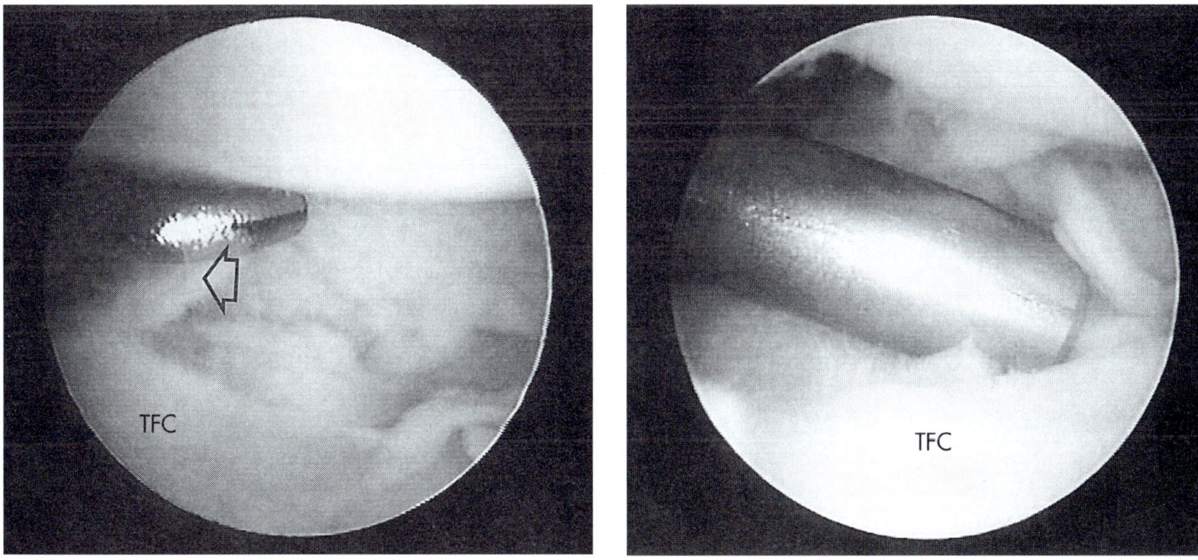

B

FIGURE 30-60 **A,** Flap tear involving the central third of the triangular cartilage *(arrow),* **B,** can be removed using a shaver or punch. *TFC,* Triangular fibrocartilage.

tears, dorsal carpal ganglia, carpal instability, and tendinitis. Treatment of the wrist condition depends on the diagnosis. In general, rest, taping and splinting of the wrist to prevent hyperextension, icing, and strengthening the flexor forearm muscles will provide varying degrees of pain relief. Arthroscopy of the wrist, débridement of the triangular fibrocartilage complex, and ulnar shortening have been used successfully to relieve ulnar-side wrist pain in a gymnast.[89,148] Preventing these conditions is difficult if not impossible, aside from stopping participation in gymnastics.

SUMMARY

A wide spectrum of wrist injuries has been discussed. Early and accurate diagnosis, appropriate treatment, and an individualized rehabilitation program will restore function to the wrist. Newer imaging techniques and arthroscopy of the wrist are valuable tools in the diagnosis and treatment of wrist disorders. Because many of these wrist injuries are potentially career ending, the treating physician and trainer must be aware of the many disorders that can occur within the wrist.

References

1. Adams BD: Partial excision of the triangular fibrocartilage complex articular disk: a biomechanical study, *J Hand Surg* 18A:334-340, 1993.
2. Adler JB, Shaftan G: Fractures of the capitate, *J Bone Joint Surg* 44A:1537-1547, 1962.
3. Alexander CE, Lichtman DM: Ulnar carpal instabilities, *Orthop Clin North Am* 15:307-320, 1984.
4. Amadio PC, Taleisnik J: Fractures of the carpal bones. In Green DP, Hotchkiss RN, editors: *Operative hand surgery,* ed 3, New York, 1993, Churchill Livingstone, pp 799-860.
5. Aronen JG: Problems of the upper extremity in gymnasts, *Clin Sports Med* 4:61-71, 1985.
6. Axelrod T et al: Limited open reduction of the lunate facet in comminuted intra-articular fractures of the distal radius, *J Hand Surg* 13A:372-377, 1988.
7. Bacorn RW, Kurtzke JF: Colles' fracture: a study of two thousand cases from the New York State Worker's Compensation Board, *J Bone Joint Surg* 35A:643-658, 1953.
8. Bartone NF, Grieco RV: Fractures of the triquetrum, *J Bone Joint Surg* 38A:353-356, 1956.
9. Beckenbaugh RD et al: Kienböck's disease: the natural history of Kienböck's disease and considerations of lunate fractures, *Clin Orthop* 149:98-106, 1980.
10. Bell MJ, Hill RJ, McMurtry RY: Ulnar impingement syndrome, *J Bone Joint Surg* 67B:126-129, 1985.
11. Bickerstaff DR, Bell MJ: Carpal malalignment in Colles' fractures, *J Hand Surg* 14B:155-160, 1989.
12. Bishop AT, Beckenbaugh RD: Fracture of the hamate hook, *J Hand Surg* 13A:135-139, 1988.
13. Blatt G: Capsulodesis in reconstructive hand surgery, *Hand Clin* 3:81-102, 1987.
14. Bora FW, Didizian NH: The treatment of injuries to the carpometacarpal joint of the little finger, *J Bone Joint Surg* 56A:1459-1463, 1974
15. Borgeskov S et al: Fracture of the carpal bones, *Acta Orthop Scand* 37:276 287, 1986.
16. Botte MJ, Gelberman RH: Fractures of the carpus, excluding the scaphoid, *Hand Clin* 3.149-161, 1987.
17. Bowers WH: The distal radio-ulnar joint. In Green DP, Hotchkiss RN, Third ED, editors: *Operative hand surgery,* New York, 1993, Churchill Livingstone, pp 973-1019.
18. Boyes JH: *Bunnell's surgery of the hand,* ed 5, Philadelphia, 1970, JB Lippincott, p 591.
19. Bradway JK, Amadio PC, Cooney WP: Open reduction and internal fixation of displaced comminuted intra-articular fractures of the distal end of the radius, *J Bone Joint Surg* 71A:839-847, 1989.
20. Brown DE, Lichtman DM: Mild carpal instability, *Hand Clin* 3:135-140, 1987.

21. Bryan RS, Dobyns JH: Fractures of the carpal bones other than lunate and navicular, *Clin Orthop* 149:107-111, 1980.
22. Bunker TD, McNamee PB, Scott TD: The Herbert screw for scaphoid fractures: a multicenter study, *J Bone Joint Surg* 69B:631-634, 1987.
23. Carter PR, Eaton RG, Littler JW: Ununited fracture of the hook of the hamate, *J Bone Joint Surg* 59A:583-588, 1977.
24. Collert S, Isacson J: Management of redislocated Colles' fractures, *Clin Orthop* 135:183-186, 1978.
25. Colles A: On the fracture of the carpal extremity of the radius, *Edinb Med Surg J* 10:182-186, 1814.
26. Cooney WP, Linscheid RL, Dobyns JH: External pin fixation for unstable Colles' fractures, *J Bone Joint Surg* 61A:840-845, 1979.
27. Cooney WP, Dobyns JH, Linscheid RL: Fractures of the scaphoid: a rational approach to management, *Clin Orthop* 149:90-97, 1980.
28. Cooney WP, Dobyns JH, Linscheid RL: Nonunion of the scaphoid: analysis of the results from bone grafting, *J Hand Surg* 5:343-354, 1980.
29. Cooney WP et al: Management of intra-articular fractures of the distal radius, *Contemp Orthop* 21:71-104, 1990.
30. Cooney WP, Dobyns JH, Linscheid RL: Complications of Colles' fracture, *J Bone Joint Surg* 62A:613-619, 1980.
31. Cooney WP et al: Scaphoid nonunion: role of anterior interpositional bone graft, *J Hand Surg* 13A:635-650, 1988.
32. Cooney WP, Linscheid RL, Dobyns JH: Carpal instability: treatment of ligament injuries of the wrist, *Instructional Course Lectures, AAOS* XLI:33-44, 1992.
33. Cordrey LJ, Ferrer-Torells M: Management of fractures of the greater multangular, *J Bone Joint Surg* 42A:1111-1118, 1960.
34. Crosby EB, Linscheid RL: Rupture of the flexor profundus tendon of the ring finger secondary to ancient fracture of the hook of the hamate: review of the literature and report of 2 cases, *J Bone Joint Surg* 56A:1076-1078, 1974.
35. Culver JE: Sports-related fractures of the hand and wrist, *Clin Sports Med* 9:85-109, 1990.
36. De Maagd RL, Engber WD: Retrograde Herbert screw fixation for treatment of proximal pole scaphoid nonunion, *J Hand Surg* 14A:996-1003, 1989.
37. Dobyns JH et al: Traumatic instability of the wrist. In: *Instructional course lectures, AAOS,* St Louis, 1975, CV Mosby, pp 182-199.
38. Dobyns JH, Gabel G: Gymnast's wrist, *Hand Clin* 6:493-505, 1990.
39. Dowling JJ, Sawyer B Jr: Comminuted Colles' fracture: evaluation of a method of treatment, *J Bone Joint Surg* 43A:657-668, 1961.
40. Egawa M, Asai T: Fracture of the hook of the hamate: report of six cases and the suitability of computerized tomography, *J Hand Surg* 8:393-398, 1983.
41. Fenton RL: The naviculo-capitate syndrome, *J Bone Joint Surg* 38A:681-684, 1956.
42. Fernandez DL: Correction of posttraumatic wrist deformity in adults by osteotomy, bone grafting and internal fixation, *J Bone Joint Surg* 64A:1164-1178, 1982.
43. Fernandez DL: A technique for anterior wedge-shaped grafts for scaphoid nonunions with carpal instability, *J Hand Surg* 9A:733-737, 1984.
44. Fernandez DL: *A practical, simplified, comprehensive and treatment oriented classification of fractures of the distal radius.* Presented at the 4th International Federation of Societies for Surgery of the Hand, Bone and Joint Injuries Committee, Paris, 1992.
45. Fernandez DL: Malunion of the distal radius: current approach to management, *Instructional Course Lectures, AAOS* 42:99-113, 1993.
46. Fisk GR: Carpal instability and the fractured scaphoid, *Ann R Coll Surg Engl* 46:63-76, 1970.
47. Ford DJ et al: The Herbert screw for fractures of the scaphoid: a review of results and technical difficulties, *J Bone Joint Surg* 69B:124-127, 1987.
48. Frykman G: Fractures of the distal radius including sequelae—shoulder hand finger syndrome, disturbance in the distal radio-ulnar joint and impairment of nerve function: a clinical and experimental study, *Acta Orthop Scand (Suppl)* 108, 1967.
49. Frykman GK et al: Treatment of nonunited scaphoid fractures by pulsed electromagnetic field and cast, *J Hand Surg* 11A:344-349, 1986.
50. Ganel A et al: Bone scanning in assessment of fractures of the scaphoid, *J Hand Surg* 4:540-543, 1979.
51. Gartland JJ Jr, Werley CW: Evaluation of healed Colles' fracture, *J Bone Joint Surg* 33A:895-907, 1951.
52. Gelberman RH, Menon J: The vascularity of the scaphoid bone, *J Hand Surg* 5:508-513, 1980.
53. Gelberman RH et al: The vascularity of the lunate bone and Kienböck's disease, *J Hand Surg* 5:272-278, 1980.
54. Gelberman RH et al: The arterial anatomy of the human carpus. I. The extraosseous vascularity, *J Hand Surg* 8:367-375, 1983.
55. Gelberman RH, Szabo RM: Kienböck's disease, *Orthop Clin North Am* 15:355-367, 1984.
56. Gelberman RH, Wolock BS, Siegel DB: Current concepts review: fractures and nonunions of the carpal scaphoid, *J Bone Joint Surg* 71A:1560-1565, 1989.
57. Green DP: The effect of avascular necrosis on Russe bone grafting for scaphoid nonunion, *J Hand Surg* 10A:597-605, 1985.
58. Green DP: Carpal dislocations and instabilities. In Green DP, Hotchkiss RN, editors: *Operative hand surgery,* New York, 1993, Churchill Livingstone, pp 861-928.
59. Hart VL, Gaynor V: Roentgenographic study of the carpal canal, *J Bone Joint Surg* 23:382-383, 1941.
60. Herbert TJ, Fisher WE: Management of the fracture scaphoid using a new bone screw, *J Bone Joint Surg* 66B:114-123, 1984.
61. Herbert TJ: Use of the Herbert bone screw, *Clin Orthop* 202:79-92, 1986.
62. Herbert TJ, Fisher WE, Leicester AW: The Herbert bone screw: a ten year perspective, *J Hand Surg* 17B:415-419, 1992.
63. Hooning Van Duyvenbode JFF et al: Pseudarthrosis of the scaphoid treated by the Matti-Russe operation, *J Bone Joint Surg* 73B:603-606, 1991.
64. Jenkins NH: The unstable Colles' fracture, *J Hand Surg* 14B:149-154, 1989.
65. Jiranek WA et al: Long-term results after Russe bone-grafting: the effect of malunion of the scaphoid, *J Bone Joint Surg* 74A:1217-1228, 1992.
66. Johnson RP: The acutely injured wrist and its residuals, *Clin Orthop* 149:33-44, 1980.
67. Jorgensen TM et al: Scanning and radiology of the carpal scaphoid bone, *Acta Orthop Scand* 50:663-665, 1979.
68. Jupiter JB: Current concepts review—fractures of the distal radius, *J Bone Joint Surg* 73A:461-469, 1991.
69. Kleinert JM et al: Complications of scaphoid silicone arthroplasty, *J Bone Joint Surg* 67A:422-427, 1985.
70. Knirk JL, Jupiter JB: Intra-articular fractures of the distal end of the radius in young adults, *J Bone Joint Surg* 68A:647-659, 1986.
71. Koman LA, Mooney JF, Poehling GG: Fractures and ligamentous injuries of the wrist, *Hand Clin* 6:477-490, 1990.
72. Kozin SH, Wood MB: Early soft-tissue complications after fractures of the distal part of the radius, *J Bone Joint Surg* 75A:144-153, 1993.
73. Lavernia CJ, Cohen M, Taleisnik J: Treatment of scapholunate dissociations by ligamentous repair and capsulodesis, *J Hand Surg* 17A:354-359, 1992.
74. Leslie IJ, Dickson RA: The fractured carpal scaphoid: natural history and factors influencing outcome, *J Bone Joint Surg* 63B:225-230, 1981.
75. Levinsohn EM, Palmar AK: Arthography of the traumatized wrist, *Radiology* 146:647-651, 1983.
76. Lichtman DM et al: Ulnar mid carpal instability: clinical and laboratory analysis, *J Hand Surg* 6:515-523, 1981.

77. Lichtman DM et al: Kienböck's disease—update on silicone replacement arthroplasty, *J Hand Surg* 343-347, 1982.
78. Lichtman DM: *The wrist and its disorders,* Philadelphia, 1988, WB Saunders.
79. Lindstrom G, Nystrom A: Natural history of scaphoid nonunion with special reference to "asymptomatic" cases, *J Hand Surg* 17B:697-700, 1992.
80. Linscheid RL et al: Traumatic instability of the wrist: diagnosis, classification and pathomechanics, *J Bone Joint Surg* 54A:1612-1632, 1972.
81. Linscheid RL, Dobyns JH: Athletic injuries of the wrist, *Clin Orthop* 198:141-151, 1985.
82. Linscheid RL, Dobyns JH: Athletic injuries of the wrist, *Clin Orthop* 198:141-151, 1985.
83. Louis DS et al: Central carpal instability-capitate lunate instability pattern: diagnosis by dynamic placement, *Orthopaedics* 7:1693-1696, 1984.
84. McClain EJ, Boyes JH: Missed fractures of the greater multangular, *J Bone Joint Surg* 48A:1525-1528, 1966.
85. McCue FC et al: Hand and wrist injuries in the athlete, *Am J Sports Med* 7:275-286, 1979.
86. McMurtry RY, Jupiter JB: Fractures of the distal radius. In Browner BO et al, editors: *Skeletal trauma,* Philadelphia, 1992, WB Saunders, pp 1063-1094.
87. McQueen MM, MacLaren A, Chalmers J: The value of remanipulating Colles' fractures, *J Bone Joint Surg* 68B:232-233, 1986.
88. Mack GR et al: The natural history of scaphoid nonunion, *J Bone Joint Surg* 66A:504-509, 1984.
89. Mandelbaum BR et al: Wrist pain syndrome in the gymnast—pathogenic, diagnostic and therapeutic considerations, *Am J Sports Med* 17:305-317, 1989.
90. Maudsley RH, Chen SC: Screw fixation in the management of fractured carpal scaphoid, *J Bone Joint Surg* 54B:432-441, 1972.
91. Mayfield JK, Johnson RP, Kilcoyne RK: Carpal dislocations: pathomechanics and progressive perilunar instability, *J Hand Surg* 5:226-241, 1980.
92. Mayfield JK: Mechanism of carpal injuries, *Clin Orthop* 149:45-54, 1980.
93. Mayfield JK: Patterns of injury to carpal ligaments: a spectrum, *Clin Orthop* 187:36-42, 1984.
94. Mazet R, Hohl M: Fractures of the carpal navicular: analysis of 91 cases and review of the literature, *J Bone Joint Surg* 45A:82-112, 1963.
95. Melone CP Jr: Articular fractures of the distal radius, *Orthop Clin North Am* 15:217-236, 1984.
96. Melone CP: Distal radius fractures: changing concepts of management, *Orthop Clin North Am* April, 1993.
97. Mikic ZD: Age changes in the triangular fibrocartilage of the wrist joint, *J Anat* 126:367-384, 1978.
98. Mino DE, Palmer AK, Levinsohn EM: Radiography and computed tomography in the diagnosis of incongruity of the distal radio-ulnar joint: a prospective study, *J Bone Joint Surg* 67A:247-252, 1985.
99. Mooney JF, Siegel DB, Koman LA: Ligamentous injuries of the wrist in athletes, *Clin Sports Med* 11:129-139, 1992.
100. Muller ME, Nazarian S, Koch P: *Classification AO des fractures les os longs,* Berlin, 1987, Springer-Verlag
101. Nakamura R et al: Sports-related Kienböck's disease, *Am J Sports Med* 19:88-91, 1991.
102. Obletz BE, Halberstein BM: Nonunions of fractures of the carpal navicular, *J Bone Joint Surg* 20:424-428, 1938.
103. Ogunro O: Fracture of the body of the hamate bone, *J Hand Surg* 8:353-355, 1983.
104. Older TM, Stabler EV, Cassebaum WH: Colles' fracture: evaluation of selection of therapy, *J Trauma* 5:469-476, 1965.
105. Palmer AK: Trapezial ridge fracture, *J Hand Surg* 6:561-564, 1981.
106. Palmer AK, Werner FW: The triangular fibro-cartilage complex of the wrist—anatomy and function, *J Hand Surg* 6:153-162, 1981.
107. Palmer AK, Levinsohn EM, Kuzma GR: Arthrography of the wrist, *J Hand Surg* 8A:15-23, 1983.
108. Palmer AK, Glisson RR, Werner FW: Relationship between ulnar variance and triangular fibrocartilage complex thickness, *J Hand Surg* 9A:681-683, 1984.
109. Palmer AK: Triangular fibrocartilage disorders: injury patterns and treatment, *Arthroscopy* 6:125-132, 1990.
110. Palmer AK: Fractures of the distal radius. In Green DP, Hotchkiss RN, editors: *Operative hand surgery,* ed 3, New York, 1993, Churchill Livingstone, pp 929-971.
111. Panagis JS et al: The arterial anatomy of the human carpus. II. The intraosseous vascularity, *J Hand Surg* 8:375-382, 1983.
112. Parker D et al: Hook of the hamate fractures in athletes, *Am J Sports Med* 14:517-523, 1986.
113. Patterson SD, Richards RS: Distal radius fractures, *Curr Opin Orthop* 4:20-28, 1993.
114. Peterson MS, Adams BD: Biomechanical evaluation of distal radio-ulnar reconstructions, *J Hand Surg* 18A:328-334, 1993.
115. Pettrone FA, Ricciardelli E: Gymnastic injuries: the Virginia experience 1982-1983, *Am J Sports Med* 15:59-62, 1987.
116. Pichora DR: Acute, nonunion and malunion of scaphoid fractures, *Curr Opin Orthop* 4:40-45, 1993.
117. Pisano SM et al: Scapho-capitate intercarpal arthrodesis, *J Hand Surg* 16A:328-333, 1991.
118. Pogue DJ et al: Effects of distal radius fracture malunion on wrist joint mechanics, *J Hand Surg* 15A:721-727, 1990.
119. Posner MA: Injuries to the hand and wrist in athletes, *Orthop Clin North Am* 8:593-618, 1977.
120. Prosser AJ, Brenkel IJ, Irvine GB: Articular fractures of the distal scaphoid, *J Hand Surg* 13B:87-91, 1988.
121. Rayhack JM, Langworthy JN, Belsole RJ: Transulnar percutaneous pinning of displaced radial fractures: a preliminary report, *J Orthop Trauma* 3:107-114, 1989.
122. Reagen DS, Linscheid RL, Dobyns JH: Luno-triquetral sprains, *J Hand Surg* 9A:502-514, 1984.
123. Rettig AC, Ryan RO, Stone JA: Epidemiology of hand injuries in sports. In Strickland JW, Rettig AC, editors: *Hand injuries in athletes,* Philadelphia, 1992, WB Saunders, pp 37-48.
124. Riester JN et al: A review of scaphoid fracture healing in competitive athletes, *Am J Sports Med* 13:159-161, 1985.
125. Ruby LK, Stinson J, Belsky MR: The natural history of scaphoid nonunion: a review of fifty-five cases, *J Bone Joint Surg* 67A:428-432, 1985.
126. Ruby L: Fractures and dislocations of the carpus. In Browner BD et al, editors: *Skeletal trauma,* Philadelphia, 1992, WB Saunders, pp 1025-1062.
127. Ruby LR: Wrist biomechanics, *Instructional Course Lecture, AAOS* XLI:25-32, 1992.
128. Ruch DS, Chabon SJ, Poehling GG. The role of arthroscopy in the treatment of scapho lunate dissociation, *Tech Orthop* 7:42-48, 1992.
129. Russe O: Fracture of the carpal navicular: diagnosis, nonoperative treatment and operative treatment, *J Bone Joint Surg* 42A:759-768, 1960.
130. Seitz WH et al: Augmented external fixation of unstable distal radius fractures, *J Hand Surg* 16A:1010-1016, 1991.
131. Short WH et al: A biomechanical study of distal radius fractures, *J Hand Surg* 12A:529-534, 1987.
132. Smaill GB: Long-term follow-up of Colles' fracture, *J Bone Joint Surg* 47B:80-85, 1965.
133. Smith DK et al: The effects of simulated unstable scaphoid fractures on carpal motion, *J Hand Surg* 14A:283-291, 1989.
134. Smith RJ, Atkinson RE, Jupiter JB: Silicone synovitis of the wrist, *J Hand Surg* 10A:47-60, 1985.
135. Solgaard S: Classification of distal radius fractures, *Acta Orthop Scand* 56:249-252, 1985.
136. Stark HH et al: Fracture of the hook of the hamate in athletes, *J Bone Joint Surg* 59A:575-582, 1977.

137. Stark HH et al:Treatment of ununited fractures of the scaphoid by iliac bone grafts and Kirschner wire fixation, *J Bone Joint Surg* 70A:982-91, 1988.
138. Stark HH et al: Fracture of the hook of the hamate, *J Bone Joint Surg* 71A:1202-1207, 1989.
139. Stein F, Siegel MW: Naviculo-capitate fracture syndrome, *J Bone Joint Surg* 51A:392-395, 1969.
140. Stewart MJ: Fractures of the carpal navicular (scaphoid): a report of 436 cases, *J Bone Joint Surg* 36A:998-1006, 1954.
141. Taleisnik J, Kelly PJ:The extraosseous and intraosseous blood supply of the scaphoid bone, *J Bone Joint Surg* 48A:1125-1137, 1966.
142. Taleisnik J:The ligaments of the wrist, *J Hand Surg* 1:110-118, 1976.
143. Taleisnik J,Watson HK: Midcarpal instability caused by malunited fractures of the distal radius, *J Hand Surg* 9:350-357, 1984.
144. Taleisnik J: *The wrist,* New York, 1985, Churchill Livingstone.
145. Taleisnik J: Current concepts review—carpal instability, *J Bone Joint Surg* 70A:1262-1268, 1988.
146. Teisen H, Hjarback J: Classification of fresh fractures of the lunate, *J Hand Surg* 13B:458-462, 1988.
147. Thiru-Pathi RG et al:Arterial anatomy of the triangular fibrocartilage of the wrist and its surgical significance, *J Hand Surg* 11A:258-263, 1986.
148. Tolat AR et al:The gymnast's wrist: acquired positive ulnar variance following chronic epiphyseal injury, *J Hand Surg* 17B:678-681, 1992.
149. Torisu T: Fracture of the hook of the hamate by a golf swing, *Clin Orthop* 83:91-94, 1972.
150. Vance RM, Gelberman RH, Evans EF: Scapho-capitate fractures, *J Bone Joint Surg* 62A:271-276, 1980.
151. Vasilas A, Grieco RV, Bartone NF: Roentgen aspects of injuries to the pisiform bone and piso-triquetral joint, *J Bone Joint Surg* 42A:1317-1328, 1960.
152. Warhold LG, Osterman AL: Scaphoid fracture and nonunion: treatment by open reduction, bone graft and a Herbert screw, *Tech Orthop* 7:7-18, 1992.
153. Watson HK, Hempton RF: Limited wrist arthrodesis: I. The triscaphoid joint, *J Hand Surg* 5A:320-327, 1980.
154. Watson HK, Rogers WD: Nonunion of the hook of the hamate: an argument for bone grafting the nonunion, *J Hand Surg* 14A:486-490, 1989.
155. Weber ER, Chao EY:An experimental approach to the mechanism of scaphoid waist fractures, *J Hand Surg* 3:142-148, 1978.
156. Weber ER: Biomechanical implications of scaphoid waist fractures, *Clin Orthop* 149:83-89, 1980.
157. Weber ER:A rational approach for recognition and treatment of Colles' fracture, *Hand Clin* 3:13-21, 1987.
158. Weiker GG: Hand and wrist problems in the gymnast, *Clin Sports Med* 11:189-202, 1992.
159. Whipple TL, Marotta JJ, Powell JH: Techniques of wrist arthroscopy, *Arthroscopy* 2:244-252, 1986.
160. Whipple TL:The role of arthroscopy in the treatment of wrist injuries in the athlete, *Clin Sports Med* 11:227-238, 1992.
161. Whipple TL: Arthroscopically assisted internal fixation of acute scaphoid fractures, *Tech Orthop* 7:19-25, 1992.
162. Zemel NP et al:Treatment of selected patients with an ununited fracture of the proximal part of the scaphoid by excision of the fragment and insertion of a curved silicone-rubber spacer, *J Bone Joint Surg* 66A:510-517, 1984.
163. Zemel NP, Stark HH: Fractures and dislocations of the carpal bones, *Clin Sports Med* 5:709-724, 1986.
164. Zemel NP:The prevention and treatment of complications from fractures of the distal radius and ulna, *Hand Clin* 3:1-11, 1987.
165. Zemel NP: Carpal fractures. In Strickland JW, Rettig AC, editors: *Hand injuries in athletes,* Philadelphia, 1992, WB Saunders, pp 155-173.

CHAPTER 31

Tendon Injuries

NORMAN P. ZEMEL

Although the flexor and extensor tendons in the hand, wrist, or forearm suffer a variety of injuries during athletic activities, certain specific injuries seem to be more prevalent. These injuries occasionally are associated with an open wound. Although they sometimes appear inconsequential at first, these tendon injuries, if not properly treated, can result in significant loss of hand or finger function.

FLEXOR TENDON INJURIES

Closed flexor tendon injuries are uncommon in the general population, but they are prevalent injuries as a result of athletic activity. Tendon ruptures occur primarily to the flexor profundus tendon of the finger, with a lesser incidence of injury to the flexor pollicis longus or flexor digitorum superficialis tendons.[4,16] The body of a tendon seldom ruptures because it is the strongest link in the musculotendinous chain.[33] The insertion, the musculotendinous origin, or the muscle itself usually will tear before the tendon. The tendon most commonly is disrupted at its distal bony insertion.

The flexor profundus tendon passes distally through the bifurcation of the flexor digitorum superficialis tendon and occupies a wide area of insertion into the distal phalanx. The tendon is intimately attached to the capsule of the distal interphalangeal joint, and its insertion into bone extends distally for about one third of the length of the distal phalanx.

The blood supply of the flexor tendons is partly through the vincular system. This vascular system is supplied by transverse communicating branches of the common digital artery. These small vessels enter the tendon dorsally. The vincula breve enter the tendons close to their respective insertions. However, the vinculum longum enters the flexor digitorum profundus tendon at the level of the proximal interphalangeal joint. This is clinically important because of possible disruption of this blood supply with proximal retraction of the profundus tendon after rupture.

Avulsion of the distal attachment of the flexor profundus tendon is a frequent sports injury. This avulsion is especially common in American football, and the ring finger is the digit most often affected[2,7,53] (Fig. 31-1).

The injury occurs when a defensive player is trying to make a tackle and forcibly grasps the opponent's jersey. If the offensive player breaks free, the defensive player loses the grasp, and the hooked ring finger is independently forcibly extended against the maximally contracting profundus muscle. The flexor profundus tendon avulses from the distal phalanx.

The exact mechanism of injury to the ring finger remains unclear. Gunther[19] and Wenger[53] attribute the injury to the lack of independent extension of the ring finger when the middle and little fingers are flexed. This is because of the common flexor muscle belly of the profundus to the middle, ring, and little fingers. Manske and Lesker[34] demonstrated that the insertion of the ring finger profundus tendon is weaker than the insertion of the profundus tendon in the adjacent fingers. They found the breaking strength of the tendon-bone junction of the profundus tendon of the ring finger to be the weakest of the four fingers. Leddy and Packer[25] reported that the arrangement of extensor tendons was a factor in the injury. Flexion of the middle, ring, and little fingers causes the extensor tendon of the ring finger to be pulled distally. This acts as a check-rein to prevent passive extension of the ring finger, making it more susceptible to a hyperextension injury.

When the athlete injures the finger, the distal segment is usually painful and swollen. The injury is often thought to be a jammed finger or a sprain. If the flexor tendon retracts proximally, the symptoms may be primarily at the proximal interphalangeal joint. The finger may be slightly swollen or ecchymotic. A tender mass will be present in the palm if the tendon retracts completely from the flexor sheath. Specific testing for active function of the profundus tendon must be done to make the correct diagnosis (Fig. 31-2). Radiographs should be done to determine whether there is an associated bony injury.[8,25] The presence of a small bony fragment in the midportion of the finger, seen on the lateral radiograph and associated with loss of active distal interphalangeal joint flexion, often shows the location of the torn profundus tendon (Fig. 31-3). However, Trumble et al[51] noted that radiographs can be misleading because the tendon can retract further than the fracture fragment. They suggested ultrasonography to help locate the retracted tendon.

Leddy and Packer[25] have described a classification of the three main types of avulsion of the flexor profundus tendon.

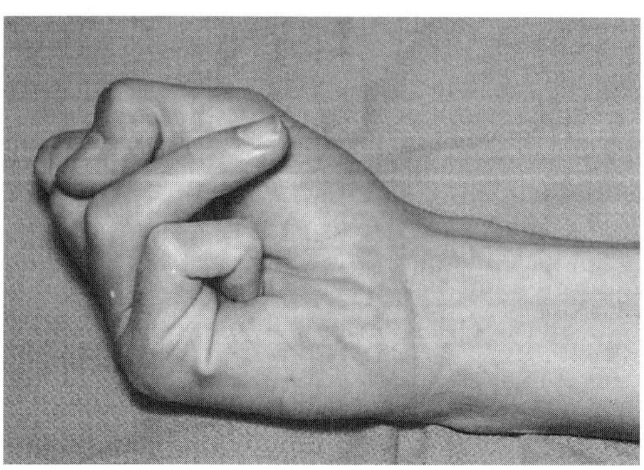

FIGURE 31-1 Loss of active flexion at the distal joint of the ring finger after avulsion of the flexor profundus tendon.

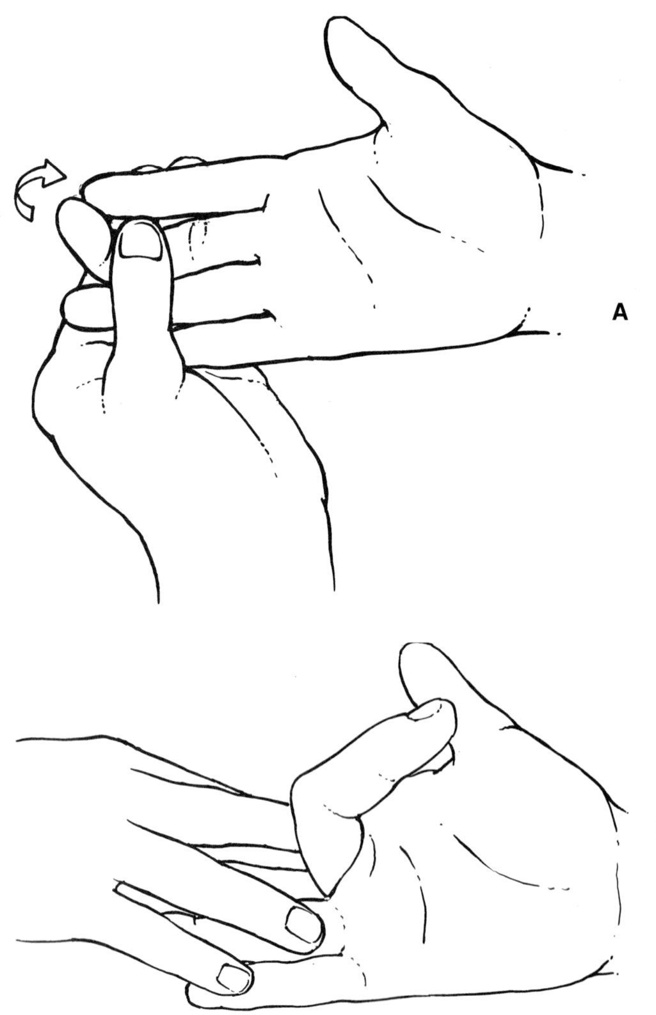

FIGURE 31-2 Method of testing for profundus **(A)** and superficialis **(B)** tendon function.

In type I, the profundus tendon retracts into the palm. Both vincula are torn. In the palm, the tendon tends to be contracted and coiled, further compromising its blood supply. The profundus tendon should be reattached within 2 to 3 weeks of injury. Further delay in treatment frequently will not allow the retracted tendon to be uncoiled and extended to reach the distal phalanx.

Type II is the most common type. The tendon, often with a small bony fragment from the distal phalanx, retracts to the level of the proximal interphalangeal joint. The tendon usually is trapped by the flexor digitorum superficialis tendon bifurcation. Because the tendon is in the flexor sheath, nutrition is provided by the synovial fluid and by the intact vincula at the proximal interphalangeal joint. Reattachment of the tendon can be done up to 8 weeks after injury, but the repair should not be delayed. The greater the delay, the greater the joint stiffness (distal interphalangeal joint and proximal interphalangeal joint) and the more difficult it is to regain good finger flexion.

In type III, the lesion has a large bony fragment attached to the profundus tendon. Because of the bone, the tendon remains within the flexor sheath and is nourished. The fragment often is trapped by the A-4 pulley. Treatment is to reduce and stabilize the bony fragment with its attached profundus tendon.

A variant of the type III injury (questionable type IV) has been described.* This variant consists of an avulsion of the flexor profundus tendon with a separate intraarticular fracture of the distal phalanx.

Avulsion

Early diagnosis and reattachment of the flexor profundus tendon is the best treatment.

*References 8, 13, 23, 37, 42, 45.

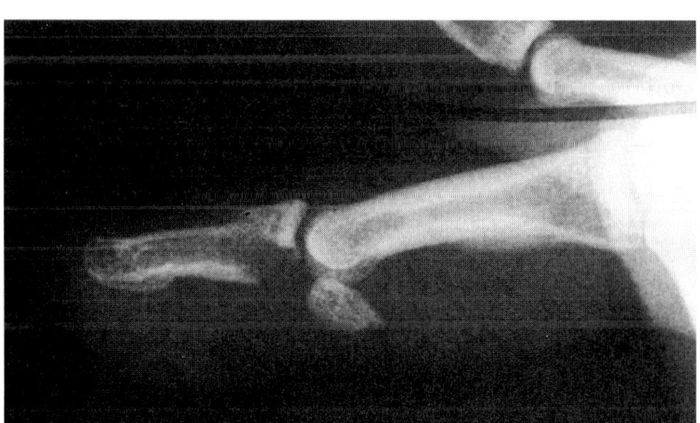

FIGURE 31-3 Fracture associated with an avulsion of the flexor profundus tendon.

Type I

The finger is opened through a mid-lateral or volar zigzag incision from just proximal to the proximal interphalangeal joint distally to the distal phalanx. If needed, the distal palm is opened through a separate incision. In the palm, the tendon is identified and freed from surrounding scar. Slight traction on the tendon will allow it to be stretched to its normal length. A small red rubber catheter can be passed retrograde into the palm. The distal end of the tendon is loosely sutured to the catheter and passed through the flexor sheath, through the decussation of the flexor digitorum superficialis tendon, and distally beneath the A-4 pulley and into the distal wound (Fig. 31-4). A Bunnell pull-out suture is used to attach the tendon to the distal phalanx. After 7 to 10 days, a dynamic splint is attached to the finger and passive and active assisted range of motion is started. The hand and wrist are protected in a splint with the wrist in slight palmar flexion. At 3 weeks, the pull-out suture is removed, and a more aggressive rehabilitation program is started.

Type II

The finger is opened as described in a type I lesion. At the A-2 level of the flexor sheath, the sheath is opened and the tendon is identified. Any granulation tissue and scar binding the tendon to its surroundings are excised.

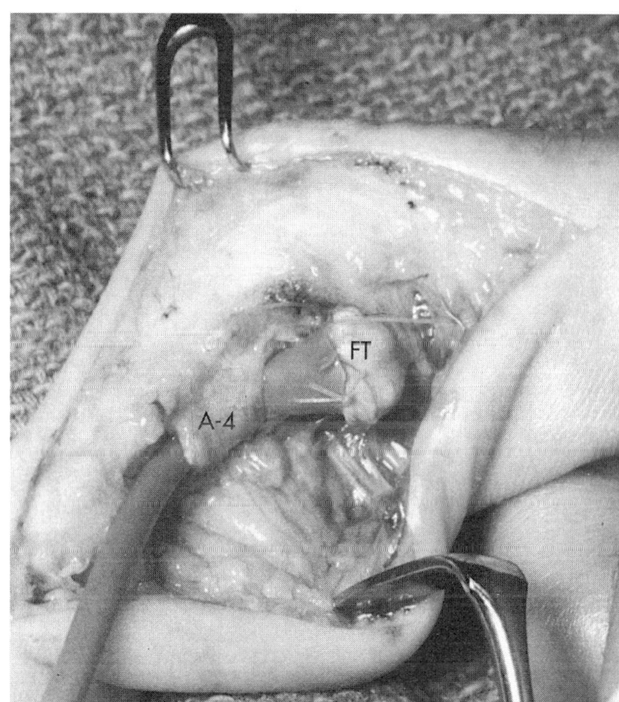

FIGURE 31-4 A small catheter is used to advance the retracted tendon from the palm, through the pulleys to the distal phalanx. *A-4,* Pulley in the middle segment of the finger; *FT,* flexor tendon.

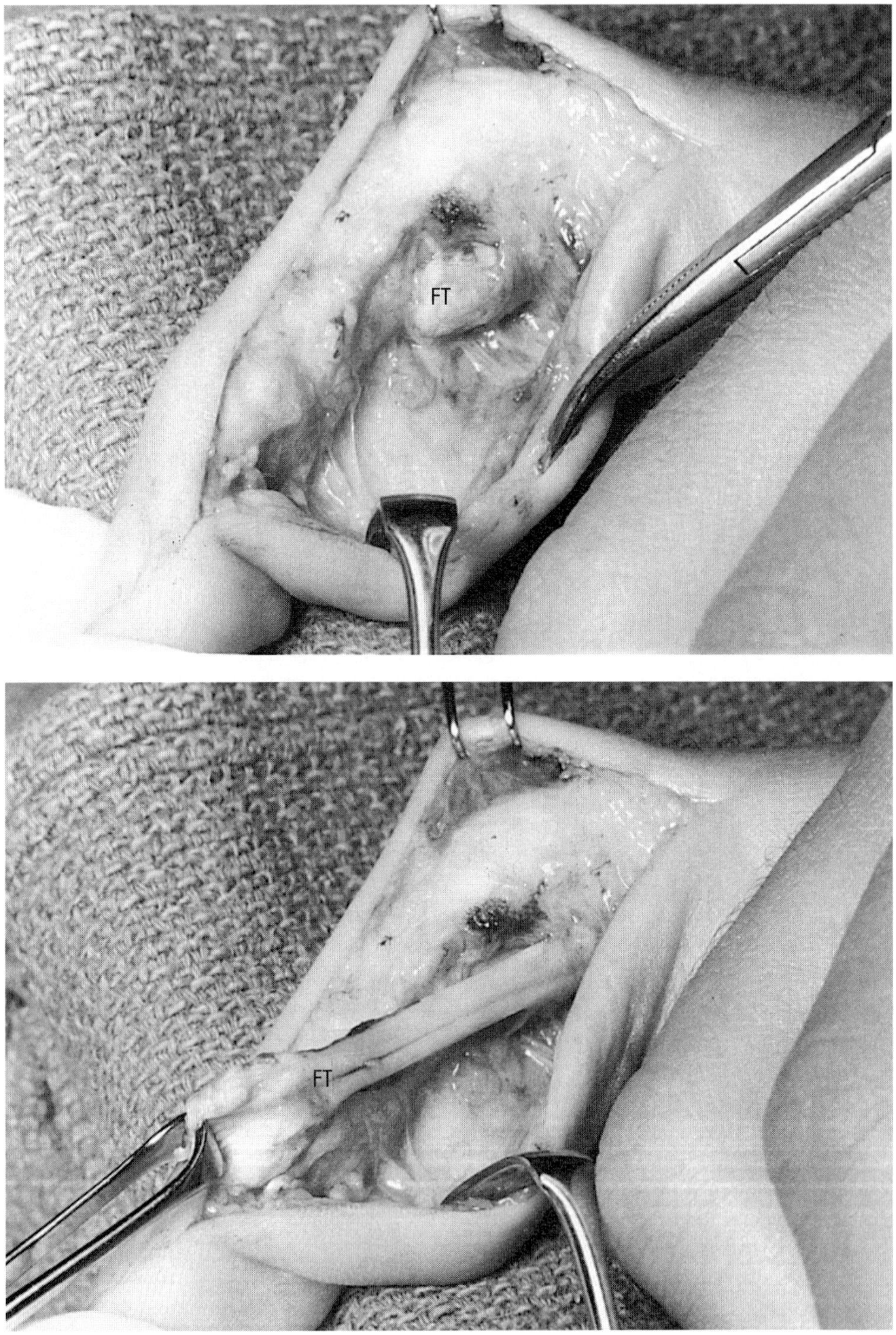

FIGURE 31-5 Type II flexor tendon avulsion. **A,** The tendon is identified within the flexor sheath, **B,** Advancement of the flexor tendon to the distal phalanx, **C,** Reattachment of the profundus tendon to bone **D,** Resting position of the ring finger (button). **E,** A dynamic splint is used to assist in the rehabilitation of the injured finger.

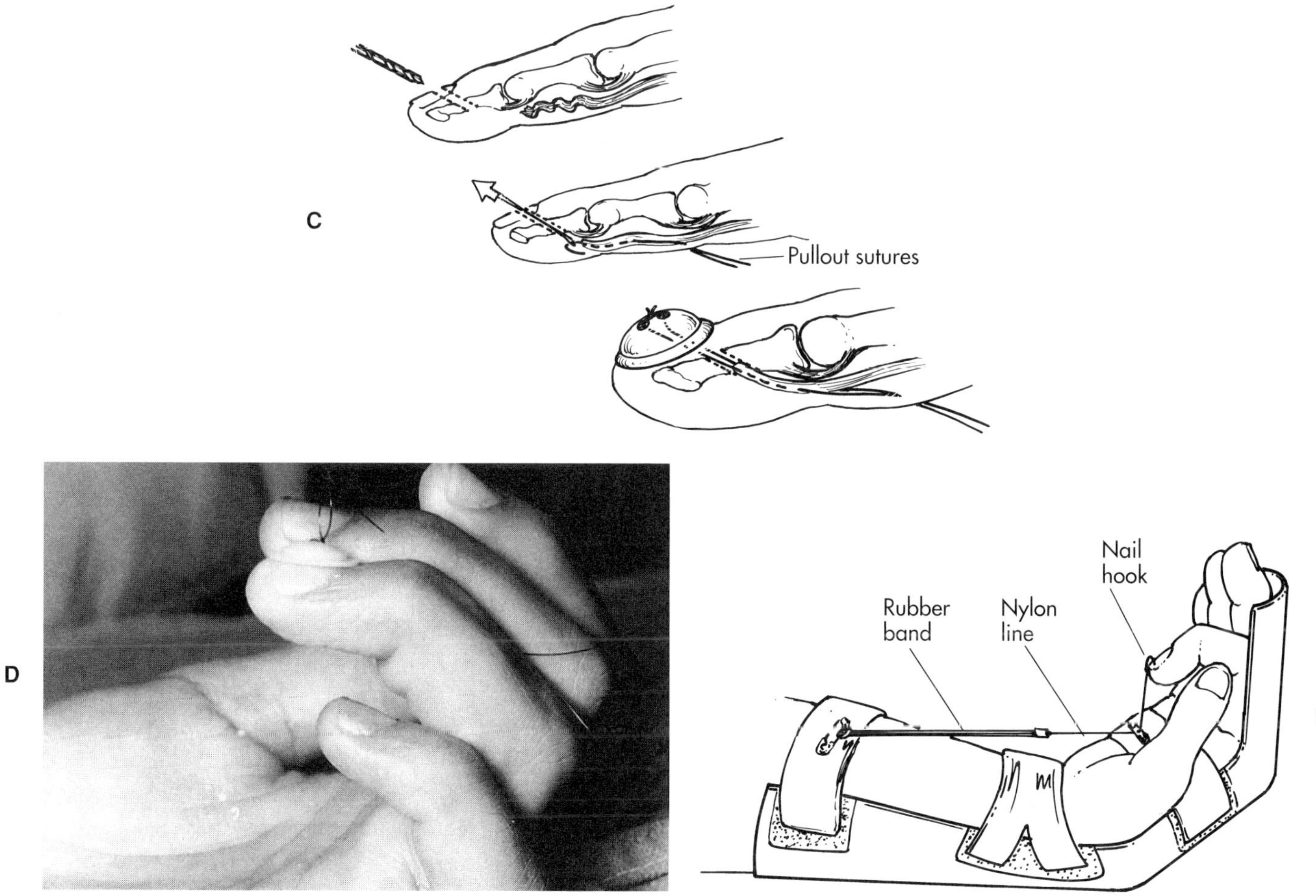

FIGURE 31-5, CONT'D.

The tendon is gently stretched to restore its length (Fig. 31-5). Carefully the tendon is passed through the sheath and pulleys to the distal phalanx and inserted into the bone. Postoperative care is the same as for a type I lesion.

Type III

Using an incision similar to that used with type II, the surgeon performs an open reduction and internal fixation of the large bony fragment. Radiographs should be taken in the operating room to ensure a proper reduction of the fracture.

If there is a separate flexor profundus avulsion in conjunction with the fracture of the distal phalanx, the bone is first reduced and then stabilized. Finally, the flexor profundus tendon is reattached to the distal phalanx (Fig. 31-6).

If the injury has been neglected or has not been properly diagnosed, several treatment options remain.[9,11,19] The functional loss is lack of active flexion of the distal joint of the ring finger. The options are the following:

1. The patient can accept the status of the finger. If there is good flexion at the proximal interphalangeal joint (more than 80°) and the distal interphalangeal joint does not hyperextend, this is a reasonable choice.
2. The distal joint can be stabilized by a tenodesis or a fusion. This is particularly useful if the distal interphalangeal joint hyperextends and gets in the way when the patient makes a fist. This author prefers a fusion. The fusion should be performed in slight flexion (20°). This provides a good, strong, stable joint, whereas a tenodesis has the potential to stretch.
3. The surgeon can perform a one-stage or two-stage flexor tendon graft to restore independent flexion to the distal interphalangeal joint of the finger. This option should be used only after considerable discussion with the patient. A one-stage flexor tendon

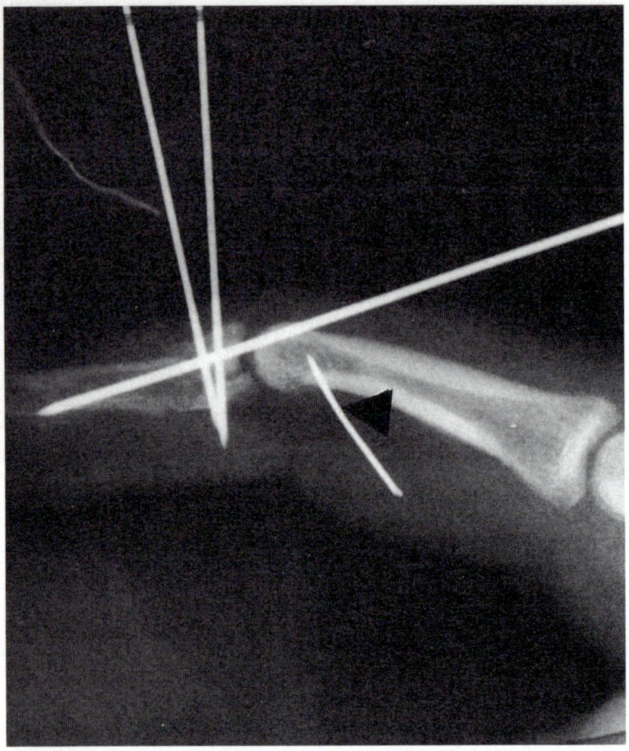

FIGURE 31-6 After the open reduction and internal fixation of the fracture, the profundus tendon, which is held in position by a needle *(arrow)*, is advanced and sutured into bone.

graft through an intact superficialis tendon has produced good results in young patients[16,18,47] and also in older patients.[27] However, the younger patient seems to be a better candidate because there is less propensity to form scar tissue. Stark et al[47] stated that the ideal age was between 10 and 21 years and that the procedure should be performed only if there was a specific need for independent flexion of the distal interphalangeal joint. Good to excellent results also have been reported with a two-stage flexor tendon graft.[55]

Any tendon graft procedure is an exacting operation. The presence of the intact superficialis tendon increases the difficulty and can compromise the result. The tendon graft can interfere with the normal function of the superficialis tendon and create a fixed flexed contracture of the finger. This finger then would have worse function than simply loss of independent flexion at the distal interphalangeal joint (Fig. 31-7).

The flexor profundus tendon can rupture within the substance of the tendon itself as a result of attrition; this usually is associated with tenosynovitis, fracture of the hook of the hamate,[4,36,48] or a Colles' fracture.[57]

An avulsion injury of the flexor digitorum superficialis tendon is extremely uncommon. Other than some discomfort after the injury, finger function usually is not impaired. This injury usually does not require treatment.

Injuries to the flexor superficialis tendon and the

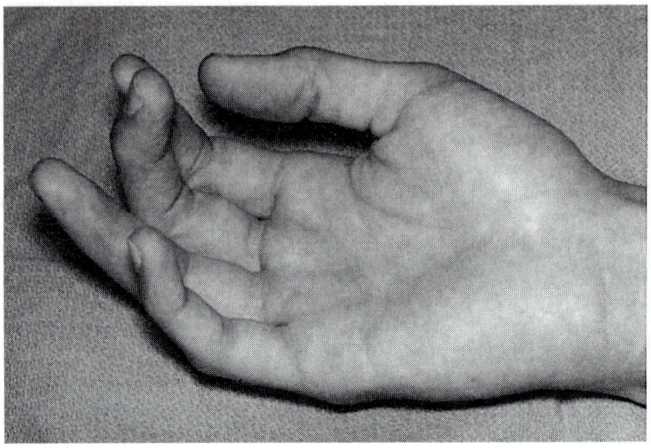

FIGURE 31-7 A flexion contracture of the middle finger after a tendon graft through the bifurcation of the flexor superficialis tendon.

flexor sheath, at the level of the proximal interphalangeal joint, have been described in competitive climbers. About one fourth of these individuals have fixed flexion deformities at the proximal interphalangeal joints.[3,50]

EXTENSOR TENDON INJURIES

Except for the occasional open wound, most athletic injuries involving the extensor tendons are closed. The injuries have a propensity to occur at the tendon insertions, particularly at the distal interphalangeal and proximal interphalangeal joints.

Distal Interphalangeal Joint

At this level, the conjoint extensor tendon is formed from the two lateral bands distal to the proximal interphalangeal joint and fibers from the oblique retinacular ligament. This tendon has an attachment to the dorsal capsule of the distal interphalangeal joint and inserts into the dorsal base of the distal phalanx.

Avulsion of the extensor tendon near its insertion (partial or complete) or avulsion of the extensor tendon with a small bony fragment attached can produce a mallet deformity of a finger or thumb[7,46] (Fig. 31-8). A "mallet finger" or "baseball finger" injury typically occurs when a sudden strong flexion force strikes the extended digit. A hyperextension mechanism at the distal interphalangeal joint resulting in an intraarticular fracture at the distal phalanx and a mallet finger deformity has been described by Land and Engber.[24] (Intraarticular fractures of the distal joint are discussed in Chapter 27.)

The patient complains of an inability to actively extend the distal interphalangeal joint. Slight active extension may indicate a partial tendon tear. Unchecked, the flexor digitorum profundus tendon maintains the distal interphalangeal joint in flexion. This injury seems to be particularly common in football receivers and baseball players, especially catchers.

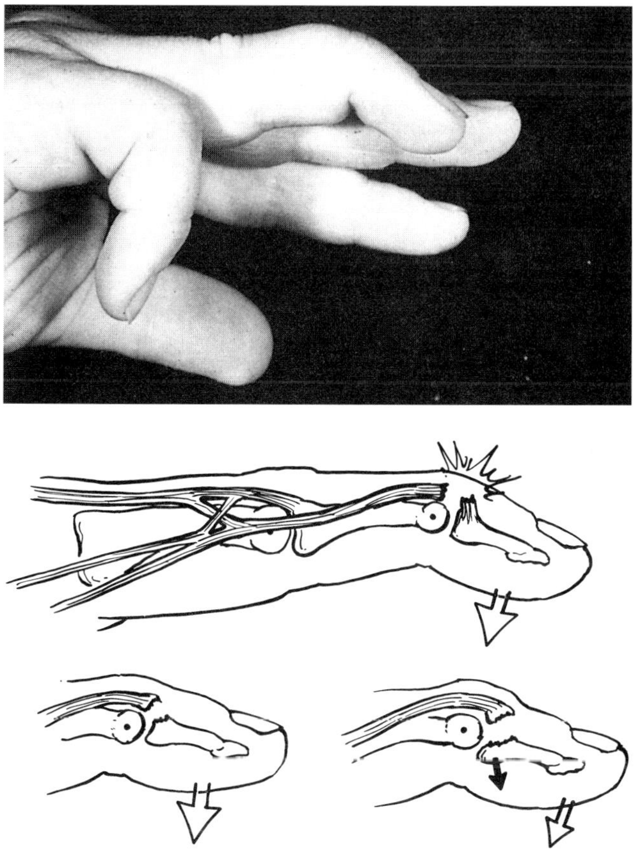

FIGURE 31-8 **A,** A mallet deformity of the right ring finger from a tendon rupture. **B,** Three injuries that can cause a mallet deformity of a finger.

A chronic mallet deformity often is associated with a hyperextension deformity at the proximal interphalangeal joint, especially in loose-jointed individuals.[31] This secondary phenomenon results from loss of continuity of the lateral bands distally, and an increased pull of the central slip of the extensor tendon at the proximal interphalangeal joint. Dorsal subluxation of the lateral bands and gradual stretching of the volar plate also can occur.

It is important to obtain radiographs of the finger to determine whether a significant intraarticular fracture also has occurred. This author believes it is rarely necessary to operate on a mallet finger caused by tendon avulsion even if a small bony fragment is attached to the tendon. This is true even if the injury is several months old.

Almost all of these fingers can be treated with a carefully applied splint to maintain the distal interphalangeal joint of the finger in extension.[31,32,38,46] The finger must remain continuously splinted for 6 to 8 weeks (Fig. 31-9). The splint should be adjusted every 2 to 3 weeks. The finger must not be hyperextended, because this can cause necrosis of the dorsal skin. Although many types of splints have been designed, a custom splint designed by a hand therapist usually best meets the needs of the athlete.

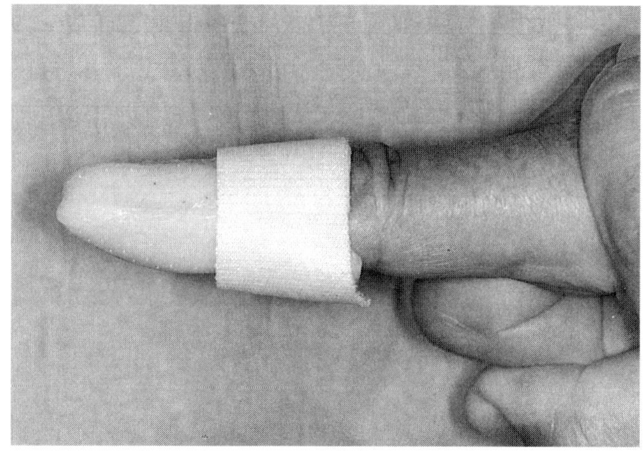

FIGURE 31-9 Mallet splint.

If the athlete cannot participate in the sport with a splint, the distal interphalangeal joint can be maintained in extension with a transarticular Kirschner wire.[10] The Kirschner wire is cut beneath the skin and removed in 6 to 8 weeks under local anesthesia.

Although surgery can be performed to repair the extensor tendon acutely or to reconstruct the extensor tendon in more chronic conditions,[14] this is rarely necessary.

Proximal Interphalangeal Joint

When the central slip of the extensor tendon is disrupted at the proximal interphalangeal joint and the lateral bands displace volarward, the resulting deformity is a boutonnière deformity. This deformity leads to a loss of extension at the proximal interphalangeal joint and hyperextension at the distal interphalangeal joint. This injury results from the finger being "jammed" or forced into flexion while the proximal interphalangeal joint is extended. Pain and swelling occur at the proximal interphalangeal joint. The injury often is treated initially as a sprain and either buddy-splinted or splinted in semiflexion.[30]

Frequently the boutonnière deformity is not immediately present and may take 2 to 3 weeks to develop into the typical posture of the finger.

Zancolli believed that the boutonnière deformity occurs in several stages.[56] Flexion of the proximal interphalangeal joint caused by disruption of the central slip occurs first. The head of the proximal phalanx buttonholes through the disrupted or stretched extensor tendon. This causes stretching of the transverse retinacular ligament and of the triangular ligament with volar migration of the lateral bands. In this position, the lateral bands become flexors of the proximal interphalangeal joint. The pull of the intrinsic muscles through the lateral bands then causes hyperextension at the distal interpha-

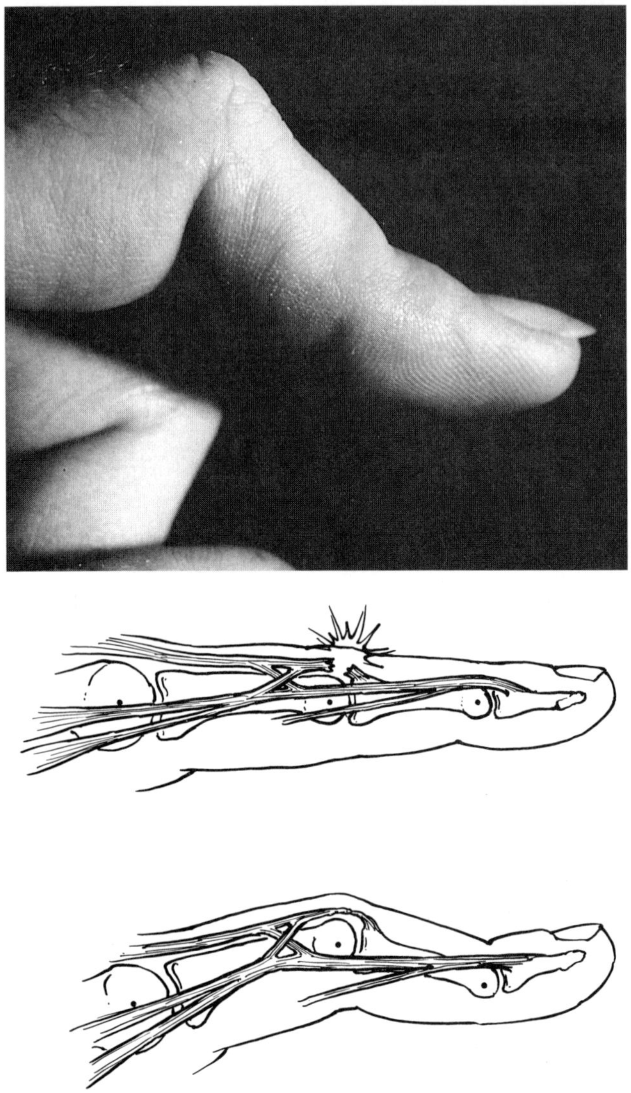

A

B

FIGURE 31-10 **A,** Boutonnière deformity of an index finger. **B,** After rupture of the central slip *(top)* the lateral bands slip volar to the axis of motion of the proximal interphalangeal joint *(bottom)*. The oblique retinacular ligament tightens and a boutonnière deformity occurs.

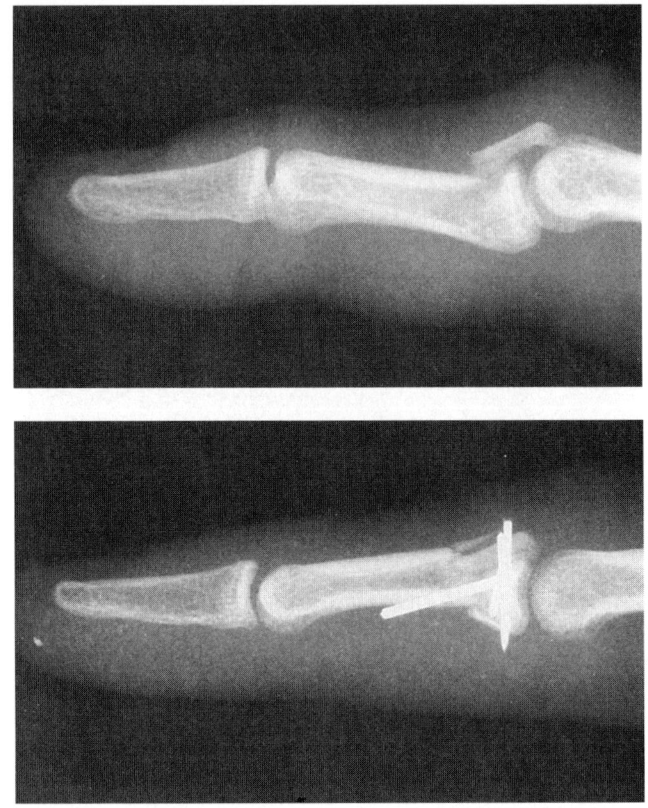

A

B

FIGURE 31-11 **A,** Dorsal intraarticular fracture with the central slip attached to the dorsal bony fragment. **B,** After open reduction and internal fixation of the fracture, the proximal interphalangeal joint should be splinted in extension.

langeal joint. Initially, the proximal interphalangeal joint and distal interphalangeal joints are flexible, and the deformities can be passively corrected. However, in time, the transverse retinacular ligament becomes tight and scarred, preventing passive relocation of the lateral bands to their dorsal position. In addition, the oblique retinacular ligament contracts and accentuates the hyperextension attitude of the distal interphalangeal joint (Fig. 31-10).

Volar dislocation of the proximal interphalangeal joint also can also tear the central slip and cause a boutonnière deformity.[44]

Radiographs of the fingers should be done to determine whether there is an associated bony injury. Occasionally a bony fragment is attached to the central slip, and if the fragment is large, an open reduction and internal fixation of the fracture is necessary (Fig. 31-11). This will be discussed more completely in Chapter 27.

Correction of the boutonnière deformity depends on whether the injury is acute or chronic.

Acute Boutonnière Deformity

The boutonnière deformity resulting from an athletic injury is invariably a closed injury. At the acute stage of injury, the proximal interphalangeal joint can be passively extended completely. The best treatment is to immobilize the digit with a safety-pin splint or a custom splint designed by a hand therapist (Fig. 31-12). As recommended by Boyes,[5] the proximal interphalangeal joint is splinted in extension, leaving the distal interphalangeal joint free. The athlete uses the splint constantly for 5 weeks and is advised to voluntarily flex the distal interphalangeal joint. The patient usually requires 5 to 6 weeks to restore balance between the components of the extensor tendon (central slip and lateral bands). If a splint cannot be used, the proximal interphalangeal joint can be maintained in extension with a transarticular Kirschner wire, cut off beneath the skin. The Kirschner

A

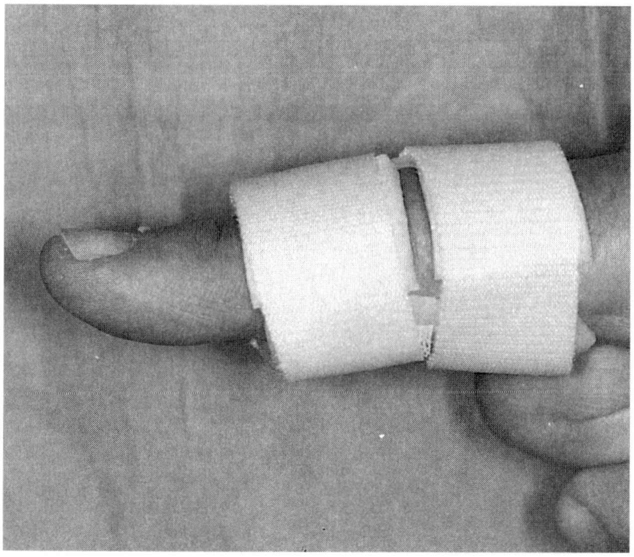

B

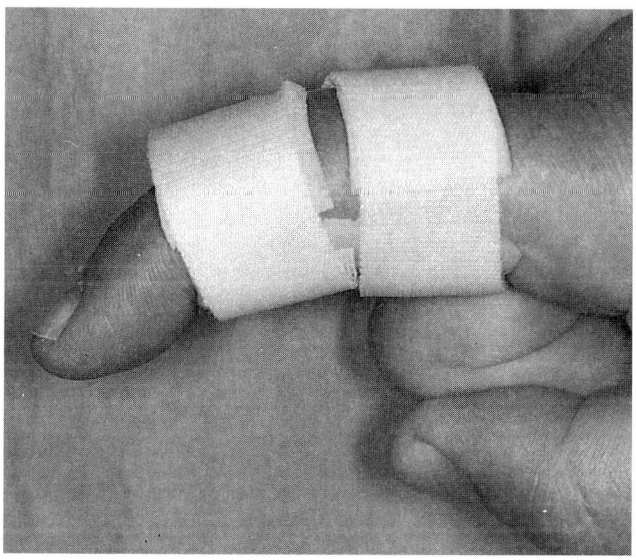

FIGURE 31-12 **A,** Boutonnière splint. **B,** Active flexion of distal joint to restore proper balance between the central slip and lateral bands of the extensor tendon.

wires should be removed in 4 to 5 weeks; otherwise an extension contracture can occur. Apparently the time interval from injury to treatment is less important than the presence or absence of a fixed contracture at the proximal interphalangeal joint.[32] The greater the amount of time since injury, the less the chance of restoring complete extension at the proximal interphalangeal joint. Frequently an extensor lag of 10° to 20° will persist, even with extended splinting. This will not greatly interfere with the individual's athletic performance.

Chronic Boutonnière Deformity

As long as the proximal interphalangeal joint is reasonably supple and the joint can be partially extended, splinting is still the treatment of choice.

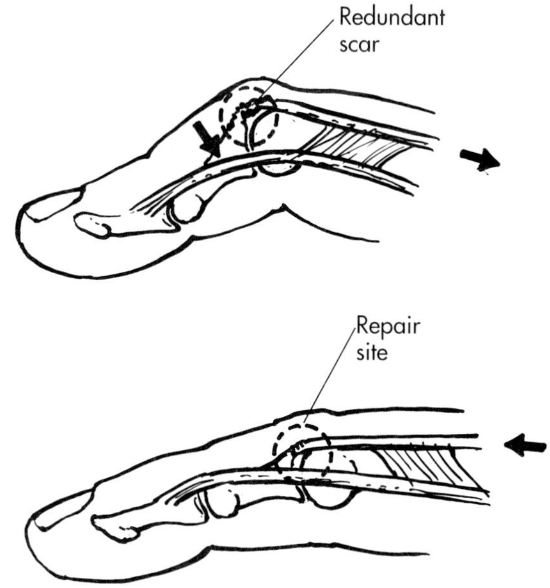

FIGURE 31-13 Reconstruction of the central slip can often be accomplished by excising the redundant scar, repairing the tendon, and lysing and relocating the lateral bands.

If the deformity is long-standing with a supple joint but without active extension at the proximal interphalangeal joint, surgical correction of the deformity can be considered. The potential complication of surgery is that the finger will become stiff in extension.

Although many operations to treat long-standing boutonnière deformities have been described,[26,35] this author prefers the direct repair or reattachment of the central slip.[14,52,58] This treatment consists of reconstruction of the central slip of the extensor tendon and lysis of the lateral bands, with these bands relocated to a dorsal position. In most instances, the appropriate tension was restored to the central slip by excision of a 2- to 4-mm segment of bridging scar and an end-to-end repair of the tendon (Fig. 31-13). The relocated lateral bands were sutured to the sides of the central slip proximal to the proximal interphalangeal joint, thereby allowing flexion of the joint. The pull-out sutures were removed in 3 weeks. A safety-pin splint was used for an additional 2 to 3 weeks. Active range-of-motion exercises then were started and splinting of the proximal interphalangeal joint was continued as needed.

In cases with an adequate distal stump of central tendon, the proximal end of the tendon was inserted directly into the base of the middle phalanx with a pull-out suture.

A fixed flexion contracture at the proximal interphalangeal joint must be corrected by either splinting before surgical reconstruction of the extensor mechanism or a surgical release of the proximal interphalangeal joint as a first-stage procedure. This is followed by a second operation to the extensor tendon after maximal passive ex-

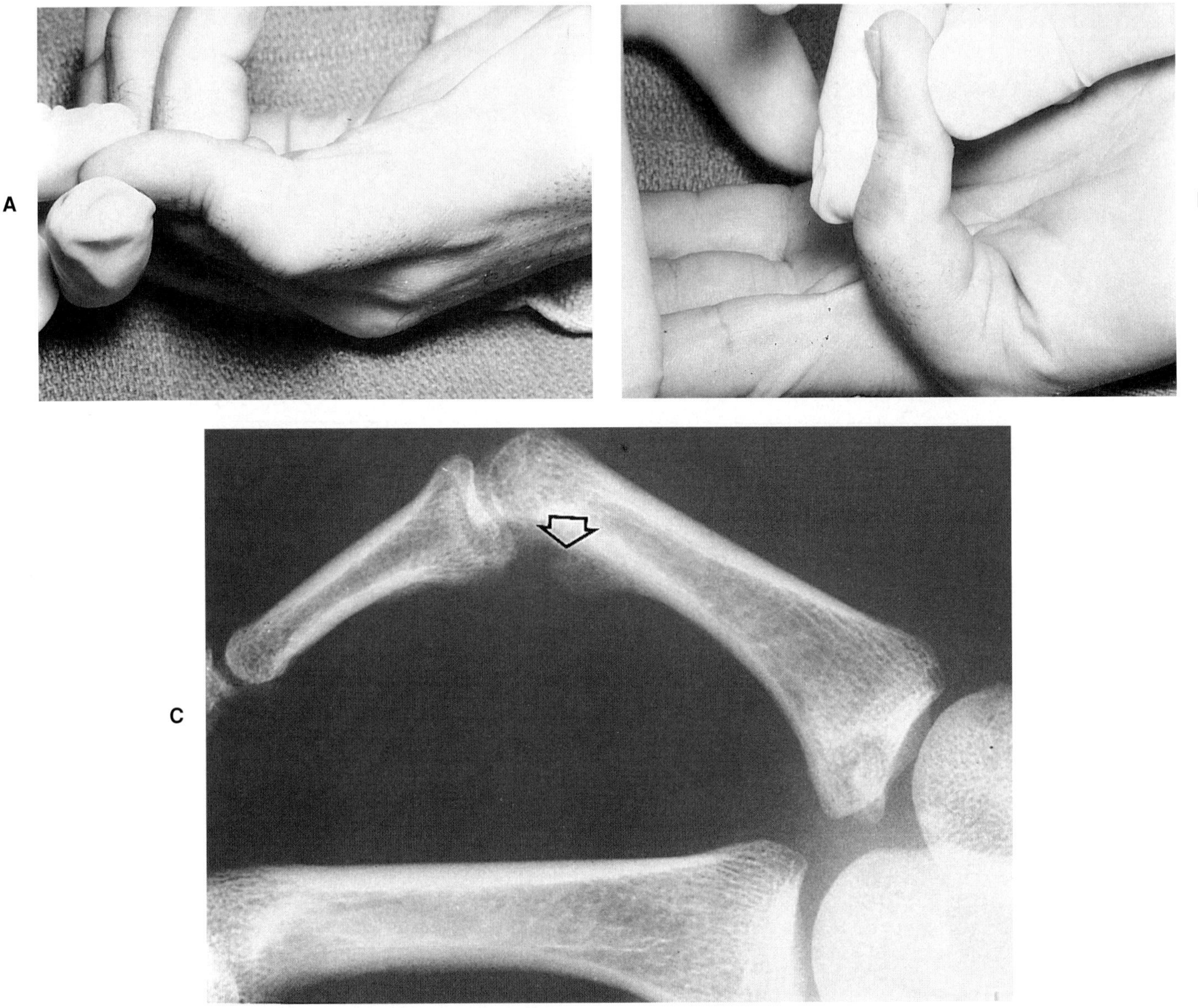

FIGURE 31-14 **A,** and **B,** A fixed flexion contracture of the middle joint of the little finger. **C,** The pseudo-boutonnière was caused by an injury to the volar plate *(arrow)*.

tension at the proximal interphalangeal joint has been restored.

Patients with a chronic boutonnière deformity often complain more of the hyperextension at the distal interphalangeal joint than the flexion contracture at the proximal interphalangeal joint. The hyperextended distal interphalangeal joint interferes with their ability to grasp. This can be corrected by dividing the conjoint extensor tendon and creating a mallet deformity.[12]

Destruction of the proximal interphalangeal joint articular cartilage is best treated by either arthrodesis or Silastic arthroplasty.

The clinician must differentiate between a boutonnière deformity and a pseudo-boutonnière deformity. The pseudo-boutonnière deformity results from an injury to the volar plate of the proximal interphalangeal joint.[29,43] This produces a flexion contracture at the proximal interphalangeal joint but only a slight extension deformity at the distal interphalangeal joint (Fig. 31-14). Radiographs may show calcification on the volar aspect of the proximal phalanx related to the volar plate injury. Treatment is the release of the scarred and contracted volar plate.

METACARPOPHALANGEAL JOINT

Direct impact injuries over the metacarpophalangeal joints of the hand occur frequently during many sporting activities and result in injury to the extensor tendon and soft tissue over the joint. These injuries often are noted in boxers and students of the martial arts. The common

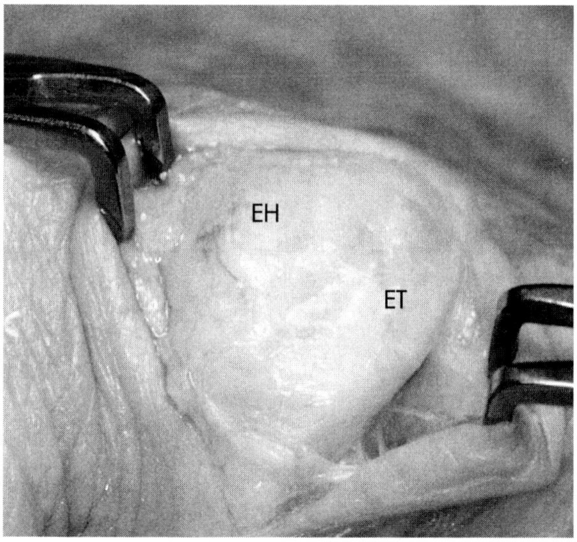

FIGURE 31-15 The extensor tendon over the proximal joint of the middle finger has subluxated ulnarward, secondary to a tear on the radial side of the extensor hood. *ET,* Extensor tendon; *EH,* extensor hood.

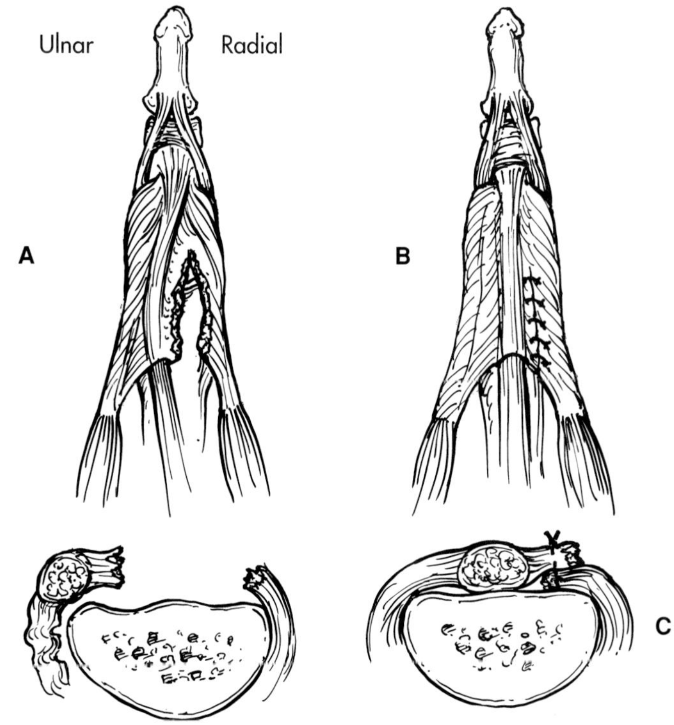

FIGURE 31-16 **A,** A tear on the radial side of the extensor hood, **B** and **C**, can be repaired by overlapping the fibers of the hood in order to centralize the extensor tendon.

injuries that occur are subluxation of the extensor tendon and a boxer's knuckle (soft knuckle).

Subluxation of the Extensor Tendon

A forceful blow to the metacarpophalangeal joint can force the finger into ulnar deviation,[1,21] or a twisting or flicking motion of the finger[20] can result in a tear of the sagittal fibers of the extensor hood and subluxation of the extensor tendon (Fig. 31-15). A longitudinal oblique tear occurs on the radial side of the extensor hood, causing the tendon to sublux ulnarward when the metacarpophalangeal joint is flexed. The middle finger is most often involved because of the peculiar anatomic relationship of the extensor tendon and extensor hood at the metacarpophalangeal joint.[21]

In the acute injury, the joint is swollen and finger motion is restricted. Careful examination usually is necessary to identify the dislocated extensor tendon. In the chronic injury, the patient presents with a painful snap of the extensor tendon with flexion of the finger. Frequently the patient must passively deviate the finger ulnarward to relocate the extensor tendon and allow extension of the finger. If the diagnosis is made acutely and the extensor tendon can be centralized by extending the metacarpophalangeal joint of the finger, the tear of the extensor hood can be treated conservatively. The metacarpophalangeal joint of the finger is splinted in extension for 3 to 4 weeks, allowing the more distal joints of the finger to flex.

If the extensor tendon cannot be reduced by extending the joint or if several weeks has elapsed since the injury, the tear of the sagittal fibers must be treated with an operation. Treatment consists of relocating the extensor tendon and reinforcing the radial fibers of the extensor hood. Frequently a direct repair of the defect is possible.[1,21] This can be performed even in the more chronic situation when thin bridging scar must be excised and the ulnar side of the extensor hood released to bring the extensor tendon over the joint.[40] The author prefers to a perform a double-layer repair of the extensor hood for greater stability (Fig. 31-16). Passive flexion of the metacarpophalangeal joint at the operating table will ensure that the repair is not too tight.

When the tissue on the radial side of the extensor hood is insufficient or of poor quality, other reconstructive procedures have been used. Wheeldon[54] used a strip of the ulnar juncturae tendinum swung over and attached to the radial side of the hood. Other methods used a radial strip of the extensor tendon looped around the lumbrical tendon[28] or the deep transverse metacarpal ligament[15] to act as a tether for the extensor tendon.

Ishizuki[20] described a superficial and deep layer of the sagittal band that attaches to the extensor tendon over the metacarpophalangeal joint of the middle finger. In the spontaneous type of dislocation of the extensor tendon, the superficial layer ruptures just radial to the tendon. However, in a traumatic dislocation, both layers of the sagittal band rupture at a site several millimeters ra-

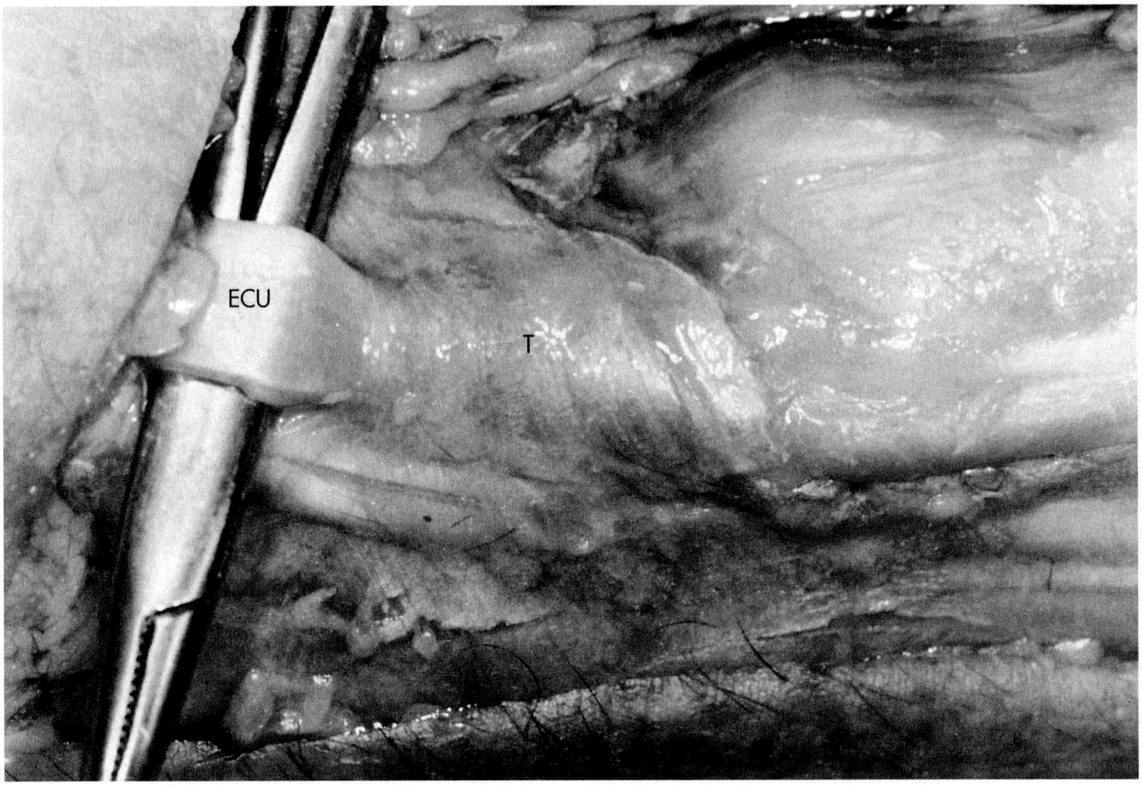

FIGURE 31-17 The dorsum of a right wrist showing the separate fibrous tunnel *(T)* of the extensor carpi ulnaris tendon *(ECU)*.

dial to the extensor tendon. The sagittal band lies just dorsal to the dorsal capsule and is separated from it by loose connective tissue.

Dorsal Capsule Injuries—Boxer's Knuckle

The term *boxer's knuckle* was used by Gladden[17] to describe a painful soft-tissue swelling usually present over the metacarpophalangeal joint of the index and middle fingers after direct injury. This injury also has been called a "soft knuckle." The painful swelling over the dorsum of the joint usually is caused by a specific event and is exacerbated by repeated injury. It occurs predominantly in boxers. In a study of 11 patients with closed crush injuries to the metacarpophalangeal joint of the fingers resulting from direct blows to the dorsum of the hand, Koniuch et al[22] noted that the patients had chronic pain and swelling without subluxation of the extensor tendon. Of the 9 patients who were examined, all had partial arcuate tears of the sagittal fibers tethered by scar tissue to the skin and dorsal capsule. In addition, 7 had lesions on the ulnar side and 2 on the radial side. A specific tear of the dorsal capsule was not identified because the average patient was seen 7 months after injury. Posner and Ambrose[39] identified a specific dorsal capsular tear in six patients (four boxers) resulting from closed injury to the

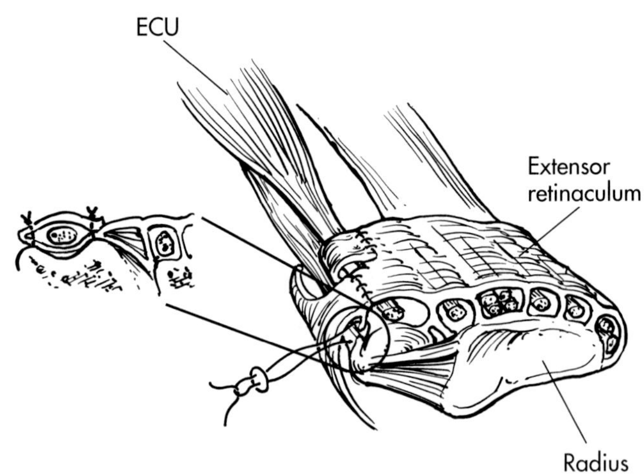

FIGURE 31-18 A strip of the extensor retinaculum is used to stabilize the extensor carpi ulnaris tendon.

metacarpophalangeal joints of the index and middle fingers. The extensor tendon may or may not be subluxated. An important clinical finding was a palpable defect over the joint that represented the tear in the dorsal capsule. This injury can be severely debilitating to an amateur or professional boxer. The patients in their study did well after operative treatment.

Boxer's knuckle seems to consist of a spectrum of injury to the extensor hood and dorsal capsule of the metacarpophalangeal joint of the index or middle fingers.

Extensor Carpi Ulnaris Subluxation—Wrist

Although subluxation of the extensor carpi ulnaris tendon often is associated with instability of the distal radioulnar joint, it also can occur as an isolated entity separate from athletic activity. The injury results from forearm hypersupination in conjunction with wrist palmar flexion and ulnar deviation.[6]

The sixth extensor compartment is anatomically very complex. Within the space covered by the retinaculum there is a separate fibrous tunnel for the tendon (Fig. 31-17). Proximal to the base of the ulnar styloid, medial containment for the extensor carpi ulnaris tendon is provided by strong longitudinal fibers that act as a dynamic block to ulnar subluxation of the tendon.[49] At the ulnar styloid, tendon containment is provided by a medial wall of transverse fibers; distal to the ulnar styloid, containment is provided by a fibrous tunnel. In supination, the extensor carpi ulnaris tendon forms an oblique angle directed medially, which results in ulnar translation stress with extensor carpi ulnaris muscle contractions, especially when the forearm is in supination and the hand is in ulnar deviation.

As a result of the injury, the extensor carpi ulnaris tendon subluxates with a painful snap with supination of the forearm and ulnar deviation of the hand. Forearm pronation restores the tendon to its groove. In many patients, this occurs every time the forearm rotates. The acute injury is rarely seen, and the patient presents for treatment because of the chronic painful condition.

Surgical treatment consists of restoration of a pulley or restraint to prevent a tendon from subluxating ulnarward. Burkhart et al[6] either repaired the ulnar septum, supplemented by a radially based sling of the extensor retinaculum, or used a portion of the flexor carpi ulnaris tendon to reconstruct the ulnar wall of the sixth dorsal compartment. They immobilized the extremity in an above-elbow cast with the forearm in neutral and the wrist in 30° of dorsiflexion for about 6 weeks. Rayan[41] recommended reconstruction of the fibroosseous sheath of the extensor carpi ulnaris tendon.

The author prefers to either create a radially based sling from the extensor retinaculum and wrap it around the extensor carpi ulnaris tendon as a restraining pulley (Fig. 31-18) or weave a strip of tendon (palmaris longus) through the medial wall of the fibrous tissue along the extensor carpi ulnaris tendon. These reconstructive procedures provide a stable restraint for the tendon, relieve the painful snap, and allow the athlete to return to competitive sports.

Although there are many other types of injuries to the flexor and extensor tendons of the wrist and hand, they are beyond the scope of this text. The reader should refer to a hand surgery textbook for the treatment of tendon lacerations.

References

1. Araki S, Ohtani T, Tanaka T: Acute dislocation of the extensor digitorum communis tendon of the metacarpophalangeal joint, *J Bone Joint Surg* 69A:616-619, 1987.
2. Blazina ME, Lane C: Rupture of the flexor digitorum profundus tendon in student athletes, *J Am Coll Health Assoc* 14:248-249, 1966.
3. Bollen SR, Gunson CK: Hand injuries in competition climbers, *Br J Sports Med* 24:16-18, 1990.
4. Boyes JH, Wilson JN, Smith JW: Flexor-tendon ruptures in the forearm and hand, *J Bone Joint Surg* 42A:637-646, 1960.
5. Boyes JH: *Bunnels surgery of the hand,* ed 5, Philadelphia, 1970, JB Lippincott, pp 439-442.
6. Burkhart SS, Wood MB, Linscheid RL: Post-traumatic recurrent subluxation of the extensor carpi ulnaris tendon, *J Hand Surg* 7:1-3, 1982.
7. Burton RI, Eaton RG: Common hand injuries in the athlete, *Orthop Clin North Am* 4:808-836, 1973.
8. Buscemi MJ, Page BJ: Flexor digitorum profundus avulsion with associated distal phalanx fractures, *Am J Sports Med* 15:366-370, 1987.
9. Carroll RE, Match RM: Avulsion of the flexor profundus tendon insertion, *J Trauma* 10:1109-1118, 1970.
10. Casscells SW, Strange TB: Intramedullary wire fixation of mallet finger, *J Bone Joint Surg* 51A:1018-1019, 1969.
11. Chang WW, Thoms OJ, White WL: Avulsion injury of the long flexor tendons, *Plast Reconstr Surg* 50:260-264, 1972.
12. Dolphin JA: Extensor tenotomy for chronic boutonnière deformity of the finger: report of two cases, *J Bone Joint Surg* 47A:161-164, 1965.
13. Eglseder WA, Russell JM: Type IV flexor digitorum profundus avulsion, *J Hand Surg* 15A:735-739, 1990.
14. Elliott RA: Injuries to the extensor mechanism of the hand, *Orthop Clin North Am* 1:335-354, 1970.
15. Elson RA: Dislocation of the extensor tendons of the hand: report of a case, *J Bone Joint Surg* 49B:324-326, 1967.
16. Folmar RC, Nelson CL, Phalen QS: Ruptures of the flexor tendons in hands of non-rheumatoid patients, *J Bone Joint Surg* 54A:579-584, 1972.
17. Gladden RJ: Boxer's knuckle, *Am J Surg* 93:388-397, 1957.
18. Goldner JL, Conrad RW: Tendon grafting of the flexor profundus in the presence of a completely or partially intact flexor sublimis, *J Bone Joint Surg* 51A:527-532, 1969.
19. Gunter GS: Traumatic avulsion of the insertion of flexor digitorum profundus, *Aust NZ J Surg* 30:1-8, 1960.
20. Ishizuki M: Traumatic and spontaneous dislocation of extensor tendon of the long finger, *J Hand Surg* 15A:967-972, 1990.
21. Kettlekamp DB, Flatt AE, Moulds R: Traumatic dislocation of the long finger extensor tendon, *J Bone Joint Surg* 53A:229-240, 1971.
22. Koniuch MP et al: Closed crush injury of the metacarpophalangeal joint, *J Hand Surg* 12A:750-757, 1987.
23. Langa V, Posner M: Unusual rupture of a flexor profundus tendon, *J Hand Surg* 11A:227-229, 1986.
24. Lange RH, Engber WD: Hyperextension mallet finger, *Orthopaedics* 6:1426-1431, 1983.
25. Leddy JP, Packer JW: Avulsion of the profundus tendon insertion in athletes, *J Hand Surg* 2:66-69, 1977.
26. Littler JW, Eaton RG: Redistribution of the forces in the correction of boutonnière deformity, *J Bone Joint Surg* 49A:1267-1274, 1967.
27. McClinton MA, Curtis RM, Wilgis EFS: One hundred tendon grafts for isolated flexor digitorum profundus injuries, *J Hand Surg* 7:224-229, 1982.

28. McCoy FJ, Winsky AJ: Lumbrical loop operation for luxation of the extensor tendons of the hand, *Plast Reconstr Surg* 44:142-146, 1969.
29. McCue FC et al: Athletic injuries of the proximal interphalangeal joint requiring surgical treatment, *J Bone Joint Surg* 52A:937, 1970.
30. McCue FC et al: The coaches' finger, *J Sports Med* 2:270-275, 1974.
31. McCue FC et al: Hand and wrist injuries in the athlete, *Am J Sports Med* 7:275-286, 1979.
32. McFarlane RM, Hampole MK: Treatment of extensor tendon injuries of the hand, *Can J Surg* 16:366-375, 1973.
33. McMaster PE: Tendon and muscle ruptures: clinical and experimental studies on the causes and location of spontaneous ruptures, *J Bone Joint Surg* 15:705-722, 1933.
34. Manske PR, Lesker PA: Avulsion of the ring finger flexor digitorum profundus tendon: an experimental study, *Hand* 10:52-55, 1978.
35. Matev I: Transposition of the lateral slips of the aponeurosis in treatment of long standing boutonnière deformity of the fingers, *Br J Plast Surg* 17:281-286, 1964.
36. Milek M, Boulas HJ: Flexor tendon ruptures secondary to hamate hook fractures, *J Hand Surg* 15-A:740-744, 1990.
37. Ostrowski DM: Avulsion of a ring finger profundus tendon with separation of the tendon from a large distal phalanx fracture fragment, *Orthopaedics* 14:1014-1017, 1991.
38. Posner MA: Injuries to the hand and wrist in athletes, *Orthop Clin North Am* 8:593-617, 1977.
39. Posner MA, Ambrose L: Boxer's knuckle—dorsal capsular rupture of the metacarpophalangeal joint of a finger, *J Hand Surg* 14A:229-236, 1989.
40. Posner MA: Hand injuries. In Nicholas JA, Hershman EB, editors: *The upper extremity in sports medicine,* Philadelphia, 1990, CV Mosby, p 495.
41. Rayan GM: Recurrent dislocation of the extensor carpi ulnaris in athletes, *Am J Sports Med* 11:183-184, 1983.
42. Robins PR, Dobysn JH: Avulsion of the insertion of the flexor digitorum profundus tendon associated with fracture of the distal phalanx. In: *AAOS symposium on tendon surgery in the hand,* St Louis, 1975, CV Mosby.
43. Rothwell AG: The pseudo-boutonnière deformity, *NZ Med J* 89:51-54, 1979.
44. Spinner M, Choi BY: Anterior dislocation of the proximal interphalangeal joint, a cause of rupture of the central slip of the extensor mechanism, *J Bone Joint Surg* 52A:1329-1336, 1970.
45. Smith JH: Avulsion of the profundus tendon with simultaneous intra-articular fracture of the distal phalanx: case report, *J Hand Surg* 6:600-601, 1981.
46. Stark HH, Boyes JH, Wilson JN: Mallet finger, *J Bone Joint Surg* 44A:1061-1068, 1962.
47. Stark HH et al: Flexor tendon graft through intact superficialis tendon, *J Hand Surg* 2:456-461, 1977.
48. Stark HH et al: Fracture of the hook of the hamate in athletes, *J Bone Joint Surg* 59A:575-582, 1977.
49. Taleisnik J: The ligaments of the wrist. In Taleisnik J, editor: *The wrist,* New York, 1985, Churchill Livingstone, pp 36-37.
50. Tropet Y et al: Closed traumatic rupture of the ring finger flexor tendon pulley, *J Hand Surg* 15A:745-747, 1990.
51. Trumble TE, Vedder NB, Benirschke SK: Misleading fractures after profundus tendon avulsions: a report of six cases, *J Hand Surg* 17A:902-906, 1992.
52. Urbaniak JR, Hayes MG: Chronic boutonnière deformity—an anatomical reconstruction, *J Hand Surg* 6:379, 1981.
53. Wenger DR: Avulsion of the profundus tendon insertion in football players, *Arch Surg* 106:145-149, 1973.
54. Wheeldon FT: Recurrent dislocation of extensor tendons in the hand, *J Bone Joint Surg* 36B:612-617, 1954.
55. Wilson RL et al: Flexor profundus injuries treated with delayed two-staged tendon grafting, *J Hand Surg* 5:74-78, 1980.
56. Zancolli E: *Structural and dynamic basis of hand surgery,* Philadelphia, 1968, JB Lippincott, pp 105-106.
57. Zemel NP: The prevention and treatment of complications from fractures of the distal radius and ulna, *Hand Clin* 3:1-11, 1987.
58. Zemel NP et al: Boutonnière deformity of the finger—long-term evaluation of splinting versus operative treatment. Presented to the American Society for Surgery of the Hand, Sept, 1988, Baltimore.

Index

A

B

C

G

H

J

K

L

O

P

Q

R

T

U

V

W

X

Y